Access to Health

Access to Health

4th Edition

Rebecca J. Donatelle
Oregon State University

Lorraine G. Davis
University of Oregon

ALLYN AND BACON

BOSTON LONDON TORONTO SYDNEY TOKYO SINGAPORE

Senior Series Editor: *Suzy Spivey*
Vice President and Publisher: *Susan Badger*
Developmental Editors: *Mark Palmer, Mary Kriener*
Series Editorial Assistant: *Lisa Davidson*
Executive Marketing Manager: *Anne Harvey*
Composition and Prepess Buyer: *Linda Cox*
Manufacturing Buyer: *Megan Cochran*
Cover Administrator: *Linda Knowles*
Cover Designer: *Susan Paradise*
Photo Researcher: *Laurel Anderson/Photosynthesis*
Production Administrator: *Susan Brown*

Copyright © 1996 by Allyn & Bacon
A Simon & Schuster Company
Needham Heights, MA 02194
Previous editions copyrighted 1994, 1991, 1988

Library of Congress Cataloging-in-Publication Data

Donatelle, Rebecca, J.
    Access to health / Rebecca J. Donatelle, Lorraine G. Davis.—4th
ed.
      p.   cm.
    Includes bibliographical references and index.
    ISBN 0-205-18170-8
    1. Health.   I. Davis, Lorraine G.   II. Title.
RA776.D66   1995   95-35599
618—dc20   CIP

Printed in the United States of America

10 9 8 7 6 5 4 3 2   99 98 97 96

Brief Contents

$\mathcal{C}$ontents

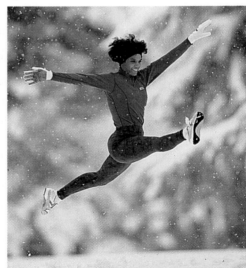

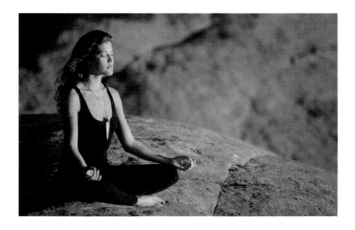

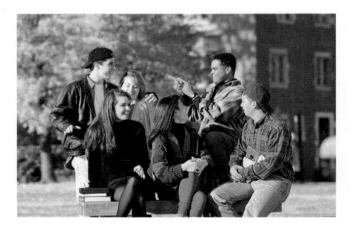

Part 2: Creating Healthy and Caring Relationships

5 Healthy Relationships: Friends, Family, and Significant Others 104

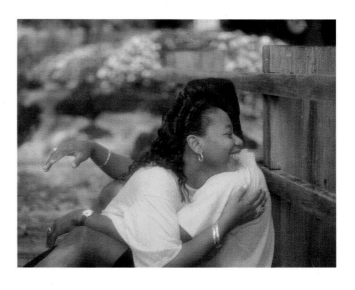

6 Sexuality: Defining Your Sexual Behavior 130

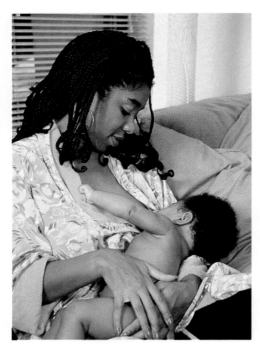

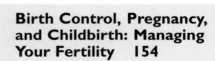

7   Birth Control, Pregnancy, and Childbirth: Managing Your Fertility   154

Part 3: Building Healthy Lifestyles

8   Nutrition: Eating for Optimum Health   192

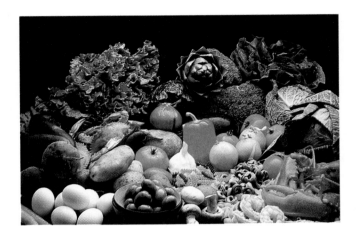

 9 Managing Your Weight: Finding a Healthy Balance   230

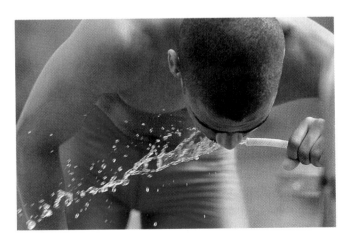

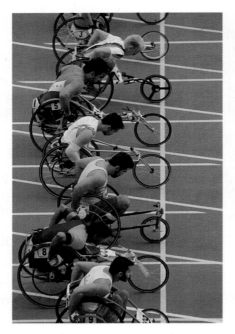

10 Personal Fitness: Improving Your Health Through Exercise 262

Part 4: Avoiding or Overcoming Harmful Habits

11 Addictions and Addictive Behavior: Threats to Wellness 290

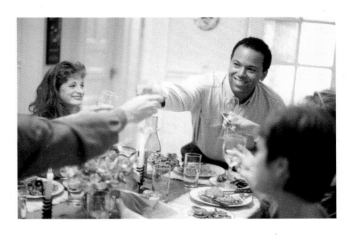

Cancer: Reducing Your Risks   432

Infectious and Sexually Transmitted Diseases: Risks and Responsibilities   462

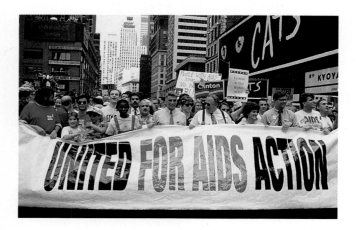

19 Noninfectious Conditions: The Modern Maladies 496

Part 6: Facing Life's Challenges

20 Healthy Aging: A Lifelong Process 520

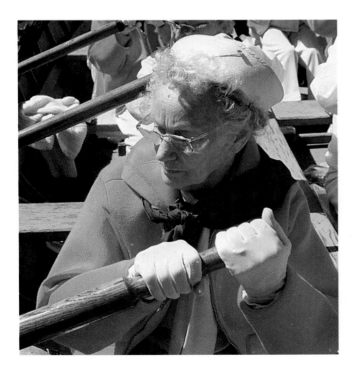

21 Dying and Death: The Final Transition 542

Part 7: Today's Health Issues

22 Violence and Abuse: An Epidemic of Fear 566

23 Environmental Health: Thinking Globally, Acting Locally 588

LETHAL WEAPON

VIOLENCE AT HOME IS WAR AGAINST WOMEN

To get help call: 415-864-4555 San Francisco Domestic Violence Consortium

Liz claiborne

24 Consumerism: Selecting Health-Care Products and Services 614

Feature Boxes

Building Communication Skills

Choices for Change

Health Headlines

Multicultural Perspectives

Rate Yourself

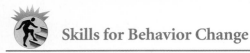

Skills for Behavior Change

Student Preface

How many times have you bought a textbook thinking that it looked interesting and might be really useful only to find it lifeless, uninteresting, and unfulfilling? You read the text, you memorize a few facts, and are left asking yourself, "SO WHAT? HOW DOES THIS RELATE TO ME?" Sound familiar?

Writing an introductory health text that would be likely to grab and hold your attention posed an enormous challenge for us. After all, most of you already have been bombarded with the importance of practicing safer sex, saying no to drugs, eating fat-free foods, and conserving the environment. Right? In fact, some of you may think that if you hear another word about those condoms or those low-fat desserts, you'll scream. So, what makes this book different? How does this book go where no personal health book has gone before? How will this book and this course be relevant to you? *Access to Health* is presented in a behavioral management, individual decision-making approach to personal health. Our goal is to give you the practical means of assessing and managing your personal health behaviors.

Chances are that if you are like most of today's college students, you already know more than any previous generation about health. Contrary to what most of us think, because health information changes quickly and there is so much to know, none of us can ever really know enough. Even if you have the basic facts, translating them into a meaningful plan of action that is personally relevant can be a difficult task. How do you stay healthy in a society where there are so many threats to health from so many sources? How does improving one aspect of your health affect your overall health? And how do you get healthy if you're not healthy right now? You have the opportunity to choose from health alternatives that were not available a few short years ago. How do you make the right choices? Where do

you go for reliable and accurate information? With so many choices available to you, how can you be sure that your everyday decisions will ultimately lead to good health? With these questions in mind, we have placed increasing emphasis on developing skills to help you make informed, responsible health decisions. Achieving good health is a process that occurs in stages. These stages include recognizing the importance of a particular health outcome, understanding the factors that contribute to the positive and negative aspects of health, contemplating how your actions affect health, and choosing to change or modify risk behaviors and develop new and improved behaviors.

When you hear someone talking about a health fact or read about a health problem, how do you react? When you are thinking about something you should do differently, how do you make your choices? When you have a health-related problem, what do you do? For many of you, it is the first time in your life that Mom, Dad, and your high school friends that you have learned to rely on are not there to give you advice. You need to develop new sources of reliable health information. *Access to Health* can be one important source. As you use the latest health information, the special features and the learning aids in the book, as well as the supplements, we hope to make your ACCESS to health fun and enlightening with long-term results of improved overall health.

New to This Edition:

- Beginning with the introduction of a **new decision-making model called DECIDE** in Chapter 1, decision making through critical thinking now forms the cornerstone of every chapter, from the "What Do You Think?" scenarios and reflective questions throughout the chapter, the boxed features, and in the "Taking

Charge" section (which includes a "Critical Thinking" decision-making situation).

- **Cancer and Cardiovascular Disease coverage has been expanded** into separate chapters to emphasize prevention and treatment of the major killing diseases. New and expanded coverage in the Cancer chapter includes options that women face in light of improved technological advances in the area of cancer treatment. In the Cardiovascular Disease chapter, a major new section on women and heart disease includes coverage of risk factors, symptoms of heart disease in postmenopausal women, why women's CVD symptoms are often neglected, and gender bias in research.

- **Expanded coverage of gender issues in health** is integrated throughout the text. Topics include areas such as: the Women's Health Initiative, gender bias in mental health treatment, women and heart disease, the Men's Health Movement, and how gender roles may affect stress levels and a person's ultimate health status.

- **The role of community in health expands coverage** beyond personal health, and demonstrates how to improve a community's health. Community coverage is integrated throughout the text and in special "Checklist for Change: Making Community Decisions" parts within the "Taking Charge" section at the end of each chapter.

- **Greater emphasis on prevention** is applied in the context of changing health behaviors. For example, the text covers how early intervention allows more options, how prevention eases the burden on the health-care system, and how prevention affects lifetime decisions.

- **Expanded coverage of multicultural issues,** now appearing in every chapter, will enhance your understanding of the diversity of the human experience and appreciation for human differences.

- **Enhanced coverage of "hot" topics** surrounding some of the new threats to health, such as Hanta Virus, Ebola, Fibromyalgia, threats to food supplies, and a host of other timely health concerns.

- With a **new pedagogical framework,** emphasis on building health skills is integrated consistently throughout the text. You'll learn specific applications in every chapter through "Rate Yourself" boxes, "Skills for Behavior Change" boxes, "Building Communication Skills" boxes, "Choices for Change" boxes, and in the "Taking Charge" section.

Special Features

Each chapter of *Access to Health* includes the following special feature boxes designed to help you build health behavior skills as well as think about and apply the concepts:

New **"Choices for Change"** boxes empower you to make more informed choices concerning your healthy lifestyle decisions. These boxes provide information to help you understand how your choices affect your health.

New **"Skills for Behavior Change"** boxes offer specific skills that you can use in improving your health behavior.

"Building Communication Skills" boxes, now appearing in every chapter, strengthen the emphasis on using communication as a tool to better health. Designed to implement the material covered in Chapter 4 on Communication, these boxes provide practical suggestions for improving communication behaviors, interpersonal relations, and social interactions, all essential components of good health.

"Multicultural Perspectives" boxes are designed to promote acceptance of diversity on college campuses and assist you in adjusting to an increasingly diverse world. These boxes increase awareness that people of differing backgrounds can have different perspectives, concerns, and solutions related to current health issues.

"Rate Yourself" (self-assessment) boxes include many assessments new to this edition. These assessments give you the chance to examine your behaviors and determine ways to improve your health. Additional assessments are available in the self-assessment manual, and in the new, comprehensive software.

"Health Headlines" boxes present newsworthy information on key health issues and provide additional information to complement facts presented in the chapter.

"Taking Charge" sections at the end of each chapter encourage you to apply the chapter material to your own life. This highly acclaimed feature, expanded to include more directed activities, now includes the following sections: *Making Decisions for You,* which outlines steps and strategies for making and implementing health decisions; *Checklists for Change,* which outlines specific actions you can take to change unhealthy behaviors, on both a personal and community level; *Critical Thinking* situations, which present a hypothetical situation in which you must make a decision—we encourage you to apply the DECIDE model to make this decision.

Learning Aids

Chapter Objectives: Each chapter begins with a list of objectives tied to the major sections of the chapter to emphasize important topics. These objectives can serve as a helpful tool for you to use when learning the key concepts presented in the chapter.

"What Do You Think" chapter opening scenarios: These scenarios prompt stimulating discussions that quickly involve you in the concepts to be presented in the chapter.

New "What Do You Think" reflective questions: These questions appear in major sections of every chapter to encourage you to think critically about important concepts as you read through the chapter.

Margin Glossary of Key Terms: For convenience and added emphasis, Key Terms are boldfaced in the text and defined in the margin on the page where they are first introduced as well as in an alphabetical glossary at the end of the text.

Chapter Summary: Linked to the chapter opening learning objectives, these summaries provide a quick, at-a-glance review of key points presented in each chapter.

New Discussion Questions: Tied to major sections of the chapter, these new questions encourage you to consider important concepts from varying angles.

New Application Exercises: These new exercises are linked to the chapter opening scenarios and expand your discussion on these points. Be sure to apply the knowledge you have obtained from the chapter.

Further Readings: An annotated bibliography of additional readings is provided at the end of each chapter for those of you who desire more in-depth coverage of selected topics.

References: Extensive listings of major sources used in researching each chapter are provided in the Reference section at the end of the text.

New Health Resource Guide and Nutritional Information for Selected Fast Food Restaurants Appendices: To provide you with more tools to use in improving your health behavior, we have included both a comprehensive health resource guide offering you access to hundreds of health services and a handy reference for determining the nutritional values of many popular fast food restaurants.

Student Supplements

Available with *Access to Health, Fourth Edition,* is a comprehensive set of ancillary material designed to enhance your learning.

Thinking About Health: A Student Resource Manual: This study guide now includes language-enrichment sections for those of you who need special language assistance or who have difficulty with health vocabulary. A valuable study tool, it also provides a wealth of learning objectives, critical thinking exercises and activities, chapter summaries, key terms, review questions, and practice tests.

Take Charge of Your Health! Self-Assessment Workbook with Practice and Review Tests: Using this self-assessment workbook along with *Access to Health* will assist you in acquiring a broader understanding of health issues, evaluate your attitudes and behaviors, and gain a clearer picture of your overall health. Also included are general review questions and two practice tests (with situations) for each chapter. (*Available free to every student.*)

New *Take Charge of Your Health! Self-Assessment Software:* This **custom-designed software** for the IBM and Macintosh computer is interactive and constitutes an excellent learning tool. You can assess your individual health behaviors and plan a risk-reduction program, all in the context of material covered in the text.

Issues in Health: Readings from The Washington Post: This brief series of timely articles from *The Washington Post* presents high-interest, topical, and provocative issues related to health. (*Available free for every student*).

Instructor Supplements

We offer the following comprehensive set of ancillary material for the instructor to facilitate classroom preparation:

Instructor's Resource Manual

Test Item File

New Computerized Testing Program

Images of Health Laserdisc

Health Transparencies

AIDS and STDs Slide Set

CNN Video

Allyn & Bacon Video Library for Health

Time-out Video

Custom Publishing Program

America Online

Acknowledgments

After writing four editions of *Access to Health,* we recognize that the publishing business is an ever-changing, dynamic process. Fortunately, we have had several highly competent editors working on *Access to Health,* over the last decade. Each of these editors and their staffs helped us develop a high-quality, cutting-edge product—one that will be useful in the short- and long-term. From the excellent initial development efforts of Joe Heider on the first edition of *Access to Health* to the outstanding project oversight of Prentice Hall's Ted Bolen on the second and third editions, we have been pleased with the efforts of our publishing teams. As we began writing this fourth edition, Allyn and Bacon acquired the book. We are again extremely grateful to be placed with another group of outstanding publishing professionals. From the initial planning vision of Susan Badger and her editorial team to the highly personalized, detailed developmental attention of Senior Editor Suzy Spivey, the revision process has been positive. Our personal thanks to all of you. Without your help and direction, *Access to Health* would not be among the leading texts in the market today.

While the publishing and production staffs have provided the direction, writing the various editions of *Access to Health* would not have been possible without the professional expertise and efforts of many of our colleagues from across the country. Whether acting as reviewers, generating new ideas, providing expert commentary, or writing chapters, each of these professionals have added their skills to our collective endeavor.

Contributors to the Fourth Edition:

Patricia Ketcham, Health Educator and Director of Student Health Education and Student Services at the University of Iowa, completed a major revision of her chapter on Drinking Responsibly. She was also responsible for significant revisions and ideas to the chapters "Birth Control, Pregnancy, and Childbirth," "Pharmaceutical Drugs," "Tobacco and Caffeine," and "Illicit Drugs." Her help in the development of the content and ideas in *Access to Health* since the first edition have been invaluable.

Rod Harter, Associate Professor in the Department of Exercise and Sport Science at Oregon State University, utilized his expertise in human physiology, training, human performance, and strength and conditioning in writing his exceptional chapter, "Personal Fitness."

Cathy Barnett, Health Educator at the University of Iowa Student Health Center, utilized her experience of working with hundreds of students with addictive-behavior problems in writing a top-notch, cutting edge, completely new section on addictive behavioral patterns.

Chris Hafner-Eaton, Assistant Professor in the Department of Public Health at Oregon State University and RAND corporation-policy analyst, used her considerable background in health services and public policy to provide a major revision of Chapter 24, "Consumerism."

Donna Champeau, Health Educator and Assistant Professor at Boise State University, offered her expertise in the areas of health policy and the rights of the dying to provide excellent revisions and updates to Chapter 21, "Dying and Death."

Peggy Pederson, Health Educator and Assistant Professor at Northern Illinois University, used her background in sexuality to submit significant editorial comment and revisions for Chapter 6, "Sexuality."

Contributors to Previous Editions:

Cheryl Graham, Health Educator in Student Health Services at Oregon State University contributed significantly to previous versions of Chapter 11, "Addictions and Addictive Behavior."

Tomina Torey, Assistant Professor in the Department of Psychology at Western Oregon State University, using her academic training in human development and interpersonal communication, wrote a strong chapter on com-

munication in the third edition of *Access to Health*. Several of her fine ideas were carried forward in the revision of the chapter.

Tom Thomas, Exercise Physiologist at the University of Missouri, provided excellent chapters on fitness and strength and conditioning in the *Brief Access to Health, Second Edition*. Several of his ideas were carried over into the revised chapter on personal fitness in *Access to Health, Third Edition*.

Marion Micke, Health Educator in the Department of Health Education at Illinois State University, offered substantive revisions to Chapter 21, "Dying and Death" in *Access to Health , Third Edition*. Her efforts paved the way for subsequent revisions of this outstanding chapter.

Anna Harding, Environmental Health Specialist in the Department of Public Health at Oregon State University, provided major revisions to Chapter 22, "Environmental Health" in *Access to Health, Third Edition*. Her efforts produced one of the most up-to-date and comprehensive environmental health chapters on the market.

Carolyn Hoover, Health Educator, Alaska Public Schools, is owed a special debt of gratitude for her authorship in the first and second editions of *Access to Health*. Without her assistance in the early years, *Access to Health* may never have materialized.

In addition, we would like to thank the many colleagues who provided recommendations in constructive reviews of previous editions and the manuscript of the fourth edition of *Access to Health*.

Reviewers of the Fourth Edition and members of the focus group:

Judith Ary, North Dakota State University
Judy Baker, East Carolina University
Rick Barnes, East Carolina University
W. Henry Baughman, Western Kentucky University
Jill Black, Cleveland State University
Donna Champeau, Boise State University
Susanne Christopher, Portland Community College
Barbara Cole, Texas Tech University
Gerald Davoli, University of Massachussetts
Lori Dewald, Shippensburg University
Nancy Geha, Columbia, Missouri
James Herauf, Northwest Missouri State University
Jim Johnson, Northwest Missouri State University
Rebecca Leas, Clarion University of Pennsylvania
Barbara Day Lockhart, Brigham Young University
Brad Lopez, Fresno City College
Judith Luebke, Mankato State University
Mickey McCowan, John A. Logan College
Jacqueline Palmer, Mt. Ida College
Carol Parker, University of Central Oklahoma
Henry Petracki, Palm Beach Community College
Connie Thorngren, Boise State University

Reviewers of previous editions and members of the Third Edition focus group:

O. Matthew Adeyanju, University of Kansas
Wes Alles, Pennsylvania State University
Judy Baker, East Carolina University
Danny Ballard, Texas A & M University
Rick Barnes, East Carolina University
W. Henry Baughman, Western Kentucky University
Ken Becker, University of Wisconsin, LaCrosse
Gerald Benn, Northeastern State University
Christine Beyer, Southern Illinois University
Fay Biles, Kent State University
John Bonugaro, Ohio University
Robert Bowers, Tallahassee Community College
Jerry Braza, University of Utah
Andrew Brennan, Metropolitan Life Corporation
Herman Bush, Eastern Kentucky University
Jean Byrne, Kent State University
Donald L. Calitri, Eastern Kentucky University
Vivien Carver, University of Southern Mississippi
Carol Cates, Cerritos College
Carol Christensen, San Jose State University
Bethann Cinelli, West Chester University
Joseph S. Darden, Jr., Kean College
Steve M. Dorman, University of Florida
Margaret Dosch, University of Wisconsin, LaCrosse
Judy Drolet, Southern Illinois University
Ruth Engs, Indiana University
William Faraclas, Southern Connecticut University
Aaron F. Felman, Southern Carolina State University
Jeff Forman, DeAnza College
Emogene Fox, University of Central Arkansas
Erika Friedman, Brooklyn College of CUNY
Bob Fries, Fresno State University
J. Frederick Garman, Kutztown University
Julie A. Gast, Southern Illinois University
Stephen Germeroth, Catonsville Community College
Ray Goldberg, SUNY College at Cortland
Susan Graham-Kresge, University of
    Southern Mississippi
William C. Gross, Western Michigan University
Rick Guyton, University of Arkansas
Steven B. Hafen, Catonsville Community College
Dickie Hill, Abilene Christian University
Marsha Hoagland, Modesto Junior College
Kathleen J. Hunter, Southern Illinois University
Phil Huntsinger, University of Kansas
John Janowiak, Appalachian State University
Jack A. Jordan, University of Wisconsin, LaCrosse
Sally D. Klein, Dutchess Community College

Alfred Kouneski, Montgomery College
Nancy LaCursia, Southern Illinois University
Charles LeRoy, Eastern Montana College
John Leavy, SUNY College at Cortland
Michael Lee, Joliet Junior College
Robert McDermott, Southern Illinois University
Richard T. Mackey, Miami University of Ohio
Richard E. Madson, Palm Beach Community College
Patrick Moffitt, University of Northern Iowa
Karen Mondrone, M. S., R. D.
L. Mike Morris, Idaho State University
Louis Munch, Ithaca College
Bikash R. Nandy, Mankato State University
Judith Nelson, Burlington Community College
Boyd L. Newman, University of North Carolina
Ian Newman, University of Nebraska, Lincoln
George Niva, Bowling Green State University
Larry Olsen, Pennsylvania State University
Gaye Osborne, Morehead State University
Robert D. Patton, East Tennessee State University
Jeanine Paz, Chabot College
Carl J. Peter, Western Illinois University
Judy Phillips, Valdosta State College
Valerie Pinhas, Nassau Community College
James Price, University of Toledo
Bruce M. Ragon, Indiana University, Bloomington
Kerry Redican, Virginia Polytechnic Institute
Harold F. Risk, St. Cloud State University
Kim Roberts, Eastern Kentucky University
Stephen Roberts, Eastern Kentucky University
Norma Schira, Western Kentucky University
John Sciacca, Northern Arizona University
Delores Seemayer, Palm Beach Junior College
Warren Smith, University of Oregon
Sherman Sowby, California State University, Fresno
Donald B. Stone, University of Illinois
S. Carol Theisen, Weber State University
Merita Lee Thompson, Eastern Kentucky University
Cheryl Tucker, Northeast Missouri State
Martin S. Turnauer, Radford University
James Tryniechi, Southern Louisiana University
J. Dale Wagoner, Chabot College
Alex Waigandt, University of Missouri, Columbia
Rita Ward, Central Michigan University
Parris R. Watts, University of Missouri, Columbia
Mark G. Wilson, University of Georgia
Janice Clark Young, Iowa State University
Lynne Young, University of District of Columbia
Verne Zellner, American River College

Access to Health

C H A P T E R

1

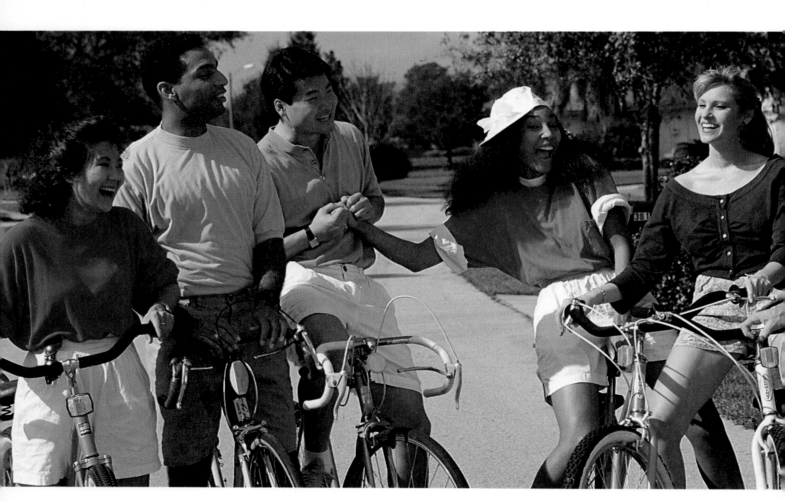

𝒞HAPTER OBJECTIVES

◆ Define health and wellness, and explain the intercon-
nected roles of the physical, social, mental, emotional,
environmental, and spiritual dimensions of health.

◆ Discuss the health status of Americans, the factors that
contribute to health, and the importance of *Healthy
People 2000* objectives in establishing national goals for
promoting health and preventing premature death and
disability.

◆ Evaluate the role of gender in health status, health
research, and health training.

◆ Identify the leading causes of death and the lifestyle
patterns associated with the reduction of risks.

◆ Examine how predisposing factors, beliefs, attitudes,
and significant others affect your behavior changes.

◆ Survey behavior change techniques, and learn how to
apply them to personal situations.

◆ Apply decision-making techniques to behavior changes.

Promoting Healthy Behavior Change

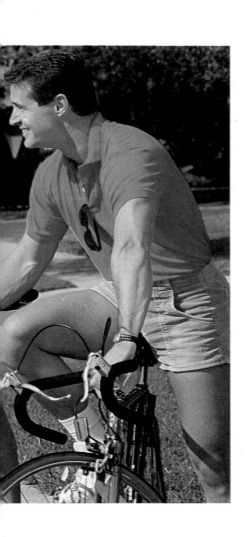

Tim is a 22-year-old sophomore who is 75 pounds overweight and does not like exercising. A sensitive, caring young man, he has many close friends and is a volunteer at many health-related agencies that help people in need. He likes to enjoy nature and the inner peace he derives from a walk on the beach or a quiet night by a campfire in the wilderness. He is a strong advocate for human rights, animal rights, and the preservation of the environment.

Miko is a first-year college student who has been paraplegic since she was in a car accident at the age of 10. She is bright and funny, and she gets along well with people. Miko spends her free time at the local homeless shelter talking to people she feels are much worse off than she is. She maintains an ideal weight, watches her fat intake, and has a close, loving relationship with her family.

Kim is a 20-year-old first-year college student who lives off campus. She tries to eat healthful foods some of the time, feels she is about 10 pounds overweight, and walks 1 to 2 miles per day. She is shy and hasn't made many friends since coming to college. During a typical day, she goes to class, studies, watches TV, and writes letters to her high school friends and family. She likes bicycle riding, but she only finds time to get out for a short ride on weekends. She is tired much of the time and wonders why she is in school. After a checkup, her doctor says, "Everything looks good. Keep up whatever you're doing, and you should be fine."

Vern is a young college professor with a wife, four children, and a home in the "burbs." He is vigilant about his fat intake, exercises two to three hours daily, and runs every 10K and marathon his schedule allows. His conversations focus on his races, his disappointment when he has failed to run well, and his daily workout performances. He is highly critical of and hostile to overweight students and does not want "unfit" students to be admitted to his classes. He is extremely thin, has a tired, drawn expression and a volatile temper, and seldom socializes with others because it takes time from his workouts.

- Do you know people who are like any of these individuals? Which of these people do you think is the healthiest? The most unhealthy? What factors may have contributed to their current behaviors? What actions could you take to help these people achieve a more balanced "healthstyle"? Where else could they go for help?

If you and your close friends were to list the most important things in your lives, you might be surprised at the differences in the responses. Some of you would probably list family, love, financial security, significant others, and happiness. Others might also list health. Raised on a steady diet of clichés—"If you have your health, you have everything," "Be all that you can be," "Use it or lose it," "Just do it"—most of us readily acknowledge that good health is a desirable goal. But what does it really mean to be healthy? How can you "get healthy" if you aren't doing so well now? How can you maintain and enhance the good health behaviors you may already have?

This text offers fundamental information that will provide you an *Access to Health* consistent with who you are and what you want to become. Health is not an entity that is always totally within your control, but there are many changes you can make in your behavior that may significantly affect your risk factors. For those risk factors beyond your control, you must learn to react, adapt, and make optimal use of your resources to create the best situation for yourself. By making informed, rational decisions, you will be able to improve both the quality and the length of your life.

𝒲HAT IS HEALTH?

The current definition of **health** has evolved over several periods of world and American history.

Health and Sickness: Defined by Extremes

Prior to the late 1800s, people viewed health as the opposite of sickness. A person was healthy if he or she wasn't suffering from a life-threatening infectious disease. When deadly epidemics such as bubonic plague, pneumonic plague, influenza, tuberculosis, and cholera killed millions of people, survivors were considered healthy and congratulated themselves on their good fortune. In the late 1800s and early 1900s, researchers slowly began to discover that victims of these epidemics were not simply unhealthy people. Rather, they were the victims of microorganisms found in contaminated water, air, and human wastes.

Public health officials moved swiftly to sanitize the environment and, as a result, many people began to think of health as *good hygiene*. Practices such as sanitary disposal of wastes and other behaviors that promoted hygiene were the harbingers of good health. Colleges offered courses in "Health and Hygiene" or "Hygiene" that were the ancestors of the course you are in today.

Health: More than a Statistic

Once scientists began to learn about the microorganisms that cause infectious diseases, dramatic changes occurred in the sickness profile of the American public. In the early 1900s, the leading causes of death were infectious diseases such as tuberculosis, pneumonia, and influenza. The average life expectancy was only 47. Improvements in sanitation brought about dramatic changes in life expectancy; the development of vaccines and antibiotics added even more years to the average life span. According to **mortality** (death rate) statistics, people are now living longer than in any previous time in our history. **Morbidity** (illness) rates also indicate that people are sick less often from the common infectious diseases that devastated previous generations. Today, because most childhood diseases are curable and because multiple public health efforts are aimed at reducing the spread of infectious diseases, many people are living well into their 70s and 80s.

However, just because we're living longer and not getting sick as often doesn't mean we're necessarily healthier. In an attempt to clarify what the term *health* meant, the World Health Organization (WHO) came up with its own definition in the 1940s: "Health is the state of complete physical, mental, and social well-being, not merely the absence of disease or infirmity."[1] Health officials viewed this as a landmark definition because it said for the first time that health was more than the absence of disease. The WHO definition also implied that health was more than just a vital statistic indicating low mortality or morbidity rates.

Although the WHO definition of health maintained currency well into the 1960s, critics argued that health is not a state that people somehow manage to achieve; rather, it is an ever-changing dimension of life. They also argued that complete health was much more than just a measure of physical, mental, and social aspects of life given growing recognition of the contributions of envi-

Responsiveness to the physical, emotional, social, spiritual, and environmental dimensions of life—not merely the presence or absence of illness—determines health status.

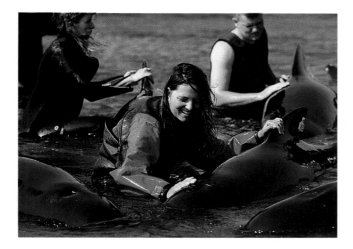

ronmental, emotional, and spiritual health to the quality of life as well as to the number of years a person lives.

Health as Wellness: Putting Quality into Years

René Dubos, biologist and philosopher, expanded the WHO definition of health: "Health is a quality of life, involving social, emotional, mental, spiritual, and biological fitness on the part of the individual, which results from adaptations to the environment."[2] As more people considered the term *health,* the concept began to include many different components and encompass many different aspects of life. Eventually the term **wellness** came to refer to the achievement of the highest level of health in each of several key dimensions. Today, *health* and *wellness* are often used interchangeably to mean the dynamic, ever-changing process of trying to achieve one's individual potential in each of several interrelated dimensions. These dimensions typically include those presented in Figure 1.1.

- **Physical Health.** Includes characteristics such as body size and shape, sensory acuity, susceptibility to disease and disorders, body functioning, and recuperative ability.

- **Social Health.** Refers to the ability to have satisfying interpersonal relationships: to interactions with others, the ability to adapt to various social situations, and daily behaviors.

- **Mental Health.** Refers to the ability to learn, the ability to grow from experience, and intellectual capabilities. Decision making is a vital component of one's mental health.

- **Emotional Health.** Refers to the feeling component; to express emotions when appropriate and to control expressing emotions either when it is inappropriate to do so or in an inappropriate manner. Feelings of self-esteem, self-confidence, self-efficacy, trust, love, and many other emotional reactions and responses are all part of emotional health.

- **Environmental Health.** Refers to an appreciation of the external environment and the role individuals play in preserving, protecting, and improving environmental conditions.

- **Spiritual Health.** May involve a belief in a supreme being or a specified way of living prescribed by a particular religion. Spiritual health also includes the feeling of unity with the environment—a feeling of oneness with others and with nature—and a guiding sense of meaning or value in life. It also may include the ability to understand and express one's purpose in life; to feel a part of a greater spectrum of existence; to experience love, joy, pain, sorrow, peace, contentment, and wonder over life's experiences; and to care about and respect all living things.

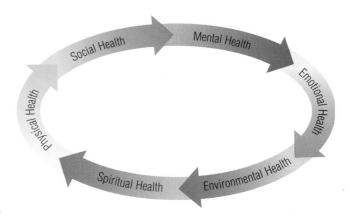

FIGURE 1.1

The Six Dimensions of Health

Health: Dynamic, ever-changing process of trying to achieve your individual potential in the physical, social, emotional, mental, spiritual, and environmental dimensions.

Mortality: Death rate.

Morbidity: Illness rate.

Wellness: The achievement of the highest level of health possible in each of several dimensions.

Whether contemporary definitions are of *health* or *wellness,* they focus on individual attempts to achieve optimal well-being within a realistic framework of individual potential.

In Figure 1.2, a continuum from illness to optimal well-being describes health and wellness. Where you are on this continuum may vary from day to day as you are buffeted by life's ups and downs. But if you persist in your attempts to change behaviors to reduce risk, your chances of remaining on the positive end of the continuum will greatly improve. The current definition of health acknowledges that each of us must attempt to achieve this optimal level of being in a sometimes hostile environment. Each of us must come to terms with the obstacles obstructing the way to optimal health in our own way by focusing on our positive attributes whenever possible, changing those negative aspects of ourselves that we can, and learning to recognize and deal with those that we cannot.

Well individuals take an honest look at their personal capabilities and limitations and make an effort to change those factors that are within their control. They try to achieve a balance in each of the health/wellness dimensions while trying to achieve a positive wellness position on an imaginary continuum. Many people believe that wellness can best be achieved by the adoption of a holistic approach in which a person emphasizes the integration of and balance between mind, body, and spirit. Persons on the illness and disability end of the continuum have failed to achieve this integration and balance and may be seriously deficient in one or more of the wellness dimensions.

But the disability component of the wellness continuum does not imply that a person with physical handicaps cannot achieve wellness. Such a person may in fact be very healthy in terms of relationships with others, level of self-confidence, environmental sensitivity, and overall attitude toward life. In contrast, a person who spends hours

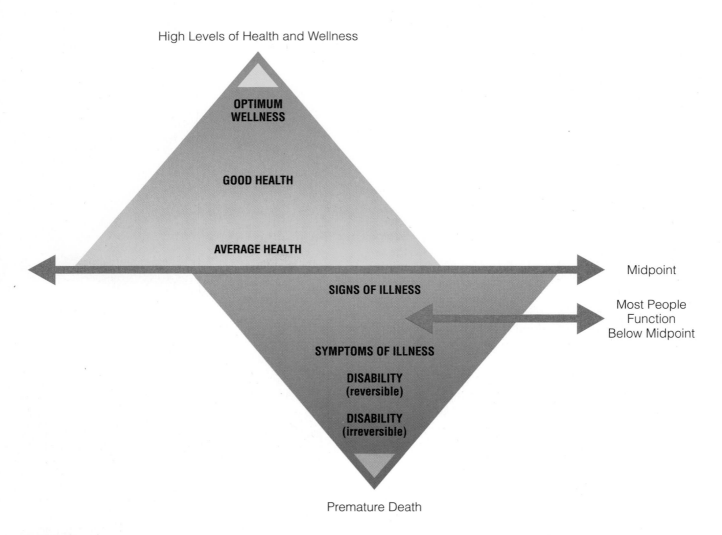

FIGURE 1.2

The Continuum from Illness to Wellness

in front of a mirror lifting weights to perfect the size and shape of each muscle may be unhealthy in these same terms. Although we often place a premium on physical attractiveness and external trappings, appearance and physical performance indicators are actually only two signs of a person's overall health.

Typically, the closer you get to your potential in the six components of health, the more well you will be. Both health and wellness are ongoing, active processes that include those positive attitudes and behaviors that continually improve the quality of your life. By completing the appraisal in the Rate Yourself box, you may gain a better perspective on how you measure up in each of the health dimensions discussed above.

*H*EALTHY PEOPLE 2000: A NEW DIRECTION

In an effort to improve the health of Americans, the United States Public Health Service and the surgeon general of the United States worked closely with many segments of the population to review years of data collected by the National Center for Health Statistics and other government agencies. These data revealed that the United States population was not as healthy as it should be and that major differences existed between various communities in terms of health problems, health status, and available health services. As a direct result, in 1990 the surgeon general proposed a national plan for promoting the health of individuals and groups. Known as *Healthy People 2000*, this plan outlined a series of long- and short-range goals and objectives:[3]

- *To increase the span of healthy years for all Americans by three years.* Although the average American lives to be 73.7, he or she spends the final 11.7 years in poor health.

- *To reduce health disparities among Americans.* Life expectancy of white Americans has steadily increased, but it has decreased for African Americans.

- *To secure all Americans' access to health systems and services, particularly preventive services.* Large numbers of Americans lack access to even the most basic health-care services due to the high cost or distant location of such services. In many areas, preventive services (such as prenatal counseling, cancer screening, and nutritional counseling) are nearly nonexistent or extremely difficult to access.

To realize these broad-based goals, *Healthy People 2000* provided hundreds of specific objectives to reach by the year 2000. For example, one goal is to reduce the average dietary-fat intake to 30 percent of calories consumed or less (currently the average is about 40 percent). Another goal is to reduce homicides to no more than 7.2 per 100,000 (currently over 8.5 per 100,000). These specific goals are then grouped into various "priority areas," based on the best way to achieve the target. Two of the most prominent priority areas are health promotion and prevention.

Health Promotion: Helping You Stay Healthy

The health promotion area of *Healthy People 2000* targets individual actions and behaviors. In discussions of health and wellness, the term **health promotion** is often used. Health promotion programs combine educational, organizational, procedural, environmental, and financial supports to help individuals and groups change negative health behaviors. In other words, health promotion

---

Having the motivation to improve the quality of your life within the framework of your unique capabilities and limitations is crucial to achieving health and wellness.

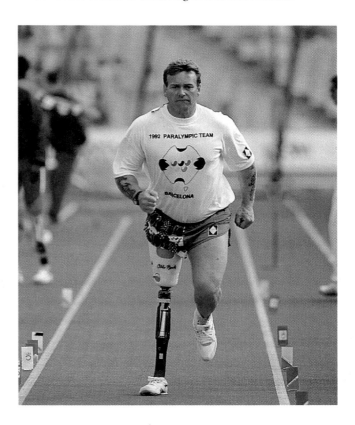

Health promotion: Combines educational, organizational, policy, financial, and environmental supports to help people change negative health behaviors.

How Healthy Are You?

Although many of us recognize the importance of healthy behaviors, we are often negligent in maintaining a healthy regimen. Rate your health status in each of the following dimensions by circling the number that best describes you.

	Very Unhealthy	Somewhat Unhealthy	Somewhat Healthy	Very Healthy
Physical Health	1	2	3	4
Social Health	1	2	3	4
Emotional Health	1	2	3	4
Mental Health	1	2	3	4
Environmental Health	1	2	3	4
Spiritual Health	1	2	3	4

After completing the above section, how healthy do you think you are? Which area(s), if any, do you think you should work on improving?

Now answer the following set of questions regarding each dimension of health. Indicate how often you think the statements describe you.

Physical Health

	Rarely, if Ever	Sometimes	Most of the Time	Always
1. I maintain a desirable weight.	1	2	3	4
2. I engage in vigorous exercises such as brisk walking, jogging, swimming, or running for at least 30 minutes per day, 3–4 times per week.	1	2	3	4
3. I do exercises designed to strengthen my muscles and joints.	1	2	3	4
4. I warm up and cool down by stretching before and after vigorous exercise.	1	2	3	4
5. I feel good about the condition of my body.	1	2	3	4
6. I get 7–8 hours of sleep each night.	1	2	3	4
7. My immune system is strong and I am able to avoid most infectious diseases.	1	2	3	4
8. My body heals itself quickly when I get sick or injured.	1	2	3	4
9. I have lots of energy and can get through the day without being overly tired.	1	2	3	4
10. I listen to my body; when there is something wrong, I seek professional advice.	1	2	3	4

(continued)

programs don't just tell people to lose weight and to eat better food: they help them learn more (*educational supports*), provide programs and services that encourage them to participate (*organizational supports*), establish rules governing their behaviors and supporting their decisions to change (*environmental supports*), and provide monetary incentives to motivate them toward healthful decision making (*financial supports*). In short, health promotion programs enhance the likelihood that, once a person decides to change a behavior, conditions are optimal for his or her success. Health promotion programs identify healthy people who are at risk for disease and attempt to motivate them to improve their health status. They encourage those whose health and wellness behaviors are already sound to maintain and improve them. But health promotion goes one step farther by modifying

Social Health

	Rarely, if Ever	Sometimes	Most of the Time	Always
1. When I meet people I feel good about the impression I make on them.	1	2	3	4
2. I am open, honest, and get along well with other people.	1	2	3	4
3. I participate in a wide variety of social activities and enjoy being with people who are different than me.	1	2	3	4
4. I try to be a "better person" and work on behaviors that have caused problems in my interactions with others.	1	2	3	4
5. I get along well with the members of my family.	1	2	3	4
6. I am a good listener.	1	2	3	4
7. I am open and accessible to a loving and responsible relationship.	1	2	3	4
8. I have someone I can talk to about my private feelings.	1	2	3	4
9. I consider the feelings of others and do not act in hurtful or selfish ways.	1	2	3	4
10. I consider how what I say might be perceived by others before I speak.	1	2	3	4

Emotional Health

	Rarely, if Ever	Sometimes	Most of the Time	Always
1. I find it easy to laugh about things that happen in my life.	1	2	3	4
2. I avoid using alcohol as a means of helping me forget my problems.	1	2	3	4
3. I can express my feelings without feeling silly.	1	2	3	4
4. When I am angry, I try to let others know in non-confrontational and non-hurtful ways.	1	2	3	4
5. I am a chronic worrier and tend to be suspicious of others.	4	3	2	1
6. I recognize when I am stressed and take steps to relax through exercise, quiet time, or other activities.	1	2	3	4
7. I feel good about myself and believe others like me for who I am.	1	2	3	4
8. When I am upset, I talk to others and actively try to work through my problems.	1	2	3	4
9. I am flexible and adapt or adjust to change in a positive way.	1	2	3	4
10. My friends regard me as a stable, emotionally well-adjusted person.	1	2	3	4

(continued)

behaviors, attitudes, and values and by introducing health-enhancing activities.

Whether we use the term *health* or *wellness,* we are talking about a person's overall responses to the challenges of living. Occasional dips into the ice cream bucket and other dietary slips, failure to exercise every day, flare-ups of anger, and other deviations from optimal behavior should not be viewed as major failures to maintain wellness. Ac-

Environmental Health

	Rarely, if Ever	Sometimes	Most of the Time	Always
1. I am concerned about environmental pollution and actively try to preserve and protect natural resources.	1	2	3	4
2. I report people who intentionally hurt the environment.	1	2	3	4
3. I recycle my garbage.	1	2	3	4
4. I reuse plastic and paper bags and tin foil.	1	2	3	4
5. I vote for pro-environmental candidates in elections.	1	2	3	4
6. I write my elected leaders about environmental concerns.	1	2	3	4
7. I consider the amount of packaging covering a product when I buy groceries.	1	2	3	4
8. I try to buy products that are recyclable.	1	2	3	4
9. I use both sides of the paper when taking class notes or doing assignments.	1	2	3	4
10. I try not to leave the faucet running too long when I brush my teeth, shave, or bathe.	1	2	3	4

Spiritual Health

	Rarely, if Ever	Sometimes	Most of the Time	Always
1. I believe life is a precious gift that should be nurtured.	1	2	3	4
2. I take time to enjoy nature and the beauty around me.	1	2	3	4
3. I take time alone to think about what's important in life—who I am, what I value, where I fit in, and where I'm going.	1	2	3	4
4. I have faith in a greater power, be it a God-like force, nature, or the connectedness of all living things.	1	2	3	4
5. I engage in acts of caring and good will without expecting something in return.	1	2	3	4
6. I feel sorrow for those who are suffering and try to help them through difficult times.	1	2	3	4
7. I feel confident that I have touched the lives of others in a positive way.	1	2	3	4
8. I work for peace in my interpersonal relationships, in my community, and in the world at large.	1	2	3	4
9. I am content with who I am.	1	2	3	4
10. I go for the gusto and experience life to the fullest.	1	2	3	4

(continued)

tually, an ability to recognize that each of us is an imperfect being attempting to adapt in an imperfect world signals individual well-being.

We must also remember to be tolerant of others who are attempting to improve their health. Rather than being warriors against pleasure in our zeal to change the health behaviors of others, we need to be supportive, understanding, and nonjudgmental in our interactions with them. *Health bashing*—intolerance or negative feelings, words, or actions aimed at people who fail to meet our

Mental Health

	Rarely, if Ever	Sometimes	Most of the Time	Always
1. I tend to act impulsively without thinking about the consequences.	4	3	2	1
2. I learn from my mistakes and try to act differently the next time.	1	2	3	4
3. I follow directions or recommended guidelines and act in ways likely to keep myself and others safe.	1	2	3	4
4. I consider the alternatives before making decisions.	1	2	3	4
5. I am alert and ready to respond to life's challenges in ways that reflect thought and sound judgment.	1	2	3	4
6. I tend to let my emotions get the better of me and I act without thinking.	4	3	2	1
7. I actively try to learn all I can about products and services before making decisions.	1	2	3	4
8. I manage my time well, rather than time managing me.	1	2	3	4
9. My friends and family trust my judgment.	1	2	3	4
10. I think about my self-talk (the things I tell myself) and then examine the real evidence for my perceptions and feelings.	1	2	3	4

Personal Checklist

Now, total your scores in each of the health dimensions and compare it to the ideal score. Which areas do you need to work on? How does your score compare with how you rated yourself in the first part of the questionnaire?

	Ideal Score	Your Score
Physical Health	40	_____
Social Health	40	_____
Emotional Health	40	_____
Social Health	40	_____
Environmental Health	40	_____
Spiritual Health	40	_____

What Your Scores Mean

Scores of 35–40: Outstanding! Your answers show that you are aware of the importance of this area to your health. More importantly, you are putting your knowledge to work for you by practicing good health habits. As long as you continue to do so this area should not pose a serious health risk. It's likely that you are setting an example for your family and friends to follow. Although you received a very high score on this part of the test, you may want to consider other areas where your scores could be improved.

Scores of 30–35: Your health practices in this area are good, but there is room for improvement. Look again at the items you answered that scored one or two points. What changes could you make to improve you score? Even a small change in behavior can often help you achieve better health.

Scores of 20–30: Your health risks are showing! Would you like more information about the risks you are facing and why it is important for you to change these behaviors? Perhaps you need help in deciding how to make the changes you desire. In either case, help is available from this book, from your professor, and from your student health services.

Scores below 20: You may be taking serious and unnecessary risks with your health. Perhaps you are not aware of the risks and what to do about them. In this book you will find the information you need to help you improve your scores and your health.

Source: Adapted from the U.S. Health and Human Services, *Health Style: A Self Test* (Washington, DC: Public Health Service, 1981).

own expectations of health—may indicate our own deficiencies in the psychological, social, and/or spiritual dimensions of the health continuum.

Prevention: The Key to Future Health

In addition to advocating health promotion, *Healthy People 2000* makes a strong case for the role of **prevention** in insuring the health of Americans. Prevention means taking positive actions now to avoid becoming sick later. Getting immunized against diseases such as polio, never starting to smoke cigarettes, practicing safer sex, and taking similar preventive measures constitute **primary prevention**—actions designed to stop health problems before they start. Another form of prevention is **secondary prevention**, or the recognition of a health problem early in its development and intervention to eliminate its underlying causes before serious illness develops. Attending health education seminars in order to stop cigarette smoking is an example of secondary prevention.

Because two of every three deaths and one of every three hospitalizations in the United States today are linked to largely preventable behaviors—tobacco use, alcohol abuse, sedentary activities, and overeating, for example—primary and secondary prevention are essential to reducing the *incidence* (number of new cases) and *prevalence* (number of existing cases) of diseases and disabilities.[4] Historically, the government has underfunded health education and health promotion activities; less than 5 percent of the total health care expenditure in the United States focuses on these preventive areas. Instead, government money has been allocated primarily for research and **tertiary prevention,** treatment and/or rehabilitation efforts made after a person has become sick. This form of prevention is both more costly and less effective in promoting health than is any other prevention method.

If the government and the health-care system are primarily interested in taking care of you only after you are sick, who is responsible for helping you remain well? Although many health agencies, programs, and public-health prevention specialists are available to assist you, much of the responsibility for your health rests with you. As costs for treatment rise in the years ahead, you may

Prevention: Actions or behaviors designed to keep you from getting sick.

Primary prevention: Actions designed to stop problems before they start.

Secondary prevention: Intervention early in the development of a health problem.

Tertiary prevention: Treatment and/or rehabilitation efforts.

have increasing difficulty in paying for them. What are your options? What are the options for those who lack health insurance or who do not have sufficient knowledge to make informed health choices?

By definition, truly healthy people possess a sense of both individual and social responsibility. Rather than focusing solely on their own personal health, healthy people are concerned about others and the greater environment. This concern translates into the taking of actions designed to help themselves as well as to help others who are less fortunate. It also means taking the time to understand the vast differences in health status between different social groups and actively promoting community actions that erase these disparities. For an example of these differences, see the Multicultural Perspectives box.

GENDER DIFFERENCES AND HEALTH STATUS

You don't have to be a health expert to know that there are physiological differences between men and women. Although much of male and female anatomy is identical, it's clear that many major medical differences exist. Many diseases—osteoporosis, thyroid disease, lupus, and Alzheimer's disease, for example—are far more common in women than in men. Diseases may show up differently in men than in women—research suggests that hypertension treatment for men may not be beneficial to white women, for example. Finally, although women live longer than men, they don't necessarily have a better quality of life.[5]

The Women's Health Initiative

Much of the current interest in exploring women's health came after a highly publicized 1990 government study raised concern about the uneven numbers of women included in clinical trial research conducted by the National Institutes of Health (NIH). The NIH established the Office of Research on Women's Health (ORWH) in 1990 to oversee the representation of women in NIH studies. According to Vivian Pinn, ORWH's director, "For too long, medicine has viewed women as 'abnormal men' when considering health problems."[6]

Researchers excluded women from clinical trials of new drugs for several reasons. The Food and Drug Administration (FDA) issued rules in the 1970s stating that women with "childbearing potential" should be excluded from most studies, due largely to the disastrous results of a study of the drug thalidomide—a large number of the pregnant women in the study went on to have deformed babies. Moreover, in order to determine the precise effects of a drug or treatment, researchers have not wanted to deal with variations caused by women's menstrual cycles.

Report on Prevention Project Is Mixed Bag

Nearly 15 years ago, the federal government launched an ambitious prevention program to increase the American lifespan. Midway through the effort, Americans have made significant gains against killers such as heart disease. But there also have been turns for the worse, most notably the rates of teenage pregnancy and homicide. Moreover, the gap in health status between white Americans and members of minority groups has widened along socioeconomic lines.

The national project, called Healthy People 2000, set specific targets for a variety of preventive strategies. Health officials estimate that about half of all deaths could be prevented. Some of the findings of this large-scale project appeared in last week's Journal of the American Medical Association.

On the plus side: Greater life expectancy. Death rates are down for all age groups, and today the typical American can expect to live a record 75.8 years.

There also are promising trends in tobacco use and in alcohol-related deaths. Prenatal care is increasing. So are childhood immunizations. The number of people who die in motor vehicle accidents is declining thanks to wider use of seat belts, air bags and child safety seats. And the number who succumb to heart disease and stroke is declining. There also are slight improvements as well in cancer deaths and solid progress against two sexually transmitted diseases: gonorrhea and syphilis.

"Generally, I see this report as positive, but at the same time, there's no question that in some critical areas we are not making progress and are even slipping," said Morehouse School of Medicine president Louis Sullivan, who started the Healthy People 2000 effort when he was secretary of health and human services in the Bush administration.

On the negative side, there is a troubling trend toward obesity. Also, there's such an increase in teenage pregnancies that "one in 10 girls ages 15 to 17 is getting pregnant in this country," notes J. Michael McGinnis, deputy assistant secretary for health of the U. S. Public Health Service. The number of homicides continues to sharply increase, particularly among young black males.

The Healthy People 2000 report shows progress for blacks in a wide variety of health categories: more prenatal care and breast-feeding and less infant death, coronary heart disease, stroke, cirrhosis and unintentional injuries. But teen pregnancies, AIDS incidence and asthma hospitalizations are all moving away from the goals, and there is nearly a seven-year gap in life expectancy between African Americans and whites.

Among Hispanics, there are increases in the number of women being screened for breast and cervical cancers, as well as higher rates of breast-feeding. There are reductions in teen pregnancy rates, infant mortality and the number of smokers. But there also is a decline in access to primary health care, as well as increased numbers of AIDS cases, TB and obesity.

"So much of the area where we have not made much progress is in addressing the health of poor people," Sullivan said. "We have always known that people who are more affluent and more educated are more successful at getting and acting on information, including health information. The health movement is a middle-class movement. Now we need to find ways to educate and motivate low-income individuals to improve their health behavior, knowledge and attitudes."

Among the mid-decade findings of the 10-year Healthy People 2000 project reported last week:

Children made some of the most significant gains as a result of reductions in infant mortality and improved childhood immunizations. In 1983, nearly 250,000 children were exposed to lead and at risk of permanent brain damage. Five years later, that number had dropped to 93,000 children, a decline of two-thirds, McGinnis said, noting that the trend is well on the way to the zero exposure targeted for the year 2000. . . .

Where children's health continues to fall short, however, is in the number of infants born weighing less than 2,500 grams (5½ pounds). They are at risk of a variety of ailments, from growth retardation and lung problems to developmental delay. Some 6.9 percent of babies were born with dangerously low birth weights in 1987. Five years later, the number rose slightly to 7.1 percent. "There's been no progress made in this area," McGinnis said. "There continues to be a persistent gap."

Adolescents saw major improvements in the area of addiction. Fewer adolescents are beginning to smoke. Fewer teens use alcohol and marijuana. But while the numbers are moving in the right direction, McGinnis said, not enough progress has been made to reach the goals by 2000.

In 1987, an estimated 6 million teenagers smoked cigarettes. Five years later, the number had declined only 3 percent, not enough to meet the target. Alcohol use has declined significantly. "But there's been some slight movement up in the last couple of years," McGinnis said, "so we have to watch it.". . .

The biggest setbacks in adolescent health involve teenage pregnancy, homicide and other violence. The plan targeted a 20 percent decrease in homicide rates, designed to reduce the 91 homicides per 100,000 found among black males aged 15 to 34 years in 1987. By comparison, 1987 homicide rates for the total U. S. population were 9 per 100,000.

Despite these efforts, however, homicide rates in 1992 rose across the board, reaching 11 per 100,000 for the total population and 134 per 100,000 for black males aged 15 to 34. Both figures are well above the year 2000 targets.

Healthy People 2000 also targeted a 30 percent reduction in teenage pregnancies by the year 2000. In 1987, there were

(continued)

71 teen pregnancies per 1,000 pregnant women; by 1993, the figure had risen to 74 per 1,000, well above the 50 per 1,000 pregnancies goal.

Adults have seen gains in reducing the risks for heart disease, still the leading killer of Americans, declining exposure to air pollutants, and increasing rates of physical activity and blood testing for colon cancer. Blood cholesterol levels dropped from an average of 213 milligrams in the four-year period from 1976 to 1980 to 205 milligrams in 1988 to 1991—well on the way to the Healthy People 2000 goal of 200 milligrams. . . .

More people are living in communities with clean air, an important way to reduce the risk of various lung diseases. About half of Americans were living in places with little air pollution in 1988. By 1993, the number had risen to more than three quarters, "well on the way to the year 2000 target," McGinnis said. "We have made striking gains in this area."

A few more people are working out, but the numbers still fall far short of the goal. By 1991 about 24 percent of Americans were exercising regularly, an increase of 2 percent since 1985.

Most distressing to health officials is that one in every three Americans is now considered overweight. In 1976, one in four Americans were overweight.

Women showed gains in screening for cervical cancer and have now met the plan's goal. In 1993, 95 percent of eligible women 18 and older were having Pap smears and pelvic exams, achieving the target goal seven years early.

Another goal nearly met is the number of women screened for breast cancer. Only one in four women aged 50 and older were regularly screened for the disease in 1987. By 1993, 55 percent of eligible women were undergoing the screening, close to the 60 percent mark set by Healthy People 2000.

The number of women who have prenatal care in the first trimester is also on the upswing, an improvement designed to reduce health risks for expectant mothers and their children. Some 76 percent of mothers received prenatal care in the first trimester of pregnancy in 1987; by 1992, the figure had risen to 78 percent, moving toward the 90 percent target for the year 2000.

Men may find the greatest potential benefit in regular exercise. Those who do about 30 minutes a day of moderate activity, such as brisk walking or stair climbing, are at significantly reduced risk of premature death (defined as dying before age 65), according to a study of nearly 10,000 men conducted by the Cooper Institute's Steven Blair and colleagues. So too are sedentary men who change their ways and engage in regular physical activity, according to the study, which was issued at the same time as the Healthy People 2000 findings.

Healthy People 2000 Report Card

Goal	Start (1983)	Update (1995)	Target (2000)
Lower cholesterol levels (avg. level)	213 mg	205 mg	200 mg
More people exercise regularly	22%	24%	30%
More people with clean air in communities	50%	76%	85%
No measles cases	3,058	312	0
Fewer youths beginning to smoke	30%	27%	15%
Reduced alcohol use among teens	25%	18%	13%
Reduced marijuana use among teens	6.4%	4.9%	3.2%
No children with blood lead	234	93	0
Fewer newborns with low birth weight	6.9%	7.1%	5%
Fewer people overweight	26%	34%	20%
Reduced homicide rate for black males, 15–34 (homicides per 100,000)	91	134	72
Fewer teen pregnancies (pregnancies per 1,000)	71	74	50

Source: Excerpted from Sally Squires, "Report on Prevention Project is Mixed Bag," *Washington Post Health,* April 18, 1995. ©1995 The Washington Post. Reprinted by permission.

Of course, men and women do vary physiologically, and the elimination of women from many studies means that the results from these studies cannot be applied to women directly. According to social psychologist Carol Tavris, "If you want to know the effects of Drug X and you throw women out of your study because the men-strual cycle affects their responses to medication, you cannot then extrapolate from your study of men to women, precisely because the menstrual cycle affects their responses to medication."[7] One of the most salient examples of this phenomenon was research suggesting that aspirin could prevent heart attacks. The research involved

Disparities in Health: Real or Imagined?

While arguments currently rage over the best system of health care for the United States, it is useful to remember the vast differences between the haves and the have-nots when it comes to certain health indicators.

Achieving a healthier United States depends on significant improvements in the health of population groups now at higher risk for premature death, disease, and disability.

Indicator of Health	White Male	Black Male	White Female	Black Female
Death rate for suicide*	19.6	12.5	4.8	2.4
Death rate for homicide and legal intervention*	8.1	61.5	2.8	12.5
Maternal death rate for complications during pregnancy and childbirth*	NA	NA	5.4	18.6
Death rate for breast cancer*	NA	NA	22.9	26.0
Infant death rate**	8.2	17.7	8.2	17.7

* Age-adjusted rates per 100,000
** Per 1,000 live births.

1. Of all the death rates listed, which shows the greatest disparity between whites and blacks? Which rates are worse for whites than for blacks? For females than for males? Why do you think these differences occur?

2. What factors do you believe have contributed to these disparities?

3. What actions could be taken to improve each of the above health indicators? Which indicators may be modified by individual actions? Which ones must be modified by community (legislative, economic, environ- mental, or health-care system) measures? By both individual and community actions?

Source: Adapted by permission of the American Public Health Association from C. Hogue and M. Hargreaves, "Class, Race, and Infant Mortality in the United States," *American Journal of Public Health,* 83, no. 1 (1993): 9–12; and from U.S. Department of Health and Human Services (1994), *Health: United States 1993 and Prevention Profile,* DHHS Publication.

a study of 22,000 male doctors. Without accounting for the physiological differences between men and women (premenopausal women have fewer heart attacks than same-aged men; postmenopausal women have more), aspirin was prescribed to women as well.

To address concerns about women's health, the NIH launched the Women's Health Initiative (WHI), a 15-year, $625 million study focusing on the leading causes of death and disease in more than 140,000 postmenopausal women. WHI researchers hope to find out how a healthful lifestyle and increased medical attention can help prevent women's cancers, heart disease, and osteoporosis. In addition, the NIH has specified that equal amounts of money and time must be spent on men's and women's health research.[8]

Medical School Training

The push for change is coming from the government as well. In 1994, a House Appropriations Committee report declared that U.S. physicians are "not adequately trained to address the needs of women." As a result, the NIH's Office of Research on Women's Health and the Health Resources and Services Administration have joined forces to find out exactly where the gaps in medical education are and to recommend a model curriculum to Congress. The new curriculum will require students to consider examples of women in all their classes, not just in obstetrics and gynecology. Eventually, medical students who learn about high cholesterol will have to consider the effects of estrogen and other previously ignored topics.[9]

WHAT DO YOU THINK?

What factors do you think may contribute to each of the disparities in men's and women's health status shown in the Health Headlines box? What actions should be taken to reduce these disparities?

IMPROVING YOUR HEALTH

Benefits of Achieving Optimal Health

Table 1.1 provides an overview of the leading causes of death in the United States today. Risks for each of these leading killers can be reduced significantly by the practice of specific lifestyle patterns—for example, consuming a diet low in saturated fat and cholesterol, exercising regularly, reducing sodium intake, and managing stress. Individual behavior is believed to be a major determinant of good health, but heredity, access to health care, and the environment are other factors that influence health status (see Figure 1.3). When these factors are combined, the net effect on health can be great.

For example, you may be predisposed to a less healthy lifestyle if you are unable to access the health-care system because you have no health insurance, if your family doesn't believe in traditional medicine, or if family members or friends smoke, drink heavily, and/or take drugs. While you can't change your genetic history, and while improving your environment and the health-care system can be difficult, you can influence your future health status by the behaviors you choose today.

Reduction in risk for major diseases is just one of the benefits that you can hope to achieve when choosing healthy behaviors. Among the others are

- improved quality of life, in addition to an increased life span

- greater energy levels and increased capacity for and interest in having fun

- a stronger immune system, which enhances your ability to fight infections

- improved self-confidence, self-concept and self-esteem, and self-efficacy

- enhanced relationships with others due to better communication and "quality" time spent with them

- an improved ability to control and manage stress

- a reduced reliance on the health-care system

- improved cardiovascular functioning

- increased muscle tone, strength, flexibility, and endurance, which results in improved physical appearance, performance, and self-esteem

- a more positive outlook on life, fewer negative thoughts, and an ability to view life as challenging and negative events as an opportunity for growth

- improved environmental sensitivity, responsibility, and behaviors

- enhanced levels of spiritual health, awareness, and feelings of oneness with yourself, others, and the environment

Health Behaviors: Making Health-Wise Choices

Although mounting evidence indicates that there are significant benefits to being healthy, many people find it difficult to become and remain healthy. Most experts believe that there are several key behaviors that will help people live longer, such as:

- getting a good night's sleep (minimum of seven hours)

TABLE 1.1 ■ Leading Causes of Death in the United States

All Ages and Races Combined	15–24 Years of Age
1. Heart disease	1. Accidents and adverse effects
2. Cancer	2. Homicide
3. Stroke	3. Suicide
4. Chronic lung diseases	4. Cancer
5. Accidents and adverse effects	5. Heart disease
6. Pneumonia and influenza	6. AIDS
7. Diabetes	7. Congenital abnormalities
8. AIDS	8. Pneumonia and influenza
9. Suicide	9. Stroke
10. Homicide and legal intervention	10. Chronic lung disease

Source: Kochanek, Kenneth, and Bettie Hudson. Advance Report of Final Mortality Statistics. *Monthly Vital Statistics Report,* Vol. 43, No. 6. March 22, 1995. Centers for Disease Control and Prevention/ National Center for Health Statistics.

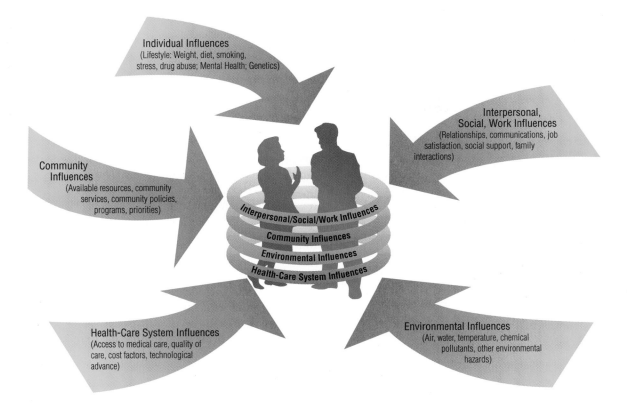

FIGURE 1.3

Factors that Influence Your Health Status

- maintaining healthy eating habits

- weight management

- physical recreational activities

- avoiding tobacco products

- practicing safe sex

- limiting intake of alcohol

- scheduling regular self-exams and medical check-ups

Although health professionals can statistically assess the health benefits of these behaviors, there are several other actions that may not cause quantifiable "years added to life," but may significantly result in "life added to years," such as

- controlling the real and imaginary stressors in life

- forming and maintaining meaningful relationships with family and friends

- making time for oneself

- participating in at least one fun activity each day

- respecting the environment and the people in it

- considering alternatives when making decisions and assessing how actions affect others

- valuing each day and making the best of each opportunity

- viewing mistakes as opportunities to learn and grow

- being as kind to oneself as to others

- understanding the health-care system and using it wisely

While it's easy to list things that one should do and even that one may really want to do, change is not easy. All people, no matter where they are on the health/wellness continuum, have to start somewhere. All people have faced personal and external challenges to their attempts to change their health behaviors—some have not done so well, some have been extremely successful, and some have made only small changes that may add up to significant improvements in how they feel and how they live their lives. The key is to decide what needs to change, determine the major actions necessary for the accomplishment of goals, set up a plan of action, and get started. But first, it is important to take a close look at those factors that may contribute to current behaviors.

PREPARING FOR BEHAVIOR CHANGE

Mark Twain said that "habit is habit, and not to be flung out the window by anyone, but coaxed downstairs a step at a time." Changing negative behavior patterns into healthy ones is often a time-consuming and difficult process. The chances of successfully changing negative behavior problems improve when you make gradual changes that give you time to unlearn negative patterns and to substitute positive ones. We have not yet developed a foolproof method for effectively changing behavior, but we do know that certain behavior changes can benefit both individuals and society. To understand how the process of behavior change works, we must first identify specific behavior patterns and attempt to understand the reasons for them.

The development and maintenance of health behaviors, however, do not necessarily conform to a model in which we can assume that if we have knowledge, our attitudes and behaviors will automatically change. If this were so, knowledgeable people would not behave in ways detrimental to their health. The reasons why people be-

Getting involved in an enjoyable physical activity is a significant step toward a healthy lifestyle and the prevention of illness.

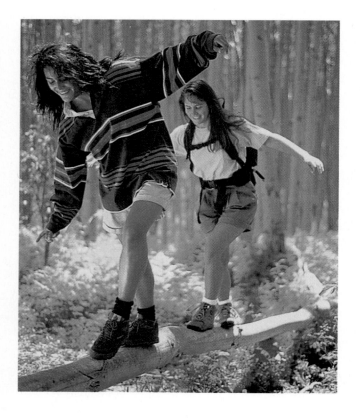

have in unhealthy ways, despite known risks, are complex and not easily understood. Health researchers have studied health behaviors for decades and continue to analyze the reasons why one person chooses to act responsibly while another ignores obvious health risks.

Factors Influencing Behavior Change

Figure 1.4 identifies the major factors that influence behavior and behavior-change decisions. These factors can be divided into three general categories: predisposing, enabling, and reinforcing factors.

Predisposing Factors. Our life experiences, knowledge, cultural and ethnic inheritance, and current beliefs and values are all *predisposing factors* influencing behavior and behavior change. Factors that may predispose us to certain conditions include our age, sex, race, income, family background, educational background, and access to health care. For example, if your parents smoked, you are 90 percent more likely to start smoking than someone whose parents didn't. If your peers smoke, you are 80 percent more likely to smoke than someone whose friends don't.

Enabling Factors. Skills or abilities; physical, emotional, and mental capabilities; and resources and accessible facilities that make health decisions more convenient or difficult are *enabling factors.* Positive enablers encourage you to carry through on your intentions. Negative enablers work against your intentions to change. For example, if you would like to join a local fitness center but discover that the closest one is 4 miles away and that the membership fee is $500, those negative enablers may convince you to stay home. On the other hand, if your school's fitness center is two blocks away, is open until midnight, and has a special student membership deal, those positive enablers will probably convince you to join the center. Identifying these positive and negative enabling factors and devising alternative plans when the negative factors outweigh the positive are part of a necessary planning strategy for behavioral change.

Reinforcing Factors. The presence or absence of support, encouragement, or discouragement that significant people in your life bring to a situation is a *reinforcing factor.* For example, if you decide to stop smoking and your family and friends smoke in your presence, you may be tempted to start smoking again. In other words, your smoking behavior was reinforced. Reinforcing factors also include policies and services that make it easier for you to maintain a particular behavior. If, however, you are overweight and you lose a few pounds and all your friends tell you how terrific you look, your positive behavior will be reinforced and you will be more likely to continue to diet. Reinforcing factors, which may influence you toward pos-

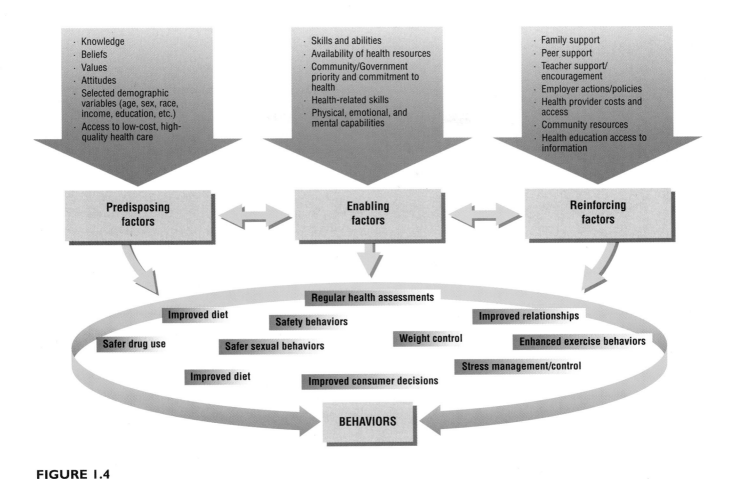

FIGURE 1.4

Factors that Influence Your Behavior-Change Decisions

itive and/or negative behaviors, include money, popularity, support and appreciation from friends, and family interest and enthusiasm for what you are doing.

The manner in which you reward or punish yourself for your own successes and failures may affect your chances of adopting healthy behaviors. Learning to accept small failures and to concentrate on your successes may foster further successes. Berating yourself because you binged on ice cream, argued with a friend, or didn't jog because it was raining may create an internal environment in which failure becomes almost inevitable. Telling yourself that you're worth the extra time and effort and giving yourself a pat on the back for small accomplishments is an often overlooked factor in positive behavior change.

It is not our intention to blame you if you are struggling with personal health behaviors or to suggest that all the variables that affect health are within your control. Our goal is to help you realize which factors are within your personal control and to show you how to maximize your decision-making powers to maintain your current good health, improve your current health, or prevent premature deterioration of your health status.

Major changes in health behavior are not made by following easy, one-step recipes. Lasting behavior changes that ultimately improve your overall health and well-being require careful thought, individual analysis, and considerable effort. Changing beliefs, attitudes, values, actions, and behaviors that have been developing from infancy is difficult. Not surprisingly, even the most strong-willed people discover that willpower alone is not enough to get them through the many adjustments usually needed to change behavior.

A joke among psychologists goes like this. Question: "How many psychologists does it take to change a light bulb?" Answer: "Only one. But the light bulb has to really want to change!" Wanting to change is a prerequisite of the change process, but there is much more to the process than motivation. Motivation must be combined with common sense, commitment, and a realistic understanding of how best to move from point A to point B. *Readiness* is the state of being that precedes behavior change. People who are ready to change possess the knowledge, attitudes, skills, and internal and external resources that make change a likely reality. For someone to be ready for change, certain basic steps and adjustments in thinking must occur.

What Do You Think?

Who do you think you could ask to help support you in your behavior change effort? What factors could make this change difficult? What can you do to avoid these difficulties? Is this the right time for you to begin this change? How ready are you? Do you think you know enough about what's involved? Do you need to have any special skills?

Your Beliefs and Attitudes

Even if you know why you should make a specific behavior change, your beliefs and attitudes about the value of your actions in making a difference will significantly af-

The support and encouragement of friends who have similar goals and interests will strengthen your commitment to develop and maintain positive health behaviors.

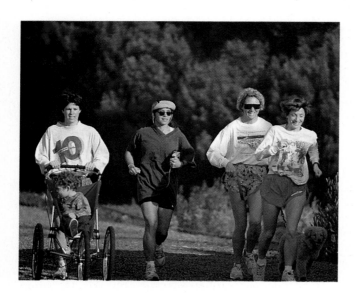

Belief: Appraisal of the relationship between some object, action, or idea and some attribute of that object, action, or idea.

Attitude: Relatively stable set of beliefs, feelings, and behavioral tendencies in relation to something or someone.

Health Belief Model (HBM): Model for explaining how beliefs may influence behaviors.

fect what you do. We often assume that when rational people realize there is a risk in what they are doing, they will act to reduce that risk. But this is not necessarily true. Consider the number of physicians and other health professionals who smoke, fail to manage stress, consume high-fat diets, and act in other unhealthy ways. They surely know better, but their "knowing" is disconnected from their "doing." Why is this so? Two strong influences on our actions are beliefs and attitudes.

A **belief** is an appraisal of the relationship between some object, action, or idea (for example, smoking) and some attribute of that object, action, or idea (for example, smoking is expensive, dirty, and causes cancer—or it is relaxing). Beliefs may develop from direct experience (for example, if you have trouble breathing after smoking for several years) or from secondhand experience or knowledge conveyed by other people (for example, if you see your grandfather die of lung cancer after he has smoked for years).[10] Although most of us have a general idea of what constitutes a belief, we may be a bit uncertain about what constitutes an attitude. We often hear or make such comments as, "He's got a rotten attitude," or, "She needs an attitude adjustment," but may still be unable to define *attitude*. An **attitude** is a relatively stable set of beliefs, feelings, and behavioral tendencies in relation to something or someone.

Do Beliefs and Attitudes Influence Behavior?

It seems logical to conclude that your beliefs will influence your behavior. If you believe (make the appraisal) that taking drugs (an action) is harmful for you (attribute of that action), you will not use drugs. If you believe that drinking and driving are incompatible, you will never drink and drive. Or will you?

Psychologists studying the relationship between beliefs and health behaviors have determined that although beliefs may subtly influence behavior, these beliefs may not actually cause people to change behavior. In 1966, psychologist I. Rosenstock developed a model for explaining how beliefs may or may not influence subsequent behaviors.[11] His **Health Belief Model (HBM)** provides a means to show when beliefs affect behavior change (see Figure 1.5). Although many other models attempt to explain the influence of beliefs on behaviors, the HBM is one of the most widely accepted models. According to the HBM, several factors must support a belief in order for change to be likely to occur:

- *Perceived seriousness of the health problem.* First, a person needs to consider how severe the medical and social consequences would be if the health problem was to develop or was left untreated. The more serious a person believes the effects will be, the more likely he or she is to take action.

The Health-Wise Consumer: Separating Fact from Fiction

One of the most difficult problems you may have when trying to inform yourself about health issues is determining what to believe and what not to believe about all the conflicting articles, reports, and televised claims about various health risks. Is beta-carotene the miracle cancer cure of the future? Can creams really rub your cellulite and wrinkles away? Does a glass of wine a day keep the doctor away? If you're puzzled by it all, you're not alone. Although no 100 percent foolproof methods exist for determining the merits of health messages, you can ask some basic questions when someone tells you, or you read about, a new "health" product or service.

1. *What is the source of the information?* Where the study was done and who paid for the research will often reveal possibly unreliable or biased research conclusions. Data supplied by independent investigators working for agencies that do not have a vested interest in the outcome may reduce potential bias.

2. *Who are the authors of the study?* Who conducted the research? What were their credentials for doing the research? Are they working at a reputable institution or agency? Have they done similar research in these areas previously? Do they stand to gain financially from the outcome of the research?

3. *What research methods were used in the study?* Familiarity with basic research terms and principles of sound research methods may help you determine the merit of a study. You should consider the following:

Sample size. Always look at the number of people involved in a study that supposedly proves a health effect. Obviously, the more people participating in the study the better, particularly if the researchers are generalizing their findings to the population. Although some studies using small numbers of subjects may be valid, they must follow certain special research protocols.

Subjects. How were the subjects selected? Are they from diverse backgrounds? Did they volunteer to participate? Were they selected at random?

Study design. Does the study have a control group (a group of people with similar characteristics who did not receive the treatment being used to study a given effect)?

4. *Is the source generally reputable?*

News magazines/newspapers. News magazines or newspapers may have a sensational twist to their reporting. They often have interesting articles written by health writers who are not necessarily knowledgeable about their subject. They may have a one-sided approach to an issue or provide inaccurate or incomplete information.

Self-help books. Reader beware. Many self-made authorities have been successful at getting people to buy their books. Just because something is published in a book doesn't make it accurate or reliable. Stick to reputable authors having degrees or academic training in the subject, check their statements against textbooks in the field, or call health professionals to verify particular points.

Professional journals. Although sometimes more difficult to read, *refereed* (peer-reviewed) journals are perhaps the most reliable sources of health information. A refereed article is reviewed by at least three experts in the field before it is accepted for publication. Do not confuse an edited journal with a refereed journal. Edited journals have paid editors who review the work for style and so forth, but these editors may not have the background required to deal with the content of a particular study. Most refereed journals publish guidelines for submitting manuscripts to their journal. These guidelines typically give information about the peer-review process. Most college and university journals are peer-reviewed.

- *Perceived susceptibility to the health problem.* Next, a person needs to evaluate the likelihood of developing the health problem. Those who perceive themselves as more likely to develop the health problem are more likely to take preventive action.

- *Cues to action.* Those who are reminded or alerted about a potential health problem are more likely to take preventive action.

Three other factors are linked to perceived risk for health problems: *demographic variables,* including age, gender, race, and ethnic background; *sociopsychological variables,* including personality traits, social class, and social pressure; and *structural variables,* including knowledge about or prior contact with the health problem.

The Health Belief Model is followed many times every day. Take, for example, smokers. Older smokers are likely to know other smokers who have developed serious heart or lung problems as a result of smoking. They are thus more likely to perceive a threat to their health connected with the behavior of smoking than is a young person who has just begun smoking. The greater the perceived threat of health problems caused by smoking, the greater the chance a person will quit smoking. However, many chronic smokers know that they have serious health problems, yet they continue to smoke. Why do people fail to

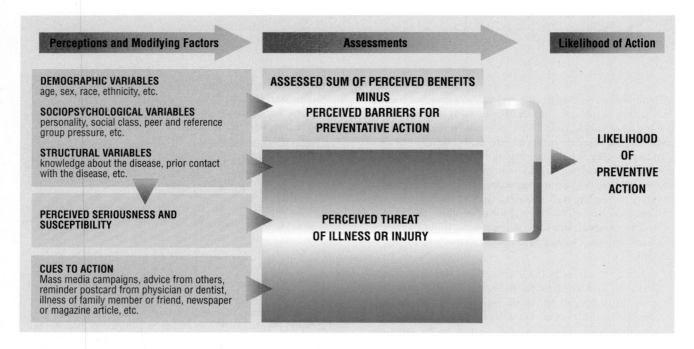

FIGURE 1.5

Health Belief Model

Source: Adapted by permission from Edward P. Sarafino, *Health Psychology: Biopsychosocial Interactions* (New York: John Wiley & Sons, 1990), p. 190. Copyright © 1990 by John Wiley & Sons.

take actions to avoid further harm? According to Rosenstock, some people do not believe that they will be affected by a severe problem—they act as if they believe they have some kind of immunity—and are unlikely to change their behaviors. In some cases, they may think that, even if they get cancer or have a heart attack, the health-care system will cure them.

Other HBM factors that affect the likelihood of behavior change are assessments about whether the benefits outweigh the costs and whether actions will actually work. If you are so addicted to smoking that the thought of quitting is not acceptable to you, or if you enjoy smoking too much, you will probably keep smoking, particularly if the consequences won't be felt for some time and the pleasure is there for the moment.

𝒲HAT DO YOU THINK?

What is one major health behavior that you believe you should change? How serious a threat to your health is this behavior right now? Do you worry much about what will happen to you if you don't make the change? What can you do right now to reduce your risks for the above health threat? List the steps that you intend to take today. This week. Is anyone influencing you to make this decision?

Your Intentions to Change

Our attitudes tend to reflect our emotional responses to situations and also tend to follow from our beliefs. According to the **Theory of Reasoned Action,** our behaviors result from our intentions to perform actions. An intention is a product of our attitude toward an action and our beliefs about what others may want us to do.[12] A behavioral intention, then, is a written or stated commitment to perform an action.

If, for example, you are out of shape and your health is important to you, you may take steps to improve your fitness level. But if your best friends tell you that you really do need to get into shape and you want to gain their respect or admiration, your intention to begin an exercise program may become stronger. In brief, the more consistent and powerful your attitudes about an action are and the more you are influenced by others to take that action, the greater will be your stated intention to do so—in this example, to exercise. The more you verbalize your commitment to exercising, the more likely it is that you will exercise.

Significant Others as Change Agents

Many people are highly influenced by the approval or disapproval (real or imagined) of close friends and loved ones and of the social and cultural groups to which they belong. Such influences can offer support for health actions, making healthy behavior all the more possible to attain; they can also affect behavior negatively, interfering with even the best intentions of making a positive change.

Your Family. From the time of your birth, your parents have influenced your behaviors by giving you strong cues about which actions are socially acceptable and which are not. Brushing your teeth, bathing, wearing deodorant, and chewing food with your mouth closed are probably all behaviors that your family instilled in you long ago. Your family culture influenced your food choices, your religious beliefs, your political beliefs, and all your other values and actions. If you deviated from your family's norms, your mother or father probably let you know fairly quickly.

Family can mean many things to a child growing up. For those who have two parents present, it may mean a mother and a father who take the time to teach respect for property and for others, and to provide the social support and comfort that a child needs to feel loved and secure. For others, it may mean a single mom or dad who uses the support of friends and relatives to create a loving and nurturing atmosphere for growth. In some cases, family is the group of loved ones that a person lives with, whether relatives, friends, or a group brought together by common bonds. No two family structures are exactly alike. What good family units have in common is a dedication to the healthful development of all family members, unconditional trust, and a commitment to work out difficulties.

When the loving family unit does not exist, when it does not provide for basic human needs, or when dysfunctional, irresponsible individuals try to build a family under the influence of drugs or alcohol, it becomes difficult for a child to learn positive health behaviors. Healthy behaviors get their start in healthy homes; unhealthy homes breed unhealthy habits. Healthy families provide the foundation for a clear and necessary understanding of what is right and wrong, what is positive and negative. Without this fundamental grounding, many young people have great difficulties.

Social Bonds. Like family, hometown environments also mold behaviors. If you deviated from the actions expected in your hometown, you probably suffered strange looks, ostracism by some high school cliques, and other negative social reactions. The more you value the opinions of other people, the more likely you are to change a behavior that offends them. If you couldn't care less what they think, you probably brush off their negative reactions or suggested changes. How often have you told yourself, "I don't care what so-and-so thinks. I'll do what I darn well please"? Although most of us have thought or said these words, we in fact all too often care too much about what even the insignificant people in our lives think. We say certain things, act in a prescribed manner, and respond in a specific way because our culture, our upbringing, and

our need to be liked by others pressure us to do what we believe they think is the right thing. In general, the lower your level of self-esteem and self-efficacy, the higher the chances that others will influence your actions.

Sometimes, the influence of others can be a powerful social support for our positive behavior changes. At other times, we are influenced to drink too much, party too hard, eat too much, or engage in some other negative action because we don't want to be left out or because we fear criticism. Learning to understand the subtle and not-so-subtle ways in which our families, friends, and other people have influenced and continue to influence our behaviors is an important step toward changing our behaviors.

BEHAVIOR CHANGE TECHNIQUES

Once you have analyzed all the factors influencing your current behavior and all the factors that may influence the direction and potential success of the behavior change you are considering, you must decide which of several possible behavior change techniques will work best for you.

Shaping: Developing New Behaviors in Small Steps

Regardless of how motivated and committed you are to change, some behaviors are almost impossible to change immediately. To reach your goal, you may need to take a number of individual steps, each designed to change one small piece of the larger behavior. This process is known as **shaping**. For example, suppose that you have not exercised for awhile. You decide that you want to get into shape and your goal is to be able to jog 3 to 4 miles every other day. You realize that you'd face a near-death experience if you tried to run even just a few blocks in your current condition. So you decide to start slowly and build up to your desired fitness level gradually. During week 1, you will walk for one hour every other day at a slow, relaxed pace. During week 2, you will walk the same amount of time but will speed up your pace and cover slightly more ground. During week 3, you will speed up even more and will try to go even farther. You will continue taking such steps until you reach your goal.

Theory of Reasoned Action: Model for explaining the importance of our intentions in determining behaviors.

Shaping: Using a series of small steps to get to a particular goal gradually.

Whatever the desired behavior change, all shaping involves

- starting slowly and trying not to cause undue stress during the early stages of the program
- keeping the steps small and achievable
- being flexible and ready to change if the original plan proves uncomfortable
- refusing to skip steps or to move to the next step until the previous step has been mastered. Behaviors don't develop overnight, so they won't change overnight.

Visualizing: The Imagined Rehearsal

Mental practice and rehearsal can help change unhealthy behaviors into healthy ones. Athletes and others have used a technique known as **imagined rehearsal** to reach their goals. By visualizing their planned action ahead of time, they were better prepared when they put themselves to the test.

For example, suppose you want to ask someone out on a date. Imagine the setting (walking together to class) for the action. Then practice exactly what you're going to say ("Minh, there's a great concert this Sunday and I was wondering if . . .") in your mind and out loud. Mentally anticipate different responses ("Oh, I'd love to but I'm busy that evening.") and what you will say in reaction ("How about if I call you sometime this week?"). Careful mental and verbal rehearsal (you could even try your scenario out on a good friend) will greatly improve the likelihood of successful behavioral consequences because you will be less likely to be flustered or to be taken by surprise.

Modeling

Modeling, or learning behaviors through careful observation of other people, is one of the most effective strategies for changing behavior. For example, suppose that you have great difficulty talking to people you don't

know very well. Effective communication is essential to achieving optimal health (see the Building Communication Skills box). One of the easiest ways to improve your communication skills is to select friends whose "gift of gab" you envy. Observe their social skills. What do they say? How do they act? Do they talk more or listen more? How do people respond to them? Why are they such good communicators? If you carefully observe behaviors you admire and isolate their components, you can model the steps of your behavior change strategy on a proven success.

Controlling the Situation

Sometimes, putting yourself in the right setting or with the right group of people will positively influence your behaviors directly or indirectly. Many situations and occasions trigger similar behaviors by different people. For example, in libraries, churches, and museums, most people talk softly. Few people laugh at funerals. The term **situational inducement** refers to an attempt to influence a behavior by using situations and occasions that are structured to exert control over that behavior.

For example, you may be more apt to stop smoking if you work in a smoke-free office, a positive situational inducement. But a smoke-filled bar, a negative situational inducement, may tempt you to resume smoking. Your

---

The success of efforts to change unhealthy behaviors often depends on conscious decisions to choose the right friends and to put oneself in constructive situations.

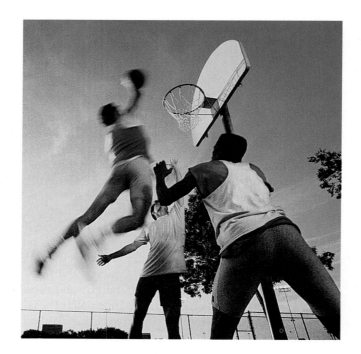

Imagined rehearsal: Practicing through mental imagery, to become better able to perform an event in actuality.

Modeling: Learning specific behaviors by watching others perform them.

Situational inducement: Attempt to influence a behavior by using situations and occasions that are structured to exert control over that behavior.

Positive reinforcement: Presenting something positive following a behavior that is being reinforced.

How to Help Someone Make a Change

In our quest to help loved ones change unhealthy behaviors, we sometimes become self-righteous. We then become "warriors against pleasure" to our loved ones and all our brilliant advice falls on deaf ears.

Why do our good intentions go up in smoke? Probably because of the way we communicate our advice. Ask yourself the following questions before offering your words of wisdom:

- Did your friend ask for your advice or help?
- Did your friend give any indication of being dissatisfied about something? Is there something that your friend indicated needed a change?
- Are you in a position to offer advice? Are you practicing what you preach?
- If you were in need of advice or help, how would you want someone to approach the subject with you?
- How honest can you be? How well do you know your friend's reactions? Can your friend take constructive advice? Is your friend very sensitive or defensive about his or her problem?

After you've asked yourself these questions,

- Go slow. Wait for some suggestion that your friend wants to talk. Don't just meet him or her in class and say, "Hey, have you thought about getting rid of that weight?"
- If your friend doesn't initiate a conversation about the problem, try to ease into it slowly. You could say, "Boy, I sure put on weight over the holidays. I really need to start working out to get rid of these extra pounds. I hate to go alone. Would you be interested in going swimming with me sometime this week?"
- **If your friend brings up the problem, be supportive.** "I know how hard it is to lose weight. I've struggled with it myself over the years, but have found that such and such works for me. I need to lose some weight myself. Let's work on it together. It'd really help me to have someone help me stay motivated."
- **If your friend is successful in getting started, regularly compliment his or her persistence in sticking to the diet/exercise program.** Don't overdo the compliments, particularly with someone who isn't comfortable with a cheerleader approach. Treat him or her as you'd normally do. Don't go overboard.
- **If your friend has a set-back, say it's okay.** Say you understand, but also encourage him or her to get back on track and stay motivated.
- **Help your friend stay interested.** Try to think of new things to do, new exercise routines, and new eating habits that will make behavior change a lifestyle change rather than an obstacle to be overcome.
- **Keep positive and offer support whenever it's asked for.** If you are brushed off or if your friend becomes angry, be patient and try another method.

---

careful consideration of which settings will help and which will hurt your effort to change, and your decision to seek the first and avoid the second, will improve your chances for successful behavior change.

Reinforcement: "Different Strokes for Different Folks"

A **positive reinforcement** seeks to increase the likelihood that a behavior will occur by presenting something positive as a reward for that behavior. Each of us is motivated by different reinforcers. While a special T-shirt may be a positive reinforcer for young adults entering a race, it would not be for a 40-year-old runner who dislikes message-bearing T-shirts.

Most positive reinforcers can be classified under five headings: consumable, activity, manipulative, possessional, and social reinforcers.

- *Consumable reinforcers* are delicious edibles such as candy, cookies, or gourmet meals.

- *Activity reinforcers* are opportunities to watch TV, to go on a vacation, to go swimming, or to do something else enjoyable.

- *Manipulative reinforcers* are such incentives as lower rent in exchange for mowing the lawn or the promise of a better grade for doing an extra-credit project.

- *Possessional reinforcers* are tangible rewards such as a new TV or a sports car.

- *Social reinforcers* are such things as loving looks, affectionate hugs, and praise.

When choosing reinforcers to help you maintain a healthy behavior or change an unhealthy behavior, you need to determine what would motivate you to act in a particular way. Your rewards or reinforcers may initially come from others (extrinsic rewards), but as you see positive changes in yourself, you will begin to reward and reinforce yourself (intrinsic rewards). Keep in mind that reinforcers should immediately follow a behavior. But beware of overkill. If you reward yourself with a movie on the VCR every time you go jogging, this reinforcer will soon lose its power. It would be better to give yourself this reward after, say, a full week of adherence to your jogging program.

What Do You Think?

What type of consumable reinforcers (food or drink) would be a healthy reward for your new behavior? If you could choose one activity reinforcer to reward yourself after you've been successful for one day in your new behavior, what would it be? If you could obtain/buy something for yourself (possessional reinforcer) after you reach your goal, what would it be? If you maintain your behavior for one week, what type of social reinforcer would you like to receive from your friends?

Changing Self-Talk

Self-talk, or the way you think and talk to yourself, can also play a role in modifying your health-related behaviors. Here are some cognitive procedures for changing self-talk.

Rational-Emotive Therapy. This form of cognitive therapy or self-directed behavior change is based on the premise that there is a close connection between what people say to themselves and how they feel. According to psychologist Albert Ellis, most everyday emotional problems and related behaviors stem from irrational statements that people make to themselves when events in their lives are different from what they would like them to be.[13]

For example, suppose that after doing poorly on an exam, you say to yourself, "I can't believe I flunked that easy exam. I'm so stupid." By changing this irrational, "catastrophic" self-talk into rational, positive statements about what is really going on, you can increase the likelihood that positive behaviors will occur. Positive self-talk could be, "I really didn't study enough for that exam, and I'm not surprised I didn't do very well. I'm certainly not stupid. I just need to prepare better for the next test." Such self-talk will help you to recover quickly from your disappointment and to take positive steps to correct the situation.

Meichenbaum's Self-Instructional Methods. In Meichenbaum's behavioral therapies, clients are encouraged to give "self-instructions" ("Slow down, don't rush") and "positive affirmations" ("My speech is going fine—I'm almost done!") to themselves instead of thinking self-defeating thoughts ("I'm talking too fast—my speech is terrible") whenever a situation seems to be getting out of control. Meichenbaum is perhaps best known for a process known as stress inoculation, in which clients are subjected to extreme stressors in a laboratory environ-

ment. Before a stressful event (e.g., going to the doctor), clients practice individual coping skills (e.g., deep breathing exercises) and self-instructions (e.g., "I'll feel better once I know what's causing my pain"). Meichenbaum demonstrated that clients who practiced coping techniques and self-instruction were less likely to resort to negative behaviors in stressful situations.

Blocking/Thought Stopping. By purposefully blocking or stopping negative thoughts, a person can concentrate on taking positive steps toward necessary behavior change. For example, suppose you are preoccupied with your ex-partner, who has recently deserted you for someone else. In blocking/thought stopping, you consciously stop thinking about the situation and force yourself to think about something more pleasant (e.g., dinner tomorrow with your best friend). By refusing to dwell on negative images and by forcing yourself to focus elsewhere, you can save wasted energy, time, and emotional resources and move on to positive change.

Making Behavior Change

Self-Assessment: Antecedents and Consequences

Behaviors, thoughts, and feelings always occur in a context—the situation. Situations can be divided into two components: the events that come before and those that come after a behavior. *Antecedents* are the setting events for a behavior; they cue or stimulate a person to act in certain ways. Antecedents can be physical events, thoughts, emotions, or the actions of other people. *Consequences*—the results of behavior—affect whether a person will repeat a behavior.[14] Consequences can also be physical events, thoughts, emotions, or the actions of other people.

For example, suppose you are shy and must give a speech in front of a large class. The antecedents are walking into the class, feeling frightened, wondering if you are capable of doing a good job, and being unable to remember a word of your speech. If the consequences are negative—if your classmates laugh and you get a low grade—your terror about speaking in public will be reinforced and you will continue to dread this kind of event. In contrast, if you receive positive feedback from the class or instructor, you may actually learn to like speaking in public.

Learning to recognize the antecedents of a behavior and acting to modify them is one method of changing behavior. A diary noting your undesirable behaviors and identifying the settings in which they occur can be a useful tool. For example, if you are gaining weight because you are snacking too much, keep a diary of when, where, and with whom you snack. If you are shoveling in the potato chips while studying, you may need to study in the library, where food isn't allowed, or to keep only low-calorie snacks in the house. If you eat more when you are angry, upset, depressed, or stressed, try to deal directly with your stressors. The positive consequences of these changes will be that you will maintain your weight. In the Choices for Change box, you may recognize several factors that can make behavior change more difficult.

Analyzing the Behavior You Want to Change

Successful behavior change requires a careful assessment of exactly what it is that you want to change. All too often we berate ourselves by using generalities: "I am not a good person, I'm lousy to my friend, I need to be a better person." Before you can begin to change a negative behavior, you must take a hard look at its specifics. Determining the specific behavior you would like to change—in contrast to the general problem—will allow you to set clear goals for change. What are you doing that makes you a lousy friend? Are you gossiping about your friend? Are you lying to your friend? Have you been a "taker" rather than a "giver" in the friendship? Or are you really a good friend most of the time?

Let's say the problem is gossiping. You can now analyze this behavior by examining the following components:

- *Frequency.* How often are you gossiping? All the time, or only once in a while?

- *Duration.* Have you been gossiping about your friend for a long period of time? How long?

- *Seriousness.* Is your gossiping just idle chatter, or are you really getting down and dirty and trying to injure the other person? What are the consequences for you? For your friend? For your friendship?

- *Basis for problem behavior.* Is your gossip based on facts, on your perceptions of facts, or on deliberate embellishments of facts?

- *Antecedents.* What kinds of situations trigger your gossiping? Do some settings or people bring out the gossip in you more than other settings and people? What triggers your feelings of dislike for or irritation toward your friend? Why are you talking behind your friend's back?

Decision Making: Choices for Change

You've assessed the antecedents and consequences of the behavior you want to change and analyzed its components. Now comes the real crunch: deciding what to do when faced with choices. Decision making is a skill that you must consciously develop. Choosing among alternatives is difficult when you are consciously and unconsciously pressured by internal and external influences. For example, "just saying no" is, of course, one choice when you are handed a glass of beer at a party. However, if you are trying desperately not to be considered a dweeb, if people with whom you identify are all drinking, or if you like the taste of beer, the decision becomes harder. By practicing the following decision-making skills prior to having that drink put into your hands, your chances of making the choice you really want to make will increase. This set of skills, referred to as **DECIDE,** can be applied to many situations in which you have to make a decision.[15]

D *Decide in advance what the problem is.* By defining the problem in advance, you will have time to decide how

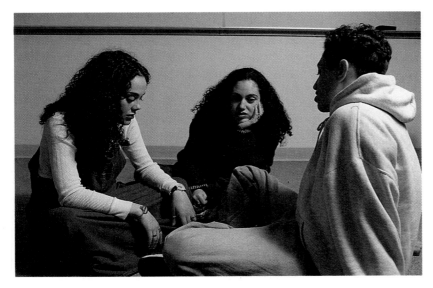

Talking with friends who have similar values can help you clarify your thinking about behaviors you want to change and provide on-going support as you attempt to reach your goals.

Overcoming Obstacles to Behavior Change: Why You May Self-Sabotage

Psychologists offer a number of explanations for why you may fail in your efforts to change your behavior:

■ *Stress.* When you are under lots of stress, it is often more difficult to get started on serious self-change projects. Symptoms of excessive stress include feeling emotionally drained, tense, or depressed; having a short reaction fuse; failing to overcome frustration quickly; and experiencing physical symptoms such as muscle tension, nausea, and headache. If you lower your stress levels, you will have a better chance of succeeding at change.

■ *Social pressures to repeat old habits.* The people around us influence us strongly. You may be trying to give up caffeine and a friend says, "Come on, have just one cup of coffee with me. I made this dessert for you, and we need coffee to go with it." One of the best things you can do when trying to change a behavior is to ask your friends to be supportive rather than to pressure you to do what you don't want to do.

■ *Not expecting mistakes.* Falling off the wagon—eating an ice-cream cone while you're on a diet, taking a drink when you've resolved not to—is almost inevitable. Unwanted behaviors that have been automatic for years are tough to change. A typical reaction to a slip-up is to become totally discouraged and to give up. This phenomenon happens so frequently that it has been given a name: the abstinence violation effect. Most experts believe that the best response to a slip-up is to forget about it and get right back on plan. Accept that slips are inevitable, but maintain control.

■ *Blaming yourself for poor coping or a weak personality.* If you blame your innate weakness when you backslide, you will tend to accept that change is impossible. Blame pres-sures from the environment or your own lack of skills instead. You will then realize that there is something you can do to make change easier.

■ *Lack of effort.* Some people really do not try hard enough. A study found that most students who fail introductory psychology courses study only about one-third as much as do students who make As and Bs even though they think they are studying just as much.

■ *Faulty beliefs/low self-efficacy.* Self-efficacy beliefs are your beliefs about your ability to deal with a specific situation. Research has shown that if people don't believe they can change behaviors, they are less likely to be successful. Developing new skills, focusing on your successes, and planning ahead for difficult situations may help you cope more effectively with behavioral challenges.

What behavior are you currently trying to change? Will it be easy or hard for you to make this change right now? Is your stress level high? What can you do to reduce or control your stress level? What will make it easier for you to stick to your behavior change? What will make it more difficult? Can you change or avoid some of the things that will make it hard for you? Are you really committed to do what it takes to change?

Do you believe you are ready to change and that you can do it this time?

Source: From *Self-Directed Behavior: Self-Modification for Personal Adjustment* by D. L. Watson and R. G. Tharp, 40–45. Copyright 1993, 1989, 1985, 1981, 1977, 1972 by Brooks/Cole Publishing Company, a division of Thomson Publishing Inc., Pacific Grove, CA 93950. Reprinted by permission of the publisher.

---

important it is. If you have really decided that drinking is not for you, or that drinking in certain situations could put you at risk, you will have set your basic criteria for acting in specific situations.

E *Explore the alternatives.* List the possible alternatives, ranging from not drinking to drinking heavily. If any of these alternatives is unacceptable to you, cross it off and work with those remaining.

C *Consider the consequences.* Think about each of the alternatives remaining. What are the possible positive and negative consequences of each? Think about what will probably happen, not just what may happen in the best and worst scenarios. How risky is each alternative?

Are the consequences of losing the friendship of a group because you refuse to drink as serious as of drinking heavily and getting into trouble sexually or of drinking and driving? Is there another alternative that could reduce your risks?

I *Identify your values.* Your beliefs and feelings about certain behaviors represent your values, and your values influence the vast majority of your behaviors. When choosing to drink or not to drink in a social setting, or when choosing how much to drink, you should base your choice on an analysis of your values.

D *Decide and take action.* If you have seriously thought about the first four DECIDE skills and decided that it's

Managing Your Behavior-Change Strategies

Having read this chapter, you should realize that health involves many dimensions of your life. Changing negative health-related behaviors is a complicated, multifaceted process requiring a great deal of commitment, personal insight, and knowledge. Very few of us could ever "just do it" as the advertisements may lead you to believe (at least not on the first try). As you read this book, you will find that each chapter lists specific activities and choices that enable you to adopt or maintain healthy behaviors. It may be helpful for you to consider the following activities and questions as you begin planning your best course of action.

Making Decisions for You

1. **List** the specific behavior that you want to change.

2. **Outline** the steps you will take to achieve this change.

3. **What reinforcers** can you give yourself along the way? Who could you call upon to help keep you motivated? Are they willing to help?

4. **What techniques** do you think will be most useful (positive reinforcement, shaping, modeling, imagined rehearsal, situational inducement, changes in self-talk, others)?

Checklist for Change: Making Personal Choices

✓ Are you ready to make this change? Are you in a healthy emotional state? Are you doing it for you or to please someone else?

✓ Have you completed a personal health history to assess your risks from various sources?

✓ Have you developed an action plan with short- and long-term goals? Have you set priorities?

✓ Have you assessed your personal resources? Who can you call on to help you? Where can you go for support and advice?

✓ Have you planned alternative actions in case you run into obstacles or begin to self-sabotage?

✓ Have you set up a list of reinforcers and supports that will keep you motivated along the way?

✓ Have you established a set of guidelines for success? Will you have small goals to achieve at selected intervals or will you only consider yourself successful if you have met your ultimate goal?

Checklist for Change: Making Community Choices

✓ Have you taken time to become educated about issues/concerns affecting others in your community?

✓ Have you prioritized the actions that you can take to make a difference in changing community behaviors? Do you have a particular goal?

✓ Do you act responsibly to preserve the environment by: consuming fewer resources? using fewer packaged items? reusing, recycling, and reducing consumption whenever possible?

✓ Do you analyze what is happening in your school, community, state, and nation by reading about issues, actively discussing problems and possible solutions, and developing personal opinions?

✓ Do you listen carefully to what your elected officials say and let them know in writing or by calling if you disagree with them?

✓ Do you vote for elected officials whose policies, rhetoric, and past histories have indicated that they support improvements in health care, the environment, education, and minority health?

✓ Do you volunteer your time to help others who are less fortunate at least once during every term?

✓ Do you purchase products and services from companies that have proven records of protecting the environment, providing safe foods and products, and supporting the health and well-being of others through their organizational practices?

Critical Thinking

Each chapter of this text will end with a decision-making situation. You may wish to use the DECIDE model introduced in this chapter to develop decision-making skills. For your first decision, let's return to the situation described when we introduced the DECIDE model: To drink or not to drink. Let's assume that you are attending a major dorm party tonight where alcohol will be served—and you have a test tomorrow afternoon. Using the decision-making model, will you drink? If so, will you set a limit? How will you respond if offered more than your limit?

okay to have one or two drinks over the course of the evening and that that is the absolute limit, this may be a reasonable decision for you. Now you must take action based upon your decision—you must actively resist temptation and stick to your limit.

E *Evaluate the consequences.* A key component of the decision-making process is a careful look backward at your decision and your resulting behavior, how you felt about them, and whether you want to do anything differently in the future. You may add other alternatives at step 2, for instance. The secret to success is to think about the problem in advance, consider your values and wants, and anticipate the choices you will have.

𝒲HAT DO YOU THINK?

Why is it sometimes hard for you to make decisions? What things influence your decisions?

Setting Goals

There are several steps you can take to develop behavior-change goals that are realistic for you. For example, suppose that you are gaining weight. Rather than saying, "I eat too much and my goal is to not eat so much," you need to be specific about your current behavior. Are you eating too many sweets? Are you gorging yourself at dinner and not eating breakfast? Perhaps a better statement of the problem would be, "I eat too many high-fat foods, particularly at dinner." A realistic goal that could follow from that statement is, "I am going to try to eat less fat during dinner every day." What strategies could you use to reach this goal? Recording all the foods you eat every day may show, for instance, that the greatest source of fat in your meals is condiments. You could reach your goal by buying low-fat dressings and other condiments, by limiting your use of condiments, or by finding fat-free substitutes. You may find you've been eating too many fried and sautéed foods. In that case, your goal would be to bake or broil as many foods as possible, thereby reducing your fat intake.

Another antecedent for your diet choices may be with whom you're eating. Do you eat as much or the same type of foods when you are with your diet-conscious, fitness-zealot friends as you do when you are with your overweight, food-loving friends? Or do you eat more fattening foods in greater quantity when you are alone? Why? Answering these kinds of questions will give you valuable insights into your behaviors.

Summary

- Health is defined as a dynamic process of trying to achieve your individual potential in the physical, social, emotional, mental, spiritual, and environmental dimensions. Wellness means achieving the highest level of health possible along several dimensions.

- Although Americans have increased average lifespan, we need to increase our span of quality life. *Healthy People 2000* establishes a national set of objectives for achieving improved lifespan and quality of life for all Americans through health promotion and prevention.

- Gender continues to play a major role in health status and care. Women have longer lives but more medical problems than do men. The recent inclusion of women in medical research and training attempts to close the gap in health care.

- The leading causes of death are heart disease, cancer, and stroke. But in the 15-to-24 age group, the leading causes are accidents, homicide, and suicide. Many of the risks associated with the leading killers can be reduced through lifestyle changes. Many of the risks associated with the 15-to-24-age-group killers can be reduced through preventive measures.

- Several factors contribute to your health status, but not all of them are within your control. Your beliefs and attitudes, your intentions to change, support from significant others, and your readiness to change are all factors over which you have some degree of control. Access to health care, genetic predisposition, health policies that are supportive of your actions, and other factors are all potential reinforcing, predisposing, and enabling factors that may influence your health decisions.

- Applying behavior change techniques such as shaping, visualizing, modeling, controlling the situation, reinforcing, and changing self-talk to your personal situations will help you to be successful in making behavior changes.

- Decision making has several key components: Defining the problem, Exploring alternatives, Considering consequences, Identifying your values, Deciding and acting, and Evaluating the consequences of your choices. Following the DECIDE model can assist you to make behavior changes.

Discussion Questions

1. How are the terms *health* and *wellness* similar? What, if any, are important distinctions between these terms?

2. How healthy are Americans today? How will health promotion and illness and accident prevention improve both lifespan and quality of life?

3. What are some of the major differences in the way males and females are treated in the health-care system? Why do you think these differences exist?

4. What are the leading causes of death when you look at all ages and races? What are the leading causes of death

for people aged 15 to 24? Why are these statistics so different? Explain why it is important to look at these statistics by age rather than just in total. What lifestyle changes can you make to lower your risks for major diseases?

5. What is the Health Belief Model? The Theory of Reasoned Action? How may each of these models be working when a young woman decides to smoke her first cigarette? Her last cigarette?

6. Explain the predisposing, reinforcing, and enabling

factors influencing the decision of a young welfare mother who is deciding to sell drugs to support her children.

7. Describe how you could use each of the behavior change techniques to change your couch-potato behavior and start an exercise program.

8. What are the key components of the decision-making process? Why is it important that you be ready to change before you try to start changing?

Application Exercise

Reread the *What Do You Think?* scenarios at the beginning of the chapter and answer the following questions.

1. From what you learned in this chapter, what steps would each of the people discussed here have to take to change their behaviors?

2. On your campus, where could students having similar problems go for help?

3. As a friend, what can you do to be more supportive of the health of someone you know who is trying to make a change?

Further Reading

Peter Conrad and Rochelle Kern, *The Sociology of Health and Illness,* 4th ed. (New York: St. Martin's Press, 1994).

Examines the many ways in which an individual's personal, social, environmental, health care, and psychological health influence his or her responses to illness. Also examines the possibility of avoiding illness through health-promoting behaviors. An outstanding collection of critical essays dealing with pertinent health topics.

Philip Lee and Carroll Estes, *The Nation's Health* (Boston: Jones and Bartlett Publishers, 1994).

Collection of critical essays covering a myriad of health topics such as health status and determinants, the health-care system, minority groups and health, health-care reform, and health-care inequities. One of the leading contemporary texts providing comprehensive information on key health issues.

D. Watson and R. Tharp, *Self-Directed Behavior: Self-Modification for Personal Adjustment* (Pacific Grove, CA: Brooks/Cole, 1993).

Scientifically based instruction in the principles and practices of self-applied psychology. Offers an opportunity for students to learn principles of psychology applicable to their own lives. The emphasis is on coping skills for personal problem solving.

U.S. Department of Health and Human Services, *Health United States: 1993* (Washington, DC: Government Printing Office, 1993).

Contains the 1993 Prevention Profile, submitted by the secretary of the Department of Health and Human Services to the president and the congress. This is the 18th report on the health status of the nation and provides vital health statistics. Published yearly in March/April.

U.S. Department of Health and Human Services, *Healthy People 2000: National Health Promotion and Disease Objectives* (Boston: Jones and Bartlett, 1992).

Contains the national strategy for significantly improving the health of the nation over the coming decade. It addresses the prevention of major chronic illnesses, injuries, and infectious diseases.

2

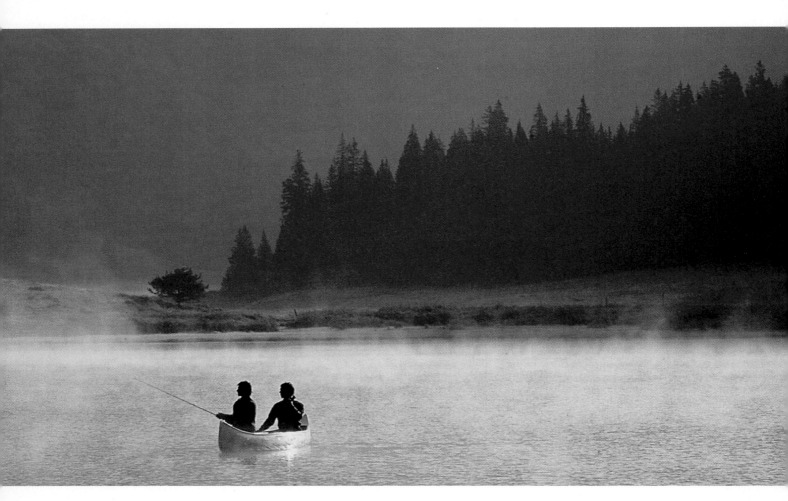

CHAPTER OBJECTIVES

◆ Define psychosocial health in terms of its mental, emotional, social, and spiritual components, and identify the basic elements shared by psychosocially healthy people.

◆ Identify the internal and external factors influencing psychosocial health.

◆ Discuss the positive steps you can take to enhance your psychosocial health.

◆ Identify and describe common psychosocial problems, and explain their causes and available treatments.

◆ Illustrate the warning signs of suicide and what actions can be taken to help a suicidal individual.

◆ Evaluate the role gender plays in diagnoses of mental health.

◆ Identify the different types of mental health professionals and the most popular types of therapy.

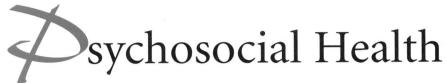

Psychosocial Health

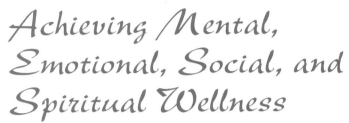

Achieving Mental, Emotional, Social, and Spiritual Wellness

W H A T   D O   Y O U   T H I N K ?

Marisol is a 19-year-old junior majoring in liberal arts. She has become increasingly bored with her classes, finds little excitement in her days, and doesn't have the energy or desire to go out with friends. One recent weekend, she stayed in bed for two days "resting," and when she got up on Monday, she was still so tired that she could barely stay awake in class. She can't concentrate, she finds herself lounging on the couch watching TV every evening, and she doesn't care whether her apartment is a mess. She has gone to the student health center, but after several tests, the doctor tells her that there is nothing physically wrong with her.

■ Have you ever felt like Marisol? What do you think has contributed to her present condition? Do you have any friends who are showing similar characteristics? Why might a typical student health professional miss such obvious symptoms? What do you think Marisol should do to help herself get better? As a friend, what could you do to help her? What services and programs are available on your campus for helping someone like her?

Mark is a senior. He describes himself as a woman-hater and is extremely hateful toward any woman he considers to be strong and outspoken. Although he is a straight A student, he is extremely unpredictable in his interactions with faculty members and other students. Sometimes he is extremely agitated and angry, sometimes he is friendly and outgoing, and sometimes he is very quiet and introverted. People tend to avoid him because they never know how he will react. He says that his family is "trash," and he recently joked about seeing his "old lady" on the street for the first time in several years. He says that his mother took one look at him, pretended she hadn't seen him, and walked away. He brags that he "doesn't need anybody." Recently, he remarked that no one would miss him if he was gone and that he might just do someone a favor and take the "short trip" off a bridge.

■ What do you think is going on with Mark? What factors may have contributed to his current situation? Have you known people who say they don't need anyone? What do you think these people are really saying? How would Mark's mother's reaction have made you feel if she were one of your parents? Without the support of family, where do people often turn for help? If you knew more about Mark's past and his family relationships, would you be more understanding when he acted irrationally? Would you worry about Mark's apparent suicide threats? Why? If you were one of Mark's friends, what would you do? Where could he go for help?

Do you ever wake up in the morning exhausted, feeling as if you've never been to bed? Does the prospect of going to classes, writing yet another paper, or talking with friends seem an enormous chore? Or have you ever found yourself slumped in front of the TV on a beautiful day, lacking the energy to go for a walk much less to clean your apartment or wash your clothes?

Most of us have felt this "down" occasionally, but we are typically able to get through the day in a reasonably productive, if not altogether exciting, way. We eventually sort through seemingly overwhelming problems, suppress our anxieties, and use our social support system (families, friends, significant others, etc.) to help us get through the low times. But for some of us, these skirmishes with the blues become persistent, nagging experiences that vary from small "downers" to "black holes" that are increasingly difficult to emerge from. Whether caused by temporary setbacks or major blows, these miserable moods can sap our energy, reduce our physical reserves, waste our time, diminish our spirit, and take the joy out of our lives. They may even lead to serious mental or emotional illness. Eventually, they may result in a shortened life expectancy. Perhaps even more important, they will almost certainly result in diminished life experiences.

On the other hand, do you ever wake up in the morning raring to go? You feel refreshed and alive, and you notice the birds chirping outside and the fresh, crisp air? Those clothes your roommates have left scattered around the house don't seem such a big deal, and you look forward to a day of studying, classes, and seeing your friends for some fun later in the day.

How we feel and think about ourselves, those around us, and our circumstances can tell us a lot about our psychosocial health. Just as important as our physical health, our psychosocial health can have a profound impact on the quality of our lives. And, just as with our physical health, we can enhance our psychosocial health by becoming aware of and working toward modifying our behaviors.

DEFINING PSYCHOSOCIAL HEALTH

Psychosocial health encompasses the mental, emotional, social, and spiritual dimensions of health. Psychosocially healthy people have managed to develop these dimensions to optimal levels (see Figure 2.1). They seem to have an endless reserve for facing life's ups and downs. They respond to challenges, disappointments, joys, frustrations, and pain by summoning up personal resources acquired through years of experience. Their resiliency is strong and they are actively involved in the process of living rather than being trapped in despondency caused by the negative events in their lives.

Psychosocial health is the result of a complex interaction between a person's history and conscious and unconscious thoughts about and interpretations of the past. Although definitions of psychosocial health vary, most authorities identify several basic elements shared by psychosocially healthy people.[1]

- *They feel good about themselves.* Psychosocially healthy people are not overwhelmed by fear, love, anger, jealousy, guilt, or worry. They estimate their abilities accurately, take life's disappointments in stride, maintain their self-respect, and accept their personal shortcomings.

- *They feel comfortable with other people.* Psychosocially healthy people have satisfying and lasting personal relationships and do not take advantage of others, nor do they allow others to take advantage of them. They can give love, consider others' interests, respect personal

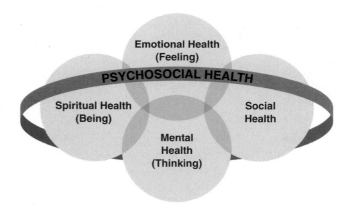

FIGURE 2.1

Psychosocial health is a complex interaction of your mental, emotional, social, and spiritual health.

differences, and feel responsible for their fellow human beings.

- *They control tension and anxiety.* Psychosocially healthy people recognize the underlying causes and symptoms of stress and anxiety in their lives and consciously struggle to avoid illogical or irrational thoughts, unnecessary aggression, hostility, excessive excuse making, and blaming others for their problems.

- *They are able to meet the demands of life.* Psychosocially healthy people try to solve problems as they arise, to accept responsibility, and to plan ahead. They set realistic goals, think for themselves, and make independent decisions. Acknowledging that change is inevitable, they welcome new experiences. They use their natural abilities to control their environment whenever possible and try to fit themselves into the environment whenever necessary.

- *They curb hate and guilt.* Psychosocially healthy people acknowledge and combat their tendencies to respond with hate, anger, thoughtlessness, selfishness, vengeful acts, or feelings of inadequacy. They do not try to knock others aside to get ahead but rather reach out to help others—even those they don't particularly care for. They attempt to understand other people's motivations for negative actions and respond with empathy and sympathy when appropriate.

- *They maintain a positive outlook.* Psychosocially healthy people try to approach each day with a presumption that things will go well. Since they believe that life is a gift, they are determined to enjoy it on a moment-to-moment basis rather than wander through it aimlessly. They block out most negative and cynical thoughts and give the good things in life star billing. They look to the future with enthusiasm rather than dread.

- *They enrich the lives of others.* Psychosocially healthy people recognize that there are others whose needs are greater than their own. They seek to ease these others' burdens by doing such simple things as giving a ride to an elderly neighbor who can't drive, bringing flowers to someone who's in pain, making dinner for someone who's too grief-stricken to cook, volunteering at a community agency, and making charitable donations.

- *They cherish the things that make them smile.* Psychosocially healthy people make a special place in their lives for memories of the past. Family pictures, high school mementos, souvenirs of past vacations, and other reminders of good experiences brighten their day. Fun is an integral part of their lives. So is making time for themselves.

- *They value diversity.* Psychosocially healthy people don't fear difference. They do not feel threatened by people who are of a different race, gender, religion, sex-

ual orientation, ethnicity, or political party. They appreciate creativity in others as well as in themselves.

- *They appreciate nature.* Psychosocially healthy people enjoy and respect natural beauty and wonders. They take the time to enjoy their surroundings and are conscious of their place in the universe.

Of course, few of us ever achieve perfection in these areas. Attaining psychosocial health and wellness involves many complex processes. We will now break these processes down into their components and focus on each in turn. We start by examining the roles that your mental, emotional, social, and spiritual health play in your overall well-being and how these interact. Then we will look at some external and internal factors that may influence your psychosocial health. You will see how the decisions you make today may significantly affect your future psychosocial health and learn how to defend yourself against some common and debilitating psychosocial problems.

Mental Health: The Thinking You

The term **mental health** is often used to describe the "thinking" part of psychosocial health. As a thinking being, you have the ability to reason, interpret, and remember events from a unique perspective; to sense, perceive, and evaluate what is happening; and to solve problems. In short, you are intellectually able to sort through the clutter of events, contradictory messages, and uncertainties of a situation and attach meaning (either positive or negative) to it. Your values, attitudes, and beliefs about your body, your family, your relationships, and life in general are usually—at least in part—a reflection of your mental health.

A mentally healthy person is likely to respond in a positive way even when things do not go as expected. For example, a mentally healthy student who receives a *D* on an exam may be very disappointed, but she will try to assess why she did poorly. Did she study enough? Did she attend class and ask questions about the things she didn't under-

---

Mental health: The "thinking" part of psychosocial health. Includes your values, attitudes, and beliefs.

Psychosocial health: The mental, emotional, social, and spiritual dimensions of health.

stand? Even though the test result may be very important to her, she will find a constructive way to deal with her frustration: She may talk to the instructor, plan to devote more time to studying before the next exam, or hire a tutor. In contrast, a mentally unhealthy person may take a distorted view and respond in an irrational manner. She may believe that her instructor is out to get her or that other students cheated on the exam. She may allow her low grade to provoke a major crisis in her life. She may spend the next 24 hours getting wasted, decide to quit school, try to get back at her instructor, or even blame her roommate for preventing her from studying.

When a person's mental health begins to deteriorate, he or she may experience sharp declines in rational thinking ability and increasingly distorted perceptions. The person may become cynical and distrustful, experience volatile mood swings, or choose to be isolated from others. The person's negative reactions to events may threaten the life and health of others. People showing such signs of extreme abnormal behavior or mental disorders are classified as having *mental illnesses,* discussed later in this chapter.

Emotional Health: The Feeling You

The term **emotional health** is often used interchangeably with *mental health.* Although emotional and mental health are closely intertwined, emotional health more accurately refers to the "feeling," or subjective, side of psychosocial health. **Emotions** are intensified feelings or complex patterns of feelings that we experience on a minute-by-minute, day-to-day basis. Loving, caring, hating, hurt, despair, release, joy, anxiety, fear, frustration, and intense anger are some of the many emotions we experience.

Psychologist Richard Lazarus believes that there are four basic types of emotions: (1) emotions resulting from harm, loss, or threats; (2) emotions resulting from benefits; (3) borderline emotions, such as hope and compassion; and (4) more complex emotions, such as grief, disappointment, bewilderment, and curiosity.[2] Each of us may experience any of these emotions in any combination at any time. As rational beings, it is our responsibility to evaluate our individual emotional responses, the environment that is causing these responses, and the appropriateness of our actions.

Emotionally healthy people are usually able to respond in a stable and appropriate manner to upsetting events. When they feel threatened, they are not likely to react in an extreme fashion, behave inconsistently, or adopt an offensive attack mode. Even when their feelings are trampled upon or they suffer agonizing pain because of a lost love, they can reach through their resentment or suffering to respond with forgiveness or to find a new love.

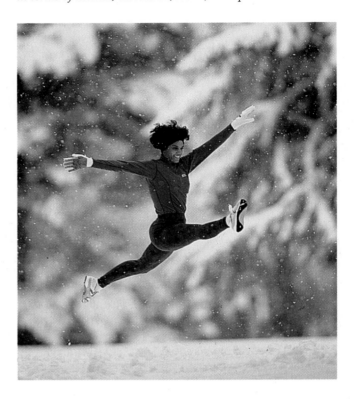

A joyful spirit and the resiliency to face life's ups and downs are measures of psychosocial health as defined in terms of mental, emotional, social, and spiritual wellness.

Emotionally unhealthy people are much more likely to let their feelings overpower them than are emotionally healthy people. Emotionally unhealthy people may be highly volatile and prone to unpredictable emotional outbursts and to inappropriate, sometimes frightening responses to events. An ex-boyfriend who becomes so angry that he begins to hit you and push you around in front of your friends because he is jealous of your new relationship is showing an extremely unhealthy and dangerous emotional reaction. Violent responses to situations have become a problem of epidemic proportions in the United States.

Emotional health also affects social health. Someone feeling hostile, withdrawn, or displaying other mood fluctuations may be avoided by others. People in the midst of emotional turmoil may be grumpy, nasty, irritable, or overly quiet; they may cry easily or demonstrate other disturbing emotional responses. Since they are not much fun to be around, their friends may avoid them at the very time they are most in need of emotional support. Social isolation is just one of the many potential negative consequences of unstable emotional responses.

For students, a more immediate concern is the impact of emotional trauma or turmoil on academic performance. Have you ever tried to study for an exam after a fight with a close friend or family member? Emotional turmoil may seriously affect your ability to think, reason, or act in a rational way. Many otherwise rational, mentally healthy people do ridiculous things when they are going through a major emotional upset. Mental functioning and emotional responses are indeed intricately connected.

Social Health: Interactions with Others

Social health is the part of psychosocial health dealing with our interactions with others and our ability to adapt to social situations. Socially healthy individuals have a wide range of social interactions with family, friends, acquaintances, and individuals with whom they may only occasionally come into contact. They are able to listen, to express themselves (see Chapter 4), to form healthy relationships, to act in socially acceptable and responsible ways, and to find a best fit for themselves in society.

Numerous studies have documented the importance of our social life in the achievement and maintenance of health, and two factors of social health have proven to be particularly important:[3]

- *Presence of strong social bonds.* **Social bonds,** or social linkages, reflect the general degree and nature of our interpersonal contacts and interactions. Social bonds generally have six major functions: (1) providing intimacy, (2) providing feelings of belonging to or integration with a group, (3) providing opportunities for giving or receiving nurturance, (4) providing reassurance of one's worth, (5) providing assistance and guidance, and (6) providing advice. In general, people who are more "connected" to others manage stress more effectively and are much more resilient when they are bombarded by life's crises.

- *Presence of key social supports.* **Social supports** refer to relationships that bring positive benefits to the individual. Social supports can be either expressive (emotional support, encouragement) or structural (housing, money). Families provide both structural and expressive support to children. Adults need to develop their own social supports. Psychosocially healthy people create a network of friends and family to whom they can give and receive support.

Social health also reflects the way we react to others around us. In its most extreme forms, a lack of social health may be represented by aggressive acts of prejudice and bias toward other individuals or groups. **Prejudice** is a negative evaluation of an entire group of people that is typically based on unfavorable (and often wrong) ideas about the group.[4] In its most obvious manifestations, prejudice is reflected in acts of discrimination against others, in overt acts of hate and bias, and in purposeful intent to harm individuals or groups.

Spiritual Health

Although mental and emotional health are key factors in your overall psychosocial functioning, it is possible for you to be mentally and emotionally healthy and still not achieve optimal levels of psychosocial well-being. What is missing? For many people, that difficult-to-describe element that gives zest to life is the spiritual dimension. What does it mean to be spiritually healthy? Spiritual health refers to possession of a belief in some unifying force that gives purpose or meaning to life or to a sense of belonging to a scheme of existence greater than the merely personal. For some people, this unifying force is nature; for others, it is a feeling of connection to other people coupled with a recognition of the eternal nature of the human race; for still others, the unifying force is a god or other spiritual symbol.

Many of us live on a rather superficial material plane throughout the formative years of our lives. We have basic human needs that must be satisfied according to a set hierarchical order. We tend to be rather egocentric, or self-oriented, during these formative years and seek immediate material and emotional gratification while denying or ignoring the spiritual aspect of our selves. Worrying about the clothes you wear, the car you drive, the appearance of your apartment, and other material possessions are examples of this type of preoccupation. According to psychologists and psychoanalysts such as Carl Jung, our materialistic Western civilization leads us to deny our spiritual needs for much of our lives (see Figure 2.2). But there comes a point, usually around midlife, when we discover that material possessions do not automatically bring a sense of happiness or self-worth.[5] Crisis may move us to this realization earlier. A failed relationship, the death of a close friend or family member, or other loss often prompts us to look for meaning in what is happening around us. We recognize that material things, prestige, money, power, and fame count for little in the larger scheme of existence, and that if we were to die

Emotional health: The "feeling" part of psychosocial health. Includes your emotional reactions to life.

Emotions: Intensified feelings or complex patterns of feelings we constantly experience.

Social bonds: Degree and nature of our interpersonal contacts.

Social supports: Structural and functional aspects of our social interactions.

Prejudice: A negative evaluation of an entire group of people that is typically based on unfavorable and often wrong ideas about the group.

tomorrow these would not give meaning to our lives. At this point, many people reach what is often called a midlife crisis, which is characterized by a sense of spiritual bankruptcy.[6] According to Jung,

> We need not be devastated by this sudden recognition, for with it comes the opportunity to reach deep within ourselves in order to resolve and integrate the polarities of our nature. Within our creative and collective unconscious we may discover a richness and a strength and a wisdom that we have not been able to utilize before.[7]

As we develop into spiritually healthy beings, we begin to recognize who we are as unique individuals. We reach a better understanding of our strengths and shortcomings and of our place in the universe. Many of us find that our families, the environment, animals, friends, strangers who are suffering, and religion assume greater significance in our lives. We become more willing to sacrifice for others or to improve the world around us. Many people do not have to wait until their middle years to experience spiritual growth. While the media regularly report horrible stories of hate, crime, violence, and global destruction, they frequently ignore the heartening stories of young people having humanistic concerns who volunteer to work with others in need and who are seriously searching for meaning in life.

Spiritual health takes time and experience to acquire. The longer you live, the more you experience. The more you ponder the meaning of your experiences, the greater your chances of achieving psychosocial health.

*F*ACTORS INFLUENCING PSYCHOSOCIAL HEALTH

Although it's relatively easy to say what psychosocial health is, it is much more difficult to assess why some people are psychosocially well virtually all the time, others are some of the time, and still others almost never are. What factors have influenced your own patterns of mental, emotional, social, and spiritual health? Are these fac-

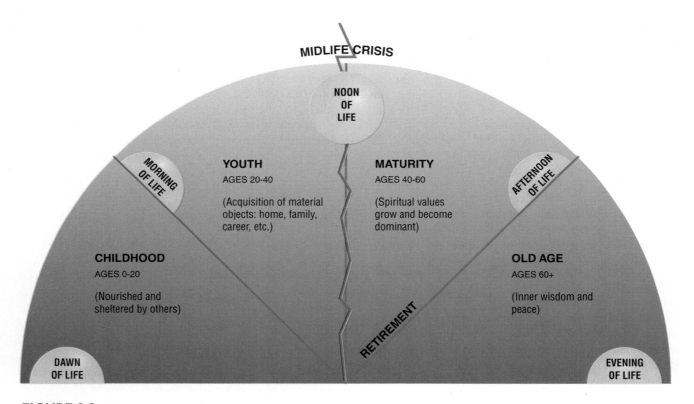

FIGURE 2.2

Jung's View of Personal Growth and Spiritual Development

Learning to Trust: The Tie that Binds

What does the word *trust* really mean to you? How many people in your social group do you trust with your innermost thoughts? Would you trust your life with them? Loan them money? Loan them your notes the day before a big exam?

By indicating how much you agree with the following statements, you may find out how much you trust the significant people in your life:

1. I know how my partner (or friend) is going to act. My partner (or friend) can always be counted on to act as I expect.

2. I am very familiar with the patterns of behavior my partner (or friend) has established, and he or she will behave in certain ways.

3. I have found that my partner (or friend) is a thoroughly dependable person, especially when it comes to things that are important.

4. My partner (or friend) has proven to be a faithful person. No matter with whom my partner (or friend) was involved in a relationship, he or she would never be unfaithful, even if there was absolutely no chance of being caught.

5. I am never concerned that unpredictable conflicts and serious tensions may damage our relationship because I know we can weather any storm.

6. I feel completely secure in facing unknown new situations because I know my partner (or friend) will never let me down.

Items 1 and 2 measure the component of *predictability,* your ability to foretell your partner's (or friend's) actions. Items 3 and 4 measure *dependability,* your feelings that your partner (or friend) is someone upon whom you can rely even when you feel vulnerable and afraid. Finally, items 5 and 6 measure *faith,* your confidence that, although the future may be uncertain and people can change, your partner (or friend) will continue to care for and respond to you.

Trust is hard-won but valuable in any relationship, intimate or not. As you face life's challenges, you learn how much you can depend on another person, not just how much you would like to expect of your relationship. Ironically, while trust may take a long time to develop, it can be utterly destroyed in moments. If you discover that your partner or best friend has betrayed you—by violating a confidence or cheating on you—your best efforts to forgive and forget may never make you completely trustful again. The pain of betrayal makes trust a risky venture.

How can trust be developed and strengthened from the start of a relationship? Here are some approaches:

- *When interpreting another's behavior, be fair and realistic.* Try to understand the behavior from his or her point of view rather than take it personally.

- *Beware of dwelling on negative memories.* Balance remembered disappointments by recalling the good and selfless things the other person has done.

- *Focus on the other person's actions instead of jumping to conclusions about his or her motives.* Many unpleasant actions are the result not of malice but of honest mistakes and human error.

- *Be trustworthy yourself.* In order to gain the trust of another person, it is important that you be a good model. Having double standards, being untrustworthy yourself, and then berating your friend or partner for slip-ups is an unhealthy response.

- *Finally, remember that trust is always risky.* However, intimacy in your social interactions is a desirable component of social and emotional health. To avoid all risk of lost trust is to lose an opportunity to grow and have meaningful interactions with others.

Taking Action

Think about how much you trust your parents, your partner, and your best friend. Why do you trust each of these people as much as you do? What things do you not trust about them? Have there been specific incidents to prove you can't trust them? Have you thought about why they may have acted as they did? What positive things have they done that may prove you can trust them? How trustworthy have you been to them? What actions can you take to be more trustworthy? What actions can you take to help your friend/partner become a more trustworthy person or to remain trustworthy in the future?

Source: Adapted from Charles G. Morris, *Understanding Psychology,* 2nd ed., © 1993, 569. Adapted by permission of Prentice-Hall, Inc., Englewood Cliffs, NJ.

---

tors changeable? Can you do anything to improve your health if you have problems? How can you enhance the positive qualities you already possess?

Most of our mental, emotional, and spiritual reactions to life are a direct outcome of our experiences and social and cultural expectations. Each of us is born with the innate capacity to experience emotions. Some of us apparently have a predisposition toward more emotionality than others. But how we express our emotions has a lot to do with our mental interpretations of events. These interpretations are often learned reactions to certain environmental and social stimuli.

External Influences

Our psychosocial health is based on how we perceive our life's experiences. While some experiences are under our control, others are not. External influences are those factors in our life that we do not control, such as who raised us and the physical environment in which we live.

Influences of the Family. Our families are a significant influence on our psychosocial development. Children raised in healthy, nurturing, happy families are more likely to become well-adjusted, productive adults. Children raised in families in which violence, sexual, physical, or emotional abuse, negative behaviors, distrust, anger, dietary deprivation, drug abuse, parental discord, or other characteristics of **dysfunctional families** are present may have a harder time adapting to life. In dysfunctional families, love, security, and unconditional trust are so lacking that the children in such families are often confused and psychologically bruised. Yet, not all people raised in dysfunctional families become psychosocially unhealthy. Conversely, not all people from healthy family environments become well-adjusted. There are obviously more factors involved in our "process of becoming" than just our family.

Influences of the Greater Environment. While isolated negative events may do little damage to psychosocial health, persistent stressors, uncertainties, and threats may cause significant problems. Children raised in environments where crime is rampant and daily safety is in question, for example, run an increased risk of psychosocial

> **Dysfunctional families:** Families in which there is violence; physical, emotional, or sexual abuse; parental discord; or other negative family interactions.
>
> **Self-efficacy:** Belief in your ability to perform a task successfully.
>
> **Personal control:** Belief that your internal resources can allow you to control a situation.
>
> **Learned helplessness:** Pattern of responding to situations by giving up because you have always failed in the past.
>
> **Id:** Our unconscious desire for immediate gratification of wants and needs.
>
> **Ego:** Personality force that seeks to restrain the id.
>
> **Superego:** Personality force that serves as our conscience.
>
> **Behavioral psychology:** Branch of psychology that posits that all behavior is learned through a system of punishments and rewards.
>
> **Developmental psychology:** Branch of psychology that focuses on the personality's development by means of progression through developmental tasks.

problems. Drugs, crime, violent acts, school failure, unemployment, and a host of other bad things can happen to good people. But it is believed that certain protective factors, such as having a positive role model in the midst of chaos or a high level of self-esteem, may help children from even the worst environments remain healthy and well-adjusted.

Another important influence on psychosocial health is access to health services and programs designed to support the maintenance and/or enhancement of psychosocial health. Going to a support group or seeing a trained counselor or therapist is often a crucial first step in prevention and intervention efforts. Individuals from poor socioeconomic environments who cannot afford such services often find it difficult to secure help in positively influencing their psychosocial health.

Internal Influences

Although your life experiences influence you in fairly obvious ways, many internal factors are also working more subtly to shape who you are and who you become. Some of these factors are your hereditary traits, your hormonal functioning, your physical health status (including neurological functioning), your physical fitness level, and selected elements of your mental and emotional health. If problems occur with any of these factors, overall psychosocial health declines.

During our formative years, our successes and failures in school, in athletics, in friendships, in our intimate relationships, in our jobs, and in every other aspect of life subtly shape our perceptions and beliefs about our own personal worth and ability to act to help ourselves. These perceptions and beliefs in turn become internal influences on our psychosocial health. Psychologist Albert Bandura used the term **self-efficacy** to describe a person's belief about whether he or she can successfully engage in and execute a specific behavior. If one has already been successful in academics, athletics, or achieving popularity, one will undoubtedly expect to be successful in these events in the future. If one has always been the last chosen to play basketball or volleyball or has never been able to make friends easily, one may tend to believe that failure is inevitable. In general, the more self-efficacious a person is and the more his or her past experiences have been positive, the more likely he or she will be to keep trying to execute a specific behavior successfully. A person having low self-efficacy may give up easily or never even try to change a behavior. People who have a high level of self-efficacy are also more likely to feel that they have **personal control** over situations, or, in other words, their own internal resources allow them to control events.

Psychologist Martin Seligman has proposed that people who continually experience failure may develop a pattern of responding known as **learned helplessness** in which they give up and fail to take any action to help

Pets: Helping to Keep You Healthy

As T. S. Eliot pointed out, animals are "such agreeable friends—they ask no questions, they pass no criticisms." Wouldn't it be wonderful if all friends were so loyal and supportive? Pets often serve a critical role as family members, trusted friends, and social supports. For the estimated 52 percent of American families who have a pet member of their homes, this service comes as no surprise.

Although pets have been a part of our lives since the earliest days of human existence, scientists have become interested in the beneficial effects that they can have on human health only in the last few decades. One way to assess pets' health effects is to measure the short-term physiological impact caused by contact with an animal. Experiments using children and college students have found that watching or petting and talking to an animal can lower blood pressure and heart rate. For college students in a laboratory setting, petting a friendly dog lowered not only blood pressure and heart rate but also anxiety level as measured by standard tests. Studies have also shown that dental patients waiting to have oral surgery who watched fish in an aquarium remained as calm and experienced as little discomfort as dental patients who underwent hypnosis.

Many epidemiological studies have focused on comparisons between people who have and people who do not have pets. These studies generally conclude that those who share their lives with animals have higher morale and lower rates of depression. Older people in particular seem to maintain their interest in and enthusiasm for life if they have a pet to care for. In a large study of pet ownership among the elderly, epidemiologist Judith Siegel determined that pet owners had fewer visits to the doctor. When family members or friends became severely ill or died, pets seemed to be a "stress buffer" for their bereaved human companions. Siegel's study also confirmed that pets provide a sense of security and love that many older persons living alone may not otherwise experience. Although there are down sides to pet ownership, as when, for instance, owners become allergic to pet dander, most experts agree that the benefits outweigh the risks in terms of health-enhancing interactions.

Source: Adapted by permission from Diana Schellenberg, "Pets: A Friend Indeed," from the December 1993 issue of the *Harvard Health Letter*, 1–3. © 1993, President and Fellows of Harvard College.

themselves. Recently, Seligman's theory has been expanded; just as we may learn to be helpless, so may we learn to be optimistic. His learned optimism research provides growing evidence for the central place of mental health in overall positive development.[8]

Personality. Our personality is the unique mix of characteristics that distinguishes us from others. Hereditary, environmental, cultural, and experiential factors influence how we develop. For each of us, the amount of influence exerted by any of these factors differs. Our personality determines how we react to the challenges of life. It also determines how we interpret the feelings we experience and how we resolve the conflicts we feel on being denied the things we need or want.

The modern effort to understand the development of the human personality began with the teachings of Sigmund Freud (1856–1939), an Austrian physician who believed that the human mind had two levels: the conscious and the unconscious.

To Freud, personality development was a psychosexual process based on the gratification of sexual impulses. He believed each person possessed three conflicting personality forces, which he labeled the id, ego, and superego. The **id** consists of our unconscious desire for immediate gratification of wants and needs without regard to laws,

rules, customs, or the needs of others. The **ego** seeks to restrain the id and to delay gratification. In addition, it consciously attempts to satisfy the id in socially acceptable ways. Finally, the **superego** acts as our conscience, or moral monitor. The moral standards and values of our parents are often used by the superego to judge the ego's intentions. Freud believed that a healthy ego was one that had figured out how to satisfy most of the id's impulses in ways that did not greatly offend the superego.

Other theories about the human mind were advanced following Freud's pioneer work. Scientist B. F. Skinner developed one of the earliest branches of psychology. As part of the precepts of **behavioral psychology,** Skinner stated that all behavior is learned through a system of rewards and punishments. According to Skinner, "right" behaviors could be encouraged through rewards, and "wrong" behaviors could be eliminated through punishments. Also, personality is learned through the types of reinforcement a child receives. Some followers of Skinner believe that a newborn baby's mind is a blank slate, waiting to be conditioned to be anything we want it to be.

A third branch of psychology is **developmental psychology.** The originators of this school of thought include Carl Jung and Erik Erikson, who taught that the development of personality and emotional health was dependent on the successful completion of a series of developmental tasks at various stages of the life cycle.

Erikson identified eight stages of psychosocial development (see Figure 2.3). He believed that at each stage we must resolve particular crises in order to continue growth. Successful resolution of each crisis gives us a new building block for developing self-fulfillment and emotional health. Erikson identified these building blocks as hope, will, purpose, competence, fidelity, love, care, and wisdom.

Abraham H. Maslow led the movement known as **humanistic psychology.** Humanistic psychologists believe that behavior is motivated by a desire for personal growth and achievement and that it involves free choice and the ability to make conscious, rational decisions. Maslow developed the theory that people achieve emotional well-being by meeting a hierarchy of needs: physiological needs (oxygen, food, water, sleep, sexual release, and exercise); security needs (a physically and emotionally safe and consistent environment); love and belonging needs (a family or other support group); self-esteem needs; and self-actualization needs (the achievement of self-fulfillment). Before achieving higher levels and eventually becoming "self-actualized," people must fulfill the needs of the previous levels (see Figure 2.4).

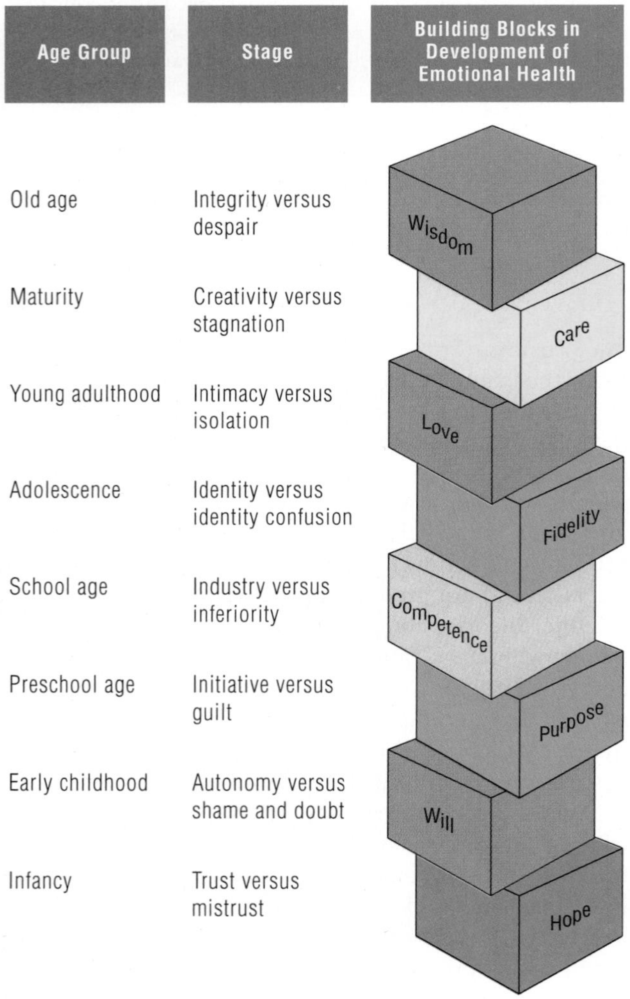

Most of the later schools of psychosocial theory promote the idea that we have the power not only to understand our behavior but also to actively change it and thus to mold our own personalities. An accurate picture of personality development probably requires combining aspects of all the personality theories. We feel conflicts and guilt over our desires and social rules, as Freud believed, and we have the capacity to learn behaviorally as well. For example, people who have been continually rejected in intimate relationships may give up trying to form such relationships because of their fear of punishment in the form of failure. We all have basic needs, as Maslow suggested, and the search for the fulfillment of those needs can certainly enrich our lives and give us life satisfaction. Most of us strive to achieve self-acceptance and self-confidence. Finally, many of us are interested in developing the ability to change and direct our own growth, as the humanistic psychologists urge us to do.

Life Span and Maturity. Although the exact determinants of personality are impossible to define, researchers do know that our personalities are not static. Rather, they change as we move through the stages of our lives. Our temperaments also change as we grow, as is illustrated by the extreme emotions experienced by many people in early adolescence. Most of us learn to control our emotions as we advance toward adulthood.

The college years mark a critical transition period for young adults and their parents. During this time, many of you move away from your families and establish yourselves as independent adults. For most, this step toward maturity entails changing the nature of your relationship with your parents. The transition to independence will be easier if you have successfully accomplished earlier developmental tasks such as learning how to solve problems, to make and evaluate decisions, to define and adhere to personal values, and to establish both casual and intimate relationships. Management of personal finances, career management strategies, interpersonal communication skills, and parenting skills (for those who choose to become parents) are among the developmental tasks college students must accomplish. Older students often have to balance the responsibilities of family, career, and school. Parents of students must accept their children's greater independence and, in some cases, adjust to being alone after years of family interaction.

Age Group	Stage	Building Blocks in Development of Emotional Health
Old age	Integrity versus despair	Wisdom
Maturity	Creativity versus stagnation	Care
Young adulthood	Intimacy versus isolation	Love
Adolescence	Identity versus identity confusion	Fidelity
School age	Industry versus inferiority	Competence
Preschool age	Initiative versus guilt	Purpose
Early childhood	Autonomy versus shame and doubt	Will
Infancy	Trust versus mistrust	Hope

FIGURE 2.3

The Major Stages in Psychosocial Development as Defined by Erikson

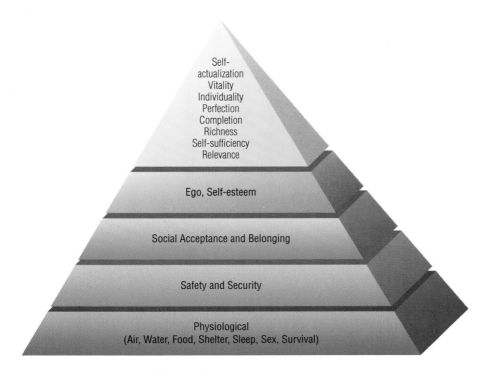

FIGURE 2.4

Maslow's Hierarchy of Needs

If you have not fulfilled earlier tasks, you will continue to grow but may find your life interrupted by recurrent "crises" left over from earlier stages. For example, if you did not learn to trust others in childhood, you may have difficulty establishing intimate relationships in late adolescence or early adulthood.

𝒲HAT DO YOU THINK?

Which factors of psychosocial health have had the greatest positive impact on your life? Any negative influences? Which are influencing your life most now?

ℰNHANCING PSYCHOSOCIAL HEALTH

You may believe that your psychosocial health is fairly well developed by the time you reach college. However, you can always take steps to change your behavior and to improve your psychosocial health. Your well-being is largely determined by your ability to respond to life's challenges and can be defined by your level of self-fulfillment or self-actualization. Attaining self-fulfillment is a lifelong, conscious process that involves building self-esteem, understanding and controlling emotions, and learning to solve problems and make decisions. Before you read on, take a few minutes to find out where you are in your road to psychosocial health by completing the Rate Yourself box.

Developing and Maintaining Self-Esteem

Self-esteem refers to one's sense of self-respect or self-confidence. It can be defined as how much one likes oneself and values one's own personal worth as an individual. People with high self-esteem tend to feel good about themselves and have a positive outlook on life. People with low self-esteem often do not like themselves, constantly demean themselves, and doubt their ability to succeed.

Our self-esteem is a result of the relationships we have with our parents and family during our formative years,

Humanistic psychology: Branch of psychology that posits that behavior is motivated by the desire to grow and achieve by making rational decisions that meet our individual needs.

Self-esteem: Sense of self-respect or self-confidence.

Respecting Who You Are

Look at each item on the scales below and write the letter *S* in the space that best represents your self-description of that trait. Use the number code 1–7 as your guide, as in the following example of the trait of fairness:

1 = extremely fair

2 = rather fair

3 = somewhat fair

4 = equally fair or unfair, or not sure

5 = somewhat unfair

6 = rather unfair

7 = extremely unfair

When you have completed your self-description, go back through each of the items and write the letter *I* in the space that best represents your ideal self, or who you think you ought to be. Using the number codes, determine the difference between your *S* score and *I* score on each trait. Your self-esteem is a measure of how well you like and respect yourself. Traits that have low discrepancy scores on this scale most likely make a positive contribution toward your self-esteem. Traits that have a large difference score may indicate areas you should work on to improve your self-esteem.

	1	2	3	4	5	6	7	
fair	___:___:___:___:___:___:___							unfair
independent	___:___:___:___:___:___:___							dependent
religious	___:___:___:___:___:___:___							irreligious
unselfish	___:___:___:___:___:___:___							selfish
self-confident	___:___:___:___:___:___:___							lacking confidence
competent	___:___:___:___:___:___:___							incompetent
important	___:___:___:___:___:___:___							unimportant
attractive	___:___:___:___:___:___:___							unattractive
educated	___:___:___:___:___:___:___							uneducated
sociable	___:___:___:___:___:___:___							unsociable
kind	___:___:___:___:___:___:___							cruel
wise	___:___:___:___:___:___:___							foolish
graceful	___:___:___:___:___:___:___							awkward
intelligent	___:___:___:___:___:___:___							unintelligent
artistic	___:___:___:___:___:___:___							inartistic
tall	___:___:___:___:___:___:___							short
obese	___:___:___:___:___:___:___							skinny

Source: Excerpts adapted from *Adjustment and Growth: The Challenges of Life,* 3rd ed., by Spencer A. Rathus and Jeffrey S. Nevid, 100–103. Copyright © 1986 by Holt, Rinehart and Winston, Inc.; reprinted by permission of the publisher.

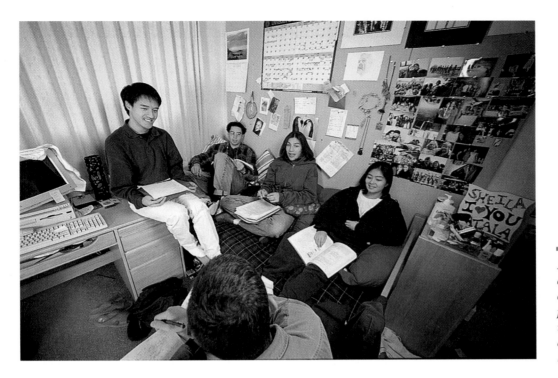

Past successes and happy experiences, which are often recalled through photos, mementos, and recollections, contribute to a person's psychosocial health.

our friends as we grow older, our significant others as we form intimate relationships, and with our teachers, co-workers, and others throughout our lives. If we felt loved and valued as children, our self-esteem may allow us to believe that we are inherently "lovable individuals" as we reach adulthood. The love and support we received from our families in childhood constitute a resource that we call on to help us deal successfully with problems at all stages of our lives (see the Skills for Behavior Change box).

Finding a Support Group.   The best way to maintain your self-esteem is through a support group. You need peers who share your values and offer you the nurturing that your family can no longer provide. The prime prerequisite for a support group is that it makes you feel good about yourself and forces you to take an honest look at your actions and the choices that you make. Members of the group should refrain from exerting negative pressures on one another. Although finding a support group seems to imply that this is always a new group, it is important to remember that old ties are often among the strongest that you will make. The friend who knew you when you were playing with crayons in grade school and who saw you through the growth years and the emotional stresses of the early teens is often a friend for life. Keeping in contact with these friends and with important family members can provide a foundation of unconditional love that may help you through the many life transitions ahead.

Try to be a support for others. Become more interesting by being more interested (in people, current events, etc.). Send news clippings to friends. Join a discussion, political action, or recreational group. Write more postcards

and "thinking of you" notes to people who matter. This will build both your own self-esteem and that of your friends.

Completing Required Tasks.   Another way to boost your self-esteem is to learn how to complete required tasks successfully. You are not likely to succeed in your studies if you leave term papers until the last minute, fail to keep up with the reading for your courses, and do not ask for clarification of points that are confusing to you. Most college campuses provide study groups for various content areas. These groups offer tips for managing time, understanding assignments, dealing with professors, and preparing for test taking. Poor grades, or grades that do not meet a student's expectations, are major contributors to diminished self-esteem and to emotional distress among college students.

Forming Realistic Expectations.   Having realistic expectations of yourself is another method of boosting self-esteem. College is a time to explore your potential. The first year is also a time to learn to feel familial love from a distance. The problems you encounter at college are different from those you had to deal with earlier in life. The stresses of college life may make your expectations for success difficult to meet. If you expect perfect grades, a steady stream of Saturday-night dates and a soap-opera-type romantic involvement, a good job, and a beautiful home and car, you may be setting yourself up for failure. Assess your current resources and the direction you are heading. Set small, incremental goals that are possible for you to meet. Don't decide, "I'm going to turn my life

Building Self-Esteem

Because self-esteem develops over many years, it cannot be wished or improved without effort in a matter of hours spent in a self-help workshop. However, there are several things you can do in your day-to-day life that may seem unimportant but, when practiced regularly and added to other actions, can have a significant impact on the way you feel about yourself.

Squelch that Inner Critic. We are often our own worse enemies. We harp at ourselves continually about how we look and how we should have behaved in certain situations. Begin squelching that inner voice now by

- *examining your faults with a "mirror" rather than a magnifying glass.* Instead of saying, "I'm stupid and I'll never get through this class," say, "I didn't do so well on this last test, but I'm going to do better. I'm doing great in another class."

- *recharacterizing your "mistakes" as opportunities to know yourself better or as growth experiences that will teach you to do things differently next time.* If you find that you made careless mistakes on a test because you rushed through it, resolve to take more time on your next test and to double-check your work.

- *saying thank you rather than mumbling something in protest next time someone compliments you.* Don't mumble "It's just my job" or "What choice did I have but to do it?" Always respond positively to a compliment.

Focus on the Positive. Don't allow yourself to wallow in self-pity. Although it's probably impossible for you to be upbeat at all times, you can do a great deal to shorten the interlude between positive thoughts:

- *Don't sulk.* When upset, allow yourself 15 minutes to worry and be upset and then force yourself to do or think something else.

- *Don't compare yourself with others.* Concentrate on improving your past performance.

- *Give yourself time to feel good.* When you reach an objective, allow time for fun before starting another project.

- *Spend time with a friend who cares about you and isn't afraid to let you know it.* Friends are crucial to positive self-esteem, say experts, because they make up your "psychic family"—an important source of support and objectivity.

- *Count your blessings.* Make a list of all of the people, events, and things in your life for which you are grateful. List your own accomplishments. Whenever you feel cheated by life, look at this list.

---

around and get better grades." Decide instead that tomorrow you will spend at least two hours studying for a class or going to the library to do research on a paper, or decide to talk to your professors to see what they recommend to help you better understand a topic.

Taking and Making Time for You. Taking time to enjoy yourself is another way to boost your self-esteem and psychosocial health. For some people, participating in a sport improves self-esteem by creating a sense of achievement. For others, meeting a new challenge, such as successfully auditioning for a university play or going to a party where they don't know anyone, is an important part of developing social skills. Viewing each new activity as something to look forward to and an opportunity to have fun is an important part of keeping the excitement in your life. Try to wake up focusing on the fun things you have to look forward to each day. Escape from the ordinary. On a clear day, rent a convertible and ride with the top down, or rent a tandem bicycle and pick up your best friend with a picnic lunch. Doing the same old thing day in and day out without having something to focus on as a reward can lead to poor coping skills and illness.

Maintaining Physical Health. Maintaining physical health also contributes to self-esteem. Regular exercise fosters a sense of well-being. Nourishing meals can help you avoid the weight gain experienced by many college students.

Examining Problems and Seeking Help. Examining your problems and seeking help when needed will also boost your self-esteem. Facing and solving problems can be one of life's most satisfying experiences. You do not necessarily have to deal with your problems alone. Help can come in the form of a friend, a group, or a mental health professional.

*W*HAT DO YOU THINK?

Which of the above tasks have you actively pursued in the past month, past six months, and past year? Are you becoming more active in enhancing your self-esteem? What steps could you take to improve your self-esteem?

Getting Adequate Amounts of Rest

Getting adequate sleep is a key contributor to positive physical and psychosocial functioning. Many of us never seem to get enough sleep. Either we don't have time to sleep or we can't seem to fall asleep once our heads hit the pillow. An estimated 20 to 40 percent of all adults have trouble sleeping. Known as *insomnia,* this sleep disorder afflicts almost everyone at one time or another. Insomnia is more common in women than in men, and its prevalence correlates with age and socioeconomic class. Though many people turn to over-the-counter sleeping pills, barbiturates, or tranquilizers to get some sleep, the following methods for conquering sleeplessness are less harmful:[9]

- *If your sleeplessness arises from worry or grief, try to correct what's bothering you.* If you can't correct it yourself, confide in a friend, join a support group, or find a qualified counselor to help you.

- *Don't drink alcohol or smoke before bedtime.* Alcohol can disrupt sleep patterns and make insomnia worse. Nicotine also makes you wakeful.

- *Avoid eating a heavy meal in the evening, particularly at bedtime.* Don't drink large amounts of liquids before retiring, either.

- *Eliminate or reduce consumption of caffeinated beverages except in the morning or early afternoon.*

- *Avoid daytime naps, even if you're tired.*

- *Spend an hour or more relaxing before retiring.* Read, listen to music, watch TV, or take a warm bath.

- *If you're unable to fall asleep, get up and do something rather than lie there.* Don't bring work to bed. If you wake up in the middle of the night and can't fall asleep again, try reading for a short time. Counting sheep or reconstructing a happy event or narrative in your mind may lull you to sleep.

- *Avoid reproaching yourself.* Don't make your sleeplessness a cause for additional worry. Insomnia is not a crime. Not everyone needs eight hours of sleep. You can feel well—and be quite healthy—on less. Don't worry that you have to make up lost sleep. One good night's sleep will reinvigorate you.

- *Don't watch the clock at night.* Turn it to the wall to avoid the temptation to worry about the night slipping away.

- *Go to bed and rise on a regular schedule.* Keep this schedule no matter how much you have or haven't slept in the recent past.

The Mind-Body Connection

Can negative emotions make a person physically sick and positive emotions boost the immune system? Researchers have explored the possible interaction between emotions and health, especially in conditions of uncontrolled, persistent stress. According to the simplest theory of this interaction, the brain of an emotionally overwrought person sends signals to the adrenal glands, which respond by secreting cortisol and epinephrine (adrenaline), the hormones that activate the body's stress response. These chemicals are also known to suppress immune functioning, so it has been surmised that the persistently overwrought person undergoes subtle immune changes. What remains to be shown is how these changes affect overall health, if they do at all. According to Marvin Stein, a professor of psychiatry at the Mount Sinai School of Medicine in New York City, "Work thus far on emotions and health adds up to little more than findings in search of meaning."[10] We still do not have conclusive proof of a relationship between emotions and health, he argues, but evidence for such a relationship is accumulating.

The notion that laughter can save your life gained wide acceptance with the 1979 publication of *Anatomy of an Illness,* by magazine editor Norman Cousins. In this book, Cousins recounted his recovery from a rheumatic disease of the spine—ankylosing spondylitis—with the aid of Marx Brothers movies and *Candid Camera* videos that made him laugh.[11] Similarly, in his 1988 best-seller, *Love, Medicine and Miracles,* surgeon Bernie Siegel argued that a fighting spirit and the determination to survive are vital adjuncts to standard cancer therapy.[12]

In the 1970s and 1980s, a number of widely publicized studies of the health of widowed and divorced people showed that their rates of illness and death are higher than those of married people. Moreover, their lab tests revealed below-normal immune-system functioning. Several follow-up studies have shown unusually high rates of cancer among depressed people.[13] But are these studies conclusive evidence of the mind-body connection? Probably not, because they do not account for many other factors known to be relevant to health. For example, some researchers suggest that people who are divorced, widowed, or depressed are more likely to drink and smoke, to use drugs, to eat and sleep poorly, and to fail to exercise—all of which may affect the immune system. Another possibly relevant factor is that such people may be less tolerant of illness and more likely to report their problems.[14]

Among the work most widely cited as proof that psychosocial treatment can help patients fight disease is an experiment involving women with advanced breast cancer. David Spiegel, professor of psychiatry at Stanford University, reported in 1989 that 50 women randomly assigned to a weekly support group lived an average of 18 months longer than 36 similarly afflicted women not in the support group. The implication of this finding is that the women in the support group cheered each other up while they endured agonizing therapy and that this allowed them to sleep and eat better, which promoted their survival. But a significant flaw in Spiegel's study was his failure to specifically measure immune functioning.[15]

In fact, the immune system changes measured in various other studies of the mind-body connection are relatively small. (They are nowhere near as large as the

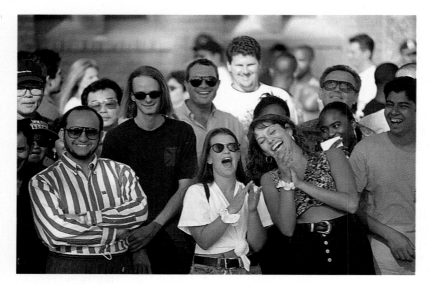

Making time for friends and activities that you enjoy and that bring laughter into your life is a powerful strategy for maintaining psychosocial health.

disruptions that occur in people with AIDS, for example.) The health consequences of such minute changes are difficult to gauge because the body can tolerate a certain amount of reduced immune function without illness resulting. The exact amount it is able to tolerate and under what circumstances are still in question.[16]

Probably the boldest theory put forward in mind-body research is the notion that certain psychosocial behaviors actually make people vulnerable to cancer. In her book on the mind-cancer link, *The Type C Connection,* psychologist Lydia Temoshok reports that among the patients she studied who had malignant melanoma (a potentially deadly skin cancer), 75 percent shared common traits. They tended to be unfailingly pleasant, to repress their negative feelings and emotions, to put others' needs ahead of their own, and to make extraordinary attempts to accommodate others. She hypothesizes that this "Type C" personality signals emotional repression, which may work to suppress the immune system.[17]

In summary, although there is a large body of evidence pointing to at least a minor association between the emotions and physical health, there is still no definitive proof of such a relationship. Another unresolved question is the actual mechanism. Does your emotional state trigger negative behaviors that in turn lead to decreased immune functioning? Or do your emotions directly affect your health by stimulating the production of hormones that tax the immune system? One more controversial issue in the mind-body theory concerns personal responsibility. If, in fact, your emotions make you sick, is it then somehow your own fault that you got sick? Some professionals argue that mind-body theorists are too quick to blame patients for succumbing to the negative emotions that supposedly made them ill. They point out that illness itself causes negative feelings of guilt and anxiety, and it is often impossible to tell which preceded and precipitated which. Clearly, we still have a lot to learn in this area. In the meantime, however, maintaining an optimistic mindset is probably sound advice.

*W*HEN THINGS GO WRONG

In spite of our own best efforts to remain psychosocially healthy, circumstances and events in our lives sometimes prove to be more than we can handle. If we have the financial and educational resources to seek help, some of these difficulties can be prevented. But in the case of other difficulties, the road to recovery may be long.

Depression

Depression is the most common emotional disorder in the United States: One of five of us will suffer from depression at some time in our lives. There are two acknowledged forms of depression: endogenous and exogenous depression. **Endogenous depression** is of biochemical origin. Neurotransmitters (chemicals that transmit nerve impulses across synapses) in the brain that are responsible for mood elevation become unbalanced for unknown reasons. A decrease in the amount of these neurotransmitters gives rise to outward expressions of depression. If not treated, endogenous depression may become chronic. **Exogenous depression,** on the other hand, is usually caused by an external event such as the loss of something or someone of great value. Victims of exogenous depression can slide into chronic depression if they are unable to work through the grieving process necessary for overcoming event-related depression.

Similar symptoms appear in both types of depression: lingering sadness; inability to find joy in pleasure-giving activities; loss of interest in work; diminished or increased appetite; unexplainable fatigue; sleep disorders, including

Cultural Differences in Emotional Terms

If you live in the United States and speak American English, your emotional life is categorized differently than if you come from Japan or Indonesia. Some words that describe emotions in the American English language, and therefore reflect the United States experience, have no real equivalent in other languages. Are there emotions that exist in English that do not exist in German, Chinese, or Japanese? If such differences exist, what do they tell us about emotion?

According to James A. Russell, who has conducted extensive research into cross-cultural comparisons of emotional terms, such differences do exist. There are 2,000 words to describe emotions in English, but only 1,500 in Dutch, 750 in Taiwanese Chinese, and 230 in Malay. More important than the number of specific terms, however, are the categories of emotion different languages allow. Some English words have no real equivalent in other languages. Russell points out that English distinguishes between *terror, horror, dread, apprehension,* and *timidity* as types of fear. However in Gidjingali, an Australian aboriginal language, one word, *guradadj,* suffices. What English treats as different emotions—for example, *anger* and *sadness*—other languages treat as one emotion. The English distinction between *shame* and *embarrassment* is only made by the people of Japan. In China, there exists no term for *anxiety;* in Sri Lanka, there exists no term for *guilt.*

These differences are important because they show researchers that emotional experience may not be the same across all cultures. Cultural differences in emotion are probably due to differences in the way each culture approaches, appraises, and responds to various life events. For example, the definition of *shameful events* among the Awlad 'Ali, a tribe of Egyptian Bedouins, is highly specific: Shameful events are those that injure one's honor; therefore, how a person codes an event is a central element in their language. In addition, just because a language does not have a particular word does not mean that the concept does not exist; it might, for example, be expressed in a phrase rather than in a single word.

From psychologists' points of view, the use of language to describe emotion is important because any discussion of emotion that names emotions uses specific words in a specific language. To describe a theory or emotion that is truly universal to all people, in all languages, a theory must be cross-culturally valid—not bound by specific word entries in a dictionary. This is an enormous challenge. Most psychologists believe that all human beings experience the same emotions, but to prove their beliefs they must first find terminology that is consistent across cultures. Most psychologists believe that all human beings experience the same emotions, but psychologists have to use terminology that is consistent across cultures in understanding and interpreting emotions. Without such consistency, cross-cultural differences will be hard to separate from cross-cultural similarities.

Source: Adapted from Lester A. Lefton, *Psychology,* 5th ed., 377. © copyright 1994 by Allyn & Bacon. Reprinted by permission.

---

insomnia or early-morning awakenings; loss of sex drive; withdrawal from friends and family; feelings of hopelessness and worthlessness; and a desire to die. A depressed person may be unable to get out of bed in the morning or may find it impossible to leave the house.

A depressed person usually suffers from low self-esteem. He or she may feel alone, separated from and unable to communicate with others. After a while, depression becomes a vicious circle. The person feels helpless and trapped, having no way out. He or she may feel that depression is a deserved punishment for real or imagined failings. Prolonged depression may cause a person to feel utterly worthless and to view suicide as the only way out.

Facts and Fallacies about Depression. Although depression appears to be one of the fastest growing psychosocial health problems, the general public is uninformed about many aspects of the disease. Myth and misperception about the disease abound. Keeping the following points in mind may help you in discussions of this problem:[18]

1. *Real depression is* not *a natural reaction to crisis and loss.* Something has happened to the mood and thinking of depressed people so that they are afflicted by pervasive pessimism, helplessness, despair, and lethargy, sometimes coupled with agitation. Victims may have diffi-

Endogenous depression: A type of depression that has a biochemical basis, such as neurotransmitter imbalances.

Exogenous depression: A type of depression that has an external cause, such as the loss of a loved one.

culty at work and have chronically negative interpersonal relationships. Symptoms may come and go and may get worse or stay stable but won't get better without treatment. Depressed people forget what it's like to feel normal.

2. *People will* not *snap out of depression by using a little willpower.* Telling a depressed person to snap out of it is like telling a diabetic to produce more insulin. Medical intervention in the form of antidepressant drugs and therapy is often necessary for recovery. Depression also tends to recur—more than half of those afflicted once will be struck down again. And although most people survive depression, it can be fatal: Depression is the leading cause of suicide in this country for both women and men.

3. *Frequent crying is* not *a hallmark of depression.* Some depressed people don't cry at all. In fact, biochemists theorize that crying may actually ward off depression by releasing chemicals that the body produces as a positive response to distress.

4. *Depression is* not *"all in the mind."* One of the best-known factors that makes one vulnerable to clinical depression is genetics. Studies of adopted children, as well as fraternal and identical twins, support the genetic link to depression. The data suggest that depressive illnesses originate with an inherited chemical imbalance in the brain. But do brain chemicals alter mood or does mood alter the balance of brain chemicals, and to what extent? Currently, no one knows for sure but it seems that each affects the other. Depression can also be a side effect of certain physiological conditions, such as thyroid disorders, Lyme disease, diabetes, multiple sclerosis, hepatitis, mononucleosis, rheumatoid arthritis, and pancreatic cancer.

5. *It is* not *true that only in-depth psychotherapy can cure long-term clinical depression.* No single psychotherapy method works for all cases of depression. But two methods are thought to be particularly well suited to this disorder, and neither of them requires years of treatment.

Treating Depression. Different types of depression require different types of treatment. Selecting the best treatment for a specific patient involves determining his or her type and degree of depression and its possible causes. Both psychotherapeutic and pharmacological modes of treatment are recommended for clinical (severe and prolonged) depression. Drugs often relieve the symptoms of depression, such as loss of sleep or appetite, while psychotherapy can improve a depressed person's social and interpersonal functioning. Treatment may be weighted toward one or the other mode depending on the specific situation. In some cases, psychotherapy alone may be the

Without appropriate treatment, depression and anxiety can become overwhelming problems that affect not only psychosocial well-being, but also physical health.

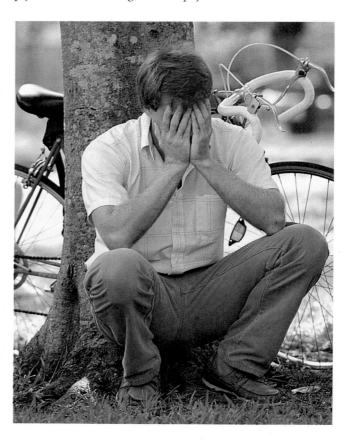

most successful treatment. The two most common psychotherapeutic therapies for depression are cognitive therapy and interpersonal therapy.

Cognitive therapy aims to help a patient look at life rationally and to correct habitually pessimistic thought patterns. It focuses on the here and now rather than analyzes a patient's past. To pull a person out of depression, cognitive therapists usually need 6 to 18 months of weekly sessions comprising reasoning and behavioral exercises.

Interpersonal therapy has also proved successful in the treatment of depression and is sometimes combined with cognitive therapy. It also addresses the present but differs from cognitive therapy in that its primary goal is to correct chronic human relationship problems. Interpersonal therapists focus on patients' relationships with their families and other people.

Antidepressant drugs relieve symptoms in nearly 80 percent of people with chronic depression. Several types of the antidepressant drugs known as tricyclics are available and work by preventing the excessive absorption of mood-lifting neurotransmitters. Tricyclics can take from six weeks to three months to become effective. Newer antidepressant drugs, called tetracyclics, work in one or two weeks.

Electroconvulsive therapy (ECT) is another treatment for depression. A patient given ECT is sedated under light general anesthesia and electric current is applied to the temples for five seconds at a time for a period of about 15 or 20 minutes. Between 10 and 20 percent of depressives who do not respond to drug therapy are responsive to ECT, but because a major risk associated with ECT is permanent memory loss, some therapists do not recommend its use under any circumstances.

Clinics have been established in large metropolitan areas to offer group support for depressed people. Some clinics treat all types of depressed people; others restrict themselves to specific groups, such as widows, adolescents, or families and friends of depressives.

Depression and Gender. For reasons that are not well understood, two-thirds of all people suffering from depression are women. Researchers have proposed biological, psychological, and social explanations for this fact. The biological explanation rests on the observation that women appear to be at greater risk for depression when their hormone levels change significantly, as during the premenstrual period, the period following the birth of a child, and the onset of menopause. Men's hormone levels appear to remain more stable throughout life. Researchers therefore theorized that women were inherently more at risk for depression. Yet evidence to support this theory is either inconsistent or contrary.

Depression is often preceded by a stressful event. Some psychologists therefore theorized that women might be under more stress than are men and thus more prone to become depressed. However, women do not report a greater occurrence of more stressful events than do men.

Finally, researches have observed gender differences in coping strategies, or the response to certain events or stimuli, and have proposed the explanation that women's strategies put them at more risk for depression than do men's strategies. Presented with "a list of things people do when depressed," college students were asked to indicate how likely they were to engage in the behavior outlined in each item on the list. Men were more likely to assert that, "I avoid thinking of reasons why I am depressed," "I do something physical," or "I play sports." Women were more likely to assert that, "I try to determine why I am depressed," "I talk to other people about my feelings," and "I cry to relieve the tension." In other words, the men tried to distract themselves from a depressed mood whereas the women tended to focus attention on it. If focusing on depressed feelings intensifies these feelings, women's response style may make them more likely than men to become clinically depressed. This hypothesis has

not been directly tested, but some supporting evidence suggests its validity.[19]

Obsessive-Compulsive Disorders

Approximately 5 million Americans suffer from obsessive-compulsive disorders. An **obsessive-compulsive disorder (OCD)** is an illness in which people have obsessive thoughts or perform habitual behaviors that they cannot control. People with obsessions have recurring ideas or thoughts that they cannot control. People with compulsions feel forced to engage in a repetitive behavior, almost as if the behavior controls them. Feeling an obsessive need for cleanliness and washing one's hands 20 times before eating, counting to a certain number while using the toilet, and checking and rechecking all the light switches in the house before leaving or going to bed are examples of compulsive behaviors. More harmful compulsive behaviors include pulling out one's hair and other forms of self-mutilation.

The causes of obsessive-compulsive disorders are difficult to isolate. Some theorists believe that sufferers engage in compulsive behaviors to distract themselves from more pressing problems. Until recently, behavioral therapy, which focuses on controlling and changing behaviors, was the common treatment for these disorders. However, research now indicates that some of these disorders may be caused by a lack of the neurotransmitter serotonin in the limbic system (an area of the brain concerned with emotion and motivation). In early 1990, a drug called clomipramine (Anafranil), which researchers believe alters the way serotonin is used in the brain, was released in the United States for prescription use. Used in conjunction with behavioral therapy, clomipramine has been found to help alleviate symptoms of obsessive-compulsive disorders.

Anxiety Disorders

Between 20 and 30 million Americans suffer from anxiety disorders. **Anxiety disorders,** in which people are plagued by persistent feelings of threat and of anxiety about everyday problems of living, are characterized by fatigue, back pains, headaches, feelings of unreality, a sensation of weakness in the legs, and fear of losing control. General-

Obsessive-compulsive disorder (OCD): A disorder characterized by obsessive thoughts or habitual behaviors that cannot be controlled.

Anxiety disorders: Disorders characterized by persistent feelings of threat and anxiety in coping with the everyday problems of living.

ized anxiety disorders can last for more than six months and typically result in excessive worry about two or more personal problems. Three major types of anxiety disorders are phobias, panic attacks, and posttraumatic stress disorder.

Phobias. A **phobia** is a deep and persistent fear of a specific object, activity, or situation, and results in a compelling desire to avoid the source of fear. Experts estimate that one of eight American adults suffers from phobias. Phobias are also thought to be more prevalent in women than in men. Simple phobias, such as fear of spiders, fear of flying, and fear of heights, can be treated successfully with behavioral therapy. Social phobias (fears that are related to interaction with others) such as fear of public speaking, fear of inadequate sexual performance, and fear of eating in public places require more extensive therapy.

Panic Attacks. A **panic attack** is the sudden onset of disabling terror. Symptoms include shortness of breath, dizziness, sweating, shaking, choking, trembling, and heart palpitations. A victim of a panic attack may feel that he or she is having a heart attack. Panic attacks may have no obvious link to environmental stimuli, or they may be learned responses to environmental stimuli. Researchers believe that panic attacks are caused by some physiological change or biochemical imbalance in the brain and are still searching for the mechanisms that trigger such attacks.

Posttraumatic Stress Disorder. Posttraumatic stress disorder (PTSD) afflicts some victims of severe traumas such as rape, assault, war, or airplane crashes. PTSD manifests itself in terrifying flashbacks to the sufferer's trauma.

When correctly diagnosed, anxiety disorders are treatable, usually through a combination of methods. Because undiagnosed diabetes, heart conditions, and endocrine disorders can mimic anxiety disorders, doctors recommend a thorough physical examination to rule out physical causes. If it is established that the causes are not physical, treatment usually consists of psychotherapy combined with medication.

Seasonal Affective Disorder

An estimated 6 percent of Americans suffer from **seasonal affective disorder** (SAD), a type of depression, and an additional 14 percent experience a milder form of the disorder known as the winter blues. SAD strikes during the winter months and is associated with reduced exposure to sunlight. People with SAD suffer from irritability, apathy, carbohydrate craving and weight gain, increases in sleep time, and general sadness. Researchers believe that SAD is caused by a malfunction in the hypothalamus, the gland responsible for regulating responses to external stimuli. Stress may also play a role in SAD.

Certain factors seem to put people at risk for SAD. Women are four times more likely to suffer from SAD than are men. Although SAD occurs in people of all ages, those between 20 and 40 appear to be most vulnerable. Certain families appear to be at risk. And people living in northern states in the United States are more at risk than are those living in southern states. During the winter, there are fewer hours of sunlight in northern regions than in southern areas. An estimated 10 percent of the population in northern states such as Maine, Minnesota, and Wisconsin experience SAD, whereas fewer than 2 percent of those living in southern states such as Florida and New Mexico suffer from the disorder.

There are some simple but effective therapies for SAD. The most beneficial appears to be light therapy, in which a patient is exposed to lamps that mimic sunlight. After being exposed to this lighting each day, 80 percent of patients experience relief from their symptoms within four days. Other forms of treatment for SAD are diet change (eating more foods high in complex carbohydrates), increased exercise, stress management techniques, sleep restriction (limiting the number of hours slept in a 24-hour period), psychotherapy, and antidepressants.

Schizophrenia

Perhaps the most frightening of all mental disorders is **schizophrenia,** a disease that affects about 1 percent of the U.S. population. Schizophrenia is characterized by alterations of the senses (including auditory and visual hallucinations); the inability to sort out incoming stimuli and to make appropriate responses; an altered sense of self; and radical changes in emotions, movements, and behaviors. Victims of this disease often cannot function in society.

For decades, scientists believed that schizophrenia was an environmentally provoked form of madness. They blamed abnormal family interactions or early-childhood traumas. Since the mid-1980s, however, when magnetic resonance imaging (MRI) and positron emission tomography (PET) began to allow scientists to study brain function more closely, scientists have recognized that schizophrenia is a biological disease of the brain. It has become evident that the brain damage involved occurs very early in life, possibly as early as in the second trimester of fetal development. However, the disease most commonly has its onset in late adolescence.

Schizophrenia is treatable but not curable at present. Treatments usually include some combination of hospitalization, medication, and supportive psychotherapy. Supportive psychotherapy, as opposed to psychoanalysis, can help the patient acquire skills for living in society.

Even though the environmental theories of schizophrenia have been discarded in favor of biological theories, a stigma remains attached to the disease. Families of schizophrenics often experience anger and guilt associated with misunderstandings about the causes of the disease. They often need help in the form of information, family counseling, and advice on how to meet the schizophrenic's needs for shelter, medical care, vocational training, and social interaction.

Gender Issues in Psychosocial Health

Studies have shown that gender bias often gets in the way of correct diagnosis of psychosocial disorders. In one study, for instance, 175 mental health professionals, of both genders, were asked to diagnose a patient based upon a summarized case history. Some of the professionals were told that the patient was male, others that the patient was female. The gender of the patient made a substantial difference in the diagnosis given (though the gender of the clinician did not). When subjects thought the patient was female, they were more likely to diagnose hysterical personality, a "women's disorder." When they believed the patient to be male, the more likely diagnosis was antisocial personality, a "male disorder."

PMS: Physical or Mental Disorder? A major controversy regarding gender bias has been the inclusion of a "provisional" diagnosis for premenstrual syndrome (PMS) in the American Psychiatric Association's *Diagnostic and Statistical Manual of Mental Disorders* (fourth edition; known as *DSM-IV*). The provisional inclusion, in an appendix to *DSM-IV,* signals that PMS should come in for further study and may be included as an approved diagnosis in future editions of the *DSM*. In other words, PMS could be considered a mental disorder in the future.

PMS is characterized by depression, irritability, and other symptoms of increased stress typically occurring just prior to menstruation and lasting for a day or two. The controversy involves the legitimacy of attaching a label indicating dysfunction and disorder to symptoms experienced only once or twice a month. Further controversy stems from the possible use (or misuse) of the diagnostic label to justify systematic exclusion of women from certain desirable jobs.[20]

𝒮UICIDE: GIVING UP ON LIFE

There are over 35,000 reported suicides each year in the United States. Experts estimate that there may actually be closer to 100,000 cases; due to the difficulty in determining many causes of suspicious deaths, many suicides are not reflected in the statistics. Suicide is often a consequence of poor coping skills, lack of social support, lack of self-esteem, and the inability to see one's way out of a bad or negative situation.

College students are more likely than the general population to attempt suicide; suicide is the third leading cause of death in people between the ages of 15 and 24.[21] The pressures, joys, disappointments, challenges, and changes of the college environment are believed to be in part responsible for these rates. However, young adults who choose not to go to college but who are searching for the directions to their career goals, relationship goals, and other life aspirations are also at risk for suicide.

Risk factors for suicide include a family history of suicide, previous suicide attempts, excessive drug and alcohol use, prolonged depression, financial difficulties, serious illness in the suicide contemplator or in his or her loved ones, and loss of a loved one through death or rejection. Although women attempt suicide at four times the rate of men, more than three times as many men as women actually succeed in ending their lives. The elderly, divorced people, former psychiatric patients, and Native Americans have a higher risk of suicide than others. In fact, the elderly make up 23 percent of those who commit suicide. Alcoholics also have a high rate of suicide.

Depression is often a precursor of suicide. People who have been suffering from depression are more likely to attempt suicide while they are recovering, when their energy level is higher, than while they are in the depths of depression. Although only 15 percent of depressed people are suicidal, most suicide-prone individuals are depressed.[22]

Due to the growing incidence of suicide, many of us will be touched by a suicide at some time. In most cases, the suicide does not occur unpredictably. In fact, between 75 and 80 percent of people who commit suicide give a warning of their intentions.

Warning Signals

Common warnings of a suicide intent include:

- a direct statement about committing suicide, such as "I can't take it anymore. I might as well end it all."

- an indirect statement about committing suicide, such as, "Soon this pain will be over," or, "You won't have to worry about me anymore."

- "final preparations," such as writing a will, repairing poor relationships with family or friends, giving away prized possessions, or writing revealing letters

Phobia: A deep and persistent fear of a specific object, activity, or situation that results in a compelling desire to avoid the source of the fear.

Panic attack: The sudden, rapid onset of disabling terror.

Seasonal affective disorder (SAD): A type of depression that occurs in the winter months, when sunlight levels are low.

Schizophrenia: A mental illness with biological origins that is characterized by irrational behavior, severe alterations of the senses (hallucinations), and, often, an inability to function in society.

- a preoccupation with themes of death

- a withdrawal from friends and family and from activities once found pleasurable

- a sudden and unexplained demonstration of happiness following a period of depression

- changes in personal appearance

- loss of interest in classes or work and an inability to concentrate

- failure to recover from a personal loss or crisis and deepening or prolonged depression

- excessive risk taking and an "I don't care what happens to me" attitude

Taking Action to Prevent a Suicide Attempt

If someone you know threatens suicide or displays any of the above warnings, take the following actions:

- *Monitor the warning signals.* Try to keep an eye on the person involved, or see that there is someone around the person as much as possible.

- *Take any threats seriously.*

- *Let the person know how much you care about him or her.* State that you are there if he or she needs help.

- *Listen.* Try not to be shocked by or to discredit what the person says to you. Empathize, sympathize, and keep the person talking.

- *Ask the person directly,* "Are you thinking of hurting or killing yourself?"

- *Do not belittle the person's feelings or say that he or she doesn't really mean it or couldn't succeed at suicide.* To

some people, these comments offer the challenge of proving you wrong.

- *Help the person think about other alternatives.* Be ready to offer choices. Offer to go for help with the person. Call your local suicide hotline and use all available community and campus resources.

- *Remember that your relationships with others involve responsibilities.* If you need to stay with the person, take the person to a health-care facility, or provide support, give of yourself and your time.

- *Tell your friend's spouse, partner, parents, brothers and sisters, or counselor.* Do not keep your suspicions to yourself. Don't let a suicidal friend talk you into keeping your discussions confidential. If your friend is successful in a suicide attempt, you will have to live with the consequences of your inaction.

*W*HAT DO YOU THINK?

If your roommate showed some of the warning signs of suicide, what action would you take? Who would you contact first? Where on campus might your friend get help? What if someone in your class that you hardly knew gave some of the warning signs? What would you then do?

*S*EEKING PROFESSIONAL HELP

Many Americans feel that seeking professional help for psychosocial problems is an admission of personal failure they cannot afford to make. Typically, any physical health problem, such as abscessed tooth or prolonged severe

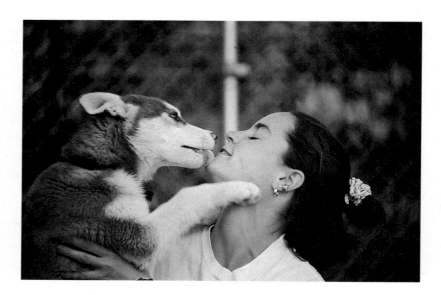

The sense of well-being that accompanies good psychosocial health helps us to remain actively involved in the process of living despite the frustrations and disappointments we may experience.

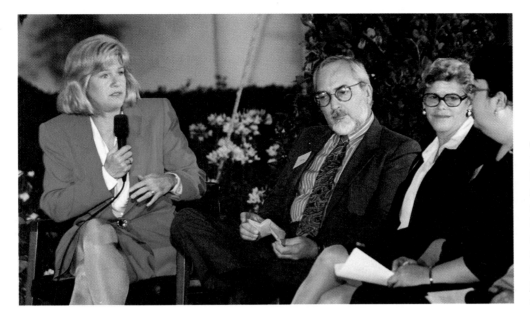

Through the efforts of well-known personalities who have stepped forward to speak on mental health, Americans are becoming increasingly aware of the symptoms of psychosocial health problems and the importance of seeking professional help with overwhelming problems.

pain, sends us to the nearest dentist or physician. On the other hand, we tend to ignore psychosocial problems until they pose a serious threat to our well-being—and even then, we may refuse to ask for the help we need. Despite this tradition, an increasing number of Americans are turning to mental health professionals for help, and in 1993, nearly one in five Americans sought such help. Researchers believe that more people want help today because "normal" living has become more hazardous. Breakdown in support systems, high expectations of the individual by society, and dysfunctional families are cited as the three major reasons more people are asking for assistance than ever before.

You should consider seeking help under the following circumstances:

- If you think you need help.

- If you experience wild mood swings.

- If a problem is interfering with your daily life.

- If your fears or feelings of guilt frequently distract your attention.

- If you begin to withdraw from others.

- If you have hallucinations.

- If you feel that life is not worth living.

- If you feel inadequate or worthless.

- If your emotional responses are inappropriate to various situations.

- If your daily life seems to be nothing but repeated crises.

- If you feel you can't "get your act together."

- If you are considering suicide.

- If you turn to drugs or alcohol to escape from your problems.

- If you feel out of control.

Types of Mental Health Professionals

Several types of mental health professionals, or providers, are available to help you. The most important criterion when choosing a provider is whether you feel you can work well with that person, not how many degrees he or she has.

Psychiatrist. A **psychiatrist** is a medical doctor. After obtaining an M.D. degree, a psychiatrist spends up to 12 years studying psychosocial health and disease. As a licensed physician, a psychiatrist can prescribe medications for various mental or emotional problems and may have admitting privileges at a local hospital. Some psychiatrists are affiliated with hospitals, while others are in private practice. Fees vary, and psychiatrists affiliated with mental health clinics may charge based on patient's financial resources on a sliding scale basis. Most insurance companies have some type of psychiatric care provision.

Psychiatrist: A licensed physician who specializes in treating mental and emotional disorders.

Psychoanalyst. A **psychoanalyst** is a psychiatrist or a psychologist having special training in psychoanalysis. Psychoanalysis is a type of therapy in which a patient is helped to remember early traumas that have blocked personal growth. Facing these traumas helps the patient to resolve the conflicts they have caused and to begin to lead a more productive life.

Psychologist. A **psychologist** usually has a Ph.D. degree in counseling or clinical psychology. In addition, many states require licensure. Psychologists are trained in various types of talk therapy. Most are trained to conduct both individual and group counseling sessions. Psychologists may also be trained in certain specialties, such as family counseling, sexual counseling, or counseling related to compulsive behaviors. Psychologists affiliated with mental health clinics often charge patients according to their ability to pay.

Clinical/Psychiatric Social Worker. A **social worker** has at least a master's degree in social work (M. S. W.) and two years of experience in a clinical setting. Many states require an examination for accreditation. Some social workers work in clinical settings, whereas others have private practices. Registered clinical social workers (R. C. S. W.)

often work in private practices, and their patients are eligible to receive insurance reimbursement.

Counselor. Persons having a variety of academic and experiential training call themselves counselors. The **counselor** often has a master's degree in counseling, psychology, educational psychology, or a related human service. Professional societies recommend at least two years of graduate coursework or supervised practice as a minimal requirement. Many counselors are trained to do individual and group counseling. They often specialize in one type of counseling, such as family, marital, relationship, children, drug, divorce, behavioral, or personal counseling.

Psychiatric Nurse Specialist. Although all registered nurses can work in psychiatric settings, some have chosen to continue their education and specialize in psychiatric practice. The psychiatric nurse specialist can be certified by the American Nursing Association in either adult, child, or adolescent psychiatric nursing.

Remember that, in most states, anyone can use the title of therapist or counselor. Before you begin treatment, you should consider the credentials of your counselor, your desired outcomes, and the expectations of you and your counselor.

Types of Therapy

Over 250 types of **therapy** exist, ranging from "traditional" individual and group therapy to "soap opera therapy" and "past lives therapy." Freudian psychoanalysis is probably the best known form of therapy, yet it is no longer practiced very widely. Because it requires from two to five sessions weekly for 2 to 15 years, many Americans reject psychoanalysis in favor of less costly, short-term therapies. In these arrangements, the patient meets the provider for from 1 to 20 sessions, during which the provider gives support and helps the patient to find positive coping devices. The four most popular types of therapy are behavioral, cognitive, family, and psychodynamic.

Behavioral Therapy. Disorders such as compulsions, phobias, and obsessive thinking are the types of problems most responsive to **behavioral therapy.** These types of behaviors are learned. Because behavioral disorders are learned, they are treated through relearning. Behavioral therapists first ask the client to define the behavior that must be changed. The client is then required to monitor old behaviors as he or she substitutes new ones. A system of client-made charts to monitor progress, along with a program of rewards and punishments, helps the client make the desired changes. The client may also be taught methods of deep relaxation and various thought-stopping techniques. Behavioral therapy usually takes from 16 to 17 weeks to complete.

Psychoanalyst: A psychiatrist or psychologist having special training in psychoanalysis.

Psychologist: A person with a Ph.D. degree and training in psychology.

Social worker: A person with an M.S.W. degree and clinical training.

Counselor: A person having a variety of academic and experiential training who deals with the treatment of emotional problems.

Therapy: One of over 250 types of treatment designed to help people overcome their personal problems.

Behavioral therapy: Therapy aimed at teaching a person to change unwanted behaviors through a system of rewards and punishments.

Cognitive therapy: Therapy aimed at teaching a person to recognize and refute the beliefs that hinder personal growth.

Family therapy: Therapy that focuses on the problems of an entire family system rather than on those of one individual in that system.

Psychodynamic therapy: Therapy that allows a person to express emotions dramatically; release comes through catharsis.

Managing Your Psychosocial Health

Psychosocial health is a complex concept. Finding the best way to help yourself achieve optimal psychosocial health requires careful introspection and planned action. Remembering the following points and acting upon them whenever possible may help you along the way.

Making Decisions for You

Psychosocial health is influenced by many factors. Why is being psychosocially healthy important to you? To the people who are close to you?

What actions can you take today that will help improve your emotional health? What steps could you take right now that could help you improve your social health? What could you do to improve your spiritual health? Finally, if you felt that you had a psychosocial problem, would you seek help? Why or why not?

Checklist for Change

- ✓ Consider life a constant process of discovery and learning.
- ✓ Accept yourself as the best that you are able to be right now.
- ✓ Remember that nobody is perfect.
- ✓ Remember that the most difficult times in life occur during transitions and can be opportunities for growth even though they are painful.
- ✓ Remember that there are other perspectives than your own.
- ✓ Recognize the sources of your own anxiety and act to reduce them.
- ✓ Ask for help when you need it; discuss your problems with others.

- ✓ Become sensitive to and aware of your own body's signals—take care of yourself.
- ✓ Find a meaning for your life and work toward achieving your goals.
- ✓ Develop strategies to get through problem situations.
- ✓ Remain open to emotional experiences—give yourself to today rather than always reserving yourself for tomorrow.
- ✓ Even when you fail, be proud of yourself for trying.
- ✓ Keep your sense of humor—learn to laugh at yourself.
- ✓ Never quit trying to grow, to experience, to love, and to live life to its fullest.

Critical Thinking

Suppose that your roommate ended a long-term relationship last month. Ever since, your roommate no longer jogs every morning, no longer attends religious services, and doesn't even want to attend school mixers to meet someone else. Worse yet, even minor mistakes lead your roommate to self-berating.

You are concerned about your roommate's psychosocial health, but unsure of what to do. You know that your roommate has in the past said that anyone who needs therapy should be "locked up and the key thrown away." But your roommate's mood is beginning to affect you. Use the DECIDE model described in Chapter 1 to decide what you would do in this situation. Explain your decision. If the action you chose did not bring about the desired result, what would you do next? Then list some ways you can show support for a friend who shows signs of psychosocial illness.

Cognitive Therapy. Cognitive therapists believe that what we feel is a reaction not to the world around us but rather to our thoughts about what is happening around us. In **cognitive therapy,** the client is taught to recognize and prevent the thoughts and beliefs that stifle growth. For example, a client who feels miserable about a poor test grade will be taught how to prevent these miserable feelings from regressing into an "I don't deserve to live" attitude. Those who benefit most from cognitive therapy are usually bright, verbal people. Cognitive therapists often use humor to refute the client's negative self-estimates. The duration of therapy is usually one session a week for six months.

Family Therapy. **Family therapy** focuses on the problems of the entire family system rather than on the problems of one individual in that system. In family therapy sessions, the members of a family play out the dynamics of their relationships. Each member is held accountable for his or her treatment of the others. Length of therapy is determined by the severity of the problem. For example, a stepfamily attempting to clarify some issues concerning living together or trying to improve communications may need only two or three sessions. For more severe problems, therapy may last up to a year.

Psychodynamic Therapy. **Psychodynamic therapy** helps the client to unearth and to scrutinize feelings and repressed memories. The client's reactions may include crying, screaming, and ranting. The client is then helped to understand the feelings and memories. Psychodynamic therapists believe that facing problems and reactions on an intellectual level frees people from emotional blocks that create maladaptive behaviors. Therapy of this type usually consists of one session a week for one to two years.

What to Expect When You Begin Therapy

The first trip to a therapist can be extremely difficult. Most of us have misconceptions about what therapy is and about what it can do. That first visit is a verbal and mental sizing up between you and the therapist. You may not accomplish much in that first hour. If you decide that the therapist is not for you, you will at least have learned how to present your problem and what qualities you need in a therapist.

1. Before meeting a therapist, briefly explain your needs to the therapist or reservations secretary. Ask what the fee is. Arrive on time. Wear comfortable clothing. Expect to spend about an hour with the therapist during your first visit.

2. The therapist will want to take down your history and details about the problems that have brought you to therapy. Answer as honestly as possible. Many therapists will ask how you feel about aspects of your life. Do not be embarrassed to acknowledge your feelings.

3. Therapists are not mind readers. They cannot tell what you are thinking. It is therefore critical to the success of your treatment that you have enough trust in your therapist that you can be open and honest.

4. Do not expect the therapist to tell you what to do or how to behave. Very few hand out behavioral prescriptions.

5. Find out if the therapist will allow you to set your own therapeutic goals and timetables. Also, find out if, later in therapy, your therapist will allow you to determine what is and what is not helping you.

6. If, after your first visit (or even after several visits), you feel you cannot work with a therapist, you must summon up the courage to say so. Do not worry about hurting the therapist's feelings. If there is a personality conflict or if you do not feel comfortable, the therapy will not be effective.

*W*HAT DO YOU THINK?

Have you ever though about seeing a therapist? What made you decide to go—or not to go? If you didn't go, did things get better quickly? Do you think you might have worked out your problem faster if you saw a therapist?

Summary

- Psychosocial health is a complex phenomenon involving mental, emotional, social, and spiritual health.

- Many factors influence psychosocial health, including life experiences, family, the environment, other people, self-esteem, self-efficacy, and personality.

- Social bonds and social support networks contribute to the ability to cope with life's challenges.

- Common psychosocial problems include depression, obsessive-compulsive disorders, anxiety disorders (including phobias, panic attacks, and posttramatic

stress syndrome), seasonal affective disorder, and schizophrenia.

- Suicide is a result of negative psychosocial reactions to life. People intending to commit suicide often give warning signs of their intentions. Such people can often be helped.

- Mental health professionals include psychiatrists, psychoanalysts, psychologists, clinical/psychiatric social workers, counselors, and psychiatric nurse specialists. Major types of therapy include behavioral, cognitive, family, and psychodynamic therapies.

Discussion Questions

1. What is psychosocial health? What indicates that you either are or aren't psychosocially healthy? Why do you think the college environment may provide a real challenge to your psychosocial health?

2. Discuss the factors that influence your overall level of psychosocial health. What factors can you change? Which ones may be more difficult to change?

3. What steps could you take today to improve your psychosocial health? Which steps require long-term effort?

4. What factors appear to contribute to psychosocial difficulties and illnesses? Which of the more common psychosocial illnesses is likely to affect people in your age group?

5. What are the warning signs of suicide? What would you do if you heard a stranger in the cafeteria say to no one in particular that he was going to "do the world a favor and end it all"?

6. Discuss the different types of health professionals and therapies. If you felt depressed about breaking off a long-term relationship, which professional and therapy do you think would be most beneficial? Explain your answer. What services are provided by your student health center? What fees are charged to students?

7. What psychosocial areas do you need to work on? Which are most important? Why?

Application Exercise

1. How psychosocially healthy are each of the individuals described in the scenarios presented in the chapter opener?

2. What factors may have contributed to their current health status?

3. What services on your campus would be available to help them improve their psychosocial health? What community services are available to nonstudents who have limited incomes?

4. As a friend, what could you do to help each of them?

Further Reading

M. McKay, P. Rogers, and J. McKay, *When Anger Hurts* (Oakland, CA: New Harbinger Publications, 1992).

Overview of the emotion called anger: why it catches us off guard, what causes it, and what we can do to control it in our lives.

A. O'Connell and V. O'Connell, *Choice and Change: The Psychology of Holistic Growth, Adjustment, and Creativity,* 4th ed. (Englewood Cliffs, NJ: Prentice Hall, 1992).

An insightful, refreshing look at options open to people trying to improve their psychosocial health. Thoughtful suggestions for action are provided.

Debora M. Haselton, *Solving the Self-Esteem Puzzle.*

Provides simple, down-to-earth suggestions for improving self-esteem one step at a time.

World Health Organization, *The ICD-IO Classification of Mental and Behavioral Disorders: Clinical Descriptions and Diagnostic Guidelines.* 1992.

An excellent reference for information on psychosocial problems. Can be used in conjunction with the DSM series.

3

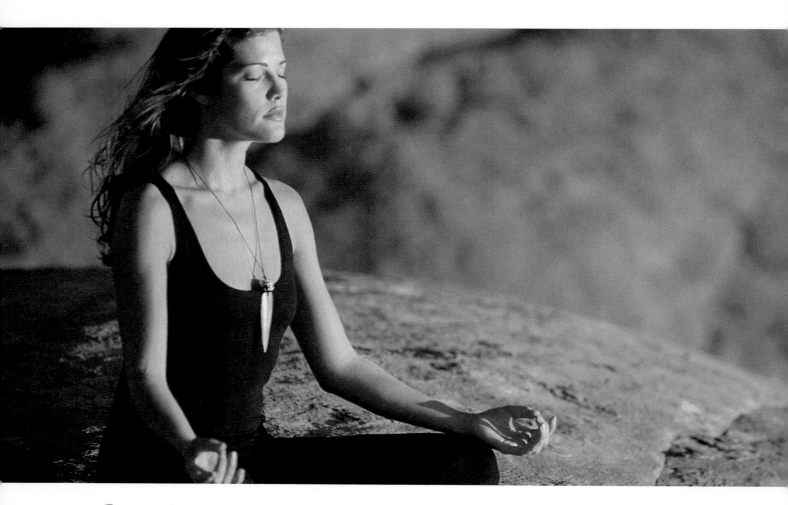

CHAPTER OBJECTIVES

◆ Define stress and examine how stress may have direct and indirect effects on your immune system and on your overall health status.

◆ Explain the three phases of the general adaptation syndrome and describe what happens physiologically when you perceive a threat.

◆ Discuss psychosocial, environmental, and self-imposed sources of stress.

◆ Examine how evolving societal expectations may cause new kinds of stress.

◆ Examine the special stressors that affect college students.

◆ Explore techniques for managing stress.

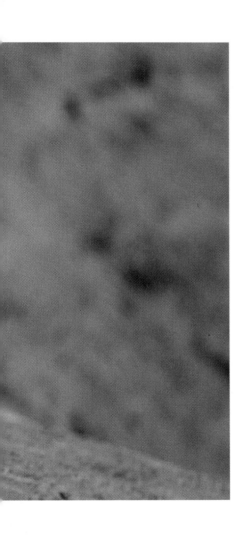

Managing Stress

Toward Prevention and Control

W H A T   D O   Y O U   T H I N K ?

Mary and DeWayne have been dating for over two years, and they have discussed their eventual marriage. Mary's whole world centers on DeWayne and she thinks about him constantly. But DeWayne has seemed less interested in the relationship recently and has broken several dates, saying he has too much work to do. But on one occasion when he is supposedly studying, Mary spots DeWayne strolling into a restaurant with another woman. When she confronts him, DeWayne tells her that the relationship is over and that he's met someone else. Mary is devastated. She stops eating, starts skipping classes, and begins to drink heavily in the early afternoon. Her friends worry that she appears listless and depressed.

■ What thoughts does Mary probably have about the significance of her relationship with DeWayne? Are her perceptions valid? If you were Mary's friend, what would you do to help her cope with her loss? Why are changes in relationships so stressful for people? Is there a way to reduce the impact of these changes? If you were to experience a painful breakup, where on your campus could you go for help?

Erica is taking 20 credits this term: Her parents are unable to help her financially, and she must graduate before her savings are depleted. She is also working 10 hours per week and is involved in several student organizations. She finds that she is usually up until 1 A.M., wakes up at dawn, and must budget every minute of the day just to keep up. In spite of her efforts, she is falling farther and farther behind, has stopped seeing her friends, and is chronically tired. She recently developed a serious cold that has lingered for two weeks. She has also had a persistent headache and finds it difficult to get to sleep at night.

■ Why is Erica so stressed? Why is she suffering from persistent illnesses? Is it possible to do everything right and still not have enough time to get everything done? What should Erica do to manage her stress? Where can she go for help?

Stress: it's hard to live with it, but it's almost impossible to live without it. We are bombarded by a host of subtle and not so subtle internal and external stresses from the moment we awake in the morning until we finally drift into deep sleep at day's end. Even during our sleeping moments, noise, temperature changes, and other activities can be sources of stress. Rarely does a day go by without someone you know talking about being under stress from homework, financial pressures, relationship demands, or other problems. Despite our best efforts to ignore it, stress cannot be run from, hidden from, or wished away. For some people, stress provides the stimulus for growth and higher levels of achievement. Yet for others, it increases the likelihood of dysfunctional or abnormal behavior or illness. Although much has been written about stress in contemporary society, understanding the complex physiological and psychological reactions to stress is no easy task. What is stress? Is it always negative? Why are some people more susceptible to stress than others? What can be done to reduce the negative consequences of stress?

The answers to these questions are complex. Stress in itself is neither positive nor negative. Rather, our reactions to stress can be positive or negative. Whether we are aware of it or not, our reactions to stress can become the habits that lead us either to health-enhancing personal growth or to debilitation in the form of migraines, alcohol and drug addiction, circulatory disorders, asthma, gastrointestinal problems, and hypertension (high blood pressure). In addition, stress can lead to psychological and social problems, including dysfunctional relationships. In this chapter, we will explore why and how these reactions take place and how we may be able to control them.

WHAT IS STRESS?

Many things that have contributed to making you who you are also have influenced how you respond to stressful events in your life. Stress reactions such as breaking out in a cold sweat before getting up in front of the class to speak, becoming anxious around people who speak too slowly or drive too cautiously, feeling nervous when meeting new people are all unique by-products of past experiences. Your family, friends, environmental conditions, general health status, personality, and support systems affect how you respond to a given event.

Stress means different things to different people. Often, we think of stress as an externally imposed factor that threatens or makes a demand on our minds and bodies. If your hard-nosed instructor tells you that you must do a 10-page paper in the next week, that's an external stressor. A more serious or life-threatening external event, such as someone breaking into your apartment while you are sleeping, is another form of external stressor. In this case, someone or something prompts a stressful response in you. Most people would agree that these situations might stress anyone out.

But, actually, most stress is self-imposed and is usually the result of an internal state of emotional tension that occurs in response to the various demands of living. Stress may manifest itself in physiological responses to the demands placed upon us, and many researchers define *stress* as these responses.[1] Most current definitions state that **stress** is the mental and physical response of our bodies to the changes in our lives.

A **stressor** is any physical, social, or psychological event or condition that causes our bodies to have to adjust to a specific situation. Stressors may be tangible, such as an angry parent or a disgruntled roommate, or intangible, such as the mixed emotions associated with meeting your significant other's parents for the first time. **Adjustment** is our attempt to cope with a given situation.[2] As we try to adjust to a stressor, strain may develop. **Strain** is the wear and tear our bodies and minds sustain during the process of adjusting to or resisting a stressor.

Stress and strain are associated with most of our daily activities. Generally, positive stress, or stress that presents the opportunity for personal growth and satisfaction is called **eustress.** Getting married, starting school, beginning a career, developing new friendships, and learning a new physical skill all give rise to eustress. **Distress,** or negative stress, is caused by those events, such as financial problems, injury or illness, the death of a loved one, trouble at work, academic difficulties, and the breakup of a relationship, that result in debilitative stress and strain.

In many cases, we cannot prevent the occurrence of distress: like eustress, it is a part of life. However, we can train ourselves to recognize the events that cause distress and to anticipate the reactions we have to them. We can

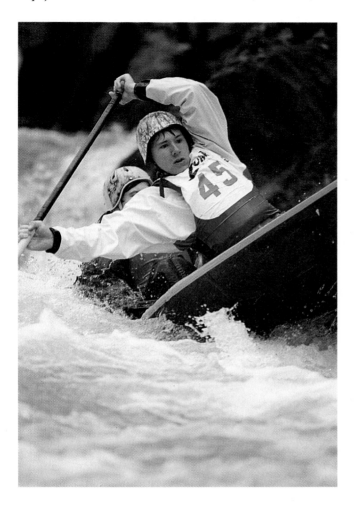

Stress is a positive factor in life when it creates opportunities for personal growth and satisfaction rather than psychological or physical wear and tear.

learn to practice prestress coping skills and to develop poststress management techniques. Development of both skills depends on our understanding of the major components of stress.

The Mind-Body Connection: Physiological Responses

Although much has been written about the negative effects of stress, researchers have only recently begun to untangle the complex web of physical and emotional interactions that actually cause the body to break down over time. As a result, stress is often described generically as a "disease of prolonged arousal" that often leads to other negative health effects. Nearly all systems of the body become potential targets for this onslaught, and the long-term effects may be devastating.

Much of the initial impetus for studying the health effects of stress came from indirect observations. Cardiolo-

gists in the Framingham Heart Study and other research projects noted that highly stressed individuals seemed to experience significantly greater risks for cardiovascular disease and hypertension.[3] Monkeys exposed to high levels of unpredictable stressors in studies showed significantly increased levels of disease and mortality.[4] In a study of susceptibility to cold viruses, subjects inhaled high doses of the virus through the nose. Those subjects who reported recent high levels of stressors were much more likely to catch a cold following exposure to virus than were their low-stress counterparts.[5] While the battle over the legitimacy of these observations continues to be waged in research labs across the country, certain factors relating too much stress over long periods of time to selected ailments has gained credibility. What does repeated stress actually do to the body? Why are health experts so concerned about stress?

Psychoneuroimmunology (PNI). Although the health effects of prolonged stress provide dramatic evidence of the direct and indirect impact of stress on body organs, researchers continue to seek more definitive answers about the exact physiological mechanisms that lead to specific diseases. The science of **psychoneuroimmunology (PNI)** attempts to analyze the relationship between the mind's response to stress and the ability of the immune system to function effectively.

Much of the preliminary PNI data on stress levels and immune functioning have focused on the hypothesis that, during periods of prolonged stress, elevated levels of adrenal hormones destroy or reduce the ability of the white blood cells known as *natural killer T cells* to aid in the immune response. When killer Ts are suppressed, illnesses have a greater chance of gaining a foothold in the body. In addition to killer T suppression, many other

Stress: Our mental and physical responses to change.

Stressor: A physical, social, or psychological event or condition that causes us to have to adjust to a specific situation.

Adjustment: Our attempt to cope with a given situation.

Strain: The wear and tear our bodies and minds sustain as we adjust to or resist a stressor.

Eustress: Stress that presents opportunities for personal growth.

Distress: Stress that can have a negative effect on health.

Psychoneuroimmunology (PNI): Science of the interaction between the mind and the immune system.

Are Black Americans More at Risk for Stress?

It's a question that has long frustrated doctors: Why do black Americans suffer high blood pressure one-third more frequently, develop it at a younger age, and have worse outcomes, than do white Americans? For years, sociologists have said that poverty is the culprit while geneticists have pointed to genetic causes. Each of these hypotheses is supported by a number of studies.

According to Dr. Elijah Saunders, of the University of Maryland's International Society on Hypertension, the cause of black Americans' higher rate of hypertension is clear: "chronic, physically debilitating stress caused not just by poverty, but by black Americans' entire social-economic status." Chronic stress incites the nervous system to release large amounts of a hormone called *norepinephrine*. Norepinephrine causes the kidneys to slow their elimination of salt from the body which in turn raises blood pressure. Saunders tested 26 black women who were on strict low salt diets by giving them extra infusions of salt and measuring their reactions. The higher their socioeconomic status, the more salt they excreted and the less their blood pressure rose. This indicates that socioeconomic status rather than genetics puts blacks at risk.

Research undertaken at the University of Georgia by Dr. Randall Tackett points to a mixed cause. His research indicates that blacks may have less flexible, more-difficult-to-dilate veins, which leads to hypertension. Tackett speculates that such rigidity could stem from the reaction of the veins' lining to prolonged onslaught by hormones released when a person is stressed. This could indicate that blacks' higher rates of hypertension are the result of higher rates of stress. But it could also indicate that these higher rates are the result of genetics: less flexible veins may be a hereditary trait. It's also possible that both these explanations are correct and that they work in tandem to raise black Americans' risk for hypertension.

Although similar research testing the socioeconomic theory on whites must be conducted, the National Institutes of Health (NIH) sees Saunders's and Tackett's research as so promising that it is investing $8.4 million dollars in a research program focusing on minority groups' older members' health.

Source: Adapted by permission of Associated Press, from "Theory Links Social Stress, Hypertension in Blacks." *Corvallis (Oregon) Gazette Times,* November 15, 1994.

---

bodily processes are disrupted and overall disease-fighting capacity is reduced. Although several studies have supported the hypothesis of a relationship between increased stress levels and greater risk of disease in times of grief, social disruption, poor mood, and so forth, there is much to be learned about possible mediating factors in this process.[6] Other studies have shown no increased risk for disease among people suffering from prolonged arousal by stressors.[7]

Homeostasis: A balanced physical state in which all the body's systems function smoothly.

Adaptive response: Form of adjustment in which the body attempts to restore homeostasis.

General adaptation syndrome (GAS): The pattern followed by our physiological responses to stress, consisting of the alarm, resistance, and exhaustion phases.

Autonomic nervous system (ANS): The portion of the central nervous system that regulates bodily functions that we do not normally consciously control.

THE GENERAL ADAPTATION SYNDROME

Every living organism tends toward a state of balance known as **homeostasis.** In homeostasis, all physical and psychological systems function smoothly, and equilibrium is maintained. When a stressor disrupts homeostasis, the body adjusts with an **adaptive response,** or an attempt to restore homeostasis. This adaptive response to stress varies in intensity and physical manifestation from person to person and from stressor to stressor.

The physiological responses to stress follow a pattern that was first recognized in 1936 by Hans Selye. The three-stage response to stress Selye outlined is called the **general adaptation syndrome (GAS)** (see Figure 3.1). The phases of the GAS are alarm, resistance, and exhaustion.[8]

Alarm Phase

During the alarm phase, a stressor disturbs homeostasis. The brain subconsciously perceives the stressor and prepares the body either to fight or to run away, a response sometimes called the *fight or flight response.* The subcon-

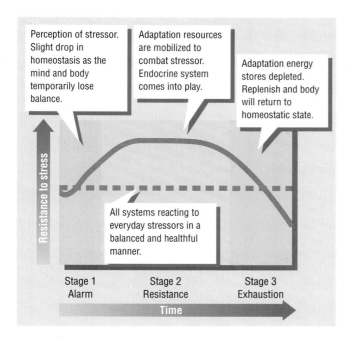

FIGURE 3.1

The General Adaptation Syndrome

Diagram labels (top to bottom, left to right):

Perception of stressor. Slight drop in homeostasis as the mind and body temporarily lose balance.

Adaptation resources are mobilized to combat stressor. Endocrine system comes into play.

Adaptation energy stores depleted. Replenish and body will return to homeostatic state.

All systems reacting to everyday stressors in a balanced and healthful manner.

Resistance to stress

Stage 1 Alarm
Stage 2 Resistance
Stage 3 Exhaustion

Time

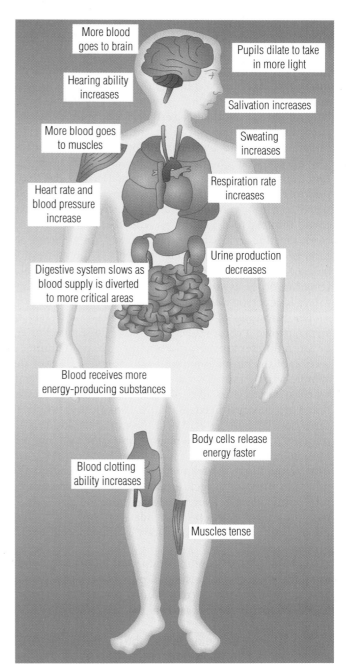

FIGURE 3.2

The General Adaptation Syndrome: Alarm Phase

Diagram labels:

More blood goes to brain

Pupils dilate to take in more light

Hearing ability increases

Salivation increases

More blood goes to muscles

Sweating increases

Heart rate and blood pressure increase

Respiration rate increases

Digestive system slows as blood supply is diverted to more critical areas

Urine production decreases

Blood receives more energy-producing substances

Body cells release energy faster

Blood clotting ability increases

Muscles tense

scious perceptions and appraisal of the stressor stimulate the areas in the brain responsible for emotions. Emotional stimulation, in turn, starts the physical reactions that we associate with stress (see Figure 3.2). This entire process usually takes only a few seconds.

Here's an example of the alarm phase. Suppose that you are walking to your car across campus at night. As you pass a particularly dark area, you sense that someone has suddenly appeared behind you. You quickly assess the situation but dismiss your anxiety as being only your imagination. You quicken your pace only to hear the footsteps quicken behind you. Your senses become increasingly alert as you note that there are no other people in the area. You speed up even more. You feel your heart and breathing rates increase, your muscles tense, and you begin sweating. Yet the stranger is getting closer and closer. In desperation you stop, clutching your keys in your hands, determined to gouge the attacker's eyes out. As you wheel around, you let out a blood-curdling yell, only to notice that it's Mrs. Jones, a woman in one of your classes, who has been following you. Fearful of the dark streets, she has tried to stay close to the only other person on the street—you. She screeches and jumps back out of the way of your swinging arms, and after a startled recognition, you both burst out in nervous laughter. You have just experienced what is commonly known as the alarm phase of the stress response.

When the mind perceives a stressor (either real or imaginary), such as a potential attacker, the *cerebral cor-*

tex, the region of the brain that interprets the nature of an event, is called to attention. If the cerebral cortex consciously or unconsciously perceives a threat, it triggers an instantaneous **autonomic nervous system (ANS)** response that prepares the body for action. The ANS is the portion of the central nervous system that regulates bodily functions that we do not normally consciously control, such as heart function, breathing, and glandular function. When we are stressed, the rate of all these bodily functions increases dramatically to give us the physical strength to protect ourselves against an attack, or to mobilize internal forces. The ANS has two branches. The **sympathetic nervous system,** one branch, begins to energize the body for either fight or flight by signaling the release of several stress hormones that speed the heart rate, increase the breathing rate, and trigger many other stress responses. The **parasympathetic nervous system,** the other branch, functions to slow all the systems stimulated by the stress response. Thus, the parasympathetic branch of the ANS serves as a system of checks and balances on the sympathetic branch. In a healthy person, these two branches work together in a balance that controls the negative effects of stress. However, long-term stress can cause this balance to become strained, and chronic physical problems can occur as stress reactions become the dominant forces in a person's body.

The responses of the sympathetic nervous system to stress involve a complex series of biochemical exchanges between different parts of the body. The **hypothalamus,** a section of the brain, functions as the control center of the sympathetic nervous system and determines the overall reaction to stressors. When the hypothalamus perceives that extra energy is needed to fight a stressor, it stimulates the adrenal glands, located near the top of the kidneys, to release the hormone **epinephrine,** also called adrenaline. Epinephrine causes more blood to be pumped with each beat of the heart, dilates the bronchioles (air sacs in the lungs) to increase oxygen intake, increases the breathing rate, stimulates the liver to release more glucose (which fuels muscular exertion), and dilates the pupils to improve visual sensitivity. The body is then poised to act immediately.

As epinephrine secretion increases, blood is diverted away from the digestive system, possibly causing nausea and cramping if the distress occurs shortly after a meal, and drying of nasal and salivary tissues, producing a dry mouth.

The stress response occurring during the alarm phase also provides for longer-term reaction to stress. The hypothalamus triggers the pituitary gland, which in turn releases another powerful hormone, **adrenocorticotrophic hormone (ACTH).** ACTH signals the adrenal glands to release **cortisol,** a hormone that makes stored nutrients more readily available to meet energy demands. Finally, other parts of the brain and body release endorphins, the body's naturally occurring opiates, which relieve pain that may be caused by a stressor.

Resistance Phase

The resistance phase of the GAS begins almost immediately after the alarm phase starts. In this phase, the body has reacted to the stressor and adjusted in a way that begins to allow the system to return to homeostasis. As the sympathetic nervous system is working to energize the body via the hormonal action of epinephrine, norepinephrine, cortisol, and other hormones, the parasympathetic nervous system is helping to keep these energy levels under control and returns the body to a normal level of functioning.

Exhaustion Phase

In the exhaustion phase of the GAS, the physical and psychological energy used to fight a stressor has been depleted. Short-term stress would probably not deplete all of a person's energy reserves, but chronic stressors, such as the struggle to get straight As, financial worries, or fights with family and friends may create continuous states of alarm and resistance. When a person no longer has the

Aerobic exercise is one way to replenish the energy stores the body uses in adapting and adjusting to negative stressors.

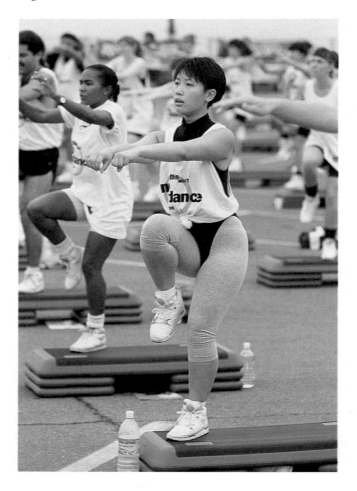

adaptation energy stores for fighting a distressor, serious illness may result.

Adaptation Energy Stores. Many stress researchers believe that each of us possesses *adaptation energy stores.* In these researchers' model, these energy stores are the physical and mental foundations of our ability to cope with stress. Two levels of adaptation energy stores exist: *deep* and *superficial.* We apparently have little control over our deep adaptation energy stores: heredity seems to be the primary influence on them and some scientists speculate that their size is preset in each of our cells. Superficial adaptation energy stores surround the deep stores. These relatively easy-to-reach stores are used before the deep energy stores beneath them and they are renewable.

Stress researchers theorize that when its deep adaptation energy stores are depleted, an organism dies. Stress management, then, is dependent on an ability to replenish superficial stores, and thereby to conserve deep stores. Superficial adaptation energy stores can be replenished by aerobic exercise (exercise that raises the heart rate), balancing work with relaxation, eliminating unnecessary drugs, maintaining a secure home environment, practicing good nutritional habits, finding challenges and adventures instead of threats in stressors, setting realistic goals, and establishing and maintaining supportive relationships.

*W*HAT DO YOU THINK?

What are the greatest sources of stress for you right now? What can you do to keep your superficial adaptation energy stores high and reduce your risks of becoming run down? Have you ever noticed that you tend to get sick more during certain times? Why might this occur?

*S*OURCES OF STRESS

Both eustress and distress have many sources. These sources include psychosocial factors, such as changes, hassles, pressure, inconsistent goals and objectives, conflict, overload, and burnout; environmental stressors, such as natural and human-made disasters; and self-imposed stress. We'll look at each factor in more detail in this section.

Psychosocial Sources of Stress

As you learned in the previous chapter, psychosocial health relates to the mental, emotional, social, and spiritual dimensions of health. These dimensions define how we perceive our lives, relate to one another, and react to

stress. Psychosocial stress refers to the factors in our daily lives that cause stress. Many factors in our daily lives cause us to be stressed. Our interactions with others, the subtle and not-so-subtle expectations we and others have of ourselves, and the social conditions we work in, play in, and live in all force us to adjust and readjust continually. Some of these stressors present very real threats to our mental and/or physical well-being; others cause us to worry about things that may never happen. Still other stressors result from otherwise good psychosocial events—being around someone you're attracted to, meeting new friends, or moving to a new and better apartment.

Change. Any time there is change in your normal daily routine, whether good or bad, you will experience stress. The more changes you experience and the more adjustments you must make, the greater the stress effects may be. In 1967, Drs. Thomas Holmes and Richard Rahe analyzed the social readjustments experienced by over 5,000 patients, noting which events seemed to occur just prior to disease onset.[9] They determined that certain events (both positive and negative) were predictive of increased risk for illness. They called their scale for predicting stress overload and the likelihood of illness the Social Readjustment Rating Scale (SRRS) and this scale has been used extensively.[10] The SRRS has since been modified for certain groups, including college-aged students, as shown in Table 3.1. Although many other factors must be considered, it is generally believed that the more of these you have, the more you need to change your behaviors or situation before problems occur. (See the Rate Yourself box.)

Hassles. While Holmes and Rahe focused on such major sources of stress as a death in the family, psychologists such as Richard Lazarus have more recently focused

Sympathetic nervous system: Branch of the autonomic nervous system responsible for stress arousal.

Parasympathetic nervous system: Part of the autonomic nervous system responsible for slowing systems stimulated by the stress response.

Hypothalamus: A section of the brain that controls the sympathetic nervous system and directs the stress response.

Epinephrine: Also called adrenaline, a hormone that stimulates body systems in response to stress.

Adrenocorticotrophic hormone (ACTH): A pituitary hormone that stimulates the adrenal glands to secrete cortisol.

Cortisol: Hormone released by the adrenal glands that makes stored nutrients more readily available to meet energy demands.

TABLE 3.1 ■ Are You Experiencing Stress?

Here are 30 life events from the Social Readjustment Rating Scale (SRRS) that may be stressful to young adults.

1. Death of a close family member
2. Death or loss of a close friend or significant other
3. Divorce of parents
4. Jail term
5. Major personal injury or illness
6. Marriage
7. Firing from job
8. Failure in an important class
9. Change in health of family member
10. Pregnancy
11. Sex problems
12. Serious argument with close friend
13. Change in financial status
14. Change in major
15. Trouble with parents
16. New girlfriend, boyfriend, or significant other
17. Increased workload or schoolwork burden
18. Outstanding personal achievement
19. First year in college
20. Change in living conditions
21. Serious argument with instructor
22. Lower grades than expected
23. Change in sleep habits
24. Change in social habits
25. Change in eating habits
26. Chronic car trouble
27. Vacation
28. Too many missed classes
29. Change of college
30. Minor traffic violations

Source: Adapted with permission of Elsevier Science Ltd., Pergamon Imprint, Oxford, England, from Thomas Holmes and Richard Rahe, "The Social Readjustment Rating Scale," *Journal of Psychosomatic Research* (1967): 213–218.

on petty annoyances, irritations, and frustrations, collectively referred to as hassles, as sources of stress.[11] Minor hassles—losing your keys, having the grocery bag rip on the way to the door, slipping and falling in front of everyone as you walk to your seat in a new class, finding that you went through a whole afternoon with a big chunk of spinach stuck in your front teeth—may seem unimportant, but the cumulative effects of these minor hassles may be harmful in the long run.

Pressure. Pressure occurs when we feel forced to speed up, intensify, or shift the direction of our behavior to meet a higher standard of performance.[12] Pressures can be based on our personal goals and expectations or on a concern about what others may think of us. Pressure can also come from outside influences. Among the most significant and consistent of these are seemingly relentless demands from society that we compete and that we be all that we can be. The forces that push us to compete for the best grades, the nicest cars, the most attractive significant others, and the highest paying jobs create significant pressure to be the personification of American success.[13] When we are pressured into doing something we don't

want to do (for example, studying when everyone else is going to a movie), significant frustration can occur.

Inconsistent Goals and Behaviors. For many of us, negative stress effects are magnified when there is a conflict between our goals (what we value or hope to obtain in life) and our behaviors (actions or activities that may or may not lead us to achieving these goals). For instance, you may want good grades, and your family may expect them. But if you party and procrastinate throughout the term, your behaviors are inconsistent with your goals, and significant stress in the form of guilt, last-minute frenzy before exams, and disappointing grades may result. On the other hand, if you want to dig in and work, and are committed to getting good grades, much of your negative stress may be eliminated or reduced. Thwarted goals may lead to frustration, and frustration has been shown to be a significant disrupter of homeostasis (see Figure 3.3).

Determining whether our behaviors are consistent with goal attainment is an essential component of our efforts to maintain a balance in our lives. If we consciously strive to attain our goals in a very direct manner, our chances of success are greatly improved. If we deviate from the plan, or if we act in a manner that is inconsistent with our goals, significant stress may result that makes our goals impossible, and they may become negative sources of stress.

Conflict. Of all life's troubles, conflict is probably one of the most common. **Conflict** occurs when we are forced to make difficult decisions concerning two or more competing motives, behaviors, or impulses or when we are forced to face two incompatible demands, opportunities, needs, or goals.[14] What if your best friends all choose to smoke

Conflict: Simultaneous existence of incompatible demands, opportunities, needs, or goals.

Overload: A condition in which we feel overly pressured by demands made on us.

Burnout: Physical and mental exhaustion caused by excessive stress.

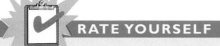

How Stressed Are You?

Each of us reacts differently to life's little challenges. Faced with a long line at the bank, most of us will get heated up for a few seconds before we shrug and move on. But for others—the one in five of us whom researchers call hot reactors—such incidents are an assault on good health. That's why rating your stress requires you both to tally your life's stressors (Part One) and to figure out whether you are particularly susceptible to stress (Part Two).

PART ONE

The Stress in Your Life

How often are the following stressful situations a part of your daily life?

1 Never
2 Rarely
3 Sometimes
4 Often
5 All the time

I work long hours	1	2	3	4	5
There are signs my job isn't secure	1	2	3	4	5
Doing a good job goes unnoticed	1	2	3	4	5
It takes all my energy just to make it through the day	1	2	3	4	5
There are severe arguments at home	1	2	3	4	5
A family member is seriously ill	1	2	3	4	5
I'm having problems with child care	1	2	3	4	5
I don't have enough time for fun	1	2	3	4	5
I'm on a diet	1	2	3	4	5
My family and friends count on me to solve their problems	1	2	3	4	5
I'm expected to keep up a certain standard of living	1	2	3	4	5

My neighborhood is crowded or dangerous	1	2	3	4	5
My home is a mess	1	2	3	4	5
I can't pay my bills on time	1	2	3	4	5
I'm not saving money	1	2	3	4	5

Your Total Score _____

Below 38:   You have a *Lower-Stress Life.*

38 & Above: You have a *High-Stress Life.*

PART TWO

Your Stress Susceptibility

Try to imagine how you would react in these hypothetical situations.

You've been waiting 20 minutes for a table in a crowded restaurant, and the host seats a party that arrived after you. You feel your anger rise as your face gets hot and your heart beats faster.

True or False

· · · · · · · · · · · · ·

Your sister calls out of the blue and starts to tell you how much you mean to her. Uncomfortable, you change the subject without expressing what you feel.

True or False

· · · · · · · · · · · · ·

You come home to find the kitchen looking like a disaster area and your spouse lounging in front of the TV. You tense up and can't seem to shake your anger.

True or False

· · · · · · · · · · · · ·

Faced with a public speaking event, you get keyed up and lose sleep for a day or more, worrying about how you'll do.

True or False

(continued)

---

marijuana and you don't want to smoke but fear rejection? Such conflicts occur every day for most of us. Worrying about the alternatives, fretting, stewing, and becoming overly anxious are common stress responses when conflict occurs.

Overload.   **Overload** occurs when you suffer from excessive time pressure, excessive responsibility, lack of support, or excessive expectations of yourself and those around you. Have you ever felt that you had so many responsibilities that you couldn't possibly begin to fulfill them all? Have you longed for a weekend when you could just curl up and read a good book or take time out with friends and not feel guilty? These feelings typically occur when a person has been under continued stress for a period of time and is suffering from overload. Students suffering from overload may experience anxiety about tests, poor self-concept, a desire to drop classes or to drop out of school, and other problems. In severe cases, in which they are unable to see any solutions to their problems, students may suffer from depression or turn to substance abuse.

Burnout.   People who regularly suffer from overload, frustration, and disappointment may eventually begin to experience **burnout**, a state of physical and mental exhaustion caused by excessive stress. People involved in the "helping professions," such as teaching, social work, drug

On Thursday your repair shop promises to fix your car in time for a weekend trip. As the hours go by, you become increasingly worried that something will go wrong and your trip will be ruined.

True or False

Two or Fewer True: You're a *Cool Reactor,* someone who tends to roll with the punches when a situation is out of your control.

Three or More True: Sorry, you're a *Hot Reactor,* someone who responds to mildly stressful situations with a "fight-or-flight" adrenaline rush that drives up blood pressure and can lead to heart rhythm disturbances, accelerated clotting, and damaged blood vessel linings. Some hot reactors can seem cool as a cucumber on the outside, but inside their bodies are silently killing them.

WHAT YOUR SCORES MEAN

Combine the results from parts one and two to get your total stress rating.

Lower-Stress Life   *Cool Reactor*

Whatever your problems, stress isn't one of them. Even when stressful events do occur—and they will—your health probably won't suffer.

Lower-Stress Life   *Hot Reactor*

You're not under stress—at least for now. Though you tend to overreact to problems, you've wisely managed your life to avoid the big stressors. Before you honk at the guy who cuts you off in rush hour traffic, remember that getting angry can destroy thousands of heart muscle cells within minutes. Robert S. Eliot, author of *From Stress to Strength,* says hot

reactors have no choice but to calm themselves down with rational thought. Ponder the fact that the only thing you'll hasten by reacting is a decline in health. "You have to stop trying to change the world," Eliot advises, "and learn to change your response to it."

High-Stress Life   *Cool Reactor*

You're under stress, but only you know if it's hurting. Even if you normally thrive with a full plate of challenges, now you might be biting off more than you can chew. Note any increase in headaches, backaches, or insomnia; that's your body telling you to lighten your load. If your job is the main source of stress, think about reducing your hours. If that's not possible, find a way to make your job more enjoyable, and stress will become manageable.

High-Stress Life   *Hot Reactor*

You're in the danger zone. Make an extra effort to exercise, get enough sleep, and keep your family and friends close. Unfortunately, even being physically fit does little to protect you if your body is in perpetual stress mode. To survive, you may need to make major changes—walking away from a life-destroying job or relationship, perhaps—as well as to develop a whole new approach to life's hourly obstacles. Such effort will be rewarded, too. In one experiment, 77 percent of hot reactors were able to cool down—lower their blood pressure and cholesterol levels—by training themselves to stay calm.

Source: Reprinted by permission of the Health Publishing Group, a division of Time Publishing Ventures, Inc., from "How Stressed Are You?" *Health,* October 1994, 47. Researched by Lora Elise Ma. © 1994.

counseling, nursing, and psychology, appear to experience high levels of burnout, as do people such as police officers and air-traffic controllers who work in high-pressure, dangerous jobs.

Other Forms of Psychosocial Stress. Other forms of psychosocial stress include problems with adaptation, difficulty in adapting to life's changes; frustration, the thwarting or inhibiting of natural or desired behaviors or goals; overcrowding, the presence of too many people in a space; discrimination, the unfavorable actions taken against people based on prejudices concerning race, religion, social status, gender, lifestyle, national origin, or physical characteristics; and such socioeconomic events as

inflation, unemployment, or poverty. People of different ethnic backgrounds may face disproportionately heavy impact from these sources of stress.

Environmental Stress

Environmental stress is stress that results from events occurring in our physical environment as opposed to our social environment. Environmental stressors include natural disasters, such as floods, earthquakes, hurricanes, and forest fires, and industrial disasters, such as chemical spills, accidents at nuclear power plants, and explosions. Often as damaging as one-time disasters are **background**

BEHAVIORS   GOALS

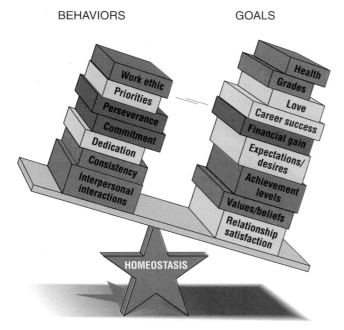

FIGURE 3.3

Stress Affects Homeostatic Balance

distressors, such as noise, air, and water pollution, although we may be unaware of them and their effects may not become apparent for decades. As with other distressors, our bodies respond to environmental distressors with the general adaptation syndrome. People who cannot escape background distressors may exist in a constant resistance phase, which may contribute to the development of stress-related disorders.

Self-Imposed Stress

Self-Concept and Stress.   How we feel about ourselves, our attitudes toward others, and our perceptions and interpretations of the stressors in our lives are all part of the psychological component of stress. Also included are the defense or coping mechanisms we have learned to use in various stressful situations.

The psychological system that governs our responses to stressors is called the **cognitive stress system.**[15] Our cognitive stress system serves to recognize stressors; evaluate them on the basis of self-concept, past experiences, and emotions; and make decisions regarding how to cope with them.

Our sensory organs serve as input channels for any information reaching the brain. From that point on, attention to the problem, memory, reasoning processes, and problem solving are organized in various parts of the brain before we act on the stressor. Because learning and memory involve the changing of various proteins in brain

We become physically and mentally exhausted—and more susceptible to illnesses and accidents—when we are unable to control the sources of stress in our lives.

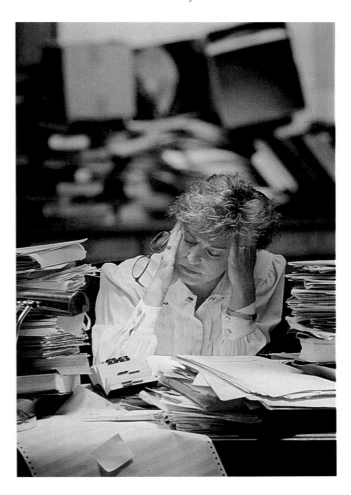

neurons, the emotions experienced during the stress response also "tickle" the memory storage neurons and contribute to our responses. Behaviorally, we will respond to the stressor in ways consistent with our memories of similar situations.

Self-esteem is closely related to the emotions engendered by past experiences. People with low self-esteem are more likely to become victims of helpless anger, an emotion experienced by people who have not learned to express anger in appropriate ways. People suffering helpless

Background distressors: Environmental stressors that we may be unaware of.

Cognitive stress system: The psychological system that governs our emotional responses to stress.

anger have usually learned that they are wrong to feel anger; therefore, instead of learning to express their anger in healthy ways, they turn it inward. They may "swallow" their anger in food, alcohol, or other drugs, or may act in other self-destructive ways.

Research indicates that self-esteem significantly affects various disease processes. People with low self-esteem create a self-imposed distressor that can impair the immune system's ability to combat disease. Some researchers believe that chronic distress can depress the immune system and thus increase the symptoms of such diseases as acquired immune deficiency syndrome (AIDS), herpes, multiple sclerosis, and Epstein-Barr syndrome.

Personality Types and Hardiness. A person's personality may contribute to the kind and degree of self-imposed stress he or she experiences. The coronary disease-prone personality was first described in 1974 by physicians Meyer Friedman and Ray Rosenman in their book *Type A Behavior and Your Heart*.[16] Although their work is now considered controversial, it is the basis for much current research.

Friedman and Rosenman identified two stress-related personality types: Type A and Type B. Type A personalities are hard-driving, competitive, anxious, time-driven, impatient, angry, and perfectionist. Type B personalities are relaxed and noncompetitive. According to Rosenman and Friedman, people with Type A characteristics are more prone to heart attacks than are their Type B counterparts.

Researchers today believe that more needs to be discovered about Type A and Type B personalities before we can say that all Type As will have greater risks for heart disease than will Type Bs. First of all, most people are not one personality type or the other all of the time. Second, there are many other unexplained variables that must be explored, such as why some Type A personalities seem to thrive in stress-filled environments. Now labeled Type C personalities, these individuals appear to succeed more often than Type B personalities and have good health even while displaying Type A patterns of behavior.

Critics of these categories for stress risk argue that attempts to explain ill health by means of personal behavioral patterns have so far been crude. For example, researchers at Duke University contend that the Type A personality may be more complex than previously described. They have identified a "toxic core" in some Type A personalities. People who have this toxic core are angry, distrustful of others, and have above-average levels of cynicism. People who are angry and hostile often have below-average levels of social support and other increased risks for ill health. It may be this toxic core rather than the hard-driving nature of the Type A personality that makes people more prone to self-imposed stress and its consequences.[17]

Psychologist Susanne Kobasa has identified **psychological hardiness** as a characteristic that has helped some people negate self-imposed stress associated with Type A behavior. Psychologically hardy people are characterized by control, commitment, and challenge.[18] People with a sense of control are able to accept responsibility for their behaviors and to make changes in behaviors that they discover to be debilitating. People with a sense of commitment have good self-esteem and understand their purpose in life. People with a sense of challenge see changes in life as stimulating opportunities for personal growth.

Modification of Type A behavior is possible because some of this behavior is "learned." Some Type A people are able to reduce their hurried behavior and become more tolerant, more patient, and better humored. Unfortunately, many people do not decide to modify their Type A habits until after they have become ill or suffered a heart attack or other circulatory system distress. Prevention of heart and circulatory disorders resulting from stress entails recognizing and changing dangerous behaviors before damage is done.

Self-Efficacy and Control. Whether people are able to cope successfully with stressful situations often depends on their level of self-efficacy, or belief in their skills and performance abilities.[19] If people have been successful in mastering similar problems in the past, they will be more likely to believe in their own effectiveness in future situations. Similarly, people who have repeatedly tried and failed may lack confidence in their abilities to deal with life's problems. In some cases, this insecurity may prevent them from trying to cope.

In addition, people who believe they lack control in a situation may become easily frustrated and give up. Those who feel they have no personal control over anything tend to have an external locus of control and a low level of self-efficacy. People who are confident their behavior will influence the ultimate outcome of events tend to have an internal locus of control. People who feel that they have limited control over their lives tend to have higher levels of stress. For some suggestions on how to gain more control in angry situations, see the Building Communication Skills box.

Gender and Stress: Changing Roles, Increasing Problems

Today, about 58 percent of mothers who have children under the age of 6 work outside the home. The figure increases to 78 percent for women whose children are between 6 and 13. But all the work that stay-at-home mothers once did still needs to be done: Children need to be dropped off and picked up at school or daycare and

Communicating Effectively to Express Anger

Expressing anger constructively is an important skill involved in learning to cope with intimate relationships, family interactions, and other stressful situations. Here are some suggestions for constructive expression of anger.

1. *Determine the real reason behind your anger.* Is it due to a real event (for example, someone you trusted is spreading malicious gossip) or to a perception you have about a situation (friends are avoiding you, so you think someone may be gossiping)?

2. *Don't let your anger build.* When you become angry, take control, and decide what actions you need to take. Try not to act rashly, but don't stew for a long time. If you choose to write a letter expressing your anger, sit down and write it, but don't mail the letter immediately. Put it away, wait a few days, and then reread it. You may choose not to send the letter, but sitting down to write may help you cool off.

3. *If you decide to confront a person, select an appropriate time and place for the meeting.* Try not to attack your target unexpectedly or in the presence of others: the person may become defensive. Give the person a general idea of what you want to discuss ahead of time.

4. *Stick to the major or most recent reason for your anger.* Bringing up a whole list of things that have made you angry over the last year will just complicate the issue and make the other person want to create his or her own list of wrongs that you have committed. Plan in advance which issue you want to discuss.

5. *Attack the problem rather than the person.* Don't get into a battle over personal characteristics. Use "I" statements to communicate resentment or disappointment ("I feel angry that we had to leave the party so early"). "You" statements often put people on the defensive.

6. *Listen carefully to what the other person has to say.* If the other person starts wandering from the issue, gently try to bring him or her back to the point. If the other person attacks you personally, stay in control and don't allow yourself to fight back.

7. *Treat the other person with respect.* Even though you may say the right things, your gestures and body language can reveal that you don't value what the other person has to say, that you are hostile, or that you are losing patience. Drumming your fingers, sighing, or rolling your eyes while the other person is talking can often increase friction.

8. *Recognize when to quit.* Sometimes even the best-laid plans go awry. No matter what you do, the problem may appear impossible to resolve. In such situations, knowing when to quit, either temporarily or permanently, is a key factor in controlling stressful anger levels.

9. *When it's over, let it be over.* After you have done all that you can do, learn to let go of your anger. Don't dwell in the past. Acknowledge your right to be angry, recognize it for what it was, and move on.

---

cared for at home, houses need to be cleaned and maintained, and shopping has to be done. Now that both parents in many families work outside the home, gender roles have blurred: The decision concerning who stays home with a sick child often has more to do with job flexibility than with gender. For some people, deviation from the gender roles they learned as children pose significant levels of stress.

*W*HAT DO YOU THINK?

Who do you think faces the greatest amounts of stress? Married men with children? Married women with children? Single men or women with children? What social institutions/services support each of the above? What social and cultural factors may increase stress for these groups? How stressed do you think your parents were/are? What actions might they take to reduce their stress levels?

*S*TRESS AND THE COLLEGE STUDENT

Stress related to college life is not caused only by pressure to excel academically. College students experience numerous distressors, including changes related to being away from home for the first time, climatic differences between home and school, pressure to make friends in a new and sometimes intimidating setting, the feeling of anonymity imposed by large classes, test-taking anxiety, and pressures related to time management.

Psychological hardiness: A personality characteristic characterized by control, commitment, and challenge.

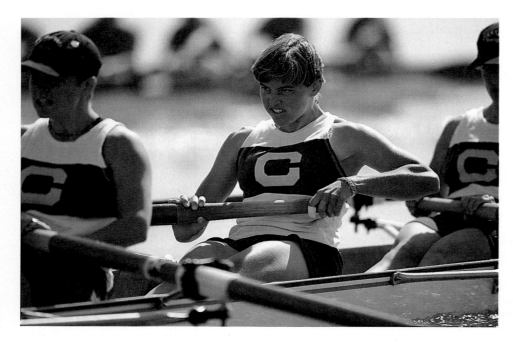

Achieving personal goals and competing at the college level can be significant sources of stress.

Some students are stressed by athletic team requirements, dormitory food, roommate habits, peers' expectations, new questions about personal values and beliefs, relationship problems, fraternity or sorority demands, or financial worries. For older students, worries about competing with 18-year-olds may also be distressful. Most colleges offer stress management workshops through their health centers or student counseling departments.

You should not ignore the following symptoms of stress overload. If you experience one or more of these symptoms, you should act promptly to reduce their impact.

- Difficulty keeping up with classes or difficulty concentrating on and finishing tasks.

- Frequent clashes with close friends, family, or intimate partners about trivial issues such as housekeeping.

- Frequent mood changes or overreaction to minor problems.

- Lethargy caused by lack of sleep or excessive frustration.

- Disinterest in social activities or tendency to avoid others.

- Avoidance of stressors through use of drugs or alcohol or through other extreme behaviors.

- Sleep disturbances, TV addiction, free-floating anxiety, or an exaggerated sense of self.

- Difficulty in maintaining an intimate relationship.

- Disinterest in sexual relationships or inability to participate in satisfactory sexual relationships.

- Tendency to be intolerant of minor differences of opinion.

- Hunger and cravings or tendency to overeat or to eat while thinking of other things.

- Lack of awareness of sensory cues.

- Inability to listen or tendency to jump from subject to subject in conversation.

- Stuttering or other speech difficulties.

- Accident proneness.

*W*HAT DO YOU THINK?

How many of these psychological and emotional reactions have you experienced? Which reactions do you think are the most damaging to you and to your relationships with others? Which ones would be the easiest to change? What actions could you take immediately to cope with these problems? What could you do to cope with these problems in the long run?

*S*TRESS MANAGEMENT

Stress can be challenging or defeating depending upon how we learn to view it. The most effective way to avoid defeat is to learn a number of skills known collectively as stress management. Stress management consists primarily of finding balance in our lives. We balance rest, relaxation, exercise, nutrition, work, school, family, finances,

Overcoming Test-Taking Anxiety

Doing well on a test is an ability needed far beyond your college days. Many careers require special exams. Tests are a fact of life in government, insurance, medicine, and other fields. And stress is a fact of tests!

But there are things you can do to get the upper hand on your anxiety. Here are some helpful hints that you will find useful now and in the future. Give them a try on your next exam.

Before the exam:

1. Manage your time. Effective management will help you find the time to study before the test. Plan to study beginning a week before your test (longer if a career exam). The more advance studying, the less anxiety you will feel. Do not wait to study until the night before the test. The final night should be limited to review. Arrive at the test a half hour early for a final run through. You will find that this will ease your anxiety and increase your confidence.

2. Build your test-taking self-esteem. Try two things. First, take a three-by-five-inch card and write down the three reasons you will pass the exam. Carry the card with you and look at it whenever you study. Second, when you get the test, write your three reasons on the test or on a piece of scrap paper. Positive affirmations such as this will help you succeed.

3. Get adequate sleep. You need to be alert, so try to get a little extra sleep for a few nights before your exam.

4. Eat well before the exam. As you'll learn in Chapter 8, sugar doesn't give you energy. In fact, it tires you. Avoid all sugary foods the day before the test and also those foods that might upset your stomach. You want to be feeling your best.

5. Take caffeine about an hour before the test. Research shows that caffeine promotes alertness, motor performance, and the capacity for work, as well as a decrease in fatigue. A cup or two of coffee, tea, or a cola drink is sufficient. Some people shouldn't use caffeine. Avoid it if you are one of the small percentage that it leaves feeling shaky and on edge for hours or if you regularly do not use caffeinated products. Test day is not the day to find our how your body reacts to caffeine.

During the test:

1. Use time management during the test. If you have 60 minutes to answer 30 multiple choice questions, you might decide to spend the first 45 minutes taking the test (1 1/2 minutes per question) and 15 minutes reviewing your answers (30 seconds per question). Hold yourself to this schedule. After 15 minutes, you should have completed the first 10 questions, etc. If you don't know an answer, or the question is taking too long, skip it and move on. Since you allotted yourself time at the end to review, you will have the time to go back.

   Test-makers usually allow sufficient time to complete and review a test. However, if you feel that you are a slow reader and may need more time, talk to your teacher or the test administrator *before* the exam.

2. Slow down. When you open your test book, always write RTFQ (Read the Full Question) at the top. Make sure you understand the question.

3. If you begin to get anxious, reread your three reasons for success. Stay on track.

and social activities. As we balance our lives, we make the choice to react constructively to our stressors. Robert Eliot, a cardiologist and stress researcher, offers two rules for people trying to cope with life's challenges: (1) "Don't sweat the small stuff," and (2) Remember that "it's all small stuff."[20]

Dealing with Stress

The first step of stress management is to examine thoroughly any problem involving stress. The Choices for Change box shows a decision-making model for stress reduction. As the model shows, dealing with stress involves assessing all aspects of a stressor, examining how you are currently responding to the stressor and how you may be able to change your response, and evaluating various methods of coping with stress. Often we cannot change the requirements at our college, unexpected distressors, or accidents. Inevitably, we will be stuck in classes that bore us and for which we find no application in real life. We feel powerless when a loved one has died. The facts themselves cannot be changed; only our reactions to the distressors in our lives can be changed.

Assessing Your Stressors. After recognizing a stressor, you need to assess it. Can you alter the circumstances in any way to reduce the amount of distress you are experiencing, or must you change your behavior and reactions to the stressor to reduce your stress levels? For example, if five term papers for five different courses are due during the semester, you will probably quickly assess that you cannot alter the circumstances: your professors are unlikely to drop their requirements. You can, however, change your behavior by beginning the papers early and spacing them over time to avoid last-minute stress. If your boss is vague about directions for assignments, you can-

Decision Making and Your Stress-Reduction Program

When trying to make decisions about how to reduce your stress levels, you must first carefully assess your situation and what you are willing and capable of doing right now to change this situation.

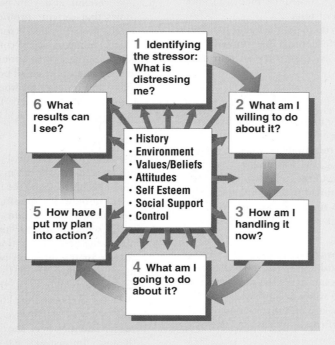

1 Identifying the stressor: What is distressing me?

2 What am I willing to do about it?

3 How am I handling it now?

4 What am I going to do about it?

5 How have I put my plan into action?

6 What results can I see?

- History
- Environment
- Values/Beliefs
- Attitudes
- Self Esteem
- Social Support
- Control

Source: Adapted from Lester A. Lefton, *Psychology,* 5th ed., 485 (Figure 13.5). © Copyright 1994 by Allyn & Bacon. Reprinted by permission.

not change the boss. You can, however, ask the boss to clarify in writing the things that are expected of you.

Changing Your Responses. Changing your responses requires practice and emotional control. If your roommate is habitually messy and this causes you stress, you can choose among several responses. You can express your anger by yelling, you can pick up the mess and leave a nasty note, or you can defuse the situation with humor. The first response that comes to mind is not always the best response. Stop before reacting to gain the time you need to find an appropriate response. Ask yourself, "What is to be gained from my response?"

Many people change their responses to potentially stressful events through *cognitive coping strategies.* These strategies help them prepare for stressors through gradual exposure to increasingly higher stress levels.

Learning to Cope. Everyone copes with stress in different ways. For some people, drinking and taking drugs helps them to cope. Others choose to get help from counselors. Still others try to keep their minds off stress or to engage in positive activities such as exercise or relaxation techniques. *Stress inoculation* is one of the newer techniques for helping people prepare for stressful events. Through stress inoculation, people are given warnings, recommendations, and reassurances that may help them to cope with impending dangers or losses. Some health experts compare stress inoculation to a vaccine given to protect against a disease. Essentially, stress inoculation

- increases the predictability of stressful events
- fosters coping skills
- generates self-talking
- encourages confidence about successful outcomes
- builds a commitment to personal action and responsibility for an adaptive course of action

Regardless of how you cope with a given situation, your conscious effort to deal with this situation is an important step in stress management.

Managing Emotional Responses

Have you ever gotten all worked up about something you thought was happening only to find that your perceptions were totally wrong or that a communication problem had caused a misinterpretation of events? If you're like most of us, this has probably happened to you. We often get upset not by realities but by our faulty perceptions. For example, suppose you found out that everyone except you is invited to a party. You might easily begin to wonder why you were excluded. Does someone dislike you? Have you offended someone? Such thoughts are typical. However, the reality of the situation may have absolutely nothing to do with your being liked or disliked. Perhaps you were sent an invitation and it didn't get to you.

Stress management requires that you examine your self-talk and your emotional responses to interactions with others. With any emotional response to a distressor, you are responsible for the emotion and the behaviors elicited by the emotion. Learning to tell the difference between normal emotions and those based on irrational beliefs can help you either to stop the emotion or to express it in a healthy and appropriate way. Admitting your feelings and allowing them to be expressed through either communication or action is a stress-management technique that can help you get through many difficult situations.

Learning to Laugh and Cry. For some people, learning to express emotions freely is a difficult task. However, it is a task worth learning. Have you ever noticed that you feel better after a good laugh or cry? It wasn't your imagination. Laughter and crying stimulate the heart and temporarily rev up many body systems. Heart rate and blood pressure then decrease significantly, allowing the body to relax.

Taking Mental Action

Stress management calls for mental action in two areas. First, positive self-esteem, which can help you cope with stressful situations comes from learned habits. Successful stress management involves mentally developing and practicing self-esteem skills.

Second, because you can't always anticipate what the next distressor will be, you need to develop the mental skills necessary to manage your reactions to stresses after they have occurred. The ability to think about and react quickly to stress comes with time, practice, experience with a variety of stressful situations, and patience. Most of all, you must strive to become more aware of potential threats to your stress levels and act quickly to avoid or to deal with potential stressors. Rather than seeing stressors as adversaries, learn to view them as exercises in life.

Changing the Way You Think. Once you realize that some of your thoughts may be irrational or overreactive, making a conscious effort to reframe or change the way you've been thinking and focus on more positive ways of

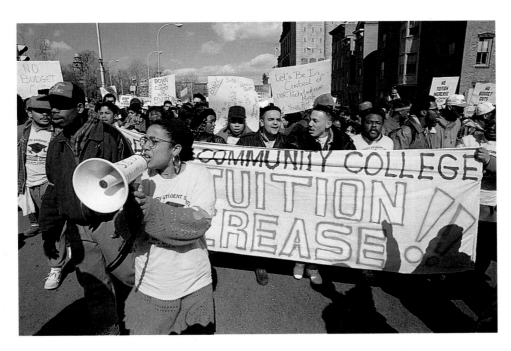

Evaluating stressors and finding a constructive way to react to them can help you cope with stressful situations and events that appear to be beyond your control.

thinking is a key element of stress management. Here are some specific actions you can take to develop these mental skills.

- *Worry constructively.* Don't waste time and energy worrying about things you can't change or things that may never happen.

- *Look at life as being fluid.* If you accept that change is a natural part of living and growing, the jolt of changes may hold much less stress for you.

- *Consider alternatives.* Remember that there is seldom only one appropriate action. Anticipating options will help you plan for change and adjust more rapidly.

- *Moderate expectations.* Aim high, but be realistic about your circumstances and motivation.

- *Weed out trivia.* Don't sweat the small stuff, and remember that most of it is small stuff.

- *Don't rush into action.* Think before you act.

Taking Physical Action

Adopting the attitudes necessary for effective stress management may seem to have little effect. However, developing successful emotional and mental coping skills is actually a satisfying accomplishment that can help you gain confidence in yourself. Learning to use physical activity to alleviate stress helps support and complement the emotional and mental strategies you employ in stress management.

Exercise. Exercise is a significant contributor to stress management. Exercise reduces stress by raising levels of endorphins, mood-elevating, pain-killing hormones, in the bloodstream. As a result, exercise often increases energy, reduces hostility, and improves mental alertness.

Most of us have experienced relief from distress at one time or another by engaging in some aggressive physical activity: chopping wood when we are angry is one example. Exercise performed as part of an immediate response to a distressor can help alleviate stress symptoms. However, a regular exercise program usually has more substantial stress management benefits than does exercise performed as an immediate reaction to a distressor. Engaging in 25 minutes of aerobic exercise three or four times a week is the most beneficial plan of action. But even simply walking up stairs, parking farther away from your destination or standing rather than sitting helps to conserve and replenish your adaptive energy stores. Plan walking breaks with friends. Stretch after prolonged periods of sitting at your desk studying. A short period of physical exercise may provide the stress break you really

need. For more information on the beneficial effects of exercise, see Chapter 10.

Relaxation. Like exercise, relaxation can help you to cope with stressful feelings, to preserve adaptation energy stores, and to dissipate the excess hormones associated with the GAS. Relaxation also helps you to refocus your energies and should be practiced daily until it becomes a habit. You may find that you even actually enjoy it. Some useful and easy relaxation techniques are demonstrated in the Skills for Behavior Change box.

Once you have learned some relaxation techniques, you can use them at any time. If you're facing a tough exam, for example, you may choose to relax before it or at intervals during it. You can also use relaxation techniques when you face stressful confrontations or assignments. When you begin to feel your body respond to distress, make time to relax, both to give yourself added strength and to help alleviate the negative physical effects of stress. As your body relaxes, your heart rate slows, your blood pressure and metabolic rate decrease, and many other body-calming effects occur, allowing you to channel energy appropriately.

Eating Right. Have you ever sat down with a glass of warm milk or a cup of hot chocolate to try to relax? Have you ever been told, "Eat—you'll feel better"? Is food really a de-stressor? Whether foods can calm us and nourish our psyches is a controversial question. Much of what has been published about hyperactivity and its relation to the consumption of candy and other sweets has been shown to be scientifically invalid. High-potency stress-tabs that are supposed to provide you with resistance against stress-related ailments are nothing more than gimmicks. But what is clear is that eating a balanced, healthful diet will help provide you with the stamina needed to get through problems and may stress-proof you in ways that are not fully understood. It is also known that undereating, overeating, and eating the wrong kinds of foods can create distress in the body. For more information about the benefits of sound nutrition in overall health and wellness, see Chapter 8.

Time Management

Time. Everybody needs more of it, especially students trying to balance the demands of classes, social life, earning money for school, family obligations, and time needed for relaxation. The following tips regarding time management should become a part of your stress management program:

- *Clean off your desk.* According to Jeffrey Mayer, author of *Winning the Fight Between You and Your Desk,* most of us spend many stressful minutes each day looking for things that are lost on our desks or in our homes.

Learning to Relax

LEARN TO BREATHE

Learning to become aware of and to control your breathing patterns can help you to relax. Deep breathing, controlled breathing, and other breathing exercises are often used to help reduce stress levels.

Example

1. Sit in a comfortable position with your hands folded over your abdomen just over your navel.

2. Keeping your eyes open, imagine a balloon lying beneath your hands.

3. Begin to inhale slowly through your nose, concentrating on the warm air entering your nose and slowly filling the imaginary balloon. When the balloon is full (this should take three to four seconds initially), slowly exhale to empty the balloon, feeling your chest and abdomen relaxing.

4. Repeat the entire process two or three times. When finished, sit quietly for a few minutes before rising. If you feel dizzy at any point, stop the procedure.

LEARN TO RELAX

Learning to relax certain muscle groups trains your muscles as well as the nerve centers that control muscles. Be cautious if you have any chronic injury or disability.

Example

Because your head, neck, and facial muscles may become very tense after you have been sitting and reading or working at a computer for a long time, relaxation of them can be very important.

ROTATION OF THE HEAD AND NECK

1. Close your eyes.

2. Roll your head slowly forward and back and then side to side. Repeat this motion.

3. When your head begins to feel heavy, stop, tilt your head forward, and rest.

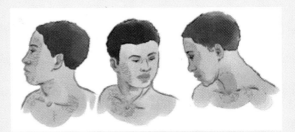

FACIAL RELAXATION

1. Clench your teeth.

2. Contract the facial muscles tightly.

3. Relax.

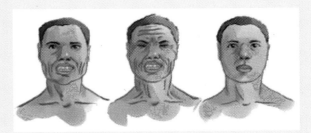

Source: Adapted from Daniel A. Girdano, George S. Everly, and Dorothy Dusek, *Controlling Stress and Tension,* 3rd ed., 219. © Copyright 1990 by Prentice-Hall, Inc. Reprinted by permission of Allyn & Bacon.

Go through the things on your desk, toss the unnecessary papers, and put papers for tasks that you must do in folders.

- *Never handle papers more than once.* When bills and other papers come in, take care of them immediately. Write out a check and hold it for mailing. Get rid of the envelopes. Read your mail and file it or toss it. If you haven't looked at something in over a year, toss it.

- *Prioritize your tasks.* Make a daily "to do" list and try to stick to it. Categorize the things you must do today, the things that you have to do but not immediately, and the things that it would be nice to do. Prioritize the Must Do Now and Have to Do Later items and put deadlines next to each. Only consider the Nice to Do items if you finish the others or if the Nice to Do list includes something fun for you. Give yourself a reward as you finish each task.

- *Avoid interruptions.* When you've got a project that requires your total concentration, schedule uninterrupted time. Unplug the phone or let your answering machine get it. Close your door and post a Do Not Disturb sign. Go to a quiet room in the library or student union where no one will find you. Guard your time and don't weaken.

- *Reward yourself for being efficient.* If you've planned to take a certain amount of time to finish a task and you finish early, take some time for yourself. Have a cup of coffee or hot chocolate. Go for a walk. Start reading something you've wanted to read but haven't had time for. Differentiate between rest breaks and work breaks. Work breaks simply mean that you switch tasks for awhile. Rest breaks get you away for yourself.

- *Reduce your awareness of time.* Rather than a slave to the clock try to ignore it. Get rid of your watch, and try to listen more to your body when deciding whether you need to eat, sleep, and so on. When you feel awake, do something productive. When you are too tired to work, take time out to sleep or to relax to try to energize yourself.

- *Remember that time is precious.* Many people learn to value their time only when they face a terminal illness. Try to value each day. Time spent not enjoying life is a tremendous waste of potential.

- *Become aware of your own time patterns.* For many of us, minutes and hours drift by without us even noticing them. Chart your daily schedule, hour by hour, for one week. Note the time that was wasted and the time spent in productive work or restorative pleasure. Assess how you could be more productive and make more time for yourself.

Making the Most of Support Groups

Support groups are an important part of stress management. Friends, family members, and co-workers can provide us with emotional and physical support. Although the ideal support group differs for each of us, you should have one or two close friends in whom you are able to confide and neighbors with whom you can trade favors. You should take the opportunity to participate in community activities at least once a week. A healthy committed relationship can also provide vital support.

> **Hypnosis:** A process that allows people to become unusually responsive to suggestion.
>
> **Meditation:** A relaxation technique that involves deep breathing and concentration.
>
> **Biofeedback:** A technique involving self-monitoring by machine of physical responses to stress.

If you do not have a close support group, you should know where to turn when the pressures of life seem overwhelming. Family members are often a steady base of support on which you can rely. But if friends or family are unavailable, most colleges and universities have counseling services available at no cost for short-term crises. Clergy members, instructors, and dorm supervisors may also be excellent resources. If university services are unavailable or if you are concerned about confidentiality, most communities offer low-cost counseling through mental health clinics.

Alternative Stress Management Techniques

The popularity of stress management as a media topic has increased the amount of advertising for various "stress fighters." We have been made aware of consumer products and services designed to fight stress: hypnosis, massage therapies, meditation, and biofeedback.

Hypnosis. Hypnosis is a process that requires a person to focus on one thought, object, or voice, thereby freeing the right hemisphere of the person's brain to become more active. The person is then unusually responsive to suggestions. Whether self-induced or induced by another person, hypnosis can reduce certain types of stress.

Massage. If you have ever had someone massage your stiff neck or aching feet, you know that massage is an excellent means of relaxation and thereby stress management. Massage therapists use techniques that vary from the more aggressive methods typical of Swedish massage to the more gentle methods associated with acupressure and Esalen massage. Before selecting a massage therapist, check his or her credentials carefully. He or she should have training from a reputable program that teaches scientific principles for anatomic manipulation.

Meditation. Another way to relax and to manage stress is through meditation. **Meditation** generally focuses on deep breathing, allowing tension to leave the body with each exhalation. There is no "right" way to meditate. Although there are several common forms of meditation, most involve sitting quietly for 15 to 20 minutes, focusing on a particular word or symbol, controlling breathing, and getting in touch with your inner self.

Biofeedback. Biofeedback involves self-monitoring by machine of physical responses to stress and attempts to subsequently control these responses. Perspiration, heart rate, respiration, blood pressure, surface body temperature, muscle tension, and other stress responses are monitored. Then, by trial and error, the person using biofeedback techniques learns to lower his or her stress responses through conscious effort. Eventually, the person develops the ability to lower his or her stress responses at will without using the machines.

Managing Stress Behaviors

Stress is not something that you can run from or wish into nonexistence. To control stress, you must meet it head on and use as many resources as you can to insure that your coping skills are fine-tuned and ready to help you. In planning your personal strategy for stress success, you should consider the following:

Making Decisions for You

Following a few simple guidelines may help you not only to enjoy more guilt-free time but also to become more productive during work hours.

- *Plan life, not time.* Determining what you want from life rather than what you can get done may help change the way you use time. Evaluate all your activities, even the most trivial, to determine whether they add to your life. If they don't, get rid of them.

- *Decelerate.* Rushing is part of the American work ethic and mind set that says that "busy is better." It can be addictive. When rushed, ask yourself if you really need to be. What's the worst that could happen if you slow down? Tell yourself at least once a day that failure seldom results from doing a job slowly or too well. Failures happen when rushing causes a lack of attention to detail.

- *Learn to delegate and share.* The need to feel in control is powerful. If you are unusually busy, leave details to someone else. Don't be afraid to ask others to help or to share the work load and responsibilities.

- *Learn to say no.* Give priority to what is most critical to your life, your job, or your current situation. Decide what things you can do, what things you must do, and what things you want to do, and delegate the rest to someone else either permanently or until you complete some of your priority tasks. Before you take on a new responsibility, finish or drop an old one.

- *Schedule time alone.* Find time each day for quiet thinking, reading, exercising, or other enjoyable activities.

Checklist for Change: Assessing Your Life Stressors

✓ Have you assessed the major stressors in your life? Are they people, events, or specific activities?

✓ Have you thought about what you may be doing to worsen your stress levels? Do you often worry about things that never happen? Are you often anxious about nothing?

✓ Have you thought about what you could change to reduce your stress levels?

✓ Do you have a network of friends and family members who can help you reduce your stress levels? Do you know where you could go to get professional advice about how to start reducing them?

✓ Have you thought about what changes you'd like to work on first? Have you developed a plan of action? When do you want to start?

Checklist for Change: Assessing Community Stressors

✓ Have you considered what in your environment may cause stress for you and the people around you?

✓ Could these stressors be changed? How could they be changed? Why would changing them make a difference?

✓ What on your campus or in your living situations causes undue stress for you or your friends? What could you do to change these stressors?

✓ What advice might you give to your school administrators to help them reduce unnecessary stress among students?

Critical Thinking

After just scraping by to pay your tuition bill in January, your college announces a large tuition hike for next year. You already work a part-time job, and seem to spend all your "free time" studying. The stress you've got now is beginning to get to you, and you realize that you will have to work another 5–10 hours per week just to pay your bills next year. And tuition is likely to go up your senior year as well. How can you manage your time and finances so that you can complete your degree?

Use the DECIDE model described in Chapter 1 to decide what you should do. Begin with your own current situation: How can you make better use of your time? Could you prioritize your week in a way that you could find the extra time to work? Finally, even if you make enough money, you need to deal with the increased stress. What will you do to keep the stress in check?

Summary

- Stress is an inevitable part of our lives. Eustress refers to stress associated with positive events, distress to negative events. Psychoneuroimmunology is the science that attempts to analyze the relationship between the mind's reaction to stress and the function of the immune system. While some evidence links disease susceptibility to stress it is not conclusive.

- The alarm, resistance, and exhaustion phases of the general adaptation syndrome involve physiological responses to both real and imagined stressors.

- Multiple factors contribute to stress and to the stress response. Psychosocial factors include change, hassles, pressure, inconsistent goals and behaviors, conflict, overload, and burnout. Other factors are environmental stressors, and self-imposed stress.

- College can be an especially stressful time. Recognition of the signs of stress is the first step in helping yourself toward better health.

- Managing stress begins with learning simple coping mechanisms: assessing your stressors, changing your responses, and learning to cope. Finding out what works best for you—probably some combination of managing emotional responses, taking mental or physical action, learning time management, or using alternative stress management techniques—will help you better cope with stress in the long run.

Discussion Questions

1. Compare and contrast distress and eustress. Are both types of stress potentially harmful?

2. Describe the alarm, resistance, and exhaustion phases of the general adaptation syndrome. During which of these phases do your perceptions and feelings about a situation often turn out to be wrong? Discuss the physiological responses that take place if you find you were wrong.

3. What are the major factors that seem to influence the nature and extent of a person's stress susceptibility?

Explain how social support, self-esteem, and personality may make you more or less susceptible to stress.

4. Why are college students often susceptible to excessive stress? What services are available on your campus to help you deal with excessive stress?

5. What can college students do to inoculate themselves against negative stress effects? What actions can you take to manage your stressors? How can you help others to manage their stressors more effectively?

Application Exercise

Reread the What Do You Think? scenarios at the beginning of the chapter and answer the following questions:

1. What could Mary and Erica have done to help inoculate themselves against or prevent their negative reactions to the stressful events in their lives? What services on your campus could they have used to help them through their troubles?

2. Why do some people have little social support? Why is social support so important to reducing stress reactions? What could Mary and Erica do to improve their interactions with others so that, in times of need, they could call on their friends for support?

3. What direct and indirect health effects of stress may these two young women experience? What symptoms of stress should particularly concern them?

4. Do you think that Mary and Erica and other college students like them are just suddenly stressed by situations like this? Or do you think that something has been leading them to these reactions for many years? Explain your answer.

Further Reading

Daniel A. Girdano, George S. Everly, and Dorothy Dusek, *Controlling Stress and Tension: A Holistic Approach* (Englewood Cliffs, NJ: Prentice Hall, 1995).

A comprehensive explanation of stress theories, methods for managing stress, and stress reduction. Includes several self-assessment guides as well as relaxation techniques and other stress interventions.

Phillip L. Rice, *Stress and Health* (Monterey, CA: Brooks/Cole, 1995).

An overview of current perspectives on stress and the influence of personal control and behavior on health. Discusses stress management as a factor in controlling pain, anxiety, and depression. An excellent resource for health professionals.

Hans Selye, *Stress Without Distress* (New York: Lippincott, 1974).

A classic work on the subject of stress. Selye was one of the first to recognize stress as a significant factor in modern life. He coined the terms *eustress* and *distress.* This book has been largely responsible for the focus placed on the subject of stress since the late 1970s.

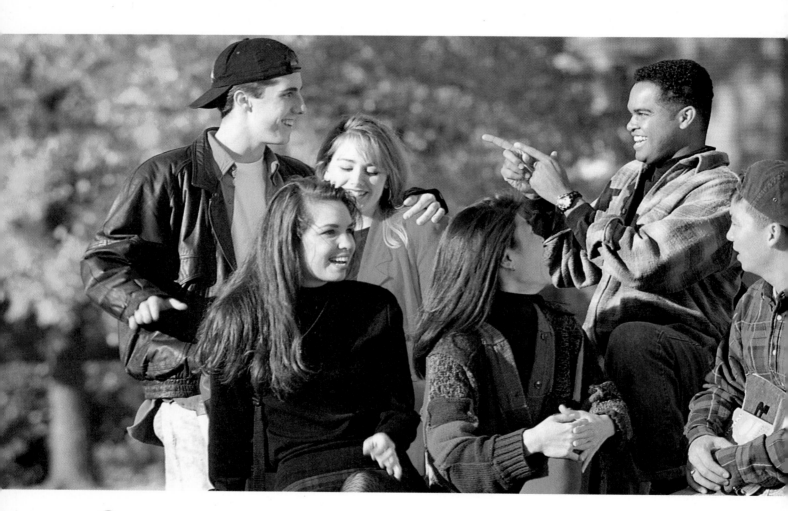

4

CHAPTER OBJECTIVES

◆ Discuss the impact that good communication skills can have on your health, including improved self-esteem, reduced stress, and increased health knowledge.

◆ Discuss the process of communication, including barriers that inhibit successful communication, and how self-disclosure enhances our lives.

◆ Discuss the importance of effective listening and speaking skills in verbal and nonverbal communication and the ways in which you can improve your own skills in these areas.

◆ Explain ways in which you can improve your communication skills through the use of "I" messages, assertive communication, establishing proper climates, and resolving conflicts.

◆ Compare and contrast the communication styles of men and women and discuss actions that you might take to help reduce potential problems.

Communicating Effectively

A Key to Interpersonal Health

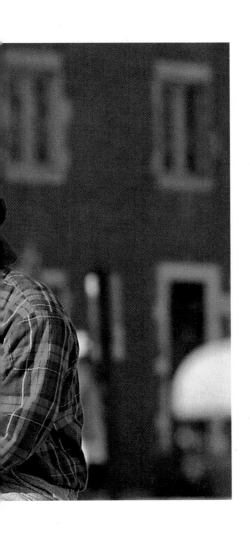

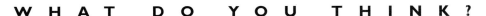

WHAT DO YOU THINK?

Marty has just gone to the doctor because he is has been passing bloody urine and experiencing a persistent pain in his groin. When the doctor comes into the examining room, he immediately begins reading Marty's chart and does not look at or speak to Marty directly. The doctor asks Marty some terse questions about his sexual history, jots down a few notes, and then begins to speak to the nurse who has accompanied him, telling her that Marty needs two different types of tests. Because he is using very technical terminology, Marty tries to ask a question about the procedures. The doctor responds in a condescending manner and abruptly tells Marty that, in his opinion, the tests are necessary and must be done immediately. The doctor then leaves the room and tells Marty to come back one week after the test results are in. Marty leaves the doctor's office feeling frustrated and angry because he feels that he was brushed off and that he still doesn't know what is wrong with him.

- Have you ever felt frustrated when trying to get information from medical personnel? What might Marty have done to improve the level of communication with his physician? If Marty's efforts had failed, what other options would he have had?

York-chi and Margaret have been roommates in a college dorm for just over one month. York-chi is increasingly finding that Margaret's annoying habits (smacking her lips, eating food with her mouth open, leaving clothes and clutter all over, and talking constantly in a loud, piercing voice) are really starting to bother her. York-chi has tried to study in the library to avoid her room but is beginning to resent having to go elsewhere to get away from her roommate. When York-chi does finally come home, Margaret pounces on her, asking a million questions, and, in general, driving York-chi crazy. Recently, York-chi told Margaret that she is a bit bothered by some of her actions, but Margaret apparently didn't get what York-chi meant. Things have gotten so bad that all York-chi has to do is to walk in the door and she immediately gets a pounding headache and feels sick to her stomach. She has tried to find another roommate and to move out, but housing officials say that there is a six-month waiting list.

- Have you ever found it difficult to confront a friend or acquaintance in this kind of situation? Is a person ever justified in hurting someone's feelings by telling her that her habits and general demeanor are offensive? If so, what do you think might be the best way to proceed? What options does York-chi have? If her actions don't work, what could she try next? How could she communicate her feelings, not hurt Margaret's feelings, and yet save herself from getting sick?

From the moment you were born, you have communicated. You communicated that you were hungry, that you needed changing, that you wanted to be held. As an infant, you used a host of subtle and not-so-subtle expressions, crying spells, gurgling sounds, and physical actions to communicate. Somehow, your parents figured out what your expressions and sounds meant and responded to your needs—with amazing accuracy and speed. As you've grown up, you've no doubt realized how important communication is to your daily life.

But why, you may be asking yourself, is communication a key topic in a health textbook? Good communication skills contribute significantly to your mental, emotional, spiritual, social, and physical dimensions of health. We spend up to three-quarters of our day communicating with others. The more we can express and understand each other's needs, the less stress we experience. Communication allows us to be included in society and to be accepted by others, increasing our self-esteem. In addition, every day we hear about new health news from various medical sources; such health communication may lead to positive behavioral changes.

The ability to communicate effectively does not just happen. Good communication requires that you learn certain basic skills. We think that communication is so important to your health that we have devoted an entire chapter to helping you find ways to improve your communication skills. Once you learn the skills, have a real interest in communicating effectively, and are willing to observe, learn from your mistakes, and keep on trying to do a better job, you will be on your way to a healthy communication style.

COMMUNICATING FOR HEALTH

In our daily interactions, good communication serves to improve our self-esteem, reduce our level of stress, and help us learn about health.

Improved Self-Esteem

We hold people who communicate well in high regard. People who are both effective and appropriate in their so-cial interactions gain approval from others. They present themselves in a manner that makes them desirable friends, lovers, or acquaintances. They probably have strong self-esteem. Those who lack communication skills, who can't make their feelings known, often suffer from self-esteem problems. Lack of self-esteem may lead to other health problems as well: Low-esteem people may blame themselves rather than seek medical attention for curable problems. People with low self-esteem don't take care of themselves as well, either.

Communication also improves our self-esteem by helping us define who we are to ourselves and others. Because self-concepts are really social concepts, they are theories of what we are like as individuals. We test these theories in interactions with others. In addition, by disclosing information about ourselves to others, we obtain feedback about what we have disclosed. If others respond to us, laugh at our attempts at humor, seek us out in social settings and generally seem to like us, our self-esteem is strengthened. The opposite is true if people seem to avoid us in spite of our best efforts to make friends. Thus, our self-esteem is closely linked to our ability to communicate.[1]

How we communicate is as important to our health as the fact that we communicate at all. For example, a pessimistic explanatory style (a habitual manner used to explain negative life events) has been linked to physical illness; the pessimistic explanatory style actually predicted poor health. While we do not know why the pessimistic style is linked with poor health, one plausible explanation may be that such people neglect health care. For example, pessimistic college students who contract colds or the flu may be less likely than their optimistic peers to take steps to ease their recovery, such as sleeping more and drinking more liquids.[2]

Reduced Stress

Difficulty in communication is a common complaint in relationships between parents and children, teachers and students, employees and employers, and partners in intimate relationships. If you listed the stressful conflicts you had during the past week, probably half would involve problems in communication.

Stress is reduced by an ability to get along better with friends, family, and co-workers. You can use communication skills to express your own needs better and to get what you want as well as to become a more effective listener and to give others what they want. Stress can also be reduced if you can use effective communication to resolve conflicts.

In addition, your ability to work out problems through communication helps you to cope better, thus reducing stress. For example, a college student upset by her roommate's inconsiderate behavior might speak to the roommate, explaining how this behavior is causing difficulty, and suggest alternative arrangements to suit both students. Such active coping skills have often been shown to reduce both the perceived and actual physiological components of stress.

Increased Health Knowledge

One of the major features of the *Healthy People 2000* national health plan (see Chapter 1) is health promotion, or health education. Many of *Healthy People 2000*'s goals are centered on the ability of the health agencies to get their messages out to the public. Thus, we regularly see ads trying to get us to stop smoking (or never to start), to get our blood pressure checked, and the like. Such mass media advertising campaigns are based on effective communication.

Take a look back at the Health Belief Model in Chapter 1, which was designed to explain how and why we take preventive health actions. As you may recall, the Health Belief Model consisted of three parts: your perception of a health problem, your perceived susceptibility to the health problem, and cues to action. In all three parts, communication plays a vital role. You may note a mole on your arm that bleeds when brushed up against the wall. But you would not suspect skin cancer if the American Cancer Society hadn't taken so much effort to get such information into the mass media (the cue for action). Knowing that it may be skin cancer may motivate you to see a doctor.

𝒲HAT DO YOU THINK?

Think for a moment about the people you hold in high esteem. Are they effective communicators? What makes them effective? What steps can you take to be more like them?

𝒲HAT IS COMMUNICATION?

You may think of communication only in terms of conversations with friends. But communication goes far beyond that. **Communication** is the transmission of information and meaning from one individual to another. The central concept here is meaning. Communication is only successful when both parties understand not only the information communicated but also the meaning of that information.

The Communication Process

When we speak of communication, we speak about a dynamic, ongoing process. Whether verbal or nonverbal, the communication process is usually described between two people: a sender and a receiver. In theory, the process has five parts: the sender has an idea, the sender encodes the message, the channel carries the message, the receiver decodes the message, and the receiver sends feedback. Let's look at an example: You (the sender) want to thank your roommate for helping you study for a midterm exam (idea). You decide how you want to send the message (encode the message), and write a note pinned to some flowers (channel). Your roommate (the receiver) decodes the message (that you appreciate her help); later she says, "I enjoyed working with you, too" (feedback).

For simple, day-to-day communication, you don't even think of the process. The simple "Hello! How are you?" would take a paragraph to describe here but takes only seconds in your daily interactions. But for more complex interactions, you do want to be aware of the process. If your communication idea, for instance, is to meet a girl in your health class, you need to think about the best way to encode your message. You could ask a mutual friend to introduce you, you could complement her (on appearance or something said in class), or you could sit next to her and ask a question about a homework assignment. How well your message progresses depends, of course, on her feedback.

Barriers to Communication

If only communication were so simple! In fact, all kinds of things can get in the way of effective communication. Barriers to communication take many forms.

Differences in Backgrounds. Age, education, social status, gender, culture, political beliefs, and many other variables can lead to differences between communicators. Your closest friends from high school, with whom you grew up, shared many similar experiences. Shared experiences contribute to shared meaning and understanding. But at college, you may suddenly find yourself among people having few shared experiences. Remember that the goal of good communication is not necessarily to have

Communication: The transmission of information and meaning from one individual to another.

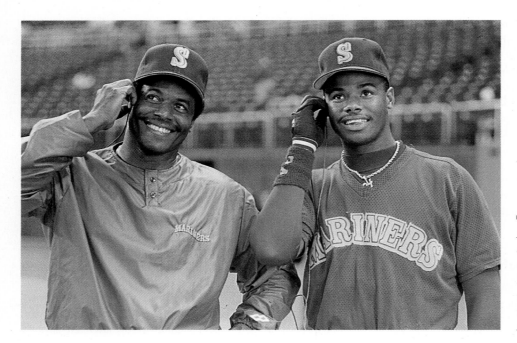

A family's ability to communicate effectively—to express and understand each other's needs—leads to the development of close relationships between family members that enhance individual self-esteem and well-being.

everyone agree with you; rather, it is to have others understand you. To find out more about how to communicate with those who are physically challenged, see the Multicultural Perspectives box.

Alcohol and Drugs.   Perhaps nothing stands in the way of effective communication more than do alcohol and drugs. With an inhibited ability to encode, you may not be understood correctly. With an inhibited ability to decode, you may interpret the message to mean anything you want. Is it any wonder that 90 percent of campus rapes take place under the influence of alcohol? Avoiding date rape depends on a woman's ability to be clear in her own mind about what she wants and then to make herself clearly understood. It also depends on a man's ability to listen. In most college campus sexual encounters that lead to date rape complaints, alcohol and drugs have interfered with thinking and communicating.

Think again about the communication process: The woman may say, "I don't think we're ready to have sex yet," meaning that the relationship is not strong enough yet. But the noise in his head created by alcohol may lead the man to hear, "Get me ready to make love." The alcohol factor affects whether or not consent has been given, whether a condom will be used, and even the ability to use a condom effectively. The Health Headlines box describes a real date rape case at Georgetown University. It is an excellent example of how miscommunication can lead to suffering for all involved.

Barriers between Patients and Medical Practitioners

As with all communication, communication between a patient and a medical practitioner is complex. When all goes well, the patient and practitioner are able to establish a good rapport, which facilitates mutual understanding. Unfortunately, several barriers often interfere with good communication.[3]

Language Specialization.   The practitioner's use of medical jargon may block communication. Terms such as *congenital, umbilicus,* and *malignant* may have little meaning to you if you don't have much experience with doctors. Hearing that a test result is negative (which is usually a positive thing) or that alcohol use during pregnancy is "contraindicative" may leave you confused as to what is actually meant.

Specialized language is common to all professions, sports—even groups of friends. In the medical field, it's necessary because medical personnel must communicate among themselves with precise terminology. When it comes to your health, there just can't be any mistakes made. Some studies have shown that some doctors may use medical jargon to impress you, gain authority, or simply to keep you quiet. However, most don't. You need to ask for clarity on any and all matters about your health.

Sociocultural Differences.   Communication may also be hindered by sociocultural differences, including differences in age, social class, ethnicity, and gender. Doctors tend to be held in high esteem because of their high degree of education, their socioeconomic status, and sometimes their age, and patients may therefore be intimidated. One study found that patients are less willing to open up to a physician of the opposite sex. Some ethnic groups may hold concepts of illness that differ dramatically from those of the medical profession; for example, Native Americans tend to view substance abuse problems as spiritual rather than medical.

Communicating with People Who Have Disabilities

Many obstacles can interfere with the communication process. People who are physically challenged have even more barriers to overcome. Here are some helpful hints.

1. Speak directly rather than through a companion or sign language interpreter who may be present.

2. Offer to shake hands when introduced. People with limited hand use or an artificial limb can usually shake hands and offering the left hand is an acceptable greeting.

3. Always identify yourself and others who may be with you when meeting someone with a visual impairment. When conversing in a group, remember to identify the person to whom you are speaking.

4. If you offer assistance, wait until the offer is accepted. Then listen or ask for instructions.

5. Treat adults as adults. Address people who have disabilities by their first names only when extending that same familiarity to all others. Never patronize people in wheelchairs by patting them on the head or shoulder.

6. Do not lean against or hang on someone's wheelchair. Bear in mind that disabled people treat their chairs as extensions of their bodies.

7. Listen attentively when talking with people who have difficulty speaking and wait for them to finish. If necessary, ask short questions that require short answers or a nod or shake of the head. Never pretend to understand if you are having difficulty doing so. Instead repeat what you have understood and allow the person to respond.

8. Place yourself at eye level when speaking with someone in a wheelchair or on crutches.

9. Tap a hearing-impaired person on the shoulder or wave your hand to get his or her attention. Look directly at the person and speak clearly, slowly, and expressively to establish if the person can read your lips. If so, try to face the light source and keep hands, cigarettes, and food away from your mouth when speaking.

10. Relax. Don't be embarrassed if you happen to use common expressions such as "See you later" or "Did you hear about this?" that seem to relate to a person's disability.

Source: From Karen Meyer, for National Center for Access Unlimited at Adaptive Environments Center, Boston, MA. Reprinted by permission.

To overcome such barriers, you need to remember that you are the best expert on your body and your health. If your doctor tells you something that contradicts what you believe, ask questions until both you and the doctor are in agreement.

Patient Anxiety. As patients, we also contribute our share to poor communication. Illnesses often stir up emotions that can impair our ability to communicate and understand what a practitioner is saying. When you are angry (from long waits) or feeling shame or helplessness (perhaps from contracting an STD), you may find it difficult to make yourself understood.

In addition, embarrassment about a situation may keep you from disclosing information. Dr. Robert E. McAffree, president of the American Medical Association, tells a story about a woman patient he saw in his office three times before he caught on that the problem was domestic violence: She came in once for a mammogram, complaining of pains in her breast. The mammogram showed no sign of cancer, so he suggested that she come again in six months. Three months later she was back, but another mammogram was negative. Again he scheduled a visit for six months later, and again she showed up much

sooner, this time with a couple of bruises. He asked her whether she bruised often. Only on certain occasions, she said. More questions led finally to a long outpouring of emotional and physical pain. The woman's husband, a prominent and respected local business leader, had been beating her for 10 years.[4]

Patient Misinterpretation. Communication is also hindered by patient misinterpretation or inability to remember instructions. Studies have shown that patients forget 56 percent of the instructions they are given and 48 percent of treatment information shortly after leaving the doctor. Another study showed that patients misinterpret up to 64 percent of the medical instructions they receive.

Overcoming Medical Barriers to Communication

Given the difficult circumstances we find ourselves in when seeking medical attention, it's doubtful that all barriers can be overcome. However, both patient and practitioner can help to remove barriers. More medical schools are now emphasizing the human side of medicine early in doctors' training. Programs like those at Harvard Univer-

Alcohol and Sex: Formula for Miscommunication

Alcohol and drugs disrupt the communication process by impairing the communicator's ability to be clear and the listener's ability to clearly understand what is meant. When you add sex to the equation, the result may be date rape. In most date rape cases, alcohol and trust built up between acquaintances have led to sexual encounters that left one student feeling violated and the other feeling unfairly accused.

Teresa Awalt, of the Campus Violence Prevention Center, says that "rape [complaints] would be dramatically decreased" if alcohol were removed from the sexual equation. In fact, about 90 percent of all campus rapes are alcohol-related. Here's the real-life story of one campus date rape case that took place in 1994. Note how alcohol impaired judgment at various points during the ordeal led each participant to perceive events differently.

Nancy DeCamara and Ajay Chitkara had been saying hi to each other for nearly four years when they went to a black-tie dance together at the end of their senior year at Georgetown University in June 1994. Both agree that they had not expected the Diplomatic Ball to be a "real date." But during the long evening, their plans changed. They had met at 8:30 P.M. and gone to two parties, the dance, and a bar before returning to Ajay's apartment at about 4:00 A.M. DeCamara's house key had been lost after she gave it to him to keep, so she agreed to go back to his apartment. She says, "I decided I wouldn't mind kissing him."

They kissed, he unzipped her dress, and they climbed into his upper bunk. She told the university police, "I know it was dumb. . . . I thought I could just lay in his bed and go to sleep and he would too." She said in an interview that she had frequently shared a bed with her previous boyfriend without having sex.

Chitkara asked whether he should get a condom. DeCamara said that they didn't know each other well enough to have sex—that he didn't even know her favorite color, for instance. This is where their stories diverge.

DeCamara said she told Chitkara, "I've never had sex before, so I don't want to have it on a whim." Then she said that, "[A]ll of a sudden, he was on top of me . . . I kept trying to push him off with my hands and squirming around, and I kept saying I didn't want to have sex."

Chitkara disclosed in an affidavit, "At no time during our sexual activity did I use any kind of physical force against Nancy. Nor did I threaten Nancy verbally."

DeCamara did not scream or wake up Chitkara's roommates, who were sleeping next door. She says, "I was in a huge daze. I was shocked at what was going on. I didn't know what to do."

DeCamara says she was raped. Chitkara says that they had consensual intercourse and that DeCamara then changed her mind.

Laura Minor, Georgetown director of student conduct, investigated the allegations, interviewing about a dozen witnesses. She said she would not comment directly on the case but says that, "[T]he facts are always difficult [in rape allegations]. I haven't had one yet where you could say it's real clear what happened."

Think about how alcohol may have impaired judgment in this case. How may a clear-headed man and woman have reacted differently? Is it possible that both sides of the story are true to some degree?

Source: Adapted from Brooke A. Masters, "In Georgetown Rape Case, One Episode, Two Stories," *Washington Post,* 5 June 1994, B1, B2. © 1994 The Washington Post. Reprinted with permission.

---

sity or the University of Missouri at Kansas City teach students to focus on the patient who has the disease rather than on the disease itself.

You as a patient can also help to overcome these barriers. If your doctor uses medical terminology, politely ask the doctor to reexplain in more common language. Or use humor to work through the experience.

In addition, you need to put yourself in your doctor's shoes. If you suspect you have an STD, you will probably place great importance on your visit to the doctor. But the doctor may see dozens of young people like yourself and may not spend as much time as you think is needed on your visit. But remember that the doctor may be pressured by other people's medical emergencies.

You may also show the doctor that you care about your health by taking notes on medical instructions or asking questions. Doctors often note those patients who seem to care about their medical care. The next time you go in, your doctor may remember you as being someone who listened and cared about what was said. That, in turn, may result in your receiving more attention.

WHAT DO YOU THINK?

Have you ever had a bad experience with a doctor or other medical practitioner? Thinking back on the experience, could it have been due to any of the above factors? Which ones? What could you change so that the same situation won't happen again?

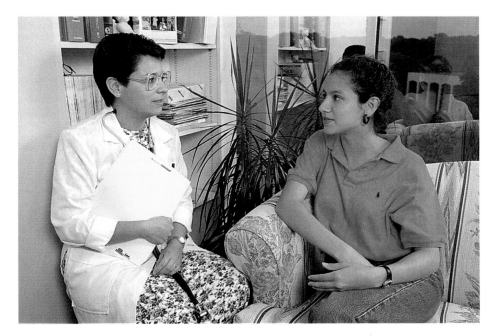

Communicating for health rests on your ability to disclose yourself to others, especially medical practitioners, without fear or embarrassment.

Self-Disclosure: Letting Others See the Real You

Self-disclosure is the sharing of personal information with others. If you are willing to share personal information with others, they will likely share personal information with you. In other words, if you want to learn more about Kathy, you have to be willing to share parts of your personal self with her. Self-disclosure is not storytelling or sharing secrets; rather, it is revealing how you are reacting to the present situation and giving any information about the past that is relevant to the other person's understanding of your current reactions.[5]

Self-disclosure can be a double-edged sword, for there is risk in divulging personal insights and feelings. If you sense that sharing feelings and personal thoughts will result in a closer relationship, you will likely take such a risk. But if you believe that the disclosure may result in rejection or alienation, you may not open up so easily. If you have had confidential chats violated before (if the person told others), then you may be hesitant to disclose yourself.[6]

However, the risk in not disclosing yourself to others is that you will lack close relationships. Psychologist Carl Rogers stressed the importance of understanding yourself and others through self-disclosure. Rogers believed that weak relationships were characterized by inhibited self-disclosure.[7]

The inability to disclose yourself to others may also affect your health. Researcher Sidney Jourard believed that people can attain health only insofar as they gain the courage to be themselves with others, that is, to self-disclose. Jourard believed that self-disclosure helped people find meaning and direction in their lives. Social health comes from self-disclosing with others. Without self-disclosure, we become estranged from other human beings.

Self-disclosure also affects our dealings within health-care settings. For example, patients may fear that self-disclosure with medical personnel could disrupt relationships they have already established. For example, a patient may have a complaint about some aspect of his or her health service but may believe that that complaint could disrupt an otherwise positive relationship with the health-care provider; it could even have a negative impact on the care received. In other words, because patients feel vulnerable, they tend to be careful about what they say to health-care professionals.[8]

*W*HAT DO YOU THINK?

What role do "white lies" play in self-disclosure? When asked a direct question, must you answer honestly?

Improving Self-Disclosure Skills

If self-disclosure is a key element in creating healthy communication, but our fears often make it a barrier to that

Self-disclosure: The process of revealing one's inner thoughts, feelings, and beliefs to another person.

process, what can we do? The following suggestions may help you overcome your fears of self-disclosure:[9]

- *Get to know yourself.* Remember that your self includes your feelings, beliefs, thoughts, and concerns. The more you know about yourself, the more likely it is that you will be able to communicate with others about yourself.

- *Become more accepting of yourself.* No one is perfect or has to be. Even the people you look up to have their flaws. Only by accepting your imperfections can you expect others to accept them, too.

- *Choose a safe context for self-disclosure.* Context refers to the setting in which the self-disclosure occurs. Choose a setting in which you feel safe to let yourself be known. When and where you disclose and to whom may greatly influence the response to your disclosure. For example, you may want to talk with your teacher about your grade problems. But you will likely wait until you can talk in a private setting, during office hours, so that your problem will remain private.

Self-Disclosure about Sex.   In a culture that puts many taboos on discussions of sex in everyday conversation, it's no wonder we find it hard to self-disclose about our sexual feelings to those whom we are intimate. However, with the soaring numbers of sexually transmitted diseases and the ever-looming threat of AIDS, there has never been a more important time to self-disclose about your sexual feelings and past.

You need to find a way to communicate about birth control, use of condoms, the possibility of pregnancy and STDs—as well as sexual satisfaction—before you start having sex. These issues don't just go away once you've started having sex. In fact, if communication is poor at the start of the sexual relationship, it probably won't improve over time. Leaving such important issues to chance will prove stressful; and that stress may harm your relationship as well as your health. The long-lasting effects of an unwanted pregnancy or the HIV virus underscore the need to communicate about sex before you start.

$\mathcal{L}$ISTENING SKILLS

How many times have you been caught not paying attention to what someone close to you is saying? After several nods and "uh-huhs," your friend finally asks you a question and you haven't the faintest idea of what he or she has just been talking about. Or how many times have you sat staring at your instructor in class, nodding occasionally and pretending that you are really into the lecture, only to be thinking about what you are going to have for dinner or what clothes you have to pack for the weekend ski trip?

When the instructor calls on you, you sit blankly and ask the instructor to repeat the question. Sound familiar? If you are like most college students, you listen to less than half of the lecture material in a class and then forget half of that within a short time. The result: students listen with a 25 percent level of listening effectiveness. If much of a course's material comes from lectures, poor listening habits can cost you your grades.[10] If you continue to be a poor listener in your interpersonal relationships, these habits may also cost you your friends.

Most of us listen more than we talk in any given situation. Because listening is such a vital part of our interpersonal communication, it is important that we develop the types of listening skills that will enhance our relationships, improve our grasp of information, and allow us to interpret what others say more effectively.

Barriers to Effective Listening

We listen best when (1) we believe that the message is somehow important to us, (2) we are interested in what is being said and it is not boring to us, and (3) we are in the mood to listen. Listening to a technical lecture on the physiology of the brain right after we have just had a major fight that ended a relationship probably would not be too productive. There are many things in our daily lives that may make listening difficult. These factors serve as barriers to the communication process and are listed in Table 4.1. Sometimes these listening barriers can become habits. Unless we consciously examine what we are doing in given situations and act to remove these habits from our behaviors, effective listening will continue to be difficult. The Rate Yourself box gives a self-assessment of your current listening skills.

$\mathcal{W}$HAT DO YOU THINK?

Are you a good listener? Do you listen more than you talk or vice versa? When do you find it difficult to listen? Is there anyone to whom you find it particularly difficult to listen? Why?

Improving Your Listening Skills

There are many things that you can do to improve your listening techniques. Among the most tried and true methods for becoming a better listener are the following:

- *Stop talking.* Accept the role of listener by concentrating on the speaker's words, not on what you want to say. Wait for logical breaks in the conversation before you try to interject your thoughts.

- *Work hard at listening.* Become actively involved and expect to learn something. Try different techniques

How Well Do You Listen?

Test your listening skills by rating yourself on a scale from 1 (lowest rating) to 5 (highest rating) in response to each of the following statements. To determine your listening score, add up the total number of points from your ratings. A score of 40 to 50 indicates that you are a terrific listener; a score of 30 to 39 indicates that you are a pretty good listener; a score of 20 to 29 indicates that you are not listening well to others; and a score of 19 or under means that you are a very poor listener. Compare your score with two friends.

1. I always attempt to give every person I speak to equal time to talk.

2. I really enjoy hearing what other people have to say.

3. I never have difficulty waiting until someone finishes talking so that I can have my say.

4. I listen even when I do not particularly like the person talking.

5. I listen even when I do not agree with what the person who is talking is saying.

6. I put away what I am doing while someone is talking.

7. I always look directly at the person who is talking and give that person my full attention.

8. I encourage other people to talk by my nonverbal messages, such as gestures, facial expressions, and posture.

9. I ask for clarification of words and ideas I do not understand.

10. I respect every person's right to his or her opinions, even if I disagree with them.

_____

Source: From the book *Communicate Like a Pro,* 77, by Nido Qubein, © 1983. Reprinted by permission of Prentice-Hall, a Division of Simon & Schuster, Inc.

such as nodding, paraphrasing, and other techniques to show the speaker that you are interested.

- *Maintain an open mind.* Know your biases and try to correct for them. Be tolerant of less-abled and different-looking speakers. When someone's communication skills really bother you, try looking for positive aspects. Focus on what you could get out of her or his conversation.

- *Provide verbal and nonverbal feedback.* Encourage the speaker with comments such as, "Yes," "I see," "Okay," and "Uh-huh." Ask polite questions without being overly sappy or sweet. Look alert.

- *Paraphrase the speaker's ideas.* Paraphrasing is a powerful listening technique. In paraphrasing, listeners restate in their own words what they understood the speaker to have said. For example, if your roommate hangs up the phone and says, "My old man really got on me about not getting a job. He just doesn't understand that I can't play football, take a full load of classes, and work at the same time. He thinks I'm lazy because I'm not putting in 80 hours per week like he used to do." You might paraphrase it by saying, "It sounds like you're frustrated by trying to live up to his expectations." This shows that you are listening and interested.

- *Take selective notes.* If you are hearing instructions or important data (e.g., at the doctor's office), record the major points; then verify your notes with the speaker. Ask for clarification of points that seem confusing.

Conversation: The Bridge to Sound Relationships

If you're like most people, your relationships begin rather informally and grow stronger over time as you and another person share more and more of your intimate thoughts, feelings, dreams, and fears. We usually form an initial impression of someone based on appearance, clothing, the apparent impressions of significant others who know the person, and other exterior factors. From these first impressions, we move to a form of scripted conversation learned through past experiences and social rules passed on from others. Typical lines of these scripted

TABLE 4.1 ■ Barriers to Listening

Mental Barriers	Physical and Other Barriers
Inattention	Hearing impairment
Prejudgment	Noisy surroundings
Frame of reference	Speaker's appearance
Closed-mindedness	Speaker's mannerisms
Faking listening	Lag time

Relationships are strengthened over time as partners develop listening skills and the ability to share their intimate thoughts and feelings.

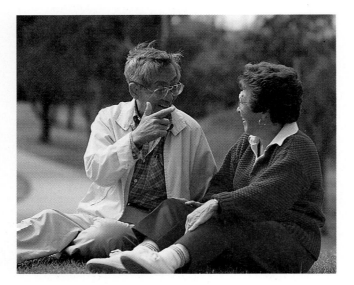

conversations include "Hi. How are you?" and "Fine, and you?" These pleasant, and often meaningless, exchanges, allow us to get past the small talk and on to more important questions about the other person. Or, if we find that we don't want to continue to get to know the person, we can stop at this rather superficial level and not place ourselves at risk by saying too much to the wrong person.

Nonverbal Communication

Understanding what someone is saying often involves much more than listening and speaking. It is often what is *not* actually said that may speak louder than any words. Rolling your eyes, looking at the floor or ceiling when speaking rather than maintaining eye contact, body movements, hand gestures—all these nonverbal clues influence the way we interpret messages.[11] Researchers have found that only 7 percent of the meaning of a message comes from the words spoken. An astounding 93 percent of the meaning, as shown in Figure 4.1, comes from nonverbal cues.[12]

Nonverbal communication includes all unwritten and unspoken messages, both intentional and unintentional.[13] Because our expressions and actions can mean so many different things and be interpreted in so many different ways, it is easy to be confused by nonverbal messages. This confusion is worse when there is a contradiction between what a person says and what he or she does. How would you interpret the following?

- Ramell assures Becky that she loves her spaghetti sauce, yet only picks at it and leaves most of it on her plate.

- Ramone tells Nicole that he loves her deeply, but whenever they go out, he constantly watches other women and acts detached and uninterested in Nicole.

- Mary tells Joselyn that she has forgiven her for gossiping about her, yet she avoids Joselyn on campus and does not look at her when Joselyn speaks to her.

- Peggy says that she is no longer angry with Pat, but she slams the door when she leaves her apartment and squeals her car tires as she pulls out of the driveway.

The nonverbal messages in the above situations appear to contradict the words of the speaker and may be difficult to interpret. In most cases, if there are differences between what is being said and what is being done, we tend to follow the line of thinking that actions speak louder than words. Effective communicators learn to observe nonverbal cues and to try to carefully differentiate between what they think someone is saying or meaning and what is really being said.

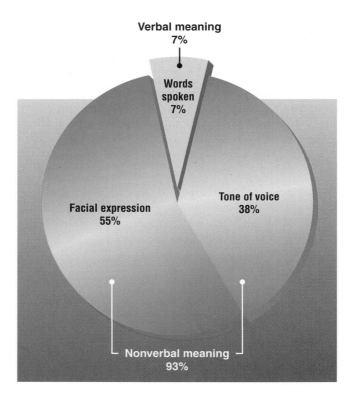

FIGURE 4.1

Elements in Message Meaning

Source: Reproduced from Mary Ellen Guffey, *Business Communication,* p. 39, with the permission of South-Western College Publishing, a division of International Thomson Publishing, Inc. Copyright 1994 Wadsworth Publishing, a division of International Thomson Publishing, Inc. All rights reserved.

WHAT DO YOU THINK?

What types of communication skills do you and your closest friend use? Do you encourage interaction? Do you use gestures and other nonverbal language?

IMPROVING YOUR COMMUNICATION SKILLS

For you to have healthy interactions with others and keep your stress levels under control, it is important that you resolve any problems that you may be having as early as possible. Learning communication skills that bring a quick resolution to fights, misunderstandings, and situations that you are fretting about can help reduce unnecessary stress and lead you to a more productive use of your time. The Skills for Behavior Change box has more helpful guidelines on improving your communication skills.

Using "I" Instead of "You" Messages

One method for improving communication with others is learning to employ "I" messages. **"I" messages** ("I like being with you." "I'm sorry that I missed practice.") are a direct, clear, and effective way to send information to others. The basic premise of using "I" messages is that each individual takes responsibility for communicating his or her own feelings, thoughts, and beliefs. People who practice using "I" messages tend to have more positive interactions and generate less defensiveness in the person receiving the communication.

The opposite of an "I" message is a "you" message. "You" messages are easy to distinguish from "I" messages because they begin with the person sending the communication saying "you" ("You made me so mad." "You never say you're sorry about anything."). "You" messages leave the receiver of the information on the defensive and ready to attack. The following example illustrates the difference between "I" and "you" messages.

Terry and Jim have been working together on a class project for most of the term. Although they are both supposed to contribute 50 percent to the final product, Jim has done very little work thus far. Terry is very angry, but rather than saying, "Jim, you're really lazy and you're not holding up your part of this assignment is really unfair to me," she decides to try another tactic. She says, "Jim, I really am feeling overburdened by all of the work I've been putting into this project. I don't want to feel 'used' in this process and I want both of us to get as much out of the ef-

fort as we can." Because Terry is putting this discussion in terms of how she is feeling (using "I" messages) rather than attacking Jim with "you" messages that make him want to defend himself, it is much more likely that the two of them will be able to continue working together. Jim may get the message and begin to contribute more to the project.

To practice using "I" messages, follow these steps:

Step 1: *"When you."* Start by thinking about a behavior or situation that you want to discuss. Make sure you are clear and specific ("When you leave your clothes all over the floor . . .").

Step 2: *"I feel."* Identify how the behavior or incident makes you feel, and state those feelings by starting your sentence with "I." Adding a feeling statement allows you to share honestly your reaction to the behavior or situation without placing blame or exerting power ("I feel frustrated and angry.").

Step 3: *"Because."* Add a statement to explain from your perspective why the feeling occurred (". . . because I spend so much time trying to keep the place looking good.").

Now let's put these steps together into one simple sentence: "When you leave your clothes on the floor, I feel frustrated and angry because I spend so much time trying to keep the place looking good."

Communicating Assertively

Communicating assertively means using direct, honest communication that maintains and defends your rights in a positive manner. **Assertive communicators** are people who get their points across while at the same time respecting the rights of others. Assertiveness demands both verbal and nonverbal skills. Verbally, assertive communicators speak calmly, directly, and clearly to those around them. Nonverbally, assertive communicators maintain direct eye contact, sit or stand facing the person they are speaking to, and sit or stand with an erect posture that

---

Nonverbal communication: All unwritten and unspoken messages, both intentional and unintentional.

"I" messages: Ways of communicating with others by taking personal responsibility for communicating our own feelings, thoughts, and beliefs.

Assertive communicators: People who use direct, honest communication that maintains and defends their rights in a positive manner.

Ways to Improve Your Communication Skills

If you find that communication is difficult, consider the following advice:

1. *Take actions to break the ice.* It isn't always easy to start a conversation, particularly about a sensitive topic. One way is just to let the other person know that talking about the subject is tough for you. Explaining why you have difficulty and sharing past experiences can help you get going and raise the comfort level for both parties.

2. *Be an active listener.* Remember that it is important to distinguish between putting on the façade of listening and really hearing what someone is saying. Being an active listener means that you are actively engaged and interested in what the other person is saying. You may nod, comment briefly, laugh, show sympathetic facial expressions, or ask questions. As you interact with people today, notice how many of them are really listening. Watch them fade in and out of the conversation. You do this, too. Observe your own listening patterns.

3. *Maintain eye contact.* Have you ever tried to talk to someone whose gaze habitually wandered to the heavens as he or she talked? It was disconcerting, wasn't it? Your eyes are one of your most sensitive conveyers of information. We frequently refer to people as having warm or sensitive eyes and say that we can tell a lot about people by their eyes. Maintaining eye contact shows that you're interested in the other person.

4. *Be supportive of others.* Just as it may be difficult for you to share your thoughts, it may be for others, also. Be sure to tell people that you appreciate their comments and acknowledge that their interest is valuable to you. Similarly, let them know that it is safe for them to talk with you and that, regardless of what they say, you'll continue to value their opinions.

5. *Paraphrase whenever possible.* By summarizing or repeating back what you think you are hearing, you increase the likelihood of good communication. Sometimes you may have to restate the message several times to get it right.

6. *Ask questions.* One of the best ways to learn what people are feeling or thinking is simply to ask them. You may sometimes be looking for a simple yes or no response. At other times, it may be best to ask questions that require more open-ended responses, which allow people more room to maneuver and to give more accurate responses.

7. *Allow responses.* You may think that another person understands that it's okay to talk about something, but you may be wrong. Saying, "I really would like you to let me know how you feel," or, "It's okay to talk about such

and such a thing," gives the other person permission to speak and affirms that it's the right time and place.

8. *Combine praise and criticism.* Obviously, it is naive to think that everyone is perfect and that criticizing others is always a bad thing to do. Under the right circumstances, criticism promotes positive growth and improvement. But without a balance of praise, it can lead to negative interactions. A good rule of thumb is always to try to temper constructive criticism with praise about the person: "I really like it that you enjoy my cooking so much. Maybe next time you could bring over the meat or main entrée so it wouldn't cost me so much to cook for you." Limiting your criticisms to one per discussion generally works better than blasting someone with everything you can think of.

9. *Be direct.* One of the hardest things to do is to learn how to say no or to be honest in your communications without feeling guilt or pressure. When you don't want to do something or feel you are being forced into something, it is generally better to be open and up-front rather than evasive or undecided. If someone asks you out on a date and you don't want to go, find a gentle, sensitive way to say no right away rather than say maybe or yes and then have to lie or make up an excuse later in order not to hurt the person's feelings. Sometimes you give mixed messages because of your own inability to hurt other people's feelings, but indecisiveness may be more destructive in the long run. Say what you think and express what you feel in as positive a way as possible.

10. *Vent anger appropriately.* While some people believe that an occasional good fight is healthy for a relationship, anger per se can be very destructive in a relationship when displayed excessively or inappropriately. Remember to avoid focusing your anger on the character of the other person. Instead, try to focus on the behavior that ticks you off. Say, "When you do such and such, I feel like you are blaming me for the bad situation and it really makes me angry. I value your company and really hope we can talk about this." Although you are telling the person that something he or she does bothers you, you are also primarily using "I" statements that express your concern but also let the other person know that you care.

Source: From "Communication in Sexual Behavior," in *Our Sexuality,* 5th ed., by Robert Crooks and Karla Baur. Copyright © 1993, 1989, 1986, 1983, 1980 by Benjamin/Cummings Publishing Company, Inc. By permission of Brooks/Cole Publishing Company, a division of International Thomson Publishing, Pacific Grove, CA 93950.

indicates confidence and control. The Choices for Change box offers suggestions on how to become an assertive communicator.

Assertiveness is often distinguished from two other styles of communication that produce poor results: *nonassertiveness* and *aggressiveness*. **Nonassertive communicators** tend to be shy and inhibited in their communication with others. Verbally, nonassertive communicators may speak too rapidly or in a voice that is too low to be heard easily or do not say directly what's on their minds. Nonverbally, their body language frequently reveals their timid nature: their shoulders slump, they don't face the person they are talking to, or they avoid direct eye contact. Nonassertive people fear that if they really express how they think or feel, it will upset others. This fear leaves them without positive ways of communicating their needs and concerns.

Aggressive communicators tend to employ an angry, confrontational, hostile manner in their interactions with others. The communications of aggressive people are typically loud and verbally abusive, and these people often blame others when things don't go their way. Someone who constantly uses "you" messages, causing the receiver of the information to feel on the defensive immediately, is usually an aggressive communicator.

---

*W*HAT DO YOU THINK?

During the last two weeks, when have you wished that you had been more assertive and direct in dealing with another person or situation? Why were you not as assertive as you should have been? What might you have done differently after reading this section?

Establishing a Proper Climate

Although selecting a safe person or place when you wish to share or self-disclose is important, it is equally important that you carefully consider your own actions in establishing such an environmental climate. How can you help put the other person or yourself at ease? Have you really established a climate for speaking freely, or are you playing an evasive game with the person you're communicating with? Are you each willing to self-disclose, or has the stage already been set for half-truths? Good communication is based on mutual respect and a sincere desire to listen founded on your caring for the other person. An open climate for communication does not simply happen. If you follow these steps when you speak, the other person is more likely to engage in an open, honest conversation with you.[14]

- *Watch judgmental statements.* Words such as *stupid, ridiculous, great, crummy,* or *fantastic* show that an evaluation has already been made. Many of these judgmental statements leave no room for another opinion. Instead, use descriptive statements that reveal your feelings without labeling them as good, bad, right, or wrong. Say, "Your borrowing my car makes me very nervous," rather than, "You stupid thing, you'll wreck my car and hurt yourself."

- *Keep an open mind.* Since absolute statements tend to close off other opinions, thereby restricting communication, use qualifying statements to give others a chance to state their opinions. Say, "This may not always be true, depending on the circumstances," or, "I could be wrong, but it's what I think."

- *Avoid projecting superiority.* If you really want someone's opinion, then respect it as having some value. As you learn to show respect for others' opinions, your opinion will become more respected. Monitor your facial expressions, voice pitch and intonation, specific words, and actions to see whether they express true interest and respect.

- *Don't ask for feedback unless you want an honest answer.* How many times have you asked people what they thought only to be hurt or to become angry when they told you? If you outwardly become upset by honest feedback, people won't give it to you. Look at such feedback as an attempt to help. No one enjoys criticism, but you can't correct a negative action unless you are aware of it.

- *Avoid people who tend to give negative feedback.* Some people have such low self-esteem that they delight in criticizing others. Try to determine the underlying motives of such people and then avoid them if at all possible.

Conflict Resolution

A **conflict** is an emotional state that arises when the behavior of one person interferes with the behavior of another. Conflicts are inevitable whenever human beings live or work together. Conflict is not automatically bad for

---

Nonassertive communicators: Individuals who tend to be shy and inhibited in their communication with others.

Aggressive communicators: People who use hostile, loud, and blaming communication styles.

Conflict: An emotional state that arises when the behavior of one person interferes with the behavior of another.

How to Be an Assertive Communicator

If you have difficulty speaking up for yourself or are an aggressive communicator, you may want to start working on your assertiveness skills. The following suggestions may help:

- *Recall a situation in which you did not act assertively.* Think about a specific situation you felt you handled nonassertively or aggressively. Reconstruct that incident. Try to remember every detail: who was there, where it occurred, and what you were thinking and feeling. Now replay the same situation step by step in your mind but this time with you acting assertively. Imagine how the original participants will respond to your new behavior.

- *Observe other people acting assertively.* Spend the day noticing other people who communicate assertively. Pay attention to both their verbal and their nonverbal behavior. On a notepad, jot down some of your observations. In addition, observe how other people respond to this type of communication. What do they say? How do they look? Imagine yourself acting as assertively as the models you have observed.

- *Role-play assertive behavior.* With a friend, think up a situation in which you would like to act assertively. Practice playing the part of the assertive communicator while your friend takes the role of the person receiving the information. Switch roles and practice until you feel comfortable with your new assertiveness.

- *Try out your new skill.* Move from the role-play situation to a real-life experiment. Choose a nonthreatening environment to practice your assertive communication skills, such as ordering a meal at a restaurant where the service is friendly. Ask the waiter or waitress to seat you at a specific table, and when ordering your meal, request that it be prepared differently from the way it appears on the menu. Use a calm, direct tone of voice and assertive nonverbals to deliver your message. Be aware of the reactions of others, for these will give you clues about your effectiveness.

a relationship or an organizational unit. Through the process of conflict resolution, relationships can actually be strengthened once the participants learn how to fight fairly.

Most conflicts revolve around two message components: content and relationship. *Content* is usually easy to discern; it is the subject of the sentences used by the participants. *Relationship* is more difficult to discern because it embodies the interactions between the people involved. Most human relationships have both spoken and unspoken rules regarding individual speaking rights and relational control.

Because of the double-pronged nature of messages, arguments can arise quite easily out of seemingly innocuous situations. For instance, one housemate may say to the other, "Mow the lawn today." The other may reply, "Why don't you mow it for a change? Stop trying to control my life." Some of us may argue that the ensuing fight was over the content—that is, over who would mow the lawn. From a relationship standpoint, however, the argument was over the right of one housemate to order the other around. The second housemate in this case quite clearly lets the first know that they are equals. The relationship between housemates in this case does not allow for "bosses."

Prolonged conflict can destroy relationships unless the participants attempt some type of conflict resolution. **Conflict resolution** is a concerted effort by all parties to resolve points of contention in a constructive manner. In relationships, whether intimate or nonintimate (see Chapter 5), it is important to build communication skills. As two people learn to negotiate and compromise concerning their various differences, the number and intensity of conflicts should diminish. Conflict resolution can therefore be a growth process for people as they learn to recognize problems and solutions based upon past experience.

Here are some strategies to consider when conflict resolution may be needed in marital or other close relationships:[15]

1. Remember to focus on one topic at a time and to make other preoccupations clear, such as in, "I may seem angry, but I had a bad day at school today and am really worried about my grades." This takes the heat off the other person.

2. Stop the action and cool down before things get out of control. One sign of major distress in a couple is escalating hostility, often in the form of nagging that provokes angry responses. The escalation seems unstoppable once it gets started.

3. Be specific in your criticisms or praises. Prevent small complaints that you may stew over. You could say, "When I see your clothes on the floor, I feel that you are not doing your share of the work in the house and I feel taken advantage of," instead of, "You're a slob."

You are more likely to feel at ease discussing important issues in a quiet, nonthreatening environment.

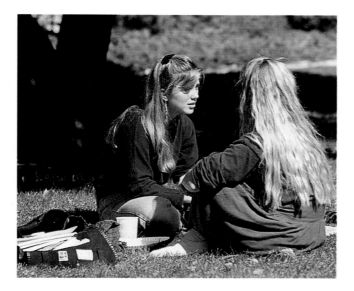

4. Learn to "edit" what you say before you say it so as to avoid saying things that would needlessly be hurtful. For example, don't dredge up past events and old grudges during a fight.

5. Try to think about possible solutions to problems that are compromises for both parties.

6. Never think in terms of winning an argument. Think instead of ways to keep an argument from happening. By doing so, both parties win.

*W*HAT DO YOU THINK?

What three steps could you take to improve your conflict resolution skills? Is there a problem you'd like to solve that you could use as practice?

*G*ENDER DIFFERENCES IN COMMUNICATION STYLES

Men and women commonly complain that they cannot really communicate with each other. But do gender differences actually exist in communication styles? If so, how may such differences cause misunderstandings between men and women? In her book *You Just Don't Understand*, Deborah Tannen describes many of the differences in conversational style between males and females in our society.[16] Tannen believes that these differences make com-

munication between the genders confusing and difficult. Tannen also believes that communication between men and women is like cross-cultural communication and as such, is prone to clashes in conversational styles. She says that men and women speak different **"genderlects"** characterized by differences in word choice, interruption patterns, questioning patterns, language interpretations and misinterpretations, and vocal inflections based on gender. Recognizing these differences and taking action to understand differences and to change weak, ineffective communication may allow men and women to communicate better and to be more satisfied with their relationships.

The following vignettes show some common complaints men and women have about the differences in their patterns of communication:[17]

- Female speaking to a male: "Why is it that when we are lost you never want to stop and ask someone for directions?"

- Male speaking to a female: "Why do you want to analyze everything I say?"

- Female speaking to a male: "You never share your feelings with me. I never know what you are thinking or feeling."

- Male speaking to a female: "Gossip, gossip, gossip. You and your friends just love to talk about other people!"

Differences in Decision Making

Moral development is another area in which males and females may differ and which may result in communication problems. According to Harvard professor Carol Gilligan, men and women may make very different decisions when facing ethical dilemmas.[18] Gilligan believes that women tend to think and speak differently from men because of the two genders' contrasting images of self. Because of these self-image differences, Gilligan believes that there is a feminine ethic of *care* and a masculine ethic of *justice*.[19] Following this line of thinking, she suggests that women view sensitivity to others, loyalty, responsibility, self-sacrifice, and peacemaking as key factors to consider in making ethical decisions. In contrast, men are more interested in individual rights, equality before law, and fair play; factors that are much more impersonal. Because

Conflict resolution: A concerted effort by all parties to resolve points in contention in a constructive manner.

Genderlect: The "dialect," or individual speech pattern and conversational style, of each gender.

such gender differences would affect both the encoding and decoding of messages, difficulties in communication might result.[20]

Sharing Feelings

Although men tend to talk about intimate issues with women more frequently than with men, females still complain that men do not communicate enough about what is really on their minds. This may reflect the powerful, different socialization processes for both sexes, which influence their communication styles. Throughout their lives, females are offered opportunities to practice sharing their thoughts and feelings with others. In contrast, males receive strong societal messages to withhold their feelings. The classic example of this training in very young males is the familiar saying "big boys don't cry." Males learn very early that certain emotions are not to be shared, with the result that they are more information-focused and businesslike in their conversations with females than females are.[21] Understandably, such differences in communication styles encourage misunderstandings and conflict between the sexes.

Although men are often perceived as being less emotional than women, the question remains whether men really feel less or just have more difficulty expressing their emotions. In one study, when men and women were shown scenes of people in distress, the men exhibited little outward emotion, whereas the women communicated feelings of concern and distress. However, physiological measures of emotional arousal (such as heart rate and blood pressure) indicated that the male subjects were actually as affected emotionally as the female subjects but inhibited the expression of their emotions, whereas the women openly expressed them. In other studies, men and women responded very differently to the same test.[22]

When men are angered, they tend to interpret the cause of their anger as something or someone in their environment and are likely to turn their anger outward in an aggressive manner. Women, on the other hand, tend to see themselves as the source of the problem and turn

their anger inward, thereby suppressing direct expression of it.[23] Such differences in expressing anger can easily lead to breakdowns in communication between men and women.

Improving Communication between Men and Women

Can communication between men and women be improved? Understanding gender differences in communication patterns, rather than casting blame at each other, may be a first step toward bettering communication between men and women. Tannen suggests that expecting persons of the opposite sex to change their style of communication is not effective in dealing with the gender gap. Instead, learning to interpret their messages, while explaining your own unique way of communicating, may be more useful in improving information transmission between you and the opposite sex. Both men and women want to be heard and understood in their conversations. Only if we begin to understand the different ways males and females use language can we gain a greater level of comfort and closeness between the genders.[24]

*W*HAT DO YOU THINK?

Do you believe that men and women really communicate in different styles? Why or why not? What can you do to improve your communication with members of the opposite sex?

Communication between Couples

Communication in intimate relationships between two adults is often a source of difficulty and can lead to an inability to solve problems and to dissatisfaction with the relationship. The following techniques can help improve communication between couples:[25]

1. **Leveling** refers to sending your partner a clear, simple, and honest message. The purposes of leveling are: (1) to make communication clear; (2) to make clear the expectations partners have of one another; (3) to clear up pleasant and unpleasant feelings and thoughts from past incidents; (4) to make clear what is relevant and what is irrelevant; and (5) to become aware of the things that draw you together or push you apart.

2. **Editing,** or censoring remarks that are meant to be hurtful or are irrelevant to the conversation, is another useful skill that improves couple communication. Often, when people are upset, they let everything fly, bringing up old issues and incidents that cause pain to their partners and put them on the defensive.

Leveling: The communication of a clear, simple, and honest message.

Editing: The process of censoring comments that would be intentionally hurtful or irrelevant to the conversation.

Documenting: Giving specific examples of issues you are discussing.

Validating: Letting your partner know that although you may not agree with his or her point of view, you still respect the fact that he or she thinks or feels that way.

Managing Your Communication Skills

As you have seen in this chapter, your interpersonal interactions with others can have an important impact on your overall health. Communication skills do not automatically arise; instead, they must be carefully cultivated in order to develop fully. There are many things you can do to help your messages get through in a nonoffensive, positive manner. Whether you are conversing with intimate partners, friends, family members, or casual acquaintances, the way in which you say things and how you act will do much to convey your message.

Making Decisions for You

Think about a situation in which you find it difficult to communicate. To learn how to improve your ability to communicate, think about people who do a great job expressing themselves in a similar situation. Who doesn't do such a good job? What is it about each of these individual's actions that make them effective or ineffective? What can you do to practice these skills so that you won't have problems next time? What must you do differently?

Checklist for Change: Making Personal Choices

✓ Have you thought about your own communication style? Are you a good listener or do you like to hold everyone's attention with your talking and other verbal interactions?

✓ Who do you admire most in terms of their interpersonal communication styles?

✓ What skills would you need to work on in order to be more like these people you admire? Are you a better listener or a better speaker? Do you feel good about how others "read" your communications? Have you ever asked someone close to you how they think you communicate?

✓ Have you thought about how you could work on the communication skills that you are not satisfied with? Have you set a time line for working on each of these skills?

✓ How will you know whether you are improving in each of the areas you have identified? What do you ultimately want to accomplish?

Checklist for Change: Making Community Choices

✓ Have you ever thought about where you get your information in your community? Does it come from spoken or written communication networks? Who is delivering the messages?

✓ Do words have meanings in your community that may differ from their meanings elsewhere? How about non-verbal actions (space between communicators, speed of speech, and the like)?

✓ Are your sources of information biased or unbiased? Who monitors the information for accuracy and completeness?

✓ When you communicate information to others in the community, do you make every attempt to be accurate, unbiased, and unemotional in your delivery?

✓ When others in your community or on your campus are presenting information that is inaccurate, biased, or incomplete, do you try to take action to improve their message?

✓ Is there a place on your campus where you can go to talk with someone about your communication problems and get feedback about how you can improve?

Critical Thinking

Mylan has never been overly keen on self-disclosure. But his girlfriend, Joyce, has gained his confidence over several months. While standing in line at a movie theater one night, Joyce starts talking about a major rock star's announcement that he was sexually abused as a child. Mylan feels so comfortable with Joyce that he tells her that he, too, was abused as a preteen by an aunt. Joyce is the first person he has ever told. A few days later, one of Joyce's friends passes Mylan in the hall and says, "I just want you to know how sorry I feel for you. It's great that you've handled it so well. Joyce says you're just a wonderful lover." Mylan is furious. Not only has Joyce exposed his biggest secret, but she has also told her girlfriends about their sex life. He decides to skip class so that he can talk to Joyce immediately.

Using the DECIDE model described in Chapter 1, decide how Mylan should approach the conversation with Joyce. Given the context in which the disclosure occurred, could Joyce have mistaken the level of intimacy of the disclosure? What can Mylan do to be better at self-disclosure?

By editing, you take the time and make the effort not to say inflammatory things. Leveling and editing help you to communicate genuinely and sensitively to your partner.

3. **Documenting** refers to giving specific examples of issues you are discussing. Documenting allows you to stay away from gross generalizations that tend to be accusatory, such as "You always" and "You never." By

your provision of specific examples of when and how an incident occurred, your partner is able to gain a concrete understanding of the issue. In documenting, you can also include specific suggestions for changing or improving the situation.

4. **Validating** means letting partners know that although you may not agree with their points of view, you still respect what they are thinking or feeling ("I don't agree with you but I can see how you might view things that way."). This does not mean that you are giving in to your partner; you are simply recognizing that your opinions differ.

To see how these techniques may help a couple discuss a sensitive issue, consider the following scenario. Cathy and Manuel are college students who have been going out for about eight months. Cathy has begun to feel that Manuel is spending too much time away from the relationship with his friends, work, and sports. The problem has been noticeable to Cathy for over a month, but she hasn't mentioned it to Manuel.

Since Cathy has been feeling hurt and frustrated for quite some time, it would be easy for her to really let Manuel have it by overwhelming him with all her pent-up feelings. But by leveling and editing, Cathy can open a dialogue with a direct communication that weeds out some extraneous material. Thus, talking to Manuel, she needs time to edit—to calm down and organize her thoughts and feelings. She could start the conversation with leveling, saying something like this: "Manuel, I was wondering if I could talk to you about something I am concerned about. It has to do with the amount of time we are spending together as a couple."

Next, Cathy might give Manuel a few specific examples (documenting) of the behavior that concerns her: "Last week I noticed that you spent Monday and Tuesday nights out with your friends, and Wednesday and Thursday nights working late. I felt like we had no time together, and I really missed you."

Finally, Cathy needs to listen to Manuel's reply in an open and caring manner and then validate his perspec-

Understanding the socialization processes that encourage women, but not men, to express their feelings can help you avoid misunderstandings and conflicts in your relationships with the opposite sex.

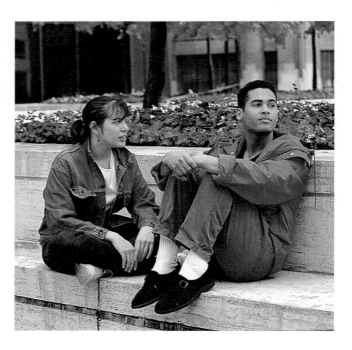

tive. For example, suppose Manuel says, "Well, you know I really have had a lot of games going on and that means spending time with my friends, and besides that I work late hours in order to make as much money as I can." Cathy's validating reply might sound like this: "I know how much your sports mean to you and how hard you work, but that doesn't leave much time for us. I would really like us to figure out a way that you can do your thing but that we also could have more time together." By using some specific techniques that improve communication between couples, Cathy is thus able to discuss with Manuel a topic that could otherwise have caused tension in their relationship.

Summary

◆ Communication improves self-esteem by building confidence and helping us to define ourselves, lowers stress by helping us to resolve interpersonal conflicts, and increases our health knowledge through health promotion efforts.

◆ Communication is an ongoing process between sender and receiver. It is often disrupted by barriers that include differences in background and alcohol and drugs. Communication with medical personnel has

special barriers: language specialization, sociocultural differences, patient anxiety, and patient misinterpretation. Self-disclosure is the sharing of personal information with others. It allows us to feel connected with others, thereby reducing stress in our lives.

◆ Listening is extremely important to good communication. Good listeners are present physically and emotionally, use paraphrasing effectively, and tend to have improved social interactions and to function more effectively in interpersonal relationships. Conversations form the basis of relationships and range from small talk to self-disclosure. Nonverbal communication provides 93 percent of the meaning of a message.

◆ Gender differences in communication include conversation styles as well as differences in decision making and in sharing feelings.

Discussion Questions

1. How are self-esteem and stress directly related to your physical well-being? How does communication improve self-esteem and reduce stress?

2. Outline the communication process. Then discuss how barriers can get in the way of effective communication.

3. What specific communication barriers may one encounter when dealing with the health-care system? Do insurance companies put up their own barriers to communication?

4. Why is self-disclosure so important to our mental well-being? Are there times when it is better not to self-disclose?

5. Is it ethical to fail to disclose information about your past sex life to a potential lover? What risks are involved in such lack of disclosure? Are white lies okay if you think they will keep the other person happy?

6. Describe some barriers to effective listening and ways to overcome them.

7. What is nonverbal communication and why is it important that you learn to enhance your skills in this area? Give examples of some things that you do to communicate without words.

8. How can you improve your interpersonal communication with the use of "I" messages? Why are assertive communicators successful in getting their message across?

9. Discuss how you would resolve a conflict with your roommate about "lights out" time.

10. Why may it be more difficult for men and women to communicate with each other than it is for two men to communicate with each other or two women to communicate with each other? What factors may have contributed to these differences? What can you do to enhance communication and interpersonal interactions between the sexes? Why is an understanding of communication-related gender differences important to couples?

Application Exercise

Reread the What Do You Think? scenarios at the beginning of the chapter and answer the following questions:

1. Discuss the specific barriers that Marty is encountering with his doctor. What could Marty do to improve his relationship with his doctor?

2. What benefit would Marty derive from improving his patient-doctor relationship?

3. Explain the problem between York-chi and Margaret in terms of what you have learned in this chapter. For example, has York-chi effectively communicated her feelings?

4. What would you recommend that York-chi try to improve her situation? If that failed, then what should she do?

Further Reading

Gerard Egan, *You and Me: The Skills of Communicating and Relating to Others* (Pacific Grove, CA: Brooks-Cole, 1993).

Focuses on skills of self-disclosure, listening, responding, challenging, and participating in groups. Presents a dynamic, step-by-step procedure for increasing self-awareness and improving communication skills.

John S. Caputo, Harry C. Hazel, and Colleen McMahon, *Interpersonal Communication* (Boston: Allyn and Bacon, 1994).

Outstanding overview of interpersonal communication, techniques for skill development, and why communication is such an important aspect of our daily interactions. Includes chapters on technology and communication, communicating with diverse and global populations, and a number of creative, innovative techniques for communicators.

Daniel J. Canary and Michael Cody, *Interpersonal Communication: A Goals-Based Approach* (St. Martin's, 1994).

Excellent text covering a wide range of interpersonal communication topics. Comprehensive, applied approach to learning new skills and improving old skills.

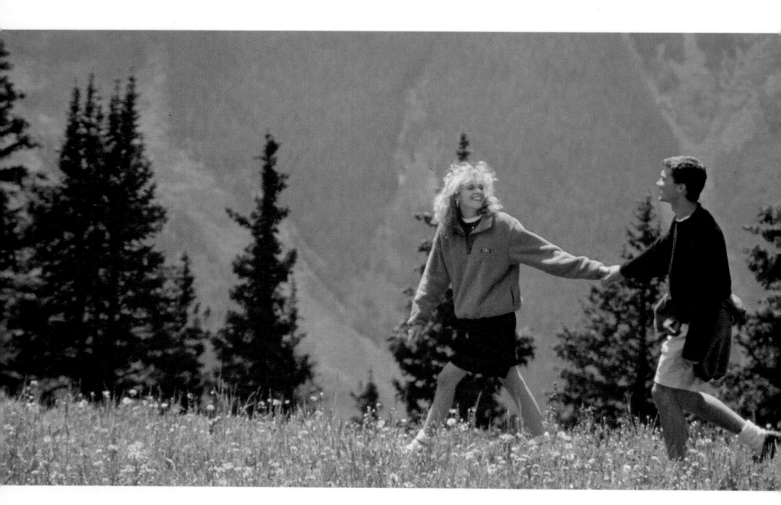

CHAPTER OBJECTIVES

◆ Explain the characteristics of intimate relationships, the purposes they serve, and the types of intimacy that each of us may be able to have.

◆ Explain how relationships develop and describe the factors that influence their formation and maintenance.

◆ Discuss the differences between men and women in relationships, partner selection, and communication styles.

◆ Discuss the barriers to intimate relationships and explain how these barriers can be overcome.

◆ Discuss the importance of commitment in each of the various types of relationships described.

◆ Examine those factors that seem to be important in determining the success of an intimate relationship.

◆ Discuss what remaining single means for many Americans.

◆ Examine child-rearing practices in the United States and the importance of a healthy family environment.

◆ Discuss the warning signs of relationship decline, where you can go to get help with a relationship crisis, and factors that ultimately lead to relationship problems.

Healthy Relationships

Friends, Family, and Significant Others

WHAT DO YOU THINK?

Roberto and Sara have been dating seriously for over two years and have talked about marriage. Sara has noticed that Roberto often seems overly possessive of her and jealous of her time spent with others. They fight regularly about who she does things with, potential threats to their relationship, and the like. Recently, Roberto took a weekend to go hunting with the guys while Sara stayed home to get caught up on her work. When Sara's friends called her to ask her to go to a party, she decided to go. She had worked hard all weekend and needed a break. When she talks to Roberto on the phone the next day, he asks her what she did the night before. Wanting to avoid a fight, she tells him that she stayed home to work. He responds angrily, "I tried to call you all night and you weren't home."

■ What should Sara do in this situation? Why do you think she felt the need to lie? Is dishonesty in a relationship ever justified? Is Roberto's jealousy a healthy aspect of their relationship? What factors may have contributed to his jealousy? Can dishonesty actually increase the likelihood of future jealous feelings? What do you think that Roberto and Sara should do if they really want to have an open and honest relationship? Where could they go for help? Can a relationship based on mistrust and half-truths survive?

Megan is a single mother who has two small children. She is divorced from the children's alcoholic father and has been dating another man for two years. Currently, Megan is working 40 hours per week and trying to take classes in the evening to complete her teaching degree. Her children spend most of their week at Megan's parents' home or in day care, but Megan makes sure that she spends quality time with each child every day. They live in a nice home and the children appear to be happy and well-adjusted and are doing very well in school. Recently, Megan's former husband's parents have successfully sued for custody of the children, saying that she is an unfit mother who is putting her needs above those of her children.

■ What makes a good parent? Do you agree or disagree with the court's decision to take Megan's children away from her simply because she is trying to get a degree and is unable to spend 24 hours a day at home? Do you think the courts would be as likely to try to intervene if a man was working the equivalent of two jobs and leaving his children with his parents? Why or why not? Is it possible for a single parent to do as good a job raising a child as a married couple? What do you believe are the essential ingredients of a healthy home environment?

Our relationships with our friends, our families, our intimate partners, people we work with, and complete strangers have been the subject of numerous articles, television programs, and a wide variety of self-help books, workshops, and counseling sessions. During recent years, psychosocial researchers, health professionals, and therapists have shown tremendous interest in the nature of interpersonal interactions. What makes a relationship with another person last? What are the characteristics of good relationships? Why are healthy relationships so vital to a healthy life?

Intense scientific investigations have attempted to unlock the mysteries of our relationships and of the effects of these relationships on our self-esteem, our health, our happiness, our individual successes and failures as human beings, and a host of other areas. We have been analyzed genetically, biologically, socially, and psychologically in an effort to determine why we behave as we do and whether there might be a better recipe for influencing later interpersonal behaviors.

Each of these studies acknowledges the importance of casual and intimate interactions in our development into well-adjusted, healthy adulthood. Friendship, close family bonds, and loving intimate and nonintimate relationships are viewed as significant factors in achieving overall health. The eternal quest to be loved and to love others appears to be one of our most basic human needs.

For many, the motivation to seek and receive love appears to be a natural result of previous life experiences and our development as sexual beings. For others, the struggle to find, develop, and maintain relationships becomes a difficult, often painful and frustrating experience, punctuated by unhappy sexual and nonsexual interactions. What makes one person more successful in his or her relationships than another? What role does friendship and the family environment have on the development of healthy relationships later in life? What effect, if any, does sexual identity have on one's ability to form healthy relationships? Taking a look at the nature of relationships (intimate and nonintimate) and our development as sexual and nonsexual beings may help provide answers to these questions.

CHARACTERISTICS OF INTIMATE RELATIONSHIPS

There are many possible definitions of **intimate relationships.** One classic definition calls these relationships "close relationships with another person in which you offer, and are offered, validation, understanding, and a sense of being valued intellectually, emotionally, and physically."[1] In this context, friends, family, lovers, partners, and even people you work with or interact with at the grocery store may be included in the sphere of intimate interactions. However, most experts today tend to focus more on family, close friendships, and romantic relationships when they discuss intimate relationships.

For the purposes of this chapter, we define intimate relationships in terms of three characteristics: *behavioral interdependence, need fulfillment,* and *emotional attachment.* Each of these three characteristics may be related to interactions with family, close friends, and romantic relationships.[2]

Behavioral interdependence refers to the mutual impact that people have on each other as their lives and daily activities become intertwined. What one person does may influence what the other person may want to do and can do. Such interdependence may become stronger over time to the point that each person would find a great void in his or her life if the other person was gone.

Another characteristic of intimate relationships is that they serve to fulfill psychological needs and so are a means of *need fulfillment.* These needs may often be met only through relationships with others:

- The need for approval and for a sense of purpose in life—requiring the sense that what we say and do counts.

Intimate relationships: "[C]lose relationships with another person in which you offer, and are offered, validation, understanding, and a sense of being valued intellectually, emotionally, and physically."[1]

Emotional availability: The ability to give to and receive from other people emotionally without being inhibited by fears of being hurt.

- The need for intimacy—requiring someone with whom we can share our feelings freely.

- The need for social integration—requiring someone with whom we can share our worries and concerns.

- The need for being nurturant—requiring someone whom we can take care of.

- The need for assistance—requiring someone to help us in times of need.

- The need for reassurance or affirmation of our own worth—requiring someone who will tell us that we matter.

In close, rewarding, intimate relationships, partners or friends meet each other's needs. They disclose feelings, share confidences, and discuss practical concerns, helping each other and providing reassurance. They serve as major sources of social support and reinforce our feelings that we are important and serve a purpose in life.

In addition to behavioral interdependence and need fulfillment, intimate relationships involve strong bonds of *emotional attachment,* or feelings of love and attachment. The intimacy level experienced by any two people cannot easily be judged by those outside the relationship. Giving advice to people who are having relationship problems is often not a great idea unless you really know both people well. Individuals share their inner selves so differently that it is impossible to assign a clear meaning to any given action. Friendship relationships can be very intimate and contribute essential elements to a person's sense of inclusion and well-being. Love relationships may be very intimate and include many aspects of intimacy in addition to sexual sharing. Often, when we hear the word *intimacy* we immediately think about a sexual relationship. A relationship may be very intimate and not be sexual, although sex may be an important part of an intimate relationship. Important relationships having high levels of intimacy may be either sexual or nonsexual. Many satisfying and lasting intimate relationships go well beyond the need for sexual contact.

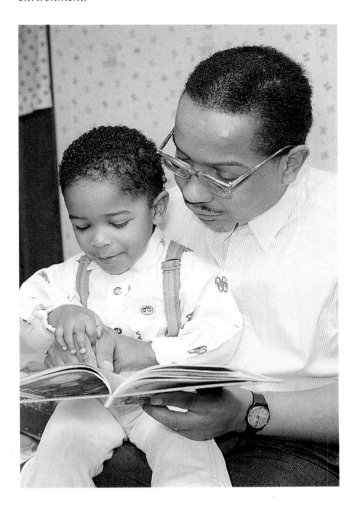

Emotional bonding and other elements of intimate relationships are rooted in a caring, supportive family environment.

ᐯHAT DO YOU THINK?

Do you have at least one person in your life right now who helps fulfill your psychological needs? Who makes you feel loved and important? Who would support you if you really needed help? Are you a source of psychological support for someone else? If you don't have this type of relationship, what could you do to develop one?

Emotional availability, the ability to give to and receive from others emotionally without fear of being hurt or rejected, is another characteristic of intimate relationships. At times, all of us may need to protect ourselves psycho-logically by making ourselves unavailable emotionally. For example, after the end of a relationship, a young woman may close down emotionally and carefully avoid letting herself feel too much. This gives her time for re-grouping and healing before she reaches out to people again. It also reduces the risk of a rebound romance that is often doomed to failure as a result of unresolved personal hurts and issues.

Types of Intimate Relationships

Balanced intimacy involves developing levels of intimacy in several dimensions. *Sexual intimacy* is one possible expression of closeness. Another dimension of intimacy is *intellectual intimacy,* the sharing of ideas. *Emotional intimacy* involves the sharing of significant meanings and feelings. *Aesthetic intimacy* refers to the sharing of experiences with one another. *Recreational intimacy* is the freedom to let the child within us come out when we are with others. *Work intimacy* is the sharing of common tasks such as housework, family responsibilities, employment, and community undertakings. *Crisis intimacy* implies the successful coping with either internal or external threats. *Commitment intimacy* involves the mutual concern for issues and philosophies that go beyond the immediate relationship (for example, a political cause). *Spiritual intimacy* is the sharing of ultimate concerns regarding the meanings of life. By achieving balanced levels in mutually selected areas of intimacy, two people contribute to *creative intimacy,* or the sharing of emotional and social factors that help each other grow and learn.

Balanced intimacy is a goal most people pursue either directly or indirectly. The chances for balanced intimacy are greater for people who were raised in an environment where close relationships were valued, where there were positive role models for friendships, close family bonds, and romantic attachments. Having nurturing relationships is an essential element of relationship modeling and a key to later successes in relationships.

$\mathcal{F}$ORMING INTIMATE RELATIONSHIPS

Throughout our lives, we go through predictable patterns of relationships. In our early years, our families are our most significant relationships. Gradually, our relationships widen to include circles of friends, co-workers, and acquaintances. Ultimately, most of us develop romantic or sexual relationships with significant others. Each of these relationships plays a significant role in psychological, social, spiritual, and physical health. Each has the potential either to serve as a growth experience or to "bring us down" as a result of unhealthy interactions. When college students are asked to identify the one person in the world to whom they feel most close, they describe one of four types of relationships.[3] Fourteen percent specify a family member, 36 percent identify a friend, and 47 percent name a romantic partner. The remaining 3 percent mention someone else, such as a fellow worker.[4]

Families: The Ties that Bind

Although many people consider the family the foundation of American society and talk about a return to "family values" as a desirable objective, it is clear that the modern American family may look quite different from families of previous generations. The *Leave It to Beaver* family type encouraged during the 1950s, composed of Mom with her apron, staying at home and content with her role as mother and spouse; Dad with his briefcase, trying to move up the corporate ladder; and two or three happy, well-adjusted children, is often not the norm. Over half of today's moms work outside the home and large

numbers of children are raised by single parents, grandparents, relatives, stepparents, nannies, day-care centers, and other "parents."

Regardless of the form or structure of each family, all families have in common one unique characteristic: the special caring, regard, and bonding that a group of people having shared interests have for each other. Whether the family is related by birth, a high level of love and regard, living arrangement, or some other factor, the family network often provides the sense of security that humans need to develop into healthy adults. In fact, because the definition of *family* changes dramatically from culture to culture and from place to place over time, no clear definition of *family* exists. Families are not inherently good or bad based on the structure or roles that people bring to the family setting. Those that result in the most positive health outcomes for all members appear to be those that offer a sense of security, safety, and love, and that provide the opportunity for members to grow as a result of positive interactions.

Today's Family Unit

The United Nations defines seven basic types of families, including single-parent families, communal families (unrelated people living together for ideological, economic, or other reasons), extended families, and others. But most Americans think of family in terms of the "family of origin" or the "nuclear family." The *family of origin* includes the people present in the household during a child's first years of life—usually parents and siblings. However, the family of origin may also include a stepparent, parents' lovers, or significant others such as grandparents, aunts, or uncles. The family of origin has a tremendous impact on the child's psychological and social development. The *nuclear family* consists of parents (usually married, but not necessarily) and their offspring.

If parents are not afraid to share feelings, affection, or love with each other and their offspring, their children are more likely to become emotionally connected adults. If the home environment provides stability and seems a safe place to be, it is likely that the children will learn to express feelings and develop intimacy skills. Sibling interactions provide a way to learn and practice interpersonal skills.[5] Brothers and sisters often experience a mixture of love and hate, closeness and rivalry; these mixed feelings recur throughout one's life because friendships, love affairs, and marriages tend to evoke the reactions originally associated with siblings.[6,7] Grandparents often serve as substitute or surrogate parents, particularly for children of divorce. Young adults from broken homes, particularly African Americans from such homes, report that it was often their grandmothers who appeared to be interested in them, loved them, and made them feel relaxed, comfortable and proud of who they were.[8,9] The family of origin and the nuclear family have the potential for encouraging significant positive interactions and growth. People can practice positive behaviors and learn the rights and wrongs of negative behaviors in a safe and nonjudgmental environment when the family itself is healthy. However, if the family is psychologically or physically unhealthy, it may pose significant barriers to later relationships, as we discuss later, in the section on dysfunctional families.

Friendships: Finding the Right Ingredients

A Friend is one who knows you as you are
understands where you've been
accepts who you've become, and
still gently invites you to grow.
Author Unknown

Although most of us have a fairly clear idea of the distinction between a friend and a lover, this difference is not always easy to verbalize. Some people believe that the major difference is that there is no intimate physical involvement between friends. Others have suggested that intimacy levels are much lower between friends than between lovers. But as we have stated, people can be intimate with each other without being sexually involved. Confused? You are probably not alone. Surprisingly, there has not been a great deal of research to clarify these terms. Psychologists Jeffrey Turner and Laurna Rubinson provide a basic overview of what friendship actually entails.[10] Beyond the fact that two people participate in a relationship as equals, friendships include the following characteristics:

- *Enjoyment.* Friends enjoy each other's company most of the time, although there may be temporary states of anger, disappointment, or mutual annoyance.

- *Acceptance.* Friends accept each other as they are, without trying to change or make the other into a different person.

- *Trust.* Friends have mutual trust in the sense that each assumes that the other will act in his or her friend's best interests.

- *Respect.* Friends respect each other in the sense that each assumes that the other exercises good judgment in making life choices.

- *Mutual assistance.* Friends are inclined to assist and support one another. Specifically, they can count on each other in times of need, trouble, or personal distress.

- *Confiding.* Friends share experiences and feelings with each other that they don't share with other people.

- *Understanding.* Friends have a sense of what is important to each and why each behaves as he or she does.

Friends are not puzzled or mystified by each other's actions.

- *Spontaneity.* Friends feel free to be themselves in the relationship rather than required to play a role, wear a mask, or inhibit revealing personal traits.

According to psychologist Dan McAdams, most of us are fortunate to develop one or two lasting friendships in a lifetime.[11] The Skills for Behavioral Change box contains tips to help you be the best friend you can be.

Significant Others, Partners, Couples

Although family and friends are necessary intimate relationships, most people choose at some point whether or not to enter into an intimate sexual relationship with another person. Numerous studies have analyzed the ways in which couples form significant partnering relationships. Most couples fit into one of four categories of significant sexual or committed relationships: married heterosexual couples, cohabiting heterosexual couples, lesbian couples, and gay male couples. These groups are discussed in greater detail later in this chapter.

Love relationships in each of these five groups typically include all the characteristics of friendship as well as other characteristics related to passion and caring:[12]

- *Fascination.* Lovers tend to pay attention to the other person even when they should be involved in other activities. They are preoccupied with the other and want to think about, look at, talk to, or merely be with the other.

- *Exclusiveness.* Lovers have a special relationship that usually precludes having the same relationship with a third party. The love relationship takes priority over all others.

- *Sexual desire.* Lovers want physical intimacy with the partner, desiring to touch, hold, and engage in sexual activities with the other. They may choose not to act on these feelings because of religious, moral, or practical considerations.

- *Giving the utmost.* Lovers care enough to give the utmost when the other is in need, sometimes to the point of extreme sacrifice.

- *Being a champion/advocate.* The depth of lovers' caring may show up as an active, unselfish championing of each other's interests and a positive attempt to ensure that the other succeeds.

For obvious reasons, the best love relationships share friendships, and the best friendships include several love components. Both relationships share common bonds of nurturance, enhancement of personal well-being, and a genuine sense of mutual regard, trust, and security.

Becoming a Better Friend

At any age, having a close network of friends is essential. As you leave the security of family in your late teens and early 20s, particularly as you move away to college, it is especially important for you to establish meaningful contact with others. Depression and suicide often flourish in settings where people are isolated. Unfortunately, friendships get low billing in the United States, far below that of torrid romances. Many of us tend to leave our friends by the wayside when our passions flare, only to find that when romance fizzles we are left alone, and our friends have gone ahead without us at a time when we most need their support. The skills that are valuable in developing friendships are the same skills needed in committed romantic relationships: trust, self-disclosure, negotiation, compromise, acceptance, respect, and understanding. And always try to remember: To have a friend, you have to be a friend. The following attitudes and behaviors will help you become that friend:

- Make time for your friends. Don't let them drift away when you meet a new love—make friends a priority.
- Be there in times of need—give of yourself.
- Maintain your friends' trust. Don't share their confidences.
- Be willing to self-disclose, share feelings, fears, anxieties, etc.

- Let friends know you appreciate them. Words, notes, cards, flowers, and other gestures go a long way.
- Be constructive, positive, and kind when providing honest feedback or criticism.
- Accept their weaknesses. Help them grow.
- Ask questions about them—show an interest in their lives and spend less time talking about you.
- Don't take them for granted or take advantage of their affection.
- Cultivate and nurture your best friendships. Recognize the difference between true friends and acquaintances.
- Don't gossip about friends behind their backs.
- Be forgiving of minor offenses. Try to understand major offenses.

What Do You Think?

Think about the above list. Who, in your view, are your best friends? What aspects of yourself can you work on to be a better friend to others? What can you do today? In the coming weeks? What things are most important to you in a best friend?

Healthy friendships and love relationships can greatly enhance overall health and lead to sustained personal growth throughout one's life (see Figure 5.1).

This Thing Called Love

What is love? Finding a definition of love may be more difficult than listing characteristics of a loving relationship. The term *love* has more entries in *Bartlett's Familiar Quotations* than does any other word except *man*.[13] This four-letter word has been written about and engraved on walls; it has been the theme of countless novels, movies, and plays. There is no one definition of *love,* and the word may mean different things to people depending on cultural values, age, gender, and situation. (Perhaps you've also wondered at some time in your life whether you felt love or just infatuation for someone. If you're still confused, see the Rate Yourself box.)

Many social scientists maintain that love may be of two kinds: *companionate* and *passionate.* Companionate love is a secure, trusting attachment, similar to what we may feel for family members or close friends. In companionate love, two people are attracted, have much in common,

care about each other's well-being, and express reciprocal liking and respect. Passionate love is, in contrast, a state of high arousal, filled with the ecstasy of being loved by the partner and the agony of being rejected.[14] The person experiencing passionate love tends to be preoccupied with his or her partner and to perceive the love object as being perfect.[15] According to Hatfield and Walster, passionate love will not occur unless three conditions are met.[16] First, the person must live in a culture in which the concept of "falling in love" is idealized. Second, a "suitable" love object must be present. If the person has been taught by parents, movies, books, and peers to seek partners having certain levels of attractiveness or belonging to certain racial groups or having certain socioeconomic status and none is available, the person may find it difficult to allow him- or herself to become involved. Finally, for passionate love to occur, there must be some type of physiological arousal that occurs when a person is in the presence of the object of desire. Sexual excitement is often the way in which such arousal is expressed.

In his article "The Triangular Theory of Love," researcher Robert Sternberg attempts to clarify further what love is by isolating three key ingredients:

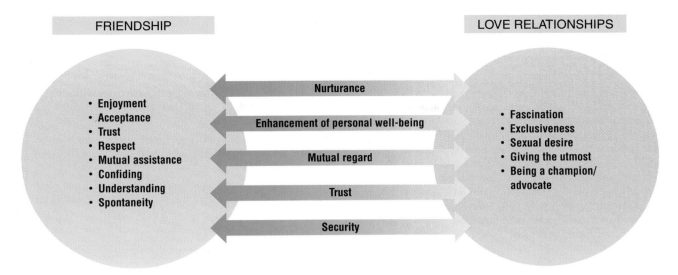

FIGURE 5.1

Common Bonds of Friends and Lovers

- *Intimacy.* The emotional component, which involves feelings of closeness.

- *Passion.* The motivational component, which reflects romantic, sexual attraction.

- *Decision/commitment.* The cognitive component, which includes the decisions you make about being in love and the degree of commitment to your partner.

According to Sternberg's model, the higher the levels of intimacy, passion, and commitment, the more likely a person is to be involved in a healthy, positive love relationship (see Table 5.1).

Anthropologist Helen Fisher, a research associate at the American Museum of Natural History and author of

Anatomy of Love: The Natural History of Monogamy, Adultery, and Divorce, has attempted to shed new light on the process of falling in love.[17] According to Fisher (and others), attraction and falling in love follow a fairly predictable pattern based on (1) *imprinting,* in which our evolutionary patterns, genetic predispositions, and past experiences trigger romantic reaction; (2) *attraction,* in which neurochemicals produce feelings of euphoria and elation; (3) *attachment,* in which endorphins—natural opiates—cause lovers to feel peaceful, secure, and calm; and (4) *production of a cuddle chemical,* in which the brain secretes the chemical oxytocin, thereby stimulating sensations during lovemaking and eliciting feelings of satisfaction and attachment[18] (see Figure 5.2).

TABLE 5.1 ■ The Triangular Theory of Love: Types of Relationships

	Intimacy	Passion	Decision and Commitment
Nonlove	Low	Low	Low
Liking	High	Low	Low
Infatuated love	Low	High	Low
Romantic love	High	High	Low
Empty love	Low	Low	High
Companionate love	High	Low	High
Fatuous love	Low	High	High
Consummate love	High	High	High

Source: R. J. Sternberg, "The Triangular Theory of Love," *Psychological Review* 93 (1986): 119–135. Copyright 1986 by the American Psychological Association. Reprinted by permission

Is It Love or Infatuation?

In the early stages, love and infatuation can be very similar emotions. They both produce a characteristic rush of excitement as well as a strong desire to have more of the loved one's time, energy, and contact. The primary difference is that with love, the feelings often grow deeper as you get to know the person better and come to appreciate him or her more. With infatuation or a crush, you begin to realize that Ms. or Mr. Right wasn't all you had thought. Taking the following test may help you determine whether it's the real thing or merely a case of infatuation. Respond YES or NO to the following statements:

1. I knew I was in love with the person almost immediately.

2. Even though I've known the person for a while, I still really love his/her personality.

3. I wonder sometimes if the person has changed a lot since I've known him/her because he/she acts differently around me now.

4. The more I'm with the person, the more I want to be around him/her.

5. I am less interested in the person sexually than I was in the beginning.

6. The more I know about the person, the more I want to know.

7. The more I know about the person, the less interested I am in him/her.

8. I feel really good associating with this person and being regarded as a couple.

9. I have begun to notice more things wrong with this person and spend a lot of time trying to get him/her to change.

10. Even though I have been with this person for a while, I am still just as sexually interested as I was in the beginning.

11. I find that I'd just as soon do things with other people as with this person because I'd probably have more fun.

12. I am able to share my feelings with this person and trust him/her completely.

13. I really love this person but don't feel good about sharing intimate feelings with him/her yet.

14. This person brings out the best in me and genuinely seems to care about me.

15. I love this person, but I don't respect him/her the way I respect others.

Scoring

There are no right or wrong responses to these statements. However, answering "yes" to the even-numbered statements may indicate that your feelings are more likely to be love-directed. In contrast, answering "yes" to the odd-numbered statements may indicate a tendency toward infatuation rather than love. Count the number of yeses to the even-numbered statements and the number of yeses to the odd-numbered statements. Look carefully at each statement. Are these things that you feel important enough to work on? Or are your responses telling you that another person may be a better choice?

Lovers who claim that they are swept away by passion may not, therefore, be far from the truth.

"A meeting of the eyes, a touch of the hands or a whiff of scent may set off a flood that starts in the brain and races along the nerves and through the blood. The familiar results—flushed skin, sweaty palms, heavy breathing—are identical to those experienced when under stress. Why? Because the love-smitten person is secreting chemical substances such as dopamine, norepinephrine, and phenylethylamine (PEA) that are chemical cousins of amphetamines."[19]

Although attraction may in fact be a "natural high," with PEA levels soaring, this hit of passion loses effectiveness over time as the body builds up a tolerance. Needing a continual fix of passion, many people may become attraction junkies, seeking the intoxication of love much as the drug user seeks a chemical high.[20]

Fisher speculates that PEA levels drop significantly over a three-to-four-year period, leading to the "four-year itch" that shows up in the peaking fourth-year divorce rates present in over 60 cultures. Those romances that last beyond the four-year decline of PEA are influenced by another set of chemicals, known as endorphins, soothing substances that give lovers a sense of security, peace, and calm.[21]

Oxytocin is also being studied for its role in the love formula. Produced by the brain, it sensitizes nerves and stimulates muscle contractions, the production of breast milk, and the desire for physical closeness between mother and infant. Scientists speculate that oxytocin may encourage similar cuddling between men and women. Oxytocin levels have also been shown to increase dramatically during orgasm for both men and women.[22]

In addition to such possible chemical influences, our past experiences may significantly affect our attractions for others. Our parents' modeling of traits we believe are

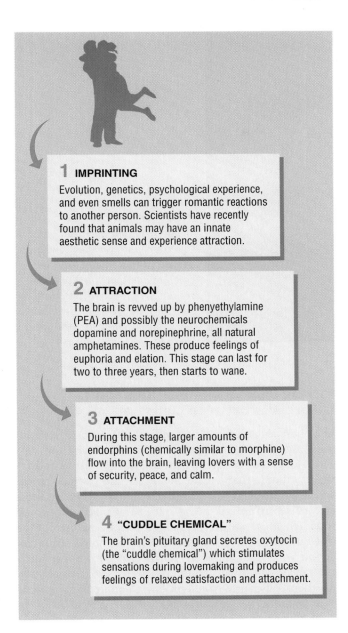

FIGURE 5.2

How do fools fall in love?

Source: Text from graphic by Nigel Holmes, "How Do Fools Fall in Love?" *Time,* February 15, 1993, 50–51. Copyright 1993 Time Inc. Reprinted by permission. Information from Helen E. Fisher, *The Anatomy of Love* (New York: Norton, 1992).

desirable or undesirable may play a role in drawing us to people with similar traits. Many researchers have investigated the possible link between males seeking their own mothers in partners and females seeking their fathers in partners. To date, research on chemical attractions and parent-seeking tendencies is inconclusive and should be viewed only as preliminary findings. Much more research

is needed to confirm these provocative new attraction theories.

GENDER ISSUES: MEN, WOMEN, AND RELATIONSHIPS

In any relationship, understanding and communication are important ingredients for success. Sometimes it may seem that the relating styles of men and women are so different that obtaining true understanding and open communication may be next to impossible. Deborah Tannen summarized the frustration often felt between men and women who are trying to relate to one another in her best-selling book *You Just Don't Understand: Women and Men in Conversation.*[23] According to Tannen, men's and women's social conditioning is so different that it is almost as if they are raised in two different cultures. Women are brought up to feel comfortable and to share freely in their intimate relationships. They tend to be more nurturing and less afraid to share their fears, anxieties, and emotions. It's okay if they cry, scream, or express wide emotional swings. Big boys, however, are not supposed to cry—at least according to popular beliefs. Unlike their female counterparts, they are not supposed to show emotions, and they are brought up to believe that being strong is often more important than having close friendships. As a result, according to research, only 1 male in 10 has a close male friend to whom he divulges his innermost thoughts.[24]

Why the Differences?

Women are usually comfortable expressing highly personal thoughts to female and male intimates, while most men express their emotions to women rather than to other men. Men's conversations with each other revolve most often around sports and sex but not relationships and feelings, whereas women seem to glide effortlessly from conversations about work to feelings and relationships.[25]

Although there are various theories about why males and females relate in the way they do, Lillian Rubin has provided the most comprehensive analysis. Rubin sees a serious barrier to intimacy in what she considers a basic difference in the development patterns of men and women.[26] In her view, men are less able to express emotions and achieve intimacy than are women owing to the process of identity development in infancy, which she sees as more difficult for males than for females. Males initially achieve intimacy with a female caregiver, usually a mother, at a preverbal stage. By the time they have developed verbal skills, boys have physically separated from the caregiver. Thus, for males, intimacy may consist of physi-

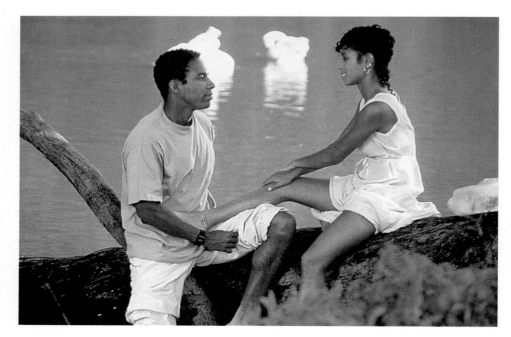

Hollywood and the media have offered countless views of what it means to "fall in love," but we need to question whether these romanticized portrayals create unrealistic expectations about the way committed relationships are formed and maintained.

cal proximity rather than verbal sharing. Because females do not need to separate themselves from a female care-giver, they do not separate their feelings of intimacy from their verbal constructs. Consequently, women are able to express intimacy verbally, whereas men are not. This male/female disparity in the ability to express emotions is both the single greatest difference between the sexes and the greatest threat to intimacy in many relationships. Rubin's theories have received widespread acceptance among sociologists and psychologists today. The disparity in the ability to express emotions may account for common female complaints about male attitudes toward sex. Rubin feels that emotion generates sexual feelings in women, whereas sexual feelings generate emotion in men. Sex, it seems, is one area in which men are allowed to contact deeper emotional states. In fact, sexual activity carries the major burden of emotional expression for many males and may explain the urgency with which some men approach sex.

𝒲HAT DO YOU THINK?

Who are the people with whom you feel most comfortable talking about very personal issues? Do you talk with both males and females about these issues, or do you tend to gravitate toward just one sex? Why do you think you do this?

Dysfunctional family: A family in which the interaction between family members inhibits rather than enhances psychological growth.

Picking Partners: Similarities and Differences between Genders

Just as males and females may find different ways to express themselves, the process of partner selection also shows distinctly different patterns. In both males and females, more than just chemical and psychological processes influence the choice of partners.[27] One of these factors is *proximity,* or being in the same place at the same time. The more you see a person in your hometown, at social gatherings, or at work, the more likely that an interaction will occur. Thus, if you live in New York, you'll probably end up with another New Yorker. If you live in northern Wisconsin, you'll probably end up with another Wisconsinite.

You also pick a partner based on *similarities* (attitudes, values, intellect, interests); the old adage that "opposites attract" usually isn't true. Even though you may initially be attracted to someone who is extremely different from you, first flames usually die quickly and there is a subliminal hunt for common ground.

If your potential partner expresses interest or liking, you may react with mutual regard known as *reciprocity.* The more you express interest, the safer it is for someone else to return the regard, and the cycle spirals onward.

Another factor that apparently plays a significant role in selecting a partner is *physical attraction.* Whether such attraction is caused by a chemical reaction or a socially learned behavior, males and females appear to have different attraction criteria. Men tend to select their mates primarily on the basis of youth and physical attractiveness. Although physical attractiveness is an important criterion for women in mate selection, they tend to place higher emphasis on partners who are somewhat older,

American society is becoming more tolerant of men sharing their emotions and feelings—vital ingredients in close friendships and intimate relationships.

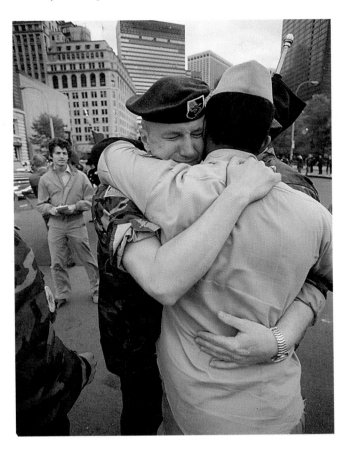

have good financial prospects, and are dependable and industrious. Good grooming is an almost universally desirable trait for both men and women. If you smell or appear less than squeaky clean, you may have problems in the partner arena regardless of your sex.

BARRIERS TO INTIMACY

Obstacles to intimacy include lack of personal identity, emotional immaturity, and a poorly developed sense of responsibility. The fear of being hurt, low self-esteem, mishandled hostility, chronic "busyness" (and its attendant lack of emotional presence), a tendency to "parentify" loved ones, and a conflict of role expectations may be equally detrimental. In addition, individual insecurities and difficulties in recognizing and expressing emotional needs can lead to an intimacy barrier. These barriers to intimacy may have many causes, including the different emotional development of men and women or an upbringing in a dysfunctional family.

Dysfunctional Families

As noted earlier, the ability to sustain genuine intimacy is largely developed in the family of origin. Unfortunately, sharing, trust, and openness do not always occur in the family. In fact, the assumption that such intimacy existed in the family of origin may actually be unrealistic. As adults, we may discover that although we thought our family encouraged emotional intimacy, it was actually judgmental, full of expectations, and, in many ways, dysfunctional. A **dysfunctional family** is one in which the interaction between family members inhibits psychological growth rather than encourages self-love, emotional expression, and individual growth. If you were to examine even the most pristine family under a microscope, you would likely find some type of dysfunction. No group of people who live together day in and day out can interact perfectly all the time. However, many people have begun to overuse the term *dysfunctional* to refer to even the smallest problems in the family unit. As such, the term becomes relatively meaningless. True dysfunctionality refers to settings where negative interactions are the norm rather than the exception. Children raised in these settings tend to face tremendous obstacles to growing up healthy. Coming to terms with past hurts may take years. However, with careful planning and introspection, support from loved ones, and counseling when needed, children from even the worst homes have proved to be remarkably resilient. Many are able to forget the past and to focus on the future, developing into healthy, well-adjusted adults. But some have problems throughout their lives.[28] For example, adults who grew up with alcoholic parents may have serious problems creating and maintaining intimate relationships. The family messages that these children receive are typically very contradictory, as the family usually tries to hide the presence of alcohol abuse in the home. It is important to note that dysfunctional families are found in every social, ethnic, religious, economic, and racial group.

Recently, social scientists have been studying the impact of the alcoholic home environment on the sexual and intimate behavior of adult children of alcoholics (ACOAs). Therapist Mary Ann Klausner has identified a number of intimacy problems as typical of ACOAs. Many ACOAs claim that they become involved in unhealthy relationships, have difficulty trusting others, have problems in communicating with partners, and have difficulty defining a healthy relationship.[29]

Another tragically large group of people struggling with intimacy problems originating in the family of origin are survivors of childhood emotional, physical, and sexual abuse. Experiencing or witnessing physical and emotional abuse as a child can have an impact on a person's intimate relations as an adult. Domestic violence, whether directed at a child or at another family member, can affect a child's ability to trust others and to maintain an intimate relationship later in life. Physical abuse may

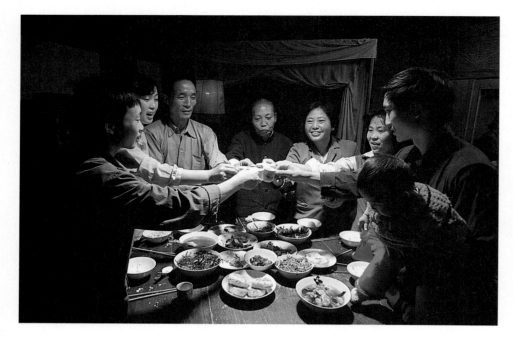

The negative interactions in dysfunctional families that damage self-esteem and deter psychosocial growth do not exist in healthy families that encourage emotional intimacy for all members throughout their lives.

vary from the use of spanking to discipline a child to violent beatings. Emotional abuse includes name-calling and other tactics that damage a child's self-esteem.

Jealousy: The Green-Eyed Monster of Relationships

"Jealousy is like a San Andreas fault running beneath the smooth surface of an intimate relationship. Most of the time, its eruptive potential lies hidden. But when it begins to rumble, the destruction can be enormous."[30] **Jealousy** has been described as an aversive reaction evoked by a real or imagined relationship involving your partner and a third person.

Contrary to what many of us may believe, jealousy is not a sign of intense devotion or of passionate love for the person who is the target of it. Instead, jealousy is often a sign of underlying problems that may prove to be a significant barrier to a healthy intimate relationship. The

Jealousy: An aversive reaction evoked by a real or imagined relationship involving a person's partner and a third person.

Monogamy: Exclusive sexual involvement with one partner.

Serial monogamy: Monogamous sexual relationship with one partner before moving on to another.

Open relationship: A relationship in which partners agree that there can be sexual involvement outside the relationship.

roots of jealous feelings and behaviors may run deep. Causes of jealousy typically include the following:

- *Overdependence on the relationship.* People who have few social ties and who rely exclusively on their significant others tend to be fearful of losing them.

- *High value on sexual exclusivity.* People who believe that sexual exclusiveness is a crucial indicator of a love relationship are more likely to become jealous. As the expectation of sexual exclusivity increases, the likelihood of becoming jealous also increases.

- *Severity of the threat.* People may feel uneasy if a person with a fantastic body, stunning good looks, and a great personality appears interested in their partners. But they may brush off the threat if they appraise the person as "unworthy" in terms of appearance or other characteristics.

- *Low self-esteem.* People who feel good about themselves are less likely to feel unworthy and to fear that someone else is going to snatch their partners away from them. The underlying question that torments people with low self-esteem is, "Why would anyone want me?" Thus, everyone other than the "beloved" becomes a threat.

- *Fear of losing control.* Some people need to feel in control of the situation. Feeling that they may be losing the attachment of or control over a partner can cause jealousy.

Although men and women react differently to jealousy, in both sexes it appears to be related to the expectation that it would be difficult to find another relationship if the current one should end. For men, jealousy is positively correlated with self-evaluative dependency, the degree to which the man's self-esteem is affected by his partner's judgments.

$\mathcal{W}$HAT DO YOU THINK?

Has anyone ever acted jealous about you spending time with or being around another person? How did it make you feel? Why do you think it made you feel that way?

$\mathcal{C}$OMMITTED RELATIONSHIPS

Feelings of love or sexual attraction are not always equated with commitment in a relationship. There can be love without commitment and there can be sex without commitment. Commitment in a relationship with another person means that there is an intent to act over time in a way that perpetuates the well-being of the other person, yourself, and the relationship. A committed relationship involves tremendous diligence on the part of both partners. Over the years, partners learn about one another and constantly adjust the direction of their relationship. The Building Communication Skills box may help you evaluate your relationship's present state and may point to positive changes you can make.

The amount of work involved in creating a successful relationship may intimidate the uncommitted person. It should be remembered that very few people have the skills and tools at the beginning of a relationship to sustain it. What separates committed from uncommitted relationships is the willingness of committed partners to dedicate themselves toward acquiring and using the skills that will ensure a lasting relationship.

Polls have shown that as many as 96 percent of Americans strive to develop a committed relationship. Many support groups are available to help couples contemplating commitments to start their journey. In the case of couples who wish to marry, some religions require premarital counseling by trained clergy or other professionals prior to arranging a wedding. Other organizations, such as Engagement Encounter, offer nondenominational weekend retreats for engaged couples to help them communicate better and define their expectations of marriage to one another.

People not wishing to involve themselves with religious organizations may find premarriage counseling or support groups through community mental health facilities.

Marriage

Marriage is the traditional committed relationship in many societies around the world. For many people, marriage is the ultimate expression of an intimate relationship. When two people marry in the United States, they enter into a legal agreement that includes shared financial plans, property, and responsibility in raising children. For religious people, marriage is also a sacrament that stresses the spirituality, rights, and obligations of each person. Close to 90 percent of all Americans marry at least once, compared to 95 percent in the 1970s. However, the United States Census Bureau reports that in recent years Americans have become more particular about commitment and more reluctant to marry young. In 1990, the median age for first marriage was higher than ever before: 26.1 years for men and 23.9 years for women, compared with 22.5 and 20.6, respectively, in 1970.[31] Nearly 80 percent of people who divorce will remarry, indicating that most married couples find marriage desirable.

Most Americans believe that marriage involves **monogamy,** or exclusive sexual involvement with one partner. The lifetime pattern for many Americans appears to be **serial monogamy,** which means that a person has a monogamous sexual relationship with one partner for the duration of a relationship before moving on to another monogamous relationship. Some people prefer to have an **open relationship,** or open marriage, in which the partners agree that there may be sexual involvement for each person outside their relationship.

Humans are not naturally monogamous; that is, most of us are capable of being sexually and/or emotionally involved with more than one person at a time. Yet, American society frowns on involvement with an outsider when we are involved in a relationship and profess to be committed. Many people find themselves being attracted to

Shared values and beliefs can help validate a committed relationship and lead to lasting contentment for both partners.

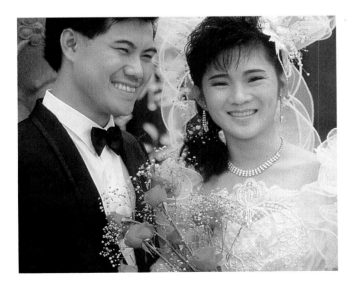

Communicating with Your Partner

How well do you and your partner know each other? Do you communicate your feelings, fears, frustrations, and hopes to one another? Completing this exercise may help you evaluate areas that you may need to work on.

1. Do you feel that your partner often does not seem to understand you? _____

2. Do you think your partner is pleased with your overall appearance? _____

3. Are you able to give constructive criticism to each other? _____

4. In appropriate places, do you openly show your affection? _____

5. When you disagree, does the same person usually give in? _____

6. Are you able to discuss money matters with each other? _____

7. Are you able to discuss religion and politics without arguing? _____

8. Do you often know what your partner is going to say before he/she says it? _____

9. Are you afraid of your partner's reactions to things that you do or say? _____

10. Do you know where your partner wants to be in five years? _____

11. Is your sense of humor basically the same as your partner's? _____

12. Do you have the persistent feeling you do not really know each other or have never really talked about important issues? _____

13. Would you be able to give an accurate biography of your partner? Do you know about his/her past experiences? _____

14. Do you know your partner's secret fantasy? _____

15. Do you feel you have to avoid discussion of many topics with your partner? _____

16. Does your partner know your biggest flaw? _____

17. Does your partner know what you are most afraid of? _____

18. Do you both take a genuine interest in each other's work? _____

19. Can you judge your partner's mood accurately by watching his/her body language? _____

20. Do you know who your partner's favorite relatives are and why? _____

21. Do you know what things you may say that could hurt your partner's feelings? _____

22. Do you know the number of children your partner would like to have? _____

Scoring

Look over your responses and give yourself one point for each "yes" response to numbers 2, 3, 4, 6, 7, 8, 10, 11, 13, 14, and 16 to 22 and one point for each "no" response to numbers 1, 5, 9, 12, and 15.

1–5: This may indicate a low level of communication/interaction between you and your partner. However, you are together, so you must be fulfilling some need through your relationship. Perhaps the two of you simply need to develop better communication.

6–9: This may indicate that your communication/interaction level is rather low, but perhaps you are trying to improve your interactions. What actions might you take?

10–14: This may indicate a moderate communication/interaction level with some room for improvement. Just keep working on the development of open and honest communication.

15–18: You seem to have a strong communication/interaction level, but you do have your differences. With open communication, you are learning to deal with your differences, which will strengthen the relationship.

19–22: You seem to have a great understanding of each other and what it takes to make a successful relationship. Keep being honest, talking, and sharing your feelings.

After rating yourself, what areas do you need to work on? What steps can you take to improve your overall level of communication and intimacy levels?

_____

Source: Adapted by permission of McGraw-Hill, Inc., from Robert F. Valois and Sandra Kammermann, *Your Sexuality: A Personal Inventory* (New York: Random House, 1984), 128–129.

others while in a relationship and consciously try to stop any subsequent interactions. Others find themselves involved unintentionally. Still others actively seek out extra-relationship affairs. Whether by choice or chance, sexual infidelity is an extremely common factor in divorces and breakups. Perhaps only those having strong self-images

and a dedication to the principles of open relationships are able to maintain nonmonogamy over a period of time.

As with all relationships, there are marriages that work well and bring much satisfaction to the partners, and there are marriages that are unhealthy for the people involved. A good marriage can yield much support and stability, not only for the couple, but also for those involved in the couple's life. Considerable research also indicates that married people live longer, are happier, remain mentally alert longer, and suffer fewer bouts with physical and mental ailments. In the late 1980s, Wood and Glenn found that modern married women may not be as happy as their parents were and that the happiness of never-married men had increased.[32] Whether due to the increasing pressures on women to work, take care of the family, and perform multiple roles, or to some other expectations, these figures may indicate future problems that must be addressed in future years. Because marriage is socially sanctioned and highly celebrated in our culture, there are numerous incentives for couples to stay together and to improve their relationships. Behavioral scientists agree that couples who make some type of formal commitment are more likely to stay together and develop the fulfilling relationship they initially sought than are those who do not commit.

Cohabitation

For various reasons, many people prefer to live together without the bonds of matrimony. Commonly called **cohabitation,** this type of relationship is defined as two people who have an intimate connection with each other who live together in the same household. The relationship can be very stable with a high level of commitment between the partners. Cohabitation that lasts a designated number of years (usually seven) constitutes a **common-law marriage** for purposes of real estate and other financial obligations in some states.

It is believed that increasing numbers of Americans will opt to cohabit in the 1990s due to loneliness, soaring housing costs, and a variety of "practical" reasons. The increase in cohabitation and the decrease in willingness to make a formal marriage commitment was a major research topic of the 1980s. According to the Census Bureau, in 1992 there were over 3.2 million cohabitors in the United States, a rise of over 80 percent since the early 1980s.[33] Elderly cohabitors and others who live together for economic reasons or for company are believed to contribute substantially to these large numbers.

This dramatic increase may be partly attributed to youth's inclination to question traditional values and to the expanding recognition that marriage may not be the only legitimate basis for sexual relations. Cheaper, more effective birth control has probably been another factor. Many couples also believe that living together simply because they want to may be more important than being bound by a legal document.

Although cohabitation is a viable alternative for some, many cohabitors eventually marry because of pressures from parents and friends, difficulties in obtaining insurance and tax benefits, legal issues over property, and a host of other reasons. In addition, many cohabitors simply decide they want to solidify their relationships.

The disadvantage of cohabitation lies in the lack of societal validation for the relationship and, in some cases, in the societal disapproval of living together without being married. Cohabiting partners do not usually experience the social incentives to stay together that they would if they were married. If they decide to separate, however, they do not experience the legal problems involved in going through a divorce. Today, several states are considering legislation to legally validate the relationship between committed partners who live together but do not marry. Eligibility for tax deductions, health insurance benefits, and other issues are among those being considered for cohabiting adults.

Gay and Lesbian Partnerships

Most people seek intimate, committed relationships during their adult years. This is no different for gay and lesbian (homosexual) couples. Lesbians and gay men are socialized like other people in our culture and tend to place a high value on relationships. They seek the same things in their primary relationships as do heterosexual partners: friendship, communication, validation, companionship, and a sense of stability. Studies of lesbian couples indicate high levels of attachment and satisfaction and a tendency toward monogamous, long-term relationships. Gay men, too, tend to form committed, long-term relationships, especially as they age.[34]

Challenges to successful lesbian and gay male relationships often stem from the discrimination they face as homosexuals and to difficulties dealing with social, legal, and religious doctrines. For lesbian and gay couples, cohabiting is usually the only available option as very few cities or states currently recognize same-sex marriages.

SUCCESS IN COMMITTED RELATIONSHIPS

Because the traditional marriage ceremony includes the vow "till death do us part," the definition of success in a relationship tends to be based on whether a couple stays together over the years. Marriage has become the model

Cohabitation: Living together without being married.

Common-law marriage: Cohabitation lasting a designated period of time (usually seven years) that is considered legally binding in some states.

that relationships must conform to in order to be considered stable or healthy. One reason for the increase in cohabitation and other alternative relationships is the need for new forms in which people can express their love and commitment to one another and still have individual needs met more adequately. Success in relating to another human being may have more to do with the quality of the interaction between two people than with the number of years they continue to live together. Many social scientists agree that the ideal in relating to another person is to develop a committed bond, the boundaries and form of which can change to allow the maximum degree of growth over time.

Partnering Scripts

Most parents love their children and want them to be happy. They often believe that their children will achieve happiness by living much as they have. They chose to marry and raise a family, and they expect their children to follow a similar pattern. These expectations usually come from wanting the best for their children rather than from an overt desire to control their lives. Accordingly, children are reared with a very strong script for what is expected of them as adults. This "scripting" is part of what maintains stability within a society. By individuals partnering with someone similar to their families of origin, groups within society remain discernible; children of upper-class parents usually remain in the upper class, children of white partners usually marry a white partner, and so forth. Each group in society has its own partnering script that includes similarities of sex, age, social class, race, religion, physical attributes, and personality types of the prospective partner. By adolescence, people generally know exactly what type of person they are expected to befriend or to date. If you are unsure of the partnering scripts by which you were raised, just picture whom you could or couldn't bring home to meet your family.

For people who select a potential mate based on the script with which they were raised, an elaboration of the concept may seem unnecessary. Yet there are two reasons why it is important to consider the concept of partnering scripts: (1) you may be among the group that has not chosen an "appropriate" partner, or (2) social approval of your mate selection may bring with it other subtle expectations of your behavior as a couple.

People who have not chosen an "appropriate" partner are subject to a great deal of external stress. Recognizing that this stress is external to the relationship can help alleviate criticism and distancing between the partners. Society provides constant reinforcement for traditional couples, but it withholds this reinforcement from couples of the same sex, mixed race, mixed religion, and mixed age. Social reinforcement includes invitations to events, inquiries about a partner who is not present, and introductions to friends and family. In addition to denying reinforcement to such a couple, friends and family often blame the "inappropriateness" of the couple if the relationship fails.

Yet, despite these obstacles, many nontraditional relationships survive and flourish. For example, the number of interracial marriages has quadrupled since the late 1960s. More than 1 of every 50 marriages in the United States is now interracial. Many interracial couples report that their lives are not much different from anyone else's, although they are still occasional targets of a dirty look or a muttered slur. These problems may arise because such marriages force people to discard stereotypes unwillingly.

People who choose an "appropriate" partner usually have plenty of validation for the relationship. The love and support they feel from friends and family is genuine. It also comes with expectations of what will occur within the relationship. Decisions that the couple feel should be exclusively theirs may provoke unsolicited advice from friends and family. The concept of "boundaries" may be helpful in learning how to minimize this external stress on a relationship. Boundaries are the lines drawn around a couple that mark them off from the rest of the social world. The lines consist of silent social agreements about the rights and privileges of two people as a couple. The marriage contract automatically establishes boundaries defining things one would or wouldn't do "because I am married."

Partners in a couple need to view themselves as a unit whose foremost consideration is the quality of their relationship, irrespective of external opinions or pressures. It is sometimes difficult, but important, to stand together on issues as a couple in the face of interference or disapproval from loved ones. Stresses inherent in relating intimately to another human being are intense enough; letting the whole world have direct input into the relationship can break it.

Most people who try to influence a couple's relationship do so out of love and respect for the people involved. It is important to remember, especially when relating to parents, that their concern usually comes from a desire for the couple's well-being. They associate well-being with living the way they lived or, in some cases, with living better than they lived. In either case, it is possible to appreciate parents' viewpoints but choose to live in a different manner if that is what the couple wants.

*W*HAT DO YOU THINK?

What characteristics are most important to you in a potential partner? Which of these would be important to your parents or friends? If your parents or friends didn't like a potential partner, how important would their opinion be?

Friends and Lovers: A Cross-Cultural Comparison

Do people of all cultures value the same traits in friends and lovers? The answer is clearly no. Two researchers from the University of Keele in England examined whether British and Hong Kong Chinese university students valued the same traits in friends and romantic partners. Half of the participants of each nationality indicated their preference for a romantic partner, and the other half indicated their preferences for a friend. The items on the questionnaires were bipolar opposites, such as "lively" versus "not lively," and students chose which items best characterized their choices for friends or romantic partners.

Results showed that, overall, romantic partners were expected to be more honest and caring than friends were expected to be. In addition, the British students stressed the importance of sensitivity and humor in both romantic partners and friends, but the Hong Kong Chinese students stressed money-mindedness and creativity.

This was a simple study using straightforward questions and methodology; however, it illustrates the complexity of human interactions and the role that our culture plays in determining our choices. It shows that we choose different people for friends and lovers; and, most important from a multicultural perspective, our choices depend on our culture.

Other results support these conclusions. When Susan Sprecher and her colleagues compared the cultural similar-ities in love attitudes and experiences among Japanese, Americans, and Russians, they found some sharp differences. For example, the Japanese were less romantic than the other groups, the Americans were more likely to associate love with marriage than were the other groups, and the Russians were the most excitable and had the most trouble staying calm when in love. Similar findings have been shown in other cross-cultural studies of mate preferences. Other studies often show gender differences in addition to cultural differences. For example, men value attractiveness more than do women; and women accord more weight than men do to socioeconomic status, ambitiousness, and character. These gender differences vary little with culture.

As these studies show, there are cultural differences in the way love is felt and expressed, especially when it comes to the importance of factors leading up to the love experience. Yet similarities abound. In the arena of love, culture seems to have a somewhat less predictable impact then we might expect. In addition, cross-cultural studies are often of college students; as researchers study a wider sample of participants, our knowledge of relationships and love will grow more comprehensive.

Source: Adapted from Lester A. Lefton, *Psychology,* 5th ed., 637.
© Copyright 1994 by Allyn & Bacon. Reprinted by permission.

The Importance of Self-Nurturance

It is often stated that you must love yourself before you can love someone else. What does this mean? Learning how you function emotionally and how to nurture yourself through all life's situations is a lifelong task. You should certainly not postpone intimate connections with others until you have achieved this state. There does, however, seem to be a certain level of individual maturity that needs to be reached before a successful intimate relationship becomes possible. In the case of marriage relationships, divorce rates are much higher for couples under the age of 30 than for older couples, as Table 5.2 shows.

Two concepts that are especially important to knowing yourself and maintaining a good relationship are "accountability" and "self-nurturance." **Accountability** means that both partners see themselves as responsible for their own decisions and actions. The other person is not held responsible for the positive or negative experiences in life. This eliminates the very common feeling of being "used" in a relationship. Each and every choice is one's own responsibility. A partner can no longer leave a relationship saying, "She ruined my life," or, "He made me do it!" When two people are accountable for their own emotional states, partners can be angry, sad, or frustrated without the other person taking it personally. Accountable people may even say something like, "This has nothing to do with you; I just happen to be angry right now."

Self-nurturance goes hand-in-hand with accountability. In order to make good choices in life, a person needs to maintain a balance of sleeping, eating, exercising, working, relaxing, and socializing. When the balance is disrupted, as it will inevitably be, self-nurturing people

Accountability: Accepting responsibility for personal decisions, choices, and actions.

Self-nurturance: Developing individual potential through a balanced and realistic appreciation of self-worth and ability.

TABLE 5.2 ■ Divorce Rates by Sex and Age, 1993*

Age	Men	Women
15–19	43.1	45.8
20–24	48.8	45.1
25–29	37.4	35.1
30–34	32.0	29.1
35–39	27.6	23.7
40–44	22.4	18.7
45–49	16.8	12.0
50–54	10.5	7.1
55–59	6.9	4.8
60–64	4.5	3.0
65 years and over	1.7	1.3

*Rates per 100 married couples.

Source: National Center for Health Statistics, *Monthly Vital Statistics Report,* May, 1993.

are patient with themselves and try to put things back on course. When they make bad choices, as all people do, self-nurturing people learn from the experience. It is a lifelong process to learn to live in a balanced and healthy way. Two people who are on a path of accountability and self-nurturance together have a much better chance of maintaining satisfying relationships.

Elements of Good Relationships

Relationships that are satisfying and stable share certain elements. Some of these are achieved through conscious efforts and communication; others evolve over time. People in healthy committed relationships trust one another. Without trust, intimacy will not develop and the relationship will experience trouble and possible failure. **Trust** can be defined as the degree of confidence felt in a relationship. Trust includes three fundamental elements: predictability, dependability, and faith.

- *Predictability* means that you can predict your partner's behavior. This sense of predictability is based on the knowledge that your partner acts in consistently positive ways.

- *Dependability* means that you can rely on your partner to give support in all situations, particularly in those in which you feel threatened with hurt or rejection.

- *Faith* means that you feel absolutely certain about your partner's intentions and behavior.

Trust can be developed even in relationships in which it is initially lacking. Trust development requires opening oneself to others, which carries the risk of hurt or rejection. The key to developing trust is learning to interpret a partner's behavior. Although changing a partner's behavior may not be possible, changing the interpretation and

reaction to it is. In good relationships, people interpret each other's behavior in the context of the current relationship. They acknowledge each other's positive qualities and allow room for mistakes. They do not overreact to behaviors that remind them of previous sensitive events that trigger emotional insecurities. For example, if a partner in an earlier relationship was continually flirting with other people and cheating on you, a current partner dancing with someone else at a party could unknowingly trigger the unpleasant memories of infidelity. Trusting people never assume that a current partner will behave as an earlier partner did.

Trust and intimacy are the foundation of healthy committed relationships. Spouses who like and enjoy one another as people and find each other interesting frequently are happier than those who don't. Many spouses describe their partners as their best friends. Although most marriages have their share of ups and downs, members of successful couples are able to talk to, listen to, and touch one another in an atmosphere of caring. They value a good sense of humor and exhibit communication, cooperation, and the ability to resolve conflicts constructively.

Sexual intimacy is also a major part of healthy relationships, but sex is not a major reason for the existence of the relationship. Some couples admit to sexual dissatisfaction within their relationships but feel the relationship is more important than sexual satisfaction. Rather than seek an outlet in an extramarital affair, those who are dissatisfied with their sex lives adjust and spend little energy worrying about it because the relationship is satisfying in other, more important ways. Many couples report that as communication and trust increase in a long-term, committed relationship, the entire sexual relationship also improves.

Spouses in happily married couples are open to and aware of one another's flaws. Having no expectations of perfection in their spouses, they are able to live with their spouses' unchangeable qualities. Couples value flexibility and openness to change in their partners. Some couples make periodic decisions to "stay married." An assumption of permanence underlines these relationships. Each partner's belief in commitment is strong. To satisfied couples, commitment means a willingness to experience periodic unhappiness because troubled times cannot be avoided in the course of human life. Furthermore, happily married couples refuse to see divorce or separation as a viable option when problems arise. Shared values, life goals, and interests are characteristic of contented couples, yet each partner pursues interests and activities individually and with other people. Happily married people seem to be secure enough in their relationships that jealousy over outside friendships is nonexistent.

One important quality of successful relationships is a shared and cherished history, including private jokes, code words and nicknames, rituals, emotions, and significant shared time and activities. Equally important is luck. Luck in choosing a partner was first, followed by luck in life events. Certain events, such as major illnesses, unemployment, career failures, family feuds, or the death of a child, can derail an otherwise good marriage. Determination to succeed as a couple can help offset these occurrences, but some couples seem destined to endure more tragedy than others and the tragedies can undermine the relationship.

Confronting Couple Issues

Couples seeking a long-term relationship have to confront a number of issues that can enhance or ruin their chances of success. Some of these issues are gender roles and power sharing.

Changing Gender Roles. Throughout history, women and men have taken on various roles in their relationships. In agricultural America, family and gender roles were determined by tradition. Each task within a family unit held equal importance. Keeping the family well fed and warmly clothed was as essential as driving a tractor or putting in the hay. There was mutual dependence between wives and husbands. With the Industrial Revolution and urbanization, many people left the farms to work in the cities. During World War II, when men went overseas, women by the thousands left their homes or other jobs to work in factories and defense plants. Many women enjoyed the independence and money that came from working outside the home, but when the war ended and the men returned from overseas, they usually reclaimed their traditional jobs. The government and advertising agencies made an effort in post-World War II America to convince women to return to the home. American women of the 1950s were portrayed in movies to be happy in their kitchens.

Unlike an agricultural culture, our modern society has very few gender-specific roles. Women and men alike drive cars, care for children, operate computers, read, do yard work, write, talk on the telephone, and perform equally well in the tasks of daily living. Because certain tasks are essential to run a family unit, couples need to devise some way to divide the labor. However, as opposed to taking on the "traditional" female and male roles, many couples find it makes more sense to divide tasks on the basis of schedule, convenience, and preference of activity. While it may make sense to divide household chores, it rarely works out that the division is equal. Even when women work full time, they tend to bear heavy family and household responsibilities. These multiple roles cause significant stress and may seriously impair health. Over time, if couples are unable to communicate about how they feel about performing certain tasks, the relationship may suffer.

Sharing Power. Power can be defined as the ability to make and implement decisions. There are many ways to exercise power, but powerful people are those who know what they want and have the ability to attain it. In tradi-

tional marriages, husbands were the wage earners and consequently had decision-making power. Wives exerted much influence, but in the final analysis they needed a husband's income for survival. But as women became wage earners in increasing numbers, the power dynamics between women and men changed. As long as men as a group earn substantially more money than women, there will continue to be greater decision-making capacity for men. Within individual households, however, the dynamics have shifted considerably, with greater numbers of women working and having their own financial resources. Part of the increase in the divorce rate undoubtedly reflects the recognition by working women that they can leave bad relationships in which they previously felt confined. In general, successful couples arrange power relationships that reflect their unique needs rather than popular marital stereotypes.

$\mathcal{S}$TAYING SINGLE

While many people choose to marry, have children, and follow in the footsteps of their ancestors, increasing numbers of young and older adults have elected to remain single. In 1970, 18.9 percent of adult men and 13.7 percent of adult women had decided that marriage wasn't for them. Their acceptance into career ladders in the work force allowed women to care for themselves financially. Large numbers of men and women gave marriage a try and found out that it wasn't for them. It became acceptable for many people to say, "No . . . sorry . . . not interested," and to pursue their lives without the stigma of being an "old maid" or a "confirmed bachelor." Grandmothers and grandfathers who had stayed together for 30 years or more for the sake of the children, religion, or "what the neighbors might think" began to say, "I've had it," and, "I want more out of life," and to set out in search of personal autonomy and a new life. Older women outlived their husbands and discovered that the number of healthy older men was limited. Many of these women decided to stay single rather than to take on a caretaker role. What were the results of all of this societal change? By the late 1980s, the proportion of adult Americans who were single by choice or by chance (often after failed marriages) had increased to slightly over 25 percent of adult men and over 20 percent of adult women. In addition,

- Americans who choose marriage now choose it much later in life (the median age for first marriages is 25.5 for men and 23.3 for women)

Trust: The degree of confidence felt in a relationship.
Power: The ability to make and implement decisions.

- it is estimated that by the year 2000, over 10 percent of all people will never marry
- people marrying today have a 50 to 55 percent chance of divorcing (some research indicates that this trend may be improving)[35]

Today, large numbers of people choose to or are forced by circumstances to remain single. While many of these people seek or have sought committed relationships, in the absence of a suitable partner, they find singlehood preferable. Singles clubs, social outings arranged by communities and churches, extended family environments, and a large number of social services support the single lifestyle. Although some research indicates that single people live shorter lives, are more unhappy, are more likely to be financially distressed, and are more prone to illnesses than their married counterparts, other studies refute these conclusions.[36] Few research studies to date have controlled for other confounding variables, such as environmental conditions, past histories, and other factors that may be more important than the married or single state. Many single people live rich, rewarding lives and maintain a large network of close friends and families. Although sexual intimacy may or may not be present, the intimacy achieved through other interactions with loved ones is a key aspect of the single person's lifestyle. Many single people use singlehood as a prelude to eventual marriage. They test the waters with potential partners and take time for individual growth, thereby maximizing their chances for successful relationships.

*H*AVING CHILDREN

The presence of children in the home necessarily changes the lives of the adults around them. When a couple decides to raise children, their relationship changes. Resources of time, energy, and money are split many ways, and the partners no longer have each other's undivided attention. Babies and young children do not time their requests for food, sleep, and care to the convenience of adults. Therefore, individuals or couples whose own basic needs for security, love, and purpose are already met make better parents. Any stresses that already exist in a relationship are further accentuated when parenting is added to the list of responsibilities. Having a child does not save a bad relationship and, in fact, only seems to compound the problems that already exist. A child cannot and should not be expected to provide the parents with self-esteem and security.

Changing patterns in family life affect the way children are raised. In modern society, it is not always clear which partner will adjust his or her work schedule to provide the primary care of children. Nearly half a million children per year become part of a blended family when their parents remarry; remarriage creates a new family of stepparents and stepsiblings. In addition, an increasing number of individuals are choosing to have children in a family structure other than a heterosexual marriage. Single women can choose adoption or alternative (formerly "artificial") insemination as a way to create a family. Single men can choose to adopt or can obtain the services of a surrogate mother. Regardless of the structure of the family, certain factors remain important to the well-being of the unit: consistency, communication, affection, and mutual respect.

Some people become parents without a lot of forethought. Some children are born into a relationship that was supposed to last and didn't. This does not mean it is too late to do a good job of parenting. Attention, consistency, and caring can be provided by other adults if a parent cannot be physically or emotionally present for a period of time. Children are amazingly resilient and forgiving if parents show respect to them and communicate about household activities that affect their lives. Even children who grew up in a household of conflict can feel loved and respected if the parents treat them fairly. This means that parents take responsibility for any of their own conflicts and make it clear to the children that they are not the reason for the conflict.

Who Will Care for Tomorrow's Babies?

In 1993, over 64 percent of mothers with children under the age of five worked outside the home. While their mothers were away, over 44 percent of these children were cared for in someone else's home, 23 to 28 percent were cared for in their own homes, 15 to 20 percent went to day-care centers, 6 to 7 percent went to preschools, and another 6 to 7 percent were cared for at work by company-sponsored programs. The average cost of day care exceeded $150 per week per child in 1993, with considerably higher costs prevailing in certain regions of the country. The burden of finding alternative means of child care, particularly on very young parents from low-income families, is very serious.[37]

The changes in the traditional family structure force society to examine alternative means of raising our children. Day-care centers, extended families, and live-in baby-sitters will all become important alternatives to the traditional parental unit.

*W*HAT DO YOU THINK?

What are the essential characteristics of a healthy "family" environment? Why is having such an environment so important to the future development of our children? Do you think that day-care centers, extended family units, and full-time baby-sitters have equal chances of providing a positive environment for personal growth? Why or why not?

$\mathcal{E}$NDING A RELATIONSHIP

The Warning Signs

The symptoms of a troubled relationship are relatively easy to recognize. Many couples choose to ignore them, however, until the situation erupts into some type of emotional confrontation. By then, the relationship may be beyond salvaging.

Breakdowns in relationships usually begin with a change in communication, however subtle. Either partner may stop listening, ceasing to be emotionally present for the other. In turn, the other feels ignored, unappreciated, or unwanted. Unresolved conflicts may increase, and unresolved anger can cause problems in sexual relations, with one partner not wanting sex and perhaps giving in and subsequently feeling used.

When a couple who previously enjoyed spending time alone together find themselves continually in the company of others or spending time apart, it may be a sign that the relationship is in trouble. Of course, individual privacy and **autonomy** (the ability to care for oneself emotionally, socially, and physically) are important. If, however, a partner decides to make a change in the amount and quality of time spent together without the input or understanding of the other, it may be a sign of hidden problems.

People with a good sense of their own identity and the ability to nurture themselves will not allow themselves to be treated poorly in a relationship. However, college students, particularly those who have remained socially isolated and who are far from family and hometown friends, may be particularly vulnerable. You may find that you have become emotionally dependent on a person for everything from eating your meals to recreational and study time. You may find yourself dependent on unhealthy relationships for shared rental arrangements, transportation, child care, and other obligations. In these situations, emotional abuse is often unidentified yet can have devastating effects on the self-esteem of both the abused and the abuser. You may mistake unwanted sexual advances for physical attraction or love and find yourself in situations that are far from the idyllic love scenes you may watch on television. Without a network of friends and supporters to talk with, to obtain validation for your feelings, and/or to share your concerns, you may find yourself in a relationship that is headed nowhere. Breaking up may be difficult and support for your breakup may not be there when you need it. Knowing how to access the services of trained counselors through your student health services or other community and campus groups is critical in these situations.

Honesty and verbal affection are usually very positive aspects of a relationship. In a troubled relationship, however, they can be used to cover up irresponsible or hurtful behavior. "At least I was honest" is not an acceptable sub-

Unresolved conflicts and frequent emotional confrontations are signs of a troubled relationship, but if the partners are committed to staying together, counseling can often bring about positive change.

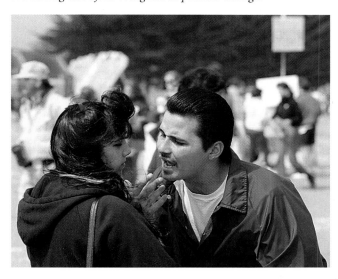

stitute for acting in a trustworthy way. The words "But I really do love you" should not be used as a license to be inconsiderate, rude, or hurtful to a partner.

Seeking Help: Where to Look

The first place some people look for help when there are problems in a relationship is a trusted friend. Although friends can offer needed support during trying times, few have the training and detachment necessary to resolve problems. Others find that they do not have the type of friendships that lend themselves to divulging deep secrets or problems.

Most communities have private practitioners trained to counsel married or committed couples. Community mental health centers usually have trained counselors as well. These practitioners may be psychiatrists, licensed psychologists, social workers, or counselors having advanced degrees. These counselors are often specially equipped to deal with the unique needs of young adults having relationship, sexual, emotional, financial, or other concerns. Most student health centers and/or counseling centers on campus have reduced student fees for students who need help. If you are unaware of such services, talk with your instructor and ask for his or her advice about where someone with your type of problem may get help.

A counselor's first step is to ascertain how much the troubled partners want to stay together. If their commit-

Autonomy: The ability to care for oneself emotionally, socially, and physically.

Developing Intimate Relationships

List the people in your life with whom you have intimate relationships. How would you rate each of these relationships in terms of need fulfillment? Emotional attachment? What kind of intimacy do you share with each person on your list? Write down some dimensions of intimacy you might like to share further, and suggest ways to make those improvements.

Think back on how your family life affected your development of personal relationships. Did the interaction between family members inhibit your psychological growth, or did it encourage self-esteem, emotional openness, and intimacy? From what you learned in your family relationships, what characteristics would you like to keep? What would you like to replace? What kinds of family relationships would you want to create when you have children? How could you make your future family network provide a sense of security and warmth?

Reflect on a love relationship of your own and describe the components of that relationship. How well do you and your partner know each other? What kinds of experiences and ideas do you need to share more fully? Do you know how to express your love verbally? Physically? If not, try to talk about these matters with your partner. Evaluate the level of trust in the relationship. If trust is lacking, list specific areas in which greater trust is needed and discuss with your partner how you might develop it.

---

ment to the relationship is strong, their chances of succeeding are greater. The counselor then interviews the partners separately and together, gradually helping them to recognize and change the behaviors and attitudes that are detrimental to the relationship. Counseling may take a few weeks, several months, or even years as couples reexamine their values and reestablish their commitment. Beware of the counselor who tells you to drop the relationship on the first visit or who tries to give advice without hearing the full story. Most good counselors will spend a good deal of time letting you tell them what you want to do and helping you work through your feelings rather than adopt theirs.

Trial Separations

Sometimes a relationship becomes so dysfunctional that even counseling cannot bring about significant change. Moving apart for a period of time may allow some preliminary healing and give both parties an opportunity to reassess themselves and their commitment to the relationship. Trial separations do not guarantee that the situation will improve, nor do they mean the relationship is ending. If both people are involved in counseling or have other support systems and mutually agree on the need for a trial separation, it may be a way to regroup and save a failing relationship.

Why Relationships End

Each year, more than a million couples in the United States end their marriages. Many others end relationships of all types. The reasons for relationship breakdown are numerous. Tragedies such as the death of a child, serious illness of one partner, severe financial reverses, and career failures certainly contribute to divorces and relationship endings. Somehow, communication and cooperation between partners break down under the additional stress of these burdens.

What about breakups between people who have never experienced these tragedies? These breakups arise from unmet expectations regarding marriage or relationships in general or personal roles within the relationship. Many people enter marriage with expectations about what marriage will be like and how they and their partner will behave. Many people enter relationships looking for someone to fill the empty spots in their lives. Failure to communicate such expectations to your partner can lead to resentment and disappointment. Because many premarital expectations may be unreasonable, early exploration of these expectations is important. This exploration may take place together or within a support program.

Differences in sexual needs may also contribute to the demise of a relationship. Many partners find that their spouses desire sex at different times or in different styles and frequencies than they do. Unless sexual differences are resolved, one or both partners may begin to feel used and resent sexual activity. In other cases, the deterioration of a relationship cannot be attributed to any one event or action. Sometimes, because people fall in love so quickly, once they really get to know the other person the initial "click" that seemed so important begins to fade. Sometimes the man or woman of your dreams may become your worst nightmare. It is often interesting to think back on the past loves of your life and to wonder how you ever could have thought that a particular person was so wonderful. Is it because you've changed? Or is it because the other person never made any changes? The bottom line is that if couples do not grow together, they often grow apart. Without a commitment to working on their differences, many find it easier to move on, and this decision may be best for all concerned.

Building Better Relationships

After you have read this chapter, it should be apparent that relationships involve complex interactions between individuals. To build strong relationships, you must carefully assess the values that you put on friendships, significant others, and other forms of interpersonal interactions. Healthy relationships involve developing intimacy in several dimensions. It may be helpful for you to take a personal inventory of your relationships to assess how healthy they are.

Making Decisions for You

Think about the most important relationship in your life. Why is this relationship important to your overall health and well-being? Are there any behaviors that you could change to strengthen this relationship? To make such a change, begin by listing the reasons that the change is important. Who will benefit from this change? What steps will you take to make this change occur? What will you do to make sure that you stay with this behavior change?

Checklist for Change: Making Personal Choices

✓ What relationships are most important to you right now?

✓ How have these relationships affected your relationships with others? Are you giving enough time to your other relationships?

✓ Have you thought about how good your relationships are from an emotional perspective? A psychological perspective? A physical perspective? Which of these factors is the most important to you? Why?

✓ What would an ideal set of relationships look like for you? How many close interactions would you want to make time for? What would the nature and extent of these relationships be?

✓ What positive things have you done for people with whom you are relating closely?

✓ What do you expect in a long-term, committed relationship? What would you be willing to accept in terms of behaviors from your committed partner?

✓ What do you think are the three most important attributes of a friend? Have you displayed these attributes when dealing with your friends?

✓ Have you considered your own values/beliefs about what is most important to you in a prospective lifelong partner? Are you asking for the same attributes that you would be able to give to a partner?

Checklist for Change: Making Community Choices

✓ Do you make a habit of putting yourself in the other person's shoes when discussing how your actions may have made that person feel or how that person may be feeling in general?

✓ Do you take time to listen to your friends? Your parents? Your acquaintances? Do you find yourself thinking about your own problems, thoughts, or issues when someone is trying to tell you about their problems?

✓ Do you reach out to friends who are having problems in their relationships?

✓ Are you supportive of couples who are having problems without being judgmental or taking sides?

✓ Do you try to work through your problems with others, or do you run from, avoid, or get angry about rather than try to talk through your difficulties?

✓ Are you supportive of counseling services and other campus/community services that offer help for people who have troubled relationships?

✓ Do you listen carefully to what your legislators propose in the way of family and individual policies and programs that may unfairly harm others?

Critical Thinking

You are in a long-term relationship with Chris and have for some time assumed that after college you would marry. However, you have noticed that Chris seems to be spending more time with a classmate. Chris says they are working on a group project. But even after the project ends, you see them talking frequently. Chris says that they are "friends, but don't share the same type of friendship we do." With jealousy boiling in your blood, you feel you need to approach Chris and discuss the matter.

Use the DECIDE model described in Chapter 1 to decide what you would do in this situation. Be sure to use the communication information you have learned to let Chris know how you feel—but without setting up a confrontation. What will you say to Chris?

Deciding to Break Up

At some point, troubled couples may feel that their relationship is not worth saving. The decision to end the relationship is usually difficult, even for couples whose relationship was over long before the decision.

For married couples, wading through divorce or dissolution proceedings may be painful as they decide child-custody issues, alimony questions, and division of property. Finding legal assistance may be difficult, because painful emotions usually affect judgment. Friends or counselors may be able to recommend lawyers who understand the emotions that follow the ending of a relationship.

Cohabiting couples also experience difficulty in separating. Legal problems involving property, children, and alimony are often more ambiguous than in a marriage. Some couples expend much time, money, and energy working out settlements with lawyers who specialize in problems following the breakup of a nonmarried committed relationship.

Aside from legal worries, many newly separated or divorced people experience painful emotions of anger, guilt, rejection, and unworthiness. No matter how miserable the relationship, feelings of failure are not uncommon or abnormal following a divorce or breakup, and the emotional wounds take varying amounts of time to heal. Counselors familiar with loss and grieving estimate that it takes at least a year and often longer to recover from the loss of a major relationship, whether by death or separation. With time, support from others, and community or professional help, most people do recover and establish new relationships.

Coping with Loneliness

Some people find establishing and maintaining relationships difficult. Others find that through death, illness, or distance, their relationships disappear or grow dim with time. Loneliness, or the unfulfilled desire to engage in a close personal relationship, is a difficult emotion to experience, even for the most determined person.

Newly single people may experience great loneliness and an intense desire for new relationships. They may deal with their loneliness through such destructive behaviors as frantic activism, superficial socializing, sexual affairs, workaholism, or abuse of drugs, alcohol, or food. When their situation appears hopeless, many people may opt for suicide. People who acknowledge the difficulty of what they are going through and share their feelings with others heal faster and more completely than those who are isolated. Cycles of anger, sadness, and resolution diminish with time until the resolution stage becomes dominant.

The loss of an important committed relationship is usually too painful for a person ever to want to repeat. Reflecting on the beginning, the course, and the ending of the relationship can help you avoid the same mistakes in the future. Concentrating on the negative aspects of past behavior of an ex-partner is a natural tendency but is only helpful in getting in touch with emotions or in learning from the situation. It is equally important to spend time remembering what was loved in the other person and what is lovable about oneself. Intimacy, love, and commitment between people always change the lives of those involved. It is through relationships that we both give and receive our greatest support and validation as worthwhile human beings. When we accept the risk and challenge of close relationships, we accept one of the greatest gifts life has to offer.

Summary

- Intimate relationships have several different characteristics, including behavioral interdependence, need fulfillment, and emotional attachment. Each of these characteristics plays a significant role in determining how happy, healthy, and well adjusted you are as you interact with others. Sexual, intellectual, emotional, aesthetic, recreational, crisis, commitment, spiritual, creative, and work intimacy are typical forms that intimacy may take.

- Family, friends, and partners or lovers provide the most common opportunities for intimacy. Each of these relationships may have healthy and/or unhealthy characteristics that may serve to influence our daily level of functioning.

- Men and women often relate very differently in intimate relationships. Gender differences exist in communicating, picking partners, sharing information, and disclosing personal facts and fears. Understanding these differences and learning how to deal with them is an important aspect of healthy relationships.

- Barriers to intimacy include the different emotional needs of men and women, jealousy, and the emotional wounds resulting from being raised in a dysfunctional family.

- Commitment is an important ingredient in relationship success for most people. The major types of committed relationships are marriage, cohabitation, and gay and lesbian partnerships.

- Success in committed relationships requires understanding the roles that partnering scripts play, the importance of self-nurturance, the elements of a good relationship, and the ability to confront couple issues.

- Remaining single is more common than ever before. Contrary to popular beliefs, most single people lead healthy, happy, and well-adjusted lives.

- The decision to have children should involve careful thought and planning, and parents should have the emotional maturity necessary to provide a healthy environment for their children. Today's family structure may look different from that of previous generations, but love, trust, and commitment to a child's welfare continue to be the cornerstones of successful child rearing.

- Before relationships fail, there are often many warning signs. By recognizing these signs and taking action to change behaviors, partners may save and/or enhance their relationships.

- There are many strategies for building better relationships. Taking a careful look at your own behaviors, those things you may need to change, and those things that you are willing to do to help develop a relationship are all important ingredients of success.

Discussion Questions

1. What are the characteristics of intimate relationships? What is behavioral interdependence, need fulfillment, and emotional attachment, and why are each of these important in subsequent relationship development?

2. What are the common types of intimate relationships? Which of these do you think is most important to you right now? Why?

3. Why are your relationships with your family important? Explain how your family unit was similar to or different from the traditional family unit in early America? Who made up your family of origin? Your nuclear family?

4. List and describe the characteristics that are important in a good friend. Who is your best friend right now? What things can you do to improve your current relationships with friends?

5. How can you tell the difference between a love relationship and one that is based primarily on attraction?

What common characteristics do love relationships share?

6. In what ways may men and women differ in their interpersonal relationships? Why may some men find it difficult to communicate their innermost feelings, fears, and emotions?

7. What can serve as barriers to intimacy? Are there actions that you can take to reduce or remove these barriers?

8. What makes a person jealous in a relationship? Is jealousy a good thing or a bad thing?

9. What types of committed relationships do most people become involved in? What factors are most likely to lead to success in these relationships?

10. What are common elements of good relationships?

11. What actions can you take to improve your own interpersonal relationships?

Application Exercise

Reread the What Do You Think? scenarios at the beginning of the chapter and answer the following questions.

1. From what you have read in this chapter, what problems do Roberto and Sara have in their relationship? Why do you think people are often forced to tell lies or half-truths in their relationships with others? Are there times when it is okay to be dishonest or to not tell the truth, or should you always be totally honest and truthful about your actions? Do you believe that you should tell your partner about all of your sexual interactions? Why or why not?

2. What factors should the judge have considered when determining Megan's suitability as a mother? Were you surprised to see a judge take children from a woman who is trying to better herself? Do you think that a judge would view a man in training for a better job, and therefore not home with his children, as negatively as a mother in the same situation? Why or why not?

Further Reading

Sharon S. Brehm, *Intimate Relationships* (New York: McGraw-Hill, 1992).

One of the most comprehensive, readable summaries of research and theory on relationships currently available.

M. A. Klausner and B. Hasselbring, *Aching for Love: The Sexual Drama of the Adult Child* (New York: Harper & Row, 1990).

Based on in-depth interviews with 100 women. Discusses the effects of growing up in alcoholic families and in sexually and emotionally abusive families.

U.S. Bureau of the Census, *Statistical Abstract of the U.S.: Current Population Reports* (Washington, DC: U.S. Government Printing Office, 1994).

Provides regular updates on vital statistics concerning births, deaths, marriages, divorce, living arrangements, and other relevant information.

6

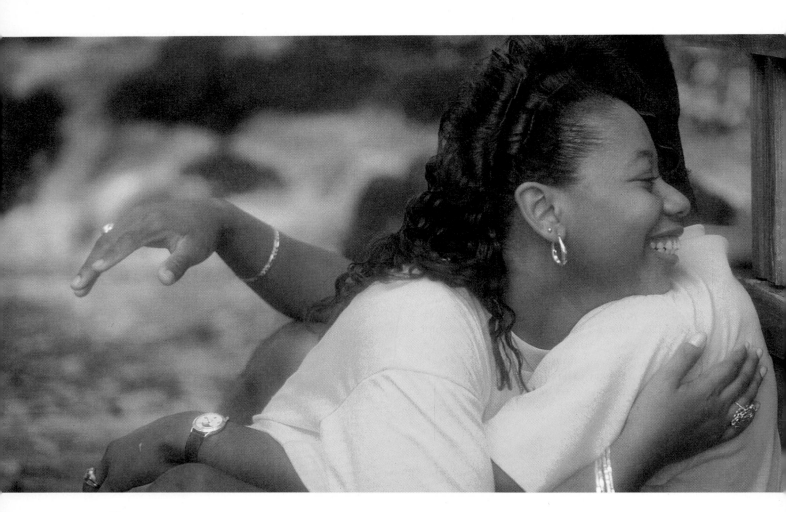

$\mathcal{C}$HAPTER OBJECTIVES

◆ Define sexual identity, and discuss the role of gender identity.

◆ Identify the components of male and female reproductive anatomy and physiology and their functions.

◆ Discuss the options available for the expression of one's sexuality.

◆ Classify sexual dysfunctions and describe each disorder.

◆ Learn to develop your own sexual identity.

$\mathcal{S}$exuality

$\mathcal{D}$efining $\mathcal{Y}$our $\mathcal{S}$exual $\mathcal{B}$ehavior

W H A T D O Y O U T H I N K ?

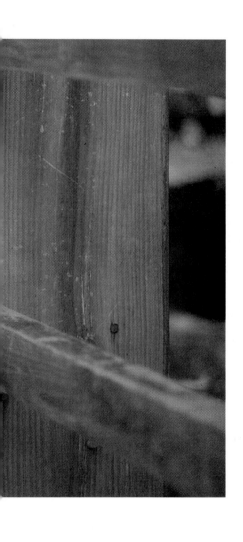

Carl and Anita, both college freshman, met in a psychology class and began dating. Neither of them has been sexually active, although many of their friends are. When the guys get together and talk, Carl is often asked, "How are things going with Anita?" He usually just smiles and says, "Great," although he knows what they are trying to get at. Carl and Anita have talked about the pressure they feel to be sexually active, but, for now, they have decided to abstain.

- Are Carl and Anita normal for wanting to wait? Is everyone else really having sex—or just talking about it?

During his freshman and sophomore years at college, Rod was quite the man about town. He dated and was sexually intimate with many women, but he knew that eventually he'd find the right girl for him. During the summer between his junior and senior years, Rod met Rachel. She was everything he had ever wanted. They dated all summer and grew closer and closer. As time passed, Rachel began asking Rod questions about his past dating history. She wanted to know if he had been serious with anyone else.

- How should Rod answer Rachel's questions? Does Rachel need to know about Rod's past sexual history? Does Rachel have the right to know about Rod's past?

You are a sexual being from birth, but, ironically, you are not born knowing all about your sexuality. Learning about and becoming comfortable with your sexual self is a lifelong process. Taboos, mores, laws, and sexual myths abound. In addition, family members, friends, the media, popular music, your religion, and the educational institutions you have attended all provide you with information about your sexuality and how you should or should not express it. In the end, it is up to you to blend all this information with your personal experience and values to create your own sexual identity.

Although we would like to believe we have made great progress in understanding and accepting our sexual selves, the dominant issues of the 1990s indicate otherwise. Sexually transmitted diseases and teen pregnancy rates are on the rise. Incidence rates for rape and violence against women continue to spiral, as do those for sexual harassment, incest, and child sexual abuse. In addition, we still struggle with the issues of abortion, prostitution, pornography, and premarital sex.

You may initially find all these problems overwhelming, but, as you seek to understand and accept yourself, you can better understand and help others. This chapter will provide information and insights to help you evaluate the various sexual messages you encounter and to sort out fact from fiction. This should aid you in making sexually responsible and healthful decisions for yourself and for those you care about.

*Y*OUR SEXUAL IDENTITY

Your **sexual identity** is determined by a complex interaction of genetic, physiological, and environmental factors. The beginning of your sexual identity occurs at conception with the combining of chromosomes that determine your sex. Actually, it is your biological father who determines whether you will be a boy or a girl. Here's how it works. All eggs (ova) carry an X sex chromosome; sperm may carry either an X or a Y chromosome. If a sperm carrying an X chromosome fertilizes an egg, the resulting combination of sex chromosomes (XX) provides the blueprint to produce a female. If a sperm carrying a Y chromosome fertilizes an egg, the XY combination produces a male (see Figure 6.1).

The genetic instructions included in the sex chromosomes lead to the differential development of male and female **gonads** at about the eighth week of fetal life. Once the male gonads (testes) and the female gonads (ovaries) are developed, they play a key role in all future sexual development because the gonads are responsible for the production of sex hormones. The primary sex hormones produced by females are estrogen and progesterone. In males, the hormone of primary importance is testosterone. The release of testosterone in a maturing fetus signals the development of a penis and other male genitals. If no testosterone is produced, female genitals form.

At the time of **puberty,** sex hormones again play major roles in development. Hormones released by the **pituitary gland,** called gonadotropins, stimulate the gonads (testes and ovaries) to make appropriate sex hormones. The increase of estrogen production in females and testosterone production in males leads to the development of **secondary sex characteristics.** The development of sec-

Sexual identity: Our recognition of ourselves as sexual creatures; a composite of gender, gender roles, sexual preference, body image, and sexual scripts.

Gonads: The reproductive organs in a male (testes) or female (ovaries).

Puberty: The period of sexual maturation.

Pituitary gland: The endocrine gland controlling the release of hormones from the gonads.

Secondary sex characteristics: Characteristics associated with gender but not directly related to reproduction, such as vocal pitch, degree of body hair, and location of fat deposits.

Gender: Your sense of masculinity or femininity as defined by the society in which you live.

Gender roles: Expression of maleness or femaleness exhibited on a daily basis.

Gender identity: Your personal sense or awareness of being masculine or feminine, a male or female.

Gender role stereotypes: Generalizations concerning how males and females should express themselves and the characteristics each possesses.

Androgyny: Combination of traditional masculine and feminine traits in a single person.

Socialization: Process by which a society identifies behavioral expectations to its individual members.

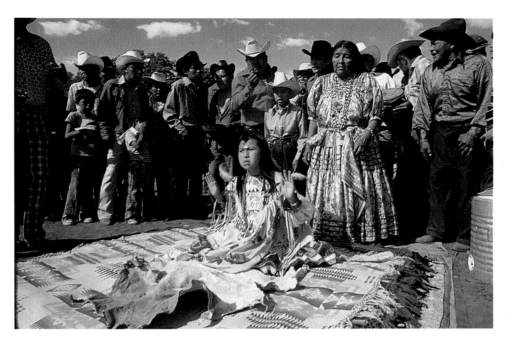

Many cultures celebrate the onset of puberty in public coming-of-age rituals that signify the changes in the young person's life.

ondary sex characteristics in males includes deepening of the voice, development of facial and body hair, and growth of the skeleton and musculature. In females, the development of secondary sex characteristics includes growth of the breasts, widening of the hips, and the development of pubic and underarm hair.

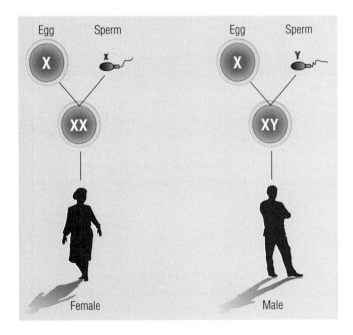

FIGURE 6.1

How Sex Is Determined

Gender Identity and Roles

Thus far, we have described sexual identity only in terms of a person's sex. Sex simply refers to the biological condition of being male or female based on physiological and hormonal differences. **Gender,** on the other hand, refers to your sense of masculinity or femininity as defined by the society in which you live. Each of us expresses our maleness or femaleness to others on a daily basis by the **gender roles** we play. **Gender identity** refers to your personal sense or awareness of being masculine or feminine, a male or a female. It may sometimes be difficult for you to express your true sexual identity because you feel bound by existing gender-role stereotypes. **Gender-role stereotypes** are generalizations about how males and females should express themselves and the characteristics each possesses. Our traditional sex roles are an example of gender-role stereotyping. Men are thought to be independent, aggressive, better in math and science, logical, and always in control of their emotions. Women, on the other hand, are traditionally expected to be passive, nurturing, intuitive, sensitive, and emotional. **Androgyny** is the combination of traditional masculine and feminine traits in a single person. Androgynous people do not always follow traditional sex roles but, rather, try to act appropriately based on the given situation. The process by which a society transmits behavioral expectations to its individual members is called **socialization.** Gender roles are shaped or socialized by our parents, peers, schools, textbooks, advertisements, and many forms of media including television, music, and movies. Think about the current television shows you watch. Do the characters play out traditional gender roles?

Sexual identity includes not only the physical features that determine one's sex, but also the healthy attitudes expressed in feminity or masculinity.

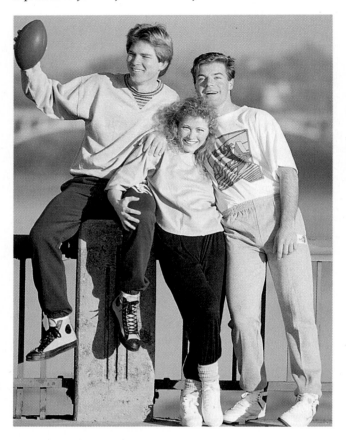

By now you can see that defining your sexual identity is not a simple matter. It is a lifelong process of growing and learning. The Skills for Behavior Change box identifies the characteristics that make up a sexually healthy adult. Your sexual identity is made up of the unique combination of your sex, gender identity, chosen gender roles, sexual preference, and personal experiences. No other person on this earth is exactly like you, and it is up to you to take every opportunity to get to know and like yourself so that you may enjoy your life to the fullest. As the saying goes, sex is what you are born with, but sexuality is who you are.

External female genitals: The mons pubis, labia majora and minora, clitoris, urethral and vaginal openings, and the vestibule of the vagina and its glands.

Vulva: The female's external genitalia.

Mons pubis: Fatty tissue covering the pubic bone in females; in physically mature women, the mons is covered with coarse hair.

The Men's Movement.   We have all heard and read about the women's movement and its part in redefining the role of women in this country. Recently, men too have begun to work toward redefining their role through the men's movement.

Traditionally, men have played the role of nurturers and protectors of land and family, but this image has been progressively shattered by a socioeconomic system that has driven men into the factory and office. Men feel as though they are losing touch with their families, their feelings, and the importance of earth and nature. This isolation is the source of great stress and may be evidenced by the higher toll that suicide, alcohol and substance abuse take on males.

Beginning in the early 1990s, men have begun to gather across the country to express their need to reconnect with their emotions and to establish friendships and emotional bonds with other men. How did men in our society get to this place of emotional isolation? Many feel it is a product of our socioeconomic system. Our culture commonly places men in the position of competing for economic resources. Men have learned not to be open and to trust other men, but rather to devote all their energies to the economic needs of their families.

The New Politics Of Masculinity.   Mountain retreats have become a popular format for gatherings of the men's movement. Some retreats have taken on the Native American traditions of drumming, chanting, dancing, and sweat lodge rituals to help men connect with their feelings and to begin to express those feeling to other men. Having the gatherings in the woods further helps to reestablish ties with nature.

While many men are supportive of this move toward greater emotional expression and bonding, some feel the movement does not go far enough. Andrew Kimbrell, an activist in the men's movement, feels that participants should go a step farther and channel energies into political action. The political platform Kimbrell would like to see supported would include such issues as support for parental-leave legislation, increase of male involvement in the raising and educating of children, support for programs promoting better health in men, support for the protection of nature, and a stand against war and military spending.[1]

WHAT DO YOU THINK?

Do you feel limited or bound by existing gender-role stereotypes? How androgynous are you? What is your opinion of the men's movement?

Characteristics of Sexually Healthy Adults

Do you have the resources and skills needed to accomplish the tasks listed below? These items have been identified as important aspects of sexual health. If you feel that one or more is beyond your current reach, make a list of the resources and skills you would need to reach this objective.

- Appreciate your own body.
- Interact with both genders in appropriate and respectful ways.
- Express love and intimacy in appropriate ways.
- Avoid exploitative relationships.
- Identify your values.
- Take responsibility for your own behavior.
- Communicate effectively with family and friends.
- Ask questions of parents and other adults about sexual issues.
- Enjoy sexual feelings without necessarily acting upon them.
- Be able to communicate and negotiate sexual limits.
- Decide what is personally "right" and act on these values.

- Understand the consequences of sexual activity.
- Talk with a partner about sexual activity before it occurs, including limits, contraceptive and condom use, and meaning in the relationship.
- Communicate desires not to have sex and accept refusals to sex.
- If sexually active, use contraception effectively to avoid pregnancy and use condoms and safer sex to avoid contracting or transmitting a sexually transmitted disease.
- Practice health-promoting behaviors, such as regular check-ups, breast or testicular self-exams.
- Demonstrate tolerance for people with different values.
- Understand the impact of media messages on thoughts, feelings, values, and behaviors related to sexuality.
- Seek further information about sexuality as needed.

Source: Reproduced with permission from D. W. Haffner, "Toward a New Paradigm on Sexual Health," *SIECUS Report,* 21, no. 2 (December 1992–January 1993). Copyright Sexuality Information and Education Council of the United States, 130 West 42nd Street, Suite 350, New York, NY 10036.

REPRODUCTIVE ANATOMY AND PHYSIOLOGY

Sexual activity is physical in nature and depends on anatomical and physiological characteristics and conditions. An understanding of the functions of the male and female reproductive systems will help you derive pleasure and satisfaction from your sexual relationships, be sensitive to your partner's wants and needs, and be more responsible in your choices regarding your own sexual health.

Female Reproductive Anatomy and Physiology

The female reproductive system includes two major groups of structures, the external genitals and the internal genitals (see Figure 6.2). The **external female genitals** include all structures that are outwardly visible and are often referred to as the vulva. Specifically, the **vulva**, or external genitalia, includes the mons pubis, the labia minora and majora, the clitoris, the urethral and vaginal openings, and the vestibule of the vagina. The **mons pubis** is a

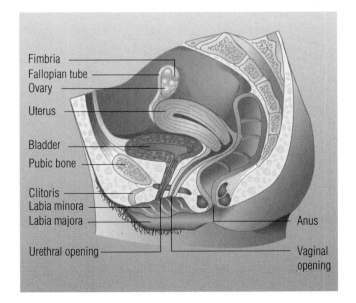

FIGURE 6.2

Side View of the Female Reproductive Organs

Source: From Jeffrey S. Turner and Laurna Rubinson, *Contemporary Human Sexuality,* © 1993, 64. Reprinted by permission of Prentice-Hall, Englewood Cliffs, NJ.

pad of fatty tissue covering the pubic bone. The mons serves to protect the pubic bone, and after puberty it becomes covered with coarse hair. The **labia minora** are folds of mucous membrane and the **labia majora** are folds of skin and erectile tissue that enclose the urethral and vaginal openings. The labia minora are found just inside the labia majora.

The female sexual organ whose only known function is sexual pleasure is called the **clitoris**. It is located at the upper end of the labia minora and beneath the mons pubis. Directly below the clitoris is the **urethral opening** through which urine leaves the body. Below the urethral opening is the vaginal opening, or opening to the **vagina**. In some women, the vaginal opening is covered by a thin membrane called the **hymen**. It is a myth that an intact hymen is proof of virginity. The **perineum** is the area between the vulva and the anus. Although not technically part of the external genitalia, the tissue is this area has many nerve endings and is sensitive to touch; it can play a part in sexual excitement.

The **internal female genitals** of the reproductive system include the vagina, uterus, fallopian tubes, and ovaries. The vagina is a tubular organ that serves as a passageway from the uterus to the outside of a female's body. This passageway allows menstrual flow to exit from the uterus during a female's monthly cycle and serves as the birth canal during childbirth. The vagina also receives the penis during intercourse. The **uterus,** also known as the womb, is a hollow, muscular, pear-shaped organ. Hormones acting on the inner lining of the uterus, called the **endometrium,** either prepare the uterus for implantation and development of a fertilized egg or signal that no fertilization has taken place, in which case the endometrium deteriorates and becomes menstrual flow.

The lower end of the uterus is called the **cervix** and extends down into the vagina. The **ovaries** are almond-sized structures suspended on either side of the uterus. The ovaries produce the hormones estrogen and progesterone and are also the reservoir for immature eggs. All the eggs a female will ever have are present in the ovaries at birth. Eggs mature and are released from the ovaries in response to hormone levels. Extending from the upper end of the uterus are two thin, flexible tubes called the **fallopian tubes.** The fallopian tubes are where sperm and egg meet and fertilization takes place. Following fertilization, the fallopian tubes serve as the passageway to the uterus, where the fertilized egg implants and development continues (see Figure 6.3).

Labia minora: "Inner lips" or folds of tissue just inside the labia majora.

Labia majora: "Outer lips" or folds of tissue covering the female sexual organs.

Clitoris: A pea-sized nodule of tissue located at the top of the labia minora.

Urethral opening: The opening through which urine is expelled.

Vagina: The passage in females leading from the vulva to the uterus.

Hymen: Thin tissue covering the vaginal opening.

Perineum: Tissue extending from the vulva to the anus.

Internal female genitals: The vagina, uterus, fallopian tubes, and ovaries.

Uterus (womb): Hollow, pear-shaped muscular organ whose function is to contain the developing fetus.

Endometrium: Soft, spongy matter that makes up the uterine lining.

Cervix: Lower end of the uterus that opens into the vagina.

Ovaries: Almond-sized organs that house developing eggs and produce hormones.

Fallopian tubes: Tubes that extend from the ovaries to the uterus.

Puberty: The maturation of the female or male reproduction system.

Pituitary gland: A gland located deep within the brain; controls reproductive functions.

Hypothalamus: An area of the brain located near the pituitary gland. The hypothalamus works in conjunction with the pituitary gland to control reproductive functions.

Gonadotropin-releasing hormone (GnRH): Hormone that signals the pituitary gland to release gonadotropins.

Follicle-stimulating hormone (FSH): Hormone that signals the ovaries to prepare to release eggs and to begin producing estrogens.

Luteinizing hormone (LH): Hormone that signals the ovaries to release an egg and to begin producing progesterone.

Estrogens: Hormones that control the menstrual cycle.

Progesterone: Hormone secreted by the ovaries; helps keep the endometrium developing in order to nourish a fertilized egg; also helps maintain pregnancy.

Menarche: The first menstrual period.

Ovarian follicles (egg sacs): Areas within the ovary in which individual eggs develop.

Ovulation: The point of the menstrual cycle at which a mature egg ruptures through the ovarian wall.

Human chorionic gonadotropin (HCG): Hormone that calls for increased levels of estrogen and progesterone secretion if fertilization has taken place.

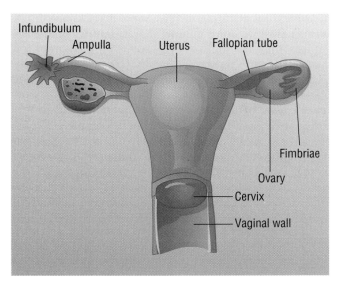

FIGURE 6.3

The Ovaries and Fallopian Tubes

The Onset of Puberty and the Menstrual Cycle. With the onset of **puberty,** the female reproductive system matures, and the development of secondary sex characteristics transforms young girls into young women. Under the direction of the endocrine system, the **pituitary gland,** the **hypothalamus,** and the ovaries all secrete hormones that act as the chemical messengers among them. Working in a feedback system, hormonal levels in the bloodstream act as the trigger mechanism for release of more or different hormones (see Figure 6.4).

At around the age of 11 or 12 in females, the hypothalamus receives the message to begin secreting **gonadotropin-releasing hormone (GnRH).** The release of GnRH in turn signals the pituitary gland to release hormones called gonadotropins. **Follicle-stimulating hormone (FSH)** and **luteinizing hormone (LH)** are two gonadotropins, and their role is to signal the gonads, in this case the ovaries, to start producing **estrogens** and **progesterone.** Increased estrogen levels assist in the development of female secondary sex characteristics. In addition, estrogens are responsible for regulating the reproductive cycle. The normal age range for the onset of the first menstrual period, termed the **menarche,** is 10 to 16 years, with the average age being 13 or 14 years.

The average menstrual cycle is 28 days long and divided into three phases, the proliferatory phase, the secretory phase, and the menstrual phase. During the proliferatory phase, the pituitary gland releases FSH and LH. The FSH acts on the ovaries to stimulate the maturation process of several **ovarian follicles (egg sacs).** These follicles secrete estrogens and, in response to this estrogen stimulation, the lining of the uterus, the endometrium, begins to grow and develop. The inner walls of the uterus become coated with a thick, spongy lining composed of blood and mucus. In the event of fertilization, the endometrial tissue will become a nesting place for the developing embryo. The increased estrogen level also signals the pituitary to slow down FSH production but to increase LH secretion. Of the several follicles developing in the ovaries, only one each month normally reaches complete maturity. Under the influence of LH, this one ovarian follicle rapidly matures, and on or about the fourteenth day of the proliferatory phase, it releases an ovum into the fallopian tube—a process referred to as **ovulation.** Just prior to ovulation, the mature egg's follicle begins to increase secretion of progesterone, the first function of which is to spur the addition of further nutrients to the developing endometrium.

After ovulation, the ovarian follicle is converted into the *corpus luteum,* or yellow body, which continues to secrete estrogen and progesterone but in decreasing amounts. In addition, FSH also falls back to its preproliferatory levels. Essentially, the woman's body is "waiting" to see whether fertilization will occur. During this time after ovulation, LH declines, and progesterone levels begin to rise, causing additional tissue growth in the endometrium. This phase of the cycle is called the secretory phase.

If fertilization takes place, cells surrounding the developing embryo release a hormone called **human chorionic gonadotropin (HCG).** This hormone leads to increased

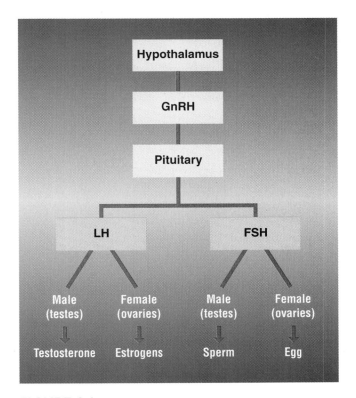

FIGURE 6.4

Hormonal Direction of the Human Reproductive System

levels of estrogen and progesterone secretion, which maintains the endometrium while signaling the pituitary gland not to start a new menstrual cycle.

When fertilization does not occur, the egg gradually disintegrates within approximately 72 hours. The corpus luteum gradually becomes nonfunctional, causing levels of progesterone and estrogen to decline. As hormonal levels decline, the endometrial lining of the uterus loses its nourishment, dies, and is sloughed off as menstrual flow. Menstruation is the third phase of the menstrual cycle.

Some issues associated with menstruation that you may be interested in reading about are premenstrual syndrome (PMS), toxic shock syndrome (TSS), and dysmenorrhea, or painful menstruation.

Menopause. Just as menarche signals the beginning of a female's potential reproductive years, **menopause**—the permanent cessation of menstruation—signals the end. Generally occurring between the ages of 50 and 55, menopause results in decreased estrogen levels, which may produce troublesome symptoms in some women. Decrease in vaginal lubrication, hot flashes, headaches, dizziness, and joint pains have all been associated with the onset of menopause. Since estrogen plays a protective role in women by guarding against heart disease and osteoporosis (loss of bone mineral density), postmenopausal women may not only reduce some of the symptoms associated with menopause but also regain some protection against heart disease and osteoporosis by going on hormone-replacement therapy (HRT), or estrogen-replacement therapy (ERT), as it is sometimes called.[2] Unfortunately, HRT/ERT is not without potential risks. Increased risk of gall bladder disease and breast cancer has been reported in some women. But overall, for most women, the benefits of hormone therapy outweigh the risks. Certainly lifestyle changes such as regular exercise and a diet low in fat and adequate in calcium can also help protect postmenopausal women from heart disease and osteoporosis.

> ### *W*HAT DO YOU THINK?
>
> Why is it so important that we understand the function of our sexual anatomy? Do men need to understand how the menstrual cycle works? Why? Some people are not comfortable using the medical terms for parts of the sexual anatomy. Why do you think this is so?

Male Reproductive Anatomy and Physiology

The structures of the male reproductive system may be divided into external and internal genitals (see Figure 6.5). The penis and the scrotum make up the **external**

Menopause: The permanent cessation of menstruation.

External male genitals: The penis and scrotum.

Internal male genitals: The testes, epididymides, vasa deferentia, ejaculatory ducts, urethra, and accessory glands.

Accessory glands: The seminal vesicles, prostate gland, and Cowper's glands.

Penis: Male sexual organ designed for releasing sperm into the vagina.

Ejaculation: The propulsion of semen from the penis.

Scrotum: Sac of tissue that encloses the testes.

Testes: Two organs, located in the scrotum, that manufacture sperm and produce hormones.

Testosterone: The male sex hormone manufactured in the testes.

Spermatogenesis: The development of sperm.

Epididymis: A comma-shaped structure atop the testis where sperm mature.

Vas deferens: A tube that transports sperm toward the penis.

Seminal vesicles: Storage areas for sperm where nutrient fluids are added to them.

Semen: Fluid containing sperm and nutrient fluids that increase sperm viability and neutralize vaginal acid.

Prostate gland: Gland that secretes nutrients and neutralizing fluids into the semen.

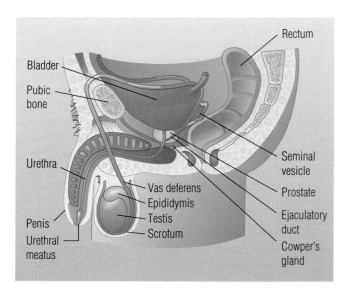

FIGURE 6.5

Side View of the Male Reproductive Organs

Source: From Jeffrey S. Turner and Laurna Rubinson, *Contemporary Human Sexuality,* © 1993, 67. Reprinted by permission of Prentice-Hall, Englewood Cliffs, NJ.

Sexuality and Aging

In our society, we often make the assumption that older adults are sexless. Here are six simple facts about sexuality and aging we should all know.

- *All older people are sexual.* They may not all be having sex, but they all do have sexual beliefs, values, memories, and feelings. To deny this sexuality is to exclude a significant part of the lives of older people.

- *Many older people have a need for a good sexual relationship.* The warmth, intimacy, and security of a good sexual relationship is as important to a 70-year-old as it is to a 20-, 30-, or 40-year-old.

- *Sexual physiology changes with age.* Older men may find that erections occur less frequently, take longer to achieve, are less firm, and are more easily lost. After menopause, older women may find decreased vaginal lubrication a problem. Estrogen replacement can alleviate this problem in most women.

- *Social attitudes are often frustrating.* Society tends to deny the sexuality of the aged, and in doing so creates complications in their sometimes already difficult lives. A good

example is the many rules, customs, and lack of privacy which severely inhibit the establishment of intimate relationships in our retirement facilities and nursing homes.

- *Use it or lose it.* Sexual activity is a physiologic function that tends to deteriorate if not exercised. It is particularly fragile in the elderly.

- *Older folks do it better.* Older people often enjoy sex more because they are experienced, they take their time, they're not goal (orgasm) oriented, and they tend to be more leisurely and relaxed.

Do you make the assumption that older people are no longer sexual? Do you treat the older people in your life as sexual beings? What can be done to change our social attitudes towards sexuality and aging?

Source: Adapted with permission from Richard J. Cross, "What Doctors Need to Know: Six Facts on Human Sexuality and Aging," *SIECUS Report,* 21, no. 5 (June–July 1993): 7–9. Copyright Sexuality Information and Education Council of the United States, 130 West 42nd Street, Suite 350, New York, NY 10036.

---

male genitals. The **internal male genitals** include the testes, epididymides, vasa deferentia, and urethra, and three other structures—the seminal vesicles, the prostate gland, and the Cowper's glands—that secrete components that, with sperm, make up semen. These three structures are sometimes referred to as the **accessory glands.**

The **penis** serves as the organ that deposits sperm in the vagina during intercourse. The urethra, which passes through the center of the penis, acts as the passageway for both semen and urine to exit the body. During sexual arousal, the spongy tissue in the penis becomes filled with blood, making the organ stiff, or erect. Further sexual excitement leads to **ejaculation,** a series of rapid spasmodic contractions that propel semen out of the penis.

Situated behind the penis and also outside the body is a sac called the **scrotum.** The scrotum serves to protect the testes and also helps control the temperature within the testes, which is vital to proper sperm production. The **testes** (singular: *testis*) are egg-shaped structures in which sperm are manufactured. The testes also contain cells that manufacture **testosterone,** the hormone responsible for the development of male secondary sex characteristics.

Spermatogenesis is the term used to describe the development of sperm. Like the maturation of eggs in the female, this process is governed by the pituitary gland. Follicle-stimulating hormone (FSH) is secreted into the bloodstream to stimulate the testes to manufacture

sperm. Immature sperm are released into a comma-shaped structure on the back of the testis called the **epididymis** (plural: *epididymides*), where they ripen and reach full maturity.

The epididymis contains coiled tubules that gradually "unwind" and straighten out to become the **vas deferens.** The two vasa deferentia, as they are called in the plural, make up the tubular transportation system whose sole function is to store and move sperm. Along the way, the **seminal vesicles** provide sperm with nutrients and other fluids that compose **semen.**

The vasa deferentia eventually connect each epididymis to the ejaculatory ducts, which pass through the prostate gland and empty into the urethra. The **prostate gland** contributes more fluids to the semen, including chemicals to aid the sperm in fertilization of an ovum, and, more importantly, a chemical that neutralizes the acid in the vagina to make its environment more conducive to sperm motility (ability to move) and potency (potential for fertilizing an ovum).

Just below the prostate gland are two pea-shaped nodules called the Cowper's glands. Their primary function is to secrete a fluid that lubricates the urethra and neutralizes any acid that may remain in the urethra after urination. Urine and semen do not come into contact with each other. During ejaculation of semen, the tube to the urinary bladder is closed off by a small valve.

Circumcision: Risk Versus Benefit. Many new parents must decide whether their male infant will be circumcised. Circumcision involves the surgical removal of the **foreskin,** a flap of skin covering the tip of the penis. Most circumcisions in the United States have traditionally been performed for religious/cultural reasons or because of concerns about hygiene. In the uncircumcised male, oily secretions and sloughed-off dead cells (smegma) can collect under the foreskin and create an irritation or set up a breeding ground for infection. Removing the foreskin makes cleansing of the penis easier. Recent studies have shown that about 1 in 10 uncircumcised male babies develops urinary tract infections. Other studies have suggested that uncircumcised males may be at slightly greater risk for penile cancer or HIV infection. These studies are not conclusive, and more research is clearly needed.

Today, infants can be given a local anesthetic, and circumcisions can be performed with little or no pain. This does not mean, however, that the procedure itself is without risk. All surgery involves some risk. If circumcision is performed later in life under a general anesthetic, the risk of complications is greater. As the most recent recommendation from the American Academy of Pediatrics points out, "Newborn circumcision has potential medical benefits and advantages as well as disadvantages and risks. When circumcision is being considered, the benefits and risks should be explained to the parents and informed consent obtained."[3]

EXPRESSING YOUR SEXUALITY

Finding healthy ways to express your sexuality is an important part of developing sexual maturity. With the many avenues of sexual expression open to you, discovering one that will bring you satisfaction can be very difficult.

Human Sexual Response

Sexual response is a physiological process that involves different stages. The biological goal of the response process is the reproduction of the species. Human psychological traits greatly influence sexual response and sexual desire. Thus, we may find relationships with one partner vastly different from those we might experience with other partners.

Foreskin: Flap of skin covering the end of the penis; it is removed during circumcision.

Vasocongestion: The engorgement of the genital organs with blood.

Sexual response generally follows a pattern. Laboratory research has delineated four or five stages within the response cycle, and researchers agree that each individual has a personal response pattern that may or may not conform to the stages observed in experimental research. Both males and females exhibit four common stages: excitement/arousal, plateau, orgasm, and resolution. In addition, some males experience a fifth stage, the refractory period. Identification of these stages was achieved in laboratory situations in which genital response was carefully measured using specially designed instruments. Regardless of the type of sexual activity (stimulation by a partner or self-stimulation), the response stages are the same. These stages are illustrated in Figure 6.6.

During the first stage, *excitement/arousal,* male and female genital responses are caused by **vasocongestion,** or increased blood flow in the genital region. Increased blood flow to these organs causes them to swell. The vagina begins to lubricate in preparation for penile penetration and the penis becomes partially erect. Both sexes may exhibit a "sex flush," or light blush all over their bodies. Excitement/arousal can be generated by touching other parts of the body, by kissing, through fantasy, by viewing films or videos, or by reading erotic literature.

The *plateau phase* is characterized by an intensification of the initial responses. Voluntary and involuntary muscle tensions increase. The female's nipples and the male's penis become erect. A few drops of semen, which may contain sperm, are secreted from the penis at this time.

During the *orgasmic phase,* vasocongestion and muscle tensions reach their peak, and rhythmic contractions occur through the genital regions. In females, these contractions are centered in the uterus, the outer vagina, and the anal sphincter. In males, the contractions occur in two stages. First, contractions within the prostate gland begin propelling semen through the urethra. In the second stage, the muscles of the pelvic floor, the urethra, and the anal sphincter contract. Semen usually, but not always, is ejaculated from the penis. In both sexes, spasms in other major muscle groups also occur, particularly in the buttocks and abdomen. Feet and hands may also contract, and facial features often contort.

Muscle tension and congested blood subside in the *resolution phase,* as the genital organs return to their prearousal states. Both sexes usually experience deep feelings of well-being and profound relaxation. In some males, a fifth, or *refractory phase,* occurs. Males experience a period of time in which their systems are incapable of subsequent arousal. This refractory period may last from a few minutes to several hours. The length of the refractory period increases with age.

Following orgasm and resolution, many females are capable of being aroused and brought to orgasm again. Males and females experience the same stages in the sexual response cycle; however, the length of time spent in any one stage is variable. Thus, one partner may be in the plateau phase while the other is in the excitement or

1. Excitement Phase

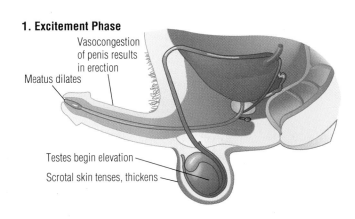

Vasocongestion of penis results in erection

Meatus dilates

Testes begin elevation

Scrotal skin tenses, thickens

1. Excitement Phase

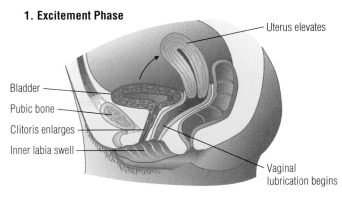

Uterus elevates

Bladder

Pubic bone

Clitoris enlarges

Inner labia swell

Vaginal lubrication begins

2. Plateau Phase

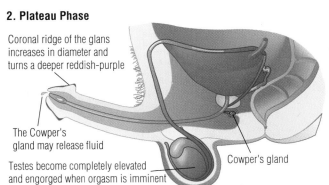

Coronal ridge of the glans increases in diameter and turns a deeper reddish-purple

The Cowper's gland may release fluid

Testes become completely elevated and engorged when orgasm is imminent

Cowper's gland

2. Plateau Phase

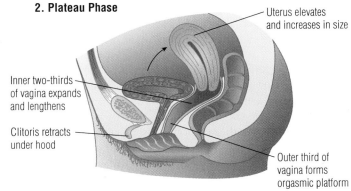

Uterus elevates and increases in size

Inner two-thirds of vagina expands and lengthens

Clitoris retracts under hood

Outer third of vagina forms orgasmic platform

3. Orgasm Phase

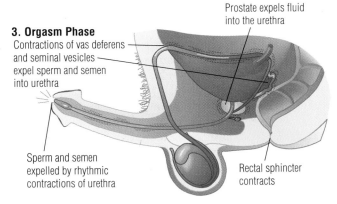

Prostate expels fluid into the urethra

Contractions of vas deferens and seminal vesicles expel sperm and semen into urethra

Sperm and semen expelled by rhythmic contractions of urethra

Rectal sphincter contracts

3. Orgasm Phase

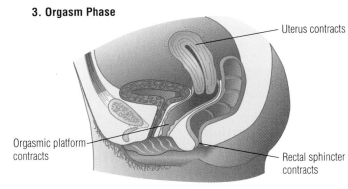

Uterus contracts

Orgasmic platform contracts

Rectal sphincter contracts

4. Resolution Phase

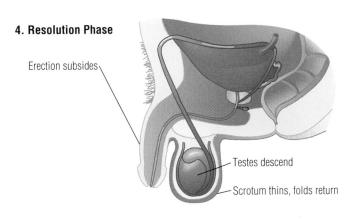

Erection subsides

Testes descend

Scrotum thins, folds return

4. Resolution Phase

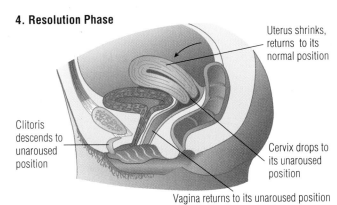

Uterus shrinks, returns to its normal position

Clitoris descends to unaroused position

Cervix drops to its unaroused position

Vagina returns to its unaroused position

FIGURE 6.6

Comparison of Sexual Reponse between Male and Female

orgasmic phase. Such variations in response rates are entirely normal. Some couples believe that simultaneous orgasm is desirable for sexual satisfaction. Although simultaneous orgasm is pleasant, so are orgasms achieved at different times.

The physical and emotional release experienced in orgasm has made this the major goal for many people in their sexual activity. These people are often more concerned with sexual performance than with the emotional and physical well-being of their partners. The pressure to perform "perfect" sex often inhibits the participants, thereby limiting pleasure.

The feelings at orgasm are not easily defined, and anyone wanting to know what orgasm feels like will receive different answers from virtually everyone who is asked. Orgasms vary in intensity and are dependent upon the individuals involved, the environment, and a host of other factors.

Sexual pleasure and satisfaction are possible without orgasm or intercourse. Achieving sexual maturity includes learning that sex is not a contest with a real or imaginary opponent. The sexually mature person enjoys sexual activity whether or not orgasm occurs. Expressing love and sexual feelings for another person involves many pleasurable activities, of which intercourse and orgasm may only be a part.

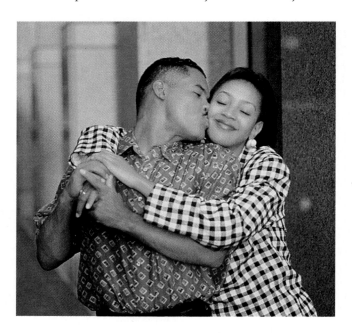

As couples become more comfortable together, they learn what pleases each other sexually and emotionally.

𝒲HAT DO YOU THINK?

Why do Americans place so much importance on the orgasmic phase of sexual response? Do you think there should be a "psychological phase" added to descriptions of the sexual response cycle?

Sexual Orientation

An essential part of your sexual identity is your sexual orientation. **Sexual orientation** refers to a person's potential to respond with sexual excitement to other persons.[4] You may be primarily attracted to members of the other sex (**heterosexual**), your same sex (**homosexual**), or both sexes (**bisexual**).

Homosexuality refers to emotional and sexual attachment to persons of your same sex. Many homosexuals prefer the use of the terms *gay* and *lesbian* to describe their sexual orientations, as these terms go beyond the exclusively sexual connotation of the term *homosexual*. The term *gay* can be applied to both men and women, but the term *lesbian* is applied only to women. Contrary to popular belief, most gays and lesbians are well adjusted and emotionally stable.[5] Some clinicians propose that when maladaptive behavior does occur in gays and lesbians, it is triggered by the social stigma our society attaches to being gay rather than by something inherently pathological in

the homosexual person.[6] **Homophobia**, as defined by Martin Weinberg, is the irrational fear of homosexuality in others, the fear of homosexual feelings within oneself, or self-loathing because of one's homosexuality.[7] Homophobia in our society is expressed in many ways subtle and not so subtle. Homophobic behavior can range from avoiding hugging same-sex friends to "gay bashing" (physical and verbal attacks on gays). The emergence of AIDS (acquired immune deficiency syndrome) seems to have magnified antihomosexual prejudice, as many people have erroneously assumed that homosexuality rather than high-risk behaviors is responsible for the epidemic.

Bisexuality refers to emotional attachment and sexual attraction to members of both sexes. Bisexuals may face great social stigma, as they are often ostracized by homosexuals as well as by heterosexuals. Little research has been done on this segment of the population, and many bisexuals remain hidden or closeted. This fear of revealing one's bisexuality to others has been increased during the current AIDS epidemic. The Centers for Disease Control (CDC) reports that 2 to 3 percent of women infected with the human immunodeficiency virus (HIV), the virus that causes AIDS, contracted that virus by engaging in sexual activity with bisexual men.[8] Many of these men are married but choose not to tell their female partners of their bisexual orientation.

Origins of Sexual Orientation. A variety of theories, both biological and psychosocial, have been proposed to explain why some people are gay or lesbian. One of the

In a society where anti-homosexual attitudes prevail, a gay person's decision to make his or her sexual preference known to the public involves courage and a strong belief in one's self.

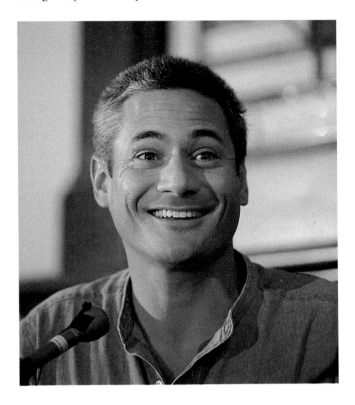

most comprehensive and well-done studies on the psychosocial origins of sexual orientation was by Bell, Weinberg, and Hammersmith. They found that (1) sexual preference appears to be largely determined before adolescence; (2) individuals seem to experience homosexual feelings for about three years prior to any open displays of homosexual activity, and these feelings play a larger role in the subject's sexual orientation than does any particular activity; (3) homosexuals tend to have a history of heterosexual experiences during childhood and adolescence but report these experiences as unsatisfying; and (4) identification with a parent of either sex appeared to play no significant role in determining one's sexual orientation.[9]

The major biological theories are based upon prenatal hormone levels, structural differences in the brain, and genetic factors. In 1991, Simon LeVay[10] found that in homosexual men, one part of the hypothalamus that influences sexual behavior was smaller than that same region of the hypothalamus in heterosexual men. Also in 1991, Bailey and Pillard[11] conducted research on the role of genetic factors in the development of sexual orientation. They studied identical twins, fraternal twins, and adoptive brothers of gay men. The researchers wanted to know the percentage of cases in which a gay orientation was present in both siblings when it was present in one sibling. They found that 52 percent of the identical twin brothers of gay men were also gay. In fraternal twins, 22 percent of the brothers were also gay. For genetically unrelated (adopted) brothers, however, it was only 11 percent. These two studies don't prove being gay or lesbian is determined strictly by biological factors, but biology may play a part.

The cause or causes of sexual orientation are complex. At present there is no single, conclusive explanation for how sexual orientation develops.[12] Most probably the determinants are a combination of various biological and environmental factors that are unique to each person.

𝒲HAT DO YOU THINK?

Why is sexual orientation such a controversial subject for some people? Do you think the origin of homosexuality is primarily biological or environmental?

Developing Sexual Relationships

Perhaps the most important part of developing mature sexuality is learning to develop rewarding sexual relationships. Like all skills, developing relationships takes time, patience, and practice. Your sexual education begins with your family. You watch the significant adults in your life and pattern your behaviors after theirs. At puberty, when extrafamilial elements, peers, and the media become more important, you adapt some of their standards to your behaviors. Your shyness, aggressiveness or assertiveness, passiveness, and levels of comfort with your sexuality come from your own personality and from what you have learned from others.

Not only do you bring your history to your sexual relationships, but you also bring your peculiar chemistry. The

Sexual orientation: Attraction to and interest in members of the opposite sex, the same sex, or both sexes in emotional, social, and sexual situations.

Heterosexual: Refers to attraction to and preference for sexual activity with people of the opposite sex.

Homosexual: Refers to attraction to and preference for sexual activity with people of the same sex.

Bisexual: Refers to attraction to and preference for sexual activity with people of both sexes.

Homophobia: Irrational hatred or fear of homosexuals or homosexuality.

human potential for passionate sexual love has been defined as **limerence**. The word *limerence* is derived from the name of the portion of the brain that controls sexual response, the limbic cortex. Limerence is what makes us feel sexually "turned on" by a person. This powerful feeling can overshadow common sense. Sexual relationships based on limerence may or may not develop into long-lasting or committed relationships. Limerence is thought to last only two years at most. Relationships based upon a love that has taken time to mature are much more likely to last. Following are some of the "symptoms" of limerence:

- Intrusive thoughts about the object of desire.

- Dependence of mood on love object's actions.

- Fear of rejection, along with almost incapacitating shyness.

- Sharp sensitivity to interpret desired person's actions favorably and ability to interpret any signs from the other as hidden passion.

- Buoyancy, walking-on-air feeling when reciprocation is evident.

- Intensity of feelings that leaves other concerns in the background.

- Ability to emphasize what is admirable in the love object and to avoid dwelling on the negative or even ability to reconceptualize the negative into a positive attribute.[13]

Learning to distinguish between love and limerence requires experience and time. The crushes you may have suffered in your early adolescent years are examples of limerence. If you allow sexual attraction to rule your relationships, you are bound to be hurt. As limerence wears off, you find yourself involved in a relationship or infatuation with an ordinary human being as opposed to a dream. If a bond based on communication and love has not been established, your obsession with your partner begins to die. The relationship collapses, and you are left to mourn and wonder why something beautiful had to end so sadly.

The advertising media constantly use limerence to sell goods. You are told you will be more sexually attractive if you do this type of exercise or drink that type of soft drink. You are also taught by family and peers that you must be sexually attractive to catch a mate. At the same time, most people want to be loved for themselves and not for their shapely bodies. You may often feel pulled by this contradiction.

In developing your sexual relationships, you must look beyond limerence. To do this, you must begin slowly, learning to recognize limerence, and realizing that the weak-kneed, heart-palpitating feelings do not have to be acted upon immediately. Taking the time to know another person helps reduce the risks involved with sexual activity. Although no sex is risk free, sex between two people who are comfortable with each other (because they have taken the time to know one another) is likely to be more satisfying.

Sexual Expression: What Are Your Options?

The range of human sexual expression is virtually infinite. What you find personally satisfying and enjoyable may not be an option for someone else. The ways you choose to meet your sexual needs today may be very different two weeks or two years from now. Knowing and accepting yourself as a sexual person with individual desires and preferences is the first step in achieving sexual satisfaction. The Health Headlines box shows some surprising results about how Americans express their sexuality.

Celibacy. **Celibacy** is avoidance of or abstention from sexual activities with others. A completely celibate person also does not engage in masturbation (self-stimulation), whereas a partially celibate person avoids sexual activities with others but may enjoy autoerotic behaviors such as masturbation. Some individuals choose to be celibate for religious or moral reasons. Others may be celibate for a period of time due to illness, the breakup of a long-term relationship, or lack of an acceptable partner. For some, celibacy is a lonely, agonizing state, but others find that it can be a time for introspection, value assessment, and personal growth.

Autoerotic Behaviors. The goal of **autoerotic behaviors** is sexual self-stimulation. Sexual fantasy and masturbation are the two most common autoerotic behaviors. **Sexual fantasies** are sexually arousing thoughts and dreams. Fantasies may reflect real-life experiences or forbidden desires or may provide the opportunity for practice of new or anticipated sexual experiences. The fact that you may fantasize about a particular sexual experience does not mean that you want to, or have to, act that experience out. Sexual fantasies are just that—fantasy. Another common autoerotic behavior is **masturbation.** Masturbation is self-stimulation of the genitals. Although many people feel uncomfortable discussing masturbation, it is a common sexual practice across the life span. Masturbation is a natural, pleasure-seeking behavior in infants and children. It is a valuable and important means for adolescent males and females, as well as adults, to explore their sexual feelings and responsiveness. In addition, masturbation is an important means of sexual expression for older adults who have lost a lifelong companion or whose companion has a prolonged illness.

The Latest Sex Survey

Recently, a group of social scientists from the University of Chicago released the results of what has been touted as the first truly scientific study of sexuality in America. The researchers' findings are based on a random sample of 3,500 Americans, ages 18 to 59. Here are some of their results.

- Americans fall into three groups. One-third have sex twice a week or more, one-third a few times a month, and one-third a few times a year or not at all.

- Americans are largely monogamous. The vast majority (83 percent) have one or zero sexual partners a year. Over a lifetime, a typical man has six partners; a woman, two.

- Married couples have the most sex and are the most likely to have orgasms when they do. Nearly 40 percent of married people say they have sex twice a week, compared with 25 percent for singles.

- Most Americans don't go in for the kinky stuff. Asked to rank their favorite sex acts, almost everyone (96 percent)

found vaginal sex "very or somewhat appealing." Oral sex ranked a distant third, after an activity that many had not realized was a sex act: "Watching partner undress."

- Adultery is the exception in America, not the rule. Nearly 75 percent of married men and 85 percent of married women said they have never been unfaithful.

- There are a lot fewer active homosexuals in America than the oft-repeated 1 in 10. Only 2.7 percent of men and 1.3 percent of women report that they had homosexual sex in the past year.

Source: List excerpted from Philip Elmer-Dewitt, "Now for the Truth about Americans and Sex," *Time,* 17 October 1994, 64. Copyright 1994 Time Inc. Reprinted by permission.

Kissing and Erotic Touching. Kissing and erotic touching are two very common forms of nonverbal sexual communication or expression. Both males and females have **erogenous zones,** or areas of the body that when touched lead to sexual arousal. Erogenous zones may include genital as well as nongenital areas, such as the earlobes, mouth, breasts, and inner thighs. Almost any area of the body can be conditioned to respond erotically to touch. Spending time with your partner exploring and learning about his or her erogenous areas is another pleasurable, safe, and satisfying means of sexual expression.

Oral-Genital Stimulation. **Cunnilingus** is the term used for oral stimulation of a female's genitals, and **fellatio** is the term used for oral stimulation of a male's genitals. Many partners find oral-genital stimulation an intensely pleasurable means of sexual expression. It is estimated that by the age of 35, 90 percent of Americans have experienced oral-genital stimulation at least once.[14] For some people, oral sex is not an option because of moral or religious beliefs. It is necessary to remember that HIV and other sexually transmitted diseases (STDs) can be transmitted via unprotected oral-genital sex. Use of an appropriate barrier device is strongly recommended if either partner's disease status is in question or unknown.

Anal Intercourse. The anal area is highly sensitive to touch, and some couples find pleasure in the stimulation of this area. **Anal intercourse** is insertion of the penis into the anus. Stimulation of the anus by mouth or with the

fingers is also practiced. As with all forms of sexual expression, anal stimulation or intercourse is not for everyone. If you do enjoy this form of sexual expression, remember to use condoms to prevent disease transmission. Also, anything inserted into the anus should not be directly inserted into the vagina, as bacteria commonly found in the anus can cause infections when introduced into the vagina.

Limerence: The quality of sexual attraction based on chemistry and gratification of sexual desire.

Celibacy: State of not being involved in a sexual relationship.

Autoerotic behaviors: Sexual self-stimulation.

Sexual fantasies: Sexually arousing thoughts and dreams.

Masturbation: Self-stimulation of genitals.

Erogenous zones: Areas in the body of both males and females that, when touched, lead to sexual arousal.

Cunnilingus: Oral stimulation of a female's genitals.

Fellatio: Oral stimulation of a male's genitals.

Anal intercourse: The insertion of the penis into the anus.

Vaginal Intercourse. The term *intercourse* is generally used to refer to **vaginal intercourse,** or insertion of the penis into the vagina. *Coitus* is another term for vaginal intercourse, which is the most often practiced form of sexual expression for most couples. A great variety of positions can be used during coitus. Examples include the missionary position (man on top facing the woman), woman on top, side by side, or man behind (rear entry). Many partners enjoy changing and experimenting with different positions. Sexual intercourse can take on different meanings under different circumstances. It can be a hurried, unplanned event involving little communication in the back seat of a car or an erotic, sensual experience including the exchange of love and mutual emotions in a private setting. Knowledge of yourself and your body, along with your ability to communicate effectively with others, will play a large part in determining the enjoyment or meaning of intercourse for you and your partner. (To check up on your communicative skills, see the Building Communication Skills box.) Whatever your circumstance, you should practice safe sex to avoid disease transmission or unwanted pregnancy.

What Is Right for Me?

Invariably, whenever people talk about the spectrum of sexual behaviors, someone in the group will bring up the issue of normality. In *The Joy of Sex,* Alex Comfort summarizes "normality" succinctly:

> Accordingly, if you must talk about "normality," any sex behavior is normal which (1) you both enjoy, (2) hurts nobody, (3) isn't associated with anxiety, (4) doesn't cut down your scope.... "Normal" implies there is something which sex ought to be. That is, it ought to be a wholly satisfying link between two affectionate people, from which both emerge unanxious, rewarded, and ready for more.[15]

Many couples worry that they don't have sex often enough. Popular magazines frequently give the "average" number of times couples engage in sex every week. Such numbers are meaningless. Rather than compare yourself to these statistics, you would be wise simply to follow your own feelings. The bottom line is that you must decide what is right or "normal" for you. The Choices for Change box may help you identify your preferred options for sexual behavior.

Variant Sexual Behavior

Although attitudes toward sexuality have changed radically since the Victorian era, some people believe that any sexual behavior other than heterosexual intercourse is abnormal, deviant, or perverted. Rather than using these negative terms, people who study sexuality prefer to use the nonjudgmental term **variant sexual behavior** to describe sexual behaviors that are not engaged in by most people. The following list of variant sexual behaviors includes behaviors that are illegal in some states and some behaviors that could be harmful to others:

- *Group sex.* Sexual activity involving more than two people. Participants in group sex run a high risk of exposure to AIDS and other sexually transmitted diseases.

- *Transvestitism.* The wearing of clothing of the opposite sex. Most transvestites are male, heterosexual, and married.

- *Transsexualism.* Strong identification with the opposite sex in which men or women feel that they are "trapped in the wrong body." In some cases, transsexuals undergo sex-change operations. Since the 1960s, 4,000 of these operations have been performed in the United States.

- *Fetishism.* Describes sexual arousal achieved by looking at or touching inanimate objects, such as underclothing or shoes.

- *Exhibitionism.* The exposure of one's genitals to strangers in public places. Most exhibitionists are seeking a reaction of shock or fear from their victims. Exhibitionism is a minor felony in most states.

- *Voyeurism.* Observing other people for sexual gratification. Most voyeurs are men who attempt to watch women undressing or bathing. Voyeurism is an invasion of privacy and is illegal in most states.

- *Sadomasochism.* Sexual activities in which gratification is received by inflicting pain (verbal or physical abuse) on a partner or by being the object of such infliction. A sadist is a person who receives gratification from inflicting pain, and a masochist is a person who receives gratification from experiencing pain.

- *Pedophilia.* Sexual activity or attraction between an adult and a child. Any sexual activity involving a minor, including possession of child pornography, is illegal.

WHAT DO YOU THINK?

How does our society decide what sexual behaviors are normal and which are variant? Are some sexual behaviors that we consider normal looked upon as abnormal or perverse in other countries or cultures? Why are some individuals very willing to try various sexual behaviors while others are not?

How Well Do You Communicate Sexually?

How well do you communicate both verbally and non-verbally with your partner? To find out, you might want to take the following communication quiz. For each question, circle the appropriate score. Compare your total score with the ratings following the questionnaire.

	Yes	No
1. Do you ever ask your sexual partner about anything he or she particularly likes or dislikes when you make love?	1	0
2. Do you find it hard to tell your partner that she or he does something you particularly like or dislike during lovemaking?	0	1
3. Are you able to tell your partner you are not in the mood for sex without making him or her feel rejected?	1	0
4. If you do not want to make love because you are hurt or upset about something, can you explain that you find it impossible to get in the mood for sex when you are upset?	1	0
5. Do you often fake orgasm or pleasure rather than tell your partner that he is not giving you the right kind of sexual stimulation?	0	1
6. Are you comfortable about making the first move when you want to make love?	1	0
7. If you had an erotic dream about your partner, could you describe it to him or her without feeling embarrassed?	1	0
8. Would you be embarrassed to tell a new partner that you wish to use a condom to reduce the risk of STDs including HIV-AIDS?	0	1
9. Are you afraid to get angry or criticize your partner because you believe that doing so would destroy the relationship?	0	1
10. When you do get angry, do your quarrels take a long time to resolve and leave you both feeling bitter?	0	1

SCORING

High Rating (8–10)

You communicate well with your partner and are able to make your needs felt and to understand his or hers.

Medium Rating (5–7)

Your score indicates that you may find it hard to talk with your partner about sexual issues without becoming embarrassed. Consequently, when sexual difficulties arise, your inhibition may lead you to ignore them, so that they become more entrenched.

Low Rating (0–4)

Your sexual communication skills need some attention. You are likely to find it hard to express your sexual needs, and you should develop new communication skills and strategies.

Source: From *Sexual Happiness: A Practical Approach* by Maurice Yaffee and Elizabeth Fenwick. Copyright © 1988 by Maurice Yaffee and Elizabeth Fenwick. Reprinted by permission of Henry Holt & Co., Inc., and Dorling Kindersley Publishers. Price $24.95.

DIFFICULTIES THAT CAN HINDER SEXUAL FUNCTIONING

Research indicates that problems that can hinder sexual functioning are quite common in this country. Table 6.1 illustrates the combined results of 23 different studies of people who reported sexual problems. The label given to the various problems that can interfere with sexual

Vaginal intercourse: The insertion of the penis into the vagina.

Variant sexual behavior: A sexual behavior that is not engaged in by most people.

Classifying Sexual Behavior

One component of behavior change is the examination of alternatives, and the values, attitudes, and beliefs we attach to those alternatives. The following activity may help you identify options for sexual behavior by realistically examining what activities you view as natural, normal, and moral.

	Natural/unnatural	Normal/abnormal	Moral/immoral
Sexual intercourse			
Oral sex			
Gay/lesbian sex			
Masturbation			
Extramarital sex			
Premarital sex			
Anal sex			

1. In the boxes above, indicate whether you believe each activity listed is "natural/unnatural," "normal/abnormal," or "moral/immoral."

2. What are your criteria for identifying a behavior as natural or unnatural?

3. What are your criteria for identifying a behavior as normal or abnormal?

4. What are your criteria for identifying a behavior as moral or immoral?

5. Do you use similar or different criteria for natural, normal, and moral? Why?

Source: Adapted by permission from Bryan Strong and Christine DeVault, *Human Sexuality,* © 1994 Mayfield Publishing Company.

---

pleasure is **sexual dysfunction.** You should not be embarrassed if you experience a sexual dysfunction at some point in your life. The sexual part of yourself does not come with a lifetime warranty. You can have breakdowns involving your sexual function just as you can have breakdowns in any of your other body systems. Sexual dysfunctions can be divided into four major classes: sexual desire disorders, sexual arousal disorders, orgasm disorders, and sexual pain disorders. We will look briefly at each of these categories. In most cases, sexual dysfunctions can be treated successfully if both partners are willing to work together to solve the problem.

Sexual Desire Disorders

The most frequent problem that causes people to seek out a sex therapist is **ISD, or inhibited sexual desire.**[16] ISD is the lack of a sexual appetite or simply a lack of interest and pleasure in sexual activity. In some instances, it can result from stress or boredom with sex. **Sexual aversion disorder** is another type of desire dysfunction, characterized by sexual phobias (unreasonable fears) and anxiety about sexual contact. The psychological stress of a punitive upbringing, rigid religious background, or a history of physical or sexual abuse may be one source of these desire disorders.

Sexual Arousal Disorders

The most common disorder in this category is erectile dysfunction. **Erectile dysfunction, or impotence,** is difficulty in achieving or maintaining a penile erection sufficient for intercourse. At some time in his life, every man experiences impotence. Causes are varied and include underlying diseases, such as diabetes or prostate problems; reactions to some medications (for example, medication for high blood pressure); depression; fatigue; stress; alcohol; performance anxiety; and guilt over real or imaginary problems (such as when a man compares himself to his partner's past lovers).

Impotence generally becomes more of a problem as men age. Statistics indicate that 2 percent of men at age 40 and 25 percent of men over age 65 experience the problem occasionally. At any given time, 10 million American men suffer from impotence.[17]

Chronic impotence (impotence lasting more than three months) should be treated by a physician. A complete medical examination and history are necessary to

TABLE 6.1 ▪ Prevalence of Sexual Problems in Nonclinical Sample

	Men	Women
Lack of sexual desire	16%	34%
Erection difficulties	4–9	—
Anorgasmia	0	5–10%
Inhibited male orgasm	4–10	—
Premature ejaculation	36–38	—
Pain during intercourse	0	8–23%

Source: Reprinted by permission of Plenum Publishing Corporation from I. Spector and H. Carey, "Incidence and Prevalence of Sexual Dysfunction: A Critical Review of the Empirical Literature," *Archives of Sexual Behavior,* 19 (1990): 389–408.

rule out physical causes. For impotence related to physical causes, new treatments are being explored. These include hormone therapy, treatment with vasoactive drugs (drugs that work on the circulatory system), and vascular surgery to correct abnormalities in the blood vessels that supply the penis.

Impotence due to psychological factors can be treated with psychotherapy. Such treatment is effective in 90 percent of cases.

Orgasm Disorders

Up to 50 percent of the male population are affected by premature ejaculation at some time in their lives. **Premature ejaculation** is ejaculation that occurs prior to or very soon after the insertion of the penis into the vagina. Another orgasm disorder in males is **retarded ejaculation,** or the inability to ejaculate once the penis is erect. Treatment for premature ejaculation involves a physical examination to rule out organic causes. If the cause of the problem is not physiological, therapy is available to help a man learn how to control the timing of his ejaculation. Fatigue, stress, performance pressure, and alcohol use can all be contributing factors to orgasmic disorders in men.

When a woman is unable to achieve orgasm with her partner, she often blames herself and learns to fake orgasm in order to preserve her partner's ego. Research has reported that up to 66 percent of women have faked an orgasm at one time or another.[18] Until recently, our society dictated that women were not supposed to enjoy sex but were to engage in it only to fulfill the "marital duty." The Kinsey reports in the 1950s and Masters and Johnson's findings in the 1960s and 1970s raised questions about these female sexual myths. We recognize today that women enjoy sexual pleasure as much as men do. In the past, women who did not experience orgasm were called frigid. This term is no longer used because it implies that the woman is at fault. Instead, the term **preorgasmic** has been substituted, since most women can be taught to become orgasmic.

For women whose sexual pleasure is hampered, therapy is available. A physical examination to rule out organic causes is generally the first step. Masturbation is usually a primary focus in teaching a woman to become orgasmic. Through masturbation, a woman can learn how her body responds sexually to various types of touch. Once a woman has become orgasmic through masturbation, she learns to communicate her needs to her partner. The investment of time and caring by both partners is usually worth the effort, for 70 percent of preorgasmic women can be helped.

Sexual Pain Disorders

Two common disorders in this category are dyspareunia and vaginismus. **Dyspareunia** is pain experienced by a female during intercourse. This pain may be caused by diseases such as endometriosis, uterine tumors, chlamydia, gonorrhea, or urinary-tract infections. Damage to tissues during childbirth and insufficient lubrication during intercourse may also cause pain or discomfort. Dyspareunia can also be psychological in origin. As with other problems, dyspareunia can be treated with good results. The first step in treatment is a thorough pelvic examination to rule out physical disease. Diseases or disorders can usually be cured with medication or surgery. Vaginal lubricants

Sexual dysfunction: Problems associated with achieving sexual satisfaction.

Inhibited sexual desire (ISD): Lack of sexual appetite or simply a lack of interest and pleasure in sexual activity.

Sexual aversion disorder: Type of desire dysfunction characterized by sexual phobias and anxiety about sexual contact.

Erectile dysfunction: Also known as impotence; difficulty in achieving or maintaining a penile erection sufficient for intercourse.

Impotence: Inability to attain or maintain an erection sufficient for intercourse.

Premature ejaculation: Ejaculation that occurs prior to or almost immediately following penile penetration of the vagina.

Retarded ejaculation: The inability to ejaculate once the penis is erect.

Preorgasmic: In women, the state of never having experienced an orgasm.

Dyspareunia: Pain experienced by women during intercourse.

can be purchased to help with inadequate lubrication. Psychologically caused dyspareunia is much more difficult to treat.

Vaginismus is the involuntary contraction of vaginal muscles, making penile insertion painful or impossible. Most cases of vaginismus are related to fear of intercourse or to unresolved sexual conflicts. Treatment of vaginismus involves teaching a woman to achieve orgasm through nonvaginal stimulation. Becoming orgasmic is important because research has indicated that treatment for vaginismus is more successful in orgasmic women. The woman and her partner are then taught methods for dilating the vagina, either with fingers or a vibrator. As dilation is achieved, the woman is taught to relax in order to effect penetration. Cure rates are close to 100 percent.

Drugs and Sex

Because psychoactive drugs affect our entire physiology, it is only logical that they affect our sexual behavior. Promises of increased pleasure make drugs very tempting to those seeking greater sexual satisfaction. Too often, however, drugs become central to sexual activities and damage the relationship. The effects of drugs on sexual performance are summarized in Table 6.2.

Alcohol is notorious for reducing inhibitions and giving increased feelings of well-being and desirability. At the same time, alcohol inhibits sexual response; thus, the mind may be willing, but not the body.

Perhaps the greatest danger associated with use of drugs during sex is the tendency to blame the drug for negative behavior. "I can't help what I did last night because I was stoned" is a response that demonstrates sexual immaturity. A sexually mature person carefully examines risks and benefits and makes decisions accordingly. If drugs are necessary to increase erotic feelings, it is likely that the partners are being dishonest about their feelings for each other. Good sex should not be dependent on chemical substances.

> **Vaginismus:** A state in which the vaginal muscles contract so forcefully that penetration cannot be accomplished.

The influence of alcohol can impair your judgment and lead to sexual encounters that are not in your best interest.

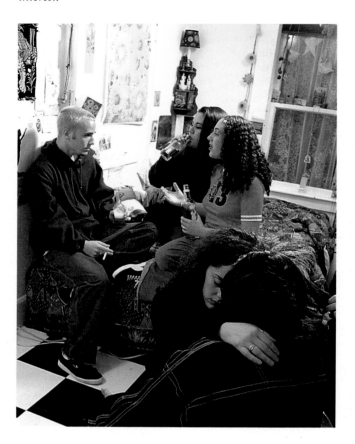

WHAT DO YOU THINK?

Why do we find it so difficult to discuss sexual dysfunction in our society? Do you think it is more difficult for men than for women to talk about dysfunction? Have you ever used alcohol or some other drug to enhance your sexual performance? Why did you feel the need to rely on something outside yourself?

Summary

◆ Sexual identity is determined by a complex interaction of genetic, physiological, and environmental factors. Gender, gender roles, and gender-role stereotypes are all blended into our sexual identity. The men's movement seeks to help men reconnect with their emotions to other men, their families, and nature.

◆ The major components of the female sexual anatomy include the mons pubis, labia minora and majora,

TABLE 6.2 ■ Drugs Affecting Sexual Performance

Name (and Street Name)	Supposed Effect	Actual Effect
Alcohol	Enhances arousal; stimulates sexual activity.	Can reduce inhibitions to make sexual behaviors less stressful. It is actually a depressant and in quantity can impair erection ability, arousal, and orgasm.
Amphetamines ("uppers"; includes Benzedrine, Dexedrine)	Elevate mood; enhance sexual experience and abilities.	Central nervous system stimulants; they reduce inhibitions. Long-term use impairs sexual functioning and can reduce vaginal lubrication in women.
Amyl nitrate ("snappers," "poppers")	Intensifies orgasms and arousal.	Dilates arteries to brain and also to genital area; produces time distortion, warmth in pelvic area. It can produce dizziness, headaches, and fainting.
Barbiturates ("barbs," "downers")	Enhance arousal; stimulate sexual activity.	Reduce inhibitions in similar fashion to alcohol. They are physically addictive, and overdose may produce severe depression and even death due to respiratory failure.
Cantharides ("Spanish fly")	Stimulates genital area, causing person to desire coitus.	Not effective as a sexual stimulant. It acts as a powerful irritant that can cause inflammation to lining of bladder and urethra; can result in permanent tissue damage and even death.
Cocaine ("coke")	Increases frequency and intensity of orgasm; heightens arousal.	Central nervous system stimulant; it loosens inhibitions and enhances sense of well-being. Regular use can induce depression and anxiety. Chronic sniffing can produce lesions and perforations of nasal passage.
LSD and other psychedelic drugs (includes mescaline, psilocybin)	Enhance sexual response.	No direct physiological enhancement of sexual response. May produce altered perception of sexual activity; frequently associated with unsatisfactory erotic experiences.
L-dopa	Sexually rejuvenates older males.	No documented benefits to sexual ability. It occasionally produces a painful condition known as priapism (constant, unwanted erection).
Marijuana	Elevates mood and arousal; stimulates sexual activity.	Enhances mood and reduces inhibitions in a way similar to alcohol. It may distort the time sense, with the resulting illusion of prolonged arousal and orgasm.
Yohimbine	Induces sexual arousal and enhances sexual performance.	Appears to have genuine aphrodisiac effect on rats. Recent evidence suggests it may enhance sexual desire or performance in some humans.

Source: From *Our Sexuality,* 5th ed., 16, by Robert Crooks and Karla Baur. Copyright © 1993, 1989, 1986, 1983, 1980 by Benjamin/Cummings Publishing Company. Reprinted by permission of Brooks/Cole Publishing Company, a division of Thomson Publishing, Pacific Grove, CA 93950.

Managing Your Sexual Behavior

By now you probably realize the importance of understanding, as well as accepting, your sexual self. Your sexuality can be one of the most complicated health issues you have to deal with. It is necessary to understand possible problems and options so that you can make informed decisions.

Making Decisions for You

Think about your sexual behaviors. Are there any behaviors in which you engage that you would like to change? What effects would that change have on you and your partner? What steps will you take to make this behavior change? What will you do to make sure that you stay with this behavior change?

Checklist for Change: Making Personal Choices

✓ Do you feel comfortable with yourself sexually? Do you know the function and location of the structures that make up the male and female sexual anatomy? Are you satisfied with your current choice(s) of sexual expression?

✓ Have you made a list of the gender roles that you have adopted to date? Do you feel limited or bound by any gender-role stereotypes? Would you like to change any of them?

✓ Do you know what resources are available to help you understand your sexual anatomy and function? Have you made a list of those components or functions that you don't understand?

✓ Do you know what your options are for expressing your sexuality? Have you reviewed the options and identified those you may be willing to try?

✓ What are your priorities? Have you set some long-term and short-term goals?

✓ Do you need to work on developing any new skills that will help you reach your goals?

✓ What are the rewards for meeting your objective(s)? What supports are available to assist you with your goals? How will you measure success?

Checklist for Change: Making Community Choices

✓ Have you taken the time to become informed about sexual issues and concerns in your community?

✓ Have you identified and prioritized concerns you would like to address? Do you know who the leaders are in the community? Have you communicated your concerns to the appropriate persons?

✓ Do you know what community resources are available to help tackle the problem? Do you know who your supporters are?

✓ Have you analyzed the risks versus the benefits for everyone involved?

✓ Are you committed to sticking with the project until its completion?

Critical Thinking

After leading what you consider a normal sexual life, which included several intimate sexual relationships, you meet that special person. When you first started dating, you learned that this person was a practicing member of an Eastern religion, but you never really gave much thought to what that meant to your relationship. Now, several months later, as you want to become intimate, you realize that this religion does not accept intercourse before marriage.

You feel sexually frustrated. But at the same time, you are sincerely in love and believe that this relationship could lead to marriage. Using the DECIDE model in Chapter 1, think about what the two of you could do to satisfy both physical and emotional feelings.

---

clitoris, urethral and vaginal openings, vagina, cervix, fallopian tubes, and ovaries. The major components of the male sexual anatomy are the penis, scrotum, testes, epididymides, vasa deferentia, ejaculatory ducts, and urethra.

◆ Sexuality can be expressed in many ways. Physiologically, males and females experience four phases of sexual response: excitement/arousal, plateau, orgasm, and resolution. In addition, men experience a fifth phase known as the refractory period. Sexual

orientation refers to a person's preference for emotional, social, and sexual attractions. Sexual activities include celibacy, autoerotic behaviors, kissing and erotic touch, oral-genital stimulation, anal intercourse, and vaginal intercourse. Numerous variant sexual behaviors also exist in our society.

◆ Sexual dysfunctions can be classified into sexual desire disorders, sexual arousal disorders, orgasm disorders, and sexual pain disorders. Various drug use can also lead to sexual dysfunction.

Discussion Questions

1. List some stereotypical gender roles. Do they still hold true in the 1990s? What positive changes could come from the men's movement? What negative changes could result?

2. What are the functions of the various hormones during puberty? What physical changes are brought about by menopause?

3. What is "normal" sexual behavior? Is sexual orientation primarily determined by biological or environmental factors? Do men and women differ in sexual response?

4. Do drugs and alcohol enhance sexual performance? What risks are involved in such experimentation?

Application Exercise

Reread the What Do You Think? scenarios at the beginning of the chapter and answer the following questions:

1. From what you have learned in this chapter, how might Carl and Anita cope with the peer pressure they feel to begin having sex? What reinforcers and supports are available to them? Is the decision that Carl and Anita have made to abstain from sex normal? Natural? Moral?

2. What sexual communication skills are Rachel and Rod lacking? If Rod wanted to change his behavior, how might he go about it?

Further Reading

Michael Robert, John Ganon, Edward Laumann, and Gina Kolata, *Sex in America: A Definitive Survey* (New York: Little, Brown, 1994).

A presentation of the results of a new and methodologically sound survey of the sexual practices and beliefs of Americans.

SIECUS (Sexuality Information and Education Council of the United States) Report. A bimonthly journal. 130 West 42nd Street, New York, NY 10036.

Highly acclaimed and readable journal. Includes timely and thought-provoking articles on human sexuality, sexuality education, and AIDS.

Boston Women's Health Collective, *The New Our Bodies, Ourselves,* 2nd ed. (New York: Simon & Schuster, 1992).

A comprehensive and progressive book dealing with all aspects of women's health, including sexual health, relationships, sexually transmitted disease, birth control, parenthood, menopause, and the politics of women's health care.

Sam Keen, *Fire in the Belly* (New York: Bantam Books, 1991).

One of several books describing the men's movement of the 1990s and a new perspective on masculinity.

Harriet Lerner, *The Dance of Intimacy* (New York: Harper & Row, 1989).

A very readable book defining intimacy and discussing how intimate relationships can thrive or be healed.

Darlene Mininni, *Sex Talk: The College Student's Guide to Sex in the 90s* (New York: Good Friends Press, 1991).

Good reference for any college student who is currently sexually active as well as any student thinking about becoming sexually active.

Jeffrey S. Nevid, Lois Fischer-Rathus, and Spencer A. Rathus, *Human Sexuality in a World of Diversity, Second Edition* (Boston: Allyn and Bacon, 1995).

A good general sexuality text for students and adults. Information covers the spectrum of sexual issues, with a particular emphasis on diversity.

Bernie Zibergeld, *The New Male Sexuality: A Guide to Sexual Fulfillment* (New York: Bantam Books, 1992).

A new and complete discussion of male sexuality, including sexual function, self-awareness, and overcoming sexuality difficulties.

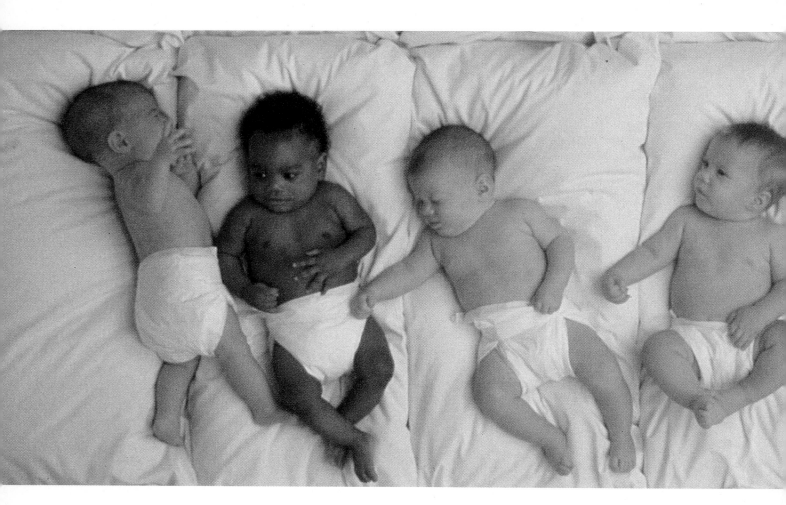

*C*HAPTER OBJECTIVES

◆ List permanent and reversible contraceptive methods, discuss their effectiveness in preventing pregnancy and sexually transmitted diseases, and describe how these methods are used.

◆ Summarize the legal decisions surrounding abortion and the various types of abortion procedures used today.

◆ Discuss emotional health, maternal health, financial evaluation, and contingency planning in terms of your

own life's goals as aspects that you should consider before becoming parents.

◆ Explain the importance of prenatal care and the process of pregnancy.

◆ Describe the basic stages of childbirth as well as some of the complications that can arise during labor and delivery.

◆ Review some of the primary causes of and possible solutions to infertility.

Birth Control, Pregnancy, and Childbirth

Managing Your Fertility

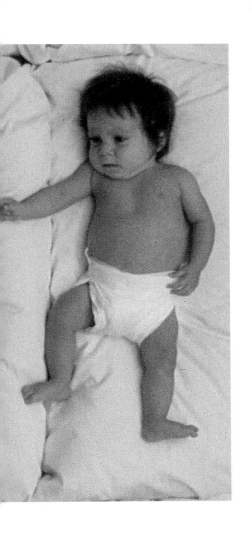

WHAT DO YOU THINK?

Anna, age 16, becomes pregnant during her sophomore year of high school. Bill, age 17, is a high-school dropout earning the minimum wage at a local gas station. They decide to marry and to keep the baby. Janet and Hank, age 23, are mentally retarded people living in a group home. When Janet becomes pregnant, they decide to marry and to get their own apartment. Sylvia is not interested in being married. She does want children, though, and so opts for alternative insemination and conceives.

- What obstacles may these people's parenting decisions present to them? What other options might they have? What potential benefits may result from their decisions?

Kari and Dave have been dating for several months. After a romantic evening, they go back to Dave's room in the residence hall with the intention of having sex. When they arrive at Dave's, Kari discovers that Dave does not have any condoms. He thought that Kari either would have a diaphragm or was taking the pill. Rather than spoil the evening, Kari and Dave have unprotected sex. The next day, they have an argument over who exactly was responsible for the birth control.

- What mistakes were made in this relationship? Who is responsible for providing birth control? What were the risks involved in having unprotected sex? What were the alternatives?

Fertility is a mixed blessing for some women. The ability to participate in the miracle of birth is an overwhelming experience for many. Yet the responsibility to control one's fertility can also seem overwhelming. Today, we not only understand the intimate details of reproduction but also possess technologies designed to control or enhance our fertility. Along with information and technological advance comes choice, and choice goes hand in hand with responsibility. Choosing if and when to have children is one of our greatest responsibilities. A woman and her partner have much to consider before planning or risking a pregnancy. Children, whether planned or unplanned, change people's lives. They require a lifelong personal commitment of love and nurturing.

Before you plan or risk a pregnancy, you have the responsibility to make certain you are physically, emotionally, and financially prepared to care for another human being. One measure of maturity is the ability to discuss reproduction and birth control with one's sexual partner before succumbing to sexual urges. Men often assume that their partners are taking care of birth control. Women often feel that if they bring up the subject, it implies that they are "easy" or "loose." You will find embarrassment-free discussion a lot easier if you understand human reproduction and contraception and honestly consider your attitudes toward these matters before you get into compromising situations.

Our culture teaches us that human life is sacred and that the creation of a new life should not be undertaken lightly. Unfortunately, the consequences of sexual activity are often ignored because people are swept along by the powerful and pleasurable feelings of the moment. Mature people have learned to control their desire for sexual gratification long enough to make rational decisions.

Fertility: A person's ability to reproduce.

Conception: The fertilization of an ovum by a sperm.

Contraception: Methods of preventing conception.

Condom: A sheath of thin latex or other material designed to fit over an erect penis and to catch semen upon ejaculation.

Methods of Fertility Control

Conception refers to the fertilization of an ovum by a sperm. The sperm enters the ovum. Its tail breaks off, and a protective chemical barrier secreted by the ovum surrounds the sperm and prevents other sperm from entering. The following conditions are necessary for conception:

1. A viable egg.

2. A viable sperm.

3. Possible access to the egg by the sperm.

Contraception refers to methods of preventing conception. Ever since people first associated sexual activity with pregnancy, society has searched for a simple, infallible, and risk-free method of preventing pregnancy. We have not yet succeeded in finding one.

Our present methods of contraception fall into two categories: *reversible methods,* such as the pill, condoms, and abstinence; and *permanent methods,* such as vasec-

---

For couples who want to avoid pregnancy, a wide variety of contraceptives are available, including male and female condoms, IUDs, cervical caps, diaphragms, and different types of pills.

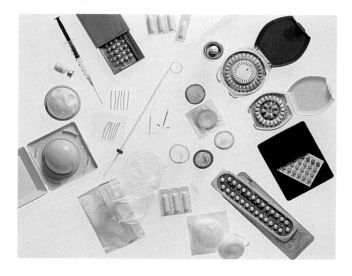

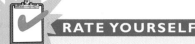
Which Contraceptive Method Is Right for You and Your Partner?

If you are sexually active, you need to use the contraceptive method that will work best for you. A number of factors may be involved in your decision. The following questions will help you sort out these factors and choose an appropriate method. Answer yes (Y) or no (N) for each statement as it applies to you and, if appropriate, your partner.

1. I like sexual spontaneity and don't want to be bothered with contraception at the time of sexual intercourse.
2. I need a contraceptive immediately.
3. It is very important that I do not become pregnant now.
4. I want a contraceptive method that will protect me and my partner against sexually transmissible diseases.
5. I prefer a contraceptive method that requires the cooperation and involvement of both partners.
6. I have sexual intercourse frequently.
7. I have sexual intercourse infrequently.
8. I am forgetful or have a variable daily routine.
9. I have more than one sexual partner.
10. I have heavy periods with cramps.
11. I prefer a method that requires little or no action or bother on my part.
12. I am a nursing mother.
13. I want the option of conceiving immediately after discontinuing contraception.
14. I want a contraceptive method with few or no side effects.

If you answered yes to the statements listed on the left, the method on the right may be a good choice for you.

1, 3, 6, 10, 11	Oral contraceptives
1, 3, 6, 8, 10, 11	Norplant
1, 3, 6, 8, 10, 11, 12	Depo-Provera
1, 3, 6, 8, 11, 12, 13	IUD
2, 4, 5, 7, 8, 9, 12, 13, 14	Condoms (male and female)
5, 7, 12, 13, 14	Diaphragm and spermicide
5, 7, 12, 13, 14	Cervical cap
2, 5, 7, 8, 12, 13, 14	Sponge
2, 5, 7, 8, 12, 13, 14	Vaginal spermicides
5, 7, 13, 14	FAM

Your answers may indicate that more than one method would be appropriate for you. To help narrow your choices, circle the numbers of the statements that are *most* important for you. Before you make a final choice, talk with your partner(s) and your physician. Consider your own lifestyle and preferences as well as characteristics of each method (effectiveness, side effects, costs, and so on). For maximum protection against pregnancy and STDs, you might want to consider combining two methods.

Source: Reprinted by permission from Bryan Strong and Christine DeVault, *Human Sexuality*, © 1994 Mayfield Publishing Company.

---

tomy (for men) and tubal ligation (for women). Let's discuss some of the methods in each category in detail so you will have the information you need to make an informed choice (also see the Rate Yourself box).

Reversible Contraception

Abstinence and "Outercourse." Strictly defined, abstinence means deliberately shunning intercourse. This strict definition would allow one to engage in such forms of sexual intimacy as massage, kissing, and solitary masturbation. But many people today have broadened the definition of abstinence to include all forms of sexual contact, even those that do not culminate in sexual intercourse.

Couples who go a step farther than massage and kissing and engage in such activities as oral-genital sex and mutual masturbation are sometimes said to be engaging

in "outercourse." Like abstinence, outercourse can be 100 percent effective for birth control as long as the male does not ejaculate near the vaginal opening. Unlike abstinence, however, outercourse is not 100 percent effective against sexually transmitted diseases (STDs). Oral-genital contact can result in transmission of an STD, although the practice can be made safer by using a condom on the penis or a dental dam on the vaginal opening.

The Condom. The **condom** is a strong sheath of latex rubber or other material designed to fit over an erect penis. The condom catches the ejaculate, thereby preventing sperm migration toward the egg. The condom is the only temporary means of birth control available for men and the only barrier that effectively prevents the spread of STDs and AIDS. Regardless of your preferred method of birth control, you should always use a condom. Condoms come in a wide variety of styles: colored, ribbed for "extra sensation," lubricated, nonlubricated, and with or without reservoirs at the tip. All may be purchased with or without spermicide in pharmacies, in some supermarkets, in some public bathrooms, and in many health clinics. A new condom must be used for each act of intercourse or oral sex.

Condoms help prevent the spread of some sexually transmitted diseases, including genital herpes and AIDS. They may also slow or reduce the development of cervical abnormalities in women that can lead to cancer. The theoretical **contraceptive effectiveness rate** for condoms is 98 percent, meaning that *when they are used correctly,* 2 women out of 100 using condoms will become pregnant in one year. In actuality, however, their effectiveness rate is only 88 percent because they are so often used incorrectly. The failure rates of contraceptives are shown in Table 7.1. Condoms should be used during every act of intercourse or oral sex. They must be rolled on the penis before the penis touches the vagina, and held in place when the penis is removed from the vagina after ejaculation (see Figure 7.1). For greatest efficacy, they should be used with a spermicide containing nonoxynol-9.

Another reason that condoms are not as effective in real life as in theory is that they can break during intercourse, especially if they are old or poorly stored. They must be stored in a cool place (not in a wallet or hip pocket) and should be inspected before use for small tears.

For some people, a condom ruins the spontaneity of sex. Stopping to put it on breaks the mood for them. Others report that the condom decreases sensation. These inconveniences contribute to improper use of the device. Couples who learn to put the condom on together as part of foreplay are generally more successful with this form of birth control.[1]

Oral Contraceptives.   **Oral contraceptive** pills were first marketed in the United States in 1960. Their convenience quickly made them the most widely used reversible method of fertility control.

Most oral contraceptives work through the combined effects of synthetic estrogen and progesterone. Because the levels of estrogen in the pill are higher than those produced by the body, the pituitary gland is never signaled to produce follicle-stimulating hormone (FSH), without which ova will not develop in the ovaries. Progesterone in the pill prevents proper growth of the uterine lining and thickens the cervical mucus, forming a barrier against sperm.

Pills are meant to be taken in a cycle. At the end of each three-week cycle, the user discontinues the drug or takes a placebo pill for one week. The resultant drop in hormones causes the uterine lining to disintegrate, and the user will have a menstrual period, usually within one to three days. The same cycle is repeated every 28 days. Menstrual flow is generally lighter than in a non-pill user because the hormones in the pill prevent thick endometrial buildup.

Today's pill is different from the one introduced more than three decades ago. The original pill contained large amounts of estrogen, which caused certain risks for the user, whereas the current pill contains the minimal amount of estrogen necessary to prevent pregnancy.

Because the chemicals in oral contraceptives change the way the body metabolizes certain nutrients, all women using the pill should check with their prescribing practitioners regarding dietary supplements. The nutrients of concern include vitamin C and the B-complex vitamins—B_2, B_6, and B_{12}. A nutritious diet that includes whole grains, fresh fruits and vegetables, lean meats, fish and poultry, and nonfat dairy products is advised.

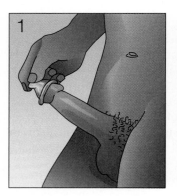 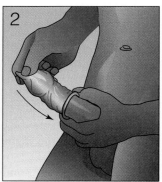 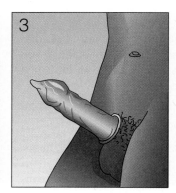 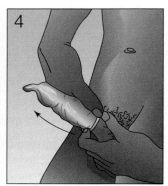

FIGURE 7.1

How To Use a Condom: The condom should be rolled over the erect penis before any penetration occurs. A small space (about 1/2") should be left at the end of the condom to collect the semen after ejaculation. Hold the tip of the condom, and unroll it all the way to the base of the penis. Hold the base of the condom before withdrawal to avoid spilling any semen.

TABLE 7.1 ■ Available Methods of Contraception and Failure Rates

Unplanned pregnancies occur at different rates in various age groups. Nearly half of unplanned pregnancies—1.7 million, or 4.7 percent—occur to women who were using contraception, mainly because of inconsistent and incorrect use. Listed below are the available methods of contraception and their ranges of failure rates.

	Percentage of Sexually Active Couples Who Use It	Failure Rate Perfect Use	Average Use
For women			
• Pill	25	0.1%	6.0%
• Diaphragm/cervical cap	5.7	6%	18%
• Sponge	1.1	8%	24%
• IUD	1.0	0.8%	4.0%
• Spermicides (foams, creams, gels)	6.0	3.0%	30%
For men and women			
• Condoms	19	2.0%	16%
• Sterilization			
Tubal ligation	27	0.2%	0.5%
Vasectomy	NA	0.1%	0.2%
• Withdrawal/rhythm	7.0	4.0%	24%

Source: Adapted with permission of Ortho-McNeil Pharmaceutical and the Alan Guttmacher Institute from Robin Herman, "Whatever Happened to the Contraceptive Revolution?" *Washington Post,* Health Section, 13 December 1994, 12–16. Contraceptive usage data from the 1993 Ortho Annual Birth Control Study; failure rate data from the Alan Guttmacher Institute.

Oral contraceptives can interact negatively with other drugs. Some antibiotics diminish the pill's effectiveness. Women in doubt should check with their prescribing practitioners, their pharmacists, or other knowledgeable health professionals. You can learn more about health methods and contraceptive choice in the Skills for Behavior Change box.

Return of fertility may be delayed after discontinuing the pill, but the pill is not known to cause infertility. Women who had irregular menstrual cycles before going on the pill are more likely to have problems conceiving, regardless of pill use.

The effectiveness rate of oral contraceptives is 97 percent, making them one of the most effective reversible methods of fertility control. Use of the pill is convenient and does not interfere with lovemaking. It may lessen menstrual difficulties, such as cramps and premenstrual syndrome (PMS). Women using oral contraceptives have lower risks for developing endometrial and ovarian cancers. They are also less likely than nonusers to develop fibrocystic breast disease. In addition, pill users have lower incidences of ectopic pregnancies, ovarian cysts, pelvic inflammatory disease, and iron deficiency anemia.[2] But possible serious health problems associated with the pill include the tendency for pill users' blood to form clots and an increased risk for high blood pressure in a few women. Clotting can lead to strokes or heart attacks. The risk is low for most healthy women under 35 who do not smoke; it increases with age and, especially, with cigarette smoking.

Outside these risk factors and certain side effects associated with the pill, its greatest disadvantage is that it must be taken every day. If a woman misses taking one pill, she is advised to use an alternative form of contraception for the remainder of that cycle. The cost of the pill may also be a problem for some women. Finally, some teenagers report that the requirement to have a complete gynecological examination in order to get a prescription for the pill is a huge obstacle. Fully 69 percent of female teenagers think that this requirement frightens their peers away from use of the pill.[3] Educating young women about what goes on in a gynecological exam would certainly help ease their anxiety.

Progestin-Only Pills. Progestin-only pills (or minipills) contain small doses of progesterone. Women who feel

Contraceptive effectiveness rate: The percentage rate of women who will become pregnant in one year when the contraceptive method is used correctly.

Oral contraceptives: Pills taken daily for three weeks of the menstrual cycle which prevent ovulation by regulating hormones.

Talking with Your Partner about Using Condoms

Knowing what's best for our health and doing something about it can be two different things. Even bringing up the subject of condoms can be hard. Here are some suggestions:

- Think about what you want to say ahead of time. Sort out your own feelings about using condoms before you talk with your partner.

- Choose a time to talk before that first intimate moment. Getting things straight before you make love means you'll both be prepared and relaxed.

- Decide how you want to start the conversation. You might say, "I need to talk with you about something that's important to both of us," or, "I've been hearing a lot lately about safer sex. Have you ever tried condoms?" or, "I feel kind of embarrassed, but I care too much about you not to talk about this."

- Remember, starting to talk is the hardest part. Don't be surprised if your partner responds with, "I'm glad you brought it up. I was worried too," or, "I like sharing the responsibility of sex. I appreciate a woman who's willing to let me."

- Once you've both agreed to use condoms, do something positive and fun. Go to the store together. Buy lots of different brands and colors. Plan a special day when you can experiment. Just talking about how you'll use all those condoms can be a turn on.

Source: Reprinted with permission from *Condoms: Talking with Your Partner,* ETR Associates, Santa Cruz, CA. For more information about this and other related materials, call 1-800-321-4407.

---

uncertain about using estrogen pills, who suffer from side effects related to estrogen, or who are nursing may want to take these pills rather than combination pills. There is still some question about the specific ways progestin-only pills work. Current thought is that they change the composition of the cervical mucus, thus impeding sperm travel. They may also inhibit ovulation in some women. The effectiveness rate of progestin-only pills is 96 percent, which is slightly lower than that of estrogen-containing pills. Also, their use usually leads to irregular menstrual bleeding.

The Morning-After Pill. The term **morning-after pill** refers to drugs that can be taken up to three days after unprotected intercourse to prevent fertilization or implantation. The most common drug prescribed is a combination of estrogen and progesterone. Other preparations include large doses of progesterone or a large dose of estrogen called **diethylstilbestrol (DES)**. Of all the drugs available to prevent pregnancy, DES is the most risky. Between 1941

and 1970, DES was given to pregnant women to prevent miscarriage. Babies born to these women are today at increased risk for developing a rare vaginal cancer (in women) or genital abnormalities (in men). Nausea or vomiting is the most likely side effect of these drugs. Other risks are the same as those associated with combination pills.

The morning-after pill is for a one-time emergency use only. It is not a method to be used regularly. The FDA has not approved any of these drugs as morning-after medications. No serious side effects have been observed when women take these drugs under medical supervision.

Foams, Suppositories, Jellies, and Creams. Like condoms, these contraceptive preparations are available without a prescription. Chemically, they are referred to as **spermicides**—substances designed to kill sperm.

Jellies and creams are packaged in tubes, and foams are available in aerosol cans. All have tubes designed for insertion into the vagina. They must be inserted far enough to cover the cervix, providing both a chemical barrier that kills sperm and a physical barrier that stops sperm from continuing toward an egg.

Suppositories are waxy capsules that are placed deep in the vagina and melt once they are inside. They must be inserted 10 to 20 minutes before intercourse to have time to melt but no longer than one hour prior to intercourse or they lose their effectiveness. Additional contraceptive chemicals must be applied for each subsequent act of intercourse (see Figure 7.2).

Jellies, creams, suppositories, and foam do not require a prescription. When used in conjunction with a condom, their effectiveness rate is nearly 98 percent. They help prevent the spread of certain sexually transmitted diseases.

Morning-after pill: Drugs taken within three days after intercourse to prevent fertilization or implantation.

Diethylstilbestrol (DES): Type of morning-after pill containing large amounts of estrogen.

Spermicides: Substances designed to kill sperm.

Female condom: A single-use polyurethane sheath for internal use by women.

Diaphragm: A latex, saucer-shaped device designed to cover the cervix and block access to the uterus; should always be used with spermicide.

Choosing a Healthy Contraceptive

Part of sexual maturity is taking responsibility for your personal health regarding contraceptives. Aside from simply worrying about contraceptive effectiveness and convenience, you need to consider the effects that your birth control method may have on your health now and in the future. Here are some things to keep in mind when you decide on your contraceptive method:

1. Talk to your medical professional about your and your family's medical history. Is there anything that would discourage use of one method or another? For example, as the Multicultural Perspectives box in this chapter points out, contraceptive methods may have serious side effects given your medical history. Someone with diabetes would not be a good candidate for Norplant.

2. Learn about the potential side effects. If you find yourself experiencing the side effects of a contraceptive, you should talk to your doctor immediately. Your doctor may suggest switching to a different contraceptive or may simply assure you that you are normal and that the "side effects" don't appear related to contraceptive use.

3. Devise a method to ensure that you can't miss using it. If you take the pill, take it at the same time every day.

Associating it with a certain time or event (for instance, taking a morning shower) will reinforce your memory. If you use condoms, you might keep some in your sport coat jacket so that they will be there when you need them. Or you might keep your diaphragm packed in your overnight bag.

4. Learn how to talk to your partner about your choice of contraception. Decisions about contraceptives should be made as a couple, taking each person's health and desires into account.

5. Learn about drug interactions with your birth control method. While we will discuss this in more detail in Chapter 12, it is important to know what medications may interact with your method of birth control. For example, reactions may occur between alcohol and contraceptive pills or between antibiotics and contraceptive pills. In other words, alcohol and antibiotics may diminish the effectiveness of birth control pills in some women. Ask your doctor about drug interactions if you receive a prescription drug. If there is a potential for diminished effectiveness of your contraceptive, ask when can you resume normal sexual relations without taking added precautions.

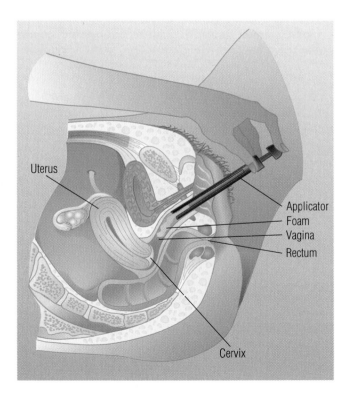

FIGURE 7.2

The Proper Method of Applying Spermicide within the Vagina

Jellies and creams are designed to be used with a diaphragm. Used alone, their effectiveness rate is only 79 percent. Foam, which is designed to be used alone, also has an effectiveness rate of 79 percent.

The Female Condom. This new contraceptive device for internal use by women has now been approved by the FDA. The **female condom** is a single-use, soft, loose-fitting polyurethane sheath. It is designed as one unit with two diaphragm-like rings. One ring, which lies inside the sheath, serves as an insertion mechanism and internal anchor. The other ring, which remains outside the vagina once the device is inserted, protects the labia and the base of the penis from infection. Tests conducted by the company that manufactures the female condom found that it was 87.6 percent effective among women in the United States. Many women like the female condom because it gives them more control over their reproduction than does the male condom. They believe that women must take full responsibility for birth control since they are the ones who become pregnant.

The Diaphragm with Spermicidal Jelly or Cream. Invented in the mid-nineteenth century, the **diaphragm** was the first widely used birth control method for women. Prior to that time, most women had to rely on their male partners to use a condom or to withdraw the penis before ejaculation.

The diaphragm is a soft, shallow cup made of thin latex rubber. Its flexible, rubber-coated ring is designed to fit snugly behind the pubic bone in front of the cervix and over the back of the cervix on the other side. Diaphragms are manufactured in different sizes and must be fitted to the woman by a trained practitioner. The practitioner should also be certain that the user knows how to insert her diaphragm correctly before she leaves the practitioner's office.

Diaphragms must be used with spermicidal cream or jelly. The spermicide is applied to the inside of the diaphragm before insertion. The jelly or cream is held in place by the diaphragm, creating a physical and chemical barrier against sperm. Additional spermicide must be applied before each subsequent act of intercourse, and the diaphragm must be left in place for six to eight hours after intercourse to allow the chemical to kill any sperm remaining in the vagina (see Figure 7.3).

The effectiveness rate of the diaphragm is only 82 percent. Using the diaphragm during the menstrual period or leaving the diaphragm in place beyond the recommended time slightly increases the user's risk of developing **toxic shock syndrome (TSS).** This condition results from the multiplication of a type of bacteria that spreads to the bloodstream and causes sudden high fever, rash, nausea, vomiting, diarrhea, and a sudden drop in blood pressure. If not treated, TSS can be fatal. The diaphragm (as well as tampons left too long in place) creates conditions conducive to the growth of these bacteria. To reduce the risk of TSS, women should wash their hands carefully with soap and water before inserting or removing the diaphragm.

Another problem with the diaphragm is that it can put undue pressure on the urethra, blocking urinary flow and predisposing the user to bladder infections. A further disadvantage is that inserting the device can be awkward, especially if the woman is rushed. When inserted incorrectly, the effectiveness rate of the diaphragm decreases.

The Contraceptive Sponge. The **contraceptive sponge** was first marketed in the United States in 1983, but was recently taken off the market. Shaped like a miniature doughnut with a depression in the center, this polyurethane device is saturated with a spermicide and inserted into the vagina. A small cord attached to the sponge aids in removal. The sponge comes in only one size.

The sponge must be dampened with water to activate the spermicide and must be inserted prior to intercourse. Once in place, it fits over the cervix, blocking the entrance, and releasing a spermicide (see Figure 7.4).

Once inserted, the sponge is effective for 24 hours. It must be left in place for six to eight hours after intercourse; 30 hours is the maximum length of time it can be left in the vagina. When removed, it is thrown away. It is good for one use only.

The effectiveness rate of the sponge is 82 percent for women who have never had a child. For women who have had a child, the effectiveness rate drops to 72 percent because of the widening of the cervix due to childbirth. To ensure effectiveness, the user should check the expiration date on each sponge, as shelf life is limited.

Some women find it difficult to remove the sponge. Some users have an allergic reaction to the spermicide,

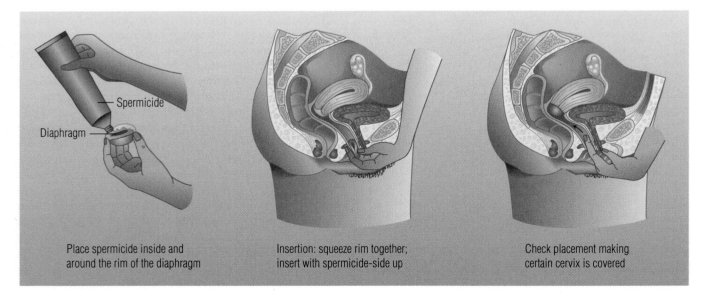

Place spermicide inside and around the rim of the diaphragm

Insertion: squeeze rim together; insert with spermicide-side up

Check placement making certain cervix is covered

FIGURE 7.3

The Proper Use and Placement of a Diaphragm

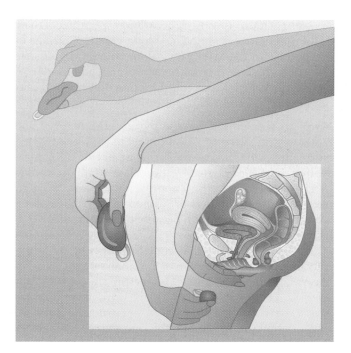

FIGURE 7.4

The Proper Placement of the Contraceptive Sponge

probably because the overall dose is significantly higher than in other spermicide products. Because of the dangers of toxic shock syndrome, the sponge should not be used during the menstrual period nor should it be left in place for longer than 30 hours. For couples who have frequent intercourse, the sponge may be expensive.

Cervical Cap. **Cervical caps** are one of the oldest methods used to prevent pregnancy. Early caps were made from beeswax, silver, or copper. The modern cervical cap has been available in Europe for several years and has been approved for use in the United States by the Food and Drug Administration (FDA) since 1988.

The cervical cap is a small cup made of latex that is designed to fit snugly over the entire cervix. It must be fitted by a practitioner and is designed for use with contraceptive jelly or cream. It is somewhat more difficult to insert than a diaphragm because of its smaller size.

The cap keeps sperm out of the uterus. It is held in place by suction created during application. Insertion may take place anywhere up to two days prior to intercourse, and the device must be left in place for six to eight hours after intercourse. The maximum length of time the cap can be left on the cervix is 48 hours. If removed and cleaned, it can be reinserted immediately.

The effectiveness rate of the cap is only 82 percent. Some women report unpleasant vaginal odors after use. Because the device can become dislodged during intercourse, placement must be checked frequently. It cannot

be used during the menstrual period or for longer than 48 hours because of the risk of toxic shock syndrome.

Intrauterine Devices. Widespread use of **intrauterine devices (IUDs)** for contraception began in the mid-1960s, when these devices were advertised as less risky and more convenient than the pill.

The devices began to fall out of favor in the mid-1970s following negative publicity about the Dalkon shield, a device associated with pelvic inflammatory disease and sterility. The manufacturer stopped making Dalkon shields in 1975.

We are not certain how IUDs work despite the fact that women have been using them since 1909. Although it was once thought that IUDs act by preventing implantation of a fertilized egg, most experts now believe that they interfere with the sperm's fertilization of the egg.

Two IUDs are currently available. The first, the Progestasert, is a T-shaped plastic device that contains synthetic progesterone. It slowly releases the progesterone. The practitioner must remove this IUD and insert a new one every year. The second, the ParaGuard, is also T-shaped, but it has copper wrapped around the shaft and does not contain any hormones. It can be left in place for four years before replacement.

A physician must fit and insert the IUD. For insertion, the device is folded and placed into a long, thin plastic applicator. The practitioner measures the depth of the uterus with a special instrument and then uses these measurements to place the IUD accurately. When in place, the arms of the T open out across the top of the uterus. One or two strings extend from the IUD into the vagina so the user can check to make sure that her IUD is in place. The device is removed by a practitioner when desired.

IUDs are 95 percent effective. But the discomfort and cost of insertion may be a disadvantage for some. When in place, the device can cause heavy menstrual flow and severe cramps. There is a risk of uterine perforation.

Toxic shock syndrome (TSS): A potentially life-threatening disease that occurs when specific bacterial toxins are allowed to multiply unchecked in wounds or through improper use of tampons or diaphragms.

Contraceptive sponge: A doughnut-shaped device moistened with water and placed in the vagina to block access to the uterus; the sponge is saturated with spermicide.

Cervical cap: A small cup made of latex that is designed to fit snugly over the entire cervix.

Intrauterine device (IUD): A T-shaped device that is implanted in the uterus to prevent pregnancy.

Women using IUDs have a higher risk of ectopic pregnancy, pelvic inflammatory disease, infertility, and tubal infections. If a pregnancy occurs while the IUD is in place, the chance of miscarriage is 25 to 50 percent. Removal of the device as soon as the pregnancy is known is advised. Doctors often offer therapeutic abortion to women who become pregnant while using an IUD because of the serious risks (including premature delivery, infection, and congenital abnormalities) associated with continuing the pregnancy.

Withdrawal. This not very effective method of birth control is most commonly used by people who have not taken the time to consider alternatives. The **withdrawal** method involves withdrawing the penis from the vagina just prior to ejaculation. Because there can be up to half a million sperm in the drop of fluid at the tip of the penis before ejaculation, this method is unreliable. Timing withdrawal is also difficult; males concentrating on accurate timing may not be able to relax and enjoy intercourse. The effectiveness rate for the withdrawal method is 82 percent.

New Methods of Birth Control

Depo-Provera. Depo-Provera is a long-acting synthetic progesterone that is injected intramuscularly every three months. Although used in other countries for years, the FDA did not approve it for use in the United States until 1992. Researchers believe that the drug prevents ovulation.

Depo-Provera encourages sexual spontaneity because the user does not have to remember to take a pill or to insert a device. Its effectiveness in preventing pregnancy is higher than 99 percent, which is better than the pill's effectiveness. Those who want to start a family can easily decide to do so without much of a waiting period. There are fewer health problems associated with Depo-Provera than with estrogen-containing pills. The main disadvantage is irregular bleeding, which can be troublesome at

first, but within a year, most women are amenorrheic (have no menstrual periods). Weight gain (an average of five pounds in the first year) is common. Other possible side effects include dizziness, nervousness, and headache. Unlike other methods of contraception, this method cannot be stopped immediately if problems arise.

Norplant. Approved for use by the FDA in 1990 and marketed since February 1991 for use in the United States, **Norplant** is one the newest forms of hormonal contraception. It has been tested by more than 1 million women in 45 countries and is now approved for use in 14 countries. Increasing numbers of women in the United States are considering this option because of its convenience, effectiveness, and safety.

Six silicon capsules that contain progestin are surgically inserted under the skin of a woman's upper arm. For five years, small amounts of progestin are continuously released. The progestin in Norplant works the same way as oral contraceptives do; it suppresses ovulation, prevents growth of uterine lining, and thickens the cervical mucus.

Norplant is one of the most effective methods of birth control ever developed. With a greater than 99 percent success rate in preventing pregnancy, its effectiveness approaches that of sterilization.[4]

Norplant can be inserted by a specially trained doctor, nurse, or nurse practitioner in 10 to 15 minutes. A local anesthetic is administered to the upper arm, a small injection is made, and, with a special needle, the six capsules are placed just under the skin in a fan shape. The capsules are similarly removed after five years or, if necessary, at any point after their insertion.

The capsules usually cannot be seen, nor does insertion leave a scar in most women. At this time, no serious side effects are known. Less serious side effects include irregular bleeding and irregular menstrual periods, acne, weight gain, breast tenderness, headaches, nervousness, and nausea.

An effectiveness rate greater than 99 percent makes Norplant one of the most effective reversible methods of fertility control. In addition to being very convenient, the implant is easy for a trained practitioner to do, so there is little chance of error. It costs less than the Pill—$550 compared to $1,180 over five years.[5] Medical assistance programs in many states will pay this cost for poor women.

Vaginal Ring. A method that is not yet approved by the FDA but that appears promising is the vaginal ring. Rings that are 2 to 3 inches in diameter and contain estrogen and progesterone or progesterone alone are placed by a woman in her vagina. They may be left in place continuously or removed every three weeks for one week to allow regular bleeding. The rate of effectiveness is similar to that of the pill.

Oral Contraceptives for Men? The development of an oral contraceptive for men has been slow. Evidently, the mechanisms involved in the manufacture and release of

Withdrawal: A method of contraception that involves withdrawing the penis from the vagina before ejaculation. Also called "coitus interruptus."

Depo-Provera: An injectable method of birth control that lasts for three months.

Norplant: A long-lasting contraceptive that consists of six silicon capsules surgically inserted under the skin in a woman's upper arm.

Fertility awareness methods (FAM): Include several types of birth control that require alteration of sexual behavior rather than chemical or physical intervention into the reproductive process.

Native American Women and Norplant Misuse

*T*hroughout this text, we stress the importance of taking health matters into your own hands. It is up to you to read the information provided about medicines or contraceptives, to ask questions of medical personnel, and to make sure that you give a full family medical history when requested. The following account of contraceptive misuse underscores the fact that you must take the time to decide which contraceptive is right for you from a medical as well as sexual standpoint.

Norplant, the implantable contraceptive that lasts up to five years, was approved in December 1990 by the Food and Drug Administration. In June 1991, Indian Health Service (IHS), a division of the United States Public Health Service, began offering the device to its clients. IHS is the primary health care provider for Native Americans living on reservations, and its clinics are often the only suppliers of health information and services. . . .

Wyeth-Ayerst Laboratories, the U.S. marketer of Norplant, lists in its pamphlet health conditions that make the contraceptive unsafe for a user. Among them: acute liver disease, unexplained vaginal bleeding, breast cancer, and blood clots. The company also lists other factors that it claims should not prevent Norplant use, but require close medical supervision. Diabetes, high blood pressure, gall bladder disease, and smoking are included.

For the average Native woman living on a reservation, Norplant is a poor contraceptive choice. Native people have the highest rates of diabetes, alcoholism and related diseases, obesity, and gall bladder disease in the U.S. They also have elevated rates of hypertension and cancer. Many are smokers and cirrhosis (a liver disease) is endemic. . . .

Two women from the Rosebud reservation, each with a family history of breast cancer, were given Norplant by IHS practitioners. Neither woman remembers being informed about the contraceptive's potential danger for women at risk for breast cancer. Similarly, an overweight smoker with occasional high blood pressure says she was not cautioned about the need for frequent checkups, nor told that Norplant's effectiveness decreases with increased weight. . . .

Because of the inadequate counseling about side effects, many women have had Norplant removed. A Yankton, South Dakota, physician, Howard Gilmore, has already extracted several implants inserted by IHS providers. Before removal, he asks the women if they know irregular bleeding was a side effect of Norplant. Too often, the answer is no. On the Rosebud reservation, about 25 percent of the women who had the device implanted later had it removed.

Source: Excerpted from The Native American Women's Health Education Resource Center, "Native American Women Uncover Norplant Abuses," *Ms.,* September–October 1993, 69. Reprinted by permission of *Ms.* Magazine, © 1993.

---

sperm are not as easy to manipulate as are the ovulatory and uterine cycles of the female. Some oral contraceptives for men have been tested, but they produced unpleasant side effects such as diminished sex drive and impotence.

At the present time, research into the development of new male contraceptives is being carried on in various countries. Many researchers expect to develop a new male contraceptive by the end of the present decade.

One compound being researched is *gossypol,* a substance derived from the cotton plant. Chinese and Canadian researchers have found that gossypol inhibits sperm production, causing infertility. Difficulties in reversing the effects of the drug are presenting problems, as are concerns over long-term health consequences and possible genetic effects.

Scientists in Sweden have pioneered research into a nasal spray containing hormones designed to inhibit sperm production. Inhalation of aerosol hormones is an alternative to injections. As with gossypol, questions regarding side effects and long-term health hazards remain unanswered.

Other researchers are investigating the possibility of using ultrasound as a male contraceptive. In this method, a high-frequency sound machine is placed in contact with the scrotum. The device emits sound waves that slow sperm production, thereby lowering sperm counts. In some cases, sperm counts have remained lowered for up to two years after the procedure. Reduced sperm count, as opposed to total destruction of sperm, may suffice as a contraceptive measure because a minimum number of sperm are needed for fertilization. Before this method can be made available, the risks for testicular cancer and genetic damage must be thoroughly explored.

Fertility Awareness Methods (FAM)

Methods of fertility control that rely upon the alteration of sexual behavior are called **fertility awareness methods (FAM).** These methods include observing female "fertile periods" by examining cervical mucus and/or keeping track of internal temperature and then abstaining from sexual intercourse (penis-vagina contact) during these fertile times.

Two decades ago, the "rhythm method" was the object of much ridicule because of its low effectiveness rates. However, it was the only method of birth control available to women belonging to religious denominations that forbid the use of oral contraceptives, barrier methods, and sterilization. Our present reproductive knowledge enables women and their partners to use natural methods of birth control with fewer risks of pregnancy, although these methods remain far less effective than others.

Fertility awareness methods of birth control rely upon basic physiology. A released ovum can survive for up to 48 hours after ovulation. Sperm can live for as long as five days in the vagina. Natural methods of birth control teach women to recognize their fertile times. Changes in cervical mucus prior to and during ovulation and a rise in basal body temperature are two indicators frequently used in natural contraceptive techniques. Another method involves charting a woman's menstrual cycle and ovulation times on a calendar. Any combination of these methods may be used to determine fertile times more accurately.

Cervical Mucus Method. The **cervical mucus method** requires women to examine the consistency and color of their normal vaginal secretions. Prior to ovulation, vaginal mucus becomes gelatinous and stringy in consistency, and normal vaginal secretions may increase. Sexual activity involving penis-vagina contact must be avoided while this "fertile mucus" is present and for several days following the mucus changes.

Body Temperature Method. The **body temperature method** relies on the fact that the female's basal body temperature rises between 0.4 and 0.8 degrees after ovulation has occurred. For this method to be effective, the woman must chart her temperature for several months to learn to recognize her body's temperature fluctuations. Abstinence from penis-vagina contact must be observed preceding the temperature rise until several days after the temperature rise was first noted.

The Calendar Method. The **calendar method** requires the woman to record the exact number of days in her menstrual cycle. Since few women menstruate with complete regularity, a record of the menstrual cycle must be kept for 12 months, during which time some other method of birth control must be used. The first day of a woman's period is counted as day 1. To determine the first fertile unsafe day of the cycle, she subtracts 18 from the number of days in the shortest cycle. To determine the last unsafe day of the cycle, she subtracts 11 from the number of days in the longest cycle. This method assumes that ovulation occurs during the midpoint of the cycle. The couple must abstain from penis-vagina contact during the fertile time.

Women interested in fertility awareness methods of birth control are advised to take supervised classes in their use. The risks of an unwanted pregnancy are great for the untrained woman. Reading a book or watching a film on the subject or talking to the proprietor of the local health food store will not provide the necessary training to ensure maximum effectiveness. Incidentally, information on these methods can be helpful to couples who are trying to conceive.

Permanent Contraception

Sterilization has become increasingly common among married couples in the United States. Since the 1970s, perfection of sterilization procedures has made this method popular. Although some of the newer surgical techniques make reversal of sterilization theoretically possible, anyone considering sterilization should assume that the operation is *not* reversible. Before becoming sterilized, people should think through such possibilities as divorce and remarriage or a future improvement in their financial status that may make them want a larger family.

Female Sterilization. One method of sterilization in females is called **tubal ligation**. It is achieved through a surgical procedure that involves tying the fallopian tubes closed or cutting them and cauterizing (burning) the edges to seal the tubes so that access by sperm to released eggs is blocked. The operation is usually done in a hospital on an outpatient basis. First, the abdomen is inflated with carbon dioxide gas through a small incision in the navel. The surgeon then inserts a *laparoscope* into another incision just above the pubic bone. This specially designed instrument has a fiber-optic light source that enables the

Cervical mucus method: A birth control method that relies upon observation of changes in cervical mucus to determine when the woman is fertile so the couple can abstain from intercourse during those times.

Body temperature method: A birth control method that requires a woman to monitor her body temperature for the rise that signals ovulation and to abstain from intercourse around this time.

Calendar method: A birth control method that requires mapping the woman's menstrual cycle on a calendar to determine presumed fertile times and abstaining from penis-vagina contact during those times.

Sterilization: Permanent fertility control achieved through surgical procedures.

Tubal ligation: Sterilization of the female that involves the cutting and tying off of the fallopian tubes.

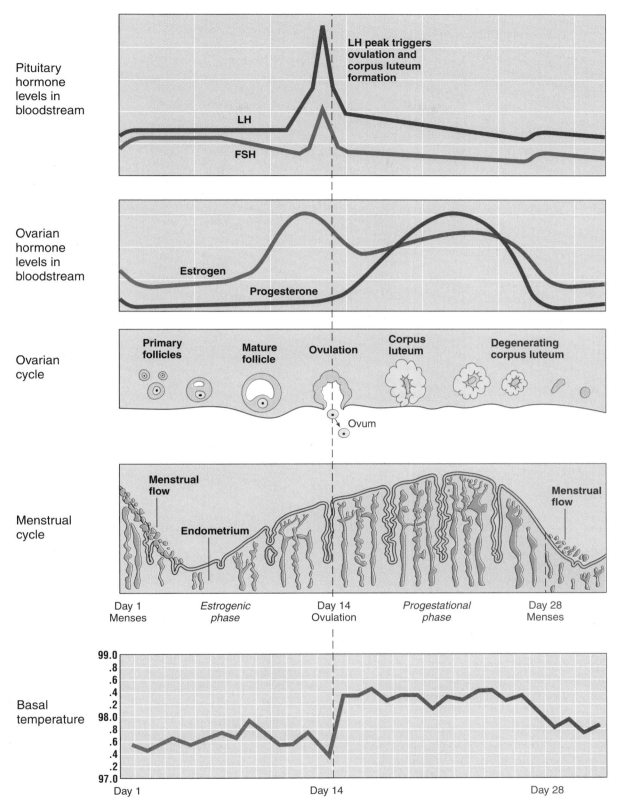

Pituitary hormone levels in bloodstream

LH peak triggers ovulation and corpus luteum formation

LH

FSH

Ovarian hormone levels in bloodstream

Estrogen

Progesterone

Ovarian cycle

Primary follicles **Mature follicle** **Ovulation** **Corpus luteum** **Degenerating corpus luteum**

Ovum

Menstrual cycle

Menstrual flow

Endometrium

Menstrual flow

Day 1
Menses

Estrogenic phase

Day 14
Ovulation

Progestational phase

Day 28
Menses

Basal temperature

99.0
.8
.6
.4
.2
98.0
.8
.6
.4
.2
97.0

Day 1

Day 14

Day 28

FIGURE 7.5

Some Bodily Changes that Occur During the Menstrual Cycle

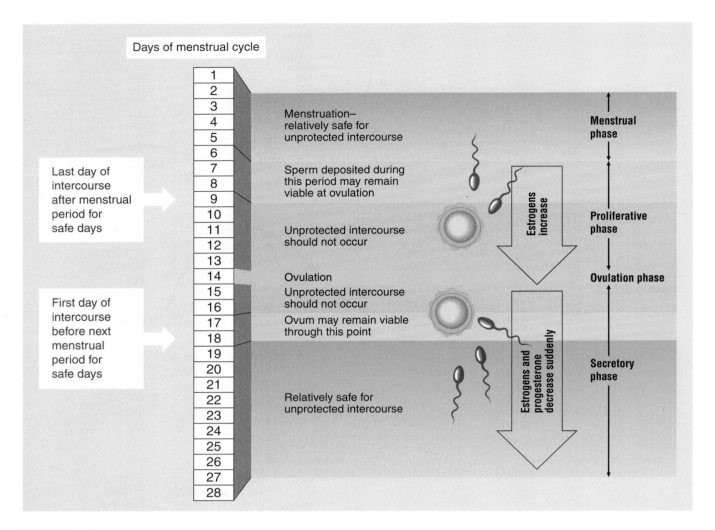

Days of menstrual cycle

| 1 |
| 2 |
| 3 | Menstruation— relatively safe for unprotected intercourse | Menstrual phase |
| 4 |
| 5 |
| 6 |
| 7 | Sperm deposited during this period may remain viable at ovulation |
| 8 |
| 9 |
| 10 |
| 11 | Unprotected intercourse should not occur | Proliferative phase |
| 12 |
| 13 |
| 14 | Ovulation | Ovulation phase |
| 15 | Unprotected intercourse should not occur |
| 16 |
| 17 | Ovum may remain viable through this point |
| 18 |
| 19 |
| 20 | Relatively safe for unprotected intercourse | Secretory phase |
| 21 |
| 22 |
| 23 |
| 24 |
| 25 |
| 26 |
| 27 |
| 28 |

Last day of intercourse after menstrual period for safe days

First day of intercourse before next menstrual period for safe days

Estrogens increase

Estrogens and progesterone decrease suddenly

FIGURE 7.6

The Fertility Cycle

physician to see the fallopian tubes clearly. Once located, the tubes are cut and tied or cauterized (see Figure 7.7).

Ovarian and uterine functions are not affected by a tubal ligation. The woman's menstrual cycle continues, and released eggs simply disintegrate and are absorbed by the lymphatic system. As soon as her incision is healed, the woman may resume sexual intercourse with no fear of pregnancy.

As with any kind of surgery, there are risks. Some patients are given general anesthesia, which presents a small risk; others receive local anesthesia. The procedure itself usually takes less than an hour, and the patient is generally allowed to return home within a short time after waking up. Women considering a tubal ligation should thoroughly discuss all the risks with their physician before the operation.

The **hysterectomy,** or removal of the uterus, is a method of sterilization requiring major surgery. It is usu-

ally done only when the patient has a disease of or damage to the uterus.

Male Sterilization. Sterilization in men is less complicated than in women. The procedure, called a **vasectomy,** is usually done on an outpatient basis using a local anesthetic. The surgeon (generally a urologist) makes an incision on each side of the scrotum. The vas deferens on each side is then located, and a piece is removed from each. The ends are usually tied or sewn shut (see Figure 7.8).

The man usually experiences some discomfort, local pain, swelling, and discoloration for about a week. In a small percentage of cases, more serious complications occur: formation of a blood clot in the scrotum (which usually disappears without medical treatment), infection, and inflammatory reactions. Because sperm are stored in other areas of the reproductive system besides the vasa deferentia, couples must use alternative methods of birth control for at least one month after the vasectomy. The man must check with his physician (who will do a semen analysis) to determine when unprotected intercourse can take place. The pregnancy rate in women whose partners have had vasectomies is about 15 in 10,000.

Many men are reluctant to consider sterilization because they fear the operation will affect their sexual performance. Such fears are unfounded (although not abnormal) and can be alleviated by talking to men who have already been vasectomized.

A vasectomy in no way affects sexual response. Because sperm constitute only a small percentage of the semen, the amount of ejaculate is not changed significantly. The testes continue to produce sperm, but the sperm are prevented from entering the ejaculatory duct because of the surgery. After a time, sperm production may diminish. Any sperm that are manufactured disintegrate and are absorbed into the lymphatic system.

Although a vasectomy should be considered a permanent procedure, surgical reversal is sometimes successful in restoring fertility. Recent improvements in microsurgery techniques have resulted in annual pregnancy rates of between 40 and 60 percent for women whose partners have had reversals. The two major factors influencing the success rate of reversal are the doctor's expertise and the time elapsed since the vasectomy.

*W*HAT DO YOU THINK?

Do you feel comfortable discussing birth control with your partner? Why or why not? Have you discussed with your partner what you would do if your method of birth control failed? What are the most important factors you and your partner considered when selecting a method of birth control?

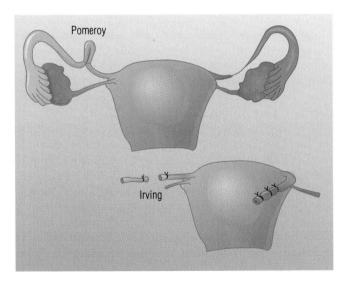

FIGURE 7.7

Two Methods of Tubal Ligation

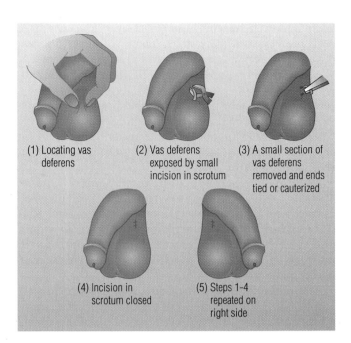

(1) Locating vas deferens

(2) Vas deferens exposed by small incision in scrotum

(3) A small section of vas deferens removed and ends tied or cauterized

(4) Incision in scrotum closed

(5) Steps 1-4 repeated on right side

FIGURE 7.8

Vasectomy

*A*BORTION

In 1973, the landmark Supreme Court decision in *Roe v. Wade* stated that the "right to privacy . . . founded on the Fourteenth Amendment's concept of personal liberty. . . is broad enough to encompass a woman's decision whether or not to terminate her pregnancy."[6] The decision maintained that during the first trimester of pregnancy, a woman and her practitioner have the right to terminate the pregnancy through **abortion** without legal restrictions. It allowed individual states to set conditions for second-trimester abortions. Third-trimester abortions were ruled illegal unless the mother's life or health was in danger.

In July 1989, in *Webster v. Reproductive Health Services,* the Supreme Court, by a vote of five to four, gave states the right to impose certain new restrictions on abortions. This decision, along with three subsequent rulings, paved the way for individual state interpretations of abortion

Hysterectomy: The removal of the uterus.

Vasectomy: Sterilization of the male that involves the cutting and tying of both vasa deferentia.

Abortion: The medical means of terminating a pregnancy.

acceptability. In recent years, strict abortion laws have been proposed in many states. There is intense political debate as abortion opponents put pressure on state and local governments to pass laws prohibiting the use of public funds for abortion as well as for abortion counseling. Abortions cannot be performed in publicly funded clinics in some states, and other states have laws requiring parental notification before a teenager can obtain an abortion. Although *Roe v. Wade* has not been overturned, it faces many future challenges.

Prior to the legalization of first- and second-trimester abortions, women wishing to terminate a pregnancy had to travel to a country where the procedure was legal, consult an illegal abortionist, or perform their own abortions. The last two methods led to death from hemorrhage or infection in some cases and to infertility from internal scarring in others.

Before the 1973 Supreme Court ruling, approximately 480,000 illegal abortions were performed in the United States each year, one-third of them on married women. Since the 1973 decision, the law has been continually challenged by groups that are convinced that the termination of a pregnancy is murder. Those who oppose abortion believe that the embryo or fetus is a human being with rights that must be protected. Although many opponents work through the courts and the political process, attacks on abortion clinics and on doctors who perform abortions are increasingly common.

More than 1.6 million abortions are performed in the United States every year, representing almost a fourth of all pregnancies.[7] It is estimated that more than 46 percent of American women will have had one abortion by the age of 45. Sixty-three percent of women obtaining abortions are single. The majority of abortions, 52 percent, are performed at less than eight weeks' gestation.

The best birth control methods can fail. Women may be raped. Pregnancies can occur despite every possible precaution. When an unwanted pregnancy does occur, the decision whether to terminate, to carry to term and keep the baby, or to carry to term and give the baby away must be made. This is a personal decision to be made by each woman based on her personal beliefs, values, and resources after careful consideration of all alternatives.

Methods of Abortion

The type of abortion procedure used is determined by how many weeks pregnant the woman is. Pregnancy length is calculated from the first day of a woman's last menstrual period.

If performed during the first trimester of pregnancy, abortion presents a relatively low risk to the mother. The most commonly used method of first-trimester abortion is **vacuum aspiration.** The procedure is usually performed with local anesthetic. The cervix is dilated with instruments or by placing *laminaria,* a sterile seaweed product, in the cervical canal. The laminaria is left in place for a few hours or overnight and slowly dilates the cervix. After it is removed, a long tube is inserted into the uterus through the cervix. Gentle suction is then used to remove the fetal tissue from the uterine walls.

Pregnancies that progress into the second trimester can be terminated through **dilation and evacuation (D&E),** a procedure that combines vacuum aspiration with a technique called **dilation and curettage (D&C).** For this procedure, the cervix is dilated with laminaria for one to two days and a combination of instruments and vacuum aspiration is used to empty the uterus (see Figure 7.9). Second-trimester abortions are frequently done under general anesthetic. Both procedures can be performed on an outpatient basis (usually in the physician's office) with or without pain medication. Generally, however, the woman is given a mild tranquilizer to help her relax. Both procedures may cause moderate to severe uterine cramping and blood loss.

The **hysterotomy,** or surgical removal of the fetus from the uterus, may be used during emergencies or when the mother's life may be in danger and when other types of abortions are deemed too dangerous.

The risks associated with abortions include infection, incomplete abortion (when parts of the placenta remain in the uterus), missed abortion (when the fetus is not actually removed), excessive bleeding, and cervical and uterine trauma. Follow-up and attention to dangerous signs decrease the chances of any long-term problems.

The mortality rate for first-trimester abortions averages out to 0.8 per 100,000. The rate for second-trimester

---

Vacuum aspiration: The use of gentle suction to remove fetal tissue from the uterus.

Dilation and evacuation (D&E): An abortion technique that combines vacuum aspiration with dilation and curettage; fetal tissue is both sucked and scraped out of the uterus.

Dilation and curettage (D&C): An abortion technique in which the cervix is dilated with laminaria for one to two days and the uterine walls are scraped clean.

Hysterotomy: The surgical removal of the fetus from the uterus.

Induction abortion: A type of abortion in which chemicals are injected into the uterus through the uterine wall; labor begins and the woman delivers a dead fetus.

RU-486: A steroid hormone that induces abortion by blocking the action of progesterone. Testing in the United States began in late 1994.

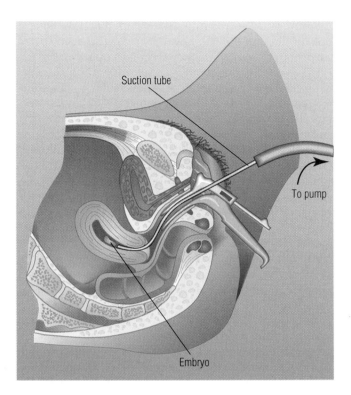

FIGURE 7.9

Vacuum Aspiration Abortion

abortions is higher, 4.3 per 100,000. This higher rate is due to the increased risk of uterine perforation, bleeding, infection, and incomplete abortion due to the fact that the uterine wall becomes thinner as the pregnancy progresses.

Two other methods used in second-trimester abortions, though less commonly than the D&E method, are prostaglandin or saline **induction abortions.** In these methods, prostaglandin hormones or a saline solution is injected into the uterus. The injected solution kills the fetus and causes labor contractions to begin. After 24 to 48 hours the fetus and placenta are expelled from the uterus.

RU-486: "The Abortion Pill"

RU-486 is a steroid hormone that induces abortion by blocking the action of progesterone, a hormone produced by the ovaries and placenta that maintains the lining of the uterus. Similar in structure to progesterone, RU-486 binds to cell receptor sites normally occupied by progesterone, causing the breakdown of the uterine lining. As a result, the uterine lining and the embryo are expelled from the uterus and the pregnancy is terminated.

Treatment consists of the ingestion of three pills of RU-486. A dose of prostaglandins must be administered 48 hours later to encourage contractions of the uterus.

Ninety-six percent of women who take these two drugs during the first nine weeks of pregnancy will experience a complete abortion. The side effects of this treatment are similar to those reported during heavy menstruation and include cramping, minor pain, and nausea. Approximately 1 in 1,000 women requires a blood transfusion because of severe bleeding. The procedure does not require hospitalization; women may be treated on an outpatient basis.

Although an estimated 150,000 European women have used RU-486, clinical trials did not begin in the United States until late October 1994. Roussel Uclaf, RU-486's European manufacturer, agreed to let the Population Council, a nonprofit group, sponsor clinical trials. Based on the results of those trials, involving 2,100 volunteers nationwide, the Food and Drug Administration will decide whether or not to approve the drug.

While RU-486's (trade name: mifepristone) nickname "the abortion pill" may imply an easy process, treatment does involve more steps for the woman than does a traditional abortion. A traditional abortion takes about 15 minutes followed by a physical recovery of about one day. For the RU-486 trials, a first visit to the clinic involves a physical exam and taking three mifepristone tablets, which may cause minor side effects such as nausea, headaches, weakness, and fatigue. The patient returns two days later for a dose of prostaglandins (trade name: misoprostal) which cause contractions of the uterus, which expel the fertilized egg. Women are required to stay under observation at the clinic for four hours. A return visit is required 12 days later because the pills fail to expel the fetus completely in 4 percent of cases, and a clinical abortion is then necessary.[8]

*W*HAT DO YOU THINK?

If you or your partner unexpectedly became pregnant, would you choose to terminate the pregnancy? How might an abortion affect your relationship? If you were married, would your decision be different? Why?

*P*LANNING A PREGNANCY

The technological ability to control your fertility gives you choices not available when your parents were born. The loosening of social restrictions in the areas of marriage and parenting also affords single men and women the opportunity to become parents. Regardless of whether you are married or single, the preparation to become a parent involves similar considerations and decisions. If you are in the process of deciding whether to have children, you need to take the time to evaluate your emotions, finances, and health.

Emotional Health

The first and foremost evaluation you should make is why you want to have a child: To fulfill an inner need to carry on the family? Out of loneliness? Any other reasons? Can you care for this new human being in a loving and nurturing manner? Are you ready to make all the sacrifices necessary to bear and raise a child? You can prepare yourself for this change in your life in several ways. Reading about parenthood, taking classes, talking to parents of children of all ages, and joining a support group are all helpful forms of preparation. If you choose to adopt, you will find many support groups available to you as well. If you and your partner agree you are ready to have a child, then consider the following as well.

Maternal Health

Before becoming pregnant, a woman should have a thorough medical examination. **Preconception care** should include assessment of possible pregnancy complications. Medical problems such as diabetes and high blood pressure should be discussed as should any genetic disorders that run in either family.

Paternal Health

It is common wisdom that mothers-to-be should steer clear of toxic chemicals that can cause birth defects. Even women who are trying to conceive are cautioned to avoid toxic environments and to eat a nourishing diet, to stop smoking and drinking alcohol, and to avoid most medications.

Now similar precautions are being urged for fathers-to-be. New research suggests that a man's exposure to chemicals influences not only his ability to father a child but also the future health of his child. Fathers-to-be have been overlooked in the past for several reasons. Researchers assumed that the genetic damage leading to birth defects and other health problems always occurred while a child was in the mother's womb. After all, they reasoned, that's where embryonic and fetal development take place. Conventional medical wisdom also held that defective-looking sperm (those with misshapen heads, crooked tails, or retarded swimming ability) were incapable of fertilizing an egg.

> **Preconception care:** Medical care received prior to becoming pregnant that helps a woman assess and address potential maternal health.

Scientists have recently discovered that how sperm look has little to do with how they act. Misshapen sperm can penetrate an egg, and they do not necessarily carry defective genetic goods. Moreover, sperm that look healthy and swim well can be the true genetic culprits. DNA fluorescent markers have identified normal-looking, yet genetically flawed, sperm that carry too many or too few chromosomes. Fathers contribute the extra chromosome 21 in about 6 percent of children with Down's syndrome, which causes mental retardation; the extra X chromosome in 50 percent of boys with Klinefelter's syndrome, which causes abnormal sexual development; and the shortened chromosome 15 in about 85 percent of children with Prader-Willi syndrome, a disorder characterized by retardation and obesity.

Although some birth defects are caused by the random errors of nature, it now appears that some disorders can be traced to sperm damaged by chemicals. Sperm are naturally vulnerable to toxic assault and genetic damage. Many drugs and ingested chemicals can readily invade the testes from the bloodstream; others ambush sperm after they leave the testes and pass through the epididymides, where they mature and are stored. By one route or another, half of 100 chemicals studied so far (including by-products of cigarette smoke) apparently harm sperm.

Some researchers believe that Vitamin C is nature's way of protecting sex cells from damage. Bad diets, exposure to toxic chemicals, cigarette smoking, and not enough foods rich in Vitamin C are probably the biggest culprits in sperm damage.[9]

Financial Evaluation

You also need to evaluate your finances. First check your medical insurance: Does it provide pregnancy benefits? If not, you can expect to pay between $1,500 and $5,000 for medical care during pregnancy and birth—and substantially more if complications arise. Both partners should find out about their employers' policies concerning parental leave including length of leave available and conditions for returning to work.

Raising a child exacts a tremendous strain on most family's finances. Expenses during the first year of life averaged $5,774 in 1990. The expense of raising a child from birth to 21 years of age is presently estimated to be over $250,000—not including the cost of a college education!

The cost and availability of quality child care should also be considered. Prospective parents should realistically assess how much family assistance they can expect with a new baby as well as the availability of nonfamily child care. While you may be aware of the federal tax credit available for child care, you may not be aware of how little assistance it provides: between a maximum of $480 for one child in a family having income of over $28,000 to a maximum of $720 for one child in a family having income

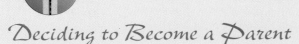
Deciding to Become a Parent

The decision to become a parent has become a choice influenced by many factors. The responsibilities of parenthood include more than financial obligations. Parents must also provide a loving and nurturing environment that supports the emotional, social, and spiritual needs of their child. Once the decision is made to have a child, a successful pregnancy involves establishing a healthy environment in which the baby can develop. If you are at a time in your life when you do not wish to have children and are sexually active, you need to give very serious consideration to choosing an effective method of pregnancy prevention. Here are some questions you should ask yourself and your partner to help guide your decision making:

1. Do I feel comfortable discussing birth control with my partner?

2. Am I comfortable using my present method of birth control?

3. Is my partner opposed to this method of birth control?

4. Have I discussed with my partner what we would do if the birth control method failed?

5. Would either of us like to have children some day?

6. How old would I like to be when I have my first child?

7. How many years of formal education would I like to complete?

8. Of all the things I could do in my life, probably the most important thing would be _____.

9. This life goal would be affected by marriage in the following ways _____. By childbearing in the following ways _____.

10. What would it mean to me if my marriage was to end in divorce?

11. Is my life plan thus far compatible with my spiritual beliefs, with the beliefs of the family and society in which I live, and with my personal code of ethics? How does it fit with what I feel is spiritually or ethically right or wrong for me? If my actions are in conflict with what I believe is right for me to be doing, how can I eliminate this potential conflict that may lead to loss of self-respect?

---

of under $10,000. A second child doubles the credit; but no further assistance is provided for a third child or more children. How much does full-time child care cost? It averages between $5,000 and $10,000 a year, depending on your location (urban areas tend to cost more).

Contingency Planning

A final consideration is how to provide for the child should something happen to you and your partner. If both of you were to die while the child is young, do you have relatives or close friends who would raise the child? If you have more than one child, would they have to be split up or could they be kept together? Unpleasant though it may be to think about, this sort of contingency planning is highly important. Children who lose their parents are usually heartbroken and confused. A prearranged plan of action may help smooth their transition into new families.

*W*HAT DO YOU THINK?

Do you think most parents plan when they will have their children? At what point in your life do you think you will be ready to take on the responsibilities of becoming a parent? What are your biggest concerns about parenthood?

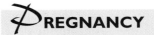

PREGNANCY

Prenatal Care

A successful pregnancy requires the mother's ability to take good care of herself and her unborn child. It is essential to have regular medical checkups, beginning as soon as possible (certainly within the first three months). Early detection of fetal abnormalities and identification of high-risk mothers and infants are the major purposes of prenatal care. On the first visit, the practitioner should obtain a complete medical history of the mother and her family and note any hereditary conditions that could put a woman or her fetus at risk.

Regular checkups to measure weight gain and blood pressure and monitor the size and position of the fetus should continue throughout the pregnancy. This early care reduces infant mortality and low birthweight. A study group for the American College of Obstetricians and Gynecologists recommends seven or eight prenatal visits for women with low-risk pregnancies. Unfortunately, prenatal care is not equally available to all pregnant women. Approximately 30 percent of pregnant teenagers and unmarried women do not have adequate access to prenatal care. Babies of mothers who received no prenatal care are about 10 times more likely to die in the first month of life than are babies of mothers who did get prenatal care.

Additional concerns include the mother's physical condition, her level of nutrition, her confidence in her ability to give birth, her use of drugs and medications, and the availability of a skilled practitioner who can oversee the pregnancy and delivery. A woman planning a pregnancy also needs a support system (spouse or partner, family, friends, community groups) willing to give her and her child the love and emotional support needed during and after her pregnancy.

Choosing a Practitioner. A woman should carefully choose a practitioner to attend her pregnancy and delivery. If possible, this choice should be made before she becomes pregnant. Recommendations from friends who were satisfied with the care they received during pregnancy may be a good starting point in the search for a practitioner. The woman's family physician may also be able to recommend a specialist. The pregnant woman needs to find a practitioner she can trust with both her own life and that of the baby and with whom she can communicate freely.

When choosing a practitioner, parents should ask a number of questions concerning credentials and professional qualifications. Besides this information, a pregnant woman must ask questions specific to her condition. Prospective parents should also inquire about the practitioner's experience in handling various complications, commitment to being at the mother's side during delivery, and beliefs and practices concerning the use of anesthesia, fetal monitoring, induced labor, and forceps delivery. What are the practitioner's attitudes toward birth control, abortion, and alternative birthing procedures? The practitioner's approach to nutrition and medication during pregnancy should be similar to the woman's own. Finally, the parents must learn under what circumstances the practitioner would perform a cesarean section.

Two types of physicians can attend pregnancies and deliveries. The *obstetrician-gynecologist* (ob-gyn) is an M.D. who specializes in obstetrics (pregnancy and birth) and gynecology (care of women's reproductive organs). These practitioners are trained to handle all types of pregnancy and delivery-related emergencies.

Teratogenic: Causing birth defects; may refer to drugs, environmental chemicals, X-rays, or diseases.

Fetal alcohol syndrome (FAS): A collection of symptoms, including mental retardation, that can appear in infants of women who drink too much alcohol during pregnancy.

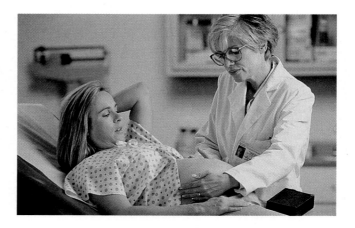

Good prenatal care involves regular medical checkups by a practitioner with whom the mother feels she can communicate freely.

A *family practitioner* is a licensed M.D. who provides comprehensive care for people of all ages. The majority of family practitioners have obstetrical experience but will refer a patient to a specialist if necessary. Unlike the ob-gyn, the family practitioner can serve as the baby's physician after attending the birth.

Midwives are also experienced practitioners who can attend both pregnancies and deliveries. *Certified nurse-midwives* are registered nurses having specialized training in pregnancy and delivery. Most midwives work in private practice or in conjunction with physicians. Those who work with physicians have access to traditional medical facilities to which they can turn in an emergency. *Lay midwives* may or may not have extensive training in handling an emergency. They may be self-taught rather than trained through formal certification procedures.

Alcohol and Drugs. A woman should avoid all types of drugs during pregnancy. Even common over-the-counter medications such as aspirin and beverages such as coffee and tea can damage a developing fetus.

During the first three months of pregnancy, the fetus is especially subject to the **teratogenic** (birth defect-causing) effects of some chemical substances. The fetus can also develop an addiction to or tolerance for drugs that the mother is using.

Of particular concern to medical professionals is the use of tobacco and alcohol during pregnancy. Women who are heavy drinkers may have normal first babies but subsequently deliver children having fetal alcohol syndrome. The symptoms of **fetal alcohol syndrome (FAS)** include mental retardation, slowed nerve reflexes, and small head size. The exact amount of alcohol necessary to cause FAS is not known, but researchers doubt that any level of alcohol consumption is safe. Therefore, total abstinence from alcohol during pregnancy is recommended.

Table 7.2 provides a list of teratogenic effects of alcohol and other drugs ingested by the mother.

Cigarette smoking during pregnancy has more predictable effects than alcohol. Studies have shown a 25 to 50 percent higher rate of fetal and infant deaths among women who smoke during pregnancy compared with those who do not.[10] Women who smoke more than 10 to 15 cigarettes a day during pregnancy have higher rates of miscarriage, stillbirth, premature births, and low-birth-weight babies than do nonsmokers. Fetal research on the effects of "secondhand" or sidestream smoke (inhaling smoke produced by others) is inconclusive, but babies whose parents smoke can be twice as susceptible to pneumonia, bronchitis, and related illnesses as other babies.

X-rays. X-rays present a clear danger to the fetus. Although most diagnostic tests produce minimal amounts of radiation, even low levels may cause birth defects or other problems, particularly if several low-dose X-rays are taken over a short time period. Pregnant women are advised to avoid X-rays unless absolutely necessary.

Nutrition and Exercise. Pregnant women have additional needs for protein, calories, and certain vitamins and minerals, so their diets should be carefully monitored by a qualified practitioner. Special attention should be paid to getting enough folic acid (found in dark leafy greens), iron (dried fruits, meats, legumes, liver, egg yolks), calcium (nonfat or lowfat dairy products, some canned fish), and fluids. Vitamin supplements can correct some deficiencies, but there is no true substitute for a well-balanced diet. Babies born to mothers whose nutrition has been poor run high risks of substandard mental and physical development (see Table 7.3).

Weight gain during pregnancy helps nourish a growing baby. For a woman of normal weight before pregnancy, the acceptable weight gain during pregnancy ranges from 25–35 pounds; a woman carrying twins needs to gain about 35–45 pounds. Usually the mother can expect to gain about 10 pounds during the first 20 weeks and about 1 pound per week during the rest of the pregnancy.

Of the total number of pounds gained during pregnancy, about 6–8 are the baby's weight. The distribution of the remaining weight is shown in Table 7.4. The baby's birth weight is important, since low weight can mean health problems during labor and the baby's first few months. Eating right and gaining enough weight helps reduce the chances of having a low birth weight baby. If a woman gains an appropriate amount of weight while pregnant, chances are that her baby will gain weight properly, too. Pregnancy is not a time to think about losing weight—doing so may endanger the baby.[11]

As in all other stages of life, exercise is an important factor in weight control during pregnancy as well as in

TABLE 7.2 ■ Teratogenic Effects of Drugs

Drug	Effect
Alcohol	Mental retardation; growth retardation; increased spontaneous abortion rate.
Amphetamines	Suspected nervous system damage.
Aspirin	Newborn bleeding.
Cocaine	Uncontrolled jerking motions; paralysis; depressed interactive behavior; poor organizational response to environmental stimuli.
Opioids	Immediate withdrawal in newborns; permanent learning disabilities.
Tetracycline	Tooth discoloration.
Sulfa drugs	Facial and skeletal abnormalities.
Barbiturates	Congenital malformations.
Streptomycin	Deafness.
Accutane	Small or absent ears; small jaw; heart defects.
Valium	Possible congenital anomalies.

Source: From Mike Samuels, M.D., and Nancy Samuels, *The Well Pregnancy Book* (New York: Summit Books, 1986), 131. Copyright 1986. Reprinted by permission of the Elaine Markson Literary Agency and Mike Samuels, M.D., and Nancy Samuels.

TABLE 7.3 ■ Nutrient Deficiency Effects

Nutrient	Deficiency Effect
Overall caloric intake	Low infant birthweight
Protein	Reduced infant head circumference
Folic acid	Miscarriage and neural tube defects
Vitamin D	Low infant birthweight
Calcium	Decreased infant bone density
Iron	Low infant birthweight and premature birth
Iodine	Varying degrees of mental and physical retardation in the infant
Zinc	Congenital malformations

Source: Reprinted by permission from *Life Cycle Nutrition: Conception through Adolescence,* by Linda Kelly Debruyne and Sharon Rady Rolfes. Copyright 1989 by West Publishing Company. All rights reserved.

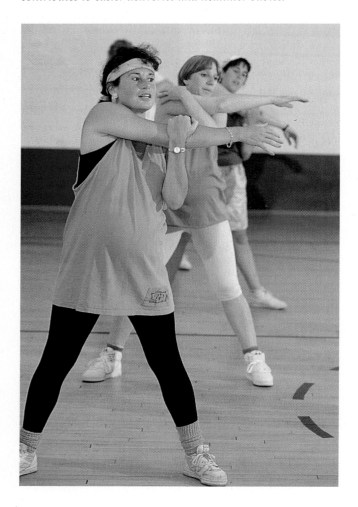

A doctor-approved exercise program during pregnancy not only helps the mother control her weight, but also contributes to easier deliveries and healthier babies.

fetus or cause blindness or hearing disorders in the infant. If the woman has ever had genital herpes, she should inform her physician. The physician may want to deliver the baby by cesarean section, especially if the woman has active lesions. Contact with an active herpes infection during birth can be fatal to the infant.

A Woman's Reproductive Years

More than half of the average American woman's expected life span is spent between menarche (first menses) and menopause (last menses), a period of approximately 40 years. During this 40-year period, she must make many decisions regarding her reproductive health. Deciding if and when to have children, as well as how to prevent pregnancy when necessary, are long-term concerns.[13]

Today, a woman over 35 who is pregnant has plenty of company. While births to women in their 20s are declining, the rate of first births to women between the ages of 30 and 39 has doubled in the past decade, and births to women over 39 have increased by more than 50 percent. Many women who wait until their 30s to consider having a child find themselves wondering, "Am I too old to have a baby?" Researchers believe that there is a decline in both the quality and viability of eggs produced after age 35. Statistically, the chances of having a baby with birth defects do rise after the age of 35. **Down's syndrome,** a condition characterized by mild to severe mental retardation and a variety of physical abnormalities, is the most common birth defect found in babies born to older mothers. The incidence of Down's syndrome in babies born to mothers aged 20 is 1 in 10,000 births; it rises to 1 in 365 births

overall maternal health. A balanced 45-minute exercise session three days per week has been associated in one study with heavier birth weight babies, fewer surgical births, and shorter hospital stays after birth.[12] Pregnant women should consult with their physicians before starting any exercise program.

Other Factors. A pregnant woman should avoid exposure to toxic chemicals, heavy metals, pesticides, gases, and other hazardous compounds. She should not clean cat-litter boxes because cat feces can contain organisms that cause a disease called toxoplasmosis. If a pregnant woman contracts this disease, her baby may be stillborn or suffer mental retardation or other birth defects.

Before becoming pregnant, a woman should be tested to determine if she has had rubella (German measles). If she has not had the disease, she should get an immunization for it and wait the recommended length of time before becoming pregnant. A rubella infection can kill the

TABLE 7.4 ■ Components of Weight Gain During Pregnancy

Development	Weight Gain (pounds)
Maternal stores (fat, protein, and other nutrients)	7
Increased fluid volume	4
Increased blood volume	4
Breast enlargement	2
Uterus	2
Baby	6–8
Amniotic fluid	2
Placenta	1 ½

Source: Reprinted by permission from American College of Obstetricians and Gynecologists, *ACOG Guide to Planning for Pregnancy, Birth, and Beyond.* Washington, DC. © 1990.

when the mother is 35, to 1 in 109 when she is 40, and to 1 in 32 when she is 45.

Women who choose to delay motherhood until their late 30s also worry about their physical ability to carry and deliver their babies. For these women, a comprehensive exercise program will assist in maintaining good posture and promoting a successful delivery.

There are some advantages to having a baby later in life. In fact, many doctors are encouraging older women to become pregnant because they find that these women tend to be more conscientious about following medical advice during pregnancy and more psychologically mature and ready to include an infant in their family than are some younger women.

Pregnancy Testing

A woman may suspect she is pregnant before she has any type of pregnancy tests. A typical sign is a missed menstrual period, yet this is not always an accurate indicator. A woman can miss her period for a variety of reasons: stress, exercise, emotional upset. Confirmation of a pregnancy can be obtained from a pregnancy test scheduled in a medical office or birth control clinic.

Women who wish to know immediately whether or not they are pregnant can purchase home pregnancy test kits. These kits, sold over the counter in drugstores, are about 85 to 95 percent reliable. A positive test is based on the secretion of **human chorionic gonadotropin (HCG)** found in the woman's urine. Home test kits come equipped with a small sample of red blood cells coated with HCG antibodies to which the user adds a small amount of urine. If the concentration of HCG is great enough, it will clump together with the HCG antibodies, indicating that the user is pregnant.

There are some problems with the accuracy of these home tests. If taken too early in the pregnancy, they may show a false negative. Other causes of false negatives are unclean test tubes, ingestion of certain drugs, and vaginal or urinary infections. Accuracy also depends on the quality of the test itself and the user's ability to perform it and interpret the results. Blood tests administered and analyzed by a medical laboratory give more accurate results.

The Process of Pregnancy

Pregnancy begins the moment a sperm fertilizes an ovum in the fallopian tubes. From there, the single cell multiplies, becoming a sphere-shaped cluster of cells as it travels toward the uterus, a journey that may last three to four days. Upon arrival, the embryo burrows into the thick, spongy endometrium and is nourished from this carefully prepared lining.

Early Signs of Pregnancy. The first sign of pregnancy is usually a missed menstrual period (although some women "spot" in early pregnancy, and such spotting may be mistaken for a period). Other signs of pregnancy include:

- Breast tenderness
- Extreme fatigue
- Sleeplessness
- Emotional upset
- Nausea
- Vomiting (especially in the morning)

Pregnancy typically lasts 40 weeks. The due date is calculated from the expectant mother's last menstrual period. Pregnancy is typically divided into three phases, or **trimesters,** of approximately three months each.

The First Trimester. During the first trimester, there are few noticeable changes in the maternal body. The expectant mother may urinate more frequently and experience morning sickness, swollen breasts, or undue fatigue. But these symptoms may not be frequent or severe, so she may not realize she is pregnant at this time unless she has a pregnancy test.

During the first two months after conception, the **embryo** differentiates and develops its various organ systems, beginning with the nervous and circulatory systems. At the start of the third month, the embryo is called a **fetus,** indicating that all organ systems are in place. For the rest of the pregnancy, growth and refinement occur in each major body system so that they can function independently, yet in coordination, at birth. The accompanying photos illustrate physical changes during fetal development.

The Second Trimester. At the beginning of the second trimester, physical changes in the mother become more visible. Her breasts swell and her waistline thickens. Dur-

Down's syndrome: A condition characterized by mental retardation and a variety of physical abnormalities.

Human chorionic gonadotropin (HCG): Hormone detectable in blood or urine samples of a mother within the first few weeks of pregnancy.

Trimester: A three-month segment of pregnancy; used to describe specific developmental changes that occur in the embryo or fetus.

Embryo: The fertilized egg from conception until the end of two months' development.

Fetus: The name given the developing baby from the third month of pregnancy until birth.

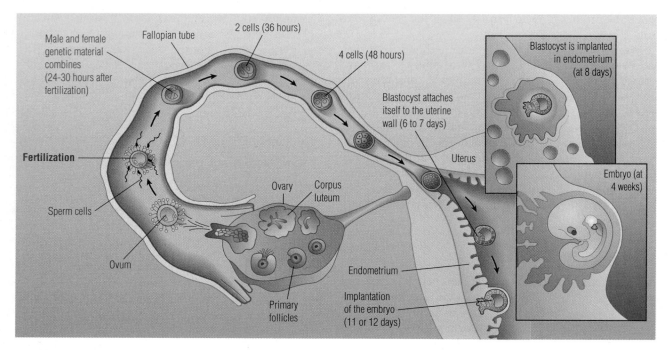

FIGURE 7.10

Fertilization

ing this time, the fetus makes greater demands upon the mother's body. In particular, the **placenta,** the network of blood vessels that carry nutrients and oxygen to the fetus and fetal waste products to the mother, becomes well established.

The Third Trimester.   From the end of the sixth month through the ninth is considered the third trimester. This is the period of greatest fetal growth. The fetus gains most of its weight during these last three months. During the third trimester, the fetus must get large amounts of calcium, iron, and nitrogen from the food the mother eats. Approximately 85 percent of the calcium and iron the mother digests goes into the fetal bloodstream.

Although the fetus may live if it is born during the seventh month, it needs the layer of fat it acquires during the eighth month and time for the organs (especially the respiratory and digestive organs) to develop to their full po-

tential. Babies born prematurely thus usually require intensive medical care.

Prenatal Testing and Screening

Modern technology has enabled medical practitioners to detect health defects in a fetus as early as the 14th to 18th weeks of pregnancy. One common testing procedure, **amniocentesis,** which is strongly recommended for women over the age of 35, involves inserting a long needle through the mother's abdominal and uterine walls into the **amniotic sac,** the protective pouch surrounding the baby (see Figure 7.11). The needle draws out 3 to 4 teaspoons of fluid, which is analyzed for genetic information about the baby. This test can reveal the presence of 40 genetic abnormalities, including Down's syndrome, Tay-Sachs disease (a fatal disorder of the nervous system common among Jewish people of Eastern European descent), and sickle-cell anemia (a debilitating blood disorder found primarily among blacks). Amniocentesis can also reveal the sex of the child, a fact many parents choose not to know until the birth. Although widely used, amniocentesis is not without risk. Chances of fetal damage and miscarriage as a result of testing are 1 in 400.

Another procedure, *ultrasound* or *sonography,* uses high-frequency sound waves to determine the size and position of the fetus. Ultrasound can also detect defects in the central nervous system and digestive system of the fetus. Knowing the position of the fetus assists practitioners in performing amniocentesis and in delivering the

---

Placenta: The network of blood vessels that carries nutrients to the developing infant and carries wastes away; it connects to the umbilical cord.

Amniocentesis: A medical test in which a small amount of fluid is drawn from the amniotic sac; it tests for Down's syndrome and genetic diseases.

Amniotic sac: The protective pouch surrounding the baby.

This series of fetoscopic photographs shows the development of a fetus from the (1) first, (2) second, and (3) third trimesters of pregnancy.

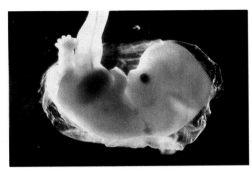

(1) First trimester

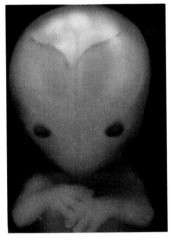

(2) Second trimester

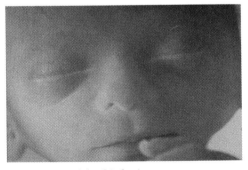

(3) Third trimester

child. In 1985, a National Institutes of Health panel found ultrasound safe for mother and child.

A third procedure, *fetoscopy,* involves making a small incision in the abdominal and uterine walls and then inserting an optical viewer into the uterus to view the fetus directly. This method is still experimental and involves some risk. It causes miscarriage in approximately 5 percent of cases.

A fourth procedure, *chorionic villus sampling (CVS),* involves snipping tissue from the developing fetal sac. CVS can be used at 10 to 12 weeks of pregnancy, and the

test results are available in 12 to 48 hours. This test is an attractive option for couples who are at high risk for having a baby with Down's syndrome or a debilitating hereditary disease.

If any of these tests reveals a serious birth defect, parents are advised to undergo genetic counseling. In the case of a chromosomal abnormality such as Down's syndrome, the parents are usually offered the option of a therapeutic abortion. Some parents choose this option; others research their unborn child's disability and decide to go ahead with the birth and offer the baby the love and support all children deserve. (See Table 7.5 for a summary of prenatal diseases and defects and the tests and treatment options available to parents.)

*W*HAT DO YOU THINK?

What are the most important concerns you have considering your choice of a health practitioner for your or your partner's pregnancy? What behaviors might you have to change if you found out that you or your partner were pregnant? In what ways would your life change if you had a child who was born with a birth defect? What type of prenatal tests would you consider before the birth of your child?

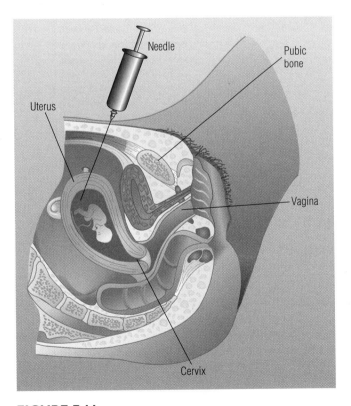

FIGURE 7.11

The process of amniocentesis can detect certain congenital problems as well as the sex of the fetus.

Chapter 7 Birth Control, Pregnancy, and Childbirth **179**

TABLE 7.5 ▪ Prenatal Testing for Diseases and Defects

Problem	Effects	Who Is at Risk	Tests and Their Accuracy	What Can Be Done
Cystic fibrosis	Body makes too much mucus, which collects in the lungs and digestive tract. Children don't grow normally and usually don't live beyond age 20.	1 in 2,000 whites.	Amniocentesis, CVS. Accuracy varies; more accurate if other family members tested for gene.	Daily physical therapy to loosen mucus.
Down's syndrome	Minor to severe mental retardation caused by an extra 21st chromosome.	1 in 350 women over age 35; 1 in 800 for all women.	Amniocentesis, CVS. Nearly 100% accurate.	Relief of symptoms through palliative therapy.
Duchenne's muscular dystrophy	Fatal disease found only in males, marked by muscle weakness. Minor mental retardation is common. Respiratory failure and death usually occur in young adulthood.	1 in 7,000 male births.	Amniocentesis, CVS. 95% accurate.	Relief of symptoms through palliative therapy.
Hemophilia	Excessive bleeding almost exclusively affecting males. In its most severe form, can lead to crippling.	1 in 1,000 families with a history of hemophilia.	Amniocentesis, CVS. 95% accurate.	Frequent transfusions of blood with clotting factors.
Anencephaly	Absence of brain tissue. Infants usually are stillborn or die soon after birth.	1 in 1,000.	Ultrasound, amniocentesis. 100% accurate.	No treatment.
Spina bifida	Incompletely closed spinal canal, resulting in muscle weakness or paralysis and loss of bladder and bowel control. Often accompanied by hydrocephalus, an accumulation of spinal fluid in the brain, which can lead to mental retardation.	1 in 1,000.	Ultrasound, amniocentesis. Test works only if the spinal cord is leaking fluid into the uterus or is exposed and visible during ultrasound.	Surgery to close spinal canal prevents further injury; shunt placed in brain drains excess fluid and prevents mental retardation.
Sickle cell anemia	Deformed, fragile red blood cells that can clog the blood vessels, depriving the body of oxygen. Symptoms include severe pain, stunted growth, frequent infections, leg ulcers, gallstones, susceptibility to pneumonia, and stroke.	1 in 500 blacks.	Amniocentesis, CVS. 95% accurate.	Painkillers, transfusions for anemia, antibiotics for infections.
Tay-Sachs disease	Degenerative disease of the brain and nerve cells, resulting in death before the age of five.	1 in 3,000 Eastern European Jews.	Amniocentesis, CVS. 100% accurate.	No treatment.

Source: Excerpted by permission of the Health Publishing Group, a division of Time Publishing Ventures, Inc., from "The Gene Screen: Looking In on Baby," *Hippocrates,* May–June 1988, 68–69. Researched by Valerie Fahey. © 1988.

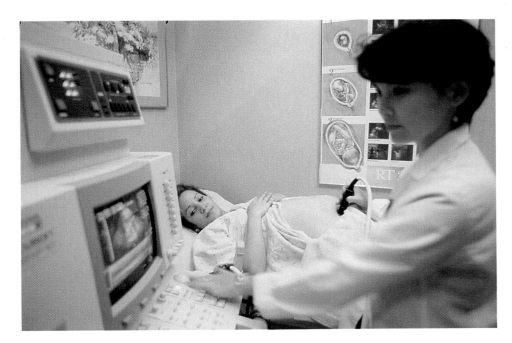

Ultrasound testing can reveal defects in the developing fetus, and, as the time of delivery nears, it can provide useful information about the size and position of the unborn child.

CHILDBIRTH

Choosing Where to Have Your Baby

Today's prospective mothers have many delivery options. These range from the traditional hospital birth to home birth. When considering birthing alternatives, parental values are important. Many couples, for instance, feel that the modern medical establishment has dehumanized the birth process; thus they choose to deliver at home or at a *birthing center,* a homelike setting outside a hospital where women can give birth and receive postdelivery care by a team of professional practitioners, including physicians and registered nurses. Financial considerations are also important, and a couple's income and insurance coverage will often dictate its choice.

Labor and Delivery

The birth process has three stages. The exact mechanisms that signal the mother's body that the baby is ready to be born are unknown. During the few weeks preceding delivery, the baby normally shifts and turns to a head-down position, and the cervix begins to dilate (open up). The junction of the pubic bones also loosens to permit expansion of the pelvic girdle during birth.

In the first stage of labor, the amniotic sac breaks, causing a rush of fluid from the vagina (commonly referred to as "breaking of the waters"). Contractions in the abdomen and lower back also signal the beginning of labor. Early contractions push the baby downward, putting pressure on the cervix and thereby causing it to dilate further. The first stage of labor may last from a couple of hours to more than a day for a first birth, but is usually much shorter during subsequent births.

The end of the first stage of labor, called **transition,** is the process when the cervix becomes fully dilated and the baby's head begins to move into the vagina, or the birth canal. Contractions usually come quickly during transition. Transition usually lasts 30 minutes or less.

The second stage of labor follows transition when the cervix has become fully dilated. Contractions become rhythmic, stronger, and more painful as the uterus works to push the baby through the birth canal. The second stage of labor (called the *expulsion stage*) may last between one and four hours and concludes when the infant is finally pushed out of the mother's body. In some cases, the attending practitioner will do an **episiotomy,** a straight incision in the mother's **perineum,** to prevent the baby's head from causing tearing of vaginal tissues and to speed the baby's exit from the vagina. Sometimes women can avoid the need for an episiotomy by exercising and getting good nutrition throughout pregnancy, by trying different birth positions, or by having an attendant massage the

Transition: The process during which the cervix becomes nearly fully dilated and the head of the fetus begins to move into the birth canal.

Episiotomy: A straight incision in the mother's perineum.

Perineum: The area between the vulva and the anus.

perineal tissue. However, the skin's natural elasticity and the baby's size are limiting factors.

After delivery, the attending practitioner cleans the baby's mucus-filled breathing passages, and the baby takes its first breath, generally accompanied by a loud wail. (The traditional "slap" on the baby's buttocks, often romanticized in old movies, is no longer a common practice because of the trauma associated with it.)

In the meantime, the mother continues into the third stage of labor, during which the placenta, or **afterbirth,** is expelled from the womb. This stage is usually completed within 30 minutes after delivery. The umbilical cord is then tied and severed. The stump of cord attached to the baby's navel dries up and drops off within a few days.

Most mothers prefer to have their new infants placed next to them following the birth. Together with their spouse or partner, they feel a need to share this time of bonding with their infant.

Birth Alternatives

Expectant parents have several options for their infant's birth and their participation in it. It is no longer necessary to turn the whole process over to a physician in the labor room. The birth methods listed below all entail preparation throughout the pregnancy. Education of both parents will help them derive emotional satisfaction from their birthing experience. Although several of these methods have decreased in popularity, all continue to be used.

Lamaze Method. This birth alternative is the most popular one in the United States. Pre-labor education classes teach the mother to control her pain through special breathing patterns, focusing exercises, and relaxation. Lamaze births usually take place in a hospital or birthing center with a physician or midwife in attendance. The husband (or labor coach) assists by giving emotional support, physical comfort (massage and ice chips), and coaching for proper breath control during contractions. Lamaze proponents discourage the use of drugs.

Harris Method. Parents using this alternative are taught by registered nurses. Gentle touching and controlled breathing are stressed. Husbands (or other partners) provide emotional support while a physician-nurse team essentially controls the labor and delivery. Drugs are not prohibited.

Childbirth without Fear. Sometimes called the Read Method, this method advocates education for understanding of the birth process. Mothers are taught to recognize that anticipation of pain creates more pain. Relaxation is stressed. The husband or other partner provides emotional support. Drugs are not prohibited.

Leboyer Method. Leboyer proponents believe that birth in the standard delivery room is a traumatic experience

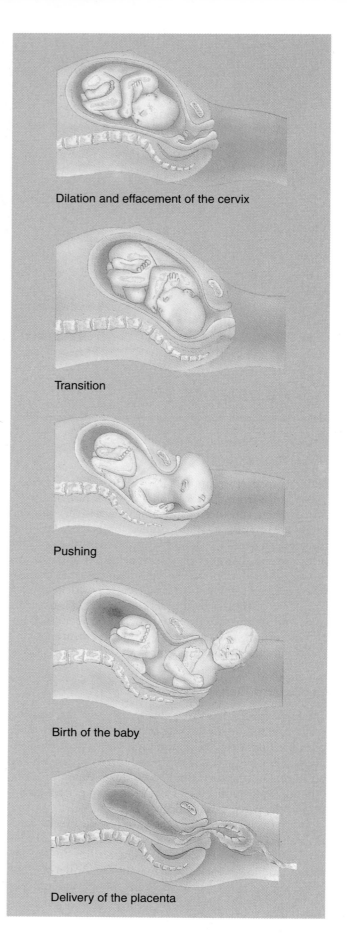

Dilation and effacement of the cervix

Transition

Pushing

Birth of the baby

Delivery of the placenta

FIGURE 7.12 The Birth Process

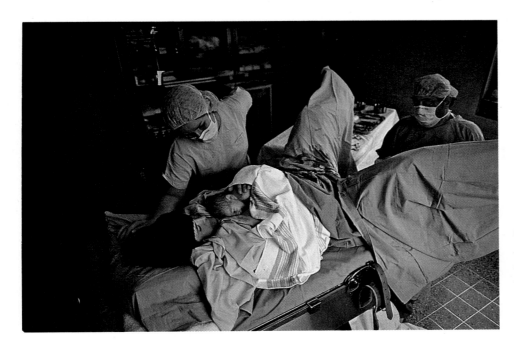

Many mothers feel more secure having their babies in a hospital environment, while others choose to deliver at home or in a birthing center that has a home-like atmosphere.

for the baby. The Leboyer method allows the mother to deliver in a dark and quiet setting. Immediately after delivery, the infant is placed in a warm bath to ease its transition to life outside the womb. Drug use is discouraged.

Drugs in the Delivery Room

Because painkilling drugs given to the mother during labor can cause sluggish responses in the newborn, many women choose drug-free labors and deliveries. Drug-free labor involves the use of exercise, massage, and controlled rhythmic breathing to control pain. Many women who choose "natural" childbirth mistakenly believe that the exercises they are taught in their classes will make their labor and delivery painless. When their time comes to give birth, they may feel inadequate because they experience the normal pain associated with childbirth. Pain is to be expected, and if it becomes too intense, the mother can be given painkilling medication.

A discussion with the attending physician before the birth of the baby will alert the mother to the practitioner's feelings about the use of painkilling drugs during delivery. Many experts believe that women should be offered the option of drugs during delivery both before and during the event. To refuse to give a mother medicine to take the edge off the pain is considered poor medical practice by some authorities.

Breast-Feeding and the Postpartum Period

Although the new mother's milk will not begin to flow for two or more days, her breasts secrete a thick yellow sub-stance called *colostrum*. Because this fluid contains vital antibodies to help fight infection, the newborn baby should be allowed to suckle.

As a result of recent scientific findings, the American Academy of Pediatrics has strongly recommended that full-term newborns be breast-fed. This recommendation does not mean that breast milk is the only adequate method of nourishing a baby. Prepared formulas can provide nourishment that allows a baby to grow and thrive.

Still, there are many advantages to breast-feeding. Breast milk is perfectly suited to a baby's nutritional needs. Breast-fed babies have fewer illnesses and a much lower hospitalization rate because breast milk contains maternal antibodies and immunological cells that stimulate the infant's immune system. When breast-fed babies do get sick, they recover more quickly. They are also less likely to be obese than babies fed on formulas, and they have fewer allergies.

When deciding whether to breast- or bottle-feed, mothers need to consider their own desires and preferences. Both feeding methods can supply the physical and emotional closeness so essential to the parent-child relationship.

The *postpartum period* lasts from four to six weeks after delivery. During this time, the mother's reproductive organs revert to a nonpregnant state. Many women experience energy depletion, anxiety, mood swings, and

Afterbirth: The expelled placenta.

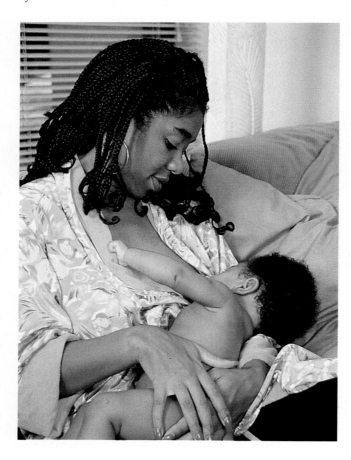

Breast feeding is one way to enhance the development of intimate bonds between mother and child.

depression during this period. This experience, known as **postpartum depression,** appears to be a normal end-product of the birth process. For most women, the symptoms gradually disappear as their bodies return to normal. For others, the symptoms, coupled with the stresses of managing a new family, can cause more severe depression that lasts for several months.

Complications

Problems and complications can occur during labor and delivery even following a successful pregnancy. Such possibilities should be discussed with the practitioner prior to labor so the mother understands what medical procedures may be necessary for her safety and for that of her child. Although pregnancy still involves a certain amount of risk, the risk is lower than for many other common activities (see Table 7.6).

Cesarean Section (C-section). If labor lasts too long or if a baby is presenting wrong (about to exit the uterus anything but head first), a **cesarean section (C-section)** may

be necessary. This surgical procedure involves making an incision across the mother's abdomen and through the uterus to remove the baby. This operation is also performed in cases in which labor is extremely difficult, maternal blood pressure falls rapidly, the placenta separates from the uterus too soon, the mother has diabetes, or other problems occur.

A cesarean section can be traumatic for the mother if she is not prepared for it. The rate of delivery by cesarean section in the United States increased from 5 percent in the mid-1960s to more than 25 percent by 1988.[14] Risks to the mother are the same as for any major abdominal surgery, and recovery from birth takes considerably longer after a C-section. Although a cesarean section may be necessary in certain cases, some physicians and critics feel that

TABLE 7.6 ▪ Putting Voluntary Risks into Perspective

Risk	Chance of Death in a Year (U.S.)
Smoking	1 in 200
Motorcycling	1 in 1,000
Automobile driving	1 in 6,000
Power boating	1 in 6,000
Rock climbing	1 in 7,500
Playing football	1 in 25,000
Having sexual intercourse	1 in 50,000
Canoeing	1 in 100,000
Using tampons (TSS)	1 in 350,000
PREVENTING PREGNANCY	
Oral contraception—nonsmoker	1 in 63,000
Oral contraception—smoker	1 in 16,000
Using IUDs	1 in 100,000
Using barrier methods	None
Using natural methods	None
UNDERGOING STERILIZATION	
Laparoscopic tubal ligation	1 in 20,000
Hysterectomy	1 in 1,600
Vasectomy	None
DECIDING ABOUT PREGNANCY	
Continuing pregnancy	1 in 10,000
Terminating pregnancy:	
Nonlegal abortion	1 in 3,000
Legal abortion:	
Before 9 weeks	1 in 400,000
Between 9 and 12 weeks	1 in 100,000
Between 13 and 16 weeks	1 in 25,000
After 16 weeks	1 in 10,000

Source: Reprinted by permission of Irvington Publishers, Manchester, New Hampshire, from *Contraceptive Technology, 1988–1989* (New York: Irvington Publishers, 1989), 11.

the option has been used too frequently in this country. The federal government's Centers for Disease Control and Prevention (CDC) believes that about one in three of the cesarean deliveries performed in 1991 were unnecessary. The CDC hopes to lower the rate of cesareans in the United States to 15 per 100 births by the year 2000, a level the agency considers to be medically appropriate.

The old adage was "once a cesarean, always a cesarean." Now, however, surgical techniques allow some women who have had a cesarean section to deliver later children vaginally. Guidelines published by the American College of Obstetricians and Gynecologists give an estimated 50 to 80 percent of women the option of a vaginal birth after cesarean (VBAC). Cesarean sections are still necessary if the original incision runs from the top to the bottom of the uterus (as opposed to across); if the baby is over 9 pounds; if the birth is multiple; or if the mother has a medical condition that would make vaginal delivery difficult or dangerous, such as a very small pelvis, chronic high blood pressure, or diabetes.

Miscarriage. One in 10 pregnancies does not end in delivery. Loss of the fetus before it is viable is called a **miscarriage** (also referred to as spontaneous abortion). An estimated 70 to 90 percent of women who miscarry eventually become pregnant again.

Reasons for miscarriage vary. In some cases, the fertilized egg has failed to divide correctly. In others, genetic abnormalities, maternal illness, or infections are responsible. Maternal hormonal imbalance may also cause a miscarriage, as may a weak cervix or toxic chemicals in the environment. In most cases, the cause is not known.

A blood incompatibility between mother and father can cause **Rh factor** problems, and sometimes miscarriage. Rh is a blood protein. Rh problems occur when the mother is Rh-negative and the fetus is Rh-positive. During a first birth, some of the baby's blood passes into the mother's bloodstream. An Rh-negative mother may manufacture antibodies to destroy the Rh-positive blood introduced into her bloodstream at the time of birth. Her first baby will be unaffected, but subsequent babies with positive Rh factor will be at risk for a severe anemia called *hemolytic disease* because the mother's Rh antibodies will attack the fetus's red blood cells.

Medical advances now offer both prevention and treatment for this condition. The mother and fetus can be tested, and if Rh incompatibility is found, intrauterine transfusions can be given or an early delivery by cesarean section can be done, depending upon the individual case. Prevention of the problem is preferable to treatment. All women with Rh-negative blood should be injected with a medication called RhoGAM within 72 hours of any birth, miscarriage, or abortion. This injection will prevent them from developing the Rh antibodies.

Another cause of miscarriage is **ectopic pregnancy,** or implantation of a fertilized egg outside the uterus. A fertilized egg may implant itself in the fallopian tube or, occasionally, in the pelvic cavity. Because these structures are not capable of expanding and nourishing a developing fetus, the pregnancy cannot continue. Such pregnancies are surgically terminated. Most often, the affected fallopian tube is also removed.

Ectopic pregnancy is generally accompanied by pain in the lower abdomen or an aching feeling in the shoulders as the blood flows up toward the diaphragm. If bleeding is significant, blood pressure drops and the woman can go into shock. If an ectopic pregnancy goes undiagnosed and untreated, the fallopian tube ruptures, and the woman is then at great risk of hemorrhage, peritonitis (infection in the abdomen), and even death.

Over the past 12 years, the incidence of ectopic pregnancy has tripled, and no one really understands why. We do know that ectopic pregnancy is a potential side effect of pelvic inflammatory disease (PID), which has become increasingly common in recent years, because the scarring or blockage of the fallopian tubes characteristic of this disease prevents the fertilized egg from passing to the uterus. About 50 percent of women who have had an ectopic pregnancy conceive again. But women who have had one ectopic pregnancy run a higher risk of having another.

Stillbirth is one of the most traumatic events a couple can face. A stillborn baby is one that is born dead, often for no apparent reason. The grief experienced following a stillbirth is usually devastating. Nine months of happy anticipation have been thwarted. Family, friends, and other children may be in a state of shock, needing comfort and

Postpartum depression: The experience of energy depletion, anxiety, mood swings, and depression that women may feel during the postpartum period.

Cesarean section (C-section): A surgical procedure in which a baby is removed through an incision made in the mother's abdominal and uterine walls.

Miscarriage: Loss of the fetus before it is viable; also called spontaneous abortion.

Rh factor: A blood protein related to the production of antibodies. If an Rh-negative mother is pregnant with an Rh-positive fetus, the mother will manufacture antibodies that can kill the fetus, causing miscarriage.

Ectopic pregnancy: Implantation of a fertilized egg outside the uterus, usually in a fallopian tube; a medical emergency that can end in death from hemorrhage for the mother.

Stillbirth: The birth of a dead baby.

not knowing where to turn. The mother's breasts produce milk, and there is no infant to be fed. A room with a crib and toys is left empty.

The grief can last for years, and both partners may blame themselves or each other at some time. In many cases, no amount of reassurance from the attending physician, relatives, or friends can assuage the grief or guilt. Well-intended comments such as, "Oh, you'll have another baby someday," may only create uncomfortable feelings.

Some communities have groups called the Compassionate Friends to help parents and other family members through this grieving process. This nonprofit organization is for parents who have lost a child of any age for any reason.

Sudden Infant Death Syndrome.   The sudden death of an infant under one year of age, for no apparent reason, is called sudden infant death syndrome (SIDS). While SIDS is the leading cause of death for children aged 1 month to 1 year, affecting about 1 in 1,000 infants in the United States each year, it is not a disease. Rather, it is ruled the cause of death after all other possibilities are ruled out. A SIDS death is sudden and silent; the death occurs quickly, often associated with sleep and no signs of suffering.

Because SIDS is a diagnosis of exclusion, doctors do not know what causes SIDS. However, research done in countries including England, New Zealand, Australia, and Norway has shown that by placing children on their backs or sides to sleep, the rate of SIDS was cut by as much as half. In 1994, the American Academy of Pediatrics began a campaign called "Back to Sleep," urging American parents to lay their infants on their backs when they put them to sleep. Additional precautions against SIDS include having a firm surface for the infant's bed, not allowing the infant to become too warm, maintaining a smoke-free environment, having regular pediatric visits, breast-feeding, and seeking prenatal care.

Any sudden, unexpected death threatens one's sense of safety and security. This is especially true in a sudden infant death. Quite simply, babies are not supposed to die. Because the death of an infant is a disruption of the natural order, it is traumatic for parents, family, and friends. The lack of a discernible cause, the suddenness of the tragedy, and the involvement of the legal system makes a SIDS death especially difficult, leaving a great sense of loss and a need for understanding.

*W*HAT DO YOU THINK?

Have you talked to your health care provider about a birth plan and arranged for it to be in your chart? What do you think would be the advantages and disadvantages of breast-feeding?

*I*NFERTILITY

An estimated one in six American couples experiences **infertility,** or difficulties in conceiving. The reasons for this phenomenon include the trend toward delaying childbirth (as a woman gets older, she is less likely to conceive), the use of IUDs, and the rise in the incidence of pelvic inflammatory disease.

Causes in Women

One cause of infertility in women is **pelvic inflammatory disease (PID),** a serious infection that scars the fallopian tubes and blocks sperm migration. Women often develop PID as a result of a gonorrhea or chlamydia infection that progresses to the fallopian tubes and the ovaries. The risk of infertility after one bout of PID is 12 percent. After two bouts, it doubles to nearly 25 percent, and following three bouts, it jumps to more than 50 percent.[15]

Endometriosis is the leading cause of infertility in women in the United States. In this disorder, parts of the endometrial lining of the uterus implant themselves outside the uterus—in the fallopian tubes, lungs, intestines, outer uterine walls, ovarian walls, and/or on the ligaments that support the uterus. The disorder can be treated surgically or with hormonal preparations. Success rates vary.

Causes in Men

Among men, the single largest fertility problem is **low sperm count.** Although only one viable sperm is needed for fertilization, research has shown that all the other sperm in the ejaculate aid in the fertilization process. There are normally 60 to 80 million sperm per milliliter of semen. When the count drops below 20 million, fertility begins to decline.

Low sperm count may be attributable to environmental factors such as exposure of the scrotum to intense heat or cold, radiation, or altitude, or even to wearing excessively tight underwear or outerwear. The mumps virus damages the cells that make sperm. Varicose veins above one or both testicles can also render men infertile. Male infertility problems account for around 40 percent of infertility cases.

Treatment

For the couple desperately wishing to conceive, the road to parenthood may be frustrating. Fortunately, medical treatment can identify the cause of infertility in about 90 percent of affected couples. The chances of becoming pregnant range from 30 to 70 percent, depending on the specific cause of the infertility. The countless tests and the invasion of privacy that characterize some couples' efforts to conceive can put stress on an otherwise strong, healthy relationship. Before starting fertility tests, the wise couple will reassess their priorities. Some will choose to undergo counseling to help them clarify their feelings about the fertility process. A good physician or fertility team will take the time to ascertain the couple's level of motivation.

Fertility work-ups can be very expensive, and the costs are not usually covered by insurance companies. Fertility work-ups for men include a sperm count, a test for sperm motility, and analysis of any disease processes present. Such procedures should only be undertaken by a qualified urologist. Women are thoroughly examined by an obstetrician/gynecologist for the composition of cervical mucus, extent of tubal scarring, and evidence of endometriosis.

Complete fertility work-ups may take four to five months and can be unsettling. The couple may be instructed to have sex "by the calendar" to increase their chances of conceiving. In some cases, surgery can correct structural problems such as tubal scarring. In others, administering hormones can improve the health of ova and sperm. Sometimes pregnancy can be achieved by collecting the husband's sperm from several ejaculations and inseminating the wife at a later time.

When all surgical and hormonal methods fail, the couple still has some options. **Fertility drugs** such as Clomid and Pergonal stimulate ovulation in women who are not ovulating. Ninety percent of women who use these drugs will begin to ovulate, and half will conceive.

Fertility drugs are associated with a great number of side effects, including headaches, irritability, restlessness, depression, fatigue, edema (fluid retention), abnormal uterine bleeding, breast tenderness, vasomotor flushes (hot flashes), and visual difficulties. Women using fertility drugs are also at increased risk of multiple ovarian cysts (fluid-filled growths) and liver damage. The drugs sometimes trigger the release of more than one egg. Thus a woman treated with one of these drugs has a 1 in 10 chance of having multiple births. Most such births are twins, but triplets and even quadruplets are not uncommon.

Alternative insemination of a woman with her partner's sperm is another treatment option. This technique has led to an estimated 250,000 births in the United States, primarily for couples in which the man is infertile. If this procedure fails, the couple may choose insemination by an anonymous donor through a "sperm bank." Many men sell their sperm to such banks. The sperm are classified according to the physical characteristics of the donor (for example, blonde hair, blue eyes), and then frozen for future use. Sperm can survive in this frozen state for up to five years. The woman being inseminated usually chooses sperm from a man whose physical characteristics resemble those of her partner or match her own personal preferences.

In the last few years, concern has been expressed about the possibility of transmitting the AIDS virus through alternative insemination. As a result, donors are routinely screened for the disease before they donate.

In vitro fertilization, often referred to as "test tube" fertilization, involves collecting a viable ovum from the prospective mother and transferring it to a nutrient medium in a laboratory, where it is fertilized with sperm from the woman's partner or a donor. After a few days, the embryo is transplanted into the mother's uterus, where, it is hoped, it will develop normally. Until 1984, in vitro fertilization was classified as "experimental." Since then, it has moved into the mainstream of standard infertility treatments. About 500 "test tube" babies are born each year.

In **gamete intrafallopian transfer (GIFT),** the egg is "harvested" from the wife's ovary and placed in the fallopian tube with her husband's sperm. Less expensive and time-consuming than in vitro fertilization, GIFT mimics nature by allowing the egg to be fertilized in the fallopian tube and to migrate to the uterus according to the normal timetable. The success rate for this procedure is approximately 20 percent.

Infertility: Difficulties in conceiving.

Pelvic inflammatory disease (PID): An infection that scars the fallopian tubes and consequently blocks sperm migration, causing infertility.

Endometriosis: A disorder in which uterine lining tissue establishes itself outside the uterus; it is the leading cause of infertility in the United States.

Low sperm count: A sperm count below 60 million sperm per milliliter of semen; it is the leading cause of infertility in men.

Fertility drugs: Hormones that stimulate ovulation in women who are not ovulating; often responsible for multiple births.

Alternative insemination: Fertilization accomplished by depositing a partner's or a donor's semen into a woman's vagina via a thin tube; almost always done in a doctor's office.

In vitro fertilization: Fertilization of an egg in a nutrient medium and subsequent transfer back to the mother's body.

Gamete intrafallopian transfer (GIFT): An egg is harvested from the female partner ovary and placed with the male partner's sperm in her fallopian tube, where it is fertilized and then migrates to the uterus for implantation.

What Are the Ethical Issues Concerning Reproductive Technology?

Recent advances in reproductive technology present ethical and legal dilemmas that appear as extremely complicated cases in our nation's courts. Many of these cases involve issues surrounding in vitro fertilization (IVF), frozen embryos, and gamete intrafallopian transfer (GIFT).

Every year, 20,000 couples undergo IVF in this country; 2,000 babies have been born using this method as of 1990. IVF costs between $8,000 and $10,000, besides the normal medical expenses associated with pregnancy and birth. One in four couples who undergo IVF choose to have some of their embryos frozen for future use. Embryos are frozen in liquid nitrogen and kept for a specified period of time (until the mother turns 45, or for 10 years, depending on the clinic). This process saves time and money.

The 200 IVF clinics throughout the United States require couples to sign elaborate agreements regarding the fate of their frozen embryos in the event of their divorce, death, or change of mind. Couples may choose to have their embryos destroyed, given to research, or donated to other couples. Challenges to these agreements are becoming more frequent and are presenting some serious ethical questions for jurists, physicians, and couples.

In 1984, a California couple named Rios left several frozen embryos in an Australian IVF clinic. The couple died in a plane crash, and their living children were concerned about how their parents' estate would be divided. Were the embryos to be considered heirs and legal issue? The judge in this first case of its kind ruled that the embryos should be distributed to other couples and that the Rioses' surviving children were the only beneficiaries of the estate.

A recent case argued in Tennessee concerned a couple named Davis who divorced, leaving seven frozen embryos in a Tennessee IVF clinic. Mrs. Davis wanted custody of the embryos in order to attempt implantation and pregnancy with one. Mr. Davis wanted the embryos to remain frozen. A Tennessee superior court justice gave custody of the frozen embryos to Mrs. Davis, ruling that life begins at conception and that all seven of the embryos had a right to be born.

These cases present interesting questions: To whom do frozen embryos belong? What, if any, are the rights of frozen embryos? If all frozen embryos have a right to be born, which should be implanted first? Should medical research be allowed on frozen embryos? If frozen embryos are alive, is destroying them the same as murder or abortion? The legal problems associated with IVF, like those associated with surrogate motherhood, are new. Lawmakers have not yet thoroughly analyzed the problems and fashioned laws governing the issues of modern reproductive technology.

Sources: Based on "Embryos in the Fridge," *Economist,* 12 August 1989, 22; "People in Petri Dishes," *Progressive,* November 1989, 38; "The Trial of an Embryonic Issue," *U.S. News and World Report,* 21 August 1989, 13.

In **nonsurgical embryo transfer,** a donor egg is fertilized by the husband's sperm and then implanted in the wife's uterus. This procedure may also be used in cases involving the transfer of an already-fertilized ovum into the uterus of another woman.

Nonsurgical embryo transfer: In vitro fertilization of a donor egg by the male partner's (or donor's) sperm and subsequent transfer to the female partner's or another woman's uterus.

Embryo transfer: Artificial insemination of a donor with male partner's sperm; after a time, the embryo is transferred from the donor to the female partner's body.

Embryo freezing: The freezing of an embryo for later implantation.

Cloning: Replacing the nucleus of an in vitro-fertilized egg with the nucleus of a donor cell.

Embryo transfer is another treatment for infertility. In this procedure, an ovum from a donor's body is artificially inseminated by the husband's sperm, allowed to stay in the donor's body for a time, and then transplanted into the wife's body.

Some laboratories are experimenting with **embryo freezing,** in which a fertilized embryo is suspended in a solution of liquid nitrogen. When desired, it is gradually thawed and implanted into the prospective mother. The first United States birth of a frozen embryo was reported in June 1986. In the future, this technique may make it possible for young couples to produce an embryo and save it for later implantation when they are ready to have a child, thus reducing the risks of fertilization of older eggs.

Cloning has been successfully used with lower animals such as toads and salamanders. In cloning, the nucleus of an in vitro-fertilized egg is replaced with the nucleus of a body cell from a donor. Offspring will be genetically identical to the donor. The possibilities of human cloning are still remote.

The ethical and moral questions surrounding experimental methods of infertility treatments are staggering. (See the Health Headlines box.) The expense of these procedures can also be astounding. Alternative insemination costs approximately $1,500 for five monthly attempts. In vitro fertilization costs $5,000 per attempt. Fewer than 50 percent of those using these procedures succeed in becoming pregnant on the first try.

Surrogate Motherhood

Between 60 and 70 percent of infertile couples are able to conceive after treatment. The rest decide to live without children, to adopt, or to attempt surrogate motherhood. In this option, the couple hires a woman to be alternatively inseminated by the husband. The surrogate then carries the baby to term and surrenders it upon birth to the couple. Surrogate mothers are reportedly paid about $10,000 for their services and are reimbursed for medical expenses. Legal and medical expenses can run as high as $30,000 for the infertile couple. Couples considering sur-

rogate motherhood are advised to consult a lawyer regarding contracts.

Most legal documents drawn up for childless couples and surrogate mothers stipulate that the surrogate must undergo amniocentesis and that if the fetus is defective, she must consent to an abortion. In that case, or if the surrogate miscarries, she is reimbursed for her time and expenses. The prospective parents must also agree to take the baby if it is carried to term, even if it is unhealthy or deformed.

---

*W*HAT DO YOU THINK?

What are the rights of surrogate mothers? What option would you most likely select if you found that you and your spouse had fertility problems? Why? Do you think cloning or embryo freezing is ethical? Why or why not? Do you think men should participate in prenatal counseling?

Summary

- Only latex condoms, when used correctly for oral sex or intercourse, are effective in preventing sexually transmitted diseases. Other contraceptive methods include abstinence, outercourse, oral contraceptives, foams, jellies, suppositories, creams, the female condom, the diaphragm, the contraceptive sponge, the cervical cap, intrauterine devices, withdrawal, Norplant, Depo-Provera, and the vaginal ring. Fertility awareness methods rely on altering sexual practices to avoid pregnancy. Sterilization is permanent contraception.

- Abortion is currently legal in the United States through the second trimester. Abortion methods include vacuum aspiration, dilation and evacuation (D&E), dilation and curettage (D&C), hysterotomy, induction abortion, and the new RU-486 "abortion pills."

- Parenting is a demanding job requiring careful planning. Emotional health, maternal health, financial evaluation, and contingency planning all need to be taken into account.

- Prenatal care includes a complete physical exam within the first trimester, avoidance of alcohol and drugs, cigarettes, X-rays, and chemicals having teratogenic effects. Full-term pregnancy covers three trimesters.

- Childbirth occurs in three stages. Birth alternatives include the Lamaze, Harris, "childbirth without fear," and Leboyer methods. Parents should jointly make decisions about labor early in the pregnancy to be better prepared for labor when it occurs. Complications of pregnancy and childbirth include miscarriage, ectopic pregnancy, stillbirth, and cesarean section.

- Infertility in women may be caused by pelvic inflammatory disease or endometriosis. In men, it may be caused by low sperm count. Treatment may include alternative insemination, in vitro fertilization, gamete intrafallopian transfer, nonsurgical embryo transfer, and embryo transfer. Surrogate motherhood involves hiring a fertile woman to be alternatively inseminated by the male partner.

Discussion Questions

1. Draw up a list of the most effective contraceptive methods. What drawbacks keep everyone from using them? What medical conditions should keep you from using them?

2. Discuss the varied methods of abortion. Do you think RU-486 should be approved by the FDA? What do you think of a method that requires three visits to a clinic?

3. What are some of the most important decisions that your parents made concerning raising you? Would you raise your child differently from how you were raised?

4. Discuss the growth of the fetus through the three trimesters. What medical checkups or tests should be done during each trimester?

Managing Your Fertility

After reading this chapter, you should realize that pregnancy, childbirth, and reproductive issues are not to be taken lightly. The choices between different types of birth control and the ethical issues surrounding fertility are complex. As you read through this chapter, we hope you were able to sort through issues and begin to contemplate some of the decisions you may have to face. We hope that you have begun the process of self-exploration and that you will be able to make informed decisions and choices.

Making Decisions for You

It's important to take control of your own fertility and to share this responsibility in your relationships. What kind of birth control do you currently use or would you use in a sexual relationship? Do you know the potential side effects? Are there any potential drug interactions? If the contraceptive has a low effectiveness rate, what further means of protection can you take? Finally, have you protected yourself from sexually transmitted diseases?

Checklist for Change: Making Personal Choices

✓ If you are in a stable relationship and are considering having a child, is it something both you and your partner want?

✓ Do you have a network of family and friends who will help if you decide to have a baby?

✓ Do you know and feel comfortable with your philosophical beliefs about children?

✓ Have you assessed your health to make sure that if you choose to get pregnant you will begin the pregnancy as healthy as possible?

✓ Do you feel comfortable discussing birth control with your partner?

✓ Do you feel comfortable choosing a method of birth control that meets the needs of both yourself and your partner?

✓ Are you familiar with the resources available if you have trouble conceiving?

✓ Have you discussed alternatives should you become or get someone pregnant?

Checklist for Change: Making Community Choices

✓ Have you taken the time to become educated about the issues and concerns related to parenting?

✓ Have you decided to become involved in issues that concern children and parenting?

✓ Do you listen with an open mind to issues involving reproduction and sexual health and then make informed decisions?

✓ When you think about having children, do you think of it in terms of long-range planning?

✓ Are you an advocate for people making choices that are in their best interest, regardless of your own personal philosophy or opinions?

✓ Do you believe in providing support for community agencies and social services that assist in meeting the sexual and reproductive health needs of your community?

✓ Do you try to volunteer your time to other people or agencies that may need your assistance?

Critical Thinking

Rebecca and Bryant are the 37-year-old parents of a 5-year-old daughter. They had always planned on having several children, but are now facing a difficult decision: Should they have another child now, wait a few more years, or perhaps not have any more children at all? Bryant thinks that they should have more children before they get to be too old. As an only child, he remembers being "lonely all the time." But Rebecca is concerned about the additional expense of having another child. With their daughter about to start school, she is considering going back to work to help out with expenses. Anyway, she recently read an article about the advantages of being an only child.

Using the DECIDE model described in Chapter 1, decide what you would do if you were Rebecca or Bryant. Is there more than one decision with which you could feel comfortable?

5. List the varied decisions that parents face when thinking about childbirth. Consider varied childbirth methods, where to have the child, and whether to use painkilling drugs during delivery. How does the first-time parent decide what to do?

6. If you and your spouse were having difficulty getting pregnant, what would your options be? If you proved infertile, what would your options be then? What would you do?

Application Exercise

Reread the What Do You Think? scenarios at the beginning of the chapter and answer the following questions.

1. From what you have read in the chapter, what pregnancy planning questions should each of the couples in the first scenario be addressing? Are the planning questions and concerns the same for each couple? Will the obstacles for some of the couples be greater? Why?

2. What concerns you most about Kari and Dave's relationship? Is it realistic that two people can date for several months and never discuss having sex? What would you have done or not done differently from Kari and Dave?

3. If you could tell incoming freshmen three personal rules about using birth control, what would they be?

Further Reading

Boston Women's Health Collective, *The New Our Bodies, Ourselves,* rev. ed. (New York: Simon & Schuster, 1993).

Like its earlier editions, *The New Our Bodies, Ourselves* contains information about women's health from a decidedly feminist angle. Every aspect of health is covered, including nutrition, emotional health, fitness, relationships, reproduction, contraception, and pregnancy.

R. A. Hatcher, *Contraceptive Technology,* 16 rev. ed. (New York: Irvington Publishers, 1994).

Perhaps the best primary reference concerning birth control for physicians, family planning centers, student health services, and educators. Contributors include many staff members of the Centers for Disease Control.

S. K. Henshaw and J. Van Vort, eds., *1992 Abortion Factbook—1992 Edition: Readings, Trends, and State and Local Data to 1988* (New York: Alan Guttmacher Institute, 1992).

A collection of articles and tables that depict abortion in the United States today, including medical services, political phenomena, and related issues.

R. F. Spark, *Male Sexual Health: A Couple's Guide* (Mount Vernon, NY: Consumer Reports Books, 1991).

A concise, up-to-date guide to male sexual problems ranging from infertility to erectile dysfunction.

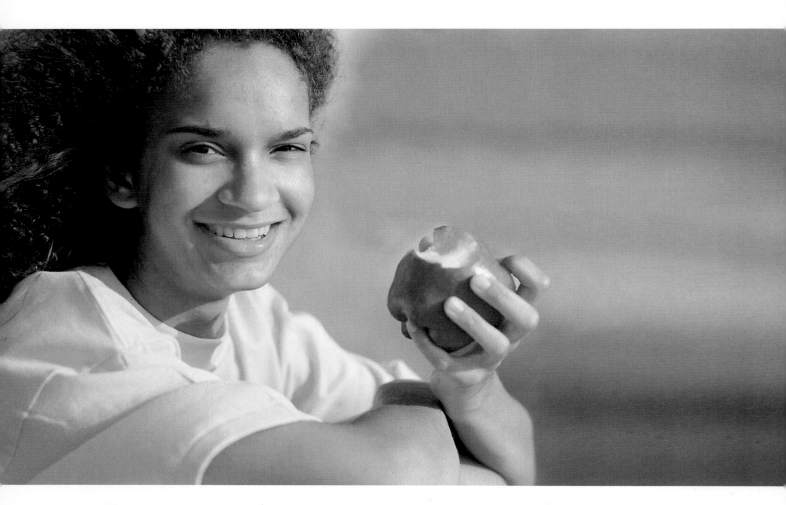

$\mathcal{C}$HAPTER OBJECTIVES

◆ Examine the factors that influence dietary decisions and discuss how the new Food Group Pyramid can be used to help break bad habits.

◆ Explain major essential nutrients (water, proteins, carbohydrates, fiber, fats, vitamins, and minerals) and indicate what purpose they serve in maintaining your overall health.

◆ Define the different types of vegetarianism and discuss possible health benefits and risks.

◆ Describe the unique problems that college students may have when trying to eat healthy foods and the actions they can take to insure compliance with the food pyramid.

◆ Explain some of the food safety concerns of which consumers should be aware, including food irradiation, food-borne illnesses, food allergies, and other food health concerns.

Nutrition

Eating for Optimum Health

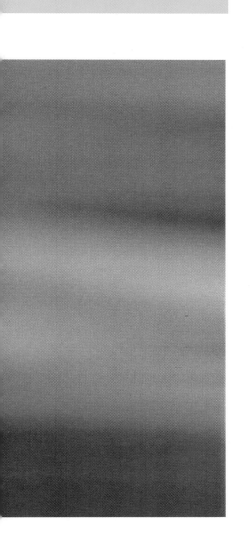

WHAT DO YOU THINK?

Bart is a senior in college and is extremely active physically, running several miles per day. He is also a vegetarian, and so eats no meat, poultry, fish, or dairy products. Salads, pasta, and breads make up almost his entire diet, and he eats very few fruits and no legumes or nuts. He can't understand why people allow themselves to get "fat" and spends a lot of time trying to tell his friends how to eat "healthy foods." He has no patience with those who are "weak willed" and just can't seem to get it together enough to eat healthful foods and get fit, and he avoids people who are "fat" and people who eat "animal flesh."

Talat is a "nutrition junkie." Every day, she completes a detailed analysis of her previous day's food intake, assessing vitamins, minerals, and all major nutrients. In addition, she takes at least 12 vitamin/mineral supplements per day, believing that she is deficient in these nutrients. She refuses to eat out because she worries about food contamination.

Jasper is a first-year student living in the dormitory of a small college. His parents opted for the food service meal plan in the hope that Jasper would eat at least one hot meal per day. This particular food service has few choices for students; foods are over-cooked, there are few salads or vegetables, and most entrees tend to be high in fat content. Jasper eats at the food service most of the time, but supplements his diet with fast food and ice cream snacks. He is gaining weight and is worried about some of the recent news stories on TV discussing high fat diets and diets lacking certain nutrients. He decides he'd better do something about his eating habits, but when he goes to the cafeteria at school, he finds he has few healthy options.

- How would you assess each of these people's dietary attitudes? Dietary habits? What problems, if any, do you think they have? What do they appear to be doing right? Why do some people find their dietary choices to be relatively easy, while others have huge problems making dietary changes? What factors may have contributed to their attitudes and behaviors? What would you suggest each of these people do to change his or her eating habits, if anything? Do you have friends who have similar problems? Where on your campus could they go for help?

*T*oday, we face dietary choices and nutritional challenges that our grandparents never dreamed of—exotic foreign foods; dietary supplements; artificial sweeteners; no-fat, low-fat, and artificial-fat alternatives; cholesterol-free, high-protein, high-carbohydrate, and low-calorie products—thousands of alternatives bombard us daily. Caught in the cross fire of advertised claims by the food industry and advice provided by health and nutrition experts, most of us find it difficult to make wise dietary decisions. Just when we think we have the answers, a new research study tells us that what we thought was true probably wasn't.

It's no wonder the typical person who is trying to do the right thing nutritionally may be left scratching his or her head in confusion. Television advertisements subtly attempt to influence us to buy "cholesterol-free" products, "high-fiber" oat bran, "stress vitamins," and a variety of items that promise to make us healthier. Newsstands overflow with books and magazines promoting health foods, weight-loss aids, and "super" diets. Many of these articles and books are written by people who have no educational background in nutrition but who claim to be nutrition experts. Their theories are based on results obtained with poorly designed research techniques and provide questionable or controversial recommendations. The ability to sift through the untruths, half-truths, and scientific realities and select a nutrition plan designed to meet your individual needs is an essential health-promoting skill.

When you are living away from home for the first time, suddenly having to make your own choices about food may be a formidable task. This is particularly true when you may not have the financial resources to buy or cook the same things that your parents did. It may be even more difficult if your parents did not prepare healthy foods and thereby provide a healthy model for your subsequent dietary choices. A 1994 study of over 2,000 college students found that they often had considerable difficulty planning their own menus, eating healthfully, and having the resources to prepare meals.[1] Did your parents fix healthy meals for you complete with green, leafy salads, vegetables, low-fat protein entrees, milk, and lots of unprocessed carbohydrates? Did you eat fried foods regularly, lots of desserts, and large quantities of food? These past patterns of eating may be influencing your current behaviors more than you realize. Understanding the reasons behind your nutritional choices may help you change negative dietary patterns and enhance positive behaviors.

*H*EALTHY EATING

Eating is one activity that most of us take for granted. We assume that we will have sufficient food to get us through the day and rarely are we forced to eat things that we do not like for the sake of staying alive. In fact, although we have all undoubtedly experienced **hunger** before mealtime, few of us have ever experienced the type of hunger that continues for days and threatens our survival. Most of us do not eat for physical survival. Instead, we eat because we feel like eating or because some inner signal tells us that it's time to eat.

Many factors influence when we eat, what we eat, and how much we eat. Sensory stimulation, such as smelling, seeing, and tasting foods, can entice us to eat. Social pressures, including family traditions, social events that involve eating, and busy work schedules, can also influence our diets. Although our ancestors typically sat down to three complete meals per day, they also labored heavily in the fields or at other work and burned off many of those calories. Today, eating three large meals per day combined with an inactive lifestyle is just the right recipe for weight gain.

Cultural factors also play a role in how we eat. People from Middle-eastern cultures tend to eat more rice, fruits, and vegetables than does the typical American. The Japanese eat more fish. Clearly, each culture has both healthy and unhealthy eating habits. The Multicultural Perspectives box suggests ethnic foods to eat and ethnic foods to avoid.

Other factors also influence our dietary choices. Our economic status may determine what types of foods we purchase; those having low incomes probably find some foods or food groups too expensive, while those having high incomes have boundless choices.

If our **appetite** for food is stimulated, we may want to eat something because it looks or smells good, even though we are not actually hungry. Finding the right balance between eating to maintain body functions (eating to live) and eating to satisfy our appetites (living to eat) is a problem for many of us.

Changing the way you think about food can mean the difference between choosing healthy foods (eating to live) and foods that satisfy your cravings (living to eat).

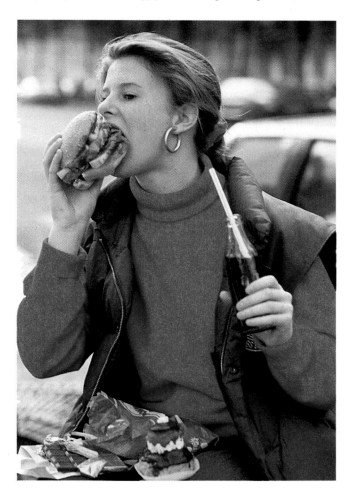

Nutrition is the science that investigates the relationship between physiological function and the essential elements of the foods we eat. With our overabundance of food, our vast number of choices, and our easy access to almost every **nutrient** (proteins, carbohydrates, fats, vitamins, minerals, and water), Americans should have few nutritional problems. But nutritionists believe that our "diets of affluence" are responsible for many of our diseases and disabilities. Our history as a land of agricultural abundance accounts for the traditional American diet: high in fats and calories and weighted toward red meats, potatoes, and rich desserts. More recent trends have indicated that Americans are changing to a white-meat diet having fewer fats and more fruits and vegetables. Some of these changes are outlined in Table 8.1.

Despite these dietary improvements, heart disease, certain types of cancer, hypertension (high blood pressure), cirrhosis of the liver, tooth decay, and chronic obesity continue to be major health risks. Why do so many of us have nutritional problems? Much of our preoccupation with food and our tendency to eat the wrong types and amounts of foods stem from our early eating habits. Find out how much you know about nutrition by taking the Rate Yourself test.

Why We Eat What We Do

If we were like most other species and ate only for survival, the likelihood of excessive food consumption would be slim. But humans learn from birth that eating is an enjoyable experience associated with warmth, pleasure, and sensory delights. Infants cry and are fed; children are rewarded with food for doing well; weddings, birthdays, and other special occasions center on eating.

These rewards carry over into times of disappointment. When we are frustrated, food often becomes our consolation. When we are busy, we reward ourselves with coffee and snack breaks. In most of these instances, we are not concerned with proper nutrition. Instead, we are concerned with fulfilling our cravings for social consumption, and the tastes of gourmet chocolate, ice cream, or pizza with the works become our "vices of choice." Many of us learn to love to eat at an early age, and we crave those foods that we have learned to enjoy. Some of us enjoy them far too much!

*W*HAT DO YOU THINK?

Think about your own eating habits. Do you eat significant amounts of red meats and dairy products? Are you a vegetarian? Would you be happy with a veggie-laden salad and some wheat bread for your evening meal or do you crave a hot, meat-and-potatoes dining experience? Why do you think you feel the way you do? How did your family eat when you were growing up? Is everyone in your family of origin still eating the same way they did when they were young? Why or why not?

Hunger: The feeling associated with the physiological need to eat.

Appetite: The desire to eat; normally accompanies hunger, but is more psychological than physiological.

Nutrition: The science that investigates the relationship between physiological function and the essential elements of foods we eat.

Nutrients: The constituents of food that sustain us physiologically: proteins, carbohydrates, fats, vitamins, minerals, and water.

Guidelines for Healthy Ethnic Eating

Ethnic Food	Healthy Ideas	Things to Avoid
Italian	■ Stick to pasta dishes with low-fat sauces; plain red and meatless marinara. Use fresh ingredients such as mushrooms. ■ Rinse pasta to remove starch. ■ Choose vegetarian pizzas. ■ Use skim-milk mozzarella.	■ Sausages, carbonara sauces, meatballs, garlic/butter breads, cream sauces, heavy-cheese pastas, pepperoni. ■ Extra cheese.
Mexican	■ Ask that cheeses and sour cream be provided on the side or left out altogether. ■ Select white-meat chicken fillings. ■ Fill up on beans, rice, and vegetables. ■ Ask what types of oils are used in stir-frying fajitas.	■ Refried beans fried in fat. ■ Fried tortillas and burrito and taco shells. ■ Pork, beef, and sausage fillings. ■ Hold the thick cheese sauces or toppings.
Chinese	■ Focus on brown rice as a major part of the meal; if unavailable, ask for steamed (*not* fried) white rice. ■ Make vegetables the key part of the meal. Stir-frying in vegetable oil is preferable to deep-frying. ■ Choose a low-fat appetizer such as wonton soup. ■ Choose chicken or fish and ask if meat content of a dish can be reduced and vegetables increased.	■ Fried rice, eggrolls, spring rolls, and crispy noodles—are all high in fat. ■ MSG and high-sodium soy sauces. ■ Rich lobster or egg dishes.
Japanese	■ Focus on steamed rice and vegetables. ■ Substitute tofu for meat; although high in fat, the fat is largely unsaturated. ■ Eat chicken or fish broiled or steamed.	■ Soy sauces. ■ Fried rice dishes. ■ Miso—it is extremely high in sodium. ■ Tempura—it is high in fat. ■ Skip sashimi and sushi (raw fish) dishes to avoid possible bacteria or parasites.
Thai	■ Choose clear broth soups. ■ Order steamed seafood in wine sauces, stir-fried chicken, vegetables, or grilled meats.	■ Coconut milk. ■ Peanut drippings/sauces. ■ Deep-fried dishes.
Cajun	■ Choose tomato-based sauces. ■ Order vegetable gumbo or jambalaya. ■ Ask for fish that is grilled. ■ Hold the salt.	■ Deep-fried foods. ■ Andouille and other sausages. ■ Hold the sauces on sandwiches.

Responsible Eating: Changing Old Habits

Americans consume more calories per person than does any other group of people in the world. A **calorie** is a unit of measure that indicates the amount of energy we obtain from a particular food. Calories are eaten in the form of *proteins, fats,* and *carbohydrates,* three of the basic nutrients necessary for life. Three other nutrients, *vitamins,*

TABLE 8.1 ■ Changes in Annual Food Consumption by Americans, 1960–1993

The following table illustrates changes in annual food consumption per person during the last three decades. Unless otherwise indicated, the amounts are presented in pounds. Are these trends generally healthy or unhealthy?

Food Product	1960	1973	1983	1993
Beef	73.7	76.5	72.0	64.0
Fish and shellfish	10.3	11.8	13.7	18.5
Chicken	24.0	26.5	34.0	50.0
Eggs (number)	334.0	285.0	260.0	235.0
Whole milk (gallons)	26.0	22.0	15.0	9.5
Lower-fat milk (2%) (gallons)	—	4.5	7.5	9.5
Nonfat milk	1.8	1.6	1.6	2.5
Fats and oils	—	56.0	63.5	68.5
Flour (white, wheat)	—	105.0	118.1	126.5
Pasta	—	7.7	11.3	30.2
Breakfast cereals	—	10.8	14.0	17.6
Sugar and corn sweeteners	111.5	126.0	125.0	140.7
Artifical sweeteners	—	5.0	10.4	23.0
Fruits (fresh)	—	91.0	103.0	118.0
Fruits (canned)	—	14.4	8.9	7.7
Vegetables (fresh)	—	82.0	86.5	104.0
Coffee (gallons)	—	33.4	26.5	27.0
Soft drinks (gallons)	—	25.5	31.0	47.0
Beer (gallons)	—	32.5	35.5	32.7
Wine (gallons)	—	2.2	3.4	4.1
Distilled spirits (gallons)	—	3.0	2.6	2.0

— = data not available

Source: U.S. Department of Agriculture. Food Consumption and Expenditures, 1960–93. Statistical Bulletin No. 915. 1994.

minerals, and *water,* are necessary for bodily function but do not contribute any calories to our diets.

Excess calorie consumption is a major factor in our tendency to be overweight. However, it is not so much the quantity of food we eat that is likely to cause weight problems and resultant diseases as it is the relative proportion of nutrients in our diets and our lack of physical activity. Americans typically get approximately 38 percent of their calories from fat, 15 percent from proteins, 22 percent from complex carbohydrates, and 24 percent from simple sugars. Nutritionists recommend that complex carbohydrates be increased to make up 48 percent of our total calories and that proteins be reduced to 12 percent, simple sugars to 10 percent, and fats to no more than 30 percent of our total diets.

It is the high concentration of fats in the American diet, particularly saturated fats (largely animal fats), that appears to increase our risk for heart disease. High concentrations of highly processed sugars seem to increase the risk for certain other diseases, particularly tooth decay. Over the years, several federal agencies have worked to modify the average American's diet through a series of dietary goals and guidelines.

The Food Guide Pyramid

Recent changes in the way we think about food groups and eating were consolidated with the development of the Food Guide Pyramid, promoted by the United States Department of Agriculture (USDA). The pyramid was designed to illustrate graphically the importance of grains, cereals, vegetables, and fruits compared to meat, fish, poultry, dairy products, and other foods. Figure 8.1 shows the Food Guide Pyramid, including recommended servings. Below are examples, each showing the equivalent of one serving from each of the major food groups.

Calorie: A unit of measure that indicates the amount of energy we obtain from a particular food.

Nutrition Quiz

Which of the following statements are true?

_____ 1. Large amounts of gelatin strengthen finger-nails.

_____ 2. Toast has fewer calories than bread.

_____ 3. Food grown on depleted soils is nutritionally inferior.

_____ 4. Commercially canned and frozen foods are nearly worthless nutritionally.

_____ 5. Athletes need more protein in their diets than does the general population.

_____ 6. Feed a cold and starve a fever.

_____ 7. Taking extra vitamins and minerals will pep you up if you are fatigued.

_____ 8. Eating certain food combinations (such as fish and milk or cucumbers and milk) is dangerous.

_____ 9. Cheese causes constipation.

_____ 10. Celery and fish are brain foods.

_____ 11. Prunes, bran, and fresh fruits are sure cures for constipation.

_____ 12. Yogurt is a nutritionally superior wonder food that will make you healthy.

_____ 13. Vitamin supplements are necessary if you are to be well-nourished.

_____ 14. Oysters and black olives are aphrodisiacs (love potions).

_____ 15. Any food craving indicates that the body needs the nutrients in that food.

_____ 16. Obesity is usually caused by glandular disorders.

_____ 17. "Health foods" are nutritionally superior to regular brands.

_____ 18. Megadoses of vitamin C help to prevent colds.

Answers: All the statements are false.

1. Many factors influence fingernail formation including disease, environment, hormones, and nutrition. Gelatin is not one of them.

2. Toasting browns and dehydrates the exterior of the bread but does not reduce its caloric value.

3. Poor soil produces poor yields. Quantity is affected, not quality. For example, depleted soil produces fewer and smaller beans, but each bean is still nutritionally complete.

4. Some methods of food preparation—including home preparation—reduce the nutrient value of certain foods. But commercial methods of processing foods are designed to preserve their nutrient values.

5. Athletes may need more calories because of increased activity, but they do not need more protein.

6. The only valid guideline with colds and fever is to increase fluid intake. With a fever, more calories are burned as a result of increase metabolic rate, but the person often eats less because of malaise and nausea.

7. Vitamins and minerals are not pep pills. They contain no calories (energy), nor are they stimulants. If fatigue persists, see a physician.

8. There are no known poisonous food combinations providing, of course, that neither food is contaminated or spoiled.

9. Generally, over 90 percent of the carbohydrate, protein, and fat in cheese is absorbed; constipation is not produced.

10. No one particular food builds any one body tissue.

11. There are several causes of constipation. If constipation is atonic, roughage may be helpful, but if it is spastic or obstructive, roughage is undesirable and the person is placed on a low-fiber diet.

12. Yogurt is a cultured milk product. It has the same nutritive value as the milk from which it was made. There are no "wonder foods."

13. A well-balanced diet provides all necessary vitamins. Hypervitaminosis can result from high amounts of ingested fat-soluble vitamins.

14. There are no known aphrodisiacs for humans.

15. Craving is a learned preference for a food rather than an indication that the body "needs" that food.

16. At the present time, it is thought that only 5 percent of obesity cases are caused by metabolic or glandular problems. The remaining 95 percent of cases are regulatory, which means too much food and too little exercise.

17. Foods claiming to be "natural" or "organic" are not superior to general foods available at the supermarket. Foods should be selected for their nutritional value, not their advertising value.

18. Many controlled and double-blind studies have been run. So far there is no statistical evidence that high doses of vitamin C help to prevent the common cold.

Source: Reprinted by permission from pages 260 and 263 of _Health Behaviors,_ 2d ed., by Rosalind Reed and Thomas A. Lang. Copyright 1986 by West Publishing Company. All rights reserved.

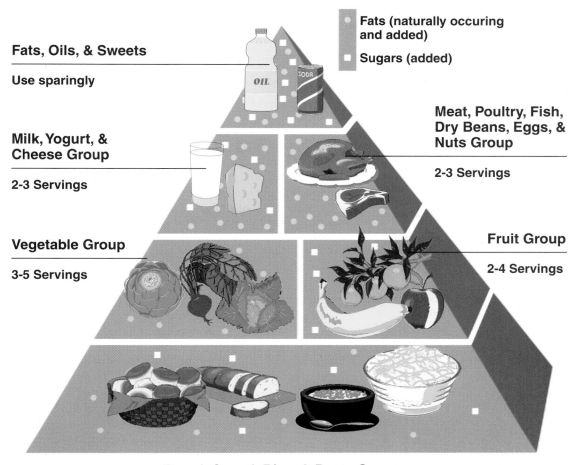

Fats, Oils, & Sweets
Use sparingly

Fats (naturally occuring and added)
Sugars (added)

Milk, Yogurt, & Cheese Group
2-3 Servings

Meat, Poultry, Fish, Dry Beans, Eggs, & Nuts Group
2-3 Servings

Vegetable Group
3-5 Servings

Fruit Group
2-4 Servings

Bread, Cereal, Rice, & Pasta Group
6-11 Servings

FIGURE 8.1

Food Guide Pyramid: A Guide to Daily Food Choices
Source: U.S. Department of Agriculture, 1993.

Breads, Cereals, Rice, and Pasta Group (6–11 servings)

- 1 slice of bread or medium dinner roll
- ½ hamburger bun, hot dog bun, bagel, or English muffin
- ½ cup cooked rice, pasta, or other grains
- 6 saltines (the small squares) or snack crackers or 3 ring pretzels
- 1 ounce ready-to-eat cereal
- ½ cup cooked cereal
- 3 cups popped popcorn
- 1 tortilla, pancake, or waffle square
- 3 graham cracker squares or small, unfrosted cookies

Fruit Group (2–4 servings)

- whole fruit such as medium apple, banana, or orange
- ½ cup of raw, cooked, or canned fruit
- ¾ cup of fruit juice
- ½ cup canned fruit
- ¼ cup dried fruit

Vegetable Group (3–5 servings)

- 1 cup leafy raw vegetables

- ½ cup chopped fresh, frozen, or canned vegetables
- ¾ cup fresh, frozen, or canned juice
- ¼ cup dried vegetables

Meat, Poultry, Fish, Dry Beans, Eggs, and Nuts Group (2–3 servings)

- 2–3 ounces lean, trimmed, and baked or roasted meat, fish, or poultry

The following can substitute for 1 ounce of meat:

- 2 tablespoons peanut butter or other nut/seed butter
- ¼ cup nuts
- ½ cup cooked legumes
- 3 oz. tofu
- 1 egg

Milk, Yogurt, and Cheese (2 servings; 3 servings for pregnant and breast-feeding women and teens; 4 servings for teens who are pregnant or breast-feeding)

- 1 cup of milk or yogurt
- 1 ½ oz. of natural cheese
- 2 oz. processed cheese
- ½ cup cottage cheese
- 1 ½ cups ice cream, ice milk, or frozen yogurt
- 1 cup sauces or puddings made with milk

Although the Food Guide Pyramid is a step in the right direction, it is not without critics. The American Dairy Association has lobbied heavily for increases in the meat and dairy product area, arguing that recommended amounts of certain substances—such as calcium for older women—are much higher than the pyramid shows. Other groups believe that the pyramid should contain higher amounts of vegetables and fruits. Modifications in the pyramid's structure and in the relative numbers of serving changes are likely in the future.

Digestive process: The process by which foods are broken down and either absorbed or excreted by the body.

Saliva: Fluid secreted by the salivary glands; enzymes in the fluid aid in the breakdown of certain foods for digestion.

Esophagus: Tube that transports food from the mouth to the stomach.

Stomach: Large muscular organ that temporarily stores, mixes, and digests foods.

Making the Pyramid Work for You

Many people are overwhelmed by their first glance at the pyramid. Most of you are probably saying to yourselves, "Eat up to 11 servings of breads, cereal, rice, and pasta? I'd have to eat like Porky Pig, and I'd end up looking the part!"

Don't despair. Take a look at what the USDA considers to be a serving: an ounce of ready-to-eat cereal, half a small hamburger bun or bagel, four to five potato chips, or one slice of bread. A normal bowl of cereal has three to four ounces of cereal. When was the last time you ate a quarter bowl of cereal? Or only half a hamburger bun? Or stopped yourself after four potato chips? When you consider breakfast, lunch, dinner, and snacks in between, it is really quite easy to get all the servings in this group that you need.

Although everyone is different, it is generally recommended that you try to consume these foods throughout the day. Try to eat at least two foods from the bread and cereal group for breakfast. A large bowl of cereal could actually take care of this for you, or you could eat a bowl of cereal and a bagel or English muffin and meet the requirements for three to four servings. Finding time for a snack of low-fat crackers could take care of another one to two servings during the day. Eating a cup of rice, a muffin, or bread at lunch could take care of two to three more servings, leaving only three to four servings for dinner. A large plate of pasta and a slice of reduced-fat, high-grain bread could just about do it. Keep in mind that with any bread, cereal, or grain product you must consider the amount of fat. Many people are duped into thinking that granola is a health food and that bran muffins are better than bagels or bread. Sometimes these products are loaded with fat, sugar, and calories. Read the labels on packaged products and opt for reduced-fat, whole-grain products when trying to meet pyramid requirements. To learn more about what information the new food labels contain, see Figure 8.2.

𝒲HAT DO YOU THINK?

Which food groups from the Food Guide Pyramid are you most likely to eat adequate amounts of during a typical day? Which ones, if any, are you most likely to skimp on? What are some simple changes that you could make right now in your diet to help you comply with pyramid recommendations?

The Digestive Process

Food provides us with the chemicals we need for energy and body maintenance. Because our bodies cannot synthesize or produce certain essential nutrients, we must

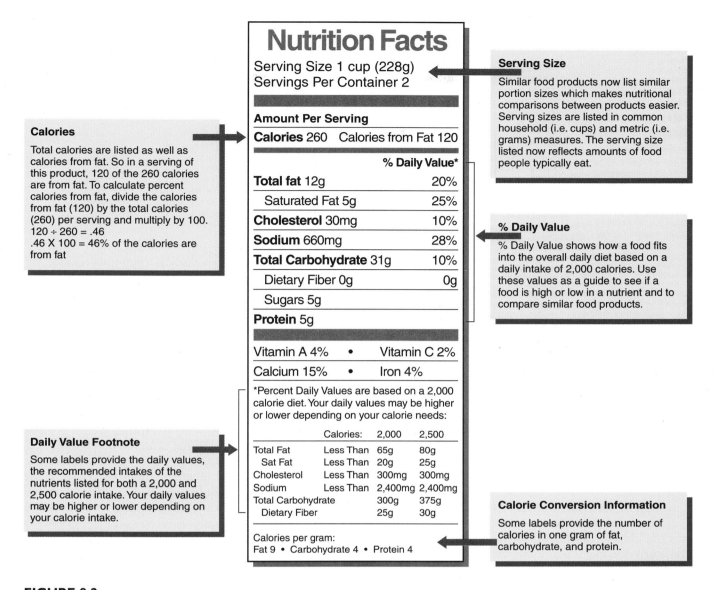

Calories

Total calories are listed as well as calories from fat. So in a serving of this product, 120 of the 260 calories are from fat. To calculate percent calories from fat, divide the calories from fat (120) by the total calories (260) per serving and multiply by 100.
120 ÷ 260 = .46
.46 X 100 = 46% of the calories are from fat

Daily Value Footnote

Some labels provide the daily values, the recommended intakes of the nutrients listed for both a 2,000 and 2,500 calorie intake. Your daily values may be higher or lower depending on your calorie intake.

Nutrition Facts

Serving Size 1 cup (228g)
Servings Per Container 2

Amount Per Serving

Calories 260   Calories from Fat 120

	% Daily Value*
Total fat 12g	20%
Saturated Fat 5g	25%
Cholesterol 30mg	10%
Sodium 660mg	28%
Total Carbohydrate 31g	10%
Dietary Fiber 0g	0g
Sugars 5g	
Protein 5g	

Vitamin A 4%	•	Vitamin C 2%
Calcium 15%	•	Iron 4%

*Percent Daily Values are based on a 2,000 calorie diet. Your daily values may be higher or lower depending on your calorie needs:

	Calories:	2,000	2,500
Total Fat	Less Than	65g	80g
Sat Fat	Less Than	20g	25g
Cholesterol	Less Than	300mg	300mg
Sodium	Less Than	2,400mg	2,400mg
Total Carbohydrate		300g	375g
Dietary Fiber		25g	30g

Calories per gram:
Fat 9 • Carbohydrate 4 • Protein 4

Serving Size

Similar food products now list similar portion sizes which makes nutritional comparisons between products easier. Serving sizes are listed in common household (i.e. cups) and metric (i.e. grams) measures. The serving size listed now reflects amounts of food people typically eat.

% Daily Value

% Daily Value shows how a food fits into the overall daily diet based on a daily intake of 2,000 calories. Use these values as a guide to see if a food is high or low in a nutrient and to compare similar food products.

Calorie Conversion Information

Some labels provide the number of calories in one gram of fat, carbohydrate, and protein.

FIGURE 8.2

The New Food Label

Source: Reprinted by permission from Darlene Zimmerman, M.S., R.D., "Hungry for a New Food Label?" *Weight Watchers Thinline* (published by The W W Group Inc.), July–August 1994, 9.

obtain them from the foods we eat. Even though we may take in adequate amounts of foods and nutrients, if our body systems are not functioning properly, much of the nutrient value in our food may be lost. Before foods can be utilized properly, the digestive system must break the larger food particles down into smaller, more usable forms. The process by which foods are broken down and either absorbed or excreted by the body is known as the **digestive process.**

Even before you take your first bite of pizza, your body has already begun a series of complex digestive responses. Your mouth prepares for the food by increasing produc-

tion of **saliva.** Saliva contains mostly water, which aids in chewing and swallowing, but it also contains important enzymes that begin the process of food breakdown, including amylase, which begins to break down carbohydrates. From the mouth, the food passes down the **esophagus,** a 9- to 10-inch tube that connects the mouth and stomach. A series of contractions and relaxations by the muscles lining the esophagus gently moves food to the next digestive organ, the **stomach.** Here food mixes with enzymes and stomach acids. Hydrochloric acid begins to work in combination with pepsin, an enzyme, to break down proteins. In most people, the stomach

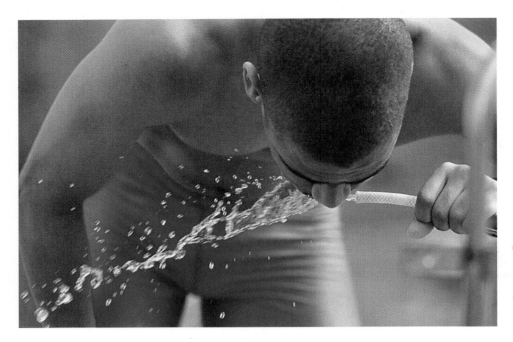

While you many not be conscious of your body's need for water until an unquenchable thirst comes along, water is actually our most necessary nutrient.

secretes enough mucus to protect the stomach lining from these harsh digestive juices. In others, there are problems with the lining that can result in ulcers or other gastric problems.

Further digestive activity takes place in the **small intestine,** a 20-foot coiled tube containing three sections: the *duodenum,* the *jejunum,* and the *ileum.* Each of these sections secretes digestive enzymes that, when combined with enzymes from the liver and the pancreas, further contribute to the breakdown of proteins, fats, and carbohydrates. Once broken down, these nutrients are absorbed into the bloodstream to supply body cells with energy. The liver is the major organ that determines whether nutrients are stored, sent to cells or organs, or excreted. Solid wastes consisting of fiber, water, and salts are dumped into the large intestine, where most of the water and salts are reabsorbed into the system and the fiber is passed out through the anus. The entire digestive process takes approximately 24 hours (see Figure 8.3).

OBTAINING ESSENTIAL NUTRIENTS

Water: A Crucial Nutrient

If you were to go on a survival trip, which would you take with you—food or water? You may be surprised to learn that you could survive for much longer periods without food than you could without water. Even in severe conditions, the average person can go for weeks without certain vitamins and minerals before experiencing serious deficiency symptoms. **Dehydration,** however, can cause serious problems within a matter of hours; after a few days without water, death is likely.

Just what function does water serve in the body? Between 50 and 60 percent of our total body weight is water. The water in our system bathes cells, aids in fluid and electrolyte balance, maintains pH balance, and transports molecules and cells throughout the body. Water is the major component of the blood, which carries oxygen and nutrients to the tissues and is responsible for maintaining cells in working order.

How much water do you need? Most experts believe that six to eight glasses of water per day are necessary. Because of high concentrations of water in most of the foods we consume, however, the actual number of glasses needed each day is somewhat less than this for the average person. Individual needs vary drastically according to dietary factors, age, size, environmental temperature and humidity levels, exercise, and the effectiveness of the individual's system. Certain diseases, such as diabetes or cystic fibrosis, cause victims to lose fluids at a rate necessitating a higher volume of fluid intake.

Proteins

Next to water, **proteins** are the most abundant substances in the human body. Proteins are major components of nearly every cell and have been called the "body builders" because of their role in the development and repair of bone, muscle, skin, and blood cells. Proteins are also the key elements of the antibodies that protect us from disease, of enzymes that control chemical activities in the body, and of hormones that regulate bodily functions. Moreover, proteins aid in the transport of iron, oxygen,

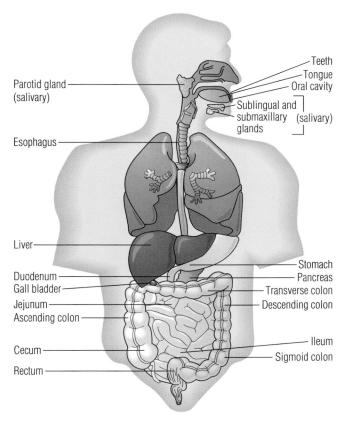

FIGURE 8.3

The illustration depicts the human digestive system. Digestion occurs throughout this system, from the mouth through the rectum.

Age (yr)		RDA (g/Kg)*
15-18 Males	=	0.9
15-18 Females	=	0.8
19 and over	=	**0.8**

* The RDA is 10 g/day higher during pregnancy, 15 g/day higher during the first six months of lactation, and 12 g/day higher during the remainder of lactation.

Calculating Your Protein RDA

40 grams

Example

① Determine your body weight

② Convert pounds to Kilograms (pounds divided by 2.2 lb/Kg equals Kilograms)

③ Multiply by 0.8 g/Kg (adult RDA) to get an RDA in Kilograms per day

① Weight = 110 lbs

② 110 ÷ 2.2 lbs/Kg = 50 Kg

③ 50 Kg x 0.8 g/Kg = 40 g

Results: a 110 lb person would have an RDA of 40 g of protein

FIGURE 8.4

Calculating Your Protein RDA

Source: Adapted by permission from p. 198 of *Nutrition Concepts and Controversies,* 6th ed., by Eva Hamilton, Eleanor Whitney, and Frances Sizer. Copyright 1994 by West Publishing Company. All rights reserved.

and nutrients to all of the body's cells and supply another source of energy to body cells when fats and carbohydrates are not readily available. In short, adequate amounts of protein in the diet are vital to many body functions and to your ultimate survival.

Few Americans suffer from protein deficiencies. The average American consumes over 90 grams of protein daily, and about 70 percent of this comes from high-fat animal flesh and dairy products.[2] The recommended protein intake for the average man is only 63 grams, while the average woman needs only 50 grams under normal circumstances. The excess is stored, like other extra calories, as fat. See Figure 8.4 to determine your own recommended daily allowance (RDA) of protein.

Proteins are made up of smaller molecules known as **amino acids.** These acids are composed of chains that link together like beads on a necklace in differing combinations. Over 22 different types of amino acids are found in animal tissue, and humans cannot synthesize all of them. The eight amino acids that the adult body cannot synthesize in adequate amounts are referred to as **essential amino acids.** They must be obtained from foods.

Small intestine: Muscular, coiled digestive organ; consists of the duodenum, jejunum, and ileum.

Dehydration: Abnormal depletion of body fluids; a result of lack of water.

Proteins: The essential constituents of nearly all body cells. Proteins are necessary for the development and repair of bone, muscle, skin, and blood, and are the key elements of antibodies, enzymes, and hormones.

Amino acids: The building blocks of protein.

Essential amino acids: Eight of the basic nitrogen-containing building blocks of protein that we must obtain from foods to ensure our personal health.

Complete (high-quality) proteins are those proteins that naturally contain all the eight essential amino acids. If we consume a food that contains protein but is deficient in some of the essential amino acids, the total amount of protein that can be synthesized by the other amino acids is decreased. It is important to remember that just because essential amino acids are present in a food does not guarantee that they will be synthesized. Quality of protein depends on the presence of amino acids in digestible form and in amounts proportional to body requirements.

The most common sources of dietary protein in the United States are red meats, poultry, fish, beans, nuts, and dairy products. In addition to providing high-quality proteins, these sources of protein (with the exception of fish, beans, and nuts) also contain high levels of saturated fat and cholesterol. Selecting leaner cuts of meat, removing the fat and skin from chicken, and choosing low-fat dairy products will enable you to get high-quality proteins without the excess calories and fat.

What about plant sources of protein? Proteins from plant sources are often **incomplete proteins** in that they are missing one or two of the essential amino acids. Nevertheless, it is relatively easy for the non-meat eater to combine plant foods effectively and to eat complementary sources of plant protein (see Figure 8.5). An excellent example of this mutual supplementation process is eating peanut butter on whole-grain bread. Although each of these foods is deficient in essential amino acids, eating them together provides high-quality protein.

Plant sources of protein fall into three general categories: legumes (beans, peas, peanuts, and soy products), grains (whole grains, corn, and pasta products), and nuts and seeds. Certain vegetables, such as leafy green vegetables and broccoli, also contribute valuable plant proteins. Mixing two or more foods from each of these categories during the same meal will provide all of the essential

Selecting from two or more of these columns will help you use a process known as *mutual supplementation*, combining two protein-rich foods to form *complementary* proteins with all of the essential amino acids. These combinations make complete proteins and help avoid possible protein deficiencies.

Grains	Legumes	Seeds and Nuts	Vegetables
Barley Bulgar Cornmeal Oats Rice Wholegrain breads Enriched pasta	Dried beans Dried lentils Dried peas Peanuts Soy products	Sesame seeds Sunflower seeds Walnuts Cashews Other nuts Nut berries	Leafy greens Broccoli Others

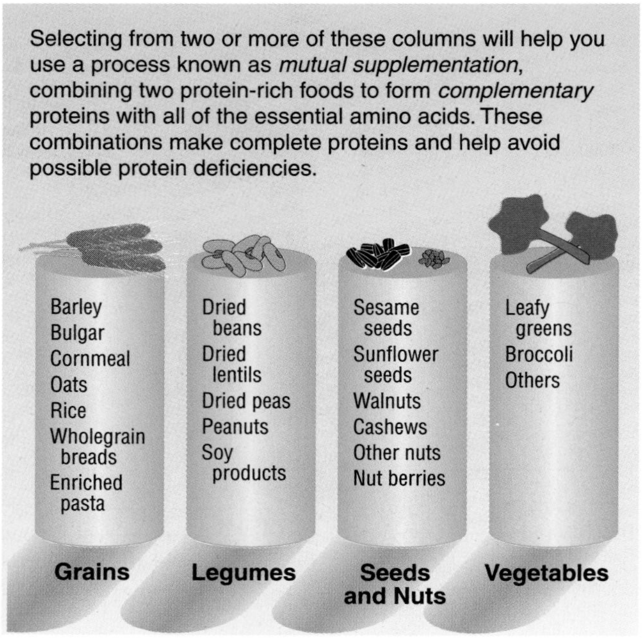

FIGURE 8.5

Complementary Proteins

Source: Adapted by permission from p. 205 of *Nutrition Concepts and Controversies*, 6th ed., by Eva Hamilton, Eleanor Whitney, and Frances Sizer. Copyright 1994 by West Publishing Company. All rights reserved.

amino acids necessary to ensure adequate protein absorption. People who are not interested in obtaining all of their protein from plants can combine incomplete plant proteins with complete low-fat animal proteins such as chicken, fish, turkey, and lean red meat. Low-fat or nonfat cottage cheese, skim milk, egg whites, and nonfat dry milk all provide high-quality proteins and have few calories and little dietary fat.

Carbohydrates: Providing Your Energy

Although the importance of proteins in the body cannot be underestimated, it is **carbohydrates** that supply us with the energy needed to sustain normal daily activity. Long maligned by weight-conscious people, carbohydrates can actually be metabolized more quickly and efficiently than can proteins. Carbohydrates are a quick source of energy for the body, being easily converted to glucose, the fuel for the body's cells. These foods also play an important role in the functioning of the internal organs, the nervous system, and the muscles. They are the best source of energy for endurance athletics because they provide both an immediate and a time-released energy source as they are digested easily and then consistently metabolized in the bloodstream.[3] For many people, a plate of pasta represents an attractive, healthy alternative to a fatty steak.

Complete (high-quality) proteins: Proteins that contain all of the eight essential amino acids.

Incomplete proteins: Proteins that are lacking in one or more of the essential amino acids.

Carbohydrates: Basic nutrients that supply the body with the energy needed to sustain normal activity.

Simple sugars: A major type of carbohydrate which provides short-term energy.

Complex carbohydrates: A major type of carbohydrate which provides sustained energy.

Monosaccharide: A simple sugar that contains only one molecule of sugar.

Disaccharide: A combination of two monosaccharides.

Does Pasta Make You Fat?

Every year, during the week before the Boston marathon, many of Boston's Italian restaurants hang signs in their windows that say, "Eat Pasta, Run Fasta!" Eating a low-fat, high-carbohydrate diet may make sense for the group of athletes running the marathon. But it now seems clear that for overweight and "insulin resistant" individuals, the sign should read, "Eat Pasta, Get Fat!"

While few researchers question the value of the low-fat, high-carbohydrate diet, many are beginning to wonder if the high-carbohydrate regime is appropriate for everyone, and particularly for the insulin-resistant, who are thought to make up 25 percent of the United States population. The insulin-resistant respond to starches or sugar by overproducing glucose, which in turn causes an overproduction of insulin, a hormone responsible for a wide range of metabolic activities, including determining how much glucose will be used immediately as energy and how much will be stored as fat; the regulation of triglycerides; and perhaps even the stimulation of appetite.

Dr. James Hill, the associate director of the Center for Human Nutrition and an obesity expert at the University of Colorado in Denver, said, "We may have gone too far with the low-fat emphasis." In the last decade, Americans cut their fat intake from 36 percent of their average daily calories to 34 percent, he said. Nevertheless, they also gained about eight pounds a person. "People can get fat on a high-fat diet," Dr. Hill said. "But people can get fat on a diet high in carbohydrates, too."

In weight-loss clinics, the anecdotal evidence is overwhelming, said Dr. Stephen Gullo, who holds a Ph.D. in psychology and is the director of the Institute for Health and Weight Sciences in Manhattan. Dr. Gullo, who has treated 10,000 overweight patients, said that over the last five years the question he has been asked most frequently is, "How did I gain weight on a low-fat diet?"

To answer this question, Dr. Gullo, along with other clinicians and obesity researchers, considered the fact that rather than replacing dietary fat with complex carbohydrates like vegetables and fruits, many were reaching for simple carbohydrates like sugar and starch. This realization led some researchers to revisit the scientific literature about the functions of insulin and to suspect that many dieters may be insulin-resistant. . . .

"Insulin resistance was helpful historically because it enabled people to survive over extended periods of caloric deprivation," said Dr. Gerald Reaven, a professor at Stanford University Medical Center who has studied insulin for three decades. Historically, he said, during times of feast, the body overproduced insulin in order to stimulate the liver to convert glucose into fat that could be stored for times of famine. Without the overproduction, the glucose would be fuel for muscles and organs, so insulin resistance allowed people to weather lean times. But in extended periods of caloric excess like the present age of abundance, Dr. Reaven said, "insulin resistance becomes a problem."

What can you do to prevent weight gain from carbohydrates? First, realize that low-fat doesn't necessarily mean low-calorie. Second, remember to limit your portions; you can't lose weight if you eat large quantities of pasta or rice. And third, try to stay away from the starches and sugars. Instead, eat complex carbohydrates like vegetables, which are rich in fiber. To take advantage of this shift in nutritional thinking, Weight Watchers has created a new Fat and Fiber program, in which members count both fat grams and fiber grams.

Source: The first two paragraphs and the last paragraph contain information from and the rest are excerpted from Molly O'Neill, "So It May Be True After All; Eating Pasta Makes You Fat," *The New York Times,* 8 February 1995, A1, B7. Copyright © 1995 by The New York Times Company. Reprinted by permission.

There are two major types of carbohydrates: **simple sugars**, which are found primarily in fruits, and **complex carbohydrates**, which are found in grains, cereals, dark green leafy vegetables, yellow fruits and vegetables (carrots, yams), *cruciferous* vegetables (such as broccoli, cabbage, and cauliflower), and certain root vegetables, such as potatoes. Most of us do not get enough complex carbohydrates in our daily diets.

A typical diet contains large amounts of simple sugars. The most common form is *glucose.* Eventually, the human body converts all types of simple sugars to glucose to provide energy to cells. In its natural form, glucose is sweet and is obtained from substances such as corn syrup, honey, molasses, vegetables, and fruits. *Fructose* is another simple sugar found in fruits and berries. Glucose and fructose are **monosaccharides** and contain only one molecule of sugar.

Disaccharides are combinations of two monosaccharides. Perhaps the best-known example is common granulated table sugar (known as sucrose), which consists of a molecule of fructose chemically bonded to a molecule of glucose. Lactose, found in milk and milk products, is another form of disaccharide, formed by the combination of glucose and galactose (another simple sugar). Disaccharides must be broken down into simple sugars before they can be used by the body.

Controlling the amount of sugar in your diet can be difficult because sugar, like sodium, is often present in food products in which you might not expect to find it. Such diverse items as ketchup, Russian dressing, Coffee-Mate, and Shake 'n' Bake derive between 30 and 65 percent of their calories from sugar. Reading labels carefully before purchasing food products is a must.

Polysaccharides are complex carbohydrates formed by the combining of long chains of saccharides. Like disaccharides, they must be broken down into simple sugars before they can be utilized by the body. There are two major forms of complex carbohydrates: *starches* and *fiber,* or **cellulose.**

Starches make up the majority of the complex carbohydrate group. Starches in our diets come from flours, breads, pasta, potatoes, and related foods. They are stored in body muscles and the liver in a polysaccharide form called **glycogen.** When the body requires a sudden burst of energy, it breaks down glycogen into glucose. While we often think of starches as an alternative to fats, the Health Headlines box points out that starches aren't better for some people.

Carbohydrates and Athletic Performance. In the last decade, carbohydrates have become the "health foods" of many people involved in athletic competition. Many fitness enthusiasts consume concentrated sugary foods or drinks before or during athletic activity, thinking that the sugars will provide extra energy. However, in some situations, they may actually be counterproductive.[4]

One possible problem involves the gastrointestinal tract. If your intestines react to activity (or the nervousness before competition) by moving material through the small intestine more rapidly than usual, undigested disaccharides and/or unabsorbed monosaccharides will reach the colon, which can result in a very inopportune bout of diarrhea.[5]

Consuming large amounts of sugar during exercise can also have a negative effect on hydration. Concentrations exceeding 24 grams of sugar per 8 ounces of fluid can delay stomach emptying and hence absorption of water. Some fruit juices, fruit drinks, and other sugar-sweetened beverages have more than this amount of sugar. If you use these products, you should dilute them with ice cubes or water.

Marathon runners and other people who require reserves of energy for demanding tasks often attempt to increase stores of glycogen in the body by a process known as *carbohydrate loading.* This process involves

---

Polysaccharide: A complex carbohydrate formed by the combination of long chains of saccharides.

Cellulose: Fiber, a major form of complex carbohydrates.

Glycogen: The polysaccharide form in which glucose is stored in the liver.

Carbo-loading with bread and pasta before an endurance event is a training strategy used by many athletes to build energy reserves for the "last mile."

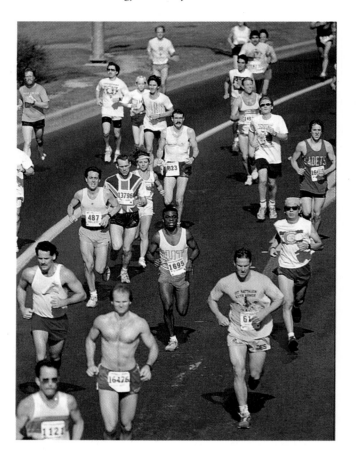

modifying the nature of both workouts and diet, usually during the week or so before competition. The athlete trains very hard early in the week while eating small amounts of carbohydrates. Right before competition, the athlete dramatically increases intake of carbohydrates to force the body to store increased levels of glycogen, to be used during endurance activities (such as the last miles of a marathon).

The Myth of Sugar and Hyperactivity. Contrary to early media reports, extensive research done in the last decade indicates that sugars *do not* cause hyperactivity.[6] In well-controlled dietary challenge studies, consumption of sugar has not been shown to have negative effects on motor activity, spontaneous behavior, performance in psychological tests, learning, memory, attention span, or problem-solving ability.

Fiber

The role fiber plays in promoting nutrition and health has been a controversial subject in recent years. What exactly is fiber? How effective is it in reducing certain health risks? Are certain types of fibers more effective than others?

Fiber, often referred to as "bulk" or "roughage," is the indigestible portion of plant foods that helps move foods through the digestive system and softens stools by absorbing water. *Insoluble fiber*, which is found in bran, whole-grain breads and cereals, and most fruits and vegetables, is associated with these gastrointestinal benefits and has also been found to reduce the risk for several forms of cancer. *Soluble fiber* appears to be a factor in lowering blood cholesterol levels, thereby reducing risk for cardiovascular disease. Major sources of soluble fiber in the diet include oat bran, dried beans (such as kidney, garbanzo, pinto, and navy beans), and some fruits and vegetables.

The best way to increase your dietary fiber is to eat more complex carbohydrates, such as whole grains, fruits, vegetables, dried peas and beans, nuts, and seeds. As with most nutritional advice, however, too much of a good thing can pose problems. Sudden increases in dietary fiber may cause flatulence (intestinal gas), cramping, or a bloated feeling. Consuming plenty of water or other liquids may reduce such side effects.

Fiber and Your Health. A few years ago, fiber was thought by some to be the remedy for just about everything. Much of this hope was exaggerated. However, current research does support many benefits of fiber, including the following:[7]

- *Protection against colon and rectal cancer.* One of the leading causes of cancer deaths in the United States, colorectal cancer is much rarer in countries having diets high in fiber and low in animal fat. Several studies have supported the theory that fiber-rich diets,

particularly those including insoluble fiber, prevent the development of precancerous growths. Whether this is because more fiber helps to move foods through the colon faster, thereby reducing the colon's contact time with cancer-causing substances, or whether some other process is at work remains unknown.

- *Protection against breast cancer.* Research into the effects of fiber on breast-cancer risks is very inconclusive. However, some studies have indicated that wheat bran (rich in insoluble fiber) reduces blood-estrogen levels, which may affect the risk for breast cancer. Another theory is that people who eat more fiber have proportionally less fat in their diets and that this is what reduces overall risk. The jury is still very much out in this area.

- *Protection against constipation.* Insoluble fiber, consumed with adequate fluids, is the safest, most effective way to prevent or treat constipation. The fiber acts like a sponge, absorbing moisture and producing softer, bulkier stools that are easily passed. Fiber also helps produce gas, which in turn, may initiate a bowel movement.

- *Protection against diverticulosis.* About 1 American in 10 over the age of 40 and at least 1 in 3 over 50 suffers from *diverticulosis*, a condition in which tiny bulges or pouches form on the large intestinal wall. These bulges become irritated and cause chronic pain if under strain from constipation. Insoluble fiber helps to reduce constipation and added pain.

- *Protection against heart disease.* Many studies have indicated that soluble fiber (as in oat bran, barley, and

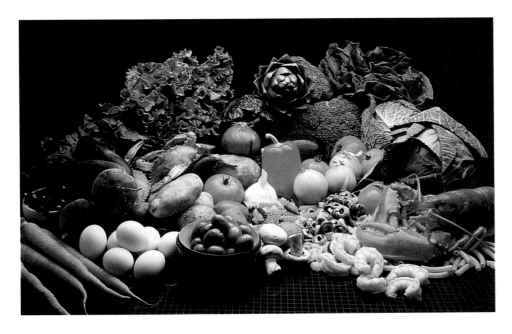

To plan a healthy diet, we can choose from among a wide range of tasty foods that are both low in fat and high in essential nutrients, including protein, and contain abundant amounts of dietary fiber.

fruit pectin) helps reduce blood cholesterol, primarily by lowering LDL ("bad") cholesterol. Whether this reduction is a direct effect or occurs instead through the displacement of fat calories by fiber calories in a high-fiber diet remains in question.

- *Protection against diabetes.* Some studies have suggested that soluble fiber improves control of blood sugar and can reduce the need for insulin or medication in people with diabetes. Exactly why isn't clear, but soluble fiber seems to delay the emptying of the stomach and slow the absorption of glucose by the intestine.

- *Protection against obesity.* Because most high-fiber foods are high in carbohydrates and low in fat, they help control caloric intake. Many take longer to chew, which slows you down at the table and makes you feel full sooner.

Most experts believe that Americans should double their current consumption of dietary fiber—to 20 to 30 grams per day for most people and perhaps to 40 to 50 grams for others. To do this, the following steps are recommended:

1. Eat a variety of foods.

2. Eat at least five servings of fruits and vegetables and three to six servings of whole-grain breads, cereals, and legumes per day.

3. Eat less processed food.

4. Eat the skins of fruits and vegetables.

5. Get your fiber from foods rather than pills or powders.

6. Spread out your fiber intake.

7. Drink plenty of liquids.

Fats

Fats (or *lipids*), another group of basic nutrients, are perhaps the most misunderstood of the body's required energy sources. Most of us do not realize that fats play a vital role in the maintenance of healthy skin and hair, insulation of the body organs against shock, maintenance of body temperature, and the proper functioning of the cells themselves. Fats make our foods taste better and carry the fat-soluble vitamins A, D, E, and K to the cells. They also provide a concentrated form of energy in the absence of sufficient amounts of carbohydrates. If fats perform all these functions, why are we constantly urged to reduce our intake of them?

Although moderate consumption of fats is essential to health maintenance, overconsumption can be dangerous. The most common form of fat circulating in the blood is the **triglyceride**, which makes up about 95 percent of total body fat. When we consume too many calories, the excess is converted into triglycerides in the liver, which are stored in all-too-obvious places on our bodies.

The remaining 5 percent of body fat is composed of substances such as **cholesterol**, which can accumulate on the inner walls of arteries, causing a narrowing of the channel through which blood flows. This buildup, called **plaque**, is a major cause of *atherosclerosis* (hardening of the arteries). At one time, the amount of circulating cholesterol in the blood was thought to be crucial. Current thinking is that the actual amount of circulating cholesterol itself is not as important as the ratio of total cholesterol to a group of compounds called **high-density lipoproteins** (HDLs). Lipoproteins are the transport facilitators for cholesterol in the blood. High-density lipoproteins are capable of transporting more cholesterol than are **low-density lipoproteins** (LDLs). Whereas LDLs transport cholesterol to the body's cells, HDLs apparently transport circulating cholesterol to the liver for metabolism and elimination from the body. People with a high percentage of HDLs therefore appear to be at lower risk for development of cholesterol-clogged arteries. Regular vigorous exercise plays a part in reduction of cholesterol by increasing high-density lipoproteins.

Fat cells consist of chains of carbon and hydrogen atoms. Those that are unable to hold any more hydrogen in their chemical structure are labeled **saturated fats**. They generally come from animal sources, such as meats and dairy products, and are solid at room temperature. **Unsaturated fats**, which come from plants and include most vegetable oils, are generally liquid at room temperature and have room for additional hydrogen atoms in their chemical structure. The terms *monounsaturated fat* and *polyunsaturated fat* refer to the relative number of hydrogen atoms that are missing. Peanut and olive oils are high in monounsaturated fats, whereas corn, sunflower, and safflower oils are high in polyunsaturated fats. There is currently a great deal of controversy about which type of unsaturated fat is most beneficial. Although polyunsaturated fats were favored by nutritional researchers in the early 1980s, today many researchers believe that polyunsaturates may decrease beneficial HDL levels while reducing LDL levels. Monounsaturated fats seem to lower only LDL levels and thus are the "preferred" fats of the 1990s. For a breakdown of the types of fats found in common vegetable oils, see Figure 8.6.

Reducing Fat in Your Diet. Finding the best ways to cut fat in your diet is largely dependent on you, your lifestyle, and determining what works for you. The following basic guidelines are a good place to start to reduce your fat intake:

- *Know what you are putting in your mouth.* Read food labels. Remember that no more than 10 percent of

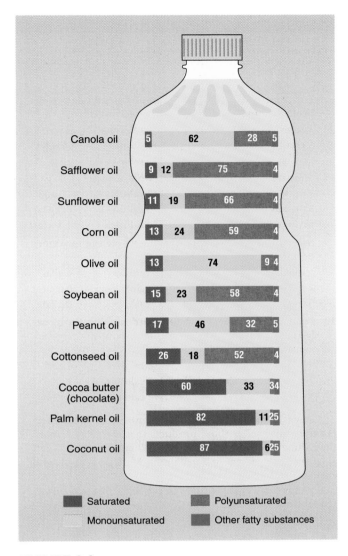

FIGURE 8.6

Percentages of Saturated, Polyunsaturated, and Monounsaturated Fats in Common Vegetable Oils

The figure shows bars for each oil with the following values:

Canola oil	5	62	28	5
Safflower oil	9	12	75	4
Sunflower oil	11	19	66	4
Corn oil	13	24	59	4
Olive oil	13	74	9	4
Soybean oil	15	23	58	4
Peanut oil	17	46	32	5
Cottonseed oil	26	18	52	4
Cocoa butter (chocolate)	60	33	3	4
Palm kernel oil	82	11	2	5
Coconut oil	87	6	2	5

■ Saturated ■ Polyunsaturated
□ Monounsaturated ■ Other fatty substances

your total calories should come from saturated fat, and no more than 30 percent should come from all forms of fat.

■ *Choose fat-free or low-fat versions of cakes, cookies, crackers, or chips.*

■ *Use olive oil for baking and sautéing.* Animal studies have shown that it doesn't raise cholesterol or promote the growth of tumors.

■ *Whenever possible, use liquid, diet, or whipped margarine: they have far less trans-fatty acids than solid fat has.*

■ *Choose lean meats, fish, or poultry.* Remove skin. Broil or bake whenever possible. In general, the more well-done the meat, the fewer the calories. Drain off fat after cooking.

■ *Choose fewer cold cuts, bacon, sausage, hot dogs, and organ meats.* Be careful of those products claiming to be "95 percent fat-free" as they may still have high levels of fat.

■ *Select nonfat dairy products whenever possible.* Part-skim-milk cheeses such as mozzarella, farmer's, lappi, and ricotta are good choices.

■ *When cooking, use substitutes for butter, margarine, oils, sour cream, mayonnaise, and salad dressings.* Chicken broths, wine, vinegar, and low-calorie dressings make good flavorings and/or cooking ingredients.

■ *Remember to think of your food intake as an average over a day or a couple of days.* If you have a high-fat breakfast or lunch, have a low-fat dinner to balance it.

For more specific ways to cut fat from your diet, see the Choices for Change box.

Trans-Fatty Acids: Still Bad? Since 1961, Americans have shown that they have heeded the dire warnings about cholesterol and saturated fat by decreasing their

Fats: Basic nutrients composed of carbon and hydrogen atoms; needed for the proper functioning of cells, insulation of body organs against shock, maintenance of body temperature, and healthy skin and hair.

Triglyceride: The most common form of fat in the body; excess calories consumed are converted into triglycerides and stored as body fat.

Cholesterol: A form of fat circulating in the blood that can accumulate on the inner walls of arteries.

Plaque: Cholesterol buildup on the inner walls of arteries, causing a narrowing of the channel through which blood flows; a major cause of atherosclerosis.

High-density lipoproteins (HDLs): Compounds that facilitate the transport of cholesterol in the blood to the liver for metabolism and elimination from the body.

Low-density lipoproteins (LDLs): Compounds that facilitate the transport of cholesterol in the blood to the body's cells.

Saturated fats: Fats that are unable to hold any more hydrogen in their chemical structure; derived mostly from animal sources; solid at room temperature.

Unsaturated fats: Fats that do have room for more hydrogen in their chemical structure; derived mostly from plants; liquid at room temperature.

How to Cut the Fat from Your Diet

The small choices you make in your daily diet can add up to a tremendous difference in how much fat you consume over time. Trimming just one teaspoon each day can cut over 5 pounds of fat from your diet in a year's time. It's still possible to eat great tasting foods and barely notice these small personal choices. Consider the following:

1. "Butter" your toast and muffins with "fruit-only" jams instead of sugary jellies and jams, butter, margarine, or other high-calorie spreads.

1 Tbsp. butter	108 calories	12 g fat
1 Tbsp. sugarless jam	18 calories	0 g fat
Savings	90 calories	12 g fat

2. Sauté meat and vegetables in chicken broth or wine (most of which burns off during cooking) rather than in oil.

1 Tbsp. oil	240 calories	27 g fat
wine or broth	0 calories	0 g fat
Savings	240 calories	27 g fat

3. Remove the skin from chicken before cooking.

3 ½ oz breast	193 calories	8 g fat
3 ½ oz. skinless breast	142 calories	3 g fat
Savings	51 calories	5 g fat

4. Use low-calorie, low-fat salad dressings on your sandwiches instead of mayonnaise.

1 Tbsp. mayonnaise	100 calories	11 g fat
1 Tbsp. low-cal dressing	7 calories	0 g fat
Savings	93 calories	11 g fat

5. When you crave ice cream, splurge instead on nonfat frozen yogurt. Today's flavors are so delicious that you may give ice cream the permanent cold shoulder.

¾ cup ice cream	400 calories	25 g fat
¾ cup nonfat yogurt	120 calories	0 g fat
Savings	280 calories	25 g fat

6. For a skinny version of cream cheese that only tastes fattening, mix three parts blenderized low-fat cottage cheese with one part nonfat yogurt and use as a delicious dip, spread, or topping.

2 Tbsp. cream cheese	99 calories	10 g fat
2 Tbsp. mock cream cheese	20 calories	0 g fat
Savings	79 calories	10 g fat

7. For a warming meal minus a lot of fat and calories, sip broth-based rather than cream-based soups.

1 cup cream of chicken soup	592 calories	15 g fat
1 cup chicken noodle soup	75 calories	2 g fat
Savings	116 calories	13 g fat

8. Substitute fish for meat at least once a week.

3 oz. top round beef	162 calories	5 g fat
3 oz. cod	70 calories	0.5 g fat
Savings	92 calories	4.5 g fat

9. Substitute two egg whites for one whole egg in recipes or omelets.

1 whole egg	79 calories	6 g fat
2 egg whites	32 calories	0 g fat
Savings	47 calories	6 g fat

10. Load up on protein without overdosing on fat by selecting meatless entrees such as lentil soup and vegetarian chili.

9 ½ oz. beef chili	256 calories	6 g fat
9 ½ oz. lentil soup	164 calories	1 g fat
Savings	92 calories	5 g fat

General Advice. Become a fat sleuth. Read food labels faithfully and select those products that contain no more than three grams of fat for every 100 calories, which will keep your fat calories to a maximum of 30 percent of total calories.

List the small changes that you can make this week to cut the fat from your diet.

1.

2.

3.

4.

5.

What other things can you do to help reduce your overall fat consumption?

Source: Adapted by permission of the author from Evelyn Tribole, "24 Ways to Trim Fat," *Shape,* July 1990, 92–93.

---

intake of butter by over 43 percent and substituting margarine, which became known as the "better butter" after reports labeled unsaturated fats the "heart-healthy" alternative. But a widely publicized study in 1990 questioned the benefits of margarine; it indicated that margarine contains fats that raise blood cholesterol at least as much as the saturated fat in butter does.[8] The culprits? **Trans-fatty acids,** fatty acids having unusual shapes that are produced when polyunsaturated oils are *hydrogenated,* a process in which hydrogen is added to unsaturated fats to make them more solid and resistant to chemical change.[9] Besides raising cholesterol levels, trans-fatty acids have been implicated in the development of certain types of cancer.[10]

While the 1990 study pointed an accusing finger at the potential "bad" margarine, researchers Walter Willet and Albert Ascherio of the Harvard School of Public Health recently provided a resounding "wake up call" for those of us who have faithfully avoided butter in favor of the healthier margarine alternative. Have we been wrong all this time? According to their analysis of several fat studies, the trans-fatty acids found in margarine may not just be potentially harmful; they may in fact pose an even greater risk for heart disease than does eating saturated fat villains such as butter and lard.[11] But before you dash out and fill your refrigerator with butter, remember that Willet and Ascherio's research is also controversial. Researchers backed by the American Heart Association say that butter, which contains both cholesterol and saturated fat, is still worse than margarine. Wondering what to do? Probably the best advice is to continue to reduce overall fat in your diet, probably to less than 30 percent of total calories. Whenever possible, opt for other condiments on your bread, using jams, fat-free cream cheeses, garlic, or other toppings whenever possible. Some experts advocate using low fat-salad dressings as toppings for bread and pasta, or using olive oil in moderation to add a bit of flavor. If you have high cholesterol, reducing all types of fat and cholesterol in the diet is still sound advice.

Vitamins

Vitamins are potent, essential, organic compounds that promote growth and help maintain life and health. Every minute of every day, vitamins help maintain your nerves and skin, produce blood cells, build bones and teeth, heal wounds, and convert food energy to body energy. And they do all of this without adding any calories to your diet.

Age, heat, and other environmental conditions can destroy vitamins in food. Vitamins can be classified as either *fat soluble*, meaning that they are absorbed through the intestinal tract with the help of fats, or *water soluble*, meaning that they are easily dissolved in water. Vitamins A, D, E, and K are fat soluble; B complex vitamins and vitamin C are water soluble. Fat-soluble vitamins tend to be stored in the body, and toxic accumulations in the liver may cause cirrhosis-like symptoms. Water-soluble vitamins are generally excreted and cause few toxicity problems (see Table 8.2).

Despite all of the media suggestions to the contrary, few Americans suffer from true vitamin deficiencies if they eat a diet containing all of the food groups at least part of the time. Nevertheless, Americans continue to purchase large quantities of vitamin supplements. For the most part, vitamin supplements are unnecessary and, in certain instances, may even be harmful. Overuse of vitamin supplements can lead to a toxic condition known as **hypervitaminosis.**

Recommended Dietary Allowances.   For over 50 years, a document called the "Recommended Dietary Allowances (RDAs)" has been the standard guide for nutrient intake in the United States.[12] Since its inception, the Food and Nutrition Board of the National Academy of Sciences has met every five years to revise RDA values. The RDAs reflect the fact that a person's actual level of need for a nutrient can be influenced by age, sex, body size, growth, and reproductive status. Thus, pregnant and lactating women have their own set of RDAs.

From the RDAs come the more familiar U.S. RDA, the U.S. Recommended *Daily* Allowance, set by the Food and Drug Administration. Up until 1993, the U.S. RDA appeared on all food labels; it is still used for vitamins and some other food products. However, the set that is typically listed is for adult males, which may be misleading for women, children, the elderly, and other groups who have different nutritional needs. The U.S. RDA is typically set at a maximum value to account for potential nutrient loss during absorption, cooking, and storage of food.

Many consumers who have grown accustomed to looking for the U.S. RDA values on food labels may be confused by the new food label that began appearing in 1993. Instead of U.S. RDA value, the new labels indicate what "% Daily Value" a particular food provides. The "% Daily Values" allow you to evaluate what percentage of an estimated total calorie diet of 2,000 or 2,500 calories your food is. See the Skills for Behavior Change box for an example of how to personalize the "% Daily Values" for a given food. Most experts believe that these "Daily Values" will be more meaningful to people trying to distinguish between certain foods as they plan their diets.

In addition to the RDAs there is another standard, known as the "Estimated Safe and Adequate Daily Dietary Intakes (ESADDI)" guide. ESADDI provides a range of recommended allowances for those nutrients on which we have insufficient data to set an RDA. It is believed that if you stay within the ESADDI range to these nutrients, you will receive adequate nutrition.

Trans-fatty acids: Fatty acids that are produced when polyunsaturated oils are hydrogenated to make them more solid.

Vitamins: Essential organic compounds that promote growth and reproduction and help maintain life and health.

Hypervitaminosis: A toxic condition caused by overuse of vitamin supplements.

TABLE 8.2 ■ A Guide to the Vitamins

Vitamin	Best Sources	Chief Roles	Deficiency Symptoms	Toxicity Symptoms
Water-soluble vitamins				
Thiamin 1.5 mg	Meat, pork, liver, fish, poultry, whole-grain and enriched breads, cereals, pasta, nuts legumes, wheat germ, oats.	Helps enzymes release energy from carbohydrate; supports normal appetite and nervous system function.	Beriberi, edema, heart irregularity, mental confusion, muscle weakness, low morale, impaired growth.	Rapid pulse, weakness, headaches, insomnia, irritability.
Riboflavin 1.7 mg	Milk, dark green vegetables, yogurt, cottage cheese, liver, meat, whole-grain or enriched breads and cereals.	Helps enzymes release energy from carbohydrate, fat, and protein; promotes healthy skin and normal vision.	Eye problems, skin disorders around nose and mouth.	None reported, but an excess of any of the B vitamins can cause a deficiency of the others.
Niacin 20 mg	Meat, eggs, poultry fish, milk, whole-grain and enriched breads and cereals, nuts, legumes, peanuts, nutritional yeast, all protein foods.	Helps enzymes release energy from energy nutrients; promotes health of skin, nerves, and digestive system.	Pellagra: skin rash on parts exposed to sun, loss of appetite, dizziness, weakness, irritability, fatigue, mental confusion, indigestion.	Flushing, nausea, headaches, cramps, ulcer irritation, heartburn, abnormal liver function, low blood pressure.
Vitamin B_6 2.0 mg	Meat, poultry, fish, shellfish, legumes, whole-grain products, green, leafy vegetables, bananas.	Protein and fat metabolism; formation of antibodies and red blood cells; helps convert tryptophan to niacin.	Nervous disorders, skin rash, muscle weakness, anemia, convulsions, kidney stones.	Depression, fatigue, irritability, headaches, numbness, damage to nerves, difficulty walking.
Folate .4 mg	Green, leafy vegetables, liver, legumes, seeds.	Red blood cell formation; protein metabolism; new cell division.	Anemia, heartburn, diarrhea, smooth tongue depression, poor growth.	Diarrhea, insomnia, irritability, may mask a vitamin B_{12} deficiency.
Vitamin B_{12} 6 µg	Meat, fish, poultry, shellfish, milk, cheese, eggs, nutritional yeast.	Helps maintain nerve cells; red blood cell formation; synthesis of genetic material.	Anemia, smooth tongue, fatigue, nerve degeneration progressing to paralysis.	None reported.
Pantothenic acid 10 mg	Widespread in foods.	Coenzyme in energy metabolism.	Rare; sleep disturbances, nausea, fatigue.	Occasional diarrhea.
Biotin .03 mg	Widespread in foods.	Coenzyme in energy metabolism; fat synthesis; glycogen formation.	Loss of appetite, nausea, depression, muscle pain, weakness, fatigue, rash.	None reported.
Vitamin C (ascorbic acid) RDA = 60 mg	Citrus fruits, cabbage-type vegetables, tomatoes, potatoes, dark green vegetables, peppers, lettuce, cantaloupe, strawberries, mangos, papayas.	Synthesis of collagen (helps heal wounds, maintains bone and teeth, strengthens blood vessels); antioxidant; strengthens resistance to infection; helps body's absorption of iron.	Scurvy, anemia, atherosclerotic plaques, depression, frequent infections, bleeding gums, loosened teeth, pinpoint hemorrhages, muscle degeneration, rough skin, bone fragility, poor wound healing, hysteria.	Nausea, abdominal cramps, diarrhea, breakdown of red blood cells in persons with certain genetic disorders, deficiency symptoms may appear at first on withdrawal of high doses.

(continued)

TABLE 8.2 ▪ A Guide to the Vitamins *(continued)*

Vitamin	Best Sources	Chief Roles	Deficiency Symptoms	Toxicity Symptoms
Fat-soluble vitamins				
Vitamin A 5,000 IU	*Retinal:* fortified milk and margarine, cream, cheese, butter, eggs, liver. *Carotene:* Spinach and other dark leafy greens, broccoli, deep orange fruits (apricots, peaches, cantaloupe) and vegetables (squash, carrots, sweet potatoes, pumpkin).	Vision, growth and repair of body tissues; reproduction; bone and tooth formation; immunity; cancer protection; hormone synthesis.	Night blindness, rough skin, susceptibility to infection, impaired bone growth, abnormal tooth and jaw alignment, eye problems leading to blindness, impaired growth.	Red blood cell breakage, nosebleeds, abdominal cramps, nausea, diarrhea, weight loss, blurred vision, irritability, loss of appetite, bone pain, dry skin, rashes, hair loss, cessation of menstruation, growth retardation.
Vitamin D 400 IU	Self-synthesis with sunlight, fortified milk, fortified margarine, eggs, liver, fish.	Calcium and phosphorus metabolism (bone and tooth formation); aids body's absorption of calcium.	Rickets in children; osteomalacia in adults; abnormal growth, joint pain, soft bones.	Raised blood calcium, constipation, weight loss, irritability, weakness, nausea, kidney stones, mental and physical retardation.
Vitamin E 30 IU	Vegetable oils, green leafy vegetables, wheat germ, whole-grain products, butter, liver, egg yolk, milk fat, nuts, seeds.	Protects red blood cells; antioxidant; stabilization of cell membranes.	Muscle wasting, weakness, red blood cell breakage, anemia, hemorrhaging, fibrocystic breast disease.	Interference with anti-clotting medication, general discomfort.
Vitamin K 70–140 µg	Bacterial synthesis in digestive tract, liver green, leafy, and cabbage-type vegetables, milk.	Synthesis of blood-clotting proteins and a blood protein that regulates blood calcium.	Hemorrhaging.	Interference with anti-clotting medication; may cause jaundice.

Source: Adapted by permission from pp. 152–153 of *Personal Nutrition,* 2d ed., by Marie Boyle and Gail Zyla. Copyright 1991 by West Publishing Company. All rights reserved.

𝒲HAT DO YOU THINK?

Of all of the nutrients discussed in this section, which one do you worry about not getting enough in your diet the most? What is the basis for your worry? Are you planning to take any action to make sure your daily intake is adequate? What steps will you take?

Minerals

Minerals are the inorganic, indestructible elements that aid physiological processes within the body. Without minerals, vitamins could not be absorbed. Minerals are readily excreted and are usually not toxic. **Macrominerals** are those minerals that the body needs in fairly large amounts: sodium, calcium, phosphorus, magnesium, potassium, sulfur, and chloride. **Trace minerals** include iron, zinc, manganese, copper, iodine, and cobalt. Only trace amounts of these minerals are needed, and serious problems may result if excesses or deficiencies occur. Specific types of minerals are listed in Table 8.3.

Minerals: Inorganic, indestructible elements that aid physiological processes.

Macrominerals: Minerals that the body needs in fairly large amounts.

Trace minerals: Minerals that the body needs in only very small amounts.

Your Guide to a Perfect-Fit Food Label

Frankly, the nutritional label [see Figure 8.2] on supermarket foods should sport a big, red warning: ONE SIZE DOES NOT FIT ALL! That's because the new "% Daily Value" for total fat, saturated fat, and total carbohydrates really fits one size only: people who eat only 2,000 calories a day. So if you eat fewer than 2,000 calories, as most women do, look out! To keep from overdoing on fat and saturated fat, for example, you need to know how far under 100 percent of the "Daily Value" your personal day's total intake should stay.

Another fat trap: The label bases each "% Daily Value" for total fat on a maximum level that's calculated at 30 percent of all calories. Yet many experts advise keeping fat even lower—to a maximum of 25 percent of calories—for top health benefits. Somehow, we need to factor this difference into how we use the "% Daily Values," too.

Feeling slightly crazed? Well, help is on the way. *Prevention* magazine designed the following Personal Label-Reference list for customizing the "% Daily Values" to fit your caloric needs *and* to fit the preferred level of 25 percent maximum fat intake. Here are the five steps to using the list:

Step 1

First, find your activity level.

Sedentary: You have a job or lifestyle that involves a lot of sitting, standing, or light walking. At most, you exercise occasionally.

Active: Your job requires more activity than light walking (for example, full-time housecleaning or construction work). Or you get 30 to 60 minutes of aerobic exercise three times every week.

Very Active: You get aerobic exercise for at least 60 minutes four or more times every week.

Step 2

Now, find the activity factor listed below that corresponds to your activity level and gender.

Sedentary woman—12

Sedentary man—14

Active woman—15

Active man—17

Very active woman—18

Very active man—20

Step 3

Determine your calorie needs by taking your activity factor from Step 2 and multiplying it by your weight in pounds (activity factor × weight in pounds = calorie needs). If overweight, use a healthy weight for this step.

Step 4

Now take your calorie level (found in Step 3) and locate it on the Calorie Customizer chart. Read across for your personal daily nutrient totals and "% Daily Value" targets for total fat, saturated fat, total carbohydrate, and protein.

Calorie customizer

Calories	Total fat (25% of calories) Grams	% DV	Saturated fat (7% of calories) Grams	% DV	Total carbohydrate (65% of calories) Grams	% DV	Protein (10% of calories) Grams
1,200	33	50	9	45	195	65	30
1,400	38	55	10	50	225	75	35
1,600	44	65	12	60	260	85	40
1,800	50	75	14	70	290	95	45
2,000	55	85	15	75	325	105	50
2,200	61	90	17	85	355	115	55
2,500	69	105	19	95	405	135	62
2,800	77	115	21	105	455	150	70
3,200	88	135	24	120	520	170	80

Step 5

Fill in the appropriate blanks on the Personal Label-Reference Card using your figures from Step 4. For each nutrient, the "% Daily Values" target tells what all the foods you eat in a day can add up to. Nice idea: Photocopy the blank form to make customized cards for family or friends.

Personal label-reference card

Name: _____

Calorie level: _____

Daily nutrient totals		% Daily Value target*
Total fat	_____ g. or less	_____ % DV ↓
Saturated fat	_____ g. or less	_____ % DV ↓
Cholesterol	300 mg. or less	100 % DV ↓
Sodium	2,400 mg. or less	100 % DV ↓
Total carbohydrate	_____ g. or more	_____ % DV ↑
Dietary fiber	20 to 35 g.	100 % DV ↑
Protein	_____ g.	**
Vitamins	***	100 % DV ↑
Minerals	***	100 % DV ↑

*For each nutrient all the foods I eat in one day can add up to this "% Daily Value."

**Most labels will not list "% Daily Value" for protein.

***Labels will list only the "% Daily Value" for vitamins and minerals.

↓ Aim Low   ↑ Aim High

TABLE 8.3 ■ A Guide to the Minerals

Mineral	Significant Sources	Chief Functions in the Body	Deficiency Symptoms	Toxicity Symptoms
Calcium RDA = 800–1,200 mg +	Milk and milk products, small fish (with bones), tofu, greens, legumes.	Principal mineral of bones and teeth; involved in muscle contraction and relaxation, nerve function, blood clotting, blood pressure.	Stunted growth in children; bone loss (osteoporosis) in adults.	Excess calcium is excreted except in hormonal imbalance states.
Phosphorus RDA = 1,000 mg	All animal tissues	Part of every cell; involved in acid-based balance.	Unknown.	Can create relative deficiency of calcium.
Magnesium RDA = 400 mg	Nuts, legumes, whole grains, dark green vegetables, seafoods, chocolate, cocoa.	Involved in bone mineralization, protein synthesis, enzyme action, normal muscular contraction, nerve transmission.	Weakness, confusion, depressed pancreatic hormone secretion, growth failure, behavioral disturbances, muscle spasms.	Not known.
Sodium RDA = 500 mg	Salt, soy sauce; processed foods; cured, canned, pickled, and many boxed foods.	Helps maintain normal fluid and acid-base balance.	Muscle cramps, mental apathy, loss of appetite.	Hypertension (in salt-sensitive persons).
Chloride RDA = 750 mg	Salt, soy sauce; processed foods.	Part of stomach acid, necessary for proper digestion, fluid balance.	Growth failure in children, muscle cramps, mental apathy, loss of appetite.	Normally harmless (the gas chlorine is a poison but evaporates from water); disturbed acid-base balance; vomiting.
Potassium RDA = 2,000 mg	All whole foods: meats, milk, fruits, vegetables, grains, legumes.	Facilitates many reactions including protein synthesis, fluid balance, nerve transmission, and contraction of muscles.	Muscle weakness, paralysis, confusion; can cause death; accompanies dehydration.	Causes muscular weakness; triggers vomiting; if given into a vein, can stop the heart.
Iodine RDA = 150 mg	Iodized salt, seafood.	Part of thyroxine, which regulates metabolism.	Goiter, cretinism.	Very high intakes depress thyroid activity.
Iron RDA = 18 mg	Beef, fish, poultry, shellfish, eggs, legumes, dried fruits.	Hemoglobin formation; part of myoglobin; energy utilization.	Anemia: weakness, pallor, headaches, reduced resistance to infection, inability to concentrate.	Iron overload: infections, liver injury.
Zinc RDA = 15 mg	Protein-containing foods: meats, fish, poultry, grains, vegetables.	Part of many enzymes; present in insulin; involved in making genetic material and proteins, immunity, vitamin A transport, taste, wound healing, making sperm, normal fetal development.	Growth failure in children, delayed development of sexual organs, loss of taste, poor wound healing.	Fever, nausea, vomiting, diarrhea.
Copper RDA = 2 mg	Meats, drinking water.	Absorption of iron; part of several enzymes.	Anemia, bone changes (rare in human beings).	Unknown except as part of a rare hereditary disease (Wilson's disease).
Fluoride 1.5–4.0 mg	Drinking water (if naturally fluoride-containing or fluoridated), tea, seafood.	Formation of bones and teeth; helps make teeth resistant to decay and bones resistant to mineral loss.	Susceptibility to tooth decay and bone loss.	Fluorosis (discoloration of teeth).

(continued)

TABLE 8.3 ■ A Guide to the Minerals *(continued)*

Mineral	Significant Sources	Chief Functions in the Body	Deficiency Symptoms	Toxicity Symptoms
Selenium 50–70 μg	Seafood, meats, grains.	Helps protect body compounds from oxidation.	Anemia (rare).	Digestive system disorders.
Chromium 50–200 μg	Meats, unrefined foods, fats, vegetable oils.	Associated with insulin and required for the release of energy from glucose.	Diabeteslike condition marked by inability to use glucose normally.	Unknown as a nutrition disorder. Occupational exposures damage skin and kidneys.
Molybdenum 75–250 μg	Legumes, cereals, organ meats.	Facilitates, with enzymes, many cell processes.	Unknown.	Enzyme inhibition.
Manganese 2.0–5.0 mg	Widely distributed in foods.	Facilitates, with enzymes, many cell processes.	In animals: poor growth, nervous system disorders, abnormal reproduction.	Poisoning, nervous system disorders.

Because we have less information about minerals than about vitamins, RDA recommendations are *estimates* of minimum requirements.

Source: Adapted by permission from pp. 178–179 of *Personal Nutrition*, 2d ed., by Marie Boyle and Gail Zyla; and pp. 298–300 of *Nutrition Concepts and Controversies*, 5th ed., by Eva Hamilton, Eleanor Whitney, and Frances Sizer. Copyright 1994 by West Publishing Company. All rights reserved.

Although minerals are necessary for body function, there are limits on the amounts of each that we should consume. Americans tend to overuse or underuse certain minerals.

Sodium. Sodium is necessary for the regulation of blood and body fluids, for the successful transmission of nerve impulses, for heart activity, and for certain metabolic functions. However, we consume much more sodium every day than we need. It is estimated that the average adult who does not sweat profusely has a need for only 500 milligrams of sodium (about ¼ teaspoon) per day; yet the average American consumes between 6,000 and 12,000 milligrams. The RDA subcommittee recommended that sodium be restricted to no more than 2,400 milligrams per day; less is better. The most common form of sodium in the American diet comes from table salt. The remainder of dietary sodium comes from the water we drink and from highly processed foods that are infused with sodium to enhance flavor. Pickles, salty snack foods, processed cheeses, many breads and bakery products, and smoked meats and sausages often contain several hundred milligrams of sodium per serving. Many fast-food entrees and convenience entrees have 500 to 1,000 milligrams of sodium per serving. Soft drinks are also likely culprits for added sodium.

Many experts believe that there is a link between excessive sodium intake and hypertension (high blood pressure). Although this theory is controversial, many organizations, including the American Heart Association, have recommended that Americans cut back on sodium consumption to reduce their risk for cardiovascular disorders.

Calcium. The issue of calcium consumption has gained national attention with the rising incidence of osteoporosis (see Chapter 20) among elderly women. Although calcium plays a vital role in building strong bones and teeth, muscle contraction, blood clotting, nerve impulse transmission, regulating heart beat, and fluid balance within cells, most Americans do not consume the 1,200 milligrams of calcium per day established by the RDA.

Improving Your Calcium Levels. Because calcium intake is so important throughout your life for a strong bone structure, it is critical that you consume the minimum required amounts each day. Over half of our calcium intake usually comes from milk, one of the highest sources of dietary calcium. Many green, leafy vegetables are good sources of calcium, but some contain oxalic acid, which makes their calcium harder to absorb. Spinach, chard, and beet greens are not particularly good sources of calcium, whereas broccoli, cauliflower, and many peas and beans offer good supplies (pinto beans and soybeans are among the best). Many nuts, particularly almonds, brazil nuts, and hazelnuts, and seeds such as sunflower and sesames contain good amounts of calcium. Molasses is fairly high in calcium. Some fruits—such as citrus fruits, figs, raisins, and dried apricots—have moderate amounts.

Of interest to those of you who drink carbonated soft drinks is the fact that the added phosphoric acid (phosphate) in these drinks can cause you to excrete extra calcium, which may result in calcium being pulled out of your bones. Calcium/phosphorous imbalances may lead to kidney stones and other calcification problems as well as to increased atherosclerotic plaque.[13]

We also know that sunlight increases the manufacture of vitamin D in the body, and is therefore like having an extra calcium source because vitamin D improves absorption of calcium. Stress, on the other hand, tends to contribute to calcium depletion. It is generally best to take calcium throughout the day, consuming protein, vitamin D, and vitamin C containing foods with it for optimum absorption. Experts vary on which type of supplemental calcium is most readily and efficiently absorbed, although bone meal, aspartate, or citrate salts of calcium are among those most often recommended. The best way to obtain calcium, like all the other nutrients is to consume it as part of a balanced diet.

Iron.   Iron is a problem mineral for millions of people. Although it is found in every cell of all living things, many humans have difficulty getting enough iron in their daily diets. Females aged 19 to 50 need about 18 milligrams per day, and males aged 19 to 50 need about 10 milligrams. Iron deficiencies can lead to **anemia,** a problem resulting from the body's inability to produce hemoglobin, the bright red, oxygen-carrying component of the blood. When this occurs, body cells receive less oxygen, and carbon dioxide wastes are removed less efficiently. These problems cause a person to feel tired and run down. Anemia can be caused by accidents, cancers, ulcers, and other conditions, but iron deficiency is a common cause. Generally, women are more likely than men to suffer from iron deficiency problems, partly because they typically eat less than men, and their diets therefore contain less iron. Also, because blood loss is the major reason for iron depletion, women having heavy menstrual flows may be prone to iron deficiency. Another problem with iron deficiency is that the immune system becomes less effective, which can lead to increased risk of illness.

Recently, researchers have speculated that too much iron in the body may increase the risk for heart disease. They point to the low risk for heart disease in premenopausal women and the striking rise in risk in postmenopausal women as a possible indicator of such an association. Men who consume high-iron diets also appear to be at increased risk. But this research is preliminary; nutrition scientists are planning further studies of this possible connection.[14] Blood donors and pregnant women may need to increase iron intake. A less common problem, iron toxicity, is caused by too much iron in the blood.

Gender Differences in Nutritional Needs

Men and women differ in body size, body composition, and overall metabolic rates. They therefore have differing

Not only do women have different nutritional needs than men, but they undergo physiological changes at different stages in life that dramatically alter their dietary requirements.

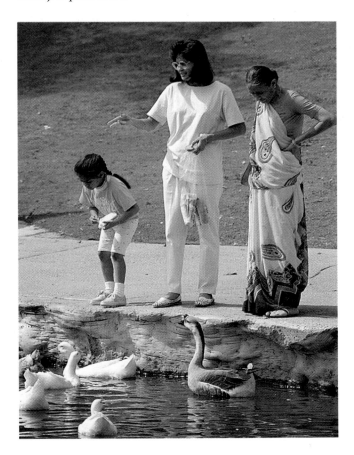

needs for most nutrients throughout the life cycle (see tables on vitamin and mineral requirements) and face unique difficulties in keeping on track with their dietary goals. Some of these differences have already been discussed. However, there are some diet/nutrition factors that need further consideration. Have you ever wondered why men can eat more than women and never seem to gain weight? Although there are many possible reasons for this apparent difference, one factor is that women have a lower ratio of lean body mass to adipose (fatty) tissue at all ages and stages of life. Also, after sexual maturation, metabolism is higher in men, meaning that they will burn more calories doing the same things as women.

Different Cycles, Different Needs.   In addition to the above differences, women have many more "landmark"

Anemia: Iron deficiency disease that results from the body's inability to produce hemoglobin.

times in their lives when their nutritional needs vary significantly from what they are at other times in their lives. From menarche to menopause, women undergo cyclical physiological changes that can have dramatic effects on metabolism, nutritional needs, and efforts to stick to a nutritional plan. For example, during pregnancy and lactation, nutritional requirements increase substantially for women. Those who are unable to follow the strict dietary recommendations of their doctors may find themselves gaining much more weight during pregnancy and retaining it afterwards. During the menstrual cycle, many women report significant food cravings that may cause them to overconsume. Later in womens' lives, with the advent of menopause, nutritional needs again change rather dramatically. With depletion of the hormone estrogen, the body's need for calcium to ward off bone deterioration becomes pronounced. Women must pay closer attention to their exercise patterns and to getting enough calcium through diet or dietary supplements or run the risk of severe osteoporosis (see Chapter 20 for a more complete description of this disease).

Changing the Meat and Potatoes Man.   Although men do not have the same cyclical patterns and dietary needs as women, they do suffer from a heritage of dietary excesses that are difficult to change. The "meat and potatoes" kind of guy has been part of the American way since our earliest agrarian years. What's wrong with all those hot dogs, steaks, and hamburgers? Heart disease, stroke, and cancer are probably the greatest threats. Add increased risks for colon and prostate cancers, and the rationale for dietary change becomes even more compelling. Consider the following:

- Men who eat red meat as a main dish five or more times a week have four times the risk of colon cancer of men who eat red meat less than once a month.

- Heavy red meat eaters are more than twice as likely to get prostate cancer and nearly 5 times more likely to get colon cancer.

- For every 3 servings of fruits or vegetables per day men can expect a 22 percent lower risk of stroke.

- High fruit and vegetable diets may lower the risk of lung cancer in smokers from 20 times the risk of nonsmokers to "only" ten times the risk. They may also protect against oral, throat, pancreas, and bladder cancers, all of which are more common in smokers.

- The fastest-rising malignancy in the U.S. is cancer of the lower esophagus, particularly in white men. While obesity seems to be a factor, fruits and vegetables are the protectors. (The average American male eats less than 3 servings/day, although 5–9 servings is recommended. Women average 3–7 servings/day.)

Is there something in the meat that makes it inherently bad? Although the fat content of meat and fried potatoes, as well as the potential carcinogenic substances produced through cooking have been implicated, it is also probably something much more basic. By eating so much protein a person fills up sooner and never gets around to the fruits and vegetables. Thus, any potential protective factors may be lost.[15]

𝒲HAT DO YOU THINK?

Think about the women that you know who seem to have weight problems. What are their ages? What factors may have influenced them to have more problems keeping weight off than you may have? What advantages, if any, do men have in controlling their eating behaviors and managing their weight?

𝒱EGETARIANISM: EATING FOR HEALTH

For aesthetic, animal rights, economic, personal, health, cultural, or religious reasons, some people choose specialized diets. Between 5 and 15 percent of all Americans today claim to be some form of vegetarian. Normally, vegetarianism provides a superb alternative to our high-fat, high-calorie, meat-based cuisine, but, without proper information, vegetarians can also have dietary problems.

The term **vegetarian** means different things to different people. Strict vegetarians, or *vegans*, avoid all foods of animal origin, including dairy products and eggs. The few people who fall into this category must work hard to ensure that they get all of the necessary nutrients. Far more common are *lacto-vegetarians*, who eat dairy products but avoid flesh foods. Their diet can be low in fat and cholesterol, but only if they consume skim milk and other low- or nonfat products. *Ovo-vegetarians* add eggs to their diet, while *lacto-ovo-vegetarians* eat both dairy products and eggs. *Pesco-vegetarians* eat fish, dairy products, and eggs, while *semivegetarians* eat chicken, fish, dairy products, and eggs. Some people in the semivegetarian category prefer to call themselves "non-red-meat eaters."

Generally, people who follow a balanced vegetarian diet have lower weights, better cholesterol levels, fewer problems with irregular bowel movements (constipation and diarrhea), and a lower risk of heart disease than do nonvegetarians. Some preliminary evidence suggests that vegetarians may also have a reduced risk for colon and breast cancer. Whether these lower risks are due to the vegetarian diet per se or to some combination of lifestyle variables remains unclear.

Although in the past vegetarians often suffered from vitamin deficiencies, the vegetarian of the 1990s is usually extremely adept at combining the right types of foods to ensure proper nutrient intake. People who eat dairy products and small amounts of chicken or fish are seldom nutrient-deficient; in fact, while vegans typically get 50 to 60 grams of protein per day, lacto-ovo vegetarians normally consume between 70 and 90 grams per day, well beyond the RDA. Vegan diets may be deficient in vitamins B_2 (riboflavin), B_{12}, and D. Riboflavin is found mainly in meat, eggs, and dairy products; but broccoli, asparagus, almonds, and fortified cereals are also good sources. Vitamins B_{12} and D are found only in dairy products and fortified products such as soy milk. Vegans are also at risk for calcium, iron, zinc, and other mineral deficiencies, but these nutrients can be obtained from supplements. Strict vegans have to pay much more attention to what they eat than the average person does, but by eating complementary combinations of plant products, they can receive adequate amounts of essential amino acids. Examples of complementary combinations are corn and beans, and peanut butter and whole-grain bread. Eating a full variety of grains, legumes, fruits, vegetables, and seeds each day will help to keep even the strictest vegetarian in excellent health. Pregnant women, the elderly, the sick, and children who are vegans need to take special care to ensure that their diets are adequate. People who are on heavy aerobic exercise programs (over three hours per week) may need to increase their protein consumption. In all cases, seek advice from a health-care professional if you have questions.

The Vegetarian Pyramid

Dr. Arlene Spark, a nutritionist at New York Medical College, devised a food guide pyramid that conveys all the essentials of a vegetarian diet in 1994 (see Figure 8.7). Modeled after the Food Guide Pyramid discussed earlier in this chapter, the vegetarian version clarifies what people who don't eat meat need to do to stay healthy. The vegetarian pyramid defines the following categories. We include examples of single servings of foods in each category.

Grains and Starchy Vegetables Group (6–11 servings/day)

- 1 slice bread
- ½ roll or bagel
- 1 tortilla (6″)
- 1 ounce cold cereal
- ½ cup cooked cereal, rice, or pasta
- 3–4 crackers
- 3 cups popcorn
- ½ cup corn
- 1 medium potato
- ½ cup green peas

Vegetable Group (3 + servings/day)

- ½ cup cooked or chopped raw vegetables

- 1 cup raw leafy vegetables
- ¾ cup vegetable juice

Fruit Group (2–4 servings/day)

- 1 medium whole piece of fruit
- ½ cup canned, chopped, or cooked fruit
- ¾ cup fruit juice

Milk and Milk Substitutes Group (3 servings/day for preteens and 4 for teens; 2–4 servings/day for adults)

- 1 cup milk or yogurt
- 1 cup calcium- and vitamin B_{12}-fortified soy milk
- 1½ ounces hard cheese
- 1½ ounces calcium- and vitamin B_{12}-fortified soy cheese

Meat/Fish Substitutes Group (2–3 servings/day)

- 1 cup cooked dry beans, peas, or lentils
- 2 eggs
- 8 ounces bean curd or tofu
- ½ cup shelled nuts
- 3–4 tablespoons peanut butter
- 3–4 tablespoons tahini
- ⅓ to ½ cup seeds

Vegans Must Consume Daily:

- 3–5 teaspoons vegetable oil + 1 tablespoon blackstrap molasses + 1 tablespoon brewer's yeast

WHAT DO YOU THINK?

Have you ever considered becoming or are you currently a vegetarian? What was your reason for making this choice? Do you find it difficult to select vegetarian foods in restaurants/eating places on your campus? What actions can you take to help insure more choices? From what you have learned here, what is one improvement you can make in your vegetarian eating behavior?

Vegetarian: A term with a variety of meanings: *vegans* avoid all foods of animal origin; *lacto-vegetarians* avoid flesh foods but eat dairy products; *ovo-vegetarians* avoid flesh foods but eat eggs; *lacto-ovo-vegetarians* avoid flesh foods but eat both dairy products and eggs; *pesco-vegetarians* avoid meat but eat fish, dairy products, and eggs; *semivegetarians* eat chicken, fish, dairy products, and eggs.

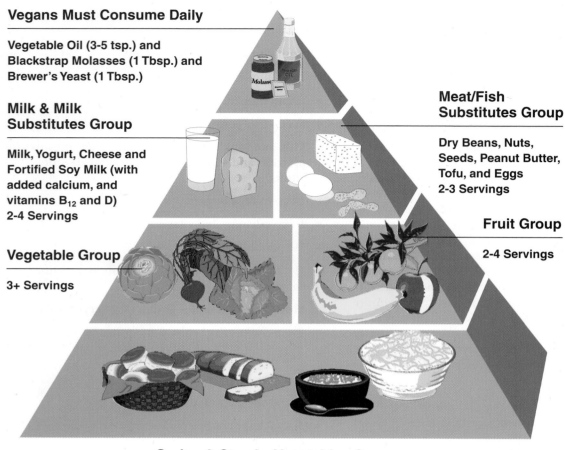

Vegans Must Consume Daily

Vegetable Oil (3-5 tsp.) and
Blackstrap Molasses (1 Tbsp.) and
Brewer's Yeast (1 Tbsp.)

Milk & Milk Substitutes Group

Milk, Yogurt, Cheese and
Fortified Soy Milk (with
added calcium, and
vitamins B$_{12}$ and D)
2-4 Servings

Vegetable Group

3+ Servings

Meat/Fish Substitutes Group

Dry Beans, Nuts,
Seeds, Peanut Butter,
Tofu, and Eggs
2-3 Servings

Fruit Group

2-4 Servings

Grains & Starchy Vegetables Group

Bread, Cereal, Rice, Pasta,
Potatoes, Corn, and Green Peas
6-11 Servings

FIGURE 8.7

New York Medical College Vegetarian Pyramid
Source: © 1994 New York Medical College. Reprinted by permission.

IMPROVED EATING FOR THE COLLEGE STUDENT

College students often face a challenge when trying to eat healthy foods. Some students live in dorms and do not have their own cooking or refrigeration facilities. Others live in crowded apartments where everyone forages in the refrigerator for everyone else's food. Still others eat at university food services where food choices are limited. Most students have time constraints that make buying, preparing, and eating healthy food a difficult task. In addition, many lack the financial resources needed to buy many foods that their parents purchased while they lived at

home. What's a student to do? While we can't come in and guard your refrigerator to make sure your roommates don't eat your food, we can offer some suggestions for choices that may make your eating experience more healthy. Basically, students should follow many of the suggestions provided in the rest of this chapter. The following sections provide advice for some of the particular problems you may face.

Fast Foods: Eating on the Run

If your campus is like many others across the country, you've probably noticed a distinct move toward fast-food restaurants in your student unions so that they now re-

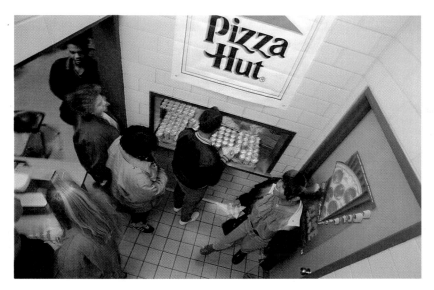

Maintaining a nutritious diet is often difficult for college students, but even fast food chains now offer possibilities for healthy eating beyond the usual pizzas and burgers that are high in fat and calories.

semble the food courts found in most major shopping malls. These new eating centers fit student's needs for a fast bite of food at a reasonable rate between classes and also bring in money to your school. Many fast foods are high in fat and sodium. But are all fast foods unhealthy?

You should recognize that not all fast foods are created equal and not all of them are bad for you. Even at the often-maligned burger chains, menus are healthier than ever before and offer excellent choices for the discriminating eater. The key word here is *discriminating*. It really is possible to eat healthy food if you follow these suggestions:

- Ask for nutritional analyses of items. Most fast-food chains now have them. For your convenience, we have included a summary of many of these analyses in an appendix at the end of this book.

- Order it "your way"—avoid mayonnaise or sauces and other add-ons. Some places even have fat-free mayonnaise if you ask.

- Hold the cheese. This extra contributes substantially to total fat while not adding a lot to taste.

- Order single, small burgers rather than large, high-calorie, bacon- or cheese-topped choices. Put on your own ketchup and keep portions small.

- Order salads and be careful how much dressing you put on. Many people think they are being health-smart by eating salad, only to load it with calorie- and fat-rich dressing. Try the vinegar and oil or low-fat alternative dressings. Stay away from eggs and other high-fat add-ons such as bacon bits.

- When ordering a chicken sandwich, order the skinless broiled version rather than the deep-fried version.

Many people think that the deep-fried chicken sandwich is a more healthy choice, when it really has more fat than the loaded double burger.

- Check to see what type of oil is used to cook fries if you must have them. Avoid lard-based or other saturated fat products.

- Order the wheat buns/bread and ask them to hold the butter.

- Avoid fried foods in general, including hot apple pies and other crust-based fried foods.

- Opt for spots where foods tend to be broiled rather than fried.

Healthy Eating When Funds Are Short

For many students, the transition from the home dinner table to the college apartment, student union, or dormitory cafeteria is often an unpleasant one. Not only are meals not prepared the way you are used to, but there also is no one to monitor what you eat and whether or not you eat. Of equal importance is the fact that grocery money may be limited.

Balancing the need for adequate nutrition with the many other activities that are part of college life can become a difficult task. Not surprisingly, it is often the nutritional part of the total picture that gets slighted. Maintaining a nutritious diet within the confines of student life is difficult. However, if you take the time to plan healthy diets, you may find that you are eating better, enjoying eating more, and actually saving money. Understanding the terminology used by the food industry may

BUILDING COMMUNICATION SKILLS

Checking Out Food Labels: Terms Used on Food Labels

Energy Terms

- **diet, dietetic** terms to indicate that a food is either a *low-calorie* or a *reduced-calorie* food.

- **low calorie** containing no more than 40 cal per serving.

- **reduced calories** containing 25 percent fewer calories per serving than a "regular" product.

Fat Terms (meat and poultry products)
extra lean contains:

- not more than 5 g of fat
- not more than 2 g of saturated fat
- not more than 95 mg of cholesterol per serving

lean* contains:

- not more than 10 g of fat
- not more than 4.5 g of saturated fat
- and less than 95 mg cholesterol per serving

Fat and Cholesterol Terms (all products)

- **fat free** containing 0.5 g or less of fat per serving

- **low cholesterol** containing fewer than 20 mg of cholesterol per serving and fewer than 2 g saturated fat per serving

- **low fat** containing 3 g or less fat per serving

- **low saturated fat** containing 1 g or less saturated fat per serving

- **percent fat free** may be used only if the product meets the definition of *low fat* or *fat free*. Requires disclosure of g fat per 100 g food.

- **reduced saturated fat** containing 25 percent or less of the saturated fat in the comparison food and reduced by more than 1 gram per serving.

- **saturated fat free** containing 0.5 g or less of saturated fat and 0.5 g or less of *trans*-fatty acids.

Other Terms

- **free, without, no, zero** containing no amount or a trivial amount. *Calorie-free* means containing fewer than 5 calories per serving; *sugar-free* or *fat-free* means containing less than half a gram per serving.

- **fresh** raw, unprocessed or minimally processed with no added preservatives.

- **good source** provides 10 to 19 percent of the Daily Value per serving.

- **healthy** a term allowable in food names, so long as the food is low in fat, saturated fat, cholesterol, and sodium.

- **high** provides 20 percent or more of the Daily Value per serving.

- **imitation food** this term must be used to describe a food intended to replace a standard food, if the replacement food lacks one or more nutrients provided by the original food. For example, imitation cheese for pizza lacks the calcium of real mozzarella cheese.

- **less, fewer** provides 25 percent less of a nutrient or calories than a reference food. This may occur naturally or as a result of altering the food. For example, pretzels, which are usually low in fat, can claim to provide less fat than potato chips, a comparable food.

- **light** this descriptor has three meanings on labels:
  1. a serving provides one-third fewer calories or half the fat of the regular product.
  2. a serving of a low-calorie, low-fat food provides half the sodium normally present.
  3. the product is light in color and texture, so long as the label makes this intent clear, as in "light brown sugar."

- **more** contains 10 percent more of the Daily Value than a comparable food. The nutrient may be added or may occur naturally.

- **reduced** altered to provide 25 percent less of a nutrient or calories than a "regular" product.

Sodium Terms

- **low sodium** containing 140 mg or fewer sodium per serving.

- **very low sodium** containing 35 mg or less sodium per serving.

---

*The word *lean* as part of the brand name (as in "Lean Supreme") indicates than the product contains fewer than 10 grams of fat per serving.
Source: "The New Food Label," *FDA Backgrounder,* 10 December 1992; "Nutrition Labeling of Meat and Poultry Products," *FSIS Backgrounder,* January 1993.

---

also help you eat a healthier diet; the Building Communication Skills box reviews some of these pertinent terms.

In addition, you can take these steps to help ensure a quality diet:

- Buy fruits and vegetables in season whenever possible for their lower cost, higher nutrient quality, and greater variety.

- Use coupons and specials whenever possible to get price reductions.

- Shop whenever possible at discount warehouse food chains; capitalize on volume discounts and no-frills products.

- Plan ahead to get the most for your dollar and avoid extra trips to the store; extra trips usually mean extra purchases. Make a list and stick to it.

- Purchase meats and other products in volume, freezing portions for future needs. Or purchase small amounts of meats and other expensive proteins and combine them with beans and plant proteins for lower total cost, lower calories, and lower fat.

- Cook large meals and freeze smaller portions for later use.

- Drain off extra fat after cooking. Save juices for use in soups and in other dishes.

- If you find that you have no money for food, talk to someone at your county/city health department. Although they often restrict subsidies such as food stamps for full-time students, they may know of some alternative ways for you to get assistance.

Healthy Eating in the Dormitory

If you're like most college students, the meals provided in the student food service or in your dormitory may provide unique nutritional challenges and opportunities. Some food services have responded exceedingly well to new guidelines for low-fat, high-carbohydrate eating. Many offer vegetarian entrees; choices between broiled, baked, or fried foods; skim milks; nonfat yogurts; and full-service salad and pasta bars. Unfortunately, there are many others that are still preparing foods as they have for years. Choices for students are limited and often provide only high- and higher-fat choices in foods.

If you find that you are in a health-conscious food service or dormitory, the guidelines and tips provided throughout this chapter should serve you well. If you are in a food service or dormitory that has a long way to go, here are some possible actions you might take to help them change their food choices and cooking practices.

- Ask your health instructor if anyone has ever done a food analysis of menu items at the food service or dorm. If they have, find out what happened to the information provided. If not, find out what you can do to get one done. Several programs are available to help you assess these foods, including a computerized program known as DINE and another known as FOOD PROCESSOR. Your student health service or local hospital may have such a program if you are unable to locate one.

- Once you've found out what the nutrient content of these meals is, talk to representatives of your student

newspaper. Ask them to run a series on food content/choices on campus. Bring your results to the student government and try to find someone who is willing to help push for food service reform.

- If you are dissatisfied with cafeteria foods, make your complaints known in writing to the director of student services or the food service administrator. Be sure to include recommendations for improvements.

- Find out what is being done on other campuses throughout the country. If you find some interesting options within your own conference, make sure it's part of the newspaper series. Competition between universities often goes beyond the playing field. You may just spur someone to action.

- Use the suggestion box provided in the cafeteria. If there isn't one, try to get one.

- Be positive in your approach. More support is gained from providing suggestions for change rather than criticism of current practice.

𝒲HAT DO YOU THINK?

What problems cause you the most difficulty when you try to eat more healthful foods? Are these problems that you noted in your family, too, or are they unique to your current situation as a student? What actions can you take that would help improve your current eating practices?

𝐼S YOUR FOOD SAFE?

Irradiation

As we become increasingly worried that the food we put in our mouths may be contaminated with potentially harmful bacteria, insects, worms, or other not-so-nice substances, the food industry has come under fire. To convince us that our products are safe for consumption, some manufacturers have come up with "new and improved" ways of protecting our foods. One of these methods, food irradiation, has become the subject of much controversy. What is food irradiation? Should you buy irradiated foods?

Food irradiation involves treating foods with gamma radiation from radioactive cobalt, cesium, or some other

---

Food irradiation: Treating foods with gamma radiation from radioactive cobalt, cesium, or some other source of X-rays to kill microorganisms.

source of X rays. The killing effect on microorganisms rises with the power of the rays, which are measured in rads (radiant energy absorbed).[16] Irradiation lengthens food products' shelf life and prevents microorganism and insect contamination. Because this results in less waste, the food industry can make higher profits while charging consumers lower prices. It is also claimed that irradiation will reduce the need to use many of the toxic chemicals now used to preserve foods and prevent contamination from external contaminants.

The following foods have already received approval for irradiation by the Food and Drug Administration: fresh produce such as strawberries, potatoes, and other perishable foods; poultry and some seafood (in which salmonella is a serious problem); and pork (to kill off the parasite trichina). Many spices and herbs have been irradiated for years, and grains, vegetables, and frozen foods are already targeted for irradiation in the near future.

The long-term side effects of irradiation are unknown. Although irradiation doesn't actually make your food radioactive, it does damage its molecular structure, creating new substances known as free radicals. Free radicals have been implicated in certain types of cancers, and diseases of the liver and kidney in animal studies, but, to date, no studies of the toxicity of irradiated foods on humans have been done. Because this radiation damages the molecular structure of foods, critics argue that it may lower the nutritional value of some foods by altering their protein structure, reducing their vitamin levels, or deactivating important enzymes. Some foods, such as apples, pears, and certain citrus fruits, have actually been shown to spoil faster after irradiation. While the health effects of irradiated food may not be known for many years, the long-term impact of the proliferation of radioactive material on our environment cannot be ignored. According to Dr. Sheldon Margen, of the University of California at Berkeley, "There are potentially serious concerns about the issues of waste disposal, engineering safety, transport of radioactive material, safe handling, etc."[17] The most serious long-term effects of irradiation, then, may come from the plants built to irradiate foods. Currently, there are only about 40 irradiation plants in the United States, most of them set up to sterilize medical equipment. If the food industry was to begin large-scale irradiation of meat, fruits, and vegetables, hundreds more plants would have to be built. Considering the enormous problems posed by current levels of radioactive waste storage and transportation, the potential threats to the environment may far outweigh the benefits of irradiation.

Food-Borne Illness

Most of us have experienced the characteristic symptoms of diarrhea, nausea, cramping, and vomiting that prompt us to say, "It must be something I ate." The number of cases of food poisoning in the United States has been growing (there are millions of cases per year), which has prompted the Food and Drug Administration to make prevention of food contamination a high priority. Deaths in the Pacific Northwest in 1994 attributed to consumption of Jack-in-the-Box hamburgers contaminated with *Escherichia coli,* a bacterial agent, increased people's fears about the overall safety of meat, poultry, and seafood.

Symptoms of food-borne illness vary tremendously, based on the type of organism and the amount of contaminant eaten. These symptoms may appear as early as a half hour after eating the food, or they may take several days or weeks to develop. In most people, they come on five to eight hours after eating and last only a day or two. In others, such as the very old and very young and those suffering from other illnesses, food-borne illness can be life-threatening.

Part of the responsibility for preventing food-borne illness lies with consumers, for over 30 percent of all such illnesses result from unsafe handling of food at home.

- When shopping, pick up your packaged and canned foods first and save frozen foods and perishables such as meat, poultry, and fish till the last. Try to put these foods in separate plastic bags so that drippings don't run onto other foods in your cart, contaminating them.

- Check for cleanliness at the salad bar and meat and fish counters. For instance, cooked shrimp lying on the same small bed of ice as raw fish can easily be contaminated.

- When shopping for fish, buy from markets that get their supplies from state-approved sources; stay clear of vendors who sell shellfish from roadside stands or the back of trucks. If you're planning to harvest your own shellfish, check the safety of the water in the area.

- Remember that most cuts of meat, fish, and poultry should be kept in the refrigerator no more than one or two days. They shouldn't be in the grocery store meat counter beyond their dated shelf life, either. If your fish smells particularly "fishy" and your meat has a dark or greenish tinge to it, use caution. Check the shelf life of all products before buying. If expiration dates are close, freeze or eat immediately.

- Leftovers should be eaten within three days.

- Keep hot foods hot and cold foods cold.

- Use a thermometer to ensure that meats are completely cooked. Remember that the rarer the steak, the greater

Learning to shop carefully for fresh, high-quality foods can help ensure that your food is safe and that you are maintaining good health.

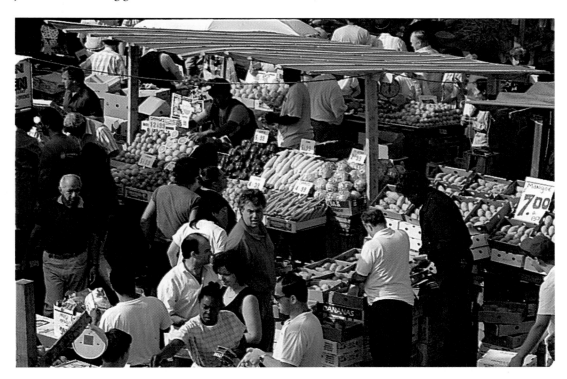

the number of bacteria swarming on the plate. Beef and lamb should be cooked to at least 140°F, pork to 150°F, and poultry to 165°F. Don't eat poultry that is pink inside.

- Fish is done when the thickest part becomes opaque and the fish flakes easily when poked with a fork.

- Cooked food should never be left standing on the stove or table for more than two hours. Disease-causing bacteria grow in temperatures between 40°F and 140°F. Cooked foods that have been left standing in this temperature range for more than two hours should be thrown away.

- Never thaw frozen foods at room temperature. Put in the refrigerator for a day to thaw, or thaw in cold water, changing the water every 30 minutes.

- Wash your hands with soap and water between courses when preparing food, particularly after handling meat, fish, or poultry. Wash the countertop and all utensils before using them for other foods.[18]

Food Allergies

Over one-third of all Americans believe that they are allergic to at least one food. Yet probably only 1 percent of adults and 3 percent of children have true (immunological) food allergies, according to Dr. Dean Metcalfe, of the National Institute of Allergy and Infectious Disease.[19] Most reactions to food have nothing to do with the immune system itself, so treatments and diets designed to prevent allergies may be not only worthless but may also shift efforts away from accurate diagnosis and appropriate actions.

True **food allergies** occur when the body overreacts to normally harmless proteins, perceiving them as allergens. The body then produces antibodies that activate immune

Food allergies: Overreaction by the body to normally harmless proteins, which are perceived as allergens. In response, the body produces antibodies, triggering allergic symptoms.

cells known as *histamines*, thus triggering a variety of allergic symptoms. Such allergic reactions vary tremendously among individuals and may range from a case of the hives or a body rash to swelling of certain body parts (especially the lips), to pain, diarrhea, nausea, or vomiting. In more severe cases, irregularities in breathing and heartbeat are experienced, along with blood pressure fluctuations, shock, and, if untreated, even death. Symptoms may occur within minutes or over a two- to three-hour period.

The most common culprits are soybeans, legumes (including peanuts), nuts, shellfish, eggs, wheat, and milk. People are often allergic to a whole family of foods; this is called **cross reactivity.** Unlike many other allergies, food allergies do not appear to be inherited. Breast-feeding babies seems to decrease their susceptibility to food allergies.

If you think you may have a food allergy, have yourself tested by a trained allergist. The most reliable method of diagnosis is the double-blind food challenge, in which you are alternately given a placebo and a minute amount of the suspected food in a capsule (or disguised in another food.) Neither you nor your doctor knows which pills are which until the test is completed.[20] Other methods in which the patient knows what food is being tested give a large number of false positive results because patients' anticipation of an allergic response trigger an imitation response. For a true food allergy, the only treatment is to eliminate the problem food from your diet.

If so many people think that they have food allergies when they really don't, what do they have? Some common reactions to food that may imitate allergies but do not involve the immune system are:

- *Food intolerance,* which occurs in people who lack certain digestive chemicals and suffer adverse effects when they consume certain substances because their bodies have difficulty breaking them down. One of the most common examples is lactose intolerance, experienced by people who do not have the digestive chemicals needed to break down the lactose in milk.

- *Reactions to food additives,* such as sulfites and MSG.

- *Reactions to substances occuring naturally in some foods,* such as tyramine in cheese, phenylethylamine in chocolate, caffeine in coffee, and some compounds in alcoholic beverages.

- *Food-borne illnesses.*

- *Unknown reactions* in people who have adverse symptoms that they attribute to foods and that may actually go away when treated as allergies but for which there is no evidence of a physiological basis for the reactions.[21]

Organic Foods

Mounting concerns about food safety have caused many people to try to protect themselves by refusing to buy processed foods and mass-produced agricultural products. Instead, they purchase foods that are **organically grown**—foods reported to be pesticide- and chemical-free. Though they are sold at premium prices, many of these products are of only average quality. They are probably not worth the money, according to most experts, for several reasons. First, whether food has been exposed to pesticides at some time in the production cycle is not as important as the residual pesticides in the food at the time you consume it. Obviously, too much of anything is potentially harmful, but if a "nonorganic" food has been sprayed and the poison has since evaporated, changed into a nontoxic compound, or been diluted below the point at which it can do any harm, the food may be no more harmful than a product labeled as "organic."[22] Second, even though so-called organic foods generally claim to be pesticide free, tests indicate that many contain pesticide residues in the same amounts as nonorganic foods.[23] These residues may be the result of pesticide drift from neighboring farms and water supplies, sneak sprays by unscrupulous producers, or soils that have residue from previous growers.

The bottom line is what is really in the food, not whether it is labeled as "organic," "natural," or "healthy." In fact, these labels are often placed on foods that are far from healthy and may actually be of very low quality. Although the ideals upon which the organic movement was founded are sound, more testing and regulation are needed before people can be assured that what they are paying high prices for is the real unadulterated thing—a pesticide-free product.

Cross reactivity: Allergic reaction to a whole family of foods.

Food intolerance: Adverse effects resulting when people who lack the digestive chemicals needed to break down certain substances eat those substances.

Organically grown: Foods that are grown without use of pesticides or chemicals.

Managing Your Eating Behavior

Let's face it. Eating for health is not easy. It takes knowledge, careful thought and analysis, and the ability to put it all together and make the best decisions for your own lifestyle and personal goals within certain budgetary limits. There are no shortcuts, and, as researchers sift through studies showing conflicting results, what is true today may turn out to be false tomorrow. But by paying attention; reading; seeking help from reputable, trained professionals; and planning ahead, you can increase your own nutritional health. The following recommendations will help you improve your nutritional status as well as the health of the environment:

Making Decisions for You

1. List the four biggest things about your current diet that you want to change.

2. Prioritize the items in the above list. Determine when you want to accomplish each item and outline a plan of action for accomplishing each goal.

3. List the little actions that you can take that may make a difference in your overall plan. List the big changes that you can make to accomplish your overall goals.

4. Based on your past history of trying to change these behaviors, what techniques do you think may be most likely to work for you? Indicate what you will use from these past tries and what you will do differently this time.

Checklist for Change: Making Personal Choices

✓ *Eat lower on the food chain.* Try to substitute fruits, vegetables, nuts, or grains for animal products at least once a day. By doing so, you will be helping to conserve the natural resources that an animal has to eat to become a table product for you.

✓ *Eat seasonal foods whenever possible.* By eating foods at the peak of harvest, you are most apt to avoid nutrient losses incurred by storage, freezing, canning, and so on. This practice will also help you avoid using high-energy (frozen, packaged) products during times of the year when it is unnecessary.

✓ *Eat lean.* The evidence against high-fat foods mounts daily. Pay attention to labels, assess your food intake, and balance high-fat meals with low-fat meals. Choose leaner cuts and bake, grill, boil, or broil whenever possible.

✓ *Increase your consumption of fruits and vegetables.* Use the real thing instead of juices and get more health for your money.

✓ *Combine foods for optimum nutrition.* Take the time to educate yourself about the best ways to combine grains, beans, fruits, vegetables, nuts, and other foods. You will

then be able to optimize dietary returns—an essential tool for eating for health. Ask your instructor for advice on this, or call your local home economics extension office for recommendations.

✓ *Practice responsible consumer safety.* Avoid unnecessary chemicals and buy, prepare, and store foods prudently to avoid food-borne illness.

✓ *Eat in moderation.* Learn to separate true hunger feelings from the food cravings that come from boredom. Recognize when your body is signaling that it is getting full, and stop eating. Don't undereat or overeat. Moderate your caloric consumption and reduce your consumption of sugars and other dietary "extras."

✓ *Keep your systems functioning well.* Even the best diets are doomed to failure if stress, drugs, lack of exercise, sleep deprivation, and other life problems are dragging your systems down, particularly your digestive system. If it doesn't operate properly, nutrients you eat may be wasted.

✓ *Keep dietary foods in balance.* Consume appropriate amounts of fats, carbohydrates, proteins, vitamins, minerals, amino acids, fatty acids, and water.

✓ *Pay attention to changing nutrient needs.* Illness, stress, aging, exercise, environmental conditions, pregnancy, and other factors in your life may require you to adjust your nutritional intake. Prepare for these changes and keep yourself informed about new, reputable sources of information concerning specific nutrient benefits and hazards.

Checklist for Change: Making Community Choices

✓ Pay attention to the types of eating establishments available on your campus. If you don't have the number of choices you think you should, take action. Involve your student newspaper and student organizations, talk with food service representatives, involve your student health service, and solicit the support of key campus representatives.

✓ Assess the priorities that your elected officials have for: nutrition in the schools, nutrition and the elderly, nutrition and pregnant women, nutrition and the homeless. Are they supporting actions to help insure adequate nutrition for high-risk groups? If not, why not? Write letters asking for clarification of their positions. Seek alternative candidates if these individuals do not represent your views.

✓ If you patronize certain food establishments, make recommendations for healthier food choices. Tell them when they are doing a good job and ask for other options.

(continued)

✓ Find out about government subsidized foods. Who is eligible for these programs? What is their purpose? What are their limitations? Strengths? Be informed about these programs. Support or refute them based on a sound information base rather than on emotional reactions.

✓ Be informed about key nutritional concepts. Speak up when you see information that is false and/or misleading. Demand accuracy in reported claims. Give advice only when you have taken the time to read and study the issues. Speak from a truly informed perspective. Read reliable nutritional sources. When in doubt, seek help from your university professors or experts in the community.

Critical Thinking

Nadeem and Sarah have been married for almost six months. Sarah came from the south and enjoys cooking large meals, many of them featuring fried foods. Nadeem, on the other hand, is from Iran. He is more used to eating dishes built around rice, fruits, and vegetables. He is concerned about their eating habits, especially the higher fat and cholesterol content. But he doesn't want to say anything that would affect their otherwise perfect marriage.

Using the DECIDE model described in Chapter 1, decide how Nadeem can open up a discussion about better eating without hurting Sarah's feelings.

Summary

◆ Recognizing that we eat for more reasons than just survival is the first step toward changing our health. The Food Guide Pyramid provides guidelines for healthy eating.

◆ The major nutrients that are essential for life and health include water, proteins, carbohydrates, fiber, fats, vitamins and minerals. RDAs and "% Daily Values" serve as guides to necessary amounts of nutrients.

◆ Vegetarianism can provide a healthy alternative for those wishing to cut fat from their diets or wanting to reduce animal consumption. The vegetarian pyramid provides dietary guidelines to help vegetarians obtain needed nutrients.

◆ College students face unique challenges in eating healthfully. Learning to make better choices at fast-food restaurants, eat healthily when funds are short, and eating nutritionally in the dorm are all possible when you use the knowledge contained in this chapter.

◆ Food irradiation, food allergies, food-borne illnesses, and other food-safety and health concerns are becoming increasingly important to health-wise consumers. Recognition of potential risks and active steps taken to prevent problems are part of a sound nutritional plan.

Discussion Questions

1. What are several factors that may influence the dietary patterns and behaviors of the typical college student? What factors have been the greatest influences on your eating behaviors? Why is it important that you know about your dietary influences as you think about changing your eating behaviors?

2. What are the six major food groups on the new Food Guide Pyramid? What groups might you find it difficult to get enough servings from? What can you do to increase/decrease your intake of selected food groups? What can you do to remember the six groups?

3. What are the major types of nutrients that you need to obtain from the foods you eat? What happens if you fail to get enough of some of these nutrients?

4. Distinguish between the different types of vegetarianism. Which types are most likely to lead to deficiencies? What can be done to insure that even the most strict vegetarian receives enough of the major nutrients?

5. What are the major problems that many college students face when trying to eat the right foods? List five actions that you and your classmates could take immediately to improve your eating.

6. What are the potential benefits and risks of food irradiation? Why is it being used? What are the major risks for food-borne illnesses and what can you do to protect yourself? How are food illnesses and food allergies different?

Application Exercise

Reread the What Do You Think? scenarios at the beginning of the chapter and answer the following questions:

1. Critique the eating habits of Bart, Talat, and Jasper. What suggestions could you make to help them? How could you make these suggestions in a way that won't offend them?

2. What do you think of Bart's attitude toward others' eating habits? What is likely to be influencing his thoughts/attitudes and behaviors?

3. What advice or help might you give to Talat? Why do people get to this stage of nutritional concern? What factors have probably influenced her thoughts/actions?

4. Is there anything Jasper can do to improve his eating situation? Do you think that his dorm food is really that unhealthy or that he just hasn't gotten used to it yet?

Further Reading

The Food and Drug Administration.

For general information, write to: Food Safety, Consumer Affairs Office (HFE-88), Food and Drug Administration, 5600 Fishers Lane, Rockville, MD 20857. For information on shellfish, write for "For Oyster and Clam Lovers, the Water Must Be Clean," a reprint from *FDA Consumer,* available from the FDA's Office of Public Affairs (HFI-40), 5600 Fishers Lane, Rockville, MD 20857.

U.S. Department of Agriculture.

For information on the proper handling of meat and poultry and other information, call the USDA's Meat and Poultry Hotline at the toll-free number (800)535-4555 between 10 A.M. and 4 P.M. on weekdays. Write to the Meat and Poultry Hotline, USDA-FSIS, Room 1165-S, Washington, DC, 20250 for a new booklet, *A Quick Consumer's Guide to Safe Food Handling.*

Nutrition Action Healthletter.

This newsletter, published 10 times a year, contains up-to-date information on diet and nutritional claims and current research issues. The newsletter can be obtained by writing to the Center for Science in the Public Interest, 1501 16th St. NW, Washington, DC 20036.

9

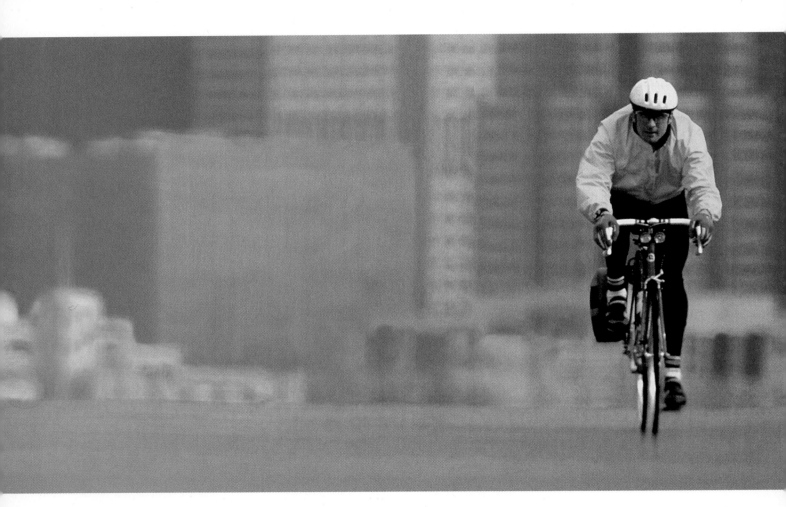

ℭHAPTER OBJECTIVES

◆ Describe how healthy weight is determined both by weight and in terms of body content; describe the major techniques for body content assessment.

◆ Describe those factors that place people at risk for problems with obesity.

◆ Discuss the roles of exercise, dieting, nutrition, "miracle diets," and other strategies in weight control.

◆ Describe the three major eating disorders and explain the health risks of these conditions.

Managing Your Weight

Finding a Healthy Balance

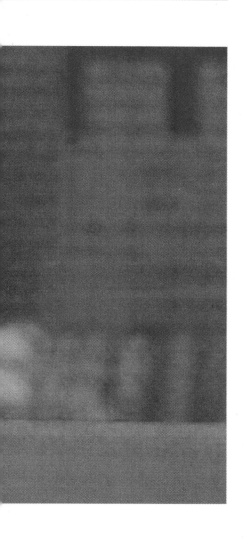

WHAT DO YOU THINK?

Ray, aged 20, is desperately trying to lose the 25 pounds he put on in his first year at college. During that year, he spent much of his time studying, made little time for exercise, and often rewarded his hard work with lunch, dinner, and snack breaks with his friends. Because he wants to lose the extra weight fast and be buff while wearing his swimsuit over spring break, Ray goes on a crash diet and begins an intense running and weight-lifting program. After three weeks on the diet, all his friends tell him how cool he is starting to look, and, bolstered by their support, Ray decides to cut his already-low food intake even more and to increase his exercise.

- What risks are associated with Ray's plan for rapid weight loss? Is his thinking typical or atypical of people you know on similar "fast" weight loss plans? What are his motivations for losing weight, and how do the opinions of others appear to influence him? As a friend, what could you do to ensure that Ray doesn't harm himself during his quest to lose weight?

Jessie is at her ideal weight and after being tested to determine her percentage of body fat, finds that she is well within the normal weight/fat range. Even after being told that she is okay, Jessie insists that she is a "fat slob" and begins a regular cycle of binging on food at the school cafeteria and coming back to her dorm room to vomit. She spends considerable amounts of time looking at her own body in the mirror and comparing herself to the models shown in fashion magazines.

- Why are so many young women in the United States preoccupied with their weight and body image? Do you know someone like Jessie? Is her preoccupation with her body like anyone else's you know? What factors do you think influence a person to have such a distorted image of what he or she really looks like? As a friend, what campus services or help might you recommend for someone in this situation? Do you know of any male friends who have similar problems? Why do women seem to be particularly vulnerable?

If you've never met a chocolate chip cookie you didn't like, you are probably one of the millions of Americans who seems to be trapped in a constant battle of the bulge. By all accounts, in spite of being part of a generation of health and fitness buffs who exercise, forsake high-fat foods, and mesmerize ourselves with self-help diet and fitness books, we are not doing better in our quest for health and fitness. In fact, according to results of a long-term National Health and Nutrition Examination Survey (NHANES III) conducted by the Centers for Disease Control and Prevention, the number of Americans who are seriously overweight, which had stayed stable for 20 years at about 25 percent of the population, exploded to about 35 percent of the population in the 1980s.[1] These data indicate that over 55 million people in the United States weigh at least 20 percent more than their ideal body weights, making them, in the unforgiving terminology of dietary science, *obese*.[2] For more of the results from the NHANES III survey, see the Health Headlines box.

All of this seems to be a slap in the face to the approximately 50 percent of American women and 25 percent of men who reported in the 1980s that they were out there dutifully trying to lose weight and get fit. What happened? Why did so many well-intentioned people obviously not succeed in their battles against the "fat monster" that seems to be stalking so many of us? Do the figures really tell the whole story? Have we really failed in our efforts?

What are all of these overweight Americans doing to shed their excess poundage? Many of them opt for nutritionally balanced diets that include sufficient amounts of exercise to burn the calories they consume. Others elect to get help from weight-loss gurus, trained professionals, or weight-loss franchises. Still others purchase questionable products and services that claim to help people "shed unsightly pounds fast and effortlessly." Some are starving themselves in pursuit of the perfect body. Finally, there is a group that has made several attempts at weight loss before giving up.

In fact, in spite of good intentions, few people get beyond the first few days of a weight-loss effort. Those who do continue on their weight-loss programs and take off a significant number of pounds tend to gain most of them back. Follow-up studies of people on controlled diets indicate that at least half of the weight lost is regained within two to four years.[3] A large national study of reports on weight-loss interventions from over 130 articles published between 1985 and 1991 found that over a typical 16-week intensive dietary regimen, people lost an average of 12.89 pounds, or less than .8 pounds per week, and that after several months, that initial weight loss had dropped to only .22 pounds per week.[4] Other research indicates that fewer than 5 percent of all those who lose weight keep it off permanently. For those of us planning to lose weight, these data are discouraging.

What's behind the American obsession with being thin? Have we become overly self-centered and preoccupied with our bodies, or are there very real health risks associated with being overweight that we should be concerned about? Why do so many of us have such a problem maintaining a healthy weight to begin with, and why are most of our efforts to lose weight doomed to failure? What does it take to take off the extra pounds and keep them off?

This chapter focuses on the American obsession with thinness and explores the reasons why so many of us seem to be trapped in overweight bodies that we can't escape from. It is designed to help you better understand what *overweight* and *obesity* really mean and why weight control is essential to your overall health. Finally, this chapter shows you how to develop strategies for controlling your own weight, losing weight, and yes, even for gaining weight if you are among that small group of underweight people who must struggle to put on needed pounds.

*B*ODY IMAGE

Most of us think of the obsession with thinness as a phenomenon of recent years. Beginning with supermodel Twiggy in the 1960s and continuing with supermodel Kate Moss in the 1990s, the thin look seems to dominate fashion ads. And not only that: Television, movies, and magazines constantly project images of lean, fit bodies. We have been led to believe that if we are thin, with shapely curves and well-defined muscles, we will be more desirable.

But the thin look has been around for a long time. Anorexia nervosa, an eating disorder, has been defined as a psychiatric disorder since 1873. During the Victorian era, corsets were used to achieve unrealistically tiny waists. By the 1920s, it was common knowledge that obesity was

Who's Getting Fatter?

Although the National Health and Nutrition Examination Survey (NHANES III) results focused mainly on adults over the age of 20, experts predict that researchers will find similar or possibly greater increases in obesity rates among children and adolescents. The percentage of teens who are overweight increased 6 percent, to a total of 21 percent by the early 1990s. Young adults in their 20s, 30s, and 40s appear to be among those who gain weight at the fastest rates. The average weight gain between ages 30 and 39 is 4 pounds for men and 9 pounds for women; these increases in weight also typically reflect increases in percentages of overall body fat. Although we often think it is the middle-aged and the elderly who are most prone to gain weight, several studies have shown that weight gain is highest for those in the 25 to 34 age group, and that women gain more weight than men in virtually all age groups.

Weight and Culture

Anyone who has ever traveled extensively has probably noted that in some places, rotund people seem to abound; in others areas, thin is definitely "in." NHANES III provided even more credence to the argument that some groups seem to have the most obese individuals. For instance, those in the lowest socioeconomic classes have nearly five times the rate of obesity as those in the highest socioeconomic classes. The groups having the highest proportion of overweight people were black, non-Hispanic women (49 percent) and Mexican-American women (47 percent). While more women of color were obese, it is important to note that both white (up 9 percent to 33.5 percent total) and nonwhite (up 4 percent among black women and 7 percent for Mexican-American women) groups have increased their weight since a similar study conducted in the 1980s. White men also showed a steep increase in obesity rates. In some Native-American communities, up to 70 percent of all adults are dangerously overweight.

Dietary experts indicate that the levels of obesity among minority women could be explained, at least in part, by culture. This notion supports the idea that there may be a greater tolerance in given cultures for a bigger body and that bigger is actually better in some settings. Other professionals suggest that obesity may be more common among lower-income and less-educated people because they eat a lower-cost diet that is higher in fat and because they lack access to parks and other safe places where they can exercise regularly. Each of these theories is controversial.

In many cultures, by contrast, the rich are fat and the poor are emaciated. George Armelagos, of Emory University, calls it the "Henry the Eighth syndrome," referring to the corpulent king of England who lived so well off the labor of his peasantry. Being rotund is still a sign of prosperity and prestige in Polynesia, parts of Africa, and other regions of the world.

Source: **Most of box adapted courtesy of the** *Boston Globe.* **From Alison Bass, "Record Obesity Levels Found,"** *Boston Globe,* **20 July 1995, 1, 10. Last paragraph adapted from Philip Elmer-Dewitt, "Fat Times,"** *Time,* **16 January 1995, 63–64.**

---

linked to poor health. The American Tobacco Company coined the phrase "reach for a Lucky instead of a sweet" to promote the idea that cigarettes dulled appetite. American Tobacco even formed the Moderation League to promote the virtues of moderation in, among other things, eating.

Today, beautiful female models in size 4 clothes and underweight Miss Americas exemplify desirability and success, delivering the subtle message that thin is in. In addition, organizations such as the American Heart Association and the American Cancer Society bombard us with straightforward warnings that being overweight increases our risk of heart disease, certain types of cancer, arthritis, gallbladder disease, diabetes, poor emotional health, and a host of other problems that decrease our life expectancy. What's a body to do?

In response to our rational and emotional quests to be thin, a multibillion-dollar diet industry has developed, purveying liquid diets, freeze-dried foods, nonfat and low-fat foods, artificial sweeteners, diet books by the hundreds, and a host of weight-loss clinics. We are offered devices that are supposed to "melt away," "burn away," and "jiggle away" fat, and pills that claim to "burn fat" while you eat whatever you like and avoid exercise. While some advertised claims are valid, others are designed to make big profits at your expense.

How do you find a safe, effective means of losing those extra pounds? A good way to start is by gathering accurate information about weight-loss products and services, learning what triggers your "eat" buttons, and analyzing your lifestyle to determine your problem areas. Developing the skills to set rational weight-loss goals and taking advantage of social and community supports are also part of the process.

Determining the Right Weight for You

The answer to whether you are overweight is somewhat subjective and depends on your body structure and how your weight is distributed. Traditionally, people have

The media, the fashion and fitness industries, health organizations, and even the food industry have all contributed to the American obsession with being thin.

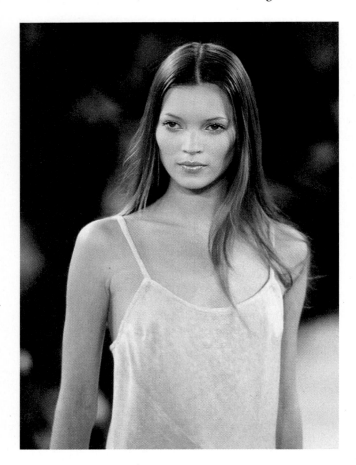

compared their weight with data from some form of standard height-and-weight chart. These charts usually give the "ideal" weight for males and females of given height and frame size. In general, if you are 20 to 30 percent above your ideal weight, as indicated by the chart, you would be classified as obese.

One of the most reliable height-weight guides is the Metropolitan Life Height and Weight Table, which is reproduced in Table 9.1. Note that the tables do not indicate a relationship between weight and quality of life, total health, vitality, or appearance. Nor do they provide an indication of the ratio of body fat to lean muscle mass,

Obesity: A weight disorder generally defined as an accumulation of fat beyond that considered normal for a person's age, sex, and body type.

which is the real indicator of how fat a person really is. Nevertheless, they are still the most commonly used measure of weight status.

Another formula for people between the ages of 18 and 25 establishes reasonable weights of 110 pounds for a 5-foot-tall man and 100 pounds for a 5-foot-tall woman. For each inch over 5 feet, men and women should add 5 pounds. In addition, a woman should subtract 1 pound for each year under 25.

Redefining Obesity: Weight versus Fat Content

In recent years, diagnosticians have revised their definition of obesity. Although body weight is certainly an important factor, they believe that the real indicator of obesity is how much fat your body contains (see Figure 9.1). A male weight lifter may be 30 to 40 percent overweight according to the charts and yet still not be obese because of the heaviness and relative density of his muscle tissue. Similarly, a 40-year-old woman who prides herself on weighing the same 130 pounds that she did in high school may be shocked to learn that her body now contains over 40 percent fat compared to 15 percent fat in

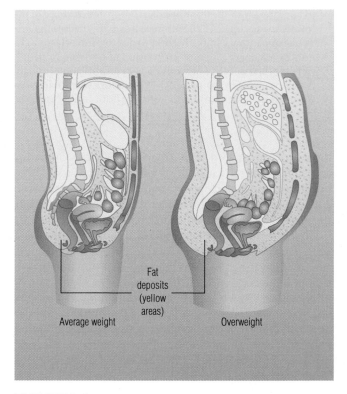

FIGURE 9.1

The figure compares an average-weight person and an overweight person. Note the fat deposits under the skin and around the internal organs.

TABLE 9.1 ■ Ideal Weights Based on Body Frame

Weights at ages 25 to 29 based on lowest mortality. Weights in pounds according to frame, in indoor clothing weighing 5 pounds for men and 3 pounds for women, shoes with 1-inch heels.

Men					Women				
Height		Small Frame	Medium Frame	Large Frame	Height		Small Frame	Medium Frame	Large Frame
Feet	Inches				Feet	Inches			
5	2	128–134	131–141	138–150	4	10	102–111	109–121	118–131
5	3	130–136	133–143	140–153	4	11	103–113	111–123	120–134
5	4	132–138	135–145	142–156	5	0	104–115	113–126	122–137
5	5	134–140	137–148	144–160	5	1	106–118	115–129	125–140
5	6	136–142	139–151	146–164	5	2	108–121	118–132	128–143
5	7	138–145	142–154	149–168	5	3	111–124	121–135	131–147
5	8	140–148	145–157	152–172	5	4	114–127	124–138	134–151
5	9	142–151	148–160	155–176	5	5	117–130	127–141	137–155
5	10	144–154	151–163	158–180	5	6	120–133	130–144	140–159
5	11	146–157	154–166	161–184	5	7	123–136	133–147	143–163
6	0	149–160	157–170	164–188	5	8	126–139	136–150	146–167
6	1	152–164	160–174	168–192	5	9	129–142	139–153	149–170
6	2	155–168	164–178	172–197	5	10	132–145	142–156	152–173
6	3	158–172	167–182	176–202	5	11	135–148	145–159	155–176
6	4	162–176	171–187	181–207	6	0	138–151	148–162	158–179

Source: Reproduced with permission of Metropolitan Life Insurance Company, *1983 Build Study,* Society of Actuaries and Association of Life Insurance Medical Directors of America, 1984.

her high school days. Weight by itself, although a useful guide, is not a valid indicator of obesity.

A more accurate assessment of total body fat requires a different type of measurement. If traditional height-weight charts do not accurately define obesity, what general guidelines should be applied for determining acceptable levels of body fat? **Obesity** is generally defined as an accumulation of fat beyond what is considered normal for a person's age, sex, and body type. The difficulty lies in defining what is normal. To date, there are no universally accepted standards for the most "desirable" or "ideal" body weight or body composition (ratio of lean body mass to fat body mass). We will discuss body composition in more detail later in the chapter.

Although sources vary slightly, most agree that men's bodies should contain between 11 and 15 percent total body fat, and women should be within the range of 18 to 22 percent body fat. A man would be considered obese if his body fat exceeded 20 percent of his total body mass. A woman would be considered obese if her body fat exceeded 30 percent of her total body mass.[5] Table 9.2 provides general guidelines for determining how adults aged 18 to 30 compare in terms of overall percentages of body fat.

Why the difference between men and women? Much of it may be attributed to the normal structure of the female body and to sex hormones. As mentioned earlier, when considering how much or how little fat a person should have, it is important to think of body composition in terms of lean body mass and body fat. Lean body mass is made up of the structural and functional elements in cells, body water, muscle, bones, and other body organs

TABLE 9.2 ■ General Ratings of Body Fat Percentages by Age and Gender

Rating	Males (ages 18–30) (percent)	Females (ages 18–30) (percent)
Athletic*	6–10	10–15
Good	11–14	16–19
Acceptable	15–17	20–24
Overfat	18–19	25–29
Obese	20 or over	30 or over

*The ratings in the athletic category are general guidelines for those athletes, such as gymnasts and long-distance runners, whose need for a "competitive edge" in selected sports may compel them to try to lose as much weight as possible. However, for the average person, such low body fat levels should be approached with caution.

such as the heart, liver, and kidneys. Body fat is composed of two types: essential fat and storage fat. Essential fat is necessary for normal physiological functioning, such as nerve conduction. Essential fat makes up approximately 3 to 7 percent of total body weight in men and approximately 15 percent of total body weight in women. Storage fat, the part that many of us are always trying to shed, makes up the remainder of our fat reserves. It accounts for only a small percentage of total body weight for very lean people and between 5 and 25 percent of body weight of most American adults. Female bodybuilders, who are among the leanest of female athletes, may have body fat percentages ranging from 8 to 13 percent, nearly all of which is essential fat.

Although most of us continually try to reduce our body fat, there are levels below which we dare not go. A minimal amount of body fat is necessary for insulation of the body, for cushioning between parts of the body and vital organs, and for maintaining body functions. In men, this lower limit is approximately 3 to 4 percent. Women should generally not go below 8 percent. Excessively low body fat in females may lead to amenorrhea, a disruption of the normal menstrual cycle. The critical level of body fat necessary to maintain normal menstrual flow is believed to be between 8 and 13 percent, but there are numerous exceptions to this rule and many additional factors that affect the menstrual cycle. Under extreme circumstances, such as starvation diets and certain diseases, the body often utilizes all available fat reserves and begins to break down muscle tissue as a last-ditch effort to obtain nourishment.

While some of us like to say that we are storing up fat to protect ourselves from the great food shortages of the future, there are limits to the plausibility of this argument! The fact is that too much fat and too little fat are both potentially harmful. The key is to find a level at which you are not at high risk for health problems and at which you are comfortable with your appearance.

Assessing Your Body Content

With all of the techniques available for calculating how fat you really are, how do you decide which is the best for you? Perhaps the best way is to ask yourself how much an exact measure of your body fat means to you. If you are interested in obtaining the most accurate measure before and after a program of diet and exercise, you may find the expense of some of the more sophisticated measures worth the investment. If you simply want a general idea of how much body fat you are carrying around, an inexpensive pinch test or skinfold measure may be all that you need. On the other hand, if you know, based on the bulges around your middle or the size and fit of your jeans, that you are obese, perhaps the exact amount of fat that you have does not matter as much as the fact that you need to take action.

Hydrostatic Weighing Techniques.   From a clinical perspective, the most accurate method of measuring body fat is through **hydrostatic weighing techniques.** This method measures the amount of water a person displaces when completely submerged. Because fat tissue has a lower density than muscle or bone tissue, a relatively accurate indication of actual body fat can be computed by comparing a person's underwater and out-of-water weights. Although this method may be subject to errors, it is one of the most sophisticated techniques currently available.

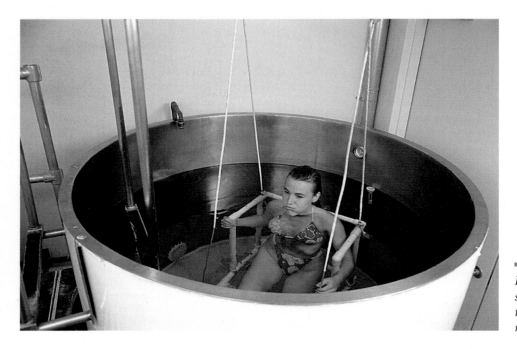

Hydrostatic weighing is the most sophisticated and accurate technique currently available to measure body fat.

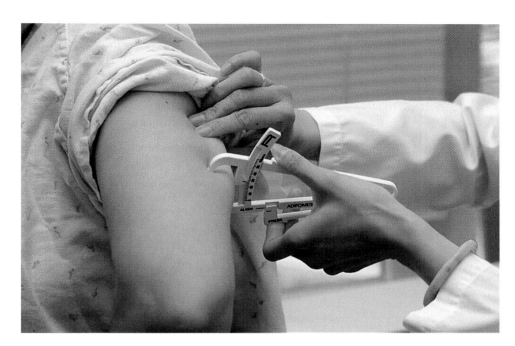

In the hands of a trained professional, the skin fold caliper can give an accurate measure of body fat for people who are not overly obese.

Pinch and Skinfold Measures. Perhaps the most commonly used method of body fat determination is the **pinch test**. Numerous studies have determined that the triceps area (located in the back of the upper arm) is one of the most reliable areas of the body for assessing the amount of fat in the subcutaneous (just under the surface) layer of the skin. In making this assessment, a person pinches a fold of skin just behind the triceps with the thumb and index finger. It is important to pinch only the fat layer and not the triceps muscle. After selecting a spot for measure, the person assesses the distance between the thumb and index finger. If the size of the pinch appears to be thicker than 1 inch, the person is generally considered overfat. Another technique, the **skinfold caliper test**, resembles the pinch test but is much more accurate. In this procedure, a person pinches folds of skin at various points on the body with the thumb and index finger. This technique uses a specially calibrated instrument called a *skinfold caliper* to take a precise measurement of the fat layer. Besides the triceps area, the points most often used in these measurements are the biceps area (front of the arm), the subscapular area (upper back), and the iliac crest (hip). Once these data points are assessed, special formulas are employed to arrive at a combined prediction of total body fat. In the hands of trained technicians, this procedure can be fairly accurate. If the person doing the test is inconsistent about the exact locations of the pinch or if there is difficulty in determining the difference between fat and muscle, the results may be inaccurate. In addition, the heavier a person is, the more prone this technique is to error. For chronically obese people, difficulties in assessment are magnified because of problems with distinguishing between flaccid muscles and fat. Also, most currently available calipers do not expand far enough to obtain accurate measurements on the moderately obese (20 to 40 percent overweight) or the morbidly obese (more than 50 percent overweight). Additional errors in skinfold assessments may occur as a result of failure to account for certain age, sex, and ethnic differences in calibrations.

Girth and Circumference Measures. Another common method of body fat assessment is the use of **girth and circumference measures**. Diagnosticians use a measuring tape to take girth, or circumference, measurements at various body sites. These measurements are then converted into constants, and a formula is used to determine relative percentages of body fat. Although this technique is inexpensive, easy to use, and commonly performed, it is not as accurate as many of the other techniques listed here.

Hydrostatic weighing techniques: Methods of determining body fat by measuring the amount of water displaced when a person is completely submerged.

Pinch test: A method of determining body fat whereby a fold of skin just behind the triceps is pinched between the thumb and index finger to determine the relative amount of fat.

Skinfold caliper test: A method of determining body fat whereby folds of skin and fat at various points on the body are grasped between thumb and forefinger and measured with calipers.

Girth and circumference measures: A method of assessing body fat that employs a formula based on girth measurements of various body sites.

Body Mass Index. One of the more widely accepted approaches to weight assessment is a technique developed by the National Center for Health Statistics called the **body mass index (BMI)**. Because the BMI is an index of the relationship of weight to height, which is based on a norm of adults between the ages of 20 and 29, it is probably one of the best assessments for most college students.

Although many people recoil in fright when they see that they have to convert pounds to kilograms and inches to meters to calculate BMI, it really is not as difficult as it may seem. To get your kilogram weight, just divide your weight in pounds (without shoes or clothing) by 2.2. To convert your height to meters squared, divide your height in inches (without shoes) by 39.4, then square this result. Sounds pretty easy and it is. Once you have these basic values, calculating your BMI involves dividing your weight in kilograms by your height in meters squared:

$$\text{BMI} = \frac{\text{Weight (in lbs)} \div 2.2 \text{ (to determine weight in Kg)}}{(\text{Height (in inches)} \div 39.4)^2 \text{ (to determine height in meters squared)}}$$

Although this formula may seem difficult for the average non–metric-oriented person, the several calculations it requires are really quite simple. In general, a BMI range of 20 to 24 is considered normal. The desirable range for females is 21 to 23; for males, it is 22 to 24. BMI values above 27.8 for men and 27.3 for women have been associated with increased health problems, including high blood pressure and diabetes. The American Dietetic Association, in an early position statement on nutrition and physical fitness, classified people having BMIs greater than 30 as obese and those having BMIs greater than 40 as morbidly obese and in need of prompt medical attention[6] (see Figure 9.2).

Soft-Tissue Roentgenogram. A relatively new technique for body fat determination, the **soft-tissue roentgenogram**, involves injecting a radioactive substance into the body and allowing this substance to penetrate muscle (lean) tissue so distinctions between fat and lean tissue can be made by means of imaging.

Bioelectrical Impedance Analysis. Another method of determining body fat levels, **bioelectrical impedance analysis (BIA)**, involves sending a small electric current through the subject's body. The amount of resistance to the current, along with the person's age, sex, and other physical characteristics, is then fed into a computer that uses special formulas to determine the total amount of lean and fat tissue.

Total Body Electrical Conductivity. One of the newest (and most expensive) assessment techniques is **total body electrical conductivity (TOBEC)**, which uses an electromagnetic force field to assess relative body fat. Although based on the same principle as impedance, this assessment requires much more elaborate, expensive equipment, and therefore is not practical for most people.

Although all of these methods can be useful, they can also be inaccurate and even harmful unless the testers are skillful and well trained. Before agreeing to any procedure, be sure you are aware of the expense, potential for accuracy, risks, and training of the tester.

*W*HAT DO YOU THINK?

Why is it important to consider your percentage of body fat rather than weight only when determining how fat you really are? Which of the above tests would you feel comfortable taking? Would any make you feel uncomfortable?

*R*ISK FACTORS FOR OBESITY

For many of us, the reason for obesity is quite simple: If you take in more calories than you burn up, you will gain weight. If you do this throughout your life, you will become increasingly obese. If we know what the cause is, we should be able to offer a simple prescription for preventing the problem. Right? Wrong.

Although the calorie explanation of obesity is certainly valid, it offers only one possible reason for a person's weight problem. It does not explain the many additional factors that contribute to the problem and that may make the possibility of permanent weight loss very unlikely. It also fails to answer many other critical questions. If we know that eating too much will cause us to gain weight, why do we continue to eat too much? Is there a metabolic explanation for obesity? Why do fewer than 5 percent of all people who go on a weight loss program achieve permanent success? Is pushing yourself away from the table the best exercise for maintaining your weight?

Heredity

Body Type and Genes. In some animal species, the shape and size of the individual's body is largely determined by the shape and size of its parents' bodies. Many scientists have explored the role of heredity in determining human body shapes. As early as 1940, Harvard psychologist William Sheldon analyzed weight problems in terms of genetically determined body types. His studies indicated that people having an ectomorphic body type, characterized by tall, slender frames, generally experienced few difficulties with weight control. People with an endomorphic body type, characterized by a rounded, soft appearance, often had a large abdomen and typically reported a history of weight problems beginning in childhood. Between these two extremes was the shorter, more

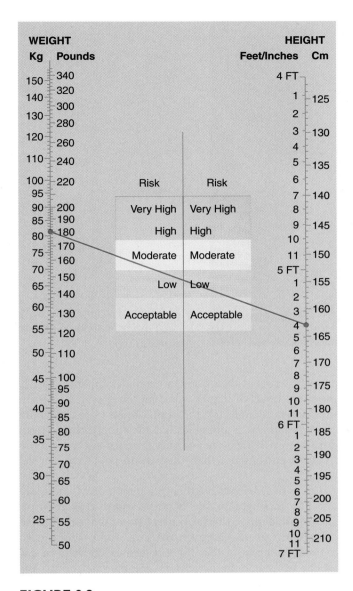

WEIGHT

Kg Pounds

HEIGHT

Feet/Inches Cm

FIGURE 9.2

Are you overweight? To find out if your current level of fatness increases your chances of dying early, angle a pencil or the edge of a piece of paper from your weight (on the left) to your height (on the right). Read your risk where the pencil crosses the center line.

muscular, and athletic-looking mesomorphic body type. Leaner and more active than endomorphs in early adulthood, mesomorphs demonstrated a strong tendency to gain weight later in life.[7]

Some researchers still support Sheldon's theories identifying body type as a major factor in the development of weight problems, but most contend that heredity plays a more subtle role in obesity. These researchers argue that obesity has a strong genetic determinant (it tends to run in families). They cite statistics showing that 80 percent of children having two obese parents are also obese.[8] But why is this the case? Can you really blame your parents for your problems with weight?

Twin Studies. Studies of identical twins who were separated at birth and raised in different environments have provided us with some of the most conclusive evidence to date that obesity may be an inherited trait. Whether raised in family environments with fat or thin family members, twins with obese natural parents tend to be obese in later life.[9] According to another study, sets of identical twins who were separated and raised in different families and who ate widely different diets still grew up to weigh about the same.[10] So, if you are overweight, you cannot blame it all on your parents for overfeeding you as a child.

These studies contain the strongest evidence yet that the genes a person inherits are the major factor determining overweight, leanness, or average weight. Although the exact mechanics remain unknown, it is believed that genes set metabolic rates, influencing how the body handles calories.

Genetic Predisposition and Environmental Factors. Health professionals are concerned that these studies will convince many overweight people that they are doomed to be fat. However, Albert Stunkard, a psychiatrist at the University of Pennsylvania and author of one of these studies, believes that, on the contrary, their conclusions offer hope to those whose extra pounds have been blamed on their lack of willpower or hidden psychological needs. In Stunkard's study, early family environment had no apparent effect on adult weight. Based on this finding, Stunkard discounts previous theories that the amount children eat early in life helps determine whether they will be fat as adults. According to Stunkard, it is not the family environment in which you were raised but the environment in which you live as an adult that determines whether you will be a fat adult. He says that people who are overweight can now be told, "It is very largely due to your genes. You are more vulnerable than others; there-

Body mass index (BMI): A technique of weight assessment based on the relationship of weight to height.

Soft-tissue roentgenogram: A technique of body fat assessment in which radioactive substances are used to determine relative fat.

Bioelectrical impedance analysis (BIA): A technique of body fat assessment in which electrical currents are passed through fat and lean tissue.

Total body electrical conductivity (TOBEC): Technique using an electromagnetic force field to assess relative body fat.

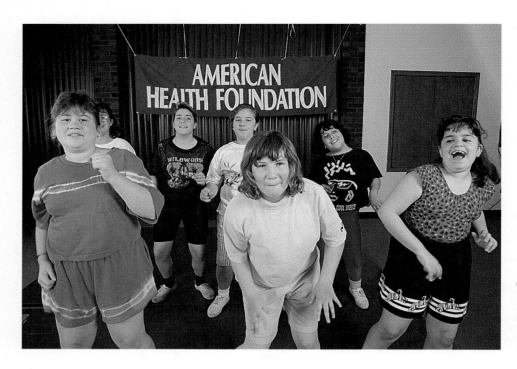

Heredity and genetic makeup, environmental factors, and learned eating patterns all play a role in obesity.

fore your actions may be even more critical than those of your genetically prone thin friends." In other words, diet and exercise will work to modify the genetic effect.[11]

Errant Eating Cues and Thrifty Genes. In November 1994, researchers at Rockefeller University reported that they had discovered a defective gene that disrupts the body's "I've had enough to eat" signaling system and may be responsible for a least some types of obesity.[12] Research on Pima Indians, who have an estimated 75 percent of their tribes that are obese and nine in ten who are overweight seems to point to an OB gene that is a *"thrifty gene."* It is theorized that as certain groups had to struggle during hard times and famines over the centuries, those people who had slower metabolic activity, which allowed them to store precious fat, survived. They passed their genes on to their descendents, which may predispose these descendents to be slow burners.[13] In times of plenty, it seems inevitable that these people will gain weight, unless they eat much less than the norm.

All studies concerning obesity and heredity are controversial because it is impossible to conduct the controlled trials that might prove heredity's role. It is still unclear whether any of these studies indicates a genetic predisposition toward obesity; learned eating habits may be just as important.

Hunger, Appetite, and Satiety

Theories abound concerning the mechanisms that regulate food intake. Some sources indicate that the hypothal-amus (the part of the brain that regulates appetite) closely monitors levels of certain nutrients in the blood. When these levels begin to fall, the brain signals us to eat. In the obese person, it is possible that the monitoring system does not work properly and that the cues to eat are more frequent and intense than they are in people of normal weight.

Other sources indicate that thin people may send more effective messages to the hypothalamus. This concept, known as **adaptive thermogenesis**, states that thin people can often consume large amounts of food without gaining weight because the appetite center of their brains speeds up metabolic activity to compensate for the increased consumption. More recent studies have indicated the possibility that specialized types of fat cells, called **brown fat cells**, may send signals to the brain, which controls the thermogenesis response.

The hypothesis that food tastes better to obese people, thus causing them to eat more, has largely been refuted. Scientists do distinguish, however, between **hunger**, an inborn physiological response to nutritional needs, and **appetite**, a learned response to food that is tied to an emotional or psychological craving for food often unrelated to nutritional need. Obese people may be more likely than thin people to satisfy their appetite and eat for reasons other than nutrition.

In some instances, the problem with overconsumption may be more related to **satiety** than to appetite or hunger. People generally feel satiated, or full, when they have satisfied their nutritional needs and their stomach signals "no more." For undetermined reasons, obese people may not feel full until much later than thin people.

Developmental Factors

Some obese people may have excessive numbers of fat cells. This type of obesity, **hyperplasia**, usually begins to develop in early childhood and perhaps, due to the mother's dietary habits, even prior to birth. The most critical periods for the development of hyperplasia seem to be the last two to three months of fetal development, the first year of life, and between the ages of 9 and 13. Parents who allow their children to eat without restrictions and to become overweight may be setting their children up for a lifelong excess of fat cells. Central to this theory is the belief that the number of fat cells in a person's body does not increase appreciably during adulthood. However, the ability of each of these cells to swell and shrink, known as **hypertrophy**, does carry over into adulthood. Weight gain may be tied to both the number of fat cells in the body and the capacity of each individual cell to enlarge.

An average-weight adult has approximately 25 billion to 30 billion fat cells, a moderately obese adult about 60 billion to 100 billion, and an extremely obese adult as many as 200 billion.[14] People who add large numbers of fat cells to their bodies in childhood may be able to lose weight by decreasing the size of each cell in adulthood, but the large numbers of cells remain, and with the next calorie binge, they fill up and sabotage weight loss efforts (see Figure 9.3). Additional research must be conducted to determine the accuracy of these theories.

Setpoint Theory

In 1982, nutritional researchers William Bennett and Joel Gurin presented a highly controversial theory concerning the difficulty some people have in losing weight. Their theory, known as the **setpoint theory**, states that a person's body has a setpoint of weight at which it is programmed to be comfortable. If your setpoint is around 160 pounds, you will gain and lose weight fairly easily within a given range of that point. For example, if you gain 5 to 10 pounds on vacation, it will be fairly easy to lose that weight and remain around the 160-pound mark for a long period of time. Some people have equated this point with the **plateau** that is sometimes reached after a person on a diet loses a certain amount of weight. The setpoint theory proposes that after losing a predetermined amount of weight, the body will actually sabotage additional weight loss by slowing down metabolism. In extreme cases, the metabolic rate will decrease to a point at which the body will maintain its weight on as little as 1,000 calories per day. Can a person change this predetermined setpoint? Proponents of this theory argue that it is possible to raise one's setpoint over time by continually gaining weight and failing to exercise. Conversely, reducing caloric intake and exercising over a long period of time can slowly decrease one's setpoint. Exercise may be

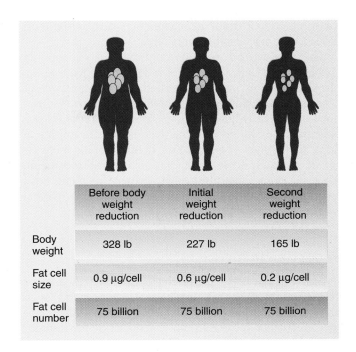

	Before body weight reduction	Initial weight reduction	Second weight reduction
Body weight	328 lb	227 lb	165 lb
Fat cell size	0.9 µg/cell	0.6 µg/cell	0.2 µg/cell
Fat cell number	75 billion	75 billion	75 billion

FIGURE 9.3

The figure depicts one person at various stages of weight loss. Note that, according to theories of hyperplasia, the number of fat cells remains constant but their size decreases.

Adaptive thermogenesis: Theoretical mechanism by which the brain regulates metabolic activity according to caloric intake.

Brown fat cells: Specialized type of fat cell that affects the ability to regulate fat metabolism.

Hunger: An inborn physiological response to nutritional needs.

Appetite: A learned response that is tied to an emotional or psychological craving for food that is often unrelated to nutritional need.

Satiety: The feeling of fullness or satisfaction at the end of a meal.

Hyperplasia: A condition characterized by an excessive number of fat cells.

Hypertrophy: The ability of fat cells to swell and shrink.

Setpoint theory: A theory of obesity causation that suggests that fat storage is determined by a thermostatic mechanism in the body that acts to maintain a specific amount of body fat.

Plateau: That point in a weight-loss program at which the dieter finds it difficult to lose more weight.

the most critical factor in readjusting your setpoint, although diet may also be important.

This theory, too, remains controversial. Perhaps its greatest impact was the sense of relief it provided for people who have lost weight, plateaued, and regained weight time and time again. It told them that their failure was not due to a lack of willpower alone. The setpoint theory also prompted nutritional experts to look more carefully at popular methods of weight loss. If the setpoint theory is correct, a low-calorie or starvation diet, besides being dangerous, may cause the body to protect the dieter from "starvation" by slowing down metabolism and making weight loss more difficult.

Endocrine Influence

Over the years, many people have attributed obesity to problems with their **thyroid glands**. They claimed that an underactive thyroid impeded their ability to burn calories. This belief substituted an organic cause for individual responsibility for obesity. How many obesity problems may justifiably be blamed on a poorly functioning thyroid? Most authorities agree that only 3 to 5 percent of the obese population have a thyroid problem.

Psychosocial Factors

The relationship of weight problems to deeply rooted emotional insecurities, needs, and wants remains uncertain. Food is often used as a reward for good behavior in childhood. As adults face unemployment, broken relationships, financial uncertainty, fears about health and other problems, the bright spot in the day is often "what's on the table for dinner," or, "we're going to that restaurant tonight." Again, the research underlying this theory is controversial. What is certain is that in mainstream America, eating tends to be a focal point of people's lives. Eating is essentially a social ritual associated with companionship, celebration, and enjoyment. The intimate dinner for two, the office party complete with snacks, and the picnic at the beach all center on eating. Is it any wonder that for many people the social emphasis on the eating experience is a major obstacle to successful dieting? Although some restaurants offer menu items designed to aid dieters, many people have difficulty choosing responsibly when confronted with an entire menu of delicious, fattening foods. Also, some people have trouble paying for health food because they associate eating out and paying with pleasurable "comfort" food that is often high in fat and calories.

Some theorists have contended that obese people tend to ignore internal cues of hunger and are more likely to use the clock as a guide for "time to eat" than real hunger cues. Other studies refute this hypothesis.

Eating Cues: Targeted by the Food Industry

At least one major factor in our preoccupation with food is the pressure placed on us by the highly sophisticated, heavily advertised "eating" campaigns launched by the food industry. There may be salad bars at the local fast-food joints, but customers have to run the gauntlet of starchy, beefy delights and tasty high-fat super-size fries to find them. According to the USDA, the food and restaurant industries spend $36 billion a year on ads designed to entice hungry people to forgo fresh fruit and sliced vegetables for Ring Dings and Happy Meals.[15] The average child, says psychologist Kelly Brownell, head of the Yale University Center for Eating and Weight Disorders, watches 10,000 food ads a year on TV. "And they're not seeing commercials for brussels sprouts," Brownell complains. "They're seeing soft drinks, candy bars, sugar-coated cereals and fast food."[16]

An increasing percentage (up over 13 percent in the 1980s) of the foods we eat are from fast-food restaurants. This is unfortunate because (1) fast food is high in calories, fat, sodium, and carbohydrates; (2) it tends to get eaten, even though portions are often much bigger than they should be; and (3) it tends to be eaten quickly, so there isn't enough time for the "I'm full" signal to get to your mouth before the last bite of food is there.[17] This is a particular problem for college students who now face the temptation of fast-food courts right on campus.

Lack of Awareness: Dietary Myth and Misperception

You've all heard the story: "I eat like a bird, but I can't lose weight." Should you believe the person who says this? Probably not, according to a recent study analyzing the self-reported and actual caloric intakes and exercise expenditures of a group of overweight adults. The researchers carefully followed obese people who had been unsuccessful following as many as 20 diets, thought they claimed that they consumed fewer than 1,200 calories per day. They blamed their failure on "metabolism." It turned out that their metabolism levels were normal, but that they were actually eating nearly twice as much as they thought they were and exercising only three-quarters as much as they reported.[18] Does this mean that obesity is simply the result of gluttony and sloth? Are obese people the only ones who underestimate their caloric intake and overestimate the amount of exercise they do? No. In fact, many studies have shown that obese individuals do not eat much more than their normal-weight counterparts. However, it should be noted that they do exercise less. The majority of overweight individuals are less active than nonobese people. Of course, it could be argued that it is their obesity that leads to their sedentary lifestyle. Much more research is necessary before scientists really have a clear profile of both the obese and nonobese.

Metabolic Changes

Even when completely at rest, the body needs a certain amount of energy. The amount of energy your body uses at complete rest is known as your **basal metabolic rate (BMR)**. About 60 to 70 percent of all the calories you consume on a given day go to support your basal metabolism: heartbeat, breathing, maintaining body temperature, and so on. So if you are consuming about 2,000 calories per day, between 1,200 and 1,400 of those calories are burned without your doing any significant physical activity. But unless you exert yourself enough to burn the remaining 600 to 800 calories, you will gain weight. Your BMR can fluctuate considerably, with several factors influencing whether it slows down or speeds up. In general, the younger you are, the higher your BMR, partly because in young people cells undergo rapid subdivision, which consumes a good deal of energy. BMR is highest during infancy, puberty, and pregnancy, when bodily changes are most rapid. BMR is also influenced by body composition. Muscle tissue is highly active—even at rest—compared to fat tissue. In essence, the more lean tissue you have, the greater your BMR and the more fat tissue you have, the lower your BMR. Men have a higher BMR than women do, at least partly because of their greater tendency toward lean tissue.

Age is another factor that may greatly affect BMR. After the age of 30, your BMR slows down by about 1 to 2 percent a year. Therefore, people over 30 commonly find that they must work harder to burn off an extra helping of ice cream than they did when they were in their teens. "Middle-aged spread," a reference to the tendency to put on weight after the age of 30, is partly related to this change. A slower BMR, coupled with an inclination to be less active and priorities (family and career) that come before fitness and weight, puts many middle-aged people's weight in jeopardy.

In addition, the body has a number of self-protective mechanisms that signal BMR to speed up or slow down. For example, when you have a fever, the energy needs of your cells increase, and this increased activity generates heat and speeds up your BMR. In starvation situations, the body tries to protect itself by slowing down BMR to conserve precious energy. Thus, when people repeatedly resort to extreme diets, their bodies "reset" their BMRs at lower rates. **Yo-yo diets**, in which people repeatedly gain weight and then starve themselves to lose the weight, lowering their BMR in the process, are doomed to failure. When they begin to eat again after the weight loss, they have a BMR that is set lower, making it almost certain that they will regain the weight they just lost. After repeated cycles of such dieting/regaining, these people find it in-creasingly hard to lose weight and increasingly easy to regain it, so they become heavier and heavier.

According to a recent study by Kelly Brownell, of Yale University, middle-aged men who maintained a steady weight (even if they were overweight) had a lower risk of heart attack than men whose weight cycled up and down in a yo-yo pattern. Brownell found that smaller, well-maintained weight losses are more beneficial for reducing cardiovascular risk than larger, poorly maintained weight losses.[19]

Finally, certain hormones, particularly the stress hormones, may cause BMR to rise in response to increased nervous activity and energy requirements by the cells.

Lifestyle

Of all the factors affecting obesity, perhaps the most critical is the relationship between activity levels and calorie intake. Obesity rates are rising. But how can this be happening? Aren't more people exercising than ever before? While it may look like it, the facts are not so positive. According to a recent Centers for Disease Control survey, 58 percent of U.S. adults said that they exercised sporadically or not at all. Inactivity was especially marked among blacks, Hispanics, low-income people, and the unemployed.[20] Meanwhile, physical education classes in schools throughout the country are the victims of budget cuts and an apparent disinterest in physical fitness accompanying the call for a return to basic skills.

You probably know someone who seems to be able to eat you under the table and does not appear to exercise more than you do, yet never seems to gain weight. You often do not understand how this person maintains a steady weight. With few exceptions, if you were to follow this person around for a typical day and monitor the level and intensity of activity, you would discover the answer to your question. Although the person's schedule may not include running or strenuous exercise, it probably includes a high level of activity. Walking up a flight of stairs rather than taking the elevator, speeding up the pace while mowing the lawn, getting up to change the TV channel

---

Thyroid gland: A two-lobed endocrine gland located in the throat region that produces a hormone that regulates metabolism.

Basal metabolic rate (BMR): The energy expenditure of the body under resting conditions at normal room temperature.

Yo-yo diet: Cycles in which people repeatedly gain weight, then starve themselves to lose weight. This lowers their BMR, which makes regaining weight even more likely.

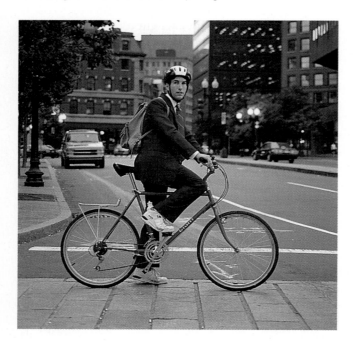

While some people do burn calories and fat better than others, exercise and an active life style are the keys to balancing caloric intake and body weight.

rather than using the remote, and doing housework vigorously all burn extra calories. (Actually, it may even go beyond that. In studies of calorie burning by individuals placed in a controlled respiratory chamber environment where calories consumed, motion, and overall activity were measured, it was found that some people are better fat burners than others. It is possible that low fat burners may not produce as many of the enzymes needed to convert fat to energy. Or they may not have as many blood vessels supplying fatty tissue, making it tougher for them to deliver fat-burning oxygen.) Or, perhaps in some subtle ways, these people just manage to burn more calories through extra motions.

A major cause of low activity levels is the abundance of laborsaving devices in the modern household. Pushing vacuum cleaners rather than sweeping floors, typing on computer keyboards rather than manual typewriters, and using remote-control buttons on television and stereo equipment cause us to expend fewer calories than previous generations did. The automobile is a great convenience, but it lowered our muscle tone and our cardiovascular efficiency.

Clearly, any form of activity that helps your body burn additional calories helps you maintain your weight. In fact, in a study conducted at Stanford University in 1987, a group of men who lost weight through exercise were far more successful at keeping the weight off than were a similar group who lost weight through dieting.

Individuality

Although researchers have learned a great deal in recent years about the factors that predispose people to gain or lose weight, controversy remains. Perhaps the most overlooked element in theories about obesity is the individual person. Just as no two people are exactly alike physiologically, no two people are psychologically identical. Each person is a unique result of genetic background, environment, lifestyle, and emotional responses to a lifetime of experiences.

It is highly possible that the causes of obesity are as varied as the people who are obese. If this is so, there can be no universal cure for weight problems. Instead, we must look for a mechanism of prevention or intervention for each individual that is based upon appropriate cultural, social, environmental, and other factors.

*W*HAT DO YOU THINK?

Based on the risk factors for obesity discussed thus far, which ones do you think pose the greatest risk for you? Which ones can you do something about? What actions can you take to reduce your risk?

Gender and Obesity

Throughout a woman's life, issues of appearance and beauty dominate her surroundings. Only recently have researchers begun to understand just how significant the quest for beauty and the perfect body really is.

In a recent study, researchers determined that being severely overweight in adolescence may predetermine one's social and economic future—particularly if you happen to be female. Researchers found that obese women complete about half a year less schooling, are 20 percent less likely to get married, and earn $6,710 on average less per year than their slimmer counterparts. Obese women also have rates of household poverty 10 percent higher than those of women who are not overweight. In contrast, the study found that overweight men were 11 percent less likely to be married than thinner men but suffer few adverse economic consequences.

It is more likely that women will suffer such consequences of obesity simply because they are more likely than men to be overweight. Compared to men, women have a lower ratio of lean body mass to fatty mass, in part due to differences in bone size and mass, muscle size, and other variables. For all ages after sexual maturity, men have higher metabolic rates, making it easier for them to burn off excess calories than it is for women. Women also face greater potential for weight fluctuation due to hormonal changes, pregnancy, and other conditions that increase the likelihood of weight gain. Also, as a group, men are more socialized into physical activity from birth.

Strenuous activity in both work and play are encouraged for men, while women's roles have typically been more sedentary and required a lower level of caloric expenditure to complete.

Not only are women more vulnerable to weight gain, but also pressures to maintain and/or lose weight make them more likely to take dramatic measures to lose weight. The predominance of eating disorders among women and the greater numbers of women than men taking diet pills is just one indicator of the female obsession with being thin and beautiful. However, males are also victims. As the male image becomes more associated with the body-builder shape and size and as men become more preoccupied with their own physical form, eating disorders, exercise addictions, and other maladaptive responses among men are on the increase.

MANAGING YOUR WEIGHT

At some point in our lives, almost all of us will decide to go on a diet. Whether dieting for vanity or for your health, it's important to begin by finding a program of exercise and healthy eating behaviors that will work for you now and in the long term. You are undoubtedly familiar with the saga of Oprah Winfrey's weight loss: Starting at 190 pounds, she quickly lost 67 pounds on a liquid diet. But failure to continue the maintenance program led to a weight gain of 84 pounds. Finally, Oprah made a lifestyle change, combining sensible eating with sensible behavior:

> This new way of eating . . . (I like to call it "clean eating") has made such a difference in my life. I feel better. But do not be misled: Changing the way you think about food is only the first step toward achieving and maintaining a desirable weight. It was only through a comprehensive plan of healthy eating, daily exercise, and changing my self-defeating behavior that I was able to release weight as an issue in my life.[21]

Are you ready to go on a weight-loss program? Take the Rate Yourself self-test and find out.

What Is a Calorie?

A *calorie* is a unit of measure that indicates the amount of energy we obtain from a particular food. One pound of body fat contains approximately 3,500 calories. So each time you consume 3,500 calories more than your body needs to maintain weight, you gain a pound. Conversely, each time your body expends an extra 3,500 calories, you lose a pound. So if you add a can of Coca-Cola (140 calories) to your diet and make no other changes in diet or activity, you would gain a pound in 25 days (3,500 calories ÷ 140 calories/day = 25 days). Conversely, if you walked for half an hour each day at a 15 minute per mile pace (172

calories burned), you would lose a pound in 20 days (3,500 calories ÷ 172 calories/day = 20.3 days).

The two ways to lose weight, then, are to lower caloric intake (through improved eating habits) and to increase exercise (expending more calories). You may want to use the Skills for Behavior Change box in Chapter 8 to help determine your daily caloric intake. Then you can determine your daily caloric intake and expenditure of calories until you reach a balance (to maintain weight), a decrease (for weight loss), or an increase (for weight gain). Table 9.3 lists the caloric output of varied activities.

Don't forget, it took time to gain weight; it will take time to lose it. As the opening of the chapter pointed out, don't plan on losing more than a pound a week if you want to be able to keep it off.

Exercise

Approximately 90 percent of the daily calorie expenditures of most people occurs as a result of the **resting metabolic rate (RMR)**. The RMR is slightly higher than the BMR; it includes the BMR plus any additional energy expended through daily sedentary activities, such as food digestion, sitting, studying, or standing. The **exercise metabolic rate (EMR)** accounts for the remaining 10 percent of all daily calorie expenditures; it refers to the energy expenditure that occurs during physical exercise. For most of us, these calories come from light daily activities, such as walking, climbing stairs, and mowing the lawn. If we increase the level and intensity of our physical activity to moderate or heavy, however, our EMR may be 10 to 20 times greater than typical resting metabolic rates and can contribute substantially to weight loss.

Increasing BMR, RMR, or EMR levels will help burn calories. An increase in the intensity, frequency, and duration of your daily exercise levels may have significant impact on your total calorie expenditure.

Physical activity makes a greater contribution to BMR when large muscle groups are used. The energy spent on physical activity is the energy used to move the body's muscles—the muscles of the arms, back, abdomen, legs, and so on—and the extra energy used to speed up heartbeat and respiration rate. The number of calories spent depends on three factors:

1. The amount of muscle mass moved.

Resting metabolic rate (RMR): The energy expenditure of the body under BMR conditions plus other daily sedentary activities.

Exercise metabolic rate (EMR): The energy expenditure that occurs during exercise.

The Diet Readiness Test

To see how well your attitudes equip you for a weight-loss program, answer the questions that follow. For each question, circle the answer that best describes your attitude. As you complete each of the six sections, tally your score and analyze it according to the scoring guide.

I. Goals, Attitudes, and Readiness

1. Compared to previous attempts, how motivated are you to lose weight this time?

1	2	3	4	5
Not at all motivated	Slightly motivated	Somewhat motivated	Quite motivated	Extremely motivated

2. How certain are you that you will stay committed to a weight-loss program for the time it will take to reach your goal?

1	2	3	4	5
Not at all certain	Slightly certain	Somewhat certain	Quite certain	Extremely certain

3. Considering all outside factors at this time in your life—stress at work, family obligations, etc.—to what extent can you tolerate the effort required to stick to a diet?

1	2	3	4	5
Cannot tolerate	Can tolerate somewhat	Uncertain	Can tolerate well	Can tolerate easily

4. Think honestly about how much weight you hope to lose and how quickly you hope to lose it. Figuring a weight loss of 1 to 2 pounds per week, how realistic is your expectation?

1	2	3	4	5
Very unrealistic	Somewhat unrealistic	Moderately unrealistic	Somewhat realistic	Very realistic

5. While dieting, do you fantasize about eating a lot of your favorite foods?

1	2	3	4	5
Always	Frequently	Occasionally	Rarely	Never

6. While dieting, do you feel deprived, angry, and/or upset?

1	2	3	4	5
Always	Frequently	Occasionally	Rarely	Never

If you scored:

6 to 16: This may not be a good time for you to start a diet. Inadequate motivation and commitment and unrealistic goals could block your progress. Think about what contributes to your unreadiness and consider changing these factors before undertaking a diet.

17 to 23: You may be close to being ready to begin a program but should think about ways to boost your readiness.

24 to 30: The path is clear: You can decide *how* to lose weight in a safe, effective way.

II. Hunger and Eating Cues

7. When food comes up in conversation or in something you read, do you want to eat, even if you are not hungry?

1	2	3	4	5
Never	Rarely	Occasionally	Frequently	Always

8. How often do you eat because of *physical hunger?*

1	2	3	4	5
Never	Rarely	Occasionally	Frequently	Always

(continued)

9. Do you have trouble controlling your eating when your favorite foods are around the house?

1	2	3	4	5
Never	Rarely	Occasionally	Frequently	Always

If you scored:

3 to 6: You might occasionally eat more than you should, but it does not appear to be due to high responsiveness to environmental cues. Controlling the attitudes that make you eat may be especially helpful.

7 to 9: You may have a moderate tendency to eat just because food is available. Dieting may be easier for you if you try to resist external cues and eat only when you are physically hungry.

10 to 15: Some or much of your eating may be in response to thinking about food or exposing yourself to temptations to eat. Think of ways to minimize your exposure to temptations so you eat only in response to physical hunger.

III. Control over Eating

If the following situations occurred while you were on a diet, would you be likely to eat *more* or *less* immediately afterward and for the rest of the day?

10. Although you planned on skipping lunch, a friend talks you into going out for a midday meal.

1	2	3	4	5
Would eat much less	Would eat somewhat less	Would make no difference	Would eat somewhat more	Would eat much more

11. You "break" your diet by eating a fattening, "forbidden" food.

1	2	3	4	5
Would eat much less	Would eat somewhat less	Would make no difference	Would eat somewhat more	Would eat much more

12. You have been following your diet faithfully and decide to test yourself by eating something you consider a treat.

1	2	3	4	5
Would eat much less	Would eat somewhat less	Would make no difference	Would eat somewhat more	Would eat much more

If you scored:

3 to 7: You recover rapidly from mistakes. However, if you frequently alternate between eating out of control and dieting very strictly, you may have a serious eating problem and should get professional help.

8 to 11: You do not seem to let unplanned eating disrupt your program. This is a flexible, balanced approach.

9 to 15: You may be prone to overeat after an event breaks your control or throws you off the track. Your *reaction* to these problem-causing events can be improved.

IV. Binge Eating and Purging

13. Aside from holiday feasts, have you ever eaten a large amount of food rapidly and felt afterward that this eating incident was excessive and out of control?

2	0
Yes	No

14. If yes to question #13, how often have you engaged in this behavior during the last year?

1	2	3	4	5	6
Less than once a month	About once a month	A few times a month	About once a week	About three times a week	Daily

(continued)

15. Have you purged (used laxatives, diuretics or induced vomiting) to control your weight?

5	0
Yes	No

16. If you answered yes to question #15, how often have you engaged in this behavior during the last year?

1	2	3	4	5	6
Less than once a month	About once a month	A few times a month	About once a week	About three times a week	Daily

If you scored:

0: It appears that binge eating and purging are not problems for you.

2 to 11: Pay attention to these eating patterns. Should they arise more frequently, get professional help.

12 to 19: You show signs of having a potentially serious eating problem. See a counselor experienced in evaluating eating disorders right away.

V. Emotional Eating

17. Do you eat more than you would like to when you have negative feelings such as anxiety, depression, anger or loneliness?

1	2	3	4	5
Never	Rarely	Occasionally	Frequently	Always

18. Do you have trouble controlling your eating when you have positive feelings—do you celebrate feeling good by eating?

1	2	3	4	5
Never	Rarely	Occasionally	Frequently	Always

19. When you have unpleasant interactions with others in your life, or after a difficult day at work, do you eat more than you'd like?

1	2	3	4	5
Never	Rarely	Occasionally	Frequently	Always

If you scored:

3 to 8: You do not appear to let your emotions affect your eating.

9 to 11: You sometimes eat in response to emotional highs and lows. Monitor this behavior to learn when and why it occurs and be prepared to find alternate activities.

12 to 15: Emotional ups and downs can stimulate your eating. Try to deal with the feelings that trigger the eating and find other ways to express them.

VI. Exercise Patterns and Attitudes

20. How often do you exercise?

1	2	3	4	5
Never	Rarely	Occasionally	Somewhat frequently	Frequently

21. How confident are you that you can exercise regularly?

1	2	3	4	5
Not at all confident	Slightly confident	Somewhat confident	Highly confident	Completely confident

22. When you think about exercise, do you develop a positive or negative picture in your mind?

1	2	3	4	5
Completely negative	Somewhat negative	Neutral	Somewhat positive	Completely positive

(continued)

23. How certain are you that you can work regular exercise into your daily schedule?

1	2	3	4	5
Not at all certain	Slightly certain	Somewhat certain	Quite certain	Extremely certain

If you scored:

4 to 10: You're probably not exercising as regularly as you should. Determine whether attitude about exercise or your lifestyle is blocking your way, then change what you must and put on those walking shoes!

11 to 16: You need to feel more positive about exercise so you can do it more often. Think of ways to be more active that are fun and fit your lifestyle.

17 to 20: It looks like the path is clear for you to be active. Now think of ways to get motivated.

After scoring yourself in each section of this questionnaire you should be able to better judge your dieting strengths and weaknesses. Remember that the first step in changing eating behavior is to understand the conditions that influence your eating habits.

Source: Reprinted from "The Diet Readiness Test," in Kelly D. Brownell, "When and How to Diet," *Psychology Today,* June 1989, 41–46. Reprinted with permission from *Psychology Today* Magazine, copyright ©1989 (Sussex Publishers, Inc.).

---

2. The amount of weight being moved.

3. The amount of time the activity takes.

An activity involving both the arms and the legs burns more calories than one involving only the legs, an activity performed by a heavy person burns more calories than one performed by a lighter person, and an activity performed for 40 minutes requires twice as much energy as the same activity performed for only 20 minutes. Thus, obese persons walking for 1 mile burn more calories than slim people walking the same distance. It may also take overweight people longer to walk the mile, which means that they are burning energy for a longer time and therefore expending more overall calories than are thin walkers.[22]

𝒲HAT DO YOU THINK?

Which of the methods for weight reduction discussed above do you think offers the lowest risk and the greatest chance for success?

Dieting: Is It Healthy?

Dieting can lead to improved health. It can also lead to serious physical problems and battered self-esteem. What seems to make the difference is whether a diet is part of an overall reappraisal of a person's attitudes about food and weight and part of an action plan that integrates improved nutrition and exercise or is just seen as a quick fix.

Most experts agree that the ultimate goal of weight-loss treatment should be improved quality of life and permanent weight control.[23] Weight goals should be set to reduce health risks and address medical problems and to help people improve their ability to perform daily tasks without undue stress and strain rather than merely to achieve an "ideal weight." In addition, experts agree that weight-loss programs that promote qualitative rather than quantitative changes in food intake improve health and long-term weight control and are more easily sustained than those that force people to severely restrict intake of calories or specific foods.[24] While the experts seem to agree on these points, many weight-loss programs fail to follow these basic premises. What happens to people who get caught up in "lose weight fast and furiously" campaigns? Researchers are increasingly concerned that

- dieting to lose weight may be more harmful than helpful in promoting health and psychological well-being[25]

- because dieting only rarely produces successful weight loss, the physical and psychological stress, damage to self-esteem, and other emotional disturbances associated with it are without purpose[26]

- dieting causes repeated cycles of weight loss and regain, changes in metabolic rates, increased risk for cardio-

TABLE 9.3 ■ Calories Expended in Various Activities

Activity	Calories per Hour*	Average Calories Used	Activity	Calories per Hour*	Average Calories Used
Sleeping	65	520 (for 8 hrs.)	Running in place or skipping rope (50–60 steps/min.)	510	255 (for ½ hr.)
Watching TV	80	80 (for 1 hr.)			
Driving a car	100	50 (for ½ hr.)	Downhill skiing	595	1,190 (for 2 hrs. on slope)
Dishwashing by hand	135	67 (for ½ hr.)			
Bowling	190	190 (for 1 hr.)			
Washing and polishing car	230	230 (for 1 hr.)	Swimming, 5.5 min./ 220 yds.	600	300 (for ½ hr.)
Dancing (waltz, rock, fox-trot)	250	105 (for 5 dances; 25 min.)	Hill climbing	600	300 (for ½ hr.)
			Touch football	600	300 (for ½ hr. actual play)
Walking, 25 min./mi.	255	127 (for ½ hr.)			
Baseball (not pitching or catching)	280	560 (for 2 hrs.)	Soccer	600	600 (for 1 hr.)
			Snow shoveling, light	610	306 (for ½ hr.)
Weight training	300	150 (for ½ hr.)	Jogging, 11 min./mi.	655	327 (for ½ hr.)
Swimming, 11 min./220 yds.	300	150 (for ½ hr.)	Cross-country skiing, 12 min./mi.	700	2,800 (for 4 hrs.)
Walking, 15 min./mi.	345	172 (for ½ hr.)	Basketball, full court	750	750 (for 1 hr.)
Volleyball, badminton	350	350 (for 1 hr.)	Squash, racquetball	775	775 (for 1 hr.)
Gardening	390	780 (for 2 hrs.)	Martial arts (judo, karate)	790	395 (for ½ hr.)
Calisthenics	415	207 (for ½ hr.)			
Bicycling, 6 min./mi.	415	207 (for ½ hr.)	Running, 7.5 min./mi.	800	400 (for ½ hr.)
Tennis	425	425 (for 1 hr.)	Ice hockey, lacrosse	900	900 (for 1 hr.)
Aerobic dancing (med.)	445	222 (for ½ hr.)			

*The bigger and more vigorous you are, the more calories your body uses for a given activity. The calories listed here are for the average, 158-pound adult. You will lose 1 pound for every 3,500 calories of exercise, as long as you eat the same amount of food.

Source: Reprinted by permission from C. Kuntzleman, *Diet Free!* (Spring Arbor, MI: Arbor Press, 1981).

vascular problems, and other conditions that are hazardous to health[27]

■ dieting contributes to the development of eating disorders such as anorexia and bulimia[28]

Most health authorities recommend that, rather than going on a diet, a person should adopt nutritional dietary changes and a program of increased activity aimed at changing metabolic rates and increasing muscle strength.

Changing Your Eating Habits

In spite of expert advice to the contrary, most of us will decide to go on a diet at some point. At any given time, 23 percent of adult men and 41 percent of adult women in the United States are trying to lose weight.[29] Whether in response to gorging ourselves on the Thanksgiving turkey and all the fixings, to noticing the "spare tire" or "love handles" on our midsections, or to other events, the attempt to lose a few pounds is a common practice in American society. Given the hundreds of different diets and

endless expert advice available, why do we fail most of the time?

Determining What Triggers Your Eating Behavior. Before you can change a given behavior, you must first determine what causes that behavior. Why do you suddenly find yourself at the refrigerator door eating everything in sight? Why do you take that second and third helping of potatoes or dessert when you know that you should be trying to lose weight?

Many people have discovered that one of the best ways of assessing their eating behavior is to chart exactly when they feel like eating, where they are when they decide to eat, the amount of time they spend eating, other activities they engage in during the meal (watching television or reading), whether they eat alone or with others, what and how much they eat, and how they felt before they took their first bite. If you keep a detailed daily log of the triggers listed in Figure 9.4 for at least a week, you will discover useful clues about what in your environment or in your emotional makeup causes you to want food. Typically, these dietary "triggers" center on problems in everyday living rather than on real hunger pangs. As you record this information, your reasons for eating will often become apparent. Many people find that they eat compulsively when stressed or when they have problems in their relationships. For other people, the exact same circumstances diminish their appetite, causing them to lose weight.

Changing Your Triggers.   Once you recognize the factors that cause you to eat, removing the triggers or substituting other activities for them will help you develop more sensible eating patterns. Here are some examples of substitute behaviors:

1. When eating dinner, turn off all distractions, including the television and radio.

2. Replace snack breaks or coffee breaks with exercise breaks.

3. Instead of gulping your food, force yourself to chew each bite slowly.

4. Vary the time of day when you eat. Instead of eating by the clock, do not eat until you are truly hungry. Allow yourself only a designated amount of time for eating—but do not rush. Try to become more aware of true feelings of hunger.

5. If you find that you generally eat all that you can cram on a plate, use smaller plates. Put your dinner plates away and use the salad plates instead.

6. If you find that you are continually seeking your favorite foods in the cupboard, stop buying them. Or place them in a spot that is very inconvenient to reach. (Having to run upstairs for the sugar bowl will probably force you to think twice before using sugar.)

These are just suggestions. After recording your daily intake for a week, you will be able to devise a list of substitutes that are geared toward your particular eating behaviors. More weight management tips can be found in the Skills for Behavior Change box.

*W*HAT DO YOU THINK?

Based on what you have read so far, what can you do to maintain your current weight if you are satisfied with it, lose weight if you need to, or gain weight if you are too thin?

Selecting a Nutritional Plan that's Right for You

Once you have discovered what factors tend to sabotage your weight-loss efforts, you will be well on your way to successful weight control. To be successful, however, you must plan for success. By setting goals that are too far in the future or unrealistic for your current lifestyle, you will doom yourself to failure. Do not try to lose 40 pounds in four months. Try, instead, to lose a healthy 1 to 2 pounds during the first week, and stay with this slow and easy regimen. Reward yourself when you lose pounds, and if you binge and go off your nutrition plan, get right back on it the next day. Remember that you did not gain 40 pounds in eight weeks, so it is unrealistic to punish your body by trying to lose that amount of weight in such a short time.

Seek assistance from reputable sources in selecting a dietary plan that is easy to follow and includes adequate amounts of the basic nutrients. Registered dietitians, some physicians (not all physicians have strong back-

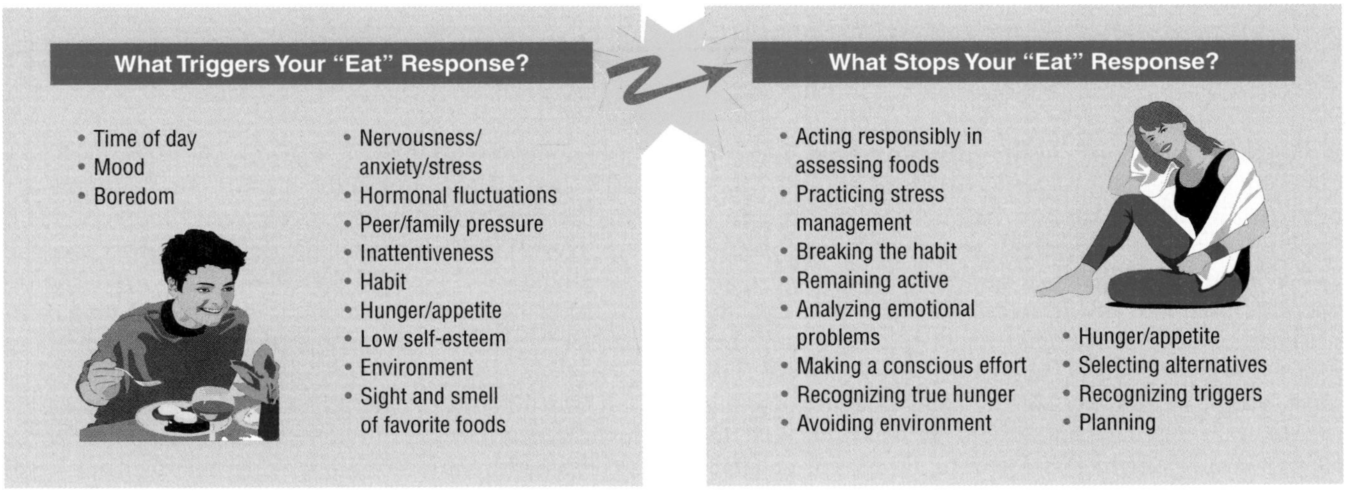

FIGURE 9.4

What Triggers Your "Eat" Response?	What Stops Your "Eat" Response?
• Time of day • Mood • Boredom • Nervousness/anxiety/stress • Hormonal fluctuations • Peer/family pressure • Inattentiveness • Habit • Hunger/appetite • Low self-esteem • Environment • Sight and smell of favorite foods	• Acting responsibly in assessing foods • Practicing stress management • Breaking the habit • Remaining active • Analyzing emotional problems • Making a conscious effort • Recognizing true hunger • Avoiding environment • Hunger/appetite • Selecting alternatives • Recognizing triggers • Planning

Learn to understand what triggers and stops your "eat" response. Keep a daily log of your responses.

General Tips for Managing Your Weight

When Eating at Home

- Eat only in the kitchen. Keep food out of your living room, bedroom, and study.
- Eat smaller meals four to five times a day rather than gorge yourself at dinner.
- Always leave some food on your plate.
- Use a smaller plate and fill it with low-calorie foods such as salad without dressing and pasta with a low-fat sauce.
- Take more time to eat; at least 20 minutes per meal is recommended. Chew each bit of food carefully, setting your fork down between bites and enjoying the taste of the food.
- Drink two to three glasses of water before a meal.
- Brush your teeth immediately after eating to avoid the temptation to take a second helping.
- Don't buy high-calorie and high-fat foods, even for guests. The temptation to eat them yourself will usually prove irresistible.
- If you must have desserts, make yourself go out for them.
- Get in tune with your true feelings of hunger. Eat only when you are really hungry, not by the clock.
- Don't skip meals or allow yourself to get too hungry before eating.
- Don't eat within three hours of going to bed.
- Put serving dishes on the counter or stove while you are eating. Leaving them on the table will only tempt you to take an extra bite.

When Eating Out

- Don't be afraid to ask for it "your way." Request that the cheese be left off, the sauce cut in half, etc.
- Ask for salad dressings, gravies, and sauces on the side. Then use only the smallest amount necessary to flavor the food.
- Ask that entrees be broiled, steamed, baked, grilled, poached, or roasted, with only a small amount of fat used for the cooking process.
- When ordering omelets, ask for a one- or two-egg-yolk version containing only the whites of the other eggs. Avoid meat and cheese fillings in favor of low-fat vegetable fillings.
- Cut down on portion size. Order à la carte if possible, with a salad or fresh vegetable on the side. Even a baked potato is fine if you waive the add-ons, such as butter and sour cream.
- Avoid the all-you-can-eat establishments. Even an all-you-can-eat salad bar is dangerous because of toppings loaded with fat and calories.
- Drink at least one glass of water before starting your meal. Try to relax while eating and make your mealtime last. Talk more, put your fork down more frequently, chew more, and generally slow down.
- Order fresh fruits in place of heavy desserts. If you have to have dessert, limit your portion size and only allow yourself to have it one or two times per week, as a special treat.
- Frequent restaurants that offer low-fat, high-complex-carbohydrate meals. All of us make better choices when there are more good options to choose from.

---

grounds in nutrition), health educators and exercise physiologists with nutritional backgrounds, and other health professionals can provide reliable information. Look out for people who call themselves "nutritionists." There is no such official designation, leaving the door open for just about anyone to call himself or herself a nutritional expert. Avoid quick weight-loss programs that promise miracle results. The majority are expensive, and most people regain the weight soon after completing the program. Ask questions about the credentials of the adviser in any weight-loss program, assess the nutrient value of the prescribed diet, verify that dietary guidelines are consistent with information from reliable dietary research, and analyze the suitability of the diet to your tastes, budget, and lifestyle to avoid putting yourself in a risky, expensive, or unhealthy dietary situation. Any diet that requires radical behavior changes is doomed to failure. Nutritional plans that do not ask you to sacrifice everything you enjoy and that allow you to make choices are generally the most successful. See Table 9.4 for a comparison of some of the most popular diet and weight loss programs.

Ultimately, the decision to practice responsible weight management is yours. To be successful, you must choose a combination of exercise and eating that fits your needs and lifestyle. Find a workable plan, stick to it, and you will succeed. The Choices for Change box offers practical advice to follow on a daily basis.

TABLE 9.4 ■ Weight Loss Diets and Programs

	Weight Loss Rate	Individ-ualized	Program	Professionals	Mainte-nance Plan	Ads/Endorse-ments	Cost
Diet Center Real-food diet with supplements (vitamins, minerals, and blood sugar stabilizer).	1 ½–2 lbs./wk.	Variations within set regimen.	One-to-one brief meetings with staff person daily, if desired.	No—contact is with Diet Center counselor.	Yes	Testimonials	Initial fee averages $400–$700 for 9-wk. program.
Diet Workshop Real-food diet without special products.	1 ½–2 lbs./wk.	Variations within set regimen.	1 hr./wk. in group setting.	No—contact is with trained graduates of program.	Yes	Testimonials	$14 membership; $9/wk. until maintenance.
Health Management Resources (HMR) Medically supervised very-low-calorie diet.	3–5 lbs./wk.	Variations within set regimen.	1 ½ hr./wk. in group setting.	Yes	Yes	Testimonials plus extensive statistics from company data.	Averages $2,775 for entire program.
Jenny Craig Real-food diet that requires prepackaged meals until maintenance phase.	1–2 lbs./wk.	Variations within set regimen.	14 1-hr. video classes plus one-to-one sessions with counselor.	No—college graduates implement program.	Yes	Celebrity testimonials and client case studies.	$185 membership; $60–$70/wk. for food.
Medifast Liquid fast dispensed from individual physician's office; program support varies greatly, depending on intensity of doctor's approach.	3–5 lbs./wk.	Variations of set plan left to M.D.'s discretion.	Lifestyle weekly group program and one-to-one counseling.	Yes	Yes	Testimonials plus information about obesity as "disease."	Averages $1,700–$1,900 ($50/wk.).
Nutri/System Real-food diet that requires prepackaged foods until maintenance phase.	1 ½–2 lbs./wk.	Variations within set regimen.	30-min. weekly group classes plus one-to-one sessions with nutrition "specialist."	No—most who implement program are college graduates.	Yes	"Dieting DJ" testimonials.	Ranges from $100 to $1,000 plus $48–$58/wk. for food.
Optifast Medically supervised very-low-calorie diet.	Up to 1–2% of body weight.	Variations within set regimen.	1 ½ hr./wk. in group setting; weekly meetings for at least 21 wks.; at least one meeting with an R.D.	Yes	Yes	Show before-and-after pictures, discuss medical team approach, and describe program.	$2,500–$3,500 for 26-week program.

TABLE 9.4 ■ Weight Loss Diets and Programs *(Continued)*

	Weight Loss Rate	Individ-ualized	Program	Professionals	Mainte-nance Plan	Ads/Endorse-ments	Cost
Slim Fast/Ultra Slim Fast Over-the-counter product.	Up to individual.	No—self-regulated.	No	No	No	Celebrity testimonials.	$8–$12/wk.
Take Off Pounds Sensibly (TOPS) Real-food diet that does not require special products.	Varies	Variations with pre-scribed ADA exchange plans.	Yes, group meetings.	No—contact is with trained graduates of program.	Yes	Newspaper announce-ment.	$12 annual fee.
Weight Loss Clinic Real-food diet that does not require special products.	2–3 lbs./wk.	Variations within set regimen.	One-to-one brief meetings with staff person up to 5 days/wk.	Yes	Yes	Testimonials.	Averages $60/wk.
Weight Watchers Real-food diet that does not require special products.	1–2 lbs./wk.	Variations within set regimen.	45-min. weekly group meeting plus question/answer period.	No—contact is with trained graduates of program.	Yes	Testimonials of "gradu-ates."	$12–$20 mem-bership plus $7–$9/wk. until maintenance.

Source: Adapted by permission from "Smart Losers' Guide to Choosing a Weight-Loss Program," *Tufts University Diet and Nutrition Letter,* August 1990.

"Miracle" Diets

Fasting, starvation diets, and other forms of **very low calorie diets** (VLCDs) have been shown to cause significant health risks. Typically, when you deprive your body of food for prolonged periods, your body makes adjustments to save you from inevitable organ shutdown. It begins to deplete its energy reserves to obtain necessary fuels. One of the first reserves the body turns to to maintain its supply of glucose is lean, protein tissue. As this occurs, you lose weight rapidly, because protein contains only half as many calories per pound as fat. At the same time, significant water stores are lost. Over time, the body begins to run out of liver tissue, heart muscle, blood, and so on, as these readily available substances are burned to supply energy. Only after the readily available proteins from these sources are depleted will your body begin to burn fat reserves. In this process, known as **ketosis**, the body adapts to prolonged fasting or carbohydrate deprivation by converting body fat to ketones, which can be used as fuel for some brain cells. Within about 10 days after the typical adult begins a complete fast, the body has used many of its energy stores and death may occur.

In very low calorie diets, powdered formulas are usually given to patients under medical supervision. These formulas have daily values of from 400 to 700 calories plus vitamin and mineral supplements. Although these diets may be beneficial for people who have failed at all conventional weight-loss methods and who face severe threats to their health that are complicated by their obesity, they should never be undertaken without strict medical supervision. Problems associated with fasting, VLCDs, and other forms of severe calorie deprivation include blood sugar imbalances, cold intolerance, constipation, decreased BMR, dehydration, diarrhea, emotional problems, fatigue, headaches, heart irregularity, ketosis, kidney infections and failure, loss of lean body tissue, weakness, and weight gain due to the yo-yo effect and other variables.

Trying to Gain Weight

Although trying to lose weight poses a major challenge for many of us, there is a smaller group of people who, for a variety of metabolic, hereditary, psychological, and other

Tips to Live by in Controlling Your Weight

The choices you make each day of your life about foods contribute to your future health and well-being. These choices are never easy, but there are actions you can take to make your decisions easier and to help yourself succeed with your dietary plan:

- Eat whatever you want. There are no good or bad foods, only bad diets. In other words, you can fit just about any food into a healthy daily eating plan if you eat that food in moderation.

- Never say *diet*. Think in terms of developing healthful eating and exercise habits. You'll lose weight more gradually, but it's more likely to stay off.

- Include weight lifting in your routine for weight maintenance as well as for physical fitness. The American College of Sports Medicine recommends undertaking strength-training activities at least two times per week. Unlike aerobic exercise, strength training builds a considerable amount of muscle, which requires more calories to sustain itself than body fat. In other words, iron pumpers burn more calories.

- Ask your doctor, health education professor, or a registered dietitian about taking vitamin and/or mineral supplements if you're adhering to a strict vegetarian diet, following a low-calorie diet, expecting a baby, or suffering from a disease that interferes with your body's ability to use nutrients.

- Take small steps, one at a time, to eliminate unhealthy habits (such as munching on chips in front of the TV). Tackling two or more deeply entrenched habits simultaneously can prove so overwhelming that it weakens resolve and sets the stage for failure.

- Always check serving sizes when comparing the nutrition labels of products. (Only 1 percent of consumers do, according to a recent survey.) This practice is important because many manufacturers have reduced their stated serving sizes to abnormally small portions, presumably to make them appear lower in calories, fat, and sodium.

- Stay off the scale. A new Food and Drug Administration survey indicates that 70 percent of dieters weigh themselves at least once per week, but most experts contend that anything more than once every other week is too much. Natural, day-to-day weight fluctuations can be misleading and discouraging. Real and lasting changes in weight take time to show up.

- Keep a journal of when you lose and when you win when battling your food cravings. Reminding yourself of what you've done before can be a great aid for avoiding problem areas and for future success.

- Review your battle plan. Make a list of your five most helpful dieting strategies, (packing your lunch, eating at the table, using smaller plates, chewing your food longer, etc.). Check the list periodically. If you aren't doing what you set out to do, make a change.

- Keep healthy snacks at hand. Rather than rushing to the refrigerator in search of something to satisfy your eating urge, keep pretzels, low-fat and low-salt popcorn, veggie sticks, and other, healthful foods close by where you'll see them first.

- Keep a log of your actual hunger pangs. Are you really eating when you are so hungry that your stomach is growling, or are you eating because it's time to eat? Try to get more in touch with your body signals. Eat only when hungry.

- Slow down when eating and never have a fork in your hand if there's food in your mouth.

- Heed the hue. According to research conducted at the Johns Hopkins Medical School, warm hues such as red, yellow, and orange make food look better and people hungrier. Cool colors such as blue and gray have the opposite effect.

---

reasons, can't seem to gain weight no matter how hard they try. If you are one of these individuals, determining the reasons for your difficulty in gaining weight is a must. Once you know what is causing you to have a daily caloric deficit, there are several things that you can do to help yourself gain extra weight:

- Control your exercise. Cut back if you are doing too much, slow down, and keep a careful record of calories burned.

- Eat more. Obviously, you are not taking in enough calories to support whatever is happening in your body. Eat more frequently, spend more time eating, eat the high-calorie foods first if you tend to fill up fast,

and always start with the main course. Take time to shop, to cook, to eat slowly. Put extra spreads such as peanut butter, cream cheese, or cheese on your foods. Make your sandwiches with extra-thick slices of bread

Very low calorie diets (VLCDs): Diets with caloric value of 400 to 700 calories.

Ketosis: A condition in which the body adapts to prolonged fasting or carbohydrate deprivation by converting body fat to ketones, which can be used as fuel for some brain activity.

and add more filling. Take seconds whenever possible and eat high-calorie snacks during the day.

- Try to relax. Many people who are underweight also suffer from anxiety and the "hurry syndrome." Slow down and try to control stress.

*E*ATING DISORDERS

Obesity itself is neither a psychiatric disorder nor an eating disorder. An **eating disorder** consists of severe disturbances in eating behavior, unhealthy efforts to control body weight, and abnormal attitudes about one's body and shape. The three main eating disorders are anorexia nervosa, bulimia nervosa, and binge eating disorder. The eating disorders are mostly associated with females.

Those with eating disorders generally suffer from low self-esteem. However, contrary to popular stereotypes, eating disorders are not restricted to middle-class white females with overprotective or over-perfectionist parents. Eating disorders span social classes and many ethnic groups.

Eating disorders have been reported to occur with roughly similar frequencies in most industrialized countries, including the United States, Canada, Europe, Australia, Japan, New Zealand, and South Africa. Emigrants from cultures in which the disorders are rare to cultures in which the disorders are more prevalent may develop anorexia nervosa as they assimilate thin-body ideals. The disorders usually begin during early adolescence, although rare cases occur even after the age of 40. Over 90 percent of cases occur in women. To learn more about why females have higher rates of eating disorders, see the Multicultural Perspectives box.

Anorexia Nervosa

Anorexia nervosa is characterized by self-starvation motivated by an intense fear of gaining weight and a severe disturbance in the perception of one's body. When

---

Eating disorder: Disorder consisting of severe disturbances in eating behavior, unhealthy efforts to control body weight, and abnormal attitudes about one's body and shape.

Anorexia nervosa: Eating disorder characterized by excessive preoccupation with food, self-starvation, and/or extreme exercising to achieve weight losses.

Bulimia nervosa: Eating disorder characterized by binge eating followed by inappropriate compensating measures taken to prevent weight gain.

---

anorexia develops in childhood or early adolescence, the symptom may be the failure to gain weight associated with normal growth rather than the loss of weight. About .5 to 1 percent of females in late adolescence or early adulthood meet the criteria for full diagnosis of anorexia nervosa.

Diagnosed anorexics weigh less then 85 percent of normal weight. Their unusual weight is accomplished primarily through reduction in total food intake. Usually, they begin by restricting high-calorie foods, and eventually exclude almost all foods from their diet. In addition, they lose weight through *purging*—self-induced vomiting or the misuse of laxatives or diuretics—and through exercise.

Individuals with this disorder have an intense fear of gaining weight or becoming fat. This intense fear is usually not alleviated by weight loss. In fact, concern about weight gain often increases as actual weight continues to decrease.

Anorexics have a distorted view of the experience and significance of body weight and shape. Some feel globally overweight; others feel that parts (particularly the abdomen, buttocks, and thighs) are "too fat." They may con-

---

The self-starvation associated with eating disorders like Anorexia nervosa can damage bones, muscles, and organs and create a host of other serious and, in some cases, life-threatening medical problems.

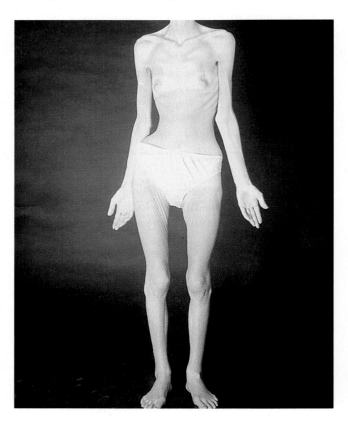

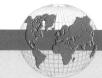
Gender and Eating Disorders

Eating disorders occur predominantly in women. Anorexia nervosa and bulimia nervosa are rare among men. What explains this striking gender difference?

At the sociocultural level, it is clear that physical attractiveness is more important for women than for men. Numerous studies have demonstrated this societal double standard. The cultural pressure to be thin influences the developmental psychology of women.

One researcher argues that two aspects of our contemporary female sex-role stereotype have particular relevance to women's risk for eating disorders. First, beauty is a central aspect of "femininity"; girls learn early on that being "pretty" is what draws attention and praise from others, and girls in books and on television focus on their appearance while boys play and "do." As early as in fourth grade, body build and self-esteem are correlated for girls but not for boys.

A second aspect is women's interpersonal orientation. Theorists about the psychology of women argue that self-worth is closely tied to the establishment and maintenance of close relationships. Thus, women's self-concept is interpersonally constructed: girls' self-descriptions at age seven have been found to be more based on the perceptions of others than are boys'. Consequently, women are said to derive self-worth from other's opinions and approval of them, and in our culture, social approval is related to physical attractiveness. Research has consistently shown a significant correlation between self-esteem and feelings about one's body, especially in women, for whom it is significantly related to how they are evaluated by others. Even lesbians, who generally take a more critical stance than other women towards sociocultural norms regarding women and female sex-role stereotypes, do not seem to differ much from heterosexual women in their attitudes about weight. In one study, self-esteem was strongly related to feelings about one's body, and the prevalence of bulimia nervosa among lesbians was similar to that among heterosexual women.

The ideal standard of physical attractiveness has become thinner over the past few decades. This has made it harder for women to meet the standard, so they resort to such extreme methods as rigid dieting rules and purging. Some men also rely on these extreme measures to achieve a leaner body; examples include jockeys and wrestlers. Both jockeys and wrestlers report some of the features of eating disorders during their competitive season. But these features disappear when they are not competing. Why do dieting and purging affect these men only temporarily but trap so many women in a life-threatening downward spiral?

There is a crucial difference between these male athletes and women. The men wish to lose weight to improve their athletic performance. Their concern with body weight is secondary to their goal of performing well. For women, dieting to achieve an ideal weight has more profound psychological meaning. It is related to their self-identity and self-evaluation. Biological factors may also help to explain the gender gap. Women not only diet more than men do, but may also suffer more serious effects of dieting than do men. Studies of dieting by normal, healthy male and female college students show a differential effect on brain serotonin function. The men were unaffected. But the women showed reduced serotonin activity.

Source: Adapted from G. Terrence Wilson, Peter Nathan, K. Daniel O'Leary, and Lee Anna Clark, *Abnormal Psychology.* © copyright 1996 by Allyn and Bacon. Reprinted by permission.

stantly weigh themselves, measure themselves, and look at themselves in the mirror to check for fat. This is because their self-esteem is highly dependent on their body shape and weight. Weight loss is viewed as an impressive achievement and a sign of extraordinary self-discipline; weight gain is perceived as unacceptable failure of self-control.[30]

The medical problems associated with anorexia are appalling. Starvation can damage the bones, the muscles, and the organs as well as the immune, nervous, and digestive systems. The acid in vomit may cause tooth enamel to dissolve. Anorexics often either lose hair or develop excessive, fine facial and body hair. Worse, between 5 and 18 percent of victims die as a result of suicide or of the medical complications of this disorder.[31]

Bulimia Nervosa

The essential features of **bulimia nervosa** are binge eating followed by inappropriate compensating measures taken to prevent weight gain. Binge eating normally occurs in secrecy and is accompanied by a lack of control. It is difficult for a person with bulimia to stop the binge once it has started. About 1 to 3 percent of adolescent and young adult females are bulimic; the rate among men is about 10 percent that among females.

As with anorexics, bulimics place an excessive emphasis on body shape and weight in their self-evaluation, and these factors are critical in determining their self-esteem. Unlike the anorexic, the bulimic's body weight is typically within the normal weight range (some may be under-

Talking to Someone with an Eating Disorder

When a family member or a friend has an eating disorder, that person needs serious medical help. You can take a proactive role in getting help. Here are some suggestions:

- Speak up. Don't encourage denial of the problem by ignoring it.

- Base what you say on your own observations and keep the tone affectionate, not accusing: "I've noticed you're skipping a lot of meals, and I'm worried about you." Or, "I can smell that you have been vomiting, and I'm concerned about your health." Make yourself available to the individual to discuss emotional concerns and anxieties.

- Inform yourself about the disorder, and share your information with the other person. For many women, recovery has started with a book or a pamphlet provided by a friend or relative. Consult an eating disorders clinic in your area. Clinics in teaching hospitals are the most likely to offer counseling and programs free or at a low cost.

- Attend a support group for help with your own pain resulting from the situation and for advice on how to interact with your family member or friend.

- If the person with the disorder agrees to seek help, be supportive in constructive ways. Offer to accompany him or her to appointments; express interest and concern without trying to take over.

- If a relative has an eating disorder, consider family therapy to explore some of the emotional roots of the disorder. Jean Rubel, Th.D., founder of Anorexia Nervosa and Related Eating Disorders, says, "Ignore tears, tantrums, and promises." If the relative is younger than 18, get him or her to a doctor and tell him or her what you suspect; this is no time for guessing games. Get educational counseling and therapy. Rubel also believes that the whole family should be involved in the therapy to deal with the root issues: "You can't send her off to be fixed like a car to a garage."

- Do not nag or bully. You can't recover for someone else, and you may create more problems by monitoring someone else's eating habits.

- Do not tell a recovering bulimic or anorexic that he or she is looking better. No matter how carefully you phrase it, he or she will hear, "You got fat."

Source: Adapted with permission from Suanne Kelman, "The Way Back," *Shape,* March 1995, 113.

---

weight or overweight). In addition, treatment of bulimia nervosa is effective in the majority of cases, with good prospects for a full and lasting recovery.[32]

Binge Eating Disorder

People afflicted with **binge eating disorder** (BED) engage in recurrent binge eating but, unlike bulimics, do not take excessive measures to lose the weight gained during binges. Neither do BED patients report abnormal attitudes about dieting or body weight and shape. Binge eating disorder occurs predominantly in obese patients. This disorder is often referred to in the popular literature as "compulsive overeating." Studies show that obese patients with BED consume significantly more food than do obese

nonbingers. Take note that, as of the date of this writing, binge eating disorder is only under consideration as a psychiatric diagnosis.[33]

Treating Eating Disorders

The most effective treatments for eating disorders combine different approaches into a package that involves the patient and his or her family and friends. Eating disorder patients usually come to the attention of medical personnel because someone else shows concern. To learn about how you could help someone you suspect has a disorder see the Building Communication Skills box.

Treatment options for eating disorders vary. Due to the medical complications brought on by dangerous weight loss, anorexia often requires hospitalization, and the first goal of treatment is to restore patients to near-normal body weight. For all eating disorders, individual psychotherapy provides an opportunity for the patient to develop self-confidence, self-esteem, and feelings of power and control. In therapy, the person learns new, more effective ways to handle stress so that it is no longer necessary to turn to or away from food to deal with problems.

Binge eating disorder (BED): Eating disorder characterized by recurrent binge eating. However, BED sufferers do not take excessive measures to lose the weight gained during binges.

Managing Your Weight

Managing your weight is not an easy task. To ensure success, you must make a real change in the way you eat and consider it a lifelong commitment rather than a diet. Analyzing where you are right now and then taking the steps outlined below will help you win the war against excess weight.

Making Decisions for You

The first step in managing your weight is an honest self-assessment of where you are. You don't need sophisticated fat-measurement techniques. What you need is a scale. Your college probably has a gym that has body-content assessment equipment available. Next you need to set a realistic goal. Ask yourself, why do I want to meet this goal? What will I do when I reach this goal? Then set out a plan to reach your goal. Keep in mind what you enjoy doing. If you like taking walks, you might make walking part of your weight-loss program. If you absolutely love chocolate chip cookies, you might consider limiting yourself to two cookies per day while eliminating some other dessert.

Checklist for Change: Making Personal Choices

✓ Design your plan for your needs. Forget the nutritional gurus who promise quick success. Your plan must fit your personality, your priorities, and your work and recreation schedules. It should allow for sufficient rest and relaxation.

✓ Plan for nutrient-dense foods. Attempt to get the most from the foods you eat by selecting foods with high nutritional value. Excellent examples of nutrient-dense foods are fruits and vegetables, whole-grain breads and cereals, and lean protein-rich foods such as fish and poultry, low-fat cottage cheese, and skim milk.

✓ Balance food intake throughout the day. Although the evidence is controversial, research indicates that the body may burn calories more efficiently in small amounts than in excessive quantities. Thus, rather than gorging yourself at one main meal, you are probably better off eating several smaller meals throughout the day.

✓ Plan for plateaus. As previously indicated, you may have an inner thermostat that attempts to set your weight at a given point. Thus, if you prepare yourself psychologically for plateaus you will be less likely to become discouraged. Exercise is probably the critical factor in getting past a plateau.

✓ Chart your progress. For many people, the daily "weigh-in" is a critical factor in maintaining their program. However, particularly for those who have reached a weight plateau, it may be necessary to think in terms of weekly weigh-ins to avoid frustration. After all, it is long-range success you are after.

✓ Chart your setbacks. Rather than thinking in terms of failure and punishment, think in terms of temporary setbacks and how to accommodate them. By carefully recording your emotional states when eating, eating habits, environmental cues, and feelings, you may determine why you needed that ice cream cone or why you chose a pizza instead of a salad. Studies suggest that the "urge" to consume more calories may be greater at certain times of the month, particularly for women during the days immediately before and after menstruation. Thus, successful weight-loss plans may have to accommodate hormonal fluctuations as an influence on dietary habits.

✓ Become aware of your feelings of hunger and fullness. For many of us, eating is time-dependent, and we stop eating only when the food is gone (the "clean your plate" syndrome). Long years of "eating when it is time" instead of eating when it is necessary cost us the ability to tell when we really are hungry and when we really are full. The message that our stomach sends to our brain signaling "full" is not immediate. Sometimes, particularly when we eat too fast, there is a delay between actual fullness and the physical awareness that we have had enough. We therefore continue to eat past the "full" point, causing discomfort and even nausea in some instances. By training yourself to become more aware of the eating process, by learning to recognize true hunger pangs and the first signals that you have eaten enough, you will be able to change your eating patterns.

✓ Accept yourself. For many people, this is the most important aspect of successful weight management. Although our culture can certainly oppress fat people, many overweight people are their own worst enemies. It is important to keep your weight in perspective. Unless you feel good about who you are inside, exterior changes will not help you very much.

✓ Exercise, exercise, exercise. Although we would all like to wish away our extra pounds, losing weight requires hard work and concentration. Different people benefit from different types of activities. Just because your friends are into jogging or jazzercise does not mean that that type of exercise program is best for you. Select an exercise program that you consider fun, not a daily form of punishment for overeating. Variety may be the key here. Planning a program that includes friends and family may also improve your chances of success. It is important to remember that every little effort contributes toward long-term results.

(continued)

Checklist for Change: Making Community Choices

✓ Have you considered volunteering at youth organizations that provide physical fitness opportunities for teens?

✓ Have you considered volunteering time at an eating disorders clinic?

✓ What opportunities for volunteering at nutrition- or weight-related programs does your campus provide?

Critical Thinking

Until college, your girlfriend Tami had taken ballet very seriously, practicing several hours a day. Now that the time pressures of college, a part-time job, and your relationship are starting to get to her, Tami rarely has time to work out on the dance floor. You notice that she has consequently been more and more concerned about her weight. She rarely eats on your dates, but she says that that's because she wants the two of you to save money for a nice trip during Spring break. When you find a laxative hidden under her pillow, she says, "Doesn't everyone get constipated now and then?" Then a mutual female friend tells you that she's heard Tami in the bathroom throwing up on several occasions after meals; Tami denies it.

Using the DECIDE model in Chapter 1, decide how you can approach Tami with your concern that she has an eating disorder. What help is available in your local area? Should you involve Tami's family? If Tami denies she has an eating disorder, what can you do?

In addition, eating disorder patients often exhibit depression and other clinical illnesses, and these problems can also be treated.

Support groups are useful for providing a social network, emotional support, and self-help techniques. Although family therapy has received a good deal of coverage by the press, the success of family therapy for eating disorder patients is not supported by scientific research.

𝒲HAT DO YOU THINK?

Why do college students in particular seem to have so many problems with eating disorders? What factors place young women at risk? Why do you think there are fewer eating disorders among men? What programs or services on your campus would you recommend for a friend with an eating disorder?

Summary

◆ Overweight, obesity, and weight-related problems appear to be on the rise in the United States. Obesity is now defined in terms of fat content rather than in terms of weight alone. There are many different methods of assessing body fat. Body fat percentages give you a more accurate indication of how fat versus lean you really are.

◆ Many factors contribute to your risk for obesity. Included among these factors are genetics, developmental factors, your setpoint, endocrine influences, psychosocial factors, eating cues, lack of awareness, metabolic changes, lifestyle, and gender.

◆ Exercise, dieting, diet pills, and other strategies are used to maintain or lose weight. However, sensible eating behavior and adequate exercise probably offer the best options.

◆ Eating disorders consist of severe disturbances in eating behaviors, unhealthy efforts to control body weight, and abnormal attitudes about body and shape. Anorexia nervosa, bulimia nervosa, and binge eating disorder are the three main eating disorders. Eating disorders occur mainly in adolescent and young adult women in industrialized countries.

Discussion Questions

1. Discuss the pressures, if any, you feel to improve your personal body image. Do these pressures come from TV shows, movies, ads, and other external sources or from concern for your personal health?

2. List the risk factors for obesity. Evaluate which seem to be most important in determining whether you will be obese in middle age.

3. Create a plan to help someone lose the "Freshman 15" over the summer vacation. Assume that the person is male, 180 pounds, and has 15 weeks to lose the excess weight.

4. Differentiate among the three eating disorders. Then give reasons why females might be more prone to anorexia and bulimia than might males.

Application Exercise

Reread the What Do You Think? scenarios at the beginning of the chapter and answer the following questions:

1. What motivates someone like Ray to try to spiff up and look good at certain times of the year? How could someone like Ray change his behaviors so as to be more healthy nutritionally and to avoid the diet syndrome so many of us find ourselves in?

2. Why is dieting to lose weight probably not such a good idea in the long run?

3. Do you know someone like Jessie? Why do you think some people have such a distorted image of what they really look like and who they really are?

4. What makes young women particularly susceptible to ads that promise quick beauty and desirability?

Further Reading

Tufts University Diet and Nutrition Letter, Tufts University Press.

Monthly newsletter covering relevant and timely information about diet and weight control. Easy to read and understand. Call (617) 482–3530 for further information.

G. Terrence Wilson, Peter Nathan, K. Daniel O'Leary, and Lee Anna Clark, *Abnormal Psychology* (Boston: Allyn and Bacon, 1996).

Includes full chapter on eating disorders by Dr. Wilson, one of the country's leading experts on eating disorders.

10

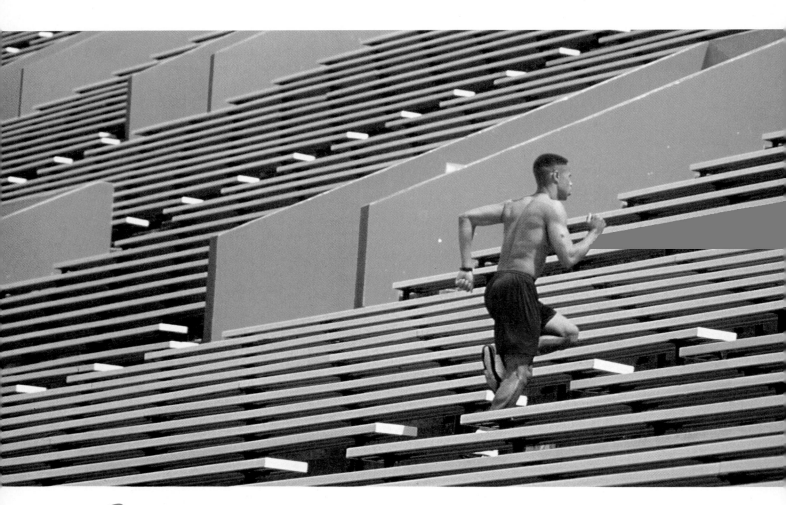

*C*HAPTER OBJECTIVES

◆ Describe the benefits of physical activity, including improved cardiorespiratory efficiency, skeletal mass, weight control, health and life span, mental health and stress management, and physical fitness.

◆ Describe the components of an aerobic exercise program and how to determine proper exercise frequency, intensity, and duration.

◆ Describe the different stretching exercises designed to improve flexibility.

◆ Compare the various types of resistance training programs, including the methods of providing external resistance and intended physiological benefits.

◆ Describe common fitness injuries, suggest ways to prevent injuries, and list the treatment process.

◆ Summarize the key components of a personal fitness program.

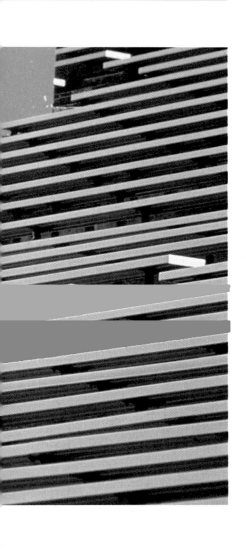

Personal Fitness

Improving Your Health Through Exercise

WHAT DO YOU THINK?

Steve has never been physically active. While growing up, he watched a lot of television and generally avoided activity that involved physical exertion. Now 19 years old and a sophomore in college, he drives his car to campus every day rather than walking the six blocks from his apartment. He always looks for a parking spot closest to the building where his class is held. Steve's idea of a great meal is a large, extra-cheese pepperoni pizza delivered to his door and washed down with a quart of soda. To relax, Steve plays one of the many computer games he owns. One day, Steve sees a TV show that describes the adverse health effects of the sedentary lifestyle—obesity, high blood pressure, increased risk of heart disease, and more. He realizes that he has made some poor choices and vows never again to be a couch potato.

- ■ Now that Steve is ready to live a more active lifestyle, how should he begin? After years of not exercising, what sorts of exercises should he begin with? Should Steve see his family physician before he starts his exercise program? How long will he need to continue a physical fitness program before he notices the positive effects of regular exercise?

While in high school, Georgia participated in many school activities, including gymnastics, soccer, and track. Among the many lifestyle changes she encountered during her first year in college was the need for much more time spent reading and writing. Georgia had seen some of her older friends struggle to control their weight during their college years; she liked the way she looked and didn't want that to change. Despite the academic and social demands of her first semester at college, Georgia was determined to make time for fitness activities and worked out at least five times a week. Instead of gaining weight, she lost 8 pounds by the end of the first semester. She studied hard and got good grades, but averaged less than six hours of sleep a night. By the end of the day, Georgia usually felt tired and stressed out.

- ■ Was Georgia overdoing it? What potential problems can you foresee if she continues her first-semester schedule? What changes should Georgia make in her life-style to reverse the effects of her first semester at college?

More than 30 years ago, the President's Council on Physical Fitness was created because of concerns about the poor fitness levels of American children. Participation in regular fitness activity gradually increased during the 1960s, 1970s, and early 1980s, but has leveled off in recent years. Research indicates that your physical activity level as a child is a good predictor of your physical activity level as an adult.[1] But if you spent your childhood or adolescence as a couch potato, don't despair. College is an excellent place to make a break with the past and develop exercise habits that can increase both the quality and duration of your life. Especially when combined with a healthy diet, regular physical activity combats obesity and thus reduces your likelihood of coronary artery disease, high blood pressure, diabetes, and other chronic diseases.[2]

Regular physical activity improves more than 50 different physiological, metabolic, and psychological aspects of human life[3]—which is why more and more Americans are getting serious about exercising. Millions are jogging, taking step aerobics classes, bicycling, swimming, or engaging in other fitness activities. Unfortunately, millions more have not abandoned their sedentary lifestyles. Only 22 percent of American adults engage in at least 30 minutes of light to moderate physical activity five or more times per week, while fewer than 10 percent exercise at the frequency and intensity needed to improve cardiorespiratory fitness.[4] This chapter will provide you with the information you need to create your own exercise program to improve or maintain your level of physical fitness now and throughout your lifetime.

BENEFITS OF PHYSICAL FITNESS

Physical activity is any force exerted by skeletal muscles that results in energy usage above the level used when the body's systems are at rest.[5] Among adults, higher levels of physical activity have been associated with a lower incidence of coronary artery disease, the leading cause of death in the United States for both men and women.[6] Regular physical activity has also been linked to lower incidence of high blood pressure (hypertension), cancers of the colon and reproductive organs, bone fractures pro-

duced by osteoporosis, and depression.[7] A recent study reported that regular exercise (four hours a week or more) beginning in adolescence and continuing into adulthood can significantly reduce the risk of breast cancer in women 40 and younger.[8]

Many of the risk factors for coronary artery disease, hypertension, and osteoporosis first appear during childhood and adolescence.[9] As many as 60 percent of American children exhibit at least one of the adult risk factors for coronary artery disease by the age of 12.[10] Fortunately, if identified during childhood, adolescence, or young adulthood, many of these risks can be reduced through exercise and modifications in diet. Unfortunately, lack of access to exercise facilities can hinder efforts by the socioeconomically disadvantaged to improve health, as the Multicultural Perspectives box discusses.

The physiological and psychological benefits of regular exercise are frequently discussed in the popular media. Some of these benefits are well established; others are controversial or not as well understood.

Improved Cardiorespiratory Efficiency

A regular program of aerobic exercise improves the efficiency of your cardiovascular and respiratory systems. As a benefit of regular exercise, the heart is able to pump more blood with each stroke, thus lowering resting heart rate. Additionally, the body's capacity to distribute oxygen to working muscles is improved while the muscles responsible for respiration are strengthened.

Reduced Risk of Heart Disease. Your heart is a muscle made up of highly specialized tissue. Because muscles become stronger and more efficient with use, regular exercise strengthens the heart, enabling it to pump more blood with each beat. This increased efficiency means that your heart requires fewer beats per minute to circulate blood throughout your body. A stronger, more efficient heart is better able to meet the ordinary and extraordinary demands of life.

Prevention of Hypertension. Hypertension is the medical term for abnormally high blood pressure. It is a significant risk factor for cardiovascular disease and stroke. Hypertension is particularly prevalent among adult African Americans, who experience it approximately 1.5

Is Exercise Accessible to the Poor?

By now you should be aware of the effect of low socioeconomic status on the health of U.S. citizens: it is associated with higher rates of heart disease and cancer, less access to health care and an increased likelihood to be overweight, to smoke, to drink, and to use drugs. As if this weren't enough of a burden to carry, the poor also lack access to exercise facilities.

Of the general population, 12 percent of people aged 18 and older and 66 percent of youth aged 10 to 17 engage in enough physical activity (three or more days per week for 20 minutes or more per occasion) to maintain cardiorespiratory fitness. Yet only 7 percent of lower-income people are this physically active. In fact, 32 percent of people with family incomes under $20,000 per year do not engage in any leisure-time physical activity.

Consider African Americans, of whom one-third live below the poverty level. Black men die of strokes at a rate four times that of the general population. A recent survey found that 49.5 percent of black women are obese compared with 33.3 percent of the population. And blacks have a lower life expectancy than the general population. Given that exercise has been shown to be effective in reducing obesity rates and improving cardiorespiratory function, why is this group so hard hit?

For inner-city residents, part of the answer lies in the lack of access to parks and other safe, affordable places to exercise. In addition, many inner-city youth lack the time for exercise because they need to work to supplement their families' earnings. Moreover, regardless of whether low-income families live in urban or rural settings, it is often difficult for them to practice good health habits such as regular exercise and proper nutrition when their attention and energy are focused on their economic struggle.

Making school and recreational facilities available at hours when low-income youth are less likely to be working is one way to improve this situation. One such successful approach to encouraging good exercise habits among inner-city youth and to providing a productive use of their time during high-crime hours is the midnight basketball program in Chicago. Similar programs that open and supervise school and recreational facilities for as many evening and weekend hours as budgets permit are needed in both rural and urban settings.

Source: Information from Alison Bass, "Record Obesity Levels Found," *Boston Globe,* 20 July 1994, 10; Jerrold S. Greenberg, George B. Dintiman, Barbee Myers Oakes, "Income Level Affects Physical Activity Level," in *Physical Fitness and Wellness* (Boston: Allyn and Bacon, 1995), 57; and Philip Elmer-Dewitt, "Fat Times," *Time,* 16 January 1995, 63.

---

times more frequently than do white adults.[11] If your resting **systolic blood pressure** is consistently 160 millimeters of mercury (mm Hg) or higher, your risk of coronary heart disease is four times greater than normal. If your resting **diastolic blood pressure** regularly exceeds 95 mm Hg, your risk of heart disease is six times greater than normal.[12] Low to moderate exercise training lowers both systolic and diastolic blood pressure by about 10 mm Hg in people with mild to moderate hypertension.[13] Regular physical activity can also reduce both systolic and diastolic blood pressure in people with normal and high blood pressures.[14]

Improved Blood Lipid and Lipoprotein Profile. Lipids are fats that circulate in the bloodstream and are stored in various places in your body. Regular exercise is known to reduce the levels of low-density lipoproteins (LDLs—"bad cholesterol") while increasing the number of high-density lipoproteins (HDLs—"good cholesterol") in the blood. Higher HDL levels are associated with lower risk for artery disease because they remove some of the "bad cholesterol" from artery walls and hence prevent clogging.

The net effect of these two physiological responses to exercise is a diminished risk of cardiovascular disease.

Improved Skeletal Mass

Osteoarthritis is a nonfatal but incurable disease characterized by degeneration of joint cartilage and irritation of surrounding bone and soft tissues. Affecting over 16 mil-

Systolic blood pressure: The pressure in the arteries during a heartbeat; abnormal if consistently 160 mm Hg or above.

Diastolic blood pressure: The pressure in the arteries during the period between heartbeats; abnormal if consistently 95 mm Hg or above.

Osteoarthritis: A disease characterized by degeneration of joint cartilage and irritation of surrounding bone and soft tissue.

lion adults, osteoarthritis is the most prevalent chronic joint condition in the United States. Women are afflicted more frequently than men.[15] Several recent studies have demonstrated that supervised fitness walking and weight-loss programs can improve physical capacity while reducing knee joint osteoarthritis symptoms.[16]

A common affliction of older women is **osteoporosis,** a disease characterized by low bone mass and deterioration of bone tissue, which increase fracture risk. One of the physical activities recommended most frequently to women wanting to improve their bone health is walking. While walking is an excellent activity for overall fitness, there is currently no evidence that it can significantly increase bone mass in healthy women.[17] Bone, like other human tissues, responds to the demands placed upon it, and unless the mechanical stresses placed on bone by a particular physical activity exceed the level of stress the bone has adapted to, there is no stimulus to increase bone mass.[18] Women (and men) have much to gain by remaining physically active as they age—bone mass levels have been found to be significantly higher among active than among sedentary women.[19] However, it appears that exercise's full benefit can only be achieved when proper hormone levels (estrogen in women, testosterone in men) are present. Regular exercise, when combined with a balanced diet containing adequate calcium, will help maintain skeletal mass, although this benefit is harder to achieve as we age.

Improved Weight Control

For many people, the desire to lose weight is the main purpose for starting an exercise program. Exercise does have a direct effect upon metabolic rate, even raising it for a few hours following a vigorous workout. According to the American College of Sports Medicine, if you are planning to lose weight through exercise alone, without decreasing the amount of food you eat, you'll have to exercise frequently (at least four days a week) for extended time periods (at least 50 minutes per workout).[20] A more effective method for losing weight combines regular endurance-type exercises with a moderate decrease (about 500 to 1,000 calories per day) in food intake. Decreasing daily caloric intake beyond this range ("severe dieting") appears to decrease metabolic rate by up to 20 percent, making weight loss more difficult.

Improved Health and Life Span

Prevention of Diabetes. Non-insulin-dependent diabetes is a complex disorder that affects 10 to 12 million Americans over the age of 20. The strongest predisposing factors for this type of diabetes are obesity, increasing age, and a family history of diabetes; lesser risk factors include high blood pressure and high cholesterol.[21] Physicians suggest exercise combined with weight reduction and

proper diet for the management of this form of diabetes. A recent large epidemiological study found that for every 2,000 calories of energy expended during leisure-time activities, the incidence of diabetes was reduced by 24 percent. Perhaps the most encouraging finding was that the protective effect of exercise was greatest among those individuals who were at the highest risk for non-insulin-dependent diabetes.[22]

Increased Longevity. Experts have long debated the relationship between exercise and longevity. For decades, most research failed to show that we could increase our life expectancy through exercise alone. Then, a landmark study conducted at the Institute for Aerobics Research in Texas found that exercise does increase longevity. More than 13,000 white middle- to upper-middle-class men and women aged 20 to 80 were followed for eight years to discover how physical fitness relates to death rates. Participants were assigned fitness levels based upon their age, sex, and results of exercise tests. The death rate in the least

Reduced risk of disease and new dimensions for living are among the benefits of physical fitness that are available to people of all ages and all capabilities.

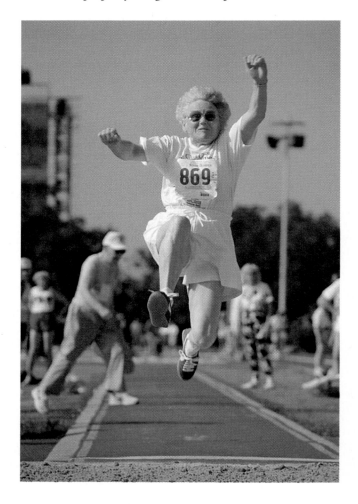

Exercise Can Reduce the Risk of Breast Cancer

Regular exercise beginning in adolescence and continuing into adulthood can significantly reduce the risk of breast cancer in younger women, according to a study published in the *Journal of the National Cancer Institute* on September 20, 1994.

In contrast to inactive women, those who exercise four hours a week or more throughout their reproductive years reduce their breast cancer risk by 60 percent, perhaps because exercise reduces levels of hormones that may promote breast cancer, the study said.

The protective effect of exercise for women 40 and under was particularly pronounced in women who have had at least one child. Women who exercised somewhat less—one to three hours per week—cut their risk by about 30 percent. And women who exercised for the first 10 years after puberty and then stopped cut their risk by 30 percent, suggesting that exercising in adolescence is critical. The particular type of exercise did not seem to matter.

The study, which an editorial in the NCI journal called "fairly convincing," shows that exercise appears to be an independent risk factor for breast cancer, which is expected to strike 182,000 women this year and kill 46,000. For women seeking to lower their breast cancer risk, the new finding is good news. Unfortunately, according to a 1990 survey, fewer than 40 percent of high school girls were enrolled in physical education classes and only 20 percent engaged in regular, vigorous physical activity.

The exercise study, led by Leslie Bernstein, an epidemiologist at the University of Southern California, looked at 1,090 women aged 40 and under—545 of them newly diagnosed breast cancer patients and 545 "controls" without cancer who were similar in age and other characteristics. All were interviewed about physical activity since puberty.

Source: Adapted courtesy of the *Boston Globe* from Judy Foreman, "Exercise Can Reduce Risk of Breast Cancer, Study Says," *Boston Globe,* 21 September 1994, 1, 14.

---

physically fit group was more than three times higher than the death rate in the most fit group. How much exercise was required to produce a difference? Participants who changed from a sedentary lifestyle to one that included a brisk 30- to 60-minute walk each day experienced significant increases in their life expectancies.[23]

Improved Immunity to Disease. Will regular exercise make you more immune to disease, and if so, how does this occur? Recent research suggests that regular moderate exercise makes people less susceptible to disease, but that this potential benefit may depend upon whether they perceive exercise as pleasurable or stressful.[24] While current evidence suggests that moderate exercise improves immunity, more extreme forms of exercise may be detrimental. For example, athletes engaging in marathon-type events or very intense physical training programs have been shown to be at increased risk of upper respiratory tract infections (e.g., colds and flu).[25] In a recent study of 2,300 marathon runners, those who ran more than 60 miles per week suffered twice as many upper respiratory tract infections as those who ran fewer than 20 miles per week.[26]

Just how exercise alters immunity is not well understood. We do know that brisk exercise temporarily increases the number of white blood cells (WBCs), the blood cells responsible for fighting infection. Generally speaking, the less fit the person and the more intense the exercise, the greater the increase in WBCs.[27] After brief periods of exercise (without injury), the number of WBCs typically returns to normal levels within one to two hours. After exercise bouts lasting longer than 30 minutes, WBCs may be elevated for 24 hours or more before returning to normal levels.[28] An increased number of WBCs suggests increased immunity to disease and infection. The Health Headlines box discusses a new study on the role of exercise in immunity to breast cancer.

If you already have a cold or the flu, is it wise to exercise? If your symptoms are "above the neck"—a runny nose, stuffy head, scratchy throat—proceed with caution. Begin exercising at about half-speed, and if after 10 minutes your head is clear and you feel better, continue to exercise. If you feel worse, stop exercising and rest. If your symptoms are "below the neck"—hacking cough, vomiting, diarrhea, muscle aches—you should not exercise.[29]

Improved Mental Health and Stress Management

People who engage in regular physical activity may be unaware of all the beneficial changes in their physiological

Osteoporosis: A disease characterized by low bone mass and deterioration of bone tissue, which increase fracture risk.

functions, but most notice the psychological benefits. While these psychological benefits are difficult to quantify, they are frequently mentioned as reasons for continuing to exercise. Regular vigorous exercise has been shown to "burn off" the chemical by-products released by our nervous system during normal response to stress. Elimination of these biochemical substances reduces our stress levels by accelerating the neurological system's return to a balanced state. For this reason, exercise should be an integral component of your stress management plan.

Regular exercise improves physical appearance by toning and developing muscles and, in combination with dieting, reducing body fat. Feeling good about personal appearance can provide a tremendous boost to self-esteem. At the same time, as people come to appreciate the improved strength, conditioning, and flexibility that accompany fitness, they often become less obsessed with physical appearance.[30] Through regular physical activity, they learn new skills and develop increased abilities in favorite recreational activities, which also help improve self-esteem.

WHAT DO YOU THINK?

Do you know your resting heart rate? Blood pressure? Cholesterol level? Who could provide you with this information? Based upon what you've read, what are the health benefits you'd like to achieve as the result of regular physical activity?

Improved Physical Fitness

Physical fitness can be defined as a set of attributes related to the ability to perform normal physical activity.[31] The individual fitness components are listed and described in Table 10.1. In contrast, **exercise** is defined as physical activity at higher-than-normal levels of exertion. **Exercise training** is the systematic performance of exercise at a specified frequency, intensity, and duration to achieve a desired level of physical fitness.[32]

The recent popularity of the quest for physical fitness has given rise to some outrageous claims about "no pain, all gain" exercise equipment and clothing (e.g., potentially fatal rubberized "sauna suits"). It has also instigated the marketing of celebrity videotapes offering the convenience of at-home exercise programs. Regular practice of the exercises demonstrated on a particular videotape may improve one or more aspects of your physical fitness; however, some of these programs are not comprehensive enough to improve overall physical fitness. Some videos suggest that following their programs will not only help you lose weight but will also transform your body contour into some "ideal" form. Almost any regular exercise program will help you lose weight, but achieving some idealized form is nearly impossible for many people. Participation in a comprehensive physical fitness program, in contrast, is healthy, realistic, and respects your own unique physical traits. It will help you to achieve a better body—*your* optimal body, not some celebrity's.

Although physical fitness has many facets, it is most commonly measured by four interdependent components: (1) cardiorespiratory endurance, (2) flexibility, (3) muscular strength, and (4) muscular endurance.

TABLE 10.1 ■ Physical Fitness Components

Agility	Speed in changing direction or in changing body positions.
Anaerobic power	Maximum rate of work performance.
Balance	Maintenance of a stable body position.
Body composition	Fatness: ratio of fat weight to total body weight.
Cardiorespiratory endurance	Ability to sustain moderate-intensity whole-body activity for extended time periods.
Flexibility	Range of motion in a joint or series of joints.
Muscular endurance	Ability to perform repeated high-intensity muscle contractions.
Muscular strength	Maximum force applied with a single muscle contraction.

Source: Reprinted by permission of Williams and Wilkins from T. Baranowski et al., "Assessment, Prevalence, and Cardiovascular Benefits of Physical Activity and Fitness in Youth," *Medicine and Science in Sports and Exercise* 24 (June 1992): supplement, S238.

People with physical disabilities can attain the levels of cardiovascular fitness and muscular strength necessary to participate in physical activities they enjoy—even competitive sports.

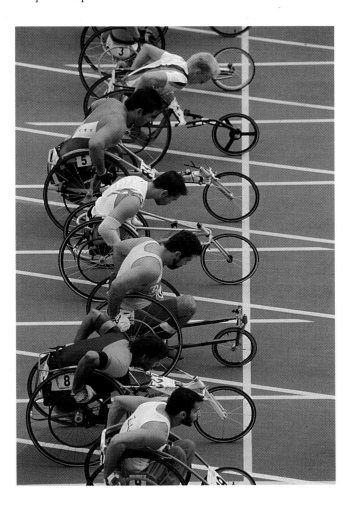

To be considered physically fit, you generally need to attain (and then maintain) certain minimum standards for each component that have been established by exercise physiologists and other fitness experts. Some people have physical limitations that make achieving one or more of these standards impossible. That doesn't mean they can't attain physical fitness. For example, a woman with limited flexibility due to arthritis in the knee and hip joints may be unable to walk or jog moderate distances without extreme pain. Yet by exercising in a swimming pool, where the buoyancy of the water will relieve much of the stress on her joints, she can improve her range of motion. She can also develop muscular strength and cardiovascular fitness by "jogging" at the deep end of a swimming pool while wearing a flotation device. Similarly, a man who needs to use a wheelchair will be unable to run or walk a mile, as is required in some fitness tests, but may achieve physical fitness by playing wheelchair basketball. Our de-

finition of physical fitness should be adapted to address individual differences in capabilities.

ᵂHAT DO YOU THINK?

Which of the key aspects of physical fitness do you currently possess? Which ones would you like to improve or develop? What types of activities will you do to improve your fitness level?

ᴵMPROVING CARDIOVASCULAR FITNESS

The number of walkers, joggers, bicyclists, step aerobics participants, and swimmers is tangible evidence of Americans' increased awareness of the most important aspect of physical fitness: **cardiovascular fitness**, which refers to the ability of your heart, lungs, and blood vessels to function efficiently. Our very lives depend on our cardiovascular system's ability to deliver oxygenated blood and nutrients to our body tissues and to remove carbon dioxide and other metabolic waste products.

The primary category of physical activity known to improve cardiovascular fitness is **aerobic exercise**. The term *aerobic* means "with oxygen" and describes any type of exercise, typically performed at moderate levels of intensity for extended periods of time, that increases your heart rate. Aerobic activities such as walking, jogging, bicycling, and swimming are among the best exercises for improving overall health status as well as cardiovascular fitness. A person said to be in "good cardiovascular shape" has an above-average *aerobic capacity*—a term used to describe the current functional status of the cardiovascular system

Physical fitness: A set of attributes related to the ability to perform normal physical activity.

Exercise: Physical activity at higher-than-normal levels of exertion.

Exercise training: The systematic performance of exercise at a specified frequency, intensity, and duration to achieve a desired level of physical fitness.

Cardiovascular fitness: The ability of the heart, lungs, and blood vessels to function efficiently.

Aerobic exercise: Any type of exercise, typically performed at moderate levels of intensity for extended periods of time (20 to 30 minutes or longer), that increases heart rate.

(i.e., heart, lungs, blood vessels). **Aerobic capacity** (commonly written $VO_{2\,max}$) is defined as the volume of oxygen consumed by the muscles during exercise.

To measure your maximal aerobic capacity, an exercise physiologist or physician will typically have you exercise on a treadmill. He or she will initially ask you to walk or run at an easy pace, and then, at set time intervals during this **graded exercise test**, will gradually increase the workload (i.e., a combination of running speed and the angle of incline of the treadmill) to the point of maximal exertion. Generally, the higher your cardiovascular fitness level, the more oxygen you can transport to exercising muscles and the longer you can maintain a high intensity of exercise prior to exhaustion. In healthy individuals, the higher the $VO_{2\,max}$ value, the higher the level of aerobic fitness. Figure 10.1 compares the aerobic capacities of healthy athletes in various sports with those of sedentary individuals.

According to the exercise testing guidelines of the American College of Sports Medicine, maximal aerobic capacity treadmill tests should not be conducted on men over 40 or women over 50 without a prior comprehensive physical examination and permission from their physicians.[33] Other less reliable, but safer, methods of measuring aerobic capacity are frequently employed to estimate $VO_{2\,max}$. These submaximal tests may use stationary bicycles, walk/run tests, or walk tests to quantify the aerobic fitness levels in people of all ages. You may have performed one of these aerobic capacity tests as part of a high school or college physical education course.

You can conduct your own submaximal test of your aerobic capacity by using either the 1.5-mile run or the 12-minute run endurance test described in the Rate Yourself box. However, you should not use these endurance-run tests when you are just beginning an exercise program.[34] Progress slowly through a walking/jogging program at low intensities before you attempt to measure your aerobic capacity with one of these tests. It is also important for you to consult a doctor before beginning an exercise program if you have certain medical conditions, such as asthma, diabetes, heart disease, or obesity.

Aerobic Fitness Programs

Researchers tell us that a physically active lifestyle is the key to improved cardiovascular health, but what level of activity is required to improve aerobic fitness? There are

> **Aerobic capacity:** The current functional status of a person's cardiovascular system; measured as $VO_{2\,max}$.
>
> **Graded exercise test:** A test of aerobic capacity administered by a physician, exercise physiologist, or other trained person; two common forms are the treadmill running test and the stationary bike test.

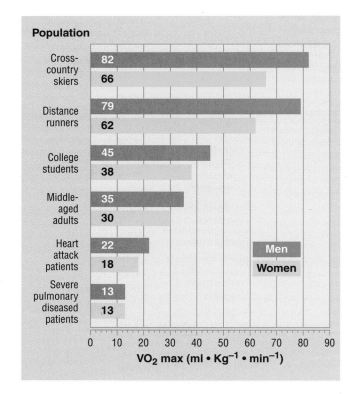

FIGURE 10.1

Various Aerobic Capacities

Source: From *Health/Fitness Instructor's Handbook* (p. 42) by Edward T. Howley and B. Don Franks. Champaign, IL: Human Kinetics Publishers, 1992. Copyright 1992 by Edward T. Howley and B. Don Franks. Reprinted by permission.

numerous variables in any particular aerobic activity, but comfortable aerobic exercise that works your heart at a moderate intensity (approximately 70 percent of your maximum heart rate, or about 140 to 160 beats per minute) for prolonged periods of time (20 to 30 minutes of continuous activity) will improve your fitness level.

The most beneficial aerobic exercises are total body activities involving all the large muscle groups of your body. If you have been sedentary for quite a while, simply initiating a physical activity program may be the hardest task you'll face. Don't be put off by the next-day soreness you are likely to feel in your long-dormant muscles. The key is to begin your exercise program at a very low intensity, progress slowly . . . and stay with it! For example, if you choose an aerobic fitness program that involves jogging, you'll need several weeks of workouts combining jogging and walking before you will reach a fitness level that enables you to jog continuously for 15 to 20 minutes.

You will need to adjust the frequency, intensity, and duration of your aerobic activity program to accommodate your level of cardiovascular fitness. As you progress, add to your exercise load by increasing exercise duration or intensity, but do not increase both at the same time. For

Self-Assessment of Cardiovascular Fitness

Once you've been exercising regularly for several weeks, you might want to assess your cardiovascular fitness level. Find a local track, typically one-quarter mile per lap, to perform your test. You may either run/walk for 1.5 miles and measure how long it takes to reach that distance, or run/walk for 12 minutes and determine the distance you covered in that time. Use the chart below to estimate your cardiovascular fitness level based upon your age and sex. Note that females have lower standards for each fitness category because of their higher levels of essential fat.

| | 1.5-Mile Run (min:sec) | | 12-Minute Run (miles) | |
Age*	Female (min:sec)	Male (min:sec)	Female (miles)	Male (miles)
Good				
15–30	<12:00	<10:00	>1.5	>1.7
35–50	<13:30	<11:30	>1.4	>1.5
55–70	<16:00	<14:00	>1.2	>1.3
Adequate for most activities				
15–30	<13:30	<11:50	>1.4	>1.5
35–50	<15:00	<13:00	>1.3	>1.4
55–70	<17:30	<15:30	>1.1	>1.3
Borderline				
15–30	<15:00	<13:00	>1.3	>1.4
35–50	<16:30	<14:30	>1.2	>1.3
55–70	<19:00	<17:00	>1.0	>1.2
Need extra work on cardiovascular fitness				
15–30	>17:00	>15:00	<1.2	<1.3
35–50	>18:30	>16:30	<1.1	<1.2
55–70	>21:00	>19:00	<0.9	<1.0

*Cardiovascular fitness declines with age.

. . . If you are now at the Good level, your emphasis should be on maintaining this level for the rest of your life. If you are now at lower levels, you should set realistic goals for improvement.

Source: From *Health/Fitness Instructor's Handbook* (p. 85) by Edward T. Howley and B. Don Franks. Champaign, IL: Human Kinetics Publishers. Copyright 1986 by Edward T. Howley and B. Don Franks. Reprinted by permission.

---

instance, if you began a 20-minute walking/jogging aerobic program at an intensity that produces a heart rate of 135 to 145 beats per minute during the first week, the following week you could add five minutes to the length of your workout while maintaining the exercise intensity. Other modifications for a beginning exercise might be to keep the exercise period fixed at 20 minutes but to walk at a faster pace or to jog for a greater percentage of your workout time. To stay mentally fresh, devise several different walking/jogging routes having varying terrain and scenery.

Determining Exercise Frequency. If you are a newcomer to regular physical activity, the frequency of your aerobic exercise bouts should be at least three times per week. If you exercise less frequently, you will achieve fewer health benefits. The proper frequency of exercise is affected by the intensity and duration of the individual exercise periods. The American College of Sports Medicine recommends three to five days per week for most aerobic exercise programs. As your fitness level improves, your goal should be to exercise five days a week. To avoid overuse injuries and monotony, vary your activities and take a day off when you need a rest.

Determining Exercise Intensity. An aerobic exercise program must employ prolonged, moderate-intensity workouts to improve cardiorespiratory fitness. The measure of such a workout is your **target heart rate**, which is a percentage of your maximum heart rate. To calculate target heart rate, subtract your age from 220 for females or from 226 for males. The result is your maximum heart rate. You determine your target heart rate by calculating a desired percentage of maximum heart rate, often 60 percent. If you are a 20-year-old female, your maximum heart rate is 200 (220 − 20). Your 60-percent target heart rate would be 120 (200 × .60). People in poor physical condition should set a target heart rate between 40 and 50 percent of maximum. As your condition improves, you can gradually increase your target heart rate. Increases should be made in small increments: Increase from 40 to 45 percent; then from 45 to 50 percent. It is not recommended that most people exceed 80 to 85 percent of maximum heart rate.

Once you know your target heart rate, you can determine how close you are to this value during your workout. You'll need to stop exercising briefly in order to measure your heart rate. To take your pulse, lightly place your index and middle fingers (don't use your thumb) over one of the major (carotid) arteries in your neck, along either side of your Adam's apple. Be sure to start counting your pulse immediately after you stop exercising, as your heart rate will decrease quickly. Using a watch or clock, take your pulse for six seconds and multiply this number by 10 (just add a zero to your count) to get the number of beats per minute. Your pulse should be within a range of about 5 bpm above or below your target heart rate. If necessary, increase or decrease the pace or intensity of your workout to achieve your target heart rate.

A target heart rate of 70 percent of maximum is sometimes called the "conversational level of exercise" because you are able to talk with a partner while exercising.[35] If you are a novice and you are breathing so hard that talking is difficult, your intensity of exercise is too high. If you can sustain a conversational level of aerobic exercise for 20

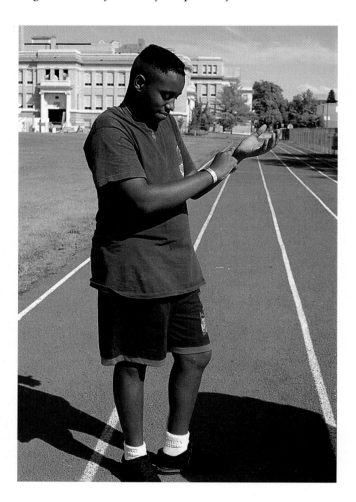

An aerobic fitness program starts with setting a target heart rate and then adjusting the frequency, intensity, and duration of exercise in order to maintain that target heart rate for a beneficial period of time.

Target heart rate: Calculated as a percentage of maximum heart rate (220 minus age); heart rate (pulse) is taken during aerobic exercise to check if exercise intensity is at the desired level (e.g., 70 percent of maximum heart rate).

Flexibility: The measure of the range of motion, or the amount of movement possible, at a particular joint.

Tai chi: An ancient, Chinese form of exercise widely practiced in the West today that promotes balance, coordination, stretching, and meditation.

Yoga: A variety of Indian forms of exercise widely practiced in the West today that promote balance, coordination, flexibility, and meditation.

to 30 minutes, you will improve your cardiovascular fitness.

Exercise at higher intensities (and therefore at higher target heart rates) results in greater fitness gains. The higher the intensity and subsequent heart rate, the less time you'll need to work out to achieve and maintain fitness. For people in excellent cardiovascular condition who exercise at a target heart rate of 90 percent of their maximum heart rate, fitness gains occur with relatively short-duration workouts.[36]

Determining Exercise Duration. Duration refers to the number of minutes of exercise performed during any one session. The Centers for Disease Control and Prevention (CDC) and the American College of Sports Medicine (ACSM) suggest that every adult accumulate 30 minutes or more of moderate-intensity physical activity over the course of most days of the week.[37] Activities that can con-

Starting Your Own Exercise Program

Beginners often start their exercise programs too rigorously. Be realistic about the amount of time you will need to get into good physical condition. Perhaps the most significant factor early on in an aerobic exercise program is personal comfort. You'll need to experiment to find an activity that you truly enjoy. Be open to exploring new activities and new exercise equipment. Try to match your exercise regimen with your target heart rate. For example, if you jog 1 mile at a local track, you may discover that running at a 6-mph pace (10:00 minutes per mile) gets you up to 60 percent of your maximum heart rate. If your target heart rate is 70 percent of your maximum heart rate, you'll need to jog a bit faster, perhaps at a 7-mph pace, to reach your goal.

It's also important to stretch the muscles you use exercising both before and after exercising, although if the activity is of very low intensity (e.g., slow walking), it is probably necessary to stretch only after exercise. Some exercise scientists believe that it is most beneficial to stretch after a muscle has undergone a warm-up. Prior to a strenuous step aerobics class, then, it may be best to do five minutes of mild aerobic exercise, such as brisk walking, and then stretch.

Following exercise, your body's physiological systems operate more efficiently if provided a cool-down period. If you have been exercising vigorously, don't stop abruptly. Instead, gradually decrease your intensity of the exercise. This strategy allows the metabolic waste products lactic acid and carbon dioxide to be removed more rapidly from the blood. If exercise is stopped abruptly, blood pools in the muscles that were active and less blood flows back to the heart. This decreases the blood output by the heart, and can result in dizziness and fainting. For a more rapid recovery after vigorous exercise, always include a cool-down period as part of your workout.

---

tribute to this 30-minute total include dancing, walking up stairs (instead of taking the elevator), gardening, and raking leaves as well as planned physical activities such as jogging, swimming, and cycling. One way to meet the CDC/ACSM recommendation is to walk 2 miles briskly.

The lower the intensity of the activity, the longer the duration you'll need to get the same caloric expenditure. For example, a 120-pound woman will burn 180 calories walking for one hour at 2.0 miles per hour, but will burn 330 calories if she walks for an hour at a 4.5-mile per hour pace. A 180-pound man will expend 288 calories per hour of playing golf if he carries his clubs, but will burn 805 calories per hour if he is cross-country skiing.[38] Your goal should be to expend 300 to 500 calories per exercise session, with an eventual weekly goal of 1,500 to 2,000 calories. As you age and your basal metabolic rate decreases, the weight-control (caloric expenditure) benefits of longer-duration, low-intensity exercise can become increasingly important.

A program of repeated bouts of exercise over several months or years—exercise training—causes changes in the way your cardiovascular system meets your body's oxygen requirements at rest and during exercise. Since many of the health benefits associated with cardiovascular fitness activities take about one year of regular exercise to achieve, you shouldn't expect an immediate reduction in your risk of cardiovascular disease when you start an exercise program.[39] However, any low-to-moderate-intensity physical activity, even if it does not meet all the cardiovascular exercise characteristics mentioned in this chapter, will benefit your overall health almost from the start. The Choices for Change box has tips for starting your workout program.

*W*HAT DO YOU THINK?

Calculate your maximum heart rate. Pick an intensity of exercise that suits your fitness level, for example, 60 percent, 70 percent, or 80 percent of your maximum heart rate. Using a familiar physical activity and monitoring your pulse, experiment by exercising at three different intensities. Do you notice any difference in the way you felt while exercising? Afterward?

*I*MPROVING YOUR FLEXIBILITY

Flexibility is a measure of the range of motion, or the amount of movement possible, at a particular joint. This component of fitness is commonly overshadowed by the muscular strength and aerobic capacity components, but muscles that lack elasticity and resiliency are more susceptible to injury. Improving your range of motion through stretching exercises will enhance your efficiency of movement and your posture.

A regular program of stretching exercises can enhance psychological as well as physical well-being. **Tai chi** is an ancient, Chinese form of exercise that combines stretching, balance, coordination, and meditation; it is widely practiced in the West today. **Yoga**, which originated in

India and also combines stretching, coordination, balance, and meditation, is even more widely practiced. Both are excellent for improving flexibility. Many factory workers in the United States now begin their workdays with simpler forms of flexibility exercises, a concept introduced from Japan.

Types of Stretching Exercises

Flexibility is enhanced by the controlled stretching of muscles that act on a particular joint. The primary strategy is to decrease the resistance to stretch (tension) within a tight muscle that you have targeted for increased range of motion.[40] To do this, you repeatedly stretch the muscle and its two tendons of attachment to elongate them. Flexibility can also be increased temporarily by having a whole-body massage that results in widespread muscle relaxation.

Two types of flexibility techniques are **static stretching** and **dynamic stretching**. Static stretching techniques involve the slow, gradual lengthening of a muscle or group of muscles. Various positions and postures are used to lengthen the tight muscle or muscle group to a point where a mild burning sensation is felt within the muscle. This end position is held for 10 to 30 seconds, and is repeated two or three times in close succession for each muscle or muscle group. With each repetition of a static stretch, range of motion improves temporarily. When static stretching is done properly, it stimulates the tension receptors within the muscle being stretched to allow the muscle to be stretched to greater length.[41]

A major goal of static stretching is to cause permanent elongation of the targeted muscle or muscle group, thus permitting greater range of motion at a given joint. To achieve this goal, a regular program of stretching exercises must be performed at least three (preferably five) days a week. If you are just beginning a program to improve your flexibility, proceed cautiously. Follow the diagrams in Figure 10.2 to stretch all the major muscle groups of your body. Hold each static stretch at the point of discomfort for 10 to 30 seconds initially.

The risk of injury with dynamic stretches is so high that this type of stretching is no longer recommended for improving flexibility. This process can be likened to taking a rubber band between two fingers, rapidly pulling it apart, and then releasing the tension again and again. And

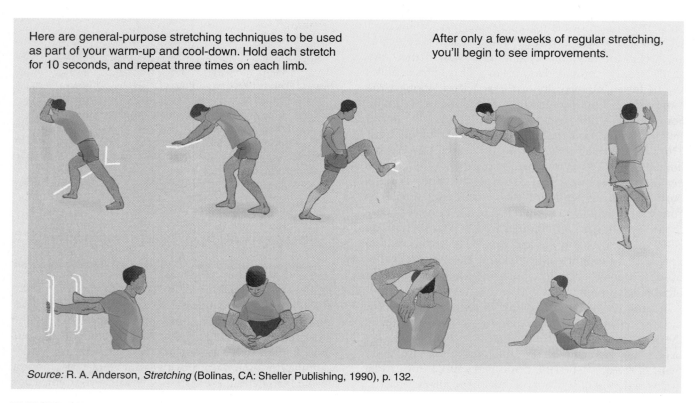

Here are general-purpose stretching techniques to be used as part of your warm-up and cool-down. Hold each stretch for 10 seconds, and repeat three times on each limb.

After only a few weeks of regular stretching, you'll begin to see improvements.

Source: R. A. Anderson, *Stretching* (Bolinas, CA: Sheller Publishing, 1990), p. 132.

FIGURE 10.2

Stretching Exercises that Will Help You Improve Your Flexibility

Source: Excerpted from *Stretching,* © 1980 by Bob and Jean Anderson. $12.00 Shelter Publications, Inc., P.O. Box 279, Bolinas, CA 94924. Distributed in bookstores by Random House. Reprinted by permission.

just as a rubber band can snap in your fingers if you apply too much tension, the muscles being stretched can be torn during these rapid movements.

𝒲HAT DO YOU THINK?

Why is it so important to have good flexibility throughout life? What are some situations in which improved flexibility would help you perform daily activities with less effort? What specific actions will you take to improve your flexibility?

𝒥MPROVING MUSCULAR STRENGTH AND ENDURANCE

Muscular strength refers to the amount of force a muscle is capable of exerting. The most common way to assess strength in a resistance exercise program is to measure the maximum amount of weight you can lift one time. This value is known as the **one repetition maximum**, and is written as **1RM**. **Muscular endurance** is defined as a muscle's ability to exert force repeatedly without fatiguing. The more repetitions of a certain resistance exercise you can perform successfully (e.g., a bench press of 100 pounds), the greater your muscular endurance.

Principles of Strength Development

There are three key principles to understand if you intend to maximize muscular strength and endurance benefits from your **resistance exercise program**.[42] Unless you follow these principles, you are likely to be disappointed in the results of your program.

The Tension Principle. The key to developing strength is to create tension within a muscle. The more tension you can create in a muscle, the greater your strength gain will be. Before our industrialized society developed, few men and women were concerned with improving their strength. The settlers of the West who farmed with horse-drawn plows, drank water from hand-dug wells, and built houses with boards made from trees they cut down by hand certainly never went looking for ways to work their muscles just for the fun of it! Today, with so many machines to do our physical labor for us, our muscles don't always have the tone we would like them to have.

The most common recreational way to create tension in a muscle is by lifting weights. While weight lifting is one method of producing tension in a muscle, any activity that creates muscle tension—for example, using weight machines with pulleys and cables or riding a bike up a steep hill—will result in greater strength. It really does not

matter what type of equipment you choose to develop tension in your muscles; what matters is that you use the equipment in such a way as to produce the desired strength and endurance.

The Overload Principle. The overload principle is the most important of the three key principles for improving muscular strength. Everyone begins a resistance training program with an initial level of strength. To increase that level of strength, you must regularly create a degree of tension in your muscles that is greater than they are accustomed to. This overloading of your muscles, most commonly accomplished with weights of some type, will cause your muscles to adapt to the level of overload. As your muscles respond to a regular program of overloading by getting larger (**hypertrophy**), they become capable of generating more tension. Figure 10.3 illustrates how a continual process of overload and adaptation to the overload improves strength. If you fail to provide an overload—if you "underload" your muscles—you will not increase your strength. But if you provide too great an overload, you may experience muscle injury, muscle fatigue, and even a loss of strength.[43]

Once you have reached your strength goal, no further overloading is necessary. Your next challenge is to maintain that level of strength by continuing to participate in a regular (at least three times per week) resistance exercise program.

The Specificity of Training Principle. This principle refers to the manner in which a specific body system responds to the physiological demands placed upon it. Ac-

Static stretching: Techniques that gradually lengthen a muscle to an elongated position (to the point of discomfort) and hold that position for 10 to 30 seconds.

Dynamic stretching: Techniques that employ the repetitive, rapid stretching of muscles with no holding of the stretch at a terminal position; not recommended because of the risk of injury to muscle and/or tendon.

Muscular strength: The amount of force that a muscle is capable of exerting.

One repetition maximum (1RM): The amount of weight/resistance that can be lifted/moved one time, but not twice; a common measure of strength.

Muscular endurance: A muscle's ability to exert force repeatedly without fatiguing.

Resistance exercise program: A regular program of exercises designed to improve muscular strength and endurance in the major muscle groups.

Hypertrophy: Increased size (girth) of a muscle.

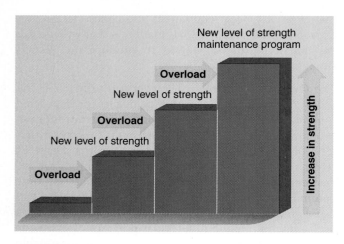

FIGURE 10.3

The overload principle contributes to an increase in strength. Notice that once the muscle has adapted to the original overload, a new overload must be placed on the muscle for subsequent gains in strength to occur.

Source: From Philip A. Sienna, *One Rep Max: A Guide to Beginning Weight Training,* Fig. 2.1, 8. Copyright © 1989. Wm. C. Brown Communications, Inc., Dubuque, Iowa. Reprinted by permission of Times Mirror Higher Education Group, Inc., Dubuque, Iowa. All rights reserved.

cording to the specificity principle, you'll get a very specific response to your chosen type of physical activity or exercise. If the specific overload you impose is designed to improve strength in the muscles of your chest and back, the response to that demand (overload) will be improved strength in those muscles only. As you can see, to get what you want and need from resistance training, you have to understand how your body is going to respond to different types of resistance exercises.

Types of Muscle Activity

When your skeletal muscles receive a stimulus from your nervous system to act, they respond by developing tension and producing a measurable force. Your skeletal muscles act in three different modes—isometric, concentric, and eccentric—to produce this force.[44] An **isometric muscle action** is one in which force is produced by the muscle without any resulting muscle movement. Isometric muscle actions do not create any joint motion. Muscles act isometrically to stabilize a particular body part while another body part is moving, or when a maximal resistance is met and the force produced by your muscles cannot overcome the resistance. Isometric exercise routines were popular in the 1960s and can develop strength, but they are not commonly used today.

One example of an isometric muscle action is the unsuccessful attempt to push a car out of snow or mud. Although you push with all your might, the car (as well as

your joints) does not move. The muscles involved are all producing forces, but in an isometric way. Another example, and one more related to resistance training, is attempting to lift a barbell too heavy for you. The more you try, the more tired your muscles become, but the barbell never leaves the floor.

A **concentric muscle action** is one in which force is produced while the muscle shortens. Joint movement is always produced during concentric muscle actions. Raising a 20-pound dumbbell in an elbow flexion movement (curl) is an example of a concentric action of the elbow flexor muscles (biceps). In general, concentric muscle actions produce movement in a direction opposite of the downward pull of gravity (Figure 10.4A).

Eccentric muscle action describes a muscle's ability to produce force while lengthening. Typically, eccentric muscle actions occur when movement is in the same direction as the pull of gravity. If you want to be sure that a given resistance exercise has an eccentric phase, you must use the type of resistance training equipment that requires you to perform an eccentric action in order to achieve the starting position prior to your next repetition. For example, with a 20-pound dumbbell biceps curl, you lower the weight slowly to the starting point of the exercise in an eccentric action of the elbow flexors. Even though the motion produced during this phase of the curl is elbow extension, it is the force exerted by the controlled lengthening of the elbow flexors (biceps) that is responsible for the motion, *not* the elbow extensor muscles (triceps) (Figure 10.4B).

All factors being equal, the greatest amount of force is produced during eccentric muscle actions, followed by isometric and then concentric muscle actions. Changes in

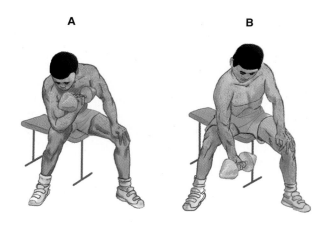

FIGURE 10.4

The figure depicts concentric and eccentric muscle actions. In A, the bicep shortens while producing tension in the upward phase of a curl. This is called a concentric muscle action. In B, the bicep lengthens while producing tension and permitting the controlled lowering of the weight. This is known as an eccentric muscle action.

muscle size and strength are affected both by the type of resistance exercise you employ and by the type of muscle action(s) you use during your workout. When using free weights (barbells, dumbbells), the typical sequential pattern of concentric-eccentric muscle actions during resistance training contributes to improved muscle strength and muscle fiber size. According to current research, if your resistance exercise program uses only concentric muscle actions, you'll need to perform at least twice as many concentric-only repetitions to achieve the same results as you would attain by using concentric-eccentric combinations.[45]

Methods of Providing Resistance

There are four commonly used methods of applying resistance to develop strength and endurance.

Body Weight Resistance. Many different techniques can be used to develop skeletal muscle fitness without relying on resistance equipment. Most of these methods use part or all of your body weight to offer the resistance during exercise. While these techniques are not as effective as external resistance in developing muscular strength, they are quite adequate for improving general muscular fitness. Many common exercises require your muscles to lift your body weight off the floor. Activities such as sit-ups, push-ups, and pull-ups use both concentric and eccentric muscle actions. These types of resistance activities are convenient—no special equipment is needed—and are generally sufficient to improve muscle tone and maintain the level of muscular strength created by this type of overload. But they do not help you to make significant strength gains.

Fixed Resistance. Fixed resistance exercises provide a constant amount of resistance throughout the full range of movement. Barbells and dumbbells provide fixed resistance because their weight (amount of resistance) does not change as you exercise. Unfortunately, due to the biomechanics of human motion, the muscle forces that must be exerted to move the weight are lower at some joint angles and higher at others. Any given muscle generates its least amount of force at the beginning and ending positions of a weight-lifting exercise and can create the most force when the joint involved in the exercise approximates a right angle (90 degrees). As a result, the disadvantage of fixed resistance exercises is that the extent to which a muscle is overloaded varies throughout the exercise, and the exercise may not fully develop the muscle. On the other hand, the advantages of fixed resistance exercise include the portability and low cost of barbells and dumbbells, the common availability of fixed resistance exercise machines at university recreation/fitness facilities and health clubs, and the existence of numerous exercises designed to strengthen all the major muscle groups in the body.

Variable Resistance. Whether found at a health club or in your home workout area, variable resistance equipment alters the resistance encountered by a muscle at various joint angles so that the effort by the muscle is more consistent throughout the full range of motion. Variable resistance machines are typically single-station devices (e.g., Nautilus), but some have multiple stations at which muscles of the upper and lower extremities can be exercised (e.g., Soloflex). While some of these machines are expensive and permanently placed, there are also inexpensive, portable forms of variable resistance devices sold for home use.

Accommodating Resistance. With accommodating resistance devices, the resistance changes according to the amount of force generated by the individual. There is no external weight to move or overcome. Resistance is provided by having the exerciser perform at maximal level of effort, while the exercise machine controls the speed of the exercise and does not allow any faster motion. The body segment being exercised must move at a rate faster than or equal to the set speed to encounter resistance. One way to distinguish between accommodating and variable resistance is to recall that with variable resistance, the resistance increases from the beginning to the end of the repetition. In contrast, accommodating resistance can become more or less difficult depending on the input (muscular force exerted by the exerciser) into the machine.[46]

Getting Started

You will find some general principles useful whatever your resistance exercise goals. If sufficient tension is generated within a muscle, it will respond by becoming stronger regardless of the type of muscle action or resistance employed. You need to determine your 1RM for each muscle or muscle group you plan to exercise in order to design your program, but the strategies you use in resistance training sessions will vary according to your specific goals.

Strength Training. There are almost as many ways to develop muscular strength as there are participants in strength-training exercise. It is important to select at least one resistance exercise for each major muscle group in the body to ensure development of comprehensive muscular strength. To develop strength, you should perform a rela-

Isometric muscle action: Force produced without any resulting muscle movement.

Concentric muscle action: Force produced while shortening the muscle.

Eccentric muscle action: Force produced while lengthening the muscle.

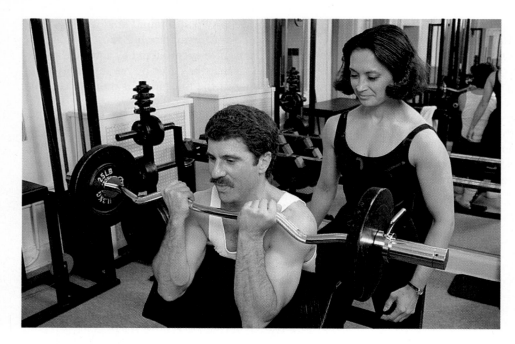

Lifting free weights to build muscular strength and endurance has many advantages, but reaching strength and endurance goals without injury requires skills that are best learned from a certified trainer.

tively low number of repetitions of each exercise using a relatively high resistance. Strength training exercises are done in a *set,* or a single series of multiple repetitions using the same resistance. Strength training with 85 percent of the 1RM increases the risk of injury, while training with 65 percent of the 1RM decreases the overload on the muscle(s) exercised.[47] Therefore, to improve strength, the amount of resistance employed is typically 70 to 80 percent of the 1RM for a given exercise, with 8 to 12 repetitions of the exercise performed per set (see Table 10.2).

Resistance training exercises cause microscopic damage (tears) to muscle fibers, and the rebuilding process that increases the size and capacity of the muscle takes about 24 to 48 hours. Thus, resistance training exercise programs require at least one day of rest (and recovery) between workouts to make overloading the same muscle group safe again.

Muscular Endurance Training. To develop muscular endurance, you should perform a relatively high number of repetitions (10 to 30 per set) using a relatively low resistance (50 to 60 percent of the 1RM for a particular exercise). Instead of using traditional resistance exercise equipment to develop muscular endurance, consider using a stationary bicycle ergometer, rowing machine, or stair-climbing machine to add variety to your training program. With these and other devices, you can control the cadence of the activity and/or adjust the amount of resistance you encounter. Performing thousands of repetitions during a 20-minute (or longer) workout using a relatively low resistance will quickly develop muscular endurance in the muscles exercised. This type of workout will also have cardiorespiratory benefits if you select an intensity that allows you to reach your target heart rate.

TABLE 10.2 ■ Resistance Training Program Guidelines

	Resistance Training Goal	
	Strength	Muscular Endurance
Repetitions (number)	8–12	10–30
Exercise sets (number per exercise)	1–3	4–8
Exercise resistance (% of 1RM)	65–85	50–60
Rest periods between sets (minutes)	1–3	1–2
Exercise frequency (days/week)	2–3	2–3

Source: Reprinted by permission from W. L. Westcott, "Muscular Strength and Endurance," in *Personal Trainer Manual—The Resource for Fitness Instructors* (San Diego: American Council on Exercise, 1991), 242–244.

Suggested Exercises for Strength Development

When you perform a series of strength exercises, we suggest that you begin each workout by exercising the larger muscle groups in the legs first and then perform exercises using the smaller muscle groups of the trunk and arms. This strategy permits performance of the most demanding exercises when muscle fatigue levels are lowest.

Days of the Week: Monday, Thursday, and Saturday (3 Times/Week)

Major Muscles/Muscle Group	Free Weight/Machine Strength Training Exercise(s)
1. Quadriceps (front of thigh)	Leg extension
2. Hamstrings (back of thigh)	Leg curl
3. Calf muscles	Heel raises
4. Quadriceps, gluteal muscles	Squat
5. Pectoralis major	Bench press
6. Deltoids	Shoulder/military press
7. Biceps	Arm curl
8. Latissimus dorsi	Lat pulldowns, bent-over row
9. Triceps	Arm extension

Days of the Week: Sunday, Tuesday, Wednesday, and Friday (4 Times/Week)

One to three sets of 25 repetitions each:

Major Muscles/Muscle Group	Body-Weight Resistance Exercises
1. Pectoralis major	Push-ups
2. Triceps	Chair or parallel bar dips
3. Abdominal muscles	Abdominal curl-ups (partial sit-ups)
4. Biceps	Chin-ups

Source: Reprinted by permission from W. L. Westcott, "Muscular Strength and Endurance," in *Personal Trainer Manual—The Resource for Fitness Instructors* (San Diego: American Council on Exercise, 1991), 250–274.

There is no one resistance exercise program perfect for everyone. Experiment with different resistance exercise devices and programs to find what works best for you. Once you gain strength and endurance, they are fairly easy to maintain. Maintenance resistance training consists of two to three workouts per week. You can consult with a fitness professional or hire a credentialed personal trainer to set up a program to meet your personal needs. The Skills for Behavior Change box gives you more tips on strength training.

WHAT DO YOU THINK?

What types of resistance equipment can you currently access? Based on what you've read, what specific actions can you take to increase your muscular strength? Muscular endurance? How would you measure your improvement?

FITNESS INJURIES

Overtraining is the most frequent cause of injuries associated with fitness activities. Enthusiastic but out-of-shape beginners often injure themselves by doing too much activity too soon. While participating in your personal fitness program, listen to your body's injury warning signs. Muscle stiffness and soreness, bone and joint pains, and whole-body fatigue are a few of the common warning signs of an impending overuse injury. One strategy to prevent overuse injury to a particular muscle group or body part is to vary your fitness activities throughout the week to give muscles and joints a rest. Setting appropriate short-term and long-term training goals is another good strategy for preventing overtraining injuries. Establishing realistic but challenging fitness goals can help you maintain a high level of motivation while ensuring that you do not attempt to do too much exercise too soon. An example of an appropriate short-term goal for a beginning runner is running an entire mile without stopping to walk. An example of an appropriate long-term goal—say, for one year after starting the running program—is completing a 3-mile race while running at an eight-minute-per-mile pace.

Overtraining injuries occur most often in repetitive activities like swimming, running, bicycling, and aerobic dance exercise. Progress slowly, set realistic exercise goals, vary your fitness activities to keep your workouts fun and fresh, and schedule rest days. Simply put, use common sense, and you're likely to remain injury-free.

Causes of Fitness-Related Injuries

There are two basic types of injuries stemming from participation in fitness-related activities: overuse and traumatic. **Overuse injuries** occur because of cumulative, day-after-day stresses placed on body parts (e.g., tendons, bones, and ligaments) during exercise. The forces that occur normally during physical activity are not enough to cause a ligament sprain or muscle strain, but when these forces are applied on a daily basis for weeks or months they can result in an injury. That is why people who sustain this type of injury typically cannot pinpoint a particular time or day when they were injured. Common sites of overuse injuries are the leg, knee, shoulder, and elbow joints.

Traumatic injuries, which occur suddenly and violently, typically by accident, are the second major type of fitness-related injuries. Typical traumatic injuries are broken bones, torn ligaments and muscles, contusions, and lacerations. Most traumatic injuries are unavoidable—for example, spraining your ankle by landing on another person's foot after jumping up for a rebound in basketball. If your traumatic injury causes a noticeable loss of function and immediate pain or pain that does not go away after 30 minutes, you should have a physician examine it.

Prevention

For personal fitness activities, the function of your exercise clothing is far more important than the fashion statement it makes. For some types of physical activity, you will need clothing that allows maximal body heat dissipation—for example, light-colored nylon shorts and mesh tank top while running in hot weather. For other types, you will need clothing that permits significant heat retention without getting you sweat-soaked—for example, layers of polypropylene and/or wool clothing while cross-country skiing.

Appropriate Footwear. When you are purchasing running shoes, look for several key components. Biomechanics research has revealed that running is a "collision"

sport—that is, the runner's foot collides with the ground with a force three to five times the runner's body weight with each stride.[48] The 150-pound runner who takes 1,000 strides per mile applies a cumulative force to his or her body of 450,000 pounds per mile. The force not absorbed by the running shoe is transmitted upward into the foot, leg, thigh, and back. Our bodies are able to absorb forces such as these, but may be injured by the cumulative effects of repetitive impacts (e.g., running 40 miles per week). Therefore, the ability of running shoes to absorb shock is a critical factor to consider when you are sampling shoes at the store.

The midsole of a running shoe must absorb impact forces, but must also be flexible (see Figure 10.5). One method used to evaluate the flexibility of the midsole is to hold the shoe between the index fingers of your right and left hand. When you push on both ends of the shoe with your fingers, the shoe should bend easily at the midsole. If the force exerted by your index fingers cannot bend the shoe, its midsole is probably too rigid and may cause irritation of your Achilles tendon, among other problems.[49] Other basic characteristics of running shoes include: a rigid plastic insert within the heel of the shoe (known as a heel counter to control the movement of your heel; a cushioned foam pad surrounding the heel of the shoe to prevent Achilles tendon irritation; and a removable thermoplastic innersole that customizes the fit of the shoe by using your body heat to mold it to the shape of your foot (see Figure 10.5). Shoes are the runner's most essential piece of equipment, so carefully select appropriate footwear before you start a running program. See Table 10.3 for more information on how to choose a running shoe.

Shoe companies also sell cross-training shoes to help combat the high cost of having to buy separate pairs of running shoes, tennis shoes, weight-training shoes, and so on. Although the cross-training shoe can be used for participation in several different fitness activities by the novice or recreational athlete, a serious long-distance runner who runs 25 or more miles per week needs a pair of specialty running shoes in order to prevent injury.

Appropriate Exercise Equipment. It is essential to use correctly fitted, appropriate athletic equipment for your personal fitness activities. For some activities, there is specialized protective equipment that will reduce your chances of injury. In tennis, for example, the use of proper equipment helps prevent the general inflammatory condition known as tennis elbow. Excessive racquet string tension, repetitive use of the forearm muscles during hours of daily practice, and poor flexibility cause this problem in experienced tennis players. To avoid tennis elbow, consult an instructor or skilled salesperson to assist you in selecting the correct tennis racquet and string tension for you.

Eye injuries can occur in virtually all fitness-related activities, though the risk of injury is much greater in some

TABLE 10.3 ■ Proper Shoe Selection for Running

- Shop in the afternoon to get the right fit.
- Try on both shoes with the same type of sock you will wear when running.
- Try on several different models to make a good comparison. Walk or jog around the store in the shoes.
- Check the quality of the shoes. Look at the stitching, eyelets, gluing. Feel for bumps inside the shoe.
- The sole should flex where your foot flexes. Look for shoes with removable insoles to accommodate orthotic devices.

- Allow a half-inch between the end of the shoe and your longest toe when you stand up.
- The heel counter should fit snugly so that there is no slipping at the heel.
- Shoes should be comfortable on the day you buy them. Don't rely on a break-in period.
- Consult the staff at running specialty stores for help in selecting the correct shoe.

Source: Reprinted by permission from Injury Prevention Information Series, "Proper Shoe Selection," American Running and Fitness Association, 1993.

activities than in others. As many as 90 percent of the eye injuries resulting from racquetball and squash are preventable with the use of appropriate eye protection—for example, goggles with polycarbonate lenses.[50] One-eyed participants should wear polycarbonate prescription or nonprescription eyeglasses for all recreational activities.[51]

According to the Bicycle Institute of America, over 90 million people in the United States rode bikes for pleasure, fitness, or competition in 1990. The selection of the right-size bicycle frame and seat height, coupled with the use of a bicycle helmet, padded grips/handlebars, and padded biking gloves, can significantly reduce the number of injuries that occur in this extremely popular activity. Head injuries used to account for 85 percent of all deaths attributable to bicycle accidents; however, the wearing of bike helmets has significantly reduced the number of skull

fractures and facial injuries among recreational cyclists.[52] Bicycle helmets that meet the standards established by the American National Standards Institute (ANSI) and the Snell Memorial Foundation (SNELL) should be worn by all cyclists.

𝒲HAT DO YOU THINK?

Given your activity level, what are some injury risks that you are exposed to on a regular basis? What changes can you make in your equipment or clothing to reduce these risks?

Common Overuse Injuries

Body movements in physical activities such as running, swimming, and bicycling are highly repetitive, so participants are susceptible to overuse injuries. In fitness activities, the joints of the lower extremities (foot, ankle, knee, and hip) tend to be injured more frequently than the upper-extremity joints (shoulder, elbow, wrist, and hand). Three of the most common injuries from repetitive overuse during exercise are plantar fasciitis, "shin splints," and "runner's knee."

Plantar Fasciitis. Plantar fasciitis is an inflammation of the plantar fascia, a broad band of dense, inelastic tissue

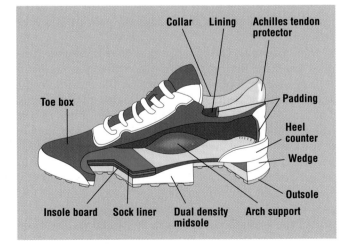

FIGURE 10.5

Anatomy of a Running Shoe
Source: Reprinted by permission of the American Council on Exercise from *Personal Trainer Manual,* 1991.

Overuse injuries: Injuries that result from the cumulative effects of day-after-day stresses placed on tendons, muscles, and joints.

Traumatic injuries: Injuries that are accidental in nature; they occur suddenly and violently (e.g., fractured bones, ruptured tendons, and sprained ligaments).

(fascia) that runs from the heel to the toe on the bottom of your foot. The main function of the plantar fascia is to protect the nerves, blood vessels, and muscles of the foot from injury. In repetitive, weight-bearing fitness activities such as walking and running, the plantar fascia may become inflamed. Common symptoms of this condition are pain and tenderness under the ball of the foot, at the heel, or at both locations. The pain of plantar fasciitis is particularly noticeable during your first steps out of bed in the morning. If not treated properly, this injury may progress in severity to the point that weight-bearing exercise is too painful to endure. Uphill running is not advised for anyone suffering from this condition, since each uphill stride severely stretches (and thus irritates) the already inflamed plantar fascia. This injury can often be prevented by regularly stretching the plantar fascia prior to exercise and by wearing athletic shoes with good arch support and shock absorbency. The plantar fascia are stretched by slowly pulling all five toes upward toward your head, holding for 10 to 15 seconds, and repeating this three to five times on each foot prior to exercise.

Shin Splints. A general term for any pain that occurs below the knee and above the ankle is shin splints. More than 20 different medical conditions have been identified within the broad description of shin splints. Problems range from stress fractures of the tibia (shinbone) to severe inflammation in the muscular compartments of the lower leg, which can interrupt the flow of blood and nerve supply to the foot. The most common type of shin splints occurs along the inner side of the tibia and is usually a combination of a muscle irritation and irritation of the tissues that attach the muscles to the bone in this region. Typically, there is pain and swelling along the middle one-third of the posteromedial tibia in the soft tissues, not the bone.

Sedentary people who start a new weight-bearing exercise program are at the greatest risk for shin splints, though well-conditioned aerobic exercisers who rapidly

increase their distance or pace may also develop shin splints.[53] Running is the most frequent cause of shin splints, but those who do a great deal of walking (e.g., waitresses) may also develop this injury.

To help prevent shin splints, wear athletic shoes that have good arch support and shock absorbency. If the severity of this lower-leg condition increases to the point that you cannot comfortably complete your desired fitness activity, see your physician. Specific pain on the tibia or on the adjacent, smaller fibula should be examined by a doctor for possible stress fracture. Reduction of the frequency, intensity, and duration of weight-bearing exercise may be required. You may be advised to substitute a non-weight-bearing activity such as swimming for weight-bearing exercise during your recovery period.

Runner's Knee. An overuse condition known as runner's knee describes a series of problems involving the muscles, tendons, and ligaments about the knee. The most common problem identified as runner's knee is abnormal movement of the patella (kneecap).[54] Women are more commonly affected by this condition than are men because their wider pelvis makes abnormal lateral pull on the patella by the muscles that act at the knee more likely. In women (and some men), this causes irritation to the cartilage on the back side of the patella as well as to the nearby tendons and ligaments.

The main symptom of this kind of runner's knee is the pain experienced when downward pressure is applied to the patella after the knee is straightened fully. Additional symptoms may include swelling, redness, and tenderness around the patella, and a dull, aching pain felt in the center of the knee.[55] If you have these symptoms in your knee, your physician will probably recommend that you stop running for a few weeks and reduce daily activities that put compressive forces on the patella (e.g., exercise on a stair-climbing machine or doing squats with heavy resistance) until you no longer have any pain around your kneecap.

Iliotibial band (ITB) friction syndrome is another runner's knee condition. It occurs when the iliotibial band rubs against the bony prominence on the outside of the knee as it is repeatedly flexed and extended, as in running. The iliotibial band is a long, dense tendon located on the lateral (outer) thigh that attaches two muscles of the hip to the knee. ITB friction syndrome is most frequently experienced by runners, but also appears in participants in fitness activities that require repetitive knee flexion and extension (e.g., cycling, rowing, and weight lifting). The condition causes pain and inflammation at the lateral aspect of the knee; minor cases can be treated with rest and the nonprescription anti-inflammatory medications ibuprofen and aspirin.[56] For more severe cases that cause a loss of function because of pain and/or swelling, consult a physician. You may substitute swimming or water exercises while unable to run. Pain-free exercise may be resumed gradually under your doctor's supervision.

RICE: Acronym for the standard first-aid treatment for virtually all traumatic and overuse injuries: rest, ice, compression, and elevation.

Heat cramps: Muscle cramps that occur during or following exercise in warm/hot conditions.

Heat exhaustion: A heat stress illness caused by significant dehydration resulting from exercise in warm/hot conditions; frequent precursor to heat stroke.

Heat stroke: A deadly heat stress illness resulting from dehydration and overexertion in warm/hot conditions; can cause body core temperature to rise from normal to 105°F to 110°F in just a few minutes.

Hypothermia: Potentially fatal condition caused by abnormally low body core temperature.

Treatment

First-aid treatment for virtually all personal fitness injuries involves **RICE**: rest, ice, compression, and elevation. *Rest,* the first component of this treatment, is required to eliminate the risk of further irritation of the injured body part. *Ice* is applied to relieve the pain of the injury and to constrict the blood vessels in order to slow and stop any internal or external bleeding associated with the injury. Never apply ice cubes, reusable gel ice packs, chemical cold packs, or other forms of cold directly to your skin. Instead, place a layer of wet toweling between the ice and your skin. Ice should be applied to a new injury for approximately 20 minutes every hour for the first 24 to 72 hours. *Compression* of the injured body part can be accomplished with a 4- or 6-inch-wide elastic bandage; this applies indirect pressure to damaged blood vessels to help stop bleeding. Be careful, though, that the compression wrap does not interfere with normal blood flow. A throbbing, painful hand or foot is an indication that the compression wrap was applied too tightly and should be loosened. *Elevation* of the injured extremity above the level of your heart also helps to control internal or external bleeding by making the blood flow uphill to reach the injured area.

Exercising in the Heat

Exercising in extreme temperatures may increase your risk for a heat-related injury. Fortunately, if you are in good physical condition and wear appropriate clothing for outdoor physical activities, you can safely withstand a wide range of temperatures and humidity levels. Heat stress, which includes several potentially fatal illnesses resulting from excessive core body temperatures, should be a constant concern when you are exercising in warm, humid weather. In these conditions, your body's rate of heat production often exceeds its ability to cool itself.

You can help prevent heat stress by following certain precautions. First, proper acclimatization to hot and/or humid climates is essential. The process of heat acclimatization, which increases your body's cooling efficiency, requires about 10 to 14 days of gradually increased exercise in a hot environment. Second, heat stress can be prevented by avoiding dehydration, accomplished through proper fluid replacement during and following exercise. Third, wear clothing appropriate for the fitness activity and the environment. Finally, use common sense when exercising in hot and humid conditions—for example, on a 95 degree, 90 percent humidity day, postpone your usual lunch-time run until the cool of evening.

The three different heat stress illnesses are progressive in their level of severity: heat cramps, heat exhaustion, and heat stroke. The least serious problem, heat-related muscle cramps (**heat cramps**), is easily prevented by adequate fluid replacement and a diet that includes the electrolytes lost during sweating (sodium and potassium).

Heat exhaustion is caused by excessive water loss resulting from intense or prolonged exercise or work in a warm and/or humid environment. Symptoms of heat exhaustion include nausea, headache, fatigue, dizziness and faintness, and, paradoxically, "goosebumps" and chills. If you are suffering from heat exhaustion, your skin will be cool and moist. Heat exhaustion is actually a mild form of shock, in which the blood pools in the arms and legs away from the brain and major organs of the body, causing nausea and fainting. **Heat stroke**, often called sunstroke, is a life-threatening emergency condition having a 20 to 70 percent death rate.[57] Heat stroke occurs during vigorous exercise when the body's heat production significantly exceeds your body's cooling capacities. Body core temperature can rise from normal (98.6°F) to 105°F to 110°F within minutes after the body's cooling mechanism shuts down. With no cooling taking place, rapidly increasing core temperatures can cause brain damage, permanent disability, and death. Common signs of heat stroke are dry, hot, and usually red skin; very high body temperature; and a very rapid heart rate.

Heat stress illnesses may occur in situations in which the danger is not obvious. Serious or fatal heat strokes may result from prolonged sauna or steam baths, prolonged total immersion in a hot tub or spa, or by exercising in a plastic or rubber head-to-toe "sauna suit." If, while exercising, you experience any of the symptoms mentioned here, you should stop exercising immediately, move to the shade or a cool spot to rest, and drink large amounts of cool fluids. See Figure 10.6 for a quick way to compute the risks of exercising under various heat and humidity conditions.

Exercising in the Cold

When you exercise in cool to cold weather, especially in windy conditions, your body's rate of heat loss is frequently greater than its rate of heat production. Under these conditions, **hypothermia**—a potentially fatal condition resulting from abnormally low body core temperature, which occurs when body heat is lost faster than it is produced—may result. Hypothermia can occur as a result of prolonged, vigorous exercise (e.g., snowboarding or rugby) in 40°F to 50°F temperatures, particularly if there is rain, snow, or a strong wind.

In mild cases of hypothermia, as your body core temperature drops from the normal 98.6°F to 93.2°F, you will begin to shiver. Shivering—the involuntary contraction of nearly every muscle in your body—is designed to increase your body temperature by using the heat given off by muscle activity. During this first stage of hypothermia, you may also experience cold hands and feet, poor judgment, apathy, and amnesia.[58] Shivering ceases in most hypothermia victims as their body core temperatures drop to between 87°F and 90°F, a sign that the body has lost its ability to generate heat. Death from hypothermia usually occurs at body core temperatures between 75°F and 80°F.

Apparent temperature (what it feels like)

Air temperature (F°)	70°	75°	80°	85°	90°	95°	100°	105°	110°	115°
0%	64°	69°	73°	78°	83°	87°	91°	95°	99°	103°
10%	65°	70°	75°	80°	85°	90°	95°	100°	105°	111°
20%	66°	72°	77°	82°	87°	93°	99°	105°	112°	120°
30%	67°	73°	78°	84°	90°	96°	104°	113°	123°	135°
40%	68°	74°	79°	86°	93°	101°	110°	123°	137°	151°
50%	69°	75°	81°	88°	96°	107°	120°	135°	150°	
60%	70°	76°	82°	90°	100°	114°	132°	149°		
70%	70°	77°	85°	93°	106°	124°	144°			
80%	71°	78°	86°	97°	113°	136°				
90%	71°	79°	88°	102°	122°					
100%	72°	80°	91°	108°						

Relative humidity (left vertical scale)

Apparent temperature	Heat stress risk with exertion
90° – 105°	Heat cramps and heat exhaustion possible.
105° – 130°	Heat cramps or heat exhaustion likely; heat stroke possible.
130° and above	Heat stroke highly likely with continued exposure.

FIGURE 10.6

The chart measures the hazards of heat and humidity. To determine the risk of exercising in the heat, locate the outside air temperature on the top horizontal scale and the relative humidity on the left vertical scale. Where these two values intersect is the *apparent temperature*. For example, on a 90°F day with 70 percent humidity, the apparent temperature is 106°F. Heat cramps or heat exhaustion are likely to occur, and heat stroke is possible during exercise under these conditions.

Source: Adapted from U.S. Department of Commerce, National Oceanic and Atmospheric Administration, "Heat Index Chart," in *Heat Wave: A Major Summer Killer* (Washington DC: Government Printing Office, 1992).

To prevent hypothermia, follow these commonsense guidelines: analyze weather conditions and your risk of hypothermia before you undertake your planned outdoor physical activity, remembering that wind and humidity are as significant as temperature; use the "buddy system"—that is, have a friend join you for your cold-weather outdoor activities; wear layers of appropriate clothing to prevent excessive heat loss (e.g., polypropylene or woolen undergarments, Gore-Tex windbreaker, and wool hat and gloves); and finally, don't allow yourself to become dehydrated.

Cross training: Regular participation in two or more types of exercises (e.g., swimming and weight lifting).

*W*HAT DO YOU THINK?

Given what you've read about the symptoms of common fitness injuries, are you currently developing any overuse injuries? If so, what specific actions can you take to prevent these problems from getting more serious?

While appropriate clothing and equipment help prevent injuries in any fitness activity, a workout partner is also an important safeguard when exercising outdoors in cold weather.

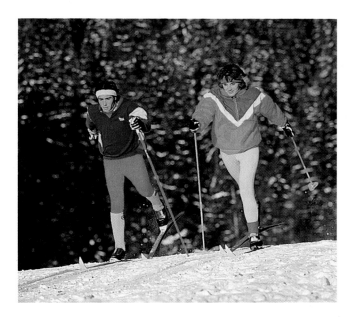

$\mathcal{P}$LANNING YOUR FITNESS PROGRAM

You now know that regular physical activity and exercise can help you avoid preventable diseases and add to both the quality and length of your life. If you are currently active, you are more aware of the benefits of regular exercise and should be motivated to continue your efforts. If you are sedentary or sporadically active, you realize that you should not delay one day longer in making the behavioral changes necessary to improve your fitness level. You should also be aware of the importance of creating a program you love and of motivating yourself through self-talk, as the Building Communication Skills box discusses.

Identifying Your Fitness Goals

Before you embark on a fitness program, analyze your personal needs, limitations, physical activity likes and dislikes, and daily schedule. Your primary reason for exercising may be to lower your risks for health problems. This goal is prudent, particularly for those of you who have a family history of cardiovascular diseases (heart attack, stroke, high blood pressure), diabetes, obesity, and/or substance abuse. If you have inherited no major risks for fatal or debilitating diseases, then your primary reason for exercising may be to improve the quality of your life. Your specific goal may be to achieve (or maintain) healthy levels of body fat, cardiovascular fitness, muscular strength and endurance, or flexibility/mobility.

Once you become committed to regular physical activity and exercise, you will observe gradual changes in your functional abilities and note progress toward your goals. Unfortunately, all the benefits gained through regular physical activity are lost if you stop exercising. You can't get fit for a couple of years while you're young and expect the positive changes to last the rest of your life. Perhaps your most vital goal is to become committed to fitness for the long haul—to establish a realistic schedule of diverse exercise activities that you can maintain and enjoy throughout your life.

Designing Your Fitness Program

Once you commit yourself to exercise, you must decide what type of fitness program is best suited to your needs. The amounts and types of exercises required to yield beneficial results vary with the age and physical condition of the exerciser. Men over 40 and women over 50 should consult their physicians before beginning a fitness program.

Good fitness programs are designed to improve or maintain cardiorespiratory endurance, flexibility, muscular strength, and muscular endurance. A comprehensive program could include a warm-up period of easy walking followed by stretching activities to improve flexibility, then selected strength development exercises, followed by performance of an aerobic activity for 20 minutes or more, and concluding with a cool-down period of gentle flexibility exercises.

The greatest proportion of your exercise time should be spent developing cardiovascular fitness, but you should not exclude the other components. Choose an aerobic activity you think you will like. Many people find **cross training**—alternate-day participation in two or more aer-

Choosing a swimming activity that suits your individual interests and level of fitness is one way to plan an enjoyable exercise program that emphasizes cardiovascular fitness and builds muscular strength.

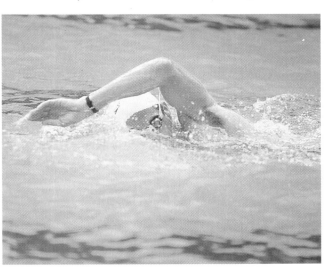

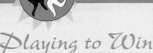

Playing to Win

Each of us has a different personal health style. Whether you are beginning or maintaining your exercise plan, it's important that it's something you believe in. Here are what three tennis professionals say about their workouts, self-motivation, and fitness and winning advice. Note how they communicate with themselves to keep going. Self-talk, introduced in Chapter 1, is an important component of your exercise program.

Gabriela Sabatini

On Working Out

I do lots of sit-ups. A couple of years ago, I started lifting weights. Since my upper body is very strong, I'm now concentrating on strength training my legs. That gives me lots of power on the court. It's made a difference. If I'm not playing tennis so much I play soccer, I run . . . I have to do something. I have lots of energy.

Self-Motivation

Of course you should talk to yourself if you're doing badly, to encourage and give yourself energy and power—but you should also talk to yourself when you're doing well—just to keep in touch so you keep going strong.

Fitness and Winning Advice

Choose tennis, choose whatever, because you love it. Run, do aerobics, play sports—it's important to do something. It takes work, but it makes you feel great. I myself have to keep active. It's the best. I highly recommend it.

Arantxa Sanchez Vicario

On Working Out

I have a personal trainer and we run and lift weights. Mostly though, I like to practice my tennis. There has never been a day yet when I haven't wanted to get out on the court. Maybe that sounds weird, but it's true. I just love the game so much.

Self-Motivation

If something goes wrong, I try to learn from it. I stop for a while, think, figure out what's happening, and then try to change. Staying positive is very important.

Fitness and Winning Advice

You have to work really hard. It takes a lot of work and a lot of sacrifice. Choose something you love, something you enjoy. That's the most important thing.

Source: All but the opening paragraph excerpted with permission from Lisa Klein, "Playing To Win," *Shape,* June 1993, 20.

---

obic activities (i.e., jogging and swimming)—less monotonous and more enjoyable than long-term participation in only one aerobic activity. Cross training is also beneficial because it strengthens a variety of muscles, thus helping you avoid overuse injuries to muscles and joints.

Jogging, walking, cycling, rowing, step aerobics, and cross-country skiing are all excellent activities for developing cardiovascular fitness. Responding to the exercise boom, fitness equipment manufacturers have made it easy for you to participate in these activities. Most colleges and universities now have recreation centers where students can use stair-climbing machines, stationary bicycles, treadmills, rowing machines, and ski-simulators. Table 10.4 describes the features of various types of aerobic exercise machines and provides tips for their use.

WHAT DO YOU THINK?

You now have the ability to design your own fitness program. What two activities would you select for a cross-training program? Do the activities you selected exercise different major muscle groups? What may happen to you if they don't?

Summary

◆ The physiological benefits of regular physical activity include reduced risk of heart attack, prevention of hypertension, improved blood profile, improved skeletal mass, improved weight control, prevention of diabetes, increased life span, improved immunity to disease, improved mental health and stress management, and improved physical fitness.

◆ An aerobic exercise program improves cardiovascular fitness. Exercise frequency begins with three days per week and eventually moves up to five. Exercise intensity

TABLE 10.4 ■ Which Aerobic-Exercise Machine Suits You?

Machine	What It Does	What to Look for	Comments
Exercise bicycle	Most models work only the lower body, but some have pumping handlebars for arms and shoulders. Some can be programmed for various workouts, such as climbing hills.	Smooth pedaling motion. Comfortable seat. Handlebars that adjust to your height. Pedal straps to keep your feet from slipping and to make your legs work on the upstroke, too. Easy-to-adjust workload. Solid construction. Some models let you pedal backward, which works your hamstring muscles (rather than quadriceps). Some have an ergometer, which calculates your work output in watts or calories.	Puts less strain on joints than running. Always adjust the seat to proper height; your knee should be only slightly bent when your leg is extended. To prevent knee problems, don't set the resistance too high: you should be able to pedal at least 60 rpm. Recumbent models let you sit back in a chairlike seat with your feet in front of you; this puts less strain on back, neck, and shoulders.
Bicycle trainer	This stand allows you to convert your regular bike for indoor use. Rear wheel typically rests on a roller.	One that is easy to mount your bike on; some don't require removal of front wheel. Wind-resistance designs simulate outdoor conditions. Magnetic-resistance models are quieter.	Since this uses your regular outdoor bike, it is likely to be comfortable. Less expensive than a stationary bike. However, it's difficult to take your hands off the handlebars, making it hard to read.
Treadmill	Some machines have adjustable inclines to simulate hills and make workouts more strenuous. Some can be programmed for various workouts. Some monitors display approximate number of calories burned, miles covered, and speed.	Easily adjustable speed and incline. Running surface that is wide and long enough for your stride and that absorbs shock well. A strong motor, which can handle high speeds and a heavy load; a weak motor may allow only for brisk walking, not running. Avoid cheap models that have no motor (your movement pushes the belt).	Many models have side or front hand rails: some people like them for balance. To prevent a mishap, straddle the machine before starting it; slow it down gradually before getting off.
Stair climber	Some larger models are like escalators and simulate real stair climbing. But most home models have pedals that work against your weight as you pump your legs; this puts less strain on your knees since you don't take real steps. Pedals may work independently or be linked (as one goes down, the other automatically goes up).	Smooth stepping action and large, comfortable pedals. Model that doesn't wobble as you step rapidly. Easily adjustable resistance. Comfortable handlebars or rails for balance. Some people prefer pedals that remain parallel to the floor; others like pivoting pedals. Models with independent pedals provide a more natural stepping motion. "Dual action" machines also have moving hand grips and thus work your upper body as well as legs. Some vertical ladder-style models simulate rock climbing.	It's easy to get a strenuous workout on one of these—in fact, beginners should be careful not to overexert themselves, since blood pressure and heart rate may rise very quickly. Start with short steps and a slow pace. Put your entire foot on the pedal, not just the ball of the foot. Try to keep your knees aligned over your toes. For an intense workout, don't lean on the rails or front monitor, since that will reduce your energy expenditure. Stair climbing may aggravate some knee problems. Most machines work your calf muscles more than real stair climbing does.

(continued)

involves working out at your target heart rate. Exercise duration should increase to 30 to 45 minutes; the longer the exercise period, the more calories burned and the bigger improvement in cardiovascular fitness.

◆ Flexibility exercises should involve static stretching exercises performed in sets of three repetitions held for 10 to 30 seconds at least three days a week in order for progress to be made.

◆ The key principles for developing muscular strength and endurance are the tension principle, the overload principle, and the specificity of training principle. The different types of muscle actions include isometric, concentric, and eccentric. Resistance training programs include fixed, variable, and accommodating resistance.

◆ Fitness injuries are generally caused by overuse or trauma; the most common are plantar fasciitis, shin splints, and runner's knee. Limited prevention can be achieved with proper footwear and equipment. Exercise in the heat or cold requires special precautions.

◆ Planning your fitness program involves setting goals and designing a program to achieve these goals.

TABLE 10.4 ■ Which Aerobic-Exercise Machine Suits You? *(continued)*

Machine	What It Does	What to Look for	Comments
Rowing machine	Provides a fuller workout than running or cycling; tones muscles in your arms, legs, abdomen, shoulders, and back. Most have hydraulic pistons to provide variable resistance; many larger models use a flywheel attached to a bar by a chain. One model actually has a flywheel in a water tank to mimic real rowing.	Piston-type models have hydraulic arms and are cheaper and more compact than flywheel models, which have smoother action that's usually more like real rowing. Look for a model that sits solidly on the floor and doesn't wobble. Smooth oar motion. Comfortable seat that moves smoothly on wheels or ball bearings to reduce friction. Pivoting foot rests. Expensive models have a monitor for speed, distance, and/or calories burned.	Proper rowing technique and cadence put little strain on body. If you have a back problem, consult your doctor before buying a rower. Make sure your legs, not your back, power your rowing motion. In early part of stroke, your arms should move forward before you bend your knees. Your grip should be relaxed. When using a flywheel model, pull the bar into your abdomen, not to your chin.
Cross-country ski machine	Works most muscle groups. Simulates the outdoor sport: feet slide back and forth in tracks; hands pull on cords or poles to copy the poling movement of skiing. Some models allow you to move your arms and legs independently; others require synchronized movements.	A base long enough to accommodate your stride. Adjustable leg and arm resistance. Smooth action. Inexpensive models tend to be flimsy and uncomfortable. Machines with cords rather than poles may provide an especially strenuous upper-body workout.	Provides perhaps the best all-around workout. It may take some practice to coordinate your movements. Puts little strain on body; shouldn't aggravate knee problems.

Source: Excerpted by permission from the *University of California at Berkeley Wellness Letter,* December 1992. © Health Letter Associates, 1992.

Application Exercise

Reread the What Do You Think? scenarios at the beginning of the chapter and answer the following questions:

1. Assume for a moment that you are Steve, thinking about starting an exercise program after a period of inactivity. Create an outline for a three-month program that starts slow and gradually progresses.

2. One of the hardest obstacles for Steve will be breaking his old habits: driving instead of walking, watching TV, playing computer games, and eating unhealthy foods. What advice would you give Steve to help him break his habits?

3. Assuming that Georgia's workouts were about 30 to 45 minutes long, five times a week, was there really anything wrong with what she was doing? What amount of workout is too much? Too little? Just right?

4. Given that Georgia is still tired and stressed out even though she regularly works out, what advice would you give her? Is stress simply a part of college life, or can it be controlled?

Further Reading

R. A. Anderson, *Stretching* (Bolinas, CA: Shelter Publishing, 1990).

S. N. Blair, *Living with Exercise* (Dallas: American Health, 1991).

B. Getchell, *Physical Fitness: A Way of Life,* 4th ed. (New York: Macmillan, 1992).

David K. Miller and T. Earl Allen, *Fitness: A Lifetime Commitment,* 5th ed. (Boston: Allyn and Bacon, 1995).

Excellent textbook providing both strategies and techniques—as well as motivation—for students to make a lifetime commitment to health fitness.

B. J. Sharkey, *New Dimensions in Aerobic Fitness* (Champaign, IL: Human Kinetics, 1991).

M. K. Williams, *Lifetime Fitness and Wellness,* 3rd ed. (Dubuque: W.C. Brown, 1993).

Managing Your Fitness Behaviors

The decision to be physically fit is an easy one to make but not always easy to put into action. Physical fitness should be enjoyable. In addition to the health benefits, you should choose activities that make you happy.

Making Decisions for You

Begin by making a list of a variety of your favorite physical activities that may increase strength, flexibility, and cardiorespiratory efficiency. Your list may include walking, gardening, or mowing the lawn, as well as athletic endeavors such as weight lifting and swimming. Which would you like to make part of your health program? Next, you need to find time to exercise. Do you have extra time you could set aside? If not, how could exercise become part of your daily activities? Could you, for example, leave a few minutes earlier to class and walk instead of taking a shuttle bus?

Checklist for Change: Making Personal Choices

✓ *Start slowly as a beginning exerciser.* For the sedentary, first-time exerciser, any type and amount of physical activity will be a step in the right direction. If you are extremely overweight or out of condition, you may only be able to walk for five minutes at a time. Don't be discouraged: you're on your way!

✓ *Make only one life change at a time.* Attempting too many major changes in your lifestyle at once invites failure. Success at one major behavior change will encourage you to make other positive changes.

✓ *Have reasonable expectations for yourself and your fitness program.* Many people become exercise dropouts because their expectations are too high to begin with. Have patience with yourself and your body. Allow sufficient time to reach your fitness goals.

✓ *Choose a specific time to exercise and stick with it.* Learning to establish priorities and keeping to a schedule are vital steps toward improved fitness. Experiment by exercising at different times of the day to learn what schedule works best for you.

✓ *Exercise with a friend.* Reneging on an exercise commitment is more difficult if you do not exercise alone. Enjoy the relaxed, social aspects of exercising with a friend. Partners can motivate and encourage one another, provided they remember that progress will not be the same for them both.

✓ *Make exercise a positive habit.* Usually, if you are able to practice a desired activity for three weeks, you will be able to incorporate it into your lifestyle. But also be aware that for some highly fit individuals exercise can become a negative habit (addiction).

✓ *Keep a record of your progress.* A personal fitness journal can be a good motivator. Your journal could include various facts about your physical activities (duration, intensity) and chronicle your emotions and personal achievements as you progress in your fitness program.

✓ *Take lapses in stride.* Physical deconditioning—a decline in fitness level—occurs at about the same rate as does physical conditioning. If you have not exercised for three or more weeks after having developed a regular exercise habit, you will notice some lower levels of cardiovascular and muscular fitness. First, renew your commitment to fitness, and then restart your exercise program.

Checklist for Change: Making Community Choices

✓ Does your college have facilities for exercise? Are there special student rates? What hours are those facilities available?

✓ What community facilities does your hometown have available for exercise? Have you ever considered using these facilities?

✓ What opportunities are available for you to volunteer at a local exercise facility? Have you considered volunteering to help out low-income individuals? Why or why not?

Critical Thinking

Your friend Joan catches everyone's eye: Five years of intense bodybuilding have created a sleek, "ripped-up," hard body. She even plans to start entering bodybuilding contests within the next year. Joan started working out in high school after her father had a heart attack at age 38. Her family doctor pointed out that her family had a history of cardiovascular disease and that she should take steps to lower her own risk. Cardiovascular exercise was his suggestion. Now Joan works out two to three hours a day in the weight room, usually powerlifting to build bigger muscles for competition. When she had a higher-than-normal blood pressure reading last week, she became convinced that she must work out harder. From what you have learned in your health class, you want to suggest that she add some elements of aerobic exercise to her workout. However, because you do little more than jog 20 minutes a day, you are afraid she won't take your suggestion seriously.

Using the DECIDE model described in Chapter 1, decide how you could approach Joan to urge her to take a more balanced approach to her workout.

11

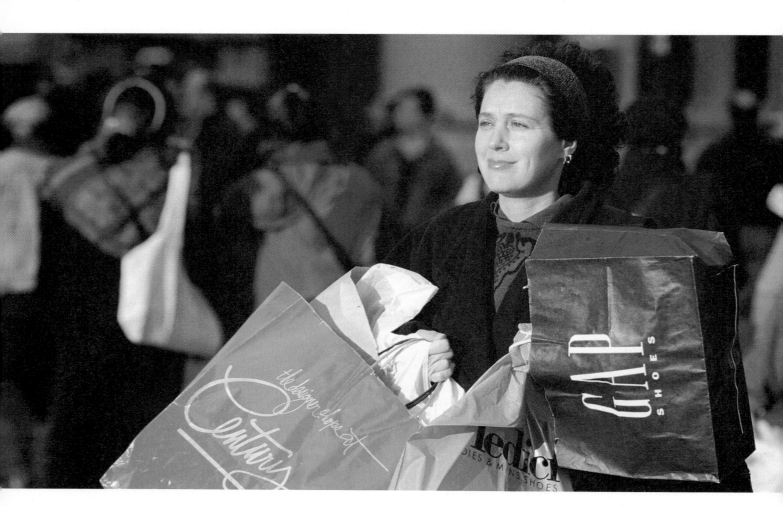

*C*HAPTER OBJECTIVES

◆ Distinguish addictions from habits and identify the signs of addiction.

◆ Discuss the addictive process, the physiology of addiction, and the biopsychosocial model of addiction.

◆ Describe the types of addictions, including money addictions, workaholism, exercise addiction, sexual addictions, and codependence.

◆ Evaluate treatment and recovery for addicts, including individual therapy, group therapy, family therapy, and 12-step programs.

Addictions and Addictive Behavior

Threats to Wellness

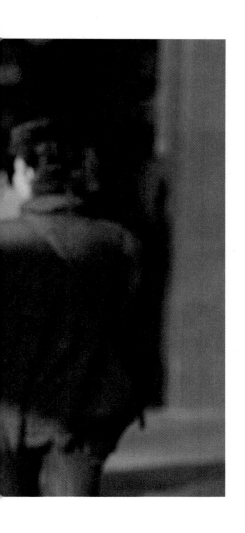

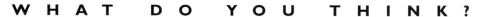

WHAT DO YOU THINK?

Jamie is an 18-year-old college freshman who has vowed she will "never be like my alcoholic parents." She has acted as a substitute mother for her younger siblings since she was nine years old. Her father was rarely around, and when he did come home, he was usually drunk and violent toward the rest of the family. Jamie is very bitter that her childhood was such a mess compared to most of her peers' nurturant upbringings. As she enters college, she finds it difficult to make friends and begins to drink socially to "fit in." Recently, she's noticed that she is uncomfortable at parties where alcohol is not present.

■ What factors in Jamie's life make her particularly vulnerable to alcoholism and other addictions? How is her relationship with alcohol likely to differ from that of her peers who grew up in healthy homes? Why is it more difficult for Jamie to drink moderately and responsibly than it may be for others? What could be done to help Jamie?

Hans' fiancée, Birgit, has begun to feel ambivalent about their upcoming marriage. Hans, a master electrician, has begun hanging out with some gamblers, and he seems to have caught the bug. He gambles most every day, hasn't shown up for scheduled construction jobs, and has spent all the money he and Birgit have saved for their honeymoon. When he doesn't answer his phone, employers call Birgit, who politely promises to pass along messages. Every week, Birgit tells Hans that she is going to break off their engagement if he won't seek joint counseling and stop associating with his gambling friends.

■ How has Birgit acted as an enabler for Hans to continue his addictive behavior? What kind of treatment should Hans turn to for his addiction? How can Birgit help Hans in his recovery?

If you pick up the newspaper, watch TV, or listen to the radio, you're certain to hear about the devastating personal and social consequences of substance abuse. Few people would challenge the idea that chemical dependency is a major health threat in the United States. But while the war on drugs rages on, it is increasingly clear that chemical dependency represents only one part of America's problem with addiction. Indeed, it seems that millions of Americans are struggling with compulsive and harmful behaviors that are not only conventional but also actually enhance the lives of people who can engage in them moderately. The most commonly recognized objects of the "other addictions" are food, sex, relationships, gambling, spending, work, and exercise.

DEFINING ADDICTION

Addiction is an unhealthy, continued involvement with a mood-altering object or activity that creates harmful consequences.[1] Addictive behaviors initially provide a sense of pleasure or stability that is beyond the addict's power to achieve otherwise. Eventually, the addictive behavior is necessary to give the addict a sense of normalcy.

Physiological dependence is only one indicator of addiction. Psychological dynamics play an important role, which explains why behaviors not related to the use of chemicals—gambling, for example—may also be addictive. In fact, psychological and physiological dependence are so intertwined that it is not really possible to separate the two. For every psychological state, there is a corresponding physiological state. In other words, everything you feel is tied to a chemical process occurring in your body.[2] Thus, addictions once thought to be entirely psychological in nature are now understood to have physiological components.

To be addictive, a behavior must have the potential to produce a positive mood change. Chemicals are responsible for the most profound addictions, not only because they produce dramatic mood changes, but also because they cause cellular changes to which the body adapts so well that it eventually requires the chemical in order to function normally. Yet other behaviors, such as gambling, spending, working, and sex, also create changes at the cellular level along with positive mood changes. Although the mechanism is not well understood, all forms of ad-

diction probably reflect dysfunction of certain biochemical systems in the brain.[3]

Traditionally, diagnosis of an addiction was limited to drug addiction and was based on three criteria: (1) the presence of an abstinence syndrome, or **withdrawal**—a series of temporary physical and psychological symptoms that occurs when the addict abruptly stops using the drug; (2) an associated pattern of pathological behavior (deterioration in work performance, relationships, and social interaction); and (3) **relapse**, the tendency to return to the addictive behavior after a period of abstinence. Furthermore, until recently, health professionals were unwilling to diagnose an addiction until medical symptoms appeared in the patient. Now we know that although withdrawal, pathological behavior, relapse, and medical symptoms are valid indicators of addiction, they do not characterize all addictive behavior.

Habit versus Addiction

What is the distinction between a harmless habit and an addiction? The stereotypical image of the addict is of someone desperately seeking a fix 24 hours a day. Conversely, people have the notion that if you aren't doing the behavior every day, then you're not addicted. The reality is somewhere between these two extremes.

Addiction certainly involves elements of **habit**, which is a repetitious behavior in which the repetition may be unconscious. A habit can be annoying, but it can be broken without too much discomfort by simply becoming aware of its presence and choosing not to do it. Addiction also involves repetition of a behavior, but the repetition occurs by compulsion and considerable discomfort is experienced if the behavior is not performed. While many people consider compulsive eating an addiction, current research shows that it is actually more of a habit, as discussed in the Health Headlines box.

It is helpful not to limit our understanding of addiction to the amount and frequency of the behavior, for what happens when a person is involved in the behavior is far more meaningful. For example, someone who drinks only rarely, and then in moderation, may experience personality changes, blackouts (drug-induced amnesia), and other negative consequences (e.g., failing a test, missing an important appointment, getting into a fight) that would never have occurred had the person not taken a few drinks. On the other hand, someone who has a few

Binge Eating: Habit or Addiction?

Can you remember a time when you meant to take just one chocolate chip cookie, only to find yourself returning to the cookie jar again, and again, and again—and again! Such behavior seems to have signs of addiction: compulsive behavior (characterized by obsession, all right!), loss of control (can't stop, can you?), withdrawal symptoms (you can taste it in your mouth, can't you?). So binge eating must be an addiction, right?

Wrong. Most leading eating-disorder specialists believe that what is being tossed around as addiction is really binge eating, a predominantly psychological, not physical, disorder. What's more, most experts are strongly opposed to the use of the word addiction in relationship to food because it suggests a physical dependence on something, which would include symptoms such as tolerance and withdrawal.

"There is no scientific support for the theory that binge eating is an addiction, and labeling it as such can have far-reaching, negative consequences on how binge eating is treated," asserts Terry Wilson, director of the Eating Disorders Clinic at Rutgers University and one of the country's leading experts on eating disorders.

It's important to remember the point made in the text: A habit is a repetitious behavior. You can break a habit without too much discomfort. While you may binge on cookies today, you may not have any for the next week. In fact, the reason that you binged on the cookies may have been that you hadn't had any cookies recently or had been on a severely restricted diet; your body simply welcomed back some of the food it had been lacking.

One problem with the suggestion that binge eating is an addiction is that treatment based on addiction theory may not only fail, it may actually do harm. According to Wilson, treatment with an antidepressant medication "doesn't help [someone] learn how to establish a regular eating pattern, to put aside weight loss as a primary goal or to develop problem-solving abilities." In addition, 12-step treatment programs (based on Alcoholics Anonymous) may encourage binge eaters to see themselves as helpless when faced with foods of abuse, reinforcing their sense of powerlessness.

Source: Quotations by Terry Wilson reprinted with permission from Janis Graham, "The Food Addicts," *Shape*, November 1994, 82, 119. See also Dr. Wilson's chapter on eating disorders in G. Terence Wilson, Peter Nathan, K. Daniel O'Leary, and Lee Anna Clark, *Abnormal Psychology* (Boston: Allyn and Bacon, 1996).

martinis every evening may never do anything out of character while under the influence of alcohol but may become irritable, manipulative, and aggressive when unable to have those regular drinks. For both of these people, alcohol appears to perform a function (mood control) that they should be able to perform without the aid of chemicals, which is a possible sign of addiction. Habits are behaviors that occur through choice. In contrast, no one decides to become addicted, even though people make choices that contribute to the development of an addiction.

Signs of Addiction

If you asked 10 people to define addiction, you would quite possibly get 10 different responses. Studies show that all animals share the same basic pleasure and reward circuits in the brain that turn on when they come into contact with addictive substances or engage in something pleasurable, such as eating or orgasm. We all engage in potentially addictive behaviors to some extent because some are essential to our survival and are highly reinforcing, such as eating, drinking, and sex. At some point along the continuum, however, some individuals are not able to engage in these or other behaviors moderately and become addicted to a substance or behavior.

Although there are different opinions as to the cause of addiction, most experts agree that there are some universal signs of addiction. All addictions are characterized by four common symptoms: (1) **compulsion**, which is characterized by **obsession**, or excessive preoccupation with the behavior and an overwhelming need to perform it;

Addiction: An unhealthy, continued involvement with a mood-altering object or activity in spite of harmful consequences.

Withdrawal: A series of temporary physical and biopsychosocial symptoms that occurs when the addict abruptly abstains from an addictive chemical or behavior.

Relapse: The tendency to return to the addictive behavior after a period of abstinence.

Habit: A repetitious behavior in which the repetition may be unconscious.

Compulsion: Obsessive preoccupation with a behavior and an overwhelming need to perform it.

Obsession: Excessive preoccupation with an addictive object or behavior.

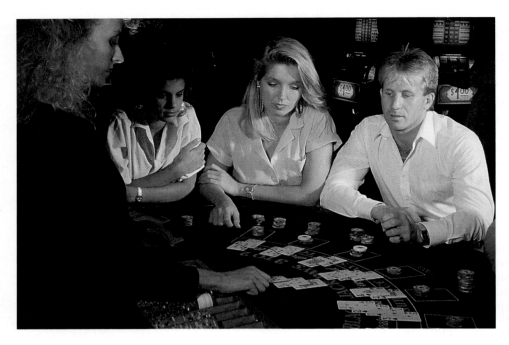

Compulsive gamblers are driven by uncontrollable urges that rule, and often ruin, their lives.

(2) **loss of control**, or the inability to predict reliably whether any isolated occurrence of the behavior will be healthy or damaging; (3) **negative consequences**, such as physical damage, legal trouble, financial problems, academic failure, and family dissolution, which do not occur with healthy involvement in any behavior; and (4) **denial**, or the inability to perceive that the behavior is self-destructive. These four components are present in all addictions, whether chemical or behavioral.

*W*HAT DO YOU THINK?

What might you do if you began to see signs of addiction in your friend? How could you be sure that what you were seeing was an addiction and not just the results of normal college stress?

*T*HE ADDICTIVE PROCESS

Addiction is a process that evolves over time. It begins when a person repeatedly seeks the illusion of relief to avoid unpleasant feelings or situations. This pattern is known as **nurturing through avoidance** and is a maladaptive way of taking care of emotional needs.[4] As a person becomes increasingly dependent on the addictive behavior, there is a corresponding deterioration in relationships with family, friends, and co-workers; in performance at work or school; and in personal life. Eventually, addicts do not find the addictive behavior pleasurable but consider it preferable to the unhappy realities they are seeking to escape.

We can also look at the progression of addiction on an emotional continuum. Vernon E. Johnson's Feeling Chart illustrates the process an addict goes through on an emotional level. For example, most of us experiment with alcohol at some point in our lives. We may have a few drinks and feel somewhat intoxicated or euphoric, learning that with time the chemical wears off and we feel "normal" again. Eventually we figure out that alcohol can induce a mood swing and that we can control the mood swing by controlling the amount of alcohol we ingest. We may even seek out the mood swing alcohol provides. At this point, most people develop rules or ideas about when, where, and how much alcohol use is appropriate. Many factors influence this decision, including one's family's use of alcohol and one's level of health in each of the six dimensions. Continuing to use alcohol in this moderate manner is referred to as "social" drinking. However if we begin to experience emotional pain as a result of our drinking, it may be a sign of problem use.

For example, consider Amy, a junior in college, who has always used alcohol moderately. Recently, she notices that she is drinking more frequently and that it helps her relax and forget about the stress of school and her problems with her roommate. One night, Amy goes to a party expecting to have a good time but instead gets into a fight with her roommate and is arrested for drunk driving on the way home. Amy will no doubt feel some emotional pain and probably feels she violated some of the rules she set for herself regarding alcohol use. If Amy continues to drink alcohol and experience negative consequences but does nothing to change her behavior, she may become addicted to alcohol. Emotionally, Amy has progressed from *phase 1—learning the mood swing* (experimenting with alcohol) to *phase 2—seeking the mood swing* (using alcohol in a moderate way) to *phase 3—harmful dependency* (forming a relationship with alcohol in which she begins to expect it to ease social awkwardness, help her relax, or have fun with friends). Depending on how often and how much alcohol Amy uses during this phase, she may experience more negative consequences which could lead to alcohol addiction. Finally, if she goes on to *phase 4—using to feel normal*, Amy may come to depend on alcohol just to feel normal[5] (See Figure 11.1).

The Physiology of Addiction

Virtually all mental, emotional, and behavioral functions occur as a result of biochemical interactions between nerve cells in the body. Biochemical messengers, called **neurotransmitters**, exert their influence at specific receptor cites on nerve cells. Drug use and chronic stress can alter these receptor sites and cause the production and breakdown of neurotransmitters.

Mood-altering chemicals, for example, fill up the receptor sites for the body's natural "feel-good" neurotransmitters (endorphins) so that nerve cells are fooled into believing they have enough neurotransmitters and shut down production of these substances temporarily. When the drug use is stopped, those receptor sites become emptied, resulting in uncomfortable feelings that remain until the body resumes neurotransmitter production or the person consumes more of the drug. Some people's bodies always produce insufficient quantities of these neurotransmitters, so they naturally seek out chemicals like alcohol as substitutes, or they pursue behaviors like exercise that increase natural production. Thus we may be "wired" to seek out substances or experiences that increase pleasure or reduce discomfort.

Mood-altering substances and experiences produce **tolerance**, a phenomenon in which progressively larger doses of a drug or more intense involvement in an experience are needed to obtain the desired effects. All of us develop some degree of tolerance to any mood-altering experience. But because addicts tend to seek intense mood-altering experiences, they eventually require amounts of mood-altering substances or experiences large enough to cause negative side effects.

Withdrawal is another phenomenon associated with mood-altering experiences. The drug or activity replaces or causes an effect that the body should normally provide on its own. If the experience is repeated often enough, the body makes an adjustment: it comes to require the drug or experience to obtain the effect it used to be able to produce itself, but no longer can. Stopping the behavior will therefore cause a withdrawal syndrome. Withdrawal symptoms of chemical dependencies are generally the opposite of the effects of the drug being withdrawn. For example, a cocaine addict experiences a characteristic "crash" (depression and lethargy), while a barbiturate addict experiences trembling, irritability, and convulsions upon withdrawal. Withdrawal symptoms for addictive behaviors are usually less dramatic. They usually involve psychic discomforts such as anxiety, depression, irritability, guilt, anger, and frustration, with an underlying preoccupation with or craving for another exposure to the behavior. Withdrawal syndromes range from mild to severe. The severest form of withdrawal syndrome is delirium tremens (DTs), which occurs in approximately 5 percent of alcoholics withdrawing from alcohol.

*W*HAT DO YOU THINK?

Since the path to addiction is most often gradual, how can you monitor your behavior in order to avoid addiction? How much is too much?

A Model of Addiction

There are many perspectives and theories concerning the cause of addictions, and most of them focus on a single causative factor. Biological or disease models have been proposed since ancient times. However, it has become clear through time that psychological, sociological, or educational factors may also be involved in the development of addiction. The most effective treatment today is being provided by those who rely on the **biopsychosocial model of addiction** to explain addiction. This theory proposes that addiction is caused by a variety of factors operating together, thereby lending a degree of credibility to all the other theories. The biopsychosocial model is not a com-

Loss of control: Inability to predict reliably whether any isolated involvement with the addictive object or behavior will be healthy or damaging.

Negative consequences: Physical damage, legal trouble, financial ruin, academic failure, family dissolution, and other severe problems associated with addiction.

Denial: Inability to perceive or accurately interpret the effects of the addictive behavior.

Nurturing through avoidance: Repeatedly seeking the illusion of relief to avoid unpleasant feelings or situations, a maladaptive way of taking care of emotional needs.

Neurotransmitters: Biochemical messengers that exert influence at specific receptor sites on nerve cells.

Tolerance: Phenomenon in which progressively larger dose of a drug or more intense involvement in a behavior is needed to produce the desired effects.

Biopsychosocial model of addiction: Theory of the relationship among an addict's biological (genetic) nature and psychological and sociocultural influences.

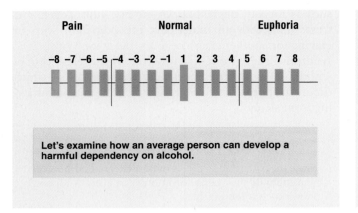

Pain — Normal — Euphoria

−8 −7 −6 −5 −4 −3 −2 −1 1 2 3 4 5 6 7 8

Let's examine how an average person can develop a harmful dependency on alcohol.

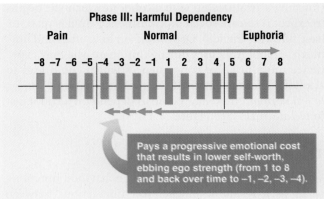

Phase III: Harmful Dependency

Pain — Normal — Euphoria

−8 −7 −6 −5 −4 −3 −2 −1 1 2 3 4 5 6 7 8

Pays a progressive emotional cost that results in lower self-worth, ebbing ego strength (from 1 to 8 and back over time to −1, −2, −3, −4).

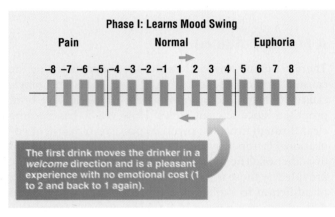

Phase I: Learns Mood Swing

Pain — Normal — Euphoria

−8 −7 −6 −5 −4 −3 −2 −1 1 2 3 4 5 6 7 8

The first drink moves the drinker in a *welcome* direction and is a pleasant experience with no emotional cost (1 to 2 and back to 1 again).

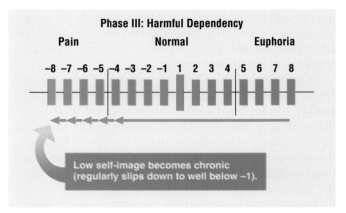

Phase III: Harmful Dependency

Pain — Normal — Euphoria

−8 −7 −6 −5 −4 −3 −2 −1 1 2 3 4 5 6 7 8

Low self-image becomes chronic (regularly slips down to well below −1).

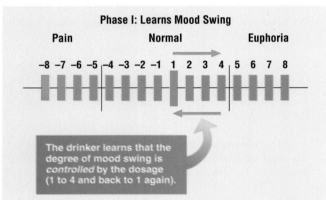

Phase I: Learns Mood Swing

Pain — Normal — Euphoria

−8 −7 −6 −5 −4 −3 −2 −1 1 2 3 4 5 6 7 8

The drinker learns that the degree of mood swing is *controlled* by the dosage (1 to 4 and back to 1 again).

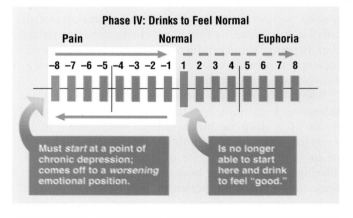

Phase IV: Drinks to Feel Normal

Pain — Normal — Euphoria

−8 −7 −6 −5 −4 −3 −2 −1 1 2 3 4 5 6 7 8

Must *start* at a point of chronic depression; comes off to a *worsening* emotional position.

Is no longer able to start here and drink to feel "good."

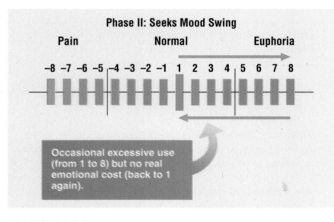

Phase II: Seeks Mood Swing

Pain — Normal — Euphoria

−8 −7 −6 −5 −4 −3 −2 −1 1 2 3 4 5 6 7 8

Occasional excessive use (from 1 to 8) but no real emotional cost (back to 1 again).

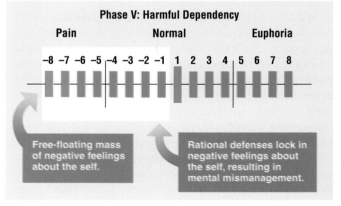

Phase V: Harmful Dependency

Pain — Normal — Euphoria

−8 −7 −6 −5 −4 −3 −2 −1 1 2 3 4 5 6 7 8

Free-floating mass of negative feelings about the self.

Rational defenses lock in negative feelings about the self, resulting in mental mismanagement.

FIGURE 11.1

The Feeling Chart

Source: Reprinted by permission from Vernon E. Johnson, *Intervention: Helping Someone Who Doesn't Want Help* (Minneapolis, MN: Johnson Institute, 1986), 16–35.

promise solution to a theoretical controversy. Rather, it represents a reasonable comprehension of all that we have learned about addiction.

Biological or Disease Influences. Studies have shown that people addicted to mood-altering substances metabolize these substances differently than nonaddicted people do. For example, studies of adult children of alcoholics have found that these people have abnormal concentrations or activity of various neurotransmitters related to mood—specifically norepinephrine, serotonin, endorphin, and enkephalin.[6] Abnormal levels of any of these neurotransmitters may create a biochemically based mood disorder. To obtain relief from the disorder, people may turn to mood-altering chemicals or behaviors.

Genetic studies support a genetic influence for addiction. It has been known for centuries that alcoholism runs in families. Research on family members and twins has repeatedly confirmed the existence of a genetic factor in alcoholism. In the last decade, other studies have shown that the children of drug-addicted parents are more likely to engage in addictive behaviors than are the children of nonaddicted parents. These findings hold true whether or not the children lived with their addicted parents.[7]

Sociocultural Influences. Cultural expectations and mores help determine whether and how people engage in certain behaviors. For example, although many native Italians use alcohol abundantly, there is a low incidence of alcoholism in this culture. Low rates of alcoholism are typically found in those cultures where children are gradually introduced to alcohol in diluted amounts, on special occasions, and within a strong family group. There is deep disapproval of intoxication, which is not viewed as socially acceptable, stylish, or funny.[8] Such cultural traditions and values are not widespread in the United States, where the incidence of alcoholism and alcohol-related problems is very high.

Societal attitudes also influence addictive behavior. The media's near-worship of youth and beauty plays a significant role in the development of eating disorders and compulsive exercise. The pervasive attitude in our society that alcohol and other drugs are necessary to have a good time makes it difficult for some people to have fun without using chemicals. The emphasis on materialism and perfectionism has made workaholism not just acceptable but admirable. Recent evidence suggests that communities that either condone substance abuse or that have unstated or unclear policies against it are likely to experience a higher incidence of substance abuse.[9]

Social learning theory proposes that people learn behaviors by watching role models—parents, caregivers, and significant others. The effects of modeling, imitation, and identification with behavior from early childhood on are well documented. Modeling is especially influential when it involves behavior that is mood-altering. Many studies show that modeling by parents and by idolized celebrities exerts a profound influence on young people.[10]

Life Events. Major and stressful life events, such as marriage, divorce, change in work status, and death of a loved one, may trigger addictive behaviors. The death of a spouse is the most common trigger event for excessive drinking in the elderly. Divorce is the most common stimulus for alcoholism in women. Traumatic events in general often instigate addictive behaviors, as the traumatized person seeks to medicate the pain of those events—pain they may not even be aware of because they've repressed it. One thing that makes addictive behaviors so powerfully attractive is that they reliably assuage personal pain.

Family Influences. Family members whose needs for love, security, and affirmation are not consistently met, who are refused permission to express their feelings, desires, or needs; and who frequently submerge their personalities in order to "keep the peace" are prone to addiction. Children whose parents are not consistently available to them (physically or emotionally); or who are subjected to sexual abuse, physical abuse, neglect, or abandonment; or who are sent inconsistent or disparaging messages about their self-worth may experience mental or physical illness or addiction in adulthood. People from dysfunctional families are more likely to die prematurely from stress-related illnesses, the physical effects of addiction, suicide, or violence.

The complexity of addiction and consistent evidence of multiple contributing factors in the lives of addicts lead to the conclusion that addiction is not the result of a single influence but rather of a variety of influences working together. Biological, psychological, sociocultural, and environmental factors all contribute to the development of addiction. Although one factor may play a larger role than another in a specific individual, a single factor is rarely sufficient to explain an addiction.

Enablers

Enablers are people who knowingly or unknowingly protect addicts from the natural consequences of their behavior. Without the benefit of having to deal with consequences, addicts are unable to see the self-destructive

---

Social learning theory: Theory that people learn behaviors by watching role models—parents, caregivers, and significant others.

Enablers: People who knowingly or unknowingly protect addicts from the natural consequences of their behavior.

---

nature of their behavior and will therefore continue it. Codependents are the primary enablers of their addicted loved ones, although anyone who has contact with an addict can be an enabler and thus contribute (perhaps powerfully) to the addictive behavior. For example, lawyers have professional relationships with addicted clients charged with illegal acts committed as a result of their addiction. It is the lawyer's role to absolve clients of responsibility for these acts, yet experiencing the consequences of these acts (e.g., jail, community service, restitution) is a powerful motivator for addicts to face the reality of their addiction.

Enablers are generally unaware that their behavior is allowing the addict to continue the addiction. In fact, enabling is rarely conscious and is certainly not intentional. But even when enablers understand what they are doing, they may not feel equipped to behave in any other way, either because they don't know how to confront the addict effectively or because they fear having to deal with the embarrassment, shame, guilt, and conflict that will result if the addictive behavior is brought out in the open. Enablers can only end their destructive contribution to the addiction if they are taught clear ways to ensure that addicts are not shielded from the consequences of their behavior.

$\mathcal{T}$YPES OF ADDICTION AND THEIR COSTS

It is difficult to document the incidence of addictions of any kind because involvement with a chemical or a behavior is not, by itself, indicative of addiction. Nevertheless, many studies on morbidity and mortality associated with consumption of a substance or performance of a behavior provide reasonable estimates. One of the best indicators of addiction in the United States is the 14 to 16 million people who attend over one-half million available self-help groups every year.[11]

Clearly, tobacco, alcohol, and other drugs are addictive, and addictions to these drugs create multiple problems for individuals, families, and society. These addictions are discussed in their own separate chapters. This chapter is devoted to the concepts and the process of addiction, as well as its associated problems. Here the discussion of specific forms of addiction will be limited to what are com-

monly called "process addictions"—behaviors known to be addictive because they are mood-altering, such as eating disorders, money addictions, workaholism, and exercise and sex addictions.

Money Addictions

Money addictions include compulsive gambling, spending, and borrowing. Money addicts tend to use drug addicts' terms to describe their experiences: *high, rush, crash.* Research has shown that the various money addictions produce in susceptible individuals profound mood elevations resulting from synthesis of the neurotransmitters that regulate stimulation, excitement, and pleasure.[12] Money addicts develop tolerance and also experience the phenomenon of withdrawal. Withdrawal symptoms include extreme restlessness, agitation, insomnia, depression, anxiety, and anger.[13]

Money addictions are common to both genders and all ages, races, religions, and socioeconomic groups. The two genders tend to select different forms of the addiction, though. For example, twice as many men as women are compulsive gamblers, while twice as many women as men are "shopaholics."[14] Men tend more than women toward compulsive borrowing, although here the gap is closing. Family backgrounds of money addicts are remarkably similar. One or both parents were typically absent or emotionally unavailable and often had addictions of their own. For ways to avoid money addictions, see the Choices for Change box.

Compulsive Gambling. Gambling is a healthy form of recreation and entertainment for millions of Americans. The majority of people gamble casually and moderately to experience the excitement of anticipating a win. But 4.2 million Americans are **compulsive gamblers** (addicted to gambling).[15] For these people, gambling is a compulsion that rules, and often ruins, their lives. While casual gamblers can stop anytime they wish and are capable of seeing the necessity to do so, compulsive gamblers are unable to control their urge to gamble even in the face of devastating consequences: high debt, legal problems, and the loss of everything meaningful, including homes, families, jobs, health—and even their lives. Cardiovascular problems affect 38 percent of compulsive gamblers and their suicide rate is 20 times higher than that of the general population.[16]

Compulsive Shopping and Borrowing. Although compulsive spending has been a pervasive problem in the United States for some time, a more insidious form of the addiction is found in the new "plastic generation." Credit card companies entice you with fantasies of having it all, right now—whether or not you can afford it. As a result of this trend toward credit, national consumer indebtedness in 1990 was twice what it was in 1981: $650 billion.[17] Moreover, the average American has seven credit cards

---

Compulsive gambler: A person addicted to gambling.

Workaholic: A person who gradually becomes emotionally crippled and addicted to control and power in a compulsive drive to gain approval and success.

Managing Your Money

These strategies are useful for everyone interested in developing and maintaining healthy habits regarding money management. If you are an addict or on your way to being one, you will need to do much more. Seeking professional help is a good place to start.

- Make a financial plan that considers *all your needs* and as many desires as your income allows. Consider the wisdom of saving for emergencies.

- If any of your money behaviors are problematic, make yourself accountable to someone you trust for your spending, borrowing, and gambling practices. This is especially important if spending or gambling causes you pleasure and excitement or if borrowing reduces the discomfort associated with indebtedness.

- Avoid purchasing items just because they are on sale or because they are a "good bargain."

- Never borrow money if you have no means of repaying it within a reasonable length of time. This includes purchasing on credit when making the payments will cause financial hardship.

- Never borrow money to pay off debts or to gamble.

- Avoid any kind of gambling activity if you are in poor financial shape—you cannot afford to lose the money, and it is unrealistic to *expect* to win.

- If you enjoy gambling, set a limit on the amount you are willing to spend (commensurate with the amount of enjoyment it provides). Resolve *never* to exceed this limit regardless of the circumstances. Be ready to acknowledge that doing so may indicate compulsion.

- Seek assistance from a consumer credit counseling service if you need help getting and staying out of debt.

- Seek assistance from a mental health specialist if you have recurring life disruptions caused by depression, anxiety, or unexplained anger.

---

and nine times the debt his or her counterpart had in 1960.[18]

The obvious "shopaholics" are people who go on wild sprees, buying things they neither want nor need. The less obvious spending addicts are those who limit purchases to single items they genuinely want and even need, but cannot afford. The critical issue in this addiction is the intangible need that is met through the behavior: the need for self-value and fulfillment. The purchases reflect qualities these people lack—power, love, and control.

Compulsive gambling and shopping frequently lead to compulsive borrowing. Irresponsible investments and purchases lead to debts that the addict tries to repay by borrowing more. Compulsive debtors borrow money repeatedly from family, friends, or institutions in spite of the problems this causes. While most people incur overwhelming debt through a combination of hardship and ignorance about financial management, compulsive debtors incur debt primarily as a result of buying or gambling behaviors in which they have engaged to relieve painful feelings.

Workaholism

Workaholism is the only addiction that wins the admiration of others. Work is, in fact, an addiction that is supported by a culture dedicated to perfectionism, power, and control.

In order to understand work addiction, we need to understand the concept of healthy work. Healthy work provides a sense of identity, helps develop our strengths, and is a means of satisfaction, accomplishment, and mastery of problems. Healthy workers may work passionately for long hours. But although they have occasional projects that keep them away from family, friends, and personal interests for short periods of time, they generally maintain balance in their lives and are in full control of their schedules. Healthy work does not "consume" the worker.

A practical definition of a **workaholic** is "a person who gradually becomes emotionally crippled and addicted to control and power in a compulsive drive to gain approval and success . . . work is an escape to an overly inflated sense of responsibility, away from true intimacy with others."[19] Work addiction is characterized by obsession, perfectionism, rigidity, fear, anxiety, feelings of inadequacy, low self-esteem, and alienation. Workaholism is more than being unable to relax when not doing something considered "productive." It is the pursuit of the "work persona"—the image workaholics wish others to have of them.

An estimated 12 million Americans are workaholics.[20] Work addiction is found in all age, racial, and socioeconomic groups, but it typically develops in people in their 40s and 50s. Male workaholics outnumber female workaholics, but women are catching up fast as they gain more equality in the workforce.

Although workaholics tend to be admired in our society and the term *workaholic* is often met with humor, the effects of this addiction on individuals and those around them are far from humorous. Workaholism is a major

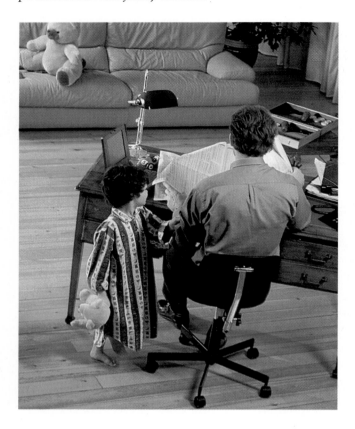

Workaholics are unable to relax and detach themselves from their "work persona"—often at the expense of personal health and family relations.

chronic fatigue. The excessive pumping of adrenaline that is part of their addiction causes fatigue, hypertension and other cardiovascular diseases, nervousness, trembling, and increased sweating. Workaholics commonly suffer from disorders of the gastrointestinal tract, and they often report a feeling of pressure in their chest, constricted breathing, dizziness, and lightheadedness.

Exercise Addiction

It may seem odd that a personal health text that advocates exercise for health-risk reduction and health maintenance would identify exercise as a potential addiction. But indeed, as a powerful mood enhancer, exercise can be addictive. Statistics on the incidence of this addiction are not available, but it is clear that a large portion of America's 2 million anorexics and bulimics use exercise as a purge instead of or in addition to self-induced vomiting. Another indirect indicator of the high incidence of addictive exercise is the explosion of fitness-related products such as videotapes, books, exercise equipment, and clothing.

Healthy exercise is done for the benefits it provides rather than as an end in itself. **Addictive exercisers** abuse exercise in the same way that alcoholics abuse alcohol or addictive spenders abuse money. They use it compulsively to try to meet needs that cannot truly be met by an object or activity: nurturance, intimacy, self-esteem, and self-competency. As a result, addictive exercise results in negative consequences similar to those found in other addictions: alienation of family and friends, injuries from overdoing it, and a craving for more (see the Rate Yourself box).

Sexual Addictions

All people need love and intimacy, but the sexual practices of sex addicts involve neither. Sex addicts confuse the intensity of sexual arousal with intimacy.[22] They do not feel nurtured by the person with whom they have sex but by the sexual activity itself. Neither are they capable of nurturing another, because sex, not the person, is the object of their affection. In fact, sex addicts do not necessarily seek partners to obtain sexual arousal; they may be satisfied by masturbation, either alone or during phone sex or while reading or watching erotica. Sex addicts may participate in a wide range of sexual activities, including affairs, sex with strangers, prostitution, voyeurism, exhibitionism, cross-dressing, rape, incest, and pedophilia.

Sex addicts frequently experience crushing episodes of depression and anxiety, fueled by the fear of discovery. Suicide is high among people who have problems with sexual control. The toll that these addictions exact is most clearly seen in loss of intimacy with loved ones, which frequently leads to family disintegration.

No group of people is more or less likely than another to become involved in sexual addictions. They affect men

source of marital discord and family breakup. In fact, most work addicts come from homes that were alcoholic, rigid, violent, or otherwise dysfunctional. A survey of grandchildren of alcoholics revealed that 64 percent identified workaholism as the most common compulsion in one or both of their parents.[21]

Whether or not they lose their families, work addicts do lose their emotional and physical health. Workaholics may become emotionally crippled, losing the communication and human interaction skills critical to living and working with other people. They are often riddled with guilt and chronic fears—of failure, of boredom, of laziness, of persecution, and of being found out. Because they are unable to relax and play, they commonly suffer from

Addictive exercisers: People who exercise compulsively to try to meet needs of nurturance, intimacy, self-esteem, and self-competency.

Codependence: A self-defeating relationship pattern in which a person is "addicted to the addict."

Are You Addicted to Exercise?

1. Do you think and talk about exercise more often than you used to?

2. Do you daydream about your workouts?

3. Do you exercise despite the weather or other negative environmental factors, such as no air conditioning at your gym on the hottest days of the year?

4. Do you exercise even when you're sick or injured?

5. Do you consistently exercise to improve your mood, to relax, or to combat depression?

6. Do you find that you get irritable on days when you can't find the time to exercise?

7. Have you ever lied about how often you exercise?

8. Do you spend more money than you can realistically afford on exercise-related equipment and/or fees?

9. Has anyone ever complained that you exercise too much?

10. Has your exercise schedule ever interfered with your ability to perform adequately at work or at school?

11. Has exercise ever damaged your relationships?

12. Do you find it difficult to relate to people who are not involved in exercise?

13. Do you find that you enjoy other activities only if you know you'll still have the opportunity to exercise?

14. Do you ever feel terrible, ugly, fat, lazy, or worthless when you don't exercise?

15. Do you feel you must exercise to keep your weight under control or to allow you to eat more?

16. Do you have trouble imagining your life without exercise?

If you answered yes to eight or more of these questions, it is possible that you are addicted to exercise. Consider those questions to which you've answered yes. What actions can you take to change your behavior? What factors influence you to act in this way? Where can you go for help?

Source: Reprinted by permission of Sanford J. Greenburger Associates from *Hooked on Exercise: How to Understand and Manage Exercise Addiction* by Rebecca Prussin, M.D., Philip Harvey, Ph.D., and Theresa Foy DiGeronimo, published by Simon & Schuster, 1992, and copyrighted by the authors.

---

and women of all ages, including married and single people, and they do not respect sexual preference. What sex addicts do usually have in common is a dysfunctional childhood family, often characterized by chemical dependency or other addictions. Many were physically and emotionally abused. Sex addicts tend to have a history of sexual abuse.

While there are no statistics on the incidence of sexual addiction, the proliferation of self-help books on the subject and support groups for sex addicts indicates that a large number of Americans are affected by this issue. Sexual abuse victims commonly manifest the pain of their abuse by engaging in sexual and other addictions. Since the number of reported cases of sexual abuse in 1988 was 60 million, we can assume that if only a small portion of these people become sex addicts, the incidence is substantial.[23]

Codependence

Codependence refers to a self-defeating relationship pattern in which a person is "addicted to the addict." It is the primary outcome of dysfunctional relationships or family systems. Four "core" symptoms are involved in codependence: Codependents have difficulty (1) experiencing appropriate levels of self-esteem, (2) setting healthy boundaries, (3) owning and expressing their own reality, and (4) taking care of their adult needs and desires.[24]

Codependence is not accurately defined by isolated incidents of characteristic behavior but rather by a pattern of characteristic behavior. Codependents tend to base their self-esteem on extrinsic factors, such as their ability to control the feelings and behaviors of others or to effect a positive outcome for precarious situations. In reality, self-esteem is intrinsic, but codependents have difficulty understanding and accepting this. Moreover, they are frequently perfectionists, which creates an even more tenuous foundation for their self-esteem.[25]

Codependents find it hard to set healthy boundaries, probably because they did not have models of healthy boundary setting when they were growing up. Healthy boundaries are "lines of demarcation that define the personal territory made up of one's feelings, thoughts, desires, needs, and rights."[26] Codependents are more likely than healthy people to have unclear, rigid, or invasive boundaries. Unclear boundaries create double messages in a relationship that give rise to tension, conflict, and uncertainty. Rigid boundaries remain immovable, even in situations where flexibility would be the healthier response. Finally, invasive boundaries are aggressive, giving rise to our behavior toward others that is inappropriate or abusive.

What does it mean to have difficulty owning and expressing our own reality? Pia Mellody refers to our reality as our bodies, thoughts, feelings, and behavior.[27] Codependents have difficulty owning all or some of their reality in the following ways: (1) they do not accurately perceive their appearance or how their body is functioning; (2) they find it hard to identify their thoughts and/or express them openly and honestly, or they perceive messages from others inaccurately; (3) they have difficulty labeling their feelings, or they feel overwhelmed by them; (4) they have difficulty perceiving how their behavior affects others or accepting that their behavior may be hurtful to others.

Codependents assume responsibility for meeting others' needs to the point where they subordinate or even cease being aware of their own needs. They may be unable to perceive their needs because they have repeatedly been told that their needs are inappropriate or less important than someone else's. Their behavior goes far beyond performing kind services for another person. Codependents feel less than human if they fail to respond to the needs of someone else, even when their help was not requested.

Because the environment in which codependents live tends to be chaotic, unpredictable, and highly stressful, they commonly resort to compulsive or addictive behaviors to medicate themselves against the pain in their lives. But while they may be able to reduce conscious awareness of their pain through these addictive behaviors, they can not "fool" their bodies. That is why codependents experience a great deal of stress-related illness, such as hypertension, headaches, asthma, and rheumatoid arthritis. Because of their difficulty in owning their own reality, they are frequently unaware of the early symptoms of an illness and thus unable to forestall more serious problems. For more on this matter, see the Skills for Behavior Change box.

Multiple Addictions

Treatment centers for addiction have discovered that most addicts are dependent on more than one chemical and/or behavior, even though they tend to have a "drug of choice" or a "behavior of choice"—one that they prefer because it is more effective at meeting their needs. As many as 60 percent of those in treatment have problems with more than one addiction, and the figure may be as high as 75 percent for people addicted to chemicals. For example, alcoholism and eating disorders are commonly paired in women, and both chemically dependent women and men frequently resort to compulsive eating to keep themselves abstinent from drugs. Anyone who has attended a meeting of Alcoholics Anonymous or Narcotics Anonymous knows that recovering alcoholics and drug addicts are often heavy smokers and/or caffeine users. One study showed that 49 percent of compulsive gamblers are also alcoholics.[28] While multiple addictions certainly complicate recovery, they do not make it impossible. As with single addictions, the place to begin recovery is with the recognition that there is a problem.

What do you think?

Based on what you've read here, do you think you have any behaviors that are unhealthy and could lead to addiction? Who could you ask to help you evaluate your behavior? Are you ready to make some changes in your attitudes or beliefs that may help you to break the cycle of the unhealthy behaviors?

Treatment and Recovery for Addiction

Treatment and recovery for any addiction begin with **abstinence**—refraining from the addictive behavior. While literal abstinence is possible for people addicted to chemicals, it obviously is not for people addicted to behaviors like work and sex. For these addicts, abstinence means restoring balance to their lives through noncompulsive engagement in the behaviors. For compulsive gamblers, abstinence may involve avoiding certain activities, such as watching sporting events, that seem to set off an uncontrollable desire to gamble. For workaholics, it may mean scheduling specific hours for work and then leaving work to participate in other aspects of life.

Detoxification refers to the early abstinence period during which an addict adjusts physically and cognitively to being free from the influence of the addiction. It occurs in virtually every recovering addict, and while it is uncomfortable for them all, it can be dangerous for some. This is primarily true for those addicted to chemicals, especially alcohol, heroin, and minor tranquilizers like Valium. For these people, early abstinence may involve such profound withdrawal symptoms that they require medical supervision. Therefore, most inpatient treatment programs provide a pretreatment component of supervised detoxification so that abstinence can be achieved safely prior to treatment.

But abstinence alone does little to change the personality and psychological dynamics or the biological and environmental influences behind the addictive behavior. Without recovery, an addict is apt to relapse time and again or simply to change addictions. Recovery involves learning new ways of looking at oneself, others, and the world. Where applicable, it requires exploration of a traumatic past so that psychological wounds can be healed to pave the way for a better future. It involves learning *interdependence* with significant others rather than independence or overdependence. It requires new ways of taking care of oneself, physically and emotionally. It involves developing communication skills and new ways of having

Preventing Codependence

If you grew up in a dysfunctional family or if you are currently in a dysfunctional relationship, seek professional help to regain confidence and skills in cultivating healthy relationships.

- End relationships with people who abuse you in any way, including those who discount your opinions about the relationship or other important issues in your life.

- Cultivate your own opinions and learn to articulate them.

- Learn how to be a clear, responsible communicator.

- Resolve to confront conflict in relationships rather than "sweep it under the rug," where tension about it builds.

- Take responsibility for your own feelings and allow others to do the same. Only accept responsibility for how others feel when you have done something hurtful to them.

- Learn to develop healthy (fluid) boundaries and to respect the boundaries of others.

- While it is okay to help people out and do nice things for them, avoid chronically subordinating your own needs in order to meet the needs of others. Recognize that your own needs are valid and important.

- Resolve never to make excuses for the inappropriate, unkind, abusive, or addictive behavior of another person. Allow others the learning experience of facing the natural negative consequences of their behavior.

- Deal with issues of low self-esteem and seek assistance for recurring episodes of painful feelings such as depression, anxiety, guilt, or unexplained anger.

---

fun. Recovery is a process, not an event. Recovery programs are the fuel that gives addicts the energy to resist relapsing. For a large number of addicts, recovery begins with a period of formal treatment involving individual, group, and family therapy.

Intervention

Denial is the hallmark of addiction. Although addicts can become master liars, denial is not the same as a lie. A lie is a deliberate falsification of the truth. *Denial is the inability to see the truth.* Denial is so powerful a part of addiction that intervention is necessary to break down the addict's denial system. **Intervention** is a planned process of confrontation by significant others—people who are important to the addict, including spouse, parents, children, boss, and friends. Its purpose is to break down the denial compassionately so that the addict can see the destructive nature of the addiction. It is not enough to get the addict to admit that he or she is addicted. The addict must come to perceive that the addiction is destructive and requires treatment. Suggestions on how to intervene are discussed in the Building Communication Skills box.

Individual confrontation is difficult and often futile. However, an addict's defenses generally crumble when significant others collectively share their observations and concerns about the addict's behavior. It is critical that those involved in the intervention communicate how they plan to end their enabling. For example, a wife may state that she will no longer cover bounced checks or make excuses for her money-addicted husband's antisocial behavior. She may even close their joint account and open a personal account so that she will not be legally responsi-

ble for his irresponsible acts. It is crucial that all parties involved in the intervention choose consequences they are ready to follow through with in the event the addict refuses treatment. Significant others must also be ready to give support if the addict is willing to begin a recovery program.

Intervention is a serious step toward helping someone who probably does not want help. It should therefore be well planned and rehearsed. Most addiction treatment centers have specialists on staff who can help plan an intervention. In addition, there are books on the subject written for families and friends who are concerned about someone who is or may be addicted.

Brief Intervention. A new approach to addiction treatment that seems to show promise is **brief intervention therapy.** The assumption underlying this approach is that

---

Abstinence: Refraining from an addictive behavior.

Detoxification: The early abstinence period during which an addict adjusts physically and cognitively to being free from the influence of the addiction.

Intervention: A planned process of confrontation by significant others.

Brief intervention therapy: Therapy based on the assumption that even very brief treatment, if designed properly, can be highly successful in treating addicts.

Confronting Addictive Behavior

Most people learn at an early age that it is impolite to confront other people about their behavior, especially if you want to be accepted. Yet the most caring thing you can do for someone who is involved in self-destructive behavior is to get involved. By not confronting the behavior, you subtly show approval.

Confrontation can be frightening. You may hit a wall of denial and hostility. You may even cause a break in the relationship. For these reasons, confrontation should always be done with an attitude of caring and concern.

It may be best to talk to the person in the company of others who are equally concerned and who have had occasion to observe the behavior. This approach reduces the risk associated with talking to the friend alone, and it eliminates some of the potential for denial.

If the person is involved with alcohol or other drugs, wait until he or she is sober so that you can discuss the situation more rationally. The only exception is when someone's safety is at stake. For example, it is appropriate to prevent an intoxicated person from driving.

The goal of the confrontation should be to inform, not to punish. This goal can best be achieved by stating your observations about the person's behavior rather than judging the person for behaving this way.

Do not get sidetracked. Someone who is involved in a harmful behavior will offer numerous explanations as to why your observations are off base. An effective denial tool is to draw attention to someone else to avoid looking bad.

If you believe that your friend has established a pattern of harmful involvement in the behavior, help is needed. It is especially important to make a referral when someone continues the behavior despite promises to stop. Before the confrontation, find out where your friend can receive help. The student health center, the counseling center, a local alcohol and drug treatment program, or a hospital are places to check out.

You can't change someone else by communicating your concern about his or her behavior. But you can increase the chances that the person will decide to change. People are more likely to change if they can understand the self-destructive nature of their behavior and see that others whom they respect do not approve of it.

---

very brief treatment, if designed properly, can be highly successful even with moderately severe addicts. Therapists use "motivational interviewing" with patients. Six key components (FRAMES) in the brief intervention therapy help patients to gain confidence in their ability to quit:

- Feedback—Specific feedback is tailored to the individual.

- Responsibility—Patients are told that recovery is up to them; they are not seen as helpless victims of a disease.

- Advice—Firm and clear recommendations are given.

- Menu—There are different ways to work out the addiction.

- Empathy—The best therapists have this and are neither too pushy nor confrontational.

- Self-efficacy—Patients are told, "You can do it," and empowered to change.

More than 30 studies in 14 countries have affirmed the value of these key components in helping addicts. Researchers report that their success lies in helping addicts to believe in their ability to quit or moderate and to retain their motivation once they do.

*W*HAT DO YOU THINK?

Have you ever watched while someone you cared about seemed to be throwing everything away because of an addiction? Did you remain quiet for fear of losing the friendship or relationship with that person? What factors do you think contributed to the person's addictive behavior?

Treatment

On TV, on any evening during prime time, you are likely to see an advertisement for facilities that offer treatment for addictive disorders. Some of them merely entice viewers with a promise of compassionate service, while others claim to be better than any other program, boasting "a number-one cure rate." Programs that claim to cure anybody are probably not worthy of your trust, since reputable treatment facilities acknowledge that addiction is never cured but only arrested through a recovery process. You probably won't be able to tell from a television or newspaper ad whether a facility is a good one. The best way to find that out is to interview key people at the facility. Here are some characteristics of a good treatment program:

- The facility employs professionals who are familiar with the specific addictive disorder for which help is being sought.

Native American Rite of Purification

The important role of spiritual health in the treatment of addictions has been clear for most of this century. Alcoholics Anonymous and other 12-step programs rely heavily on spiritual belief to help the addict maintain control. Culturally specific religious beliefs and rituals can also play a role both in the healing process and in gaining acceptance by the addict for the medical portions of therapy.

At the St. Cloud Veterans Hospital, therapists take a novel approach in the treatment of alcoholism among Native Americans. The Native American *onikane,* or sweat lodge, is used in conjunction with the 12 steps of the Alcoholics Anonymous program. The sweat lodge is the setting for a rite of purification that Native Americans believe can purge their past and reunite them with the earth and its goodness.

The sweat lodge itself is a small tent covered with blankets and tarpaulins. A group of five or six Native Americans enter the sweltering tent, followed by a "spiritual advisor"—called a "medicine man" by hospital officials. The spiritual advisor uses a pair of reindeer antlers (only natural objects are allowed in the tent) to rake red-hot rocks into a small pit in the center of the tent. Pouring water on the rocks, the medicine man transforms the darkened tent into a steamy oven, with temperatures soaring to over 100 degrees.

Participants are first urged to block out impure thoughts and to imagine that they are returning to their mothers' wombs to recall their very first thoughts. If that fails, "impure thoughts" are considered to be blocking their minds. The men remain in the tent for more than two hours, chanting songs in their native tongues, confessing to misdeeds in English, and imploring "the Great Spirit" to help them return to their traditional roots. It is a demanding ordeal.

The ceremony is an attempt to help addicted Native Americans to deal with themselves. It harkens back to tribal traditions and helps them touch base with their heritage. Most importantly, it makes them more receptive to the medical therapy offered in conjunction with the traditional part of the hospital's therapy.

Source: Adapted from Bill McAllister, "At VA Hospital, 'Medicine Man' Helps Indians Try to Beat an Old Nemesis," *Washington Post,* 9 June 1991, A3. © 1991 The Washington Post. Reprinted with permission.

- The facility provides both inpatient and outpatient services according to various, but structured, schedules. Recommendations for inpatient or outpatient treatment are based on thorough assessment of the addict.

- The facility employs medical personnel or has a working relationship with medical personnel who assess the addict's medical status and provide treatment for medical problems, whether or not they were caused by the addictive behavior.

- The facility provides or makes arrangements for medical supervision of addicts who are at high risk for a complicated detoxification (e.g., delirium tremens).

- The facility encourages family therapy for clients who have intact families.

- The facility offers a team approach to treatment of the addictive disorders (e.g., medical personnel, counselors, psychotherapists, social workers, clergy, educators, dietitians, and fitness counselors).

- The facility provides both group and individual therapy.

- The facility integrates peer-led support groups into its programs (e.g., Alcoholics Anonymous) and encourages the addict to continue in the support groups after treatment ends.

- The facility provides structured after-care and relapse-prevention programs.

- The physical structure, regardless of how old or new it is, is clean and attractive.

- The staff is cordial and willing to answer all your questions, including those about costs and financial arrangements.

- The facility is accredited by the Joint Commission for the Accreditation of Healthcare Organizations (JCAHO) and is licensed by the state in which it operates.

Treatment programs are highly structured programs that help their clients get started on a lifetime program of personal recovery. They include wellness programs to teach critical self-care skills, educational programs to formulate a deep understanding of the addiction, self-help groups to provide a foundation of self-help after treatment, and several forms of therapy, as described below. Some treatment centers also integrate cultural issues into the patient's treatment, as discussed in the Multicultural Perspectives box.

Individual Therapy. Therapy in the company of a trained addictions specialist provides a safe environment in which recovering addicts can identify and experience feelings they have been chronically medicating with their addictive behavior. In therapy, addicts begin to deal with issues related to their addiction. Individual therapy is the safest place for people to allow painful, perhaps traumatic, memories to surface so they can be resolved and left behind. Individual therapy also helps addicts deal with unhealthy boundaries and other issues, such as the need to control, that make intimate relationships difficult for them.

Group Therapy. The standard of care in the addictions field is to combine group therapy with individual therapy. While individual therapy is necessary, it is ineffective by itself. Group therapy is a safe environment in which to relearn relationship skills that were lost during addiction or that were never developed. A critical skill developed in group therapy is learning how to give and receive feedback. Addicts ask for others' perspectives about issues they bring up for discussion. Giving respectful and caring feedback is a skill that is lost during addictive acting out, because addicts tend to treat others as objects. Group therapy is a laboratory for developing the communication skills and respect that enable addicts to restore others to their rightful place as equals. Most of all, group therapy offers an environment where addicts learn how to be honest with themselves and others. Addicts are very adept at perceiving the dishonesty of other addicts, so group members keep one another in touch with the reality of their addictions and limitations.

Family Therapy. Addiction affects the addict's entire family. If the family receives no attention during the addict's recovery process, family members will continue to function as codependents because codependency is all they know. Even if they do receive therapy, families may dissolve when an addict member begins to recover. But whether the family dissolves or stays together, family therapy helps individual family members recover. Like therapy for addicts, therapy for family members is provided in individual and group settings, and it serves the same functions.

12-Step Programs. Recovery continues after treatment in an ongoing process that includes self-help programs and reeducation (e.g., reading, workbooks). Ideally, all recovering addicts develop personal recovery programs that they follow indefinitely and attend meetings of peer groups, such as 12-step programs. These **12-step programs** are peer support groups patterned after Alcoholics Anonymous (see Table 11.1). They are designed to keep addicts free of their addictions through honest acknowledgment of their shortcomings and through the mutual support of others who have had similar experiences. There are 12-step programs for every addiction, as well as for families and others who have a relationship with an addict. They have the reputation of providing the most

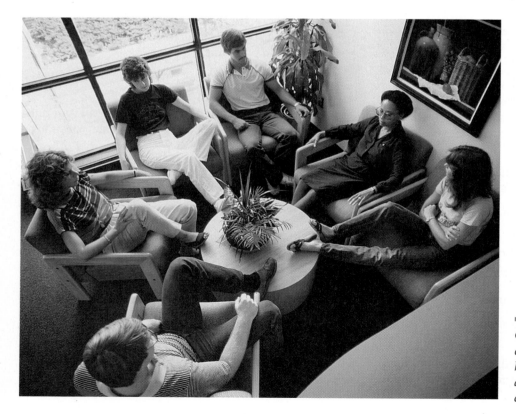

Group therapy provides a safe environment for people to learn how to be honest with themselves and others about the reality and consequences of their addictions.

TABLE 11.1 ■ The Twelve Steps

1. We admitted we were powerless over alcohol—that our lives had become unmanageable.

2. Came to believe that a Power greater than ourselves could restore us to sanity.

3. Made a decision to turn our will and our lives over to the care of God *as we understood Him.*

4. Made a searching and fearless moral inventory of ourselves.

5. Admitted to God, to ourselves and to another human being the exact nature of our wrongs.

6. Were entirely ready to have God remove all of these defects of character.

7. Humbly asked Him to remove our shortcomings.

8. Made a list of all persons we had harmed and became willing to make amends to them all.

9. Made direct amends to such people wherever possible, except when to do so would injure them or others.

10. Continued to take personal inventory and when we were wrong promptly admitted it.

11. Sought through prayer and meditation to improve our conscious contact with God *as we understand Him,* praying only for knowledge of His will for us and the power to carry that out.

12. Having had a spiritual awakening as the result of these Steps, we tried to carry this message to others, and to practice these principles in all our affairs.

Source: The Twelve Steps are reprinted with permission of Alcoholics Anonymous World Services, Inc. Permission to reprint the Twelve Steps does not mean that AA has reviewed or approved the contents of this publication, nor that AA agrees with the views expressed herein. AA is a program of recovery from alcoholism—use of the Twelve Steps in connection with programs and activities which are patterned after AA, but which address other problems, does not imply otherwise.

successful strategy for daily recovery. All use a series of 12 steps to guide recovering addicts or significant others through a process of personal growth.

Many factors contribute to the far-reaching success of 12-step programs:

■ They are accessible. Groups are available at no cost to anyone in practically every community of the nation and in many other countries.

■ Meetings are nonthreatening—no one is required to speak, but anyone who feels comfortable doing so is treated with respect and guaranteed confidentiality.

■ Members believe they will overcome their addiction with the help of God, or a higher power.

■ The shared experiences provide a sense of community and connectedness. The process of telling one's story is encouraging and inspiring to others in the group who have not yet come as far.

■ The programs emphasize abstinence and the adoption of a whole new way of life to support it. They teach that abstinence can only be maintained through an all-pervasive lifestyle change.

■ They provide a simple, organized set of priorities. These priorities are defined in the form of "slogans" that help addicts slowly restructure their lives. The most common slogans are "Easy does it," "Keep it simple," and "Live and let live." To the outsider, these slogans sound trite and even corny, but for an addict who has become confused, guilt-ridden, anxious, and depressed, they are very helpful.

Alternatives to 12-Step Programs. It is naive to think that all addicts will feel comfortable pursuing a spiritually based recovery program that refers to a godlike power. In recent years, alternative peer support programs for addiction have developed throughout the country. SOS (Secular Organizations for Sobriety; Save Our Selves), an abstinence–human support movement, is similar to 12-step programs in that it (1) addresses a variety of addictive behaviors, (2) endorses the need for abstinence in

12-step programs: Peer support groups patterned after Alcoholics Anonymous.

order to maintain recovery, and (3) encourages personal growth. But SOS is critically different from 12-step programs in that it (1) does not acknowledge the existence of or need for a higher power, (2) does not accept that the addict is powerless, and (3) rejects the notion that addiction has anything to do with character defects. The SOS program is directed toward teaching the addict to understand the cycle of addiction (chemical need, learned habit, and denial of both) and to replace it with the cycle of sobriety (daily acknowledgment of the addiction, daily acceptance of one's disease or habit, and making recovery the primary issue in one's life).[29]

Relapse

Relapse is an isolated occurrence of or full return to addictive behavior. It is one of the defining characteristics of addiction. A person who does not relapse or have powerful urges to do so was probably not addicted in the first place. Relapse is proof that a person is addicted and has abandoned the practice of an ongoing recovery program. Addicts are set up to relapse long before they actually do so because of their tendency to meet change and other forms of stress in their lives with the same kind of denial they once used to justify their addictive behavior (e.g., "I don't have a problem, I can handle this"). This sets off a series of events involving immediate or gradual abandonment of their structured recovery plans. For example, the addict may quit attending support group meetings and slip into situations that previously triggered the addictive behavior.

Because treatment programs recognize this strong tendency to relapse, they routinely teach clients and significant others concepts of relapse prevention. Relapse prevention teaches people how to recognize the signs of imminent relapse and to develop a plan for responding to these signs. Without a relapse prevention plan, recovering addicts are likely to relapse more frequently, more completely, and perhaps more permanently than do their counterparts who have plans. Relapse should not be interpreted as failure to change or lack of desire to stay well. The appropriate response to relapse is to remind addicts that they are addicted and to redirect them to the recovery strategies that have previously worked for them.

WHAT DO YOU THINK?

If you were asked to help someone find a treatment program, what features would you expect a good program to have? What makes it difficult for people with addictions to ask for help and to enter treatment programs? How would you support a friend who is recovering from an addiction?

Barriers to Women in Need of Treatment

Women in need of recovery from addictions often have barriers at the individual, family, and societal levels. Many treatment programs and, more importantly, the philosophy driving treatment programs are based on what is most helpful to men. This is simply because only in the last few decades have we as a society recognized that women become addicts just as men do. As we continue to struggle for answers regarding how to treat both men and women effectively, we must remember that gender plays an important role in the way an addict participates in and enters a treatment program. In addition, there are several physiological differences in the way men and women react to alcohol and other drugs that play a role in identifying them as addicts. Here are some obstacles that may affect whether or not women receive the help they need.

Individual Level. Women in our society have been exposed to many traditional expectations regarding the way they are "supposed" to act as women, or, in other words, to gender role socialization. While it is true that not all women subscribe to these beliefs, they remain an important factor in their development as human beings. Women are expected to be nurturing, beautiful, sexy, moody, frivolous, and passive. Women who are addicts, particularly alcohol and drug addicts, are often perceived to be bad mothers and sexually promiscuous and to have low moral standards. This presents the stigma of being both female and alcoholic. Because the female addict may be more likely to use substances as a way of managing conflict—in this case, to deal with her stigma—this double stigma may act as a strong factor in her continuing the addiction.

Women are not as readily identified as substance abusers or addicts because they do not typically act out in ways that are aggressive or public. For example, women usually come to alcohol treatment programs with histories of suicide attempts, previous psychiatric treatment, and abuse of prescription drugs, whereas men's histories include legal problems, job absenteeism, or occupational impairment. Because women's patterns of addiction do not match the male standard of addiction, they are often not identified as addicts in need of help.[30]

Family Level. Even when a women wants to enter a treatment program, she is faced with the problem of child care. Lack of child care is the most frequently reported barrier to treatment among alcoholic women. Many alcoholic women with children are single mothers or don't have family members who can care for the children.

In addition, women alcoholics are 25 percent more likely than men to encounter resistance by family and friends to the idea that they enter treatment. As a result,

Confronting Addictive Behaviors

After reading this chapter, you know that addictions can be devastating to both the addict's life and the lives of his or her family and friends. Addictions usually progress gradually, and it is difficult to know for certain when a person crosses the line from habit to addiction. Keep in mind that a behavior or chemical is problematic when it causes a person to incur negative consequences. If a person continues to perform the behavior or use the chemical despite these negative consequences, chances are that he or she is addicted. If you or someone you know is addicted or heading in that direction, the checklist below may provide some strategies to help.

Making Decisions for You

Stop and think about your own behaviors for a minute. Do you have any of the habits discussed in this chapter? What can you do to make sure that they don't turn into addictions? If you are an enabler for anyone, what can you do to help that person break out of his or her addictive behavior?

Checklist for Change: Making Personal Choices

✓ Are you ready to change or modify your behavior or substance use? Who can help support your decision?

✓ Have you thought about what impact your decision will have on your lifestyle? Are you ready to give up friends, activities, and environments that do not support your efforts?

✓ Rehearse things you may say or do if you find yourself in a situation that makes it difficult to stick with your behavior change.

✓ Remember that your motivation will decrease. During the times you are tempted, think about the reasons you decided to give up the behavior or substance.

✓ Realize that relapses happen. If you relapse, do not let the relapse serve as an excuse to slip back into old patterns of addiction. Talk with someone you trust and start again. Recovery is difficult—give yourself a break.

✓ Join a self-help group. There are lots of 12-step groups that are free and confidential. Your university or college counseling service is another place to seek help.

Checklist for Change: Making Community Choices

✓ Are you educated about the ways our society consciously or unconsciously supports addictions? Do you sometimes participate or look the other way when someone you know engages in behavior that may lead to an addiction?

✓ Do you support policies, such as laws against drunk driving, that serve to protect the community from the effects of addictive behaviors?

✓ Do you speak out against stories that glamorize potentially harmful or addictive behavior, such as binge drinking?

✓ Are you aware of what's happening in your own environment regarding identification of and help for addicts? Do you discuss alternatives or solutions to unhealthy behavior?

Critical Thinking

Think back to the opening scenario about Birgit and Hans. As Birgit's best friend (and maid-of-honor in her upcoming wedding), you are concerned about her. Birgit's self-esteem seems to be falling lower and lower as she watches Hans's addictive behavior get the better of him. Yet you think that she almost seems to be supporting him. She covers when employers call, she lets him gamble away the wedding funds, and she doesn't seem able to carry through on her threat to call off the wedding. You want to help.

Using the DECIDE model described in Chapter 1, decide how you can approach Birgit and help her break out of her codependency.

---

women have fewer family and friends involved in their treatment than do men in treatment. Another significant barrier for women is that female problem drinkers are much more likely than are male heavy drinkers to have a significant other who is also a heavy drinker. This can result in a lack of support for recovery at best and, at worst, a sabotage of recovery efforts.[31]

Societal Level. Employers are less likely to refer a women than a man to their Employee Assistance Programs—programs designed to help people with problems affecting job performance. Some employers report having more difficulty confronting women than men. Also, in today's workplace, women (more so than men) hold jobs that are below their capabilities, making impairment due to addictions more difficult to detect.[32] As if that weren't enough, women are also less likely than men to have jobs that afford them employee assistance programs and health insurance.

If a women does find herself in a treatment center for an addiction, she will likely be placed in groups with men and women. The ratio imbalance can heighten the visibility of women and increase stereotyping. In mixed groups, on average, men benefit more while women benefit less. Women are interrupted more often and tend to give in to men's opinions or decisions. Unfortunately, even counselors have been shown to be influenced by the gender role socialization of women. Counselors may view a woman's appearance from a more critical standpoint than they view a man's. And, when asked about the prognosis of a woman versus a man in treatment, alcohol treatment personnel tended to see a woman alcoholic's prognosis as worse than the man's, even though, in reality, women and men have similar outcomes.[33]

Strategies for Overcoming Gender-Based Treatment Barriers. Treatment centers should try to overcome gender-based treatment barriers by:

- addressing issues regarding sexual abuse, incest, and rape without men present. Therapists should help women to recognize that a high percentage of women are victims of this type of abuse and that it is not their fault.

- providing lectures on self-worth, assertiveness, and anger management. Therapists should direct women to be more internally focused rather than externally focused.

- encouraging recovering women to network with other women in recovery. If attending a 12-step program, women should seek out female sponsors rather than male sponsors.

- setting ground rules for interrupting and expectations regarding group participation.

- having gender-specific programming whenever possible. This is particularly important in group therapy.

*W*HAT DO YOU THINK?

What would you look for in a treatment program if you were helping an addicted woman? Are you influenced by gender role socialization in the way you consider a person's skills or faults? What steps can you take to decrease this influence?

Summary

◆ Habits are repetitive behaviors whereas addiction is behavior resulting from compulsion; without the behavior, the addict experiences withdrawal. Addicts have four common symptoms: compulsion, loss of control, negative consequences, and denial.

◆ Addiction is a process, evolving over time through a pattern known as nurturing through avoidance. Mood-altering substances and experiences produce biochemical reactions that make the body feel good; when absent, the person feels a withdrawal effect. The biopsychosocial model of addiction takes into account biological (genetic) factors as well as social and

psychological influences in understanding the addiction process.

◆ Addictions include the money addictions (compulsive gambling, spending, and borrowing), workaholism, exercise addiction, sexual addictions, and codependency. Codependents are "addicted to the addict." These behaviors are all addictive because they are mood-altering.

◆ Treatment begins with abstinence from the addictive behavior, usually instituted through intervention by significant others. Treatment programs may include individual, group, or family therapy, as well as 12-step programs.

Discussion Questions

1. What factors distinguish a habit from an addiction? Is it possible for you to tell if someone else is really addicted?

2. Explain why the biopsychosocial model is a more effective model for treatment than is a single-factor model.

3. List all the types of addictions described in the chapter. Can any behavior become an addiction? For example, is

it possible to become a "studyaholic"? Or a "chocaholic"? Why or why not?

4. Compare and contrast the varied methods of treatment. Which do you think would be most effective for you? For your best friend? For your parents? What accounts for the differences?

Application Exercise

Reread the What Do You Think? scenarios at the beginning of the chapter and answer the following questions:

1. Think about the biological, social, and psychological factors involved in Jamie's desire for alcohol. Which do you believe is playing a predominant role in her desire to drink?

2. In what ways have Jamie and Birgit acted as enablers? What could they do to improve their own situations? To help their loved ones? Why is it so hard for a codependent to make addicts stop their behavior?

Further Reading

C. D. Kasl, *Women, Sex, and Addiction* (New York: Harper and Row, 1990).

An exploration of the roots of sexual addiction among women and the journey back to wholeness.

B. Killinger, *Workaholics: The Respectable Addiction* (New York: Simon and Schuster, 1991).

Examines the causes and effects of work addiction and outlines the process of recovery for workaholics and their families.

R. Prussin, P. Harvey, and T. F. DiGeronimo, *Hooked on Exercise* (Park Ridge, IL: Parkside Publishing, 1992).

Confirms the value of moderate exercise for health improvement and maintenance but asserts that compulsive exercise can cause physical and emotional damage and lead to a cycle of dependency.

A. Washton and D. Boundy, *Willpower's Not Enough: Recovering from Addictions of Every Kind* (New York: HarperCollins, 1990).

Discusses the unifying factor in all addictive disorders, which the authors see as the need to change mood. Offers concrete approaches to personal recovery, asserting that mere exercise of willpower is inadequate.

B. Yoder, *The Recovery Resource Book: Information on Addictions and Codependence* (New York: Simon and Schuster, 1990).

A comprehensive workbook on recovery for people addicted either to substances, such as drugs or food, or to activities, such as sex, gambling, and work.

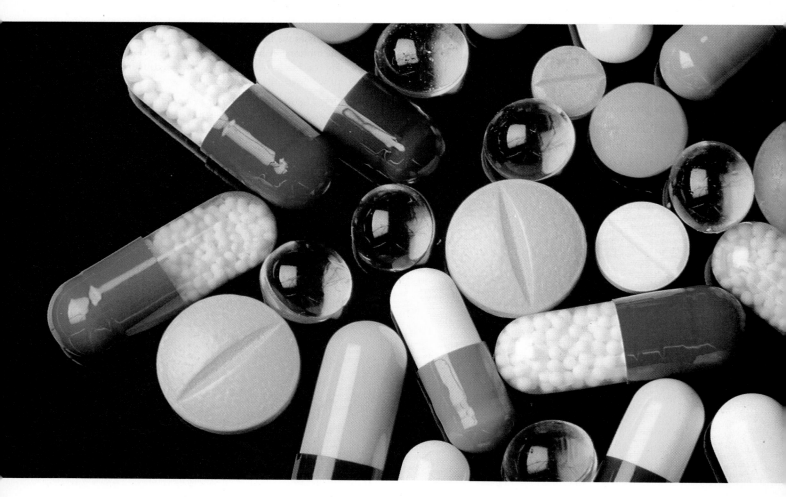

CHAPTER OBJECTIVES

◆ List the six categories of drugs and explain the routes of administration that drugs take into the body.

◆ Discuss proper drug use and explain how hazardous drug interactions occur.

◆ Describe the various kinds of prescription drugs and the advantages that generic drugs may provide to consumers.

◆ Discuss the types of over-the-counter drugs and general precautions to be taken with them.

◆ Discuss the key questions you should ask in order to make intelligent decisions about drug use.

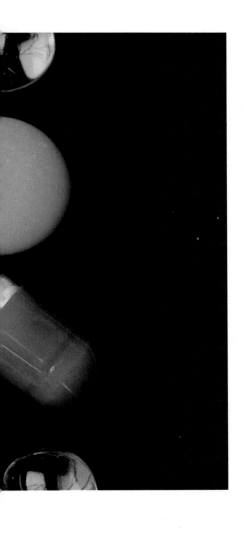

Pharmaceutical Drugs

Safe and Responsible Use

Wendy had been experiencing vaginal irritation and itching for about a week. She had seen numerous ads on TV for Gyne-Lotrimin (an over-the-counter vaginal antifungal) and decided that she must have had a yeast infection. She went to her local drugstore, purchased some Gyne-Lotrimin, and carefully followed the directions on the package. A week passed and Wendy was still having the same symptoms with no relief.

■ Should Wendy see a physician, or should she give the over-the-counter medication some more time to work? Did she compile enough information to make a responsible self-diagnosis? What other condition(s) may be the cause of Wendy's symptoms?

Donna is currently taking birth control pills and she was recently prescribed antibiotics for a bacterial infection. One of her friends has mentioned that the antibiotic she was prescribed may reduce the effectiveness of her oral contraceptive.

■ Is this true? Who should Donna consult to find out the facts? If it is true, what are her options?

Have you ever walked into a drugstore looking for some cough syrup or an antacid and become overwhelmed by the number of choices available? Although there are literally tens of thousands of drugs at our disposal, these choices cannot be made lightly. All drugs are chemical substances that have the potential to alter the structure and function of our bodies. Quite simply, any drug use involves risks. You can best minimize the risks by asking appropriate questions of health-care providers and by being an educated consumer of over-the-counter (OTC) drugs. This chapter focuses on prescription and OTC drugs, how they work, and how you can make responsible and healthy decisions about the use of these drugs. Before reading this chapter, read the accompanying box called "Rate Yourself" and spend a few moments testing your knowledge of drug interactions.

DRUG DYNAMICS

Drugs work because they physically resemble the chemicals produced naturally within the body (see Figure 12.1). For example, many painkillers resemble the endorphins

Receptor sites: Specialized cells to which drugs can attach themselves.

Psychoactive drugs: Drugs that have the potential to alter mood or behavior.

Prescription drugs: Medications that can be obtained only with the written prescription of a licensed physician.

Over-the-counter (OTC) drugs: Medications that can be purchased in pharmacies or supermarkets without a physician's prescription.

Recreational drugs: Legal drugs that contain chemicals that help people to relax or socialize.

("morphine within") that are manufactured in the body. Most bodily processes result from chemical reactions or from changes in electrical charge. Because drugs possess an electrical charge and a chemical structure similar to chemicals that occur naturally in the body, they can affect physical functions in many different ways.

A current explanation of drug actions is the *receptor site* theory, which states that drugs attach themselves to specific **receptor sites** in the body. These sites are specialized cells to which a drug is able to attach because of its size, shape, electrical charge, and chemical properties. Most drugs can attach at multiple receptor sites located throughout the body in such places as the heart and blood system, the lungs, liver, kidneys, brain, and gonads (testicles or ovaries). The physiology of drug activity and its effect on human behavior is very complex.

Types of Drugs

Scientists divide drugs into six categories: prescription drugs, OTC preparations, recreational substances, herbal preparations, illicit drugs, and commercial drugs. These classifications are based primarily upon drug action, although some classifications are based on the source of the chemical in question. Each category includes some drugs that stimulate the body, some that depress body functions, and others that produce hallucinations. Each category also includes **psychoactive drugs**, which have the potential to alter a person's mood or behavior.

- **Prescription drugs** are those substances that can be obtained only with the written prescription of a licensed physician. More than 40,000 types of prescription drugs are currently available, and a person should use these drugs only when under the care of a licensed medical practitioner. The physician determines the dosage for the individual patient at the time the prescription is written. Taking someone else's prescription can be dangerous, and deliberately sharing a prescription with another person is illegal.

- **Over-the-counter (OTC) drugs** can be purchased in pharmacies, supermarkets, and discount stores. Each year, Americans spend over $10 billion on OTC products, and the market is increasing at the rate of 20

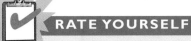

Test Your Drug Interaction IQ

Just how savvy are you about using medicine? Take this true–false quiz. Be sure you understand the answers—someday they may save your life.

1. An antacid will cause a blood-thinning (anticoagulant) drug to be absorbed too slowly.　　　　T　F

2. Drinking milk impairs the absorption of tetracycline, a widely used antibiotic.　　T　F

3. Citrus fruits and juices impair the absorption of iron from iron supplements.　　T　F

4. Fruit and vegetable juices with high acid contents (such as grape, apple, orange, or tomato juice) cause some drugs to dissolve in the stomach instead of in the intestines where they can be more readily absorbed.　　　　T　F

5. Because they contain vitamin K, eating large amounts of liver and leafy vegetables speeds the effectiveness of anticoagulants (blood-thinning drugs).　　　　T　F

6. A hazardous food–drug interaction occurs when drugs containing MAO inhibitors (sometimes prescribed for high blood pressure) are mixed with foods containing tyramine (aged cheese, sour cream, and yogurt, among others).　　T　F

7. Generic drugs are exactly the same as brand name drugs.　　　　T　F

8. You should stop taking prescribed medication when you feel better.　　T　F

9. Oral contraceptives lower blood levels of folic acid (a member of the vitamin B family) and vitamin B6.　　　　T　F

10. Taking large doses of vitamin C may lead to false results in a urinary glucose test for diabetes.　　　　T　F

Answers:

1. True. Additionally, aspirin greatly increases the blood-thinning effect of anticoagulants.

2. True. The calcium in dairy products impairs the absorption.

3. False. The ascorbic acid in citrus fruits and drinks speeds the absorption of iron from iron supplements.

4. True. Carbonated beverages have the same effect.

5. False. The vitamin K in foods such as liver and leafy vegetables promotes blood clotting which may *hinder* the effectiveness of anticoagulants.

6. True. Mixing MAO-inhibiting drugs with tyramine can raise blood pressure to dangerous levels.

7. False. Not all generic drugs are therapeutically equivalent. In other words, varied generic brands of the same drug may not act in the same way in the body. The FDA publishes lists of drugs identifying those that can be substituted safely.

8. False. You should take the prescription as directed. Although you may feel better, some of the antigens may still be active in your system. Failing to complete medication may help the antigens become resistant to the original medication.

9. True. However, the depletion is usually not serious enough to cause any symptoms. Women who use oral contraceptives would be wise to include dark green leafy vegetables in their diet.

10. True. Many drugs can alter test results. For example, taking penicillin can result in false readings of protein in the urine, a sign of kidney disease. Excessive use of laxatives can alter results of tests to determine calcium or bone metabolism. Make sure your doctor knows what drugs you are taking before having any tests done.

This self-assessment was deliberately designed to be hard, in the hope that you would learn to be more cautious about using medicine. If any of these drug interactions affects you, ask your doctor for more information.

Source: Adapted from *FDA Consumer,* transmitted on American On-Line by Health ResponseAbility Systems (File: "Medications, Precautions"), downloaded February 17, 1995.

percent annually. OTC drugs do not require a physician's prescription because they are considered safe when the user follows manufacturer's instructions correctly. Common examples of OTC drugs are analgesics (pain relievers), cold- and flu-symptom relievers, some appetite suppressants, laxatives, sleeping aids, sunscreens, and various ointments. More than 300,000 OTC products are available in stores and pharmacies.

■ **Recreational drugs** belong to a somewhat vague category whose boundaries depend upon how people define *recreation.* Generally, drugs in this category

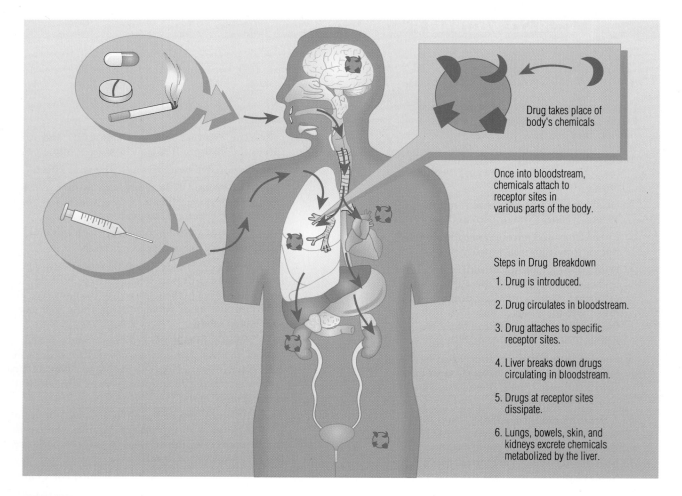

FIGURE 12.1

How the Body Metabolizes Drugs

contain chemicals used to help people relax or socialize. Most of them are legally sanctioned even though they are psychoactive. Alcohol, tobacco, coffee, tea, and chocolate products are usually included in this category.

- **Herbal preparations** form another vague category. Included among these approximately 750 substances are herbal teas and other products of botanical origin that are believed to have medicinal properties.

- **Illicit (illegal) drugs** are the most notorious substances. Although laws governing their use, possession, cultivation, manufacture, and sale differ from state to state, illicit drugs are generally recognized as harmful. Some people consider all illegal drugs to be harmful, whereas others regard certain illegal drugs, such as marijuana, as safe. Illegal drugs include heroin and other opium derivatives, cocaine, LSD, mescaline, PCP ("angel dust"), amphetamines, and marijuana. All of these substances are psychoactive.

- **Commercial preparations** are the most universally used yet least commonly recognized chemical substances having drug action. More than 1,000 of these substances exist, including such seemingly benign items as perfumes, cosmetics, household cleansers, paints, glues, inks, dyes, gardening chemicals, pesticides, and industrial by-products.

Routes of Administration of Drugs

Route of administration refers to the way in which a given drug is taken into the body. Common routes are oral ingestion, injection, inhalation, inunction, and suppository.

Oral ingestion is the most common route of administration. Drugs that you swallow include tablets, capsules, and liquids. Oral ingestion of a drug generally results in relatively slow absorption compared to other methods of administration because the drug must pass through the

People with diabetes, a disorder in which the body produces little or no insulin, learn to administer daily doses of replacement insulin by subcutaneous injection.

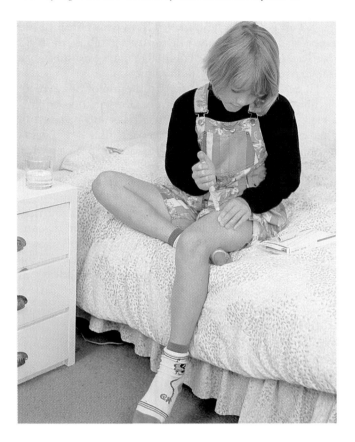

stomach, where it is acted on by digestive juices, and then move on to the small intestine before it enters the bloodstream.

Many oral preparations are coated to keep them from being dissolved by corrosive stomach acids before they reach the intestine as well as to protect the stomach lining from irritating chemicals in the drugs. If your stomach contains food, absorption will be slower than if your stomach is empty. Some drugs must not be taken with certain foods because the food will inhibit the drug's action. Others must be taken with food to prevent stomach irritation.

Depending on the drug and the amount of food in the stomach, drugs taken orally produce their effects within 20 minutes to 1 hour after ingestion. The only exception is alcohol, which takes effect sooner because some of it is absorbed directly into the bloodstream from the stomach.

Injection, another common form of drug administration, involves the use of a hypodermic syringe to introduce a drug into the body. This method can result in rapid absorption, depending on the type of injection. Intra-

venous injection, or injection directly into a vein, puts the chemical in its most concentrated form directly into the bloodstream. Effects will be felt within three minutes, making this route extremely effective, particularly in medical emergencies. But injection of many substances into the bloodstream may cause serious or even fatal reactions. In addition, some serious diseases, such as hepatitis and AIDS, can be transferred in this way. For this reason, intravenous injection can be one of the most dangerous routes of administration.

Intramuscular injection results in much slower absorption than intravenous injection. This type of injection places the hypodermic needle into muscular tissue, usually in the buttocks or the back of the upper arm. Normally used to administer antibiotics and vaccinations, this route of administration ensures a slow and consistent dispersion of the drug into the body tissues.

Subcutaneous injection puts the drug into the layer of fat directly beneath the skin. Its common medical uses are for administration of local anesthetics and for insulin replacement therapy. A drug injected subcutaneously will circulate even more slowly than an intramuscularly injected drug because it takes longer to be absorbed into the bloodstream.

Inhalation refers to administration of drugs through the nostrils. This method transfers the drug rapidly into the bloodstream through the alveoli (air sacs) in the lungs. Some examples of illicit inhalation are cocaine

Herbal preparations: Substances that are of plant origin that are believed to have medicinal properties.

Illicit (illegal) drugs: Drugs whose use, possession, cultivation, manufacture, and/or sale are against the law because they are generally recognized as harmful.

Commercial preparations: Commonly used chemical substances including cosmetics, household cleaning products, and industrial by-products.

Route of administration: The manner in which a drug is taken into the body.

Oral ingestion: Intake of drugs through the mouth.

Injection: The introduction of drugs into the body via a hypodermic needle.

Intravenous injection: The introduction of drugs directly into a vein.

Intramuscular injection: The introduction of drugs into muscles.

Subcutaneous injection: The introduction of drugs into the layer of fat directly beneath the skin.

Inhalation: The introduction of drugs through the nostrils.

sniffing and the inhalation of aerosol sprays, gases, or fumes from solvents. Effects are frequently noticed immediately after inhalation, but they do not last as long as with the slower routes of administration because only small amounts of a drug can be absorbed and metabolized in the lungs.

Inunction introduces chemicals into the body through the skin. A common example of this method of drug administration is the small adhesive patches that are used to alleviate motion sickness. These patches, which contain a prescription medicine, are applied to the skin behind one ear, where they slowly release their chemicals to provide relief for nauseated travelers. Another example is the nicotine patch.

Suppositories are drugs that are mixed with a waxy medium designed to melt at body temperature. The most common type of suppository is inserted into the anus until it is past the rectal sphincter muscles, which hold it in place. As the wax melts, the drug is released and absorbed through the rectal walls into the bloodstream. Since this area of the anatomy contains many blood vessels, the effects of the drug are usually felt within 15 minutes. Some OTC laxatives and hemorrhoid treatments are administered by suppository. In hospital settings, anal suppositories may be the chosen route of administration of painkillers for patients unable to tolerate ingestion or injection. Other types of suppositories are for use in the vagina. Vaginal suppositories usually release drugs, such as antifungal agents, that treat problems in the vagina itself as opposed to drugs meant to travel in the bloodstream.

*W*HAT DO YOU THINK?

What types of drugs have you used or experimented with? Why are some drugs administered differently than others?

*D*RUG USE, ABUSE, AND INTERACTIONS

Many people fail to take the time needed to make intelligent decisions when considering the use of a drug. They adopt the attitude that, "The doctor knows best," or, "Joe down the hall uses it, and he's fine," or even, "I can handle myself; I know what I'm doing" (when they clearly don't). This kind of casual approach can endanger their personal safety.

Using, Misusing, and Abusing Drugs

Although drug abuse is usually referred to in connection with illicit and recreational psychoactive drugs, many people abuse and misuse prescription and over-the-counter medications. **Drug misuse** is generally considered to be the use of a drug for a purpose for which it was not intended. For example, using a friend's high-powered prescription painkiller for your headache is a misuse of that drug. This is not too far removed from **drug abuse**, or the excessive use of any drug. The misuse and abuse of drugs may lead to *addiction,* the habitual reliance on a substance or behavior to produce a desired mood.

There are risks and benefits to the use of any type of chemical substance. Intelligent decision making requires a clear-headed evaluation of these risks and benefits. If, after considering all the facts, you feel that the benefits outweigh the potential problems associated with a particular drug, you may decide to use it. But sometimes unforeseeable reactions or problems arise even after the most careful deliberation.

In order to compare drug risks to benefits, you may want to create a profile for each drug you use or are considering using. A *drug profile* consists of a set of answers to specific questions about a drug. The Skills for Behavior Change box indicates key questions you should ask in preparing such a profile.

Individual Response to Psychoactive Drugs: Set and Setting

Individuals differ in how they respond to psychoactive drugs. Two environmental factors that bear on both the main effects and the side effects of psychoactive drugs are set and setting. **Set** is the total internal environment, or mindset, of a person at the time a drug is taken. Physical, emotional, and social factors work together or against one another to influence the drug's effect on that particular person. Expectations of what the drug will or will not do are also part of the set. For example, a young woman who reads two pages of reported side effects for a particular drug may experience more side effects after taking that drug than someone who was not exposed to this information. In other cases, set may be related to the user's mood. A depressed person using marijuana for a lift may find that the drug actually deepens the depression. Similarly, someone who is already giddy may become even sillier after using the drug. In addition, drugs do not necessarily have the same effect on the elderly (see the accompanying Multicultural Perspectives box).

If set refers to the internal environment, **setting** is the drug user's total external environment. It encompasses both the physical and social aspects of that environment at the time the person takes the psychoactive drug. If the user is surrounded by wild colors, heavy-metal rock music, and a noisy crowd of people, the drug will generally produce a very different effect than when it is taken in a quiet place with soft music and relaxed company.

Creating a Drug Profile

In order to compare the risks and benefits of a particular drug intelligently, you may want to create a drug profile—a set of key questions to be answered about that drug before you decide to use it.

1. *What is the chemical in the drug?* Intelligent consumers find out (from their doctors if it is a prescription drug or by reading the label if it is an OTC drug) whether a drug contains something they may be allergic to.

2. *Where within the body are the receptor sites?* Drugs are transported by the blood to receptor sites, where they interact with other chemicals in the body to influence many different bodily processes. If you learn what receptor sites are targeted by the drug you are considering, you will know whether or not that drug will do what you want it to do.

3. *What are the main effects of the drug?* It is important to know the intended actions(s) or effect(s) of the drug. Is it intended to have a stabilizing effect, a stimulating effect, a depressing effect, or what? Are the effects systemic, or are they target-specific?

4. *What are the side effects of the drug?* This question is crucial. Because all drugs have multiple receptor sites within the body, all drugs produce side effects. For example, the main effect of anticancer drugs is the killing of cancer cells, but the side effects are the destruction of intestinal and hair follicle cells, which results in nausea and hair loss.

5. *What are possible adverse reactions to the drug?* Besides their main and side effects, drugs have the potential to create adverse reactions in people who are allergic to the chemicals they contain. The body's immune system identifies a chemical in a drug as a foreign invader and seeks to destroy it, causing damage to healthy tissue.

Common allergic reactions to drugs include skin rashes, itching, swelling, watery eyes, runny nose, skin discoloration, and hives. A much more serious reaction is anaphylactic shock, which involves respiratory failure and cardiac arrest. Doctors can frequently prescribe an alternative medicine for patients allergic to a prescription drug. If a drug has a high potential for causing allergic reaction (e.g., penicillin), most physicians monitor the patient carefully.

Drug Interactions

Sharing medications, using outdated prescriptions, taking higher doses than recommended, or using medications as a substitute for dealing with personal problems may result in serious health consequences. But so may engaging in **polydrug use**: taking several medications or illegal drugs simultaneously may result in very dangerous problems associated with drug interactions. The most hazardous interactions are synergism, antagonism, inhibition, and intolerance. Hazardous interactions may also occur between drugs and nutrients (see Table 12.1 for some of the more common drug–nutrient interactions).

Synergism, also known as potentiation, is an interaction of two or more drugs in which the effects of the individual drugs are multiplied beyond what would normally be expected if they were taken alone. Synergism can be expressed mathematically as: $2 + 2 = 10$.

A synergistic interaction is most likely to occur when *central nervous system depressants* are combined. Included in this category are alcohol, opiates (morphine, heroin), antihistamines (cold remedies), sedative hypnotics (Quaaludes), minor tranquilizers (Valium, Librium, and Xanax), and barbiturates. The worst possible combination is alcohol and barbiturates (sleeping preparations such as Seconal and phenobarbital) because the combination of these depressants leads to a slowdown of the brain centers that normally control vital functions. Respiration, heart rate, and blood pressure can drop to the point of inducing coma and even death.

Prescription drugs carry special labels warning the user not to combine the drug with certain other drugs or with alcohol. Many OTC preparations carry similar warning

Inunction: The introduction of drugs through the skin.

Suppositories: Mixtures of drugs and a waxy medium designed to melt at body temperature that are inserted into the anus or vagina.

Drug misuse: The use of a drug for a purpose for which it was not intended.

Drug abuse: The excessive use of a drug.

Set: The total internal environment, or mindset, of a person at the time a drug is taken.

Setting: The total external environment of a person at the time a drug is taken.

Polydrug use: The use of multiple medications or illicit drugs simultaneously.

Synergism: An interaction of two or more drugs that produces more profound effects than would be expected if the drugs were taken separately.

Psychoactive Drugs and the Elderly

A 10-milligram dose of Valium (diazepam) taken by a 35-year-old man might relax his muscles. However, the same dose taken by a 75-year-old woman might make her so relaxed that her muscles lose coordination, causing her to fall and break her hip.

A therapeutic dose of many medications for a younger person may be too strong for an older person. Bodies change with age: muscle tissue declines and fat accumulates, the liver slows down, brain cells change in sensitivity, and kidneys do not work as efficiently as they did when they were younger. In fact, the kidney loses one-third of its function between the ages of 30 and 90, and about one-third of people develop a much larger loss than that. Because of these changes in organs that metabolize drugs, drugs may stay in the bodies of older people longer.

Recommended doses of a particular drug are based on pre-market clinical testing evaluating the drug's effectiveness in a few thousand people. Though many people have the impression that drug companies have tested drugs exclusively in young individuals, older people have been included in clinical studies. In the past, however, there was little attempt to see whether older people responded differently to tested drugs than did younger people.

To encourage the gathering of reliable data on the effect of drugs on the elderly, the FDA has issued guidelines for pharmaceutical firms. The guidelines ask that when doing drug studies manufacturers determine whether a drug is likely to have significant use by the elderly. If so, elderly patients should be included in clinical studies. These studies should then include additional analysis of the effectiveness or adverse effects of the drug due to a patient's age.

The studies need to answer two basic questions about how a drug acts in the elderly. First, what does the body do to the drug in terms of metabolism, absorption, distribution, excretion? Older individuals react differently to medications, not necessarily because they are older but because they may have other illnesses. For example, decreased kidney function, liver function, or diminished muscle mass can affect the body's metabolism of a medication. Also, the elderly are more likely to be taking other medications that can interact with the metabolism of additional drugs. Second, what does the drug do to the body? Older people may be more responsive to sedating drugs being more likely to get dizzy or confused.

In addition to studies involving older and younger patients, the new guidelines suggest that "in some cases . . . especially for drugs targeted to older patients or where age-related differences or problems are anticipated, trials might be carried out specifically in the elderly." The guideline adds that attempts should also be made specifically to include people over 75 and urges attention to possible interactions of the drug being studied with other drugs elderly patients might use.

For instance, many drugs alter the pharmacokinetics of digoxin, a heart drug that is widely prescribed for the elderly. Because this interaction is potentially toxic, evaluation of how a drug affects digoxin is important. The FDA is developing regulations to require drug manufacturers to include a special geriatric use section in the physician's labeling of all drugs.

Source: FDA Consumer, transmitted on American On-Line by Health ResponseAbility Systems (File: "Medications, Precautions"), downloaded February 19, 1995.

---

labels. Because the dangers associated with synergism are so great, you should always verify any possible drug interactions before using a prescribed or OTC drug. Pharmacists, physicians, drug information centers, or community drug education centers can answer your questions. Even if one of the drugs in question is an illegal substance, you should still attempt to determine the dangers involved in combining it with other drugs. Health-care professionals are legally bound to maintain confidentiality even when they know that a client is using illegal substances. The Building Communication Skills box suggests questions you should ask before taking any drug.

Antagonism, although not usually as serious as synergism, can produce unwanted and unpleasant effects. In an antagonistic reaction, drugs work at the same receptor site so that one drug blocks the action of the other. The "blocking" drug occupies the receptor site, preventing the other drug from attaching, and this creates alterations in absorption and action.

Inhibition is a type of interaction in which the effects of one drug are eliminated or reduced by the presence of

Antagonism: A type of interaction in which two or more drugs work at the same receptor site.

Inhibition: A type of interaction in which the effects of one drug are eliminated or reduced by the presence of another drug at the receptor site.

TABLE 12.1 ■ Examples of Drug–Nutrient Interactions for Commonly Used Drugs

Drug	Possible Effect on Nutrition Status				
	Reduces Absorption	Raises Blood Concentrations	Lowers Blood Concentrations	Increases Excretion	Other
Antacids (aluminum-containing)	Iron			Phosphorus Calcium	Thiamin*
Antibiotics	Fats Amino acids Carbohydrates Folate Vitamin B_{12} Fat-soluble vitamins Calcium Iron Potassium Magnesium Zinc			Potassium Niacin Riboflavin Folate Vitamin C	Vitamin K†
Aspirin			Folate	Vitamin C Thiamin Vitamin K	Iron‡
Caffeine				Calcium Magnesium	Cholesterol§
Diuretics		Zinc Calcium	Potassium Chloride Magnesium Phosphorus Folate Vitamin B_{12}	Calcium Sodium Thiamin Potassium Chloride Magnesium	Zinc¶
Laxatives	Fat Glucose Vitamin D Calcium Potassium Fat-soluble vitamins Carotene				
Oral contraceptives	Folate	Vitamin A Copper Iron	Vitamin B_6 Riboflavin Folate Vitamin B_{12} Vitamin C		Riboflavin‖ Vitamin B_6‖ Calcium**

*Antacids may accelerate the destruction of thiamin.
†Some antibiotics may interfere with intestinal synthesis of vitamin K.
‡Aspirin use may cause blood loss, thus compromising iron status.
§Large doses of caffeine may raise blood cholesterol concentrations.
¶Some diuretics may interfere with zinc storage in the liver.
‖Some oral contraceptives may augment the requirements for riboflavin and vitamin B_6.

**Some oral contraceptives may improve the absorption of calcium.
Source: Information from R. E. Hodges, *Nutrition in Medical Practice* (Philadelphia: Saunders, 1980), 323–331; R. C. Theuer and J. J. Vitale, "Drug and Nutrient Interactions," in *Nutritional Support of Medical Practice,* ed. H. A. Schneider, C. F. Anderson, and D. B. Coursin (Hagerstown, MD: Harper & Row, 1977), 297–305; D. A. Roe, *Drug Induced Nutritional Deficiencies* (Westport, CT: AVI, 1985).

Asking the Right Questions

At one time or another you will probably use prescriptions or OTC drugs to help restore or maintain your health. How can you be certain that you need a medication in the first place, that you are taking the right mediation for you, and that your medication is not robbing you of vital nutrients or being rendered ineffective by other products or foods you are ingesting? Only by asking the right questions of the right people can you be sure. Listed below are 13 questions to pose to your physician, your pharmacist, or yourself before you begin to take any drug.

1. Do you know the diagnosis of your condition?

2. Is your doctor or pharmacist aware of all other drugs that you are taking, both prescription and/or OTC? (Don't forget that birth control pills are drugs.)

3. Do you know the name of the medication you are taking? Is it the chemical name, a generic name, or a brand name?

4. Are you certain of how often you should take the medication, how long you should take it, and in what dosage?

5. Do you know when your medication should be taken in relation to meals?

6. Do you know if you can drink alcohol while on your medication?

7. What are the known side effects of the medication? What should you do if you experience any of the side effects?

8. Can you stop taking your medication when you start feeling better, or is it important that you continue taking the drug until the prescription is finished?

9. Do you know what you should do if you forget to take your medication at the scheduled time?

10. Do you know what signs and symptoms signal that you are allergic to the medication?

11. Do you know how and where to store your medication properly?

12. Are there any drug-nutrient interactions that you should be aware of with your medication?

13. Are there any adverse consequences of long-term use of the medication?

---

another drug at the receptor site. One common inhibitory reaction occurs between antacid tablets and aspirin. The antacid inhibits the absorption of aspirin, making it less effective as a pain reliever. Other inhibitory reactions occur between alcohol and contraceptive pills and between antibiotics and contraceptive pills. Alcohol and antibiotics may diminish the effectiveness of birth control pills in some women.

Intolerance occurs when drugs combine in the body to produce extremely uncomfortable reactions. The drug Antabuse, used to help alcoholics give up alcohol, works by producing this type of interaction. It binds liver enzymes (the chemicals the liver produces to break down alcohol), making it impossible for the body to metabolize alcohol. As a result, the user of Antabuse who drinks

alcohol experiences nausea, vomiting, and, occasionally, fever.

Cross-tolerance occurs when a person develops a physiological tolerance to one drug and shows a similar tolerance to selected other drugs as a result. Taking one drug may actually increase the body's tolerance to another drug. For example, cross-tolerance can develop between alcohol and barbiturates, two depressant drugs.

What Do You Think?

What are common expectations college students have when using drugs? What is the difference between drug abuse and drug misuse? Are people who abuse or misuse drugs addicts?

Intolerance: A type of interaction in which two or more drugs produce extremely uncomfortable symptoms.

Cross-tolerance: The development of a tolerance to one drug that reduces the effects of another, similar drug.

Antibiotics: Prescription drugs designed to fight bacterial infection.

Gender and Medications: What Every Woman Should Know

Women menstruate, can become pregnant, and go through menopause. These normal conditions all affect how women's bodies react to medication. On average,

Whenever you take more than one medication at a time, you should consider how the medications will interact. For example, women who rely on oral contraceptives need to understand that dosage instructions must be strictly followed and that medicines such as penicillin can alter the contraceptive's effectiveness. Asking a pharmacist is a good way to learn about drug interactions.

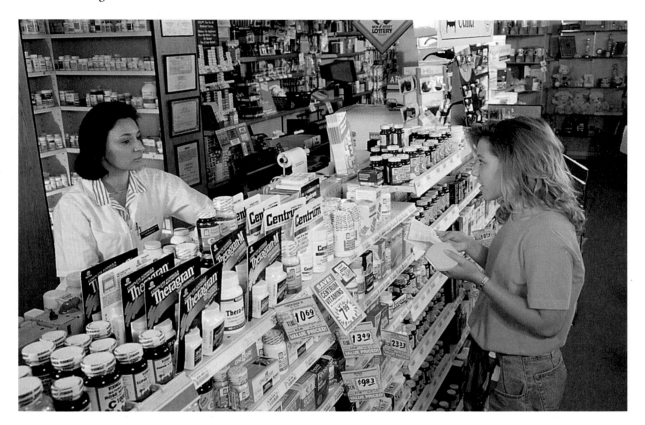

women take more prescription and nonprescription medications than do men. For these reasons, women should be especially concerned about what medications they take and about how and when they take them.

Many women take oral contraceptives, commonly known as the pill. Failure to take the pill each day can result in pregnancy, yet 25 percent of women taking the pill miss or skip days. Women may also become pregnant accidentally because some medicines—such as penicillin, some sleeping pills, tuberculosis medicines, and anxiety medicines—can keep birth control pills from working. When a woman is prescribed a new medication, she should inform her health-care provider that she is on the pill.

Medications taken when a woman is pregnant or breast-feeding may be passed to her fetus or child. If a woman is taking medication while pregnant or breast-feeding, she should make sure to inform her physician. The physician may be able to prescribe a different medication or a different way to take the medication that will not affect the fetus or baby.

ᴾRESCRIPTION DRUGS

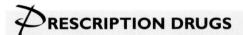

Even though prescription drugs are administered under medical supervision, the wise consumer still takes precautions. Hazards and complications arising from the use of prescription drugs are common. Responsible decision making about prescription drug use requires the consumer to acquire basic drug knowledge.

Types of Prescription Drugs

Prescription drugs can be divided into dozens of categories. Those of most interest to college students are discussed later; others are explored in the chapters on birth control, infectious and sexually transmitted diseases, cancer, and cardiovascular disease. Some of the most common are discussed here.

Antibiotics are drugs used to fight bacterial infection. They may be dispensed by intramuscular injection or in tablet or capsule form. Some, called broad-spectrum antibiotics, are designed to control disease caused by a number of bacterial species. These medications may also kill off helpful bacteria in the body, thus triggering secondary infections. For example, some types of vaginal infections are related to long-term use of antibiotics.

Analgesics are pain relievers. The earliest pain relievers were made of derivatives manufactured from the opium poppy. Most pain relievers work at receptor sites by interrupting pain signals. Some analgesics are available as OTC drugs.

Some analgesics are called **prostaglandin inhibitors**. Prostaglandins are chemicals that resemble hormones and are released by the body in response to pain. When a painful stimulus such as a cut or scrape occurs, nerve cells near the site of the pain release prostaglandins. (Scientists believe that the additional pain caused by the release of prostaglandins signals the body to begin the healing process.) Prostaglandin inhibitors restrain the release of prostaglandins, thereby reducing the pain. The most commonly used prostaglandin inhibitors are ibuprofen (Motrin) and sodium naprosyn (Anaprox). Both are used in prescription strength to relieve arthritis pain and menstrual cramps.

Most analgesics have side effects, the most common of which is drowsiness due to the depression of the central nervous system. Label warnings are, as usual, important. Some labels caution specifically against driving or operating heavy machinery when using the drug, and most state that analgesics should not be taken with alcohol.

Analgesics: Pain relievers.

Prostaglandin inhibitors: Drugs that inhibit the production and release of prostaglandins associated with arthritis or menstrual pain.

Sedatives: Central nervous system depressants that induce sleep and relieve anxiety.

Tranquilizers: Central nervous system depressants that relax the body and calm anxiety.

Antidepressants: Prescription drugs used to treat clinically diagnosed depression.

Amphetamines: Prescription stimulants not commonly used today because of the dangers associated with them.

Rebound effects: Severe withdrawal effects experienced by users of stimulants, including depression, nausea, and violent behavior.

Generic drugs: Drugs marketed by their chemical name rather than by a brand name.

Sedatives are central nervous system depressants that induce sleep and relieve anxiety. Used heavily in the 1950s and 1960s in the form of phenobarbital or Seconal, they gradually fell out of favor because of the risks associated with their use. The potential for addiction is high. Detoxification can be life-threatening and must be medically supervised. Because doctors do not prescribe sedatives as frequently as they did in past decades, users often purchase them illegally.

Methaqualone is another type of sedative that was overprescribed when it was first manufactured. Sometimes known as " 'ludes" (derived from Quaaludes, a trade name), methaqualone is a powerful central nervous system depressant that can produce dangerous synergistic effects when mixed with other depressants. In 1983, legal production of the drug was stopped and stockpiles of the pills were destroyed.

Tranquilizers are another form of central nervous system depressant. They are classified as major tranquilizers and minor tranquilizers. The most powerful tranquilizers are used in the treatment of major psychiatric illnesses. When used appropriately, these strong sedatives are capable of reducing violent aggressiveness and self-destructive impulses.

The so-called minor tranquilizers gained much notoriety in the late 1960s and early 1970s when consumer groups discovered that these drugs—known by their trade names Valium, Librium, and Miltown—were the most commonly prescribed medication in the United States. They were often prescribed for women who suffered from anxiety. These drugs have a high potential for addiction, and many people became physically and psychologically dependent on them. When the media reported on the widespread and casual prescribing of these drugs, physicians were forced to reevaluate the practice. Today a doctor is more likely to suggest psychotherapy or counseling for patients suffering from anxiety.

Antidepressants are powerful substances used to treat clinically diagnosed cases of depression. These drugs inhibit the release of certain neurotransmitters in the brain, thereby elevating the user's mood.

Amphetamines are stimulants that are prescribed less commonly now than in the past. Like many psychoactive drugs, they are purchased both legally and illegally. Amphetamines suppress appetite and elevate respiration, blood pressure, and pulse rate. Ritalin and Cylert are prescription amphetamines that are used in the treatment of attention-deficit/hyperactivity disorder in children. A newer prescription drug used in the treatment of obesity is Pondimin.

Tolerance to these powerful stimulants develops rapidly, and the user trying to cut down or quit may experience unpleasant **rebound effects**. These severe withdrawal symptoms, peculiar to stimulants, include depression, irritability, violent behavior, headaches, nausea, and deep fatigue.

Use of Generic Drugs

Generic drugs, medications sold under a chemical name rather than under a brand name, have gained popularity in recent years. These alternatives to more expensive brand-name drugs contain the same active ingredients as their brand-name counterparts.

There is some controversy about the effectiveness of some generic drugs because substitutions are often made in minor ingredients and these can affect the way the drug is absorbed, causing discomfort or even an allergic reaction in some users. Therefore, you must note any allergic reactions you have to medications and tell your doctor, who can prescribe an alternative drug. A list of medicines that can be interchanged has been approved in some states.

Generic drugs can help to reduce health-care costs because their price is often less than half that of the brand-name drugs they are substitutes for. But not all drugs are available as generics, and generic equivalents are not always recommended. For example, people taking Dilantin for control of seizures are advised to avoid generic equivalents.

If your doctor or pharmacist fails to offer you the option of using a generic drug, you should ask if such a substitute exists and if it would be safe for you to use it.

OVER-THE-COUNTER (OTC) DRUGS

Over-the-counter (OTC) drugs are nonprescription drugs we use in the course of self-diagnosis and self-medication. Many of us, in our eagerness to save on an office visit to a physician, diagnose our own illness and go to the nearest discount pharmacy to stock up on the latest and best-advertised cure for what we think ails us.

In an effort to cure themselves, American consumers spend in excess of $10 billion yearly on OTC preparations for relief of everything from runny noses to ingrown toenails. There are 40,000 OTC drugs and more than 300,000 brand names for those drugs. Most OTC drugs are manufactured from a basic group of 1,000 chemicals. The many different OTC drugs available to us are produced by combining as few as 2 and as many as 10 substances.

Despite a common belief that OTC products are both safe and effective, indiscriminate use and abuse can occur with these drugs just as with all others. In fact, many OTC drugs have the potential to produce dependency, tolerance, and addiction as well as adverse toxic reactions.

How Prescription Drugs Become OTC Drugs

Americans have become more aware of and vocal about the need for better drugs to self-medicate in recent years. In response to consumer pressures, the Food and Drug Administration (FDA) has adopted a switching policy whereby it regularly reviews prescription drugs to evaluate how suitable they would be as OTC products. For a drug to be switched from prescription to OTC status, it must meet the following criteria:

1. The drug has been marketed as a prescription drug for at least three years.

2. The use of the drug has been relatively high during the time it was available as a prescription drug.

3. Adverse drug reactions are not alarming, and the frequency of side effects has not increased during the time the drug was available to the public.

Since this policy has been in effect, the FDA has switched approximately 50 drugs from prescription to OTC status. Some examples are ibuprofen (Advil, Nuprin), the analgesic/anti-inflammatory medicine naproxen sodium (Aleve), the antihistamine Benadryl, the vaginal antifungal Gyne-Lotrimin, the bronchodilator Bronkaid Mist, and the hydrocortisone Cortaid. Many more prescription drugs are currently being considered for OTC status, including the ulcer medications Tagament and Zantac, and the antihistamine Seldane. It is estimated that by 1997 the FDA will have considered more than 170 different drugs for switching.

Types of OTC Drugs

The FDA has categorized 26 types of OTC preparations. Those most commonly used are analgesics, cold/cough/allergy and asthma relievers, stimulants, sleeping aids and relaxants, and dieting aids.

Analgesics. Although these pain relievers come in several forms, aspirin and acetaminophen are the two most commonly used ingredients in OTC analgesics.

Aspirin, or acetylsalicylic acid, is a member of the group of chemical compounds called salicylates. Acetylsalicylic acid was first synthesized in a laboratory in 1853 by the French chemist Charles Gerhardt. Although willow bark, the herbal equivalent of aspirin that is converted by the body to a salicylate, had been used as a pain reliever since ancient times, aspirin's medicinal value was not recognized until 1899, when Heinrich Dreser, a German scientist, wrote about its effectiveness in reducing pain and fever.

More and more prescription drugs are becoming available over the counter as a result of public pressure on the Food and Drug Administration, which has developed criteria for changing a drug's status based on its use and safety while available by prescription only.

Aspirin relieves pain by inhibiting the body's production of prostaglandins. It brings down fever by increasing the flow of blood to the skin surface, which causes sweating and therefore cooling of the body. Aspirin has also long been used to reduce the inflammation and swelling of arthritis. Recently it has been discovered that aspirin's anticoagulant (interference with blood clotting) effects make it a useful medication for reducing the chances of repeat heart attacks in people who have already had one heart attack.

Despite the fact that aspirin has been commonly used as a medication for nearly a century, it is not as harmless as many people think. Possible side effects include allergic reactions, ringing in the ears, stomach bleeding, and ulcers. Combining aspirin with alcohol can compound aspirin's gastric irritant properties.

In addition, research has linked aspirin to a potentially fatal condition called Reye's syndrome. Children, teenagers, and young adults (up to age 25) who are treated with aspirin while recovering from the flu or chicken pox are at risk for developing the syndrome. Aspirin substitutes are recommended for people in these age groups.

Acetaminophen is an aspirin substitute found in Tylenol and related medications. Like aspirin, acetaminophen is an effective analgesic and antipyretic (fever-reducing drug). It does not, however, provide relief from inflamed or swollen joints. The side effects associated with acetaminophen are generally minimal, though overdose can cause liver damage.

In 1985, certain drugs containing ibuprofen (prostaglandin inhibitors) were switched from prescription to OTC status. Generally marketed as arthritis or menstrual cramp relievers, these drugs are milder versions of the prescription varieties. Examples are Nuprin and Advil.

In 1994, Aleve, the first new type of nonprescription analgesic to become available in a decade, was introduced onto the market. Aleve is a version of the prescription drug Anaprox, a fast-acting, slightly less strong form of the analgesic naproxen. Compared with the other OTC analgesics, Aleve's main distinction is its lasting effect: while the others need to be taken every 4 to 6 hours, once every 8 to 12 hours is sufficient for Aleve. The four OTC analgesics are compared in Table 12.2.

Cold, Cough, Allergy, and Asthma Relievers. These substances are popular OTC remedies for the symptoms that affect millions of sufferers. The operative word in their titles is *reliever*. Most of these medications are designed to alleviate some or all of the discomforting symptoms associated with these upper-respiratory-tract maladies. Unfortunately, no drugs exist to cure the actual diseases. The drugs available provide only temporary relief until the sufferer's immune system prevails over the disease. Aspirin or acetaminophen is used in some cold preparations, as are several other ingredients. Both aspirin and acetaminophen are on the government's **GRAS** and **GRAE lists** (see the Health Headlines box).

The basic types of OTC cold, cough, and allergy relievers are:

- *Expectorants.* These drugs are formulated to loosen phlegm, allowing the user to cough it up and clear congested respiratory passages. GRAS and GRAE reviewers found no expectorants to be both safe and effective.

- *Antitussives.* These OTC drugs are used to calm or curtail the cough reflex. They are most effective when the cough is "dry," or does not produce phlegm. Oral codeine, dextromethorphan, and diphenhydramine are the most common antitussives that are on both the GRAE and GRAS lists.

- *Antihistamines.* These are central nervous system depressants that dry runny noses, clear postnasal drip, clear sinus congestion, and reduce tears.

- *Decongestants.* These remedies are designed to reduce nasal stuffiness due to colds.

- *Anticholinergics.* These substances are often added to cold preparations to reduce nasal secretions and tears. None of the preparations tested was found to be GRAE/GRAS. Some cold compounds contain alcohol in concentrations that may exceed 40 percent.

Stimulants. Nonprescription stimulants are sometimes used by college students who have neglected assignments and other obligations until the last minute. The active ingredient in OTC stimulants is caffeine (see Chapter 14). It acts to heighten wakefulness, increase alertness, and relieve fatigue. None of the OTC stimulants has been judged GRAS or GRAE.

Sleeping Aids and Relaxants. These drugs are often used to induce the drowsy feelings that precede sleep. The principal ingredient in OTC sleeping aids is an antihistamine called pyrilamine maleate. Chronic reliance on sleeping aids may lead to addiction; people accustomed to using these products may find it impossible to sleep without them. Relaxant aids advertised as "tension relievers" (e.g., Compoz) have been determined to be neither GRAE nor GRAS.

Dieting Aids. Many drugs designed to help people lose weight are available over the counter. Some of these drugs are advertised as "appetite suppressants." Their active chemical is phenylpropanolamine. Its stimulant effects can cause dangerous reactions in people suffering from diabetes or heart or thyroid ailments.

> **GRAS list:** A list of drugs generally recognized as safe; they seldom cause side effects when used properly.
>
> **GRAE list:** A list of drugs generally recognized as effective; they work for their intended purpose when used properly.

TABLE 12.2 ■ A Comparison of the Major OTC Analgesics

	Aspirin	Acetaminophen	Ibuprofen	Naproxen Sodium
Examples of brand names	Bayer, Anacin	Tylenol, Panadol	Advil, Nuprin	Aleve
Generic available	yes	yes	yes	no
Lowest cost per regular-strength dose	2¢	3–5¢	3¢	9¢
Introduced over the counter	around 1900	1960	1984	1994
Reduces pain and fever?	yes	yes	yes	yes
Reduces inflammation?	yes	no	yes	yes
Good choice for . . .	Aches and pains, fever, swelling, toothaches, pain from inflammation	Aches and pains, especially if aspirin is not tolerated	Menstrual cramps, toothaches, arthritis pain	Menstrual cramps, toothaches, arthritis pain
Side effects	Digestive tract bleeding, upset stomach, ulcers	None if taken as directed for short periods	Digestive tract bleeding, upset stomach, ulcers, dizziness, drowsiness	Digestive tract bleeding, upset stomach, ulcers
Precautions	Avoid if allergic to aspirin or have a bleeding disorder. Don't give to children or teenagers with chicken pox or flu.	Overdoses can damage the liver.	Avoid if allergic to aspirin or have heart failure or kidney problems.	Avoid if allergic to aspirin or have heart failure or kidney problems.

Source: Data (not including cost information) reprinted by permission of Prof. Janet Engle, Clinical Associate Professor of Pharmacy Practice, College of Pharmacy, University of Illinois at Chicago, from *U.S. News & World Report,* 1 August 1994, 62–63.

Phenylpropanolamine ia a **sympathomimetic**, a drug that affects the sympathetic nervous system, causing reactions similar to those we experience when we are angry or excited. These reactions include a dry mouth and a lack of appetite. There is a $200 million market for these diet aids in the United States.

Most manufacturers of appetite suppressants include a written diet to complement their drug. The majority of these diets contain 1,200 calories. On this number of calories, most people will lose weight without appetite suppressants.

Some people rely on **laxatives** and **diuretics** ("water pills") to aid weight reduction. Frequent use of laxatives to aid weight loss disrupts the body's natural elimination patterns and may cause constipation or even obstipation (inability to have a bowel movement). The use of laxatives to produce weight loss has generally unspectacular results and can rob the body of needed fluids, salts, and minerals.

Use of diuretics as part of a weight-loss plan is also dangerous. Not only will the user gain the weight back upon drinking fluids, but diuretic use may contribute to dangerous chemical imbalances. The potassium and sodium eliminated by diuretics play important roles in maintaining electrolyte balance. Depletion of these vital minerals may cause weakness, dizziness, fatigue, and sometimes death. (See Table 12.3 for a description of possible side effects of OTC drugs.)

Sympathomimetics: Drugs found in appetite suppressants that affect the sympathetic nervous system.

Laxative: Medications used to soften stool and relieve constipation.

Diuretic: Drugs that increase the excretion of urine from the body.

Some Medical Terms and What They Mean

1. **What do the initials GRAS stand for?**

   Generally Recognized as Safe. Drugs on the GRAS list have a low incidence of adverse reactions or undesirable side effects.

2. **What do the initials GRAE stand for?**

   Generally Recognized as Effective. Drugs on the GRAE list, when taken properly, work for their intended purpose.

3. **What do the initials PDR stand for?**

   Physicians' Desk Reference, a book that lists drugs by chemical (generic) name, manufacturer, and common trade name. Each description includes a synopsis of rules for use and all potential side effects. Members of the AMA (American Medical Association) receive an update of the PDR every year.

4. **What is *overmedicating*?**

   When physicians rely too much on prescribing drugs to treat medical problems, they are said to be overmedicating their patients.

5. **How does *multiprescribing* differ from *overmedicating*?**

   Multiprescribing involves the use of several different drugs at the same time for different conditions. It is often a valid practice.

6. **What is an *iatrogenic disease*?**

   An iatrogenic disease is a medical problem that results from some form of treatment by a health-care professional.

General Precautions for OTC Users

Manufacturers of OTC pharmaceuticals spend millions of dollars each year to promote their products. Up to 20 percent of the dollar sales of these products is used for advertising. Approximately 13 percent of all television advertising is for OTC preparations. Such commercials try to pressure us by appealing to our psychological needs. Most commercials promise physical attractiveness, status, health, security, or mastery of some type of skill.

The cost of promoting and advertising prescription drugs ranges from between $2 billion to $3 billion annually. Although the pharmaceutical companies have re-

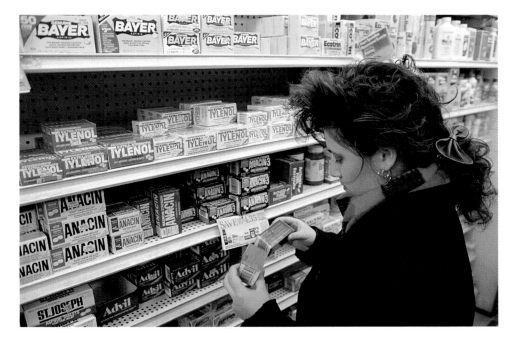

When considering over-the-counter drugs, carefully read—and heed—the directions for use, dosages, warnings, and conditions for which the product is intended that are printed on labels and packages.

TABLE 12.3 ■ Some Side Effects of OTC Drugs

Drug	Possible hazards
Acetaminophen	• Bloody urine, painful urination, skin rash, bleeding and bruising, yellowing of the eyes or skin (even for normal doses) • Difficulty in diagnosing overdose because reaction may be delayed up to a week • Severe liver damage and death (for dose of about 50 tablets) • Liver damage from chronic low-level use
Antacids	• Reduced mineral absorption from food • Possible concealment of ulcer • Reduction of effectiveness for anticlotting medications • Prevention of certain antibiotics' functioning (for antacids that contain aluminum) • Worsening of high blood pressure (for antacids that contain sodium) • Aggravation of kidney problems
Aspirin	• Stomach upset and vomiting, stomach bleeding, worsening of ulcers • Enhancement of the action of anticlotting medications • Potentiation of hearing damage from loud noise • Severe allergic reaction • Association with Reye's syndrome in children and teenagers • Prolonged bleeding time (when combined with alcohol)
Cold medications	• Loss of consciousness (if taken with prescription tranquilizers)
Diet pills, caffeine, decongestants	• Organ damage or death from cerebral hemorrhage
Ibuprofen	• Allergic reaction in some people with aspirin allergy • Fluid retention or edema • Liver damage similar to that from acetaminophen • Enhancement of action of anticlotting medications • Digestive disturbances (half as often as with aspirin)
Laxatives	• Reduced absorption of minerals from food • Creation of dependency
Toothache medications	• Destruction of the still-healthy part of a damaged tooth (for medications that contain clove oil)

cently started to advertise some of these medications directly to the public, most prescription drug advertising is still directed at health professionals who can prescribe these products.

Most of us are self-medicators at one time or another. We find it easier to function, for example, if the headache and stuffiness of the common cold do not interfere with our studies or work. Most of us can use OTC products safely with adequate precautions.

Over-the-counter precautions are based on the principles of drug dynamics introduced earlier in this chapter. Consumers must know the product, read the label, and follow instructions precisely. Single-ingredient preparations are generally safer and less expensive than combination products. They are especially safe for people who wish to minimize the chances of hypersensitive reactions because there is no need to try to isolate an offending substance.

Finally, people who decide to use OTC products with other drugs of any type must realize the risks inherent in this practice. When in doubt, consult a pharmacist or a drug information center about different drug combinations (see the Choices for Change box).

Accepting Responsibility

Visiting a physician does not exempt you from exercising responsibility for your own health. Doctors are generally aware of patients' needs, and some may be too willing to please their patients. All too frequently, this pleasing involves giving the patient a prescription. You can help by rethinking your expectations. At times, a short talk with the physician is more useful than medication. If your present physician will not take the time to talk to you, seek out one who will.

If you are contemplating the use of prescription drugs, take the following precautions:

1. Take medication only for the problem for which it has been prescribed. Treating self-diagnosed problems with leftover prescription drugs can be dangerous, as can using someone else's prescription.

2. Follow the physician's and pharmacist's instructions precisely. For example, if directed to take the medication for 30 days, take it for 30 days and not simply until symptoms disappear. A therapeutic dose is the minimum amount necessary to gain the desired effect.

3. Heed label warnings put on the bottle at the pharmacy. Ask the pharmacist about any unclear labels or directions.

4. If you experience an adverse reaction, stop taking the medication and notify your physician at once.

5. Pay particular attention to the type of liquid recommended to wash down tablets and capsules. Most medications should be taken with water, although some must be taken with food or milk. Juices and carbonated beverages may cause a tablet or capsule to dissolve too early, thereby reducing its effectiveness.

6. Discard unused medications as directed, after therapy, or after the expiration date. Keep all medications out of the reach of children. This can be accomplished by keeping such items in a locked cabinet or drawer.

7. Make sure you inform your physician if you are taking any other medications or if you have had adverse reactions to certain drugs in the past.

In the case of prescription medications, you owe it to yourself and your physician to be well informed. You also must be honest in your responses to physicians' questions about your symptoms and any other drugs or medications you use regularly. When taking a prescription medication, you also must tell the physician about any side effects or adverse reactions you experience. An alternative drug can usually be prescribed.

Summary

◆ The six categories of drugs are prescription drugs, OTC drugs, recreational drugs, herbal preparations, illicit drugs, and commercial preparations. Routes of administration include oral ingestion, injection (intravenous, intramuscular, and subcutaneous), inhalation, inunction, and suppositories.

◆ Proper drug use begins with creating a drug profile, including knowing the name of the drug, its receptor sites, its main and side effects, possible adverse reactions, methods of administration, potential for addiction and dependency, legality, and possible alternatives. Hazardous drug interactions may occur when a person takes several medications or illegal drugs simultaneously. The most hazardous

interactions are synergism, antagonism, inhibition, and intolerance.

◆ Prescription drugs are administered under medical supervision. Categories include antibiotics, analgesics, prostaglandin inhibitors, sedatives, tranquilizers, antidepressants, and amphetamines. Generic drugs can often be substituted for more expensive brand-name drugs.

◆ Over-the-counter drug categories include analgesics; cold, cough, allergy, and asthma relievers; stimulants; sleeping aids and relaxants; and dieting aids. Consumers should exercise personal responsibility by reading directions for OTC drugs and asking their pharmacist or doctor if any special precautions are advised when taking these substances.

Discussion Questions

1. What is the current theory of how drugs work?

2. What environmental factors influence the main effects and side effects of psychoactive drugs?

Making Healthy Medication Choices

While reading this chapter, you have found that the use of prescription or OTC drugs can help restore or maintain your health. As with any drugs, these drugs must be used responsibly. As you now know, there are things that you can do that will provide you with the maximum benefit if you take prescription or OTC medications.

Making Decisions for You

When you have a medical problem (even a minor one such as a headache), you need to decide how best to treat it. What are the medical symptoms from which you are seeking relief? What questions would you like to ask your pharmacist or physician? What drugs (legal or illegal) are you currently using that could cause interactions? What are the pros and cons of each alternative? Which alternative is the best solution for you?

Checklist for Change: Making Personal Choices

✓ Do you know what key questions to ask to create a drug profile for any drugs you may decide to use?

✓ Do you read the warning labels on the medications that you use?

✓ Do you take medication only for the problem for which it is being prescribed?

✓ Do you ask your doctor or pharmacist if you should avoid alcohol—or any foods, beverages such as coffee or caffeinated soft drinks, or other medications—while taking a drug?

✓ Do you purchase generic medications instead of brand-name products?

✓ Do you volunteer time at a local agency that assists those less fortunate than yourself to use medications responsibly?

✓ Do you know what resources in the community to access to help yourself and others answer questions about medications?

Critical Thinking

A recent college graduate, Ella is working at an indoor children's playground while looking for a job. She has no health insurance. She begins to get severe headaches at night, which she attributes to the stress of job hunting, listening to screaming children all day, and a side effect of her oral contraceptive. OTC pain relievers do not help Ella. To make matters worse, she has a big job interview in the morning. Her roommate offers her the prescription drug Valium, telling Ella it will relieve the pain and help her sleep. It works the first night, so her roommate offers her the rest of the prescription.

What are Ella's options? What community resources exist in your area where people without insurance can receive medical attention? Find the discussion of Valium in this chapter and debate whether or not Ella should self-medicate. Are there any potential interactions? If you were in Ella's situation, what would you do?

---

3. What are *prostaglandin inhibitors*? What are some examples of these analgesics?

4. What are rebound effects? What are the severe symptoms of withdrawal from stimulants?

5. What general precautions should OTC users consider?

Application Exercise

Reread the What Do You Think? scenarios at the beginning of this chapter and answer the following questions:

1. When is it appropriate to self-medicate? What guidelines should you follow? Is it possible to construct a drug profile from OTC medications?

2. If instead Wendy had a bad cold and had self-medicated with OTC cold medicine, would you have the same concerns? How long should one wait before going to the doctor with a cold?

3. Given that Donna needs the antibiotic, what added protection could she use in any sexual relations? How can she find out when the pill will again be effective for her?

4. When Donna started on the pill, whose responsibility was it to inform her of the possible drug interactions? Should a doctor take time with every patient to review every side effect? Or should the patient be responsible? Given the technical nature of drug literature, is it possible for the patient to understand?

Further Reading

The PDR® Family Guide to Women's Health and Prescription Drugs™ Medical Economics (Montvale, NJ: 1994).

A book of solutions—a tool for keeping health at its peak. Tells why problems develop, how best to prevent them, and what you and your doctor can do to make them right. Divided into two major parts, Part 1: A Woman's Special Health Concerns and Part 2: A Woman's Handbook of Medicines.

W. H. Griffith, *Complete Guide to Prescription and Nonprescription Drugs* (New York: The Body Press/Pedigree, 1993).

Outlines proper uses, possible dangers, effective ingredients, and relative costs of both prescription and OTC medications.

R. A. Julien, *A Primer of Drug Action,* 5th ed. (New York: W. H. Freeman, 1992).

Meant for people with a background in biochemistry. An excellent source for those wishing to know how various drugs affect the body.

J. W. Long, *The Essential Guide to Prescription Drugs* (New York: HarperCollins, 1993).

Provides detailed and comprehensive information about the most important drugs currently in use. Contains some of the most detailed information available to the general public.

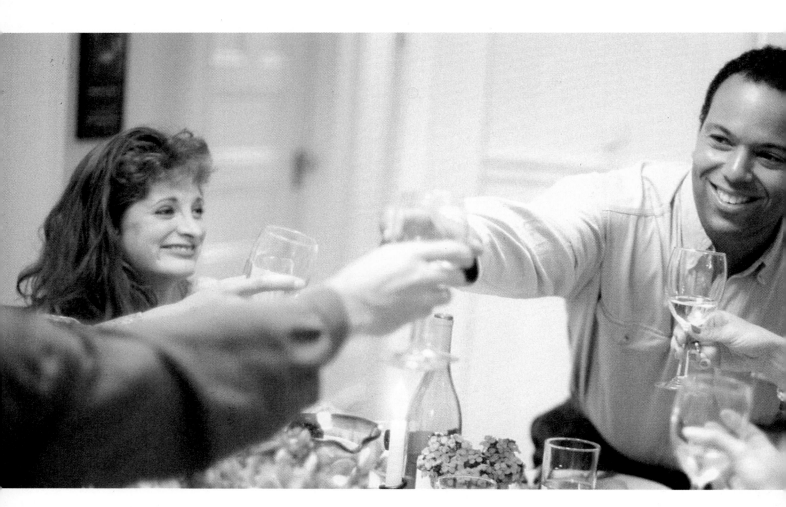

*C*HAPTER OBJECTIVES

◆ Summarize the alcohol use patterns of college students and discuss overall trends in consumption.

◆ Explain the physiological and behavioral effects of alcohol, including blood alcohol concentration, absorption, metabolism, and immediate and long-term effects of alcohol consumption.

◆ Explain the symptoms and causes of alcoholism, its cost to society, and its effects on the family.

◆ Explain the treatment of alcoholism, including the family's role, varied treatment methods, and whether or not alcoholics can be cured.

Drinking Responsibly

A Lifestyle Challenge

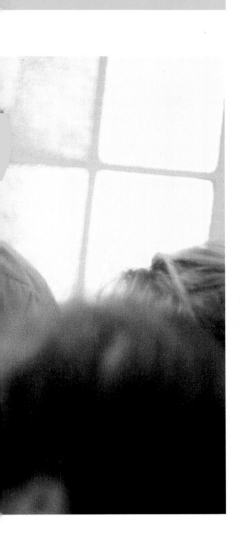

WHAT DO YOU THINK?

Dave, age 18, is a first-year student at a large university. Prior to coming to the university, Dave had never really had much alcohol. His expectation was that when he came to college he would need to learn to like to drink. Dave now lives in the residence halls where he perceives that everyone is drinking a lot of alcohol all the time. While Dave doesn't really like the taste of alcohol or the feel he gets after drinking, he feels pressured into drinking anyway. What Dave does not realize is that everyone thinks that everyone else is doing more of everything than they really are.

■ Is Dave's situation unusual for a college student? What messages do students who live in residence halls receive about drinking? From whom and where do they get this information? What can be done in the residence halls to change the perception that "everyone drinks"?

Teresa is a waitress at a restaurant. In the entryway of the building, there is a large warning sign about the dangers of drinking alcohol while pregnant. While taking a drink order from a woman, Teresa notices that she is in maternity clothes and in the advanced stages of pregnancy. Teresa takes the order and tells the restaurant manager that she feels uneasy serving alcohol to a pregnant woman. The manager says, "Mind your own business," and orders her to bring the woman the drink. Teresa delivers the drink. During the course of the evening, she brings several more drinks to the same woman.

■ Should Teresa refuse to serve the pregnant woman? Why? If the baby is born with alcohol-related problems, should the mother be sued for endangering her child?

When you hear references to the dangers of drugs, what usually comes to mind? Usually the term *drugs* conjures up images of people abusing cocaine, heroin, marijuana, LSD, PCP, and other illegal substances. We conveniently use the word *drugs* to refer to one set of dangerous substances, but we steadfastly refuse to categorize alcohol as a drug, primarily because it is socially accepted. Most of us think of alcohol the way it is portrayed in ads or in the movies: a way of having fun in company, an important adjunct to a romantic dinner or a cozy evening in front of the fireplace. Moderate use of alcohol can enhance celebrations or special times. Research shows that very low levels of use may actually lower some health risks. But you should remember that alcohol is a chemical substance that affects your physical and mental behavior. The tragedies associated with alcohol addiction receive far less attention than cocaine-related deaths, drug busts, and efforts to eradicate marijuana crops. Nevertheless, they are more common and may have devastating effects on people of all ages.

The drinking of alcoholic beverages is interwoven with our traditions. We use alcohol to celebrate everything from christenings to retirements. We use it to help ease the pain caused by rejection or loss. We are certainly not unique in this regard; people all over the world and throughout history have used alcohol for everything from social gatherings to religious ceremonies.

ALCOHOL: AN OVERVIEW

An estimated 70 percent of Americans consume alcoholic beverages regularly, though consumption patterns are unevenly distributed throughout the drinking population. Ten percent are heavy drinkers, and they account for half of all the alcohol consumed. The remaining 90 percent of the drinking population are infrequent, light, or moderate drinkers.

Alcohol and College Students

Alcohol is the most widely used (and abused) recreational drug in our society. It is also the most popular drug on college campuses, where approximately 85 percent of students consume alcoholic beverages.[1] Some 20 to 25 percent abuse alcohol. Exactly how much alcohol does a typical college student consume? According to a recent

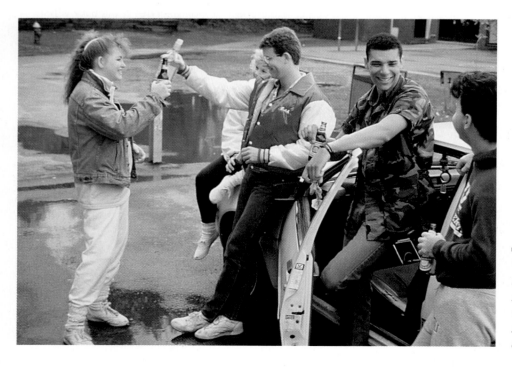

While alcohol has long been seen as a "social lubricant" by college students, alcohol abuse and reckless driving have become serious problems on many campuses.

Alcohol Use and College Students

- Two out of three college student suicide victims were legally intoxicated at the time of death.

- In a 1991 survey of 56,000 students, 42 percent reported having gone on a drinking binge (consuming five or more drinks on one occasion) at least once during the past two weeks.

- In a nationwide survey of college first-year students, 22.9 percent of the males and 14.4 percent of the females reported having engaged in unplanned sexual activity associated with alcohol use.

- Students who enter college having never consumed alcohol are three times as likely to drink in college, and consume greater quantities, if they become a member of a fraternity or sorority.

- One survey found that 60 percent of college women diagnosed with a sexually transmitted disease had been drunk at the time of infection.

- Alcohol plays a role in approximately 40 percent of all academic problems and 28.3 percent of dropouts have alcohol-related problems.

- A survey of college administrators indicated that more than half of campus crime incidents, ranging from violent behavior to damage of residence halls and other property, were directly related to alcohol use.

- Acquaintance rape is related to alcohol use by one or both parties at least 70 percent of the time.

- In 1990, college students spent more on alcohol than the combined total costs of maintenance (salaries, purchase of books, etc.) of all U.S. college and university libraries and all financial aid extended to American college students that year.

- Factors predicting which students were most likely to abuse alcohol during a two-year period were expectations of lower inhibitions for male students and expectations of positive personal effects for female students.

- First-year students are more likely to drink, to drink more, and to drink more often than seniors. For example, the most recent large-scale national survey found that 25 percent of first-year students admitted to binge drinking three or more times in the last two weeks compared to 20 percent of seniors.

- Surveys have found that one in three college students drinks primarily to get drunk.

survey, the average student consumes approximately five drinks per week, and the number of female drinkers is now close to equaling the number of male drinkers.[2] A very conservative estimate is that over 34 gallons of alcoholic beverages are consumed per college student annually. For the more than 12 million college students in the United States, the annual consumption of alcoholic beverages totals a staggering 430 million gallons. To visualize this, imagine 3,500 Olympic-sized swimming pools— roughly one for every college and university in the country—filled with beer, wine, and liquor. And that would only last our college student body a single year.[3] (See the Health Headlines box.)

College is a critical time to become conscious of and responsible about your drinking. A number of social factors are involved in campus drinking. There is little doubt that alcohol is a part of college culture and tradition. It is used to help relieve tensions and to celebrate. Its ability to lower inhibitions makes it the "social lubricant" of choice for many students, giving them an easy way to initiate conversations and create friendships. In a recent study of college student drinking, it was found that almost all male bonding took place over alcoholic beverages; in fact, that was the main purpose for male drinking.[4] Unfortunately, students also drink for a variety of reasons that are much less positive, such as to escape negative feelings, to release otherwise unacceptable emotions, or simply to get drunk.

How do students view the drinking patterns of their peers? Students consistently report that their friends drink much more than they do and that average drinking within their own social living group is higher than actual self-reports. Such misinformation may promote or be used to excuse excessive drinking practices among college students. In a survey of students at a large midwestern university, 42 percent reported not having a hangover in the past six months. Yet that same group of surveyed students believed that only 3 percent of their peers had not had a hangover in the past month. Overattending to misbehavior leads to overperception of misbehavior as the norm. Thus, pressure to misbehave is created because misbehavior allows students to perceive themselves as normal.

Binge drinking on college campuses has become a big problem. **Binge drinking** is defined as the consumption of five drinks in a row by men or four in a row by women on a single occasion. The express purpose of binge drinking is to become intoxicated. A recent study found that heavy

Binge drinking: Drinking for the express purpose of becoming intoxicated; five drinks in a single sitting for men and four drinks in a sitting for women.

drinking on college campuses is a problem even for students who do not drink.[5]

According to a 1994 Harvard Medical School study, 44 percent of students were found to be binge drinkers, and 19 percent were found to be frequent binge drinkers. Compared with nonbingers, frequent bingers were more likely to have an array of problems on campus (see Table 13.1). At schools where binge drinking is common, 9 of every 10 students endured problems as a result of someone else's drinking. One in 6 had personal property damaged, 1 in 4 experienced an unwanted sexual advance, 1 in 3 was "insulted or humiliated," more than half had to take care of a drunk, and 2 in 3 had had their sleep interrupted.[6]

Although everyone is at some risk for alcoholism and alcohol-related problems, college students seem to be particularly vulnerable:

- Alcohol exacerbates their already high risk for suicide, automobile crashes, and falls.

- Many college and university customs, norms, traditions, and mores encourage certain dangerous practices and patterns of alcohol use.

- University campuses are heavily targeted by advertising and promotions from the alcoholic beverage industry.

- It is more common for college students than their noncollegiate peers to drink recklessly and to engage in drinking games and other dangerous drinking practices.

- College students are particularly vulnerable to peer influences and have a strong need to be accepted by their peers.

In an effort to prevent alcohol abuse, many colleges and universities are instituting strong policies against drinking. At the same time, they are making more help available to students with drinking problems. Today, both individual and group counseling are offered on most campuses, and more attention is being directed toward the prevention of alcohol abuse.[7] Student organizations such as BACCHUS (Boost Alcohol Consciousness Concerning the Health of University Students) promote responsible drinking and responsible party hosting. For more on how to control your own use of alcohol, see the Choices for Change box.

Trends in Consumption

A downward trend in per capita consumption of alcoholic beverages was reported in the general population between

---

Vigorous campaigns promoting the responsible use of alcohol have lowered the alcohol consumption rate and reduced the number of drinking-and-driving fatalities in recent years.

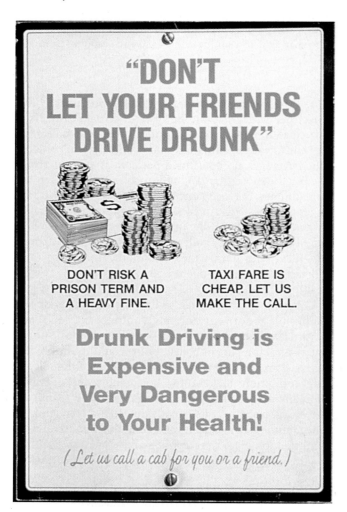

TABLE 13.1 ■ The Negative Effects of Alcohol on Student Behavior

Campus Problems Experienced in the Past Year	Non-binge Drinkers	Frequent Binge Drinkers
Had a hangover	30%	90%
Did something regrettable	14%	63%
Missed a class	8%	61%
Engaged in unplanned sex	8%	41%
Was injured	2%	23%
Damaged property	2%	22%
Got in trouble with police	1%	11%

Source: Data reprinted by permission from H. Wechsler, "Health and Behavioral Consequences of Binge Drinking in College," *Journal of the American Medical Association,* vol. 272 (1994): 1675 (Table 2). Copyright 1994 American Medical Association. Data appeared in "The Disruptions of Campus Drunkenness," *U.S. News & World Report,* 19 December 1994, 12.

Managing Your Drinking Behaviors

If you can make the safe and wise choice to drink moderately or to abstain from alcohol altogether, you will enhance your health and avoid the alcohol-related problems that some college students experience. Here are a few guidelines to help you think. Careful consideration of each of these factors will help you choose the course of action that is most appropriate for you.

1. The use of alcohol is a personal choice.

You should not feel pressured to drink or allow yourself to feel uneasy or embarrassed because of a personal choice. Many of you will choose to use alcohol safely, moderately, and appropriately. Others will simply have no desire to experience the effects of alcohol. Some students with a family history of chemical dependency or alcoholism may decide not to risk any use of alcohol. The bottom line is that you should never feel that you have to drink to be accepted.

2. Alcohol use is not essential for enjoying social events.

The real value of parties and other social activities is being with friends and taking time out from the pressures of school and work. Drinking alcohol should not be necessary for having fun and socializing. Alcohol should be regarded as an enjoyable and optional complement to other activities, not the major reason for socializing. When alcohol is made the main reason for a party, people often get intoxicated and/or sick. People who are unable to carry on a conversation or who pass out generally aren't much fun to be with after a while.

3. Know when to abstain from alcohol:

- When recovering from chemical dependency.
- When under the legal drinking age.
- When pregnant or breast-feeding.
- When operating equipment such as cars, motorcycles, boats, or firearms.
- When studying or working.
- When performing in fine arts or competing in athletics.
- When taking certain medications.

4. Drinking that leads to impairment or intoxication is unhealthy and risky.

Getting drunk is not a condition to be admired or taken lightly. Rude, destructive, or just plain foolish behavior triggered by alcohol use is socially unacceptable. It may also indicate an alcohol use problem. Drinking games often lead to drunkenness and serious risks for all involved.

5. Know your personal limit.

If you choose to drink, learn your personal limit and resolve to keep to it on every occasion that you do drink. Remember, your judgment can be affected even after a small amount of alcohol.

1981 and 1990. In 1987, the estimated per capita consumption was the equivalent of 2.54 gallons of pure alcohol per person.[8] (This measure indicates the amount of alcohol that a person would obtain by drinking approximately 50 gallons of beer, 20 gallons of wine, or more than 4 gallons of distilled spirits.) In addition, between 1982 and 1987, the proportion of fatally injured drivers who were legally intoxicated dropped from 46 percent to 40 percent.[9]

Most of us recognize the dangers associated with alcohol consumption in general, yet we tend to deny that such things could happen to us. We are aware of the relationship between alcohol and traffic accidents, spouse battering and child abuse, violent crimes, and family disruption, but we like to believe that these tragedies happen only to other people.

People who drink often argue that drinking is their inalienable right. Many refuse to acknowledge that alcohol is a drug simply because they do not wish to see themselves as drug users. Our society condones, approves, and often encourages the consumption of alcoholic beverages but neglects to teach us how to use alcohol responsibly.

Some drug educators even argue that alcohol cannot be consumed responsibly. The National Institute on Alcohol Abuse and Alcoholism (NIAAA), for example, has eliminated the phrase "responsible use of alcohol" from its educational materials.

If you make the choice to drink, you should do so judiciously, with complete information about the risks (see the Skills for Behavior Change box). The physiological and psychological reactions of the human organism to alcohol are strong. For this reason, you should approach the drug carefully. To avoid the devastating effects of alcohol abuse, you must adhere to the same principles of prevention that apply to any potentially harmful substance.

WHAT DO YOU THINK?

Have you ever thought about how much you drink in comparison to your friends? If you are not drinking more than your friends, does that mean that your drinking is not a problem?

How to Drink Responsibly in Social Situations

Because society has few rules for drinking, you would be wise to establish your own rules and limits. These rules should be based on a knowledge of the effects of alcohol and your own common sense.

Many people choose not to drink for religious, health, or personal reasons. No one should have to defend the decision to abstain from alcohol. Social pressure to consume alcoholic beverages is said to be a major influence on the drinking behaviors of people of all ages. These pressures are frequently blatant in adolescence and young adulthood and become more subtle in maturity. The first commonsense rule regarding drinking behavior is to honor anyone's decision not to consume alcoholic beverages.

Some rules to follow if you are a guest:

- Know your limits and stay within them. If others are pushing alcohol at you, you can fill your glass with ice or your beer can with water and pretend to continue drinking. You can also simply tell the truth: "Thank you, but I prefer not to drink."
- Stick to the limit of one ounce of alcohol in one hour. This will not only reduce the possibility of drunkenness but may also leave you legally able to drive home.
- Wine, beer, and other mixed drinks are easier to "nurse" than straight liquor. Stick to these rather than the higher-proof beverages.
- Eating and drinking simultaneously will promote a slower absorption rate of alcohol. Never drink on an empty stomach.
- Alternate alcoholic beverages with nonalcoholic drinks.
- If you are unfit to drive home, have your host or hostess call a cab, or ride with someone who has not been drinking. (Sometimes people go to parties with people who do not drink, secure in the knowledge they will have a safe way to get home.)
- If you're going with friends, always designate a driver who will not drink at all during the evening.

- Understand that being drunk does not excuse your behavior.
- Remember that it is easy to enjoy yourself without becoming inebriated. If you like to get drunk just to act silly, try acting silly without the alcohol—it might just be more fun.

If you are the party host:

- Be sure there is adequate food and that it is readily available to all guests.
- Serve beverages that are lighter in alcoholic content than straight liquors.
- Limit the availability of alcohol to your guests. Do not insist on refilling glasses; wait until asked.
- In preparing a mixed drink, measure the alcohol exactly. It is very easy to underestimate how much alcohol you are putting into a mixed drink.
- Limit the time of drinking.
- Plan the party to focus on something other than alcohol.
- Have coffee, tea, or other nonalcoholic beverages readily available throughout the gathering. Put alcoholic beverages away toward the end of the party.
- If a guest is too drunk to drive home, arrange alternative transportation or allow the guest to stay the night. Never accept a guest's word that he or she is sober enough to drive.

Caution!

If a friend passes out after drinking too much, be sure to monitor him or her. Place your friend on his or her side with legs bent, head turned to the side. Because alcohol is a gastric irritant, vomiting is a possibility. An intoxicated person asleep in a face-down or face-up position could inhale his or her own vomit and suffocate.

PHYSIOLOGICAL AND BEHAVIORAL EFFECTS OF ALCOHOL

Alcohol's Chemical Makeup

The intoxicating substance found in beer, wine, liquor, and liqueurs is **ethyl alcohol,** or **ethanol.** It is produced during a process called **fermentation,** whereby plant sugars are broken down by yeast organisms, yielding ethanol and carbon dioxide. Fermentation continues until the solution of plant sugars (called mash) reaches a concentration of 14 percent alcohol. At this point, the alcohol kills the yeast and halts the chemical reactions that produce it.

For beers and ales, which are fermented from malt barley, the process stops when the alcohol concentration is 14 percent. Manufacturers then add other ingredients that dilute the alcohol content of the beverage. Other alcoholic beverages are produced through further processing called **distillation,** during which alcohol vapors are released from the mash at high temperatures. The vapors are then condensed and mixed with water to make the final product.

The **proof** of an alcoholic drink is a measure of the percentage of alcohol in the beverage. "Proof" comes from

TABLE 13.2 ■ Beverages and Their Alcohol and Calorie Content

Beverage	Alcohol by Volume (approx. %)	Calories (per serving approx.)
Nonalcoholic beer	0.5	75
Beer, regular	4.5	170
Beer, light	3	70–134
Wine, light beverage	10–14	90 calories per 4 fluid ounces
Sherry and other fortified wines	17–21	140 calories per 3.5 fluid ounces
Champagne	11–12	71 calories per 3 fluid ounces
Sake wine	14–16	39 calories per 1 fluid ounce
Gin	40	120 calories per 1.5 fluid ounces
Brandy	35–40	60 calories per 4 fluid ounces
Vodka	40	95 calories per 1.5 fluid ounces
Rum	40	135 calories per 1.5 fluid ounces
Whiskey	40–54	130 calories per 1.5 fluid ounces

Source: Reprinted with the permission of Simon & Schuster, Inc., from the Macmillan College text *Drugs and the Human Body,* 4th ed., by Ken Liska. Copyright © 1994 by Macmillan Publishing Company, Inc.

"gunpowder proof," a reference to the gunpowder test, whereby potential buyers would test the distiller's product by pouring it on gunpowder and attempting to light it. If the alcohol content was at least 50 percent, the gunpowder would burn; otherwise the water in the product would put out the flame. Thus, alcohol percentage is 50 percent of the given proof. For example, 80 proof whiskey or scotch is 40 percent alcohol by volume, and 100 proof vodka is 50 percent alcohol by volume. The proof of a beverage provides an indication of its strength. Lower-proof drinks will produce fewer alcohol effects than the same amounts of higher-proof drinks.

Most wines are between 12 and 15 percent alcohol, and ales are between 6 and 8 percent (see Table 13.2). The alcoholic content of beers is between 2 and 6 percent, varying according to state laws and type of beer. Since the early 1980s, many breweries and wineries have been marketing "light" (low-calorie) and alcohol-reduced beers and wines. In an effort to alert consumers to the dangers of alcohol consumption, the government requires that warning labels be placed on alcoholic beverages.

Behavioral Effects

Behavioral changes caused by alcohol vary with the setting and with the individual. Alcohol may make shy people less inhibited and more willing to talk to others. It may make a depressed person even more depressed. In people reluctant to share emotions, it may bring out violence and aggression. In many cases, alcohol will do for the drinker what the drinker expects and wants it to do, making it possible for the user to blame his or her inappropriate behavior on the alcohol.

Blood alcohol concentration (BAC) is the ratio of alcohol to total blood volume. It is the factor used to measure the physiological and behavioral effects of alcohol. Despite individual differences, alcohol produces some general behavior effects depending on BAC (see Table 13.3). At a BAC of 0.02, a person feels slightly relaxed and in a good mood. At 0.05, relaxation increases, there is some motor impairment, and a willingness to talk

Ethyl alcohol (ethanol): An addictive drug produced by fermentation and found in many beverages.

Fermentation: The process whereby yeast organisms break down plant sugars to yield ethanol.

Distillation: The process whereby mash is subjected to high temperatures to release alcohol vapors, which are then condensed and mixed with water to make the final product.

Proof: A measure of the percentage of alcohol in a beverage.

Blood-alcohol concentration (BAC): The ratio of alcohol to total blood volume; the factor used to measure the physiological and behavioral effects of alcohol.

becomes apparent. At 0.08, the person feels euphoric and there is further motor impairment. At 0.10, the depressant effects of alcohol become apparent, drowsiness sets in, and motor skills are further impaired, followed by a loss of judgment. Thus a driver may not be able to estimate distances or speed, and some drinkers lose their ability to make value-related decisions and may do things they would not do when sober. As BAC increases, the drinker suffers increased physiological and psychological effects. All these changes are negative. No skills or functions are enhanced because of alcohol ingestion. Rather, physical and mental functions are all impaired.

People can acquire physical and psychological tolerance to the effects of alcohol through regular use. The nervous system adapts over time, so greater amounts of alcohol are required to produce the same physiological and psychological effects. Some people can learn to modify their behavior so that they appear to be sober even when their BAC is quite high. This ability is called **learned behavioral tolerance.**

Absorption and Metabolism

Unlike the molecules found in most other ingestible foods and drugs, alcohol molecules are sufficiently small and fat-soluble to be absorbed throughout the entire length of the gastrointestinal system. A negligible amount of alcohol is absorbed through the lining of the mouth. Approximately 20 percent of ingested alcohol is diffused through the stomach lining into the bloodstream. Nearly 80 percent of the liquid passes through the linings of the upper third of the small intestine. Absorption into the bloodstream is rapid and complete.

How quickly your body will absorb alcohol is influenced by several factors: the alcohol concentration in your drink, the amount of alcohol you consume, the amount of food in your stomach, pylorospasm, and your mood. The concentration of your drink and the amount of food in your stomach when you begin drinking are the two major factors affecting how quickly your system will absorb alcohol. The higher the concentration of alcohol, the more rapidly it is absorbed in your digestive tract. As a rule, wine and beer are absorbed more slowly than distilled beverages. Carbonated alcoholic beverages are absorbed more rapidly than those containing no sparkling additives, or fizz. Carbonated beverages such as champagne, carbonated wines, and drinks served with mixers cause the pyloric valve—the opening from the stomach into the

small intestine—to relax, thereby emptying the contents of the stomach more rapidly into the small intestine. Since the small intestine is the site of the greatest absorption of alcohol, carbonated beverages increase the rate of absorption. On the other hand, if your stomach is full, absorption is slowed because the surface area exposed to alcohol is smaller. A full stomach also retards the emptying of alcoholic beverages into your small intestine.

In addition, the more alcohol you consume, the longer absorption takes. Alcohol can irritate the digestive system, causing a spasm in the pyloric valve (pylorospasm). When the pyloric valve is closed, nothing can move from the stomach to the upper third of the small intestine, so absorption is slowed. If the irritation continues, it can cause vomiting.

Mood is another influence on the rate of absorption, since emotions affect how long it takes for the contents of the stomach to empty into the intestine. Powerful moods, such as stress and tension, are likely to cause the stomach to "dump" its contents into the small intestine. That is why alcohol is absorbed much more rapidly when people are tense than when they are relaxed.

Alcohol is metabolized in the liver, where it is converted by the enzyme alcohol dehydrogenase to acetaldehyde. It is then rapidly oxidized to acetate, converted to carbon dioxide and water, and eventually excreted from the body. Acetaldehyde is a toxic chemical that can cause immediate symptoms such as nausea and vomiting as well as long-term effects such as liver damage. A very small portion of alcohol is excreted unchanged by the kidneys, lungs, and skin.

When drinking alcohol, it is important to remember that choosing wine or beer and keeping food in the stomach are ways to minimize alcohol's negative effects on the mind and body.

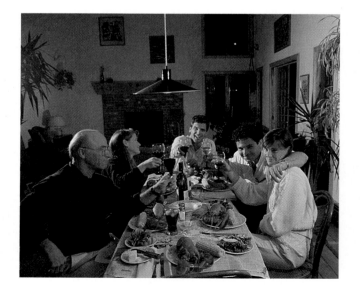

> **Learned behavioral tolerance:** The ability of heavy drinkers to modify their behavior so that they appear to be sober even when they have high BAC levels.

TABLE 13.3 ■ Psychological and Physical Effects of Various Blood-Alcohol Concentration Levels*

Number of Drinks†	Blood-alcohol Concentration	Psychological and Physical Effects	Common Effects on Driving Ability
1	0.02%–0.03%	No overt effects, slight mood elevation.	Mild changes occur. Many drivers experience slight change in feelings. Existing mood (anger, elation, etc.) may be heightened. Bad driving habits are slightly pronounced.
2	0.05%–0.06%	Feeling of relaxation, warmth; slight decrease in reaction time and in fine-muscle coordination.	Driver takes too long to decide what to do in an emergency. Inhibitions may be influenced. Shows a "so what" attitude, exaggerated behavior, and what appears to be loss of finger skills. In most states, 0.05% blood-alcohol concentration may be considered, with other competent evidence, in determining whether the person is legally under the influence of alcohol.
3	0.08%–0.09%	Balance, speech, vision, and hearing slightly impaired; feelings of euphoria, increased confidence; loss of motor coordination.	Driver exhibits exaggerated emotions and behavior—less concern, mental relaxation. Inhibitions, self-criticism, and judgment‡ are seriously affected. Shows impairment of skills of coordination. At this blood-alcohol level, a driver is presumed to be "under the influence" in all states.
	0.10%	Legal intoxication in most states; some have lower limits.	Shows serious and noticeable impairment of physical and mental functions; clumsy, uncoordinated, should wait 9 to 10 hours before driving.
4	0.11%–0.12%	Coordination and balance becoming difficult; distinct impairment of mental faculties, judgment.	
5	0.14%–0.15%	Major impairment of mental and physical control; slurred speech, blurred vision, lack of motor skills.	
7	0.20%	Loss of motor control—must have assistance in moving about; mental confusion.	
10	0.30%	Severe intoxication; minimum conscious control of mind and body.	At this point most drivers have "passed out" (unconsciousness, clammy skin, dilated pupils).
14	0.40%	Unconsciousness, threshold of coma.	
17	0.50%	Deep coma.	
20	0.60%	Death from respiratory failure.	

*For each hour elapsed since the last drink, subtract 0.015 percent blood-alcohol concentration, or approximately one drink.

†One drink = one beer (4 percent alcohol, 12 ounces), one highball (1 ounce whiskey), or one glass table wine (5 ounces).

‡The effect of alcohol on judgment, inhibitions, and self-control, even in the lower blood-alcohol levels, is serious because: (1) since self-criticism is affected early, the drinker often is unlikely to recognize any change in his or her behavior; and (2) the drinker often feels more perceptive and skillful and is therefore likely to take more chances in passing, speeding, or negotiating curves (self-confidence increases as skill decreases).

Source: Modified from data given in Ohio State Police Driver Information Seminars and the National Clearinghouse for Alcohol and Alcoholism Information, Rockville, MD.

Like food, alcohol contains calories. Proteins and carbohydrates (starches and sugars) each contain 4 kilocalories (kcal) per gram. Fat contains 9 kcal per gram. Alcohol, although similar in structure to carbohydrates, contains 7 kcal per gram. The body uses the calories in alcohol in the same manner it uses those found in carbohydrates: for immediate energy or for storage as fat if not immediately needed.

When compared to the variable breakdown rates of foods and other beverages, the breakdown of alcohol occurs at a fairly constant rate of 0.5 ounces per hour. This amount of alcohol is equivalent to 12 ounces of 5 percent beer, 5 ounces of 12 percent wine, or 1.5 ounces of 40 percent (80 proof) liquor. Legal limits of BAC for operating motor vehicles vary from state to state. Most states set the legal limit at 0.08 to 0.10 percent. A driver whose level of BAC exceeds the state's legal limit is considered legally intoxicated.

A drinker's BAC depends on weight and body fat, the water content in body tissues, the concentration of alcohol in the beverage consumed, the rate of consumption, and the volume of alcohol consumed. Heavier people have larger body surfaces through which to diffuse alcohol; therefore, they have lower concentrations of alcohol in their blood than do thin people after drinking the same amount. Because alcohol does not diffuse as rapidly into body fat as into water, alcohol concentration is higher in a person with more body fat. Because a woman is likely to have more body fat and less water in her body tissues than a man of the same weight, she will be more intoxicated than a man after drinking the same amount of alcohol.

𝒲HAT DO YOU THINK?

Have you thought that BAC is only based upon the amount of alcohol you drink? What other factors contribute to BAC? Are these factors different for men and women?

Women and Alcohol.   Body fat is not the only contributor to the differences in alcohol's effects on men and women. Compared to men, women appear to have half as much alcohol hydrogenase, the enzyme that breaks down alcohol in the stomach before it has a chance to get to the bloodstream and the brain. Therefore, if a man and a woman both drink the same amount of alcohol, the woman's BAC will be approximately 30 percent higher than the man's, leaving her more vulnerable to slurred speech, careless driving, and other drinking-related impairments. In female alcoholics, virtually none of the alcohol ingested is broken down in the stomach before it enters the bloodstream. Table 13.4 compares blood-alcohol levels by sex, weight, and consumption. Although this table can provide an estimate of probable BAC levels, many additional factors may cause considerable variation in these rates. For this reason, you should always err on the side of caution when gauging your blood alcohol level.

Breathalyzer and Other Tests.   The breathalyzer tests used by law enforcement officers are designed to determine BAC based on the amount of alcohol exhaled in the breath. Urinalysis can also yield a BAC based on the concentration of unmetabolized alcohol in the urine. Both breath analysis and urinalysis are used to determine whether a driver is legally intoxicated, but blood tests are more accurate measures. An increasing number of states are requiring blood tests for people suspected of driving under the influence of alcohol. In some states, refusal to take either the breath or the urine test results in immediate revocation of the person's driver's license.

Immediate Effects

The most dramatic effects produced by ethanol occur within the central nervous system (CNS). The primary

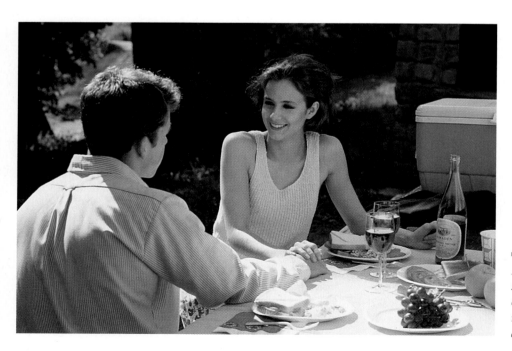

Physiological factors, such as body size, amount of body fat, and type of body chemistry, make women more vulnerable to the effects of alcohol than men.

TABLE 13.4 ■ Calculation of Estimated Blood-Alcohol Concentration (BAC) for Men and Women

Males					Number of Drinks					
Body Weight (lbs)	1	2	3	4	5	6	7	8	9	10
100	.043	0.87	.130	.174	.217	.261	.304	.348	.391	.435
125	.034	.069	.103	.139	.173	.209	.242	.278	.312	.346
150	.029	.058	.087	.116	.145	.174	.203	.232	.261	.290
175	.025	.050	.075	.100	.125	.150	.175	.200	.225	.250
200	.022	.043	.065	.087	.108	.130	.152	.174	.195	.217
225	.019	.039	.058	.078	.097	.117	.136	.156	.175	.195
250	.017	.035	.052	.070	.087	.105	.122	.139	.156	.173

Females					Number of Drinks					
Body Weight (lbs)	1	2	3	4	5	6	7	8	9	10
100	.050	.101	.152	.203	.253	.304	.355	.406	.456	.507
125	.040	.080	.120	.162	.202	.244	.282	.324	.364	.404
150	.034	.068	.101	.135	.169	.203	.237	.271	.304	.338
175	.029	.058	.087	.117	.146	.175	.204	.233	.262	.292
200	.026	.050	.076	.101	.126	.152	.177	.203	.227	.253
225	.022	.045	.068	.091	.113	.136	.159	.182	.204	.227
250	.020	.041	.061	.082	.101	.122	.142	.162	.182	.202

Body weight: Calculations are for people who have a normal body weight for their height, who are free of drugs or other affecting medications, and who are neither unusually thin nor obese.

Drink equivalents: 1 drink equals:
1 ½ oz. of rum, rye, scotch, brandy, gin, vodka, etc.
1 12-oz. bottle of normal-strength beer
3 oz. of fortified wine
5 oz. of table wine

Using the chart: Find the appropriate figure using the proper chart (male or female), body weight, and number of drinks consumed. Then subtract the time factor (see Time Factor Table below) from the figure on the chart to obtain the approximate BAC. For example, for a 150-lb. man who has had 4 drinks in 2 hours, take the figure .116 (from the chart for males) and subtract .030 (from the Time Factor Table) to obtain a BAC of .086%.

Time Factor Table

Hours since first drink	1	2	3	4	5	6
Subtract from BAC	.015	.030	.045	.060	.075	.090

Source: From *The Encyclopedia of Alcoholism* by Glen Evans and Robert O'Brien. Copyright © 1991 Facts On File and Greenspring Inc. Reprinted with permission of Facts On File, Inc., New York.

action of the drug is to reduce the frequency of nerve transmissions and impulses at synaptic junctions. This reduction of nerve transmissions results in a significant depression of CNS functions, with resulting decreases in respiratory rate, pulse rate, and blood pressure. As CNS depression deepens, vital functions become noticeably depressed. In extreme cases, coma and death can result.

Alcohol is a diuretic, causing increased urinary output. Although this effect might be expected to lead to automatic **dehydration** (loss of water), the body actually retains water, most of it in the muscles or in the cerebral tissues. This is because water is usually pulled out of the **cerebrospinal fluid** (fluid within the brain and spinal cord), leading to what is known as mitochondrial dehydration at the cell level within the nervous system. Mitochondria are miniature organs within cells that are

responsible for specific functions. They rely heavily upon fluid balance. When mitochondrial dehydration occurs from drinking, the mitochondria cannot carry out their normal functions, resulting in symptoms that include the "morning-after" headaches suffered by some drinkers.

Alcohol is also an irritant to the gastrointestinal system and may cause indigestion and heartburn if taken on an empty stomach. Long-term use of alcohol causes repeated irritation that has been linked to cancers of the esophagus

Dehydration: Loss of fluids from body tissues.

Cerebrospinal fluid: Fluid within and surrounding the brain and spinal cord tissues.

and stomach. In addition, people who engage in brief drinking sprees during which they consume unusually high amounts of alcohol put themselves at risk for irregular heartbeat or even total loss of heart rhythm, which can cause disruption in blood flow and possible damage to the heart muscle.

A **hangover** is often experienced the morning after a drinking spree. The symptoms of a hangover are familiar to most of you who drink: headache, upset stomach, anxiety, depression, thirst, and, in severe cases, an almost overwhelming desire to crawl into a hole and die. People who get hangovers often also smoke too much, stay up too late, or engage in other behaviors likely to leave them feeling unwell the next day. The causes of hangovers are not well known, but the effects of **congeners** are suspected. Congeners are forms of alcohol that are metabolized more slowly than ethanol and are more toxic. Your body metabolizes the congeners after the ethanol is gone from your system, and their toxic by-products are thought to contribute to the hangover. In addition, alcohol upsets the water balance in the body, resulting in excess urination and thirst the next day. Muscle aches, nausea caused by increased production of hydrochloric acid irritating the stomach lining, and muscle aches from overdoing on the drinking spree can all be part of a hangover. It usually takes 12 hours to recover from a hangover. Bed rest, solid food, and aspirin may help relieve the discomforts of a hangover, but unfortunately, nothing cures it but time.

Drug Interactions. When you use any drug (and alcohol is a drug), you need to be aware of the possible interactions with any prescription drugs, over-the-counter drugs, or other drugs you are taking or considering taking. Table 13.5 summarizes some possible interactions. Note that alcohol may cause a negative interaction even with aspirin.

Long-Term Effects

Doctors have sobering news for those who think a little alcohol is good for their health. According to a 1994 Harvard Medical School study, anything more than a drink a day may be too much of a good thing. Men who had two to four drinks a week had the lowest rate of death from all causes during an 11-year study. Beyond a drink a day, the risk went up sharply. Those who averaged two or more drinks a day had a death rate that was 63 percent higher than that of nondrinkers.

Researchers found that the lower risk of dying from heart disease was offset by an increase in cancer in those who had more than one drink a day. This new study suggests that the current definition of one to three drinks a

---

TABLE 13.5 ■ Drugs and Alcohol: Actions and Interactions

Drug Class/Trade Name(s)	Effects with Alcohol
Antialcohol Antabuse	Severe reactions to even small amounts: headache, nausea, blurred vision, convulsions, coma, possible death.
Antibiotics Penicillin, Cyantin	Reduces therapeutic effectiveness.
Antidepressants Elavil, Sinequan, Tofranil, Nardil	Increased central nervous system (CNS) depression, blood pressure changes. Combined use of alcohol and MAO inhibitors, a specific type of antidepressant, can trigger massive increases in blood pressure, even brain hemorrhage and death.
Antihistamines Allerest, Dristan	Drowsiness and CNS depression. Impairs driving ability.
Aspirin Anacin, Excedrin, Bayer	Irritates stomach lining. May cause gastrointestinal pain, bleeding.
Depressants Valium, Ativan, Placidyl	Dangerous CNS depression, loss of coordination, coma. High risk of overdose and death.
Narcotics heroin, codeine, Darvon	Serious CNS depression. Possible respiratory arrest and death.
Stimulants caffeine, cocaine	Masks depressant action of alcohol. May increase blood pressure, physical tension.

Source: Reprinted by permission from *Drugs and Alcohol: Simple Facts About Alcohol and Drug Combinations* (Phoenix: DIN Publications, 1988), no. 121.

TABLE 13.6 ■ Drinking and Death Rates

Amount	Overall Death Rate	Heart Disease Death Rate	Cancer Death Rate
1 drink/week	16% lower than average	11% lower than average	21% lower than average
2–4 drinks/week	22% lower than average	20% lower than average	5% lower than average
5–6 drinks/week	21% lower than average	46% lower than average	7% higher than average
1 drink/day	1% higher than average	4% lower than average	12% higher than average
2 or more/day	63% higher than average	62% higher than average	123% higher than average

Source: Reprinted by permission from H. Wechsler, "Health and Behavioral Consequences of Binge Drinking in College," *Journal of the American Medical Association* 272 (1994): 1672–1677. Copyright 1994, American Medical Association.

day as healthy, moderate drinking should be lowered considerably. The study was conducted only on men, so the results may not hold true for women. However, this should not be taken as a rationale for women to drink more in the name of good health. For a summary of the Harvard study, see Table 13.6.[10]

Effects on the Nervous System. The nervous system is especially sensitive to alcohol. Even people who drink moderately experience shrinkage in brain size and weight and a loss of some degree of intellectual ability. The damage that results from alcohol use is localized primarily in the left side of the brain, which is responsible for written and spoken language, logic, and mathematical skills. The degree of shrinkage appears to be directly related to the amount of alcohol consumed. In terms of memory loss, the evidence suggests that having one drink every day is better than saving up for a binge and consuming seven or eight drinks in a night. The amount of alcohol consumed at one time is critical. Alcohol-related brain damage can be partially reversed with good nutrition and staying sober.

Cardiovascular Effects. The cardiovascular system is affected by alcohol in a number of ways. Evidence suggests that the effect of alcohol on the heart is not all bad. Studies by the National Heart, Lung, and Blood Institute suggest that moderate drinkers suffer fewer heart attacks, have less cholesterol buildup in their arteries, and are less likely to die of heart disease than either nondrinkers or heavy drinkers.[11] However, drinking is not recommended as a preventive measure against heart disease because there are many more cardiovascular health hazards than benefits from alcohol consumption. Alcohol contributes to high blood pressure and slightly increased heart rate and cardiac output. Those who report drinking three to five drinks a day, regardless of race or sex, have higher blood pressure than those who drink less.

People who engage in brief drinking sprees, during which they consume unusually large amounts of alcohol, also suffer some risks, including irregular heartbeat or total loss of heart rhythm. This condition has been called *holiday heart syndrome* because it typically occurs after such holidays as Thanksgiving, Christmas, and New Year's Eve, occasions when drinkers are likely to overindulge. It can cause disruption in blood flow and possible damage to the heart muscle. Prolonged drinking can also lead to deterioration of the heart muscle, a condition called *cardiomyopathy.*

Liver Disease. One of the most common diseases related to alcohol abuse is **cirrhosis** of the liver. It is among the top 10 causes of death in the United States. One result of heavy drinking is that the liver begins to store fat—a condition known as *fatty liver.* If there is insufficient time between drinking episodes, this fat cannot be transported to storage sites and the fat-filled liver cells stop function-

Hangover: The physiological reaction to excessive drinking, including such symptoms as headache, upset stomach, anxiety, depression, diarrhea, and thirst.

Congeners: Forms of alcohol that are metabolized more slowly than ethanol and produce toxic by-products.

Cirrhosis: The last stage of liver disease associated with chronic heavy use of alcohol during which liver cells die and damage is permanent.

ing. Continued drinking can cause a further stage of liver deterioration called *fibrosis,* in which the damaged area of the liver develops fibrous scar tissue. Cell function can be partially restored at this stage with proper nutrition and abstinence from alcohol. If the person continues to drink, however, cirrhosis results. At this point, the liver cells die and the damage is permanent. **Alcoholic hepatitis** is a serious condition resulting from prolonged use of alcohol. A chronic inflammation of the liver develops, which may be fatal in itself or progress to cirrhosis.

Cancer. Heavy drinkers are at higher risk for certain types of cancer, particularly cancers of the gastrointestinal tract. The repeated irritation caused by long-term use of alcohol has been linked to cancers of the esophagus, stomach, mouth, tongue, and liver. Research has also shown a link between breast cancer and moderate levels of alcohol consumption in women. A study conducted in 1987 found that women between the ages of 34 and 59 who consumed between three and nine drinks a week were 30 percent more likely than nondrinkers to develop breast cancer.[12] A 1994 study by the Harvard Medical School of male drinkers showed a 12 percent increased risk for cancer for those who had only one drink a day and 123 percent for those who had two drinks a day (see Table 13.6). It is unclear how alcohol exerts its carcinogenic effects, though it is thought that it inhibits the absorption of carcinogenic substances, permitting them to be taken to sensitive organs.

Other Effects. An irritant to the gastrointestinal system, alcohol may cause indigestion and heartburn if ingested on an empty stomach. It also damages the mucous membranes and can cause inflammation of the esophagus, chronic stomach irritation, problems with intestinal absorption, and chronic diarrhea.

Alcohol abuse is a major cause of chronic inflammation of the pancreas, the organ that produces digestive

enzymes and insulin. Chronic abuse of alcohol inhibits enzyme production, which further inhibits the absorption of nutrients. Drinking alcohol can block the absorption of calcium, a nutrient that strengthens bones. This should be of particular concern to women, for as women age their risk for osteoporosis (bone thinning and calcium loss) increases. Heavy consumption of alcohol worsens this condition.

Evidence also suggests that alcohol impairs the body's ability to recognize and fight foreign bodies such as bacteria and viruses. The relationship between alcohol and AIDS is unclear, especially since some of the populations at risk for AIDS are populations that are also at risk for alcohol abuse. But any stressor like alcohol with a known effect on the immune system would probably contribute to the development of the disease.

Alcohol and Pregnancy

Of the 30 known teratogens in the environment, alcohol is one of the most dangerous and common. Alcohol can have harmful effects on fetal development. A disorder called **fetal alcohol syndrome (FAS)** is associated with alcohol consumption throughout pregnancy. Alcohol consumed during the first trimester poses the greatest threat to organ development; exposure during the last trimester, when the brain is developing rapidly, is most likely to affect CNS development. FAS is the third most common birth defect and the second leading cause of mental retardation in the United States. One of every 750 newborns has a cluster of physical and mental symptoms classified as fetal alcohol syndrome.

FAS occurs when alcohol ingested by the mother passes through the placenta into the infant's bloodstream. Because the fetus is so small, its BAC will be much higher than that of the mother. Thus, consumption of alcohol during pregnancy can affect the infant far more seriously than it does the mother. Among the symptoms of FAS are mental retardation, small head, tremors, and abnormalities of the face, limbs, heart, and brain.

Children with a history of prenatal alcohol exposure, but without all the physical or behavioral symptoms of FAS, may be categorized as having **fetal alcohol effects (FAE)**. FAE is estimated to occur three to four times as often as FAS, although it is much less recognized. The signs of FAE in newborns are low birth weight and irritability, and there may be permanent mental impairment. Infants whose mothers habitually consumed more than 3 ounces of alcohol (approximately six drinks) in a short time period when pregnant are at high risk for FAS. Risk levels for babies whose mothers consume smaller amounts are uncertain.

Alcohol can also be passed to a nursing baby through breast milk. For this reason, most doctors advise nursing

Alcoholic hepatitis: Condition resulting from prolonged use of alcohol in which the liver is inflamed. It can result in death.

Fetal alcohol syndrome (FAS): A disorder that may affect the fetus when the mother consumes alcohol during pregnancy. Among its effects are mental retardation, small head, tremors, and abnormalities of the face, limbs, heart, and brain.

Fetal alcohol effects (FAE): A syndrome describing children with a history of prenatal alcohol exposure but without all the physical or behavioral symptoms of FAS. Among its symptoms are low birth weight, irritability, and possible permanent mental impairment.

mothers not to drink for at least four hours before nursing their babies and preferably to abstain altogether.

ᵂHAT DO YOU THINK?

Why do we hear so little about FAS in this country when it is the third most common birth defect and second leading cause of mental retardation? Is this a reflection of our society's denial of alcohol as a dangerous drug?

Drinking and Driving

The leading cause of death for all age groups from 5 to 34 years old (including college students) is traffic accidents. Approximately 44 percent of all traffic fatalities are alcohol-related.[13] Nationally, we have approximately 20,000 automobile crashes per year.[14] Unfortunately, college students are overrepresented in alcohol-related crashes. A poll of undergraduates found that two out of three admitted to driving while intoxicated.[15] Furthermore, it is estimated that two out of every five Americans will be involved in an alcohol-related accident at some time in their lives (see Figure 13.1).[16] Studies show that those involved in car crashes who had been drinking have a 40 to 50 percent higher chance of dying than nondrinkers involved in car crashes.

From 1982 to 1993, the number of alcohol-related traffic fatalities (ARTFs) declined almost 14 percent,[17] and fatalities decreased among all age groups, with the largest decline among 15- to 20-year-olds. Several factors proba-

With two out of three undergraduates admitting to having driven while intoxicated, it is not surprising that college students are overrepresented in alcohol-related auto accidents.

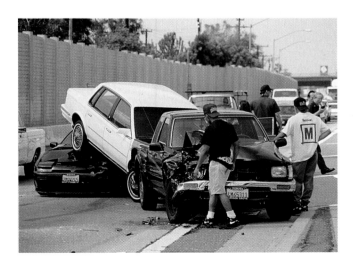

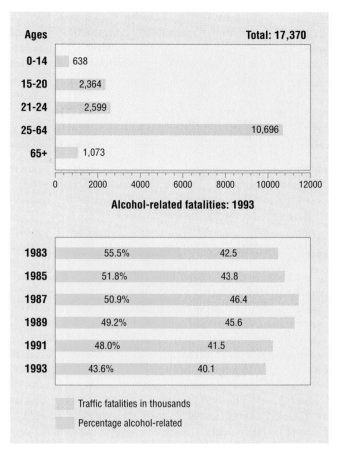

Ages		Total: 17,370
0-14	638	
15-20	2,364	
21-24	2,599	
25-64		10,696
65+	1,073	

Alcohol-related fatalities: 1993

Year	Percentage alcohol-related	Traffic fatalities in thousands
1983	55.5%	42.5
1985	51.8%	43.8
1987	50.9%	46.4
1989	49.2%	45.6
1991	48.0%	41.5
1993	43.6%	40.1

Traffic fatalities in thousands
Percentage alcohol-related

FIGURE 13.1

Traffic Fatalities and Alcohol Consumption

Source: Data for the years 1985–1991 appeared in the *New York Times*, February 15, 1993; data for the years 1992–1994 from U.S. Centers for Disease Control, *Morbidity and Mortality Weekly Report*, 3 December 1993, and 4 December 1994.

bly contributed to these reductions in ARTFs: the enactment of laws raising the drinking age to 21 and stricter enforcement of these laws; increased emphasis on zero tolerance (laws prohibiting those under 21 from driving with *any* detectable BAC); and the educational and other prevention programs designed to discourage drinking and driving. National groups such as MADD (Mothers Against Drunk Driving), started by a mother whose child was killed by a drunk driver, go as far as tracking drunk driving cases through the court systems to ensure that drunk drivers are punished. Members of the high school group SADD (Students Against Drunk Driving) educate their peers about the dangers of drinking and driving.

Despite all these measures, the risk of being involved in an alcohol-related automobile crash remains substantial. Researchers have shown a direct relationship between the amount of alcohol in a driver's bloodstream and the likelihood of a crash occurring. A driver with a BAC level of 0.10 percent has approximately 10 times the likelihood of being involved in a car accident as a driver who has not been drinking. At a BAC of 0.15, the probability increases to 25 times.

Alcoholism

Alcohol use becomes **alcohol abuse** or **alcoholism** when it interferes with work, school, or social and family relationships or when it entails any violation of the law, including driving under the influence (DUI).

How, Why, Who?

As with other drug addicts, tolerance, psychological dependence, and withdrawal symptoms must be present to qualify a drinker as an addict. Addiction results from chronic use over a period of time that may vary from person to person. Problem drinkers or irresponsible users are not necessarily alcoholics. The stereotype of the alcoholic on skid row applies to only 5 percent of the alcoholic population. The remaining 95 percent of alcoholics live in some type of extended family unit. They can be found at all socioeconomic levels and in all professions, ethnic groups, geographical locations, religions, and races. You have a 1 in 10 risk of becoming an alcoholic. Moreover, 25 percent of the American population (50 million people) is affected by the alcoholism of a friend or family member. In all, some 18 million American adults are either alcoholics or have alcohol abuse problems.[18]

Recognition of an alcohol problem is often extremely difficult. Alcoholics themselves deny their problem, often making such statements as, "I can stop any time I want to. I just don't want to right now." Their families also tend to deny the existence of a problem, saying things like, "He really has been under a lot of stress lately. Besides, he only drinks beer." The fear of being labeled a "problem drinker" often prevents people from seeking help.

Alcoholics tend to have a number of behaviors in common. Some of the indicators of this disease are listed in the Rate Yourself box. People who recognize one or more of these behaviors in themselves may wish to seek professional help to determine whether alcohol has become a controlling factor in their lives.

Women are the fastest-growing component of the population of alcohol abusers. They tend to become alcoholic at a later age and after fewer years of heavy drinking than do male alcoholics. Women at highest risk for alcohol-related problems are those who are unmarried but living with a partner, are in their 20s or early 30s, or have a husband or partner who drinks heavily.

The Causes of Alcoholism

We know that alcoholism is a disease with biological, psychological, and social/environmental components, but we do not know what role each of these components plays in the disease.

Biological and Family Factors. Research into the hereditary and environmental causes of alcoholism has found higher rates of alcoholism among family members of alcoholics. In fact, according to researchers, alcoholism is four to five times more common among the children of alcoholics than in the general population.

Male alcoholics, especially, are more likely than nonalcoholics to have alcoholic parents and siblings. Two distinct subtypes of alcoholism have provided important information about the inheritance of alcoholism. *Type 1 alcoholics* are drinkers who had at least one parent of either sex who was a problem drinker and who grew up in an environment that encouraged heavy drinking. Their drinking is reinforced by environmental events during which there is heavy drinking. Type 1 alcohol abusers share certain personality characteristics. They avoid novelty and harmful situations and are concerned about the thoughts and feelings of others. *Type 2 alcoholism* is seen in males only. These alcoholics are typically the biological sons of alcoholic fathers who have a history of both violence and drug use. Type 2 alcoholics display the opposite characteristics of Type 1 alcoholics. They do not seek social approval, they lack inhibition, and they are prone to novelty-seeking behavior.[19]

A 1984 study found a strong relationship between alcoholism and alcoholic patterns within the family.[20] Children with one alcoholic parent had a 52 percent chance of becoming alcoholics themselves. With two alcoholic parents, the chances of becoming alcoholic jumped to 71 percent. The researchers felt that both heredity and environment were significant factors in the development of alcoholism, but were reluctant to specify precisely how these factors worked.

Scientists are on the trail of an "alcohol gene," but so far they have not managed to find one. In 1990, it appeared that a specific gene linked to alcoholism had been discovered. The gene was reportedly a receptor for dopamine, a chemical that plays a crucial role in cell communication and pleasure-seeking behavior. It turned out, however, that not only was the gene not found consistently in every alcoholic studied but that it also existed in some individuals who were not alcoholics.[21]

> **Alcohol abuse (alcoholism):** Use of alcohol that interferes with work, school, or personal relationships or that entails violations of the law.

Warning Signs of Alcoholism

Knowing the facts about alcohol is only one prerequisite for making responsible decisions about alcohol use. It is also important to learn to recognize the warning signs of alcoholism in yourself and others around you. Analyze your attitudes and behavior by taking the following self-assessment.

1. Are you unable to stop drinking after a certain number of drinks?
2. Do you need a drink to get motivated?
3. Do you often forget what happened while you were partying (have blackouts)?
4. Do you drink or party alone?
5. Have others annoyed you by criticizing your alcohol use?
6. Have you been involved in fights with your friends or family while you were drunk or high?
7. Have you done or said anything while drinking that you later regretted?
8. Have you destroyed or damaged property while drinking?
9. Do you drive while high or drunk?
10. Have you been physically hurt while drinking?
11. Have you been in trouble with the school authorities or the campus police because of your drinking?
12. Have you dropped or chosen friends based on their drinking habits?
13. Do you think you are a normal drinker despite friends' comments that you drink too much?
14. Have you ever missed classes because you were too hungover to get up on time?
15. Have you ever done poorly on an exam or assignment because of drinking?
16. Do you think about drinking or getting high a lot?
17. Do you feel guilty or self-conscious about your drinking?

If you answered yes to three or more of these questions, or if your answer to any of the questions concerns you, you may be using alcohol in ways that are harmful. Do not waste time blaming yourself for past binges or other alcohol-related behavior. If you think you have or might be developing problems in which drinking plays a part, act now. You can get help.

For more information and counseling, contact your campus health or counseling center, community mental health facility, or Alcoholics Anonymous (AA). Information about local AA meetings may be available from your local library or telephone directory as well as from the national AA office at P.O. Box 459, Grand Central Station, New York, NY 10163; telephone: (212) 686–1100.

Source: From "Alcohol: Decisions on Tap," by permission of American College Health Association, P.O. Box 28937, Baltimore, MD 21240–8937 (phone 410/859–1500).

Because the effects of heredity and environment are so difficult to separate, some scientists have chosen to examine the problem through twin and adoption studies. So far, these studies have produced inconclusive results, although a slightly higher rate of similar drinking behaviors has been demonstrated among identical twins. Moreover, sons living away from their alcoholic parents tend to more nearly resemble them in drinking behavior than they do their adoptive or foster parents.

Social and Cultural Factors. Although a family history of alcoholism may predispose a person to problems with alcohol, there are numerous other factors that may mitigate or exacerbate that tendency. Furthermore, researchers now believe that social and cultural factors may trigger the affliction for many people who are not genetically predisposed to alcoholism. Some people begin drinking as a way to dull the pain of an acute loss or an emotional or social problem. For example, college students may drink to escape the stress of college life, disap-

pointment over unfulfilled expectations, difficulties in forming relationships, or loss of the security of home, loved ones, and close friends. Involvement in a painful relationship, death of a family member, and other problems may trigger a search for an anesthetic. Unfortunately, the emotional discomfort that causes many people to turn to alcohol also ultimately causes them to become even more uncomfortable as the depressant effect of the drug begins to take its toll. Thus, the person who is already depressed may become even more depressed, antagonizing friends and other social supports until they begin to turn away. Eventually, the drinker becomes physically dependent on the drug.

Family attitudes toward alcohol also seem to influence whether or not a person will develop a drinking problem. It has been clearly demonstrated that people who are raised in cultures in which drinking is a part of religious or ceremonial activities or in which alcohol is a traditional part of the family meal are less prone to alcohol dependency. In contrast, in societies in which alcohol purchase

The likelihood of alcohol dependency diminishes for people raised in cultures where alcohol is a traditional part of family meals or religious ceremonies.

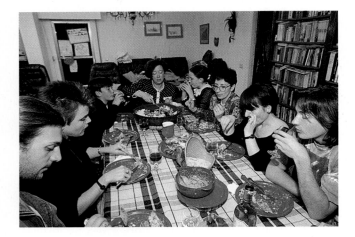

is carefully controlled and drinking is regarded as a rite of passage to adulthood, the tendency for abuse appears to be greater.[22]

Certain social factors have been linked with alcoholism as well. These include urbanization, the weakening of links to the extended family and a general loosening of kinship ties, increased mobility, and changing religious and philosophical values. Apparently, then, some combination of heredity and environment plays a decisive role in the development of alcoholism. Certain ethnic and racial groups also have special alcohol abuse problems (see the Multicultural Perspectives box).

*W*HAT DO YOU THINK?

What were the attitudes in your family toward drinking? Are those attitudes reflected in your current drinking behavior?

Effects of Alcoholism on the Family

Only recently have people begun to recognize that it is not only the alcoholic but the alcoholic's entire family that suffers from the disease of alcoholism. Although most research focuses on family effects during the late stages of alcoholism, the family unit actually begins to react early on as the person starts to show symptoms of the disease.

An estimated 30 million Americans (one out of eight) come from an alcoholic household.[23] Twenty-one million members of alcoholic families are 18 or older, and many have carried childhood emotional scars into adulthood.[24]

An estimated 7 million children who are under 18 live in an atmosphere of anxiety, tension, confusion, and denial.

In dysfunctional families, children learn certain rules from a very early age: Don't talk, don't trust, and don't feel. These unspoken rules allow the family to avoid dealing with real problems and real issues.

Dealing with the far-reaching effects of alcoholism strains the alcoholic's entire family. Many families affected by alcoholism have no idea what normal family life is like. Family members unconsciously adapt to the alcoholic's behavior by adjusting their own behavior. To minimize their feelings about the alcoholic or out of love for him or her, family members take on various abnormal roles. Unfortunately, these roles actually help keep the alcoholic drinking. Children in such dysfunctional families generally assume at least one of the following roles:

- *Family hero:* tries to divert attention from the problem by being too good to be true.

- *Scapegoat:* draws attention away from the family's primary problem through delinquency or misbehavior.

- *Lost child:* becomes passive and quietly withdraws from upsetting situations.

- *Mascot:* disrupts tense situations by providing comic relief.

For children in alcoholic homes, life is a struggle. They have to deal with constant stress, anxiety, and embarrassment. Because the alcoholic is the center of attention, the children's wants and needs are often ignored. It is not uncommon for these children to be victims of violence, abuse, neglect, or incest. As we have seen, when such children grow up, they are much more prone to alcoholic behaviors themselves than are children from nonalcoholic families.

In the last decade, we have come to recognize the unique problems of adult children of alcoholics whose difficulties in life stem from a lack of parental nurturing during childhood. Among these problems are an inability to develop social attachments, a need to be in control of all emotions and situations, low self-esteem, and depression.

Fortunately, not all individuals who have grown up in alcoholic families are doomed to have lifelong problems. Many of these people as they mature develop a resiliency in response to their families' problems. They thus enter adulthood armed with positive strengths and valuable career-oriented skills, such as the ability to assume responsibility, strong organizational skills, and realistic expectations of their jobs and others.

Costs to Society

The entire society suffers the consequences of individuals' alcohol abuse. Half of all traffic fatalities are attributable to

Drinking among Certain Ethnic and Racial Groups

Racial and ethnic minority groups appear to have their own characteristic patterns of alcohol abuse.

African Americans

Although African Americans on average drink less per person than white Americans do, alcoholism is one of the most significant problems in the African-American community. It is a major factor in blacks' higher death rates due to homicide, cirrhosis of the liver, heart disease, and the various cancers associated with heavy drinking. Black women are more likely to abstain from alcohol use than are white women; but among black women who drink, there is a higher percentage of heavy drinkers.

Malt liquor advertisements are targeted almost exclusively at African-American communities. Malt liquor contains almost twice as much alcohol as regular beer, which is why it is often referred to as "liquid crack." Nearly every inner-city black neighborhood is plastered with malt liquor ads projecting images meant to appeal to blacks. Schlitz Malt Liquor Bull, for instance, conveys an image of virility and power that is attractive to many black males, while St. Ides uses rap music, which appeals primarily to young blacks.

Hispanic Americans

Hispanic-American males have a higher than average rate of alcohol abuse and alcohol-related physical problems, such as cirrhosis of the liver. There are many theories about why this is so, but most researchers agree that a major factor is the key role heavy drinking plays in Hispanic culture, which tends to regard getting drunk as an innocently enjoyable thing to do. Other factors include low socioeconomic status, the difficulty many Hispanic immigrants have adjusting to American culture, and the concentration of liquor outlets in Hispanic neighborhoods. Like blacks, Hispanics are heavily targeted by alcohol advertisers.

Native Americans and Alaskan Natives

Alcohol is by far the most widely abused drug in the Native-American and Alaskan-Native populations, whose overall rate of alcoholism is two to three times the national average. The death rate from alcohol-related causes is about eight times higher than the national average. The problem exists among all age groups, although some Native-American women do not drink at all. Contributing factors seem to be often abysmal economic conditions and the cultural belief that alcoholism is not a physical disease but a spiritual problem. Native Americans suffer very high mortality rates from alcohol-related injuries, homicides, suicides, and cirrhosis.

Asians

Asians have very low rates of alcoholism. Social and cultural influences, such as strong kinship ties, are thought to discourage heavy drinking in Asian groups.

---

alcohol. The annual cost of alcohol-related crimes, medical expenses, accidents, and treatment programs is nearly $117 billion, and it is expected to rise to $150 billion by 1995.[25] Direct health-care costs of alcoholics are estimated to exceed $20 billion yearly, and alcoholism is directly and indirectly responsible for over 25 percent of the nation's medical expenses and lost earnings. Well over 50 percent of all child abuse cases are the result of alcohol-related problems. Finally, the costs in emotional health are impossible to measure.[26] Figure 13.2 highlights some of society's alcohol-related problems.

Women and Alcoholism

In the past, women have consumed less alcohol and have had fewer alcohol-related problems than have men. But now, greater percentages of women, especially college-aged women, are choosing to drink and are drinking more heavily.

Studies indicate that there are now almost as many female as male alcoholics. However, there appear to be differences between men and women when it comes to alcohol abuse.[27]

1. Women attribute the onset of problem drinking to a specific life stress or traumatic event more frequently than do men.

2. Women's alcoholism starts later and progresses more quickly than men's alcoholism, a phenomenon called telescoping.

3. Women tend to be prescribed mood-altering drugs more often than are men; women thus face the risks of drug interaction or cross-tolerance more often.

4. Nonalcoholic males tend to divorce their alcoholic spouses nine times more often than they do their nonalcoholic spouses; alcoholic women are thus not as likely to have a family support system to aid them in their recovery attempts.

5. Female alcoholics do not tend to receive as much social support as do males in their treatment and recovery.

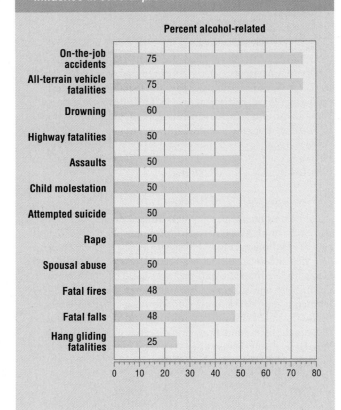

Percent alcohol-related

On-the-job accidents	75
All-terrain vehicle fatalities	75
Drowning	60
Highway fatalities	50
Assaults	50
Child molestation	50
Attempted suicide	50
Rape	50
Spousal abuse	50
Fatal fires	48
Fatal falls	48
Hang gliding fatalities	25

0 10 20 30 40 50 60 70 80

FIGURE 13.2

Alcohol's Grip on Society

Source: Reprinted by permission of the University of California at San Diego Extension from "Alcohol and Injuries: Problems and Responses," *Prevention File*, vol. 7, no. 5 (Special Edition 1992), 3. Copyright © 1992 by the Regents of the University of California.

6. Unmarried, divorced, or single-parent women tend to have significant economic problems that may make entry into a treatment program especially difficult.[28]

WHAT DO YOU THINK?

Why have women started to drink more heavily? Do we look at men's and women's drinking problems in the same way? Can you think of ways to increase support for women in their recovery process?

Intervention: A planned confrontation with an alcoholic in which family members or friends express their concern about the alcoholic's drinking.

RECOVERY

Despite the growing recognition of our national alcohol problem, fewer than 10 percent of alcoholics in the United States receive any care. Factors contributing to this low figure include an inability or unwillingness to admit to an alcohol problem; the social stigma attached to alcoholism; breakdowns in referral and delivery systems (failure of physicians or psychotherapists to follow up on referrals, client failure to follow through with recommended treatments, or failure of rehabilitation facilities to give quality care); and failure of the professional medical establishment to recognize and diagnose alcoholic symptoms among their patients.

Most alcoholics and problem drinkers who seek help have experienced a turning point or dramatic occurrence: a spouse walks out, taking children and possessions; the boss issues an ultimatum to dry out or ship out; the courtroom judge offers the alternatives of prison or a treatment center; a teenage child confesses embarrassment about bringing friends home; a friend or colleague confronts the person about drinking behavior. Regardless of the reasons for seeking help, the alcoholic ready for treatment has, in most cases, reached a low point. Devoid of hope, physically depleted, and spiritually despairing, the alcoholic has finally recognized that alcohol controls his or her life. The first step on the road to recovery is to regain that control and to begin to assume responsibility for personal actions.

The Family's Role

Family members of an alcoholic sometimes take action before the alcoholic does. They may go to an organization or a treatment facility to seek help for themselves and their relative. An effective method of helping an alcoholic to confront the disease is a process called **intervention.** Essentially, an intervention is a planned confrontation with the alcoholic that involves several family members plus professional counselors. For more on how to plan an intervention, see the Building Communication Skills box. The family members express their love and concern, telling the alcoholic that they will no longer refrain from acknowledging the problem and affirming their support for appropriate treatment. A family intervention is the turning point for a growing number of alcoholics.

Treatment Programs

The alcoholic ready for help has several avenues for treatment: psychologists and psychiatrists specializing in the treatment of alcoholism, private treatment centers, hospitals specifically designed to treat alcoholics, community mental health facilities, and support groups such as Alcoholics Anonymous.

Talking to the Drinker

Friendship is not all fun and games. There are tough times in any relationship. Sometimes that means directly confronting a problem and giving support when your friend is having trouble coping. If you think a friend has a drinking problem, it may mean getting involved in some embarrassing discussions or situations. But you can help. Don't step back and pretend it's none of your business. Many problem drinkers say that talking with friends helped them seek professional guidance or gain better control of their drinking.

Do You Know Someone with a Drinking Problem?

If you are trying to figure out whether a friend has a drinking problem you need to evaluate:

- changes in his or her drinking behavior
- the reasons for his or her drinking
- the impact of your friend's drinking on his or her relationships, studies, and goals

Your friend doesn't have to get falling down drunk or drink every night to be in trouble with alcohol. Focusing on the reasons for your friend's drinking and the impact of the drinking will often help you determine whether your friend has a drinking problem.

How to Talk to the Drinker

If you care, show your concern. Don't be too polite to bring up the topic, but be tactful. Ask whether the person feels he or she has a drinking problem and continue asking questions that encourage frankness. Avoid sermons, lectures, and verbal attacks. Keep an open mind about how the person evaluates his or her situation.

Dealing with Defensiveness. Make it clear to the problem drinker that you dislike the behavior, not the person. Understand that the person's defensiveness is based on fear of facing the problem and isn't directed at you.

Dealing with Denial. If your discussions have no effect on your friend's drinking behavior, you should still tell him or her how the drinking problem affects you. For example, you can say how hard it is for you to enjoy going out together to a party because you are afraid he or she will get sick, pass out, or otherwise embarrass you both.

Dealing with Agreement. If at some point your friend agrees that drinking is creating personal problems, you may want to ask:

1. Why do you think you have a problem with alcohol?
2. What do you think you can do about it?
3. What are you going to do about it?
4. What kinds of support do you need from me to stop or limit your drinking?

You may also want to have some referrals ready for your friend. Most campuses and communities have discussion groups and/or counseling services.

Progress, Not Perfection

In some cases, even though the drinker agrees there is a problem, he or she may be unable or unwilling to act as quickly or directly as you'd like. Keep in mind that alcohol-related habits are hard to end or control. If your friend is struggling, try to

- remain supportive by recognizing the effort the person puts into even small attempts to limit drinking
- be prepared for some steps backward as well as forward
- help your friend make contact with recovering alcoholics
- encourage nondrinking behavior by planning activities not related to alcohol and by curbing your own drinking when you are with your friend

Source: From "How to Help a Friend with a Drinking Problem," by permission of American College Health Association, P.O. Box 28937, Baltimore MD 21240–8937 (phone 410/859–1500).

Private Treatment Facilities. Private treatment facilities have been making concerted efforts to attract patients through radio and television advertising. Upon admission to the treatment facility, the patient is given a complete physical exam to determine whether there are underlying medical problems that will interfere with treatment. Alcoholics who decide to quit drinking will experience withdrawal symptoms, including:

- Hyperexcitability
- Confusion
- Sleep disorders
- Convulsions
- Agitation
- Tremors of the hands
- Brief hallucinations
- Depression

- Headache

- Seizures

In a small percentage, alcohol withdrawal results in a severe syndrome known as **delirium tremens (DTs)**. Delirium tremens is characterized by confusion, delusions, agitated behavior, and hallucinations.

For any long-term addict, medical supervision is usually necessary. *Detoxification,* the process by which addicts end their dependence on a drug, is commonly carried out in a medical facility, where patients can be monitored to prevent fatal withdrawal reactions. Withdrawal takes from 7 to 21 days. Shortly after detoxification, alcoholics begin their treatment for psychological addiction. Most treatment facilities keep their patients from three to six weeks. Treatment at private treatment centers costs several thousand dollars, but some insurance programs or employers will assume most of this expense.

Family Therapy, Individual Therapy, and Group Therapy. Various individual and group therapies are also available. In family therapy, the person and family members gradually examine the psychological reasons underlying the addiction. In individual and group therapy with fellow addicts, alcoholics learn positive coping skills for use in situations that have regularly caused them to turn to alcohol. On some college campuses, the problems associated with alcohol abuse are so great that student health centers are opening their own treatment programs.

Other Types of Treatment. Two other treatments are drug and aversion therapy. Disulfiram (trade name: Antabuse) is the drug of choice for treating alcoholics. If alcohol is consumed, the drug causes such unpleasant effects as headache, nausea, vomiting, drowsiness, and hangover. These symptoms discourage the alcoholic from drinking. Aversion therapy is based on conditioning therapy. It works on the premise that the sight, smell, and taste of alcohol will acquire aversive properties if repeatedly paired with a noxious stimulus. For a period of 10 days, the alcoholic takes drugs that induce vomiting when combined with several drinks. These treatments work best in conjunction with some type of counseling.

Alcoholics Anonymous (AA) is a private, nonprofit, self-help organization founded in 1935. The organization, which relies upon group support to help people stop

For many alcoholics and their families, the support found in organizations like Alcoholics Anonymous can mean the difference between recovery and relapse.

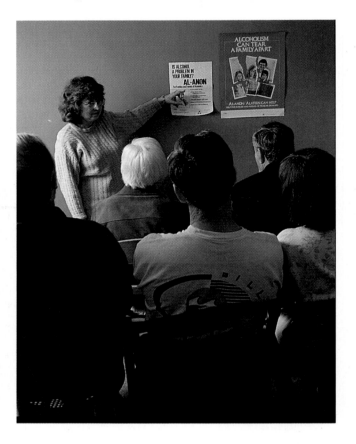

drinking, currently has over 1 million members and has branches all over the world. People attending their first AA meeting will find that no last names are ever used. Neither is anyone forced to speak. Members are taught to believe that their alcoholism is a lifetime problem. They are told that they may never use alcohol again. In meetings, they share their struggles with one another. They talk about the devastating effects alcoholism has had on their personal and professional lives. All members are asked to place their faith and control of the habit into the hands of a "higher power." The road to recovery is taken one step at a time. AA offers specialized meetings for gay, atheist, HIV-positive, and professional individuals with alcohol problems.

Alcoholics Anonymous also has auxiliary groups to help spouses or partners, friends, and children of alcoholics. *Al-Anon* is the group dedicated to helping adult relatives and friends of alcoholics understand the disease and learn how they can contribute to the recovery process. Spouses and other adult loved ones often play an unwitting role in perpetuating the alcoholic's problems. For example, the adult relative may call the alcoholic's boss and

Delirium tremens (DTs): A state of confusion brought on by withdrawal from alcohol. Symptoms include hallucinations, anxiety, and trembling.

Alcoholics Anonymous: An organization whose goal is to help alcoholics stop drinking; includes auxiliary branches such as Al-Anon and Alateen.

Managing Your Drinking Behaviors

After reading this chapter, you probably realize that the use of alcohol affects many aspects of your life. Assuming your religion doesn't forbid it, there is nothing wrong with using alcohol as long as you use it responsibly. But you must understand the possible problems and options regarding the use of alcohol and how it affects those around you in order to make informed decisions.

Making Decisions for You

Societal pressure to drink is everywhere. It's not enough that you are bombarded with ads showing the appeal of alcohol. It also seems that most college social events feature alcohol. As you walk in the door, you're handed a beer. Because of the easy availability of alcohol (especially after you turn 21), you need to take extra time to decide how *you* want to behave in situations where alcohol is being served. Can you set a drinking limit per social event? Can you set a drinking limit per week? If enticed, how can you stick with your decisions?

Checklist for Change: Making Personal Choices

✓ Do you feel comfortable with how you currently use alcohol? Would you like to change any of your current drinking behaviors?

✓ Do you know the rules to follow for responsible drinking if you are either a party guest or host?

✓ Do you know what resources are available to help yourself or others who might be experiencing a problem with alcohol? Would you know how to access these resources if you needed to?

✓ Have you examined your family's relationship with alcohol? Are there any reasons why you should be concerned about the role of alcohol in your family?

✓ Have you established responsible drinking guidelines for yourself?

✓ Have you found activities that don't involve alcohol that provide you some relief from stress?

✓ Do you really know what your long- and short-term health risks related to alcohol use are?

Checklist for Change: Making Community Choices

✓ Have you taken the time to become informed about how alcohol impacts others in your community?

✓ Have you prioritized the actions you can take to change the drinking environment on your campus? Do you know who the leaders on your campus are? Have you communicated your concerns to them?

✓ Do you act responsibly on your campus when you drink by not destroying property, hurting yourself or others, or drinking and driving?

✓ Do you voice your dissatisfactions to friends and others around you who display inappropriate behavior when they are drinking?

Critical Thinking

Here's a situation that you will encounter some day: You are giving a party at your apartment, during which you serve beer and wine. One of your closest friends seems to be drinking a lot; in fact, you think he's had five large glasses of wine over the past two hours. When he comes back for another, you suggest coffee. Your friend calmly explains that, because he is heavyset, he is able to absorb more alcohol than your thin friends. When you again suggest coffee, he becomes upset and says he is leaving the party. You think he arrived alone by car.

Using the DECIDE model described in Chapter 1, decide what you would do next. Think through the facts in the above situation before deciding: Is your friend legally intoxicated? In your state, will you be held responsible if he gets in an accident (whether or not legally intoxicated)? What options do you have?

---

lie about why the alcoholic missed work. At Al-Anon, these people's roles in their loved one's alcoholism are examined and explored, and alternative behaviors are suggested.

The support gained from talking with others who have similar problems is one of the greatest benefits derived from participation in Al-Anon. Many members learn how to exert greater control over their own lives. Some are able to rid themselves of the guilt they feel about their participation in their loved one's alcoholism.

Alateen, another AA-related organization, is designed to help adolescents live with an alcoholic parent or parents. They are taught that they are not at fault for their parents' problems. They learn skills to develop their self-esteem so they can function better socially. Alateen also helps them to overcome their guilt feelings.

Another self-help group is Women for Sobriety. This program was developed in 1975 out of a movement that recognized the differing needs of female alcoholics, who frequently have more severe problems than male alcoholics. Unlike AA meetings, where attendance can be quite large, each Women for Sobriety group has no more than 10 members. Another alternative to AA is Secular Organizations for Sobriety (SOS), which was founded in 1986 for people who cannot accept AA's spiritual emphasis.

Relapse

Success in recovery from alcoholism varies with the individual. A return to alcoholic habits often follows what appears to be a successful recovery. Some alcoholics never recover. Some partially recover and improve other parts of their lives, but remain dependent on alcohol. Many alcoholics refer to themselves as "recovering" throughout their lifetime; they never use the word *cured*.

Roughly 60 percent of alcoholics relapse (resume drinking) within the first three months of treatment. Why is the relapse rate so high? Treating an addiction requires more than getting the addict to stop using; it also requires getting the person to break a pattern of behavior that has dominated his or her life.

People who are seeking to regain a healthy lifestyle must not only confront their addiction, but must also guard against the tendency to relapse. Drinkers with compulsive personalities need to learn to understand themselves and take control. Others need to view treatment as a long-term process that takes a lot of effort beyond attending a weekly self-help group meeting. In order to work, a recovery program must offer the alcoholic ways to increase self-esteem and resume personal growth.

Can Recovering Alcoholics Take a Drink? During the mid-1970s, some scientists believed that recovering alcoholics could return to drinking on a limited social basis. Several studies supported this notion, but they have since been refuted. Research conducted over a period of 5 to 10 years has shown that less than 1 percent of recovering alcoholics are able to resume drinking on a limited basis. To prevent the return to the bottle, abstinence is the safest and sanest path for reformed alcoholics to follow.[29]

A comprehensive treatment approach that includes drug therapy, group support, family therapy, and personal counseling designed to improve living and coping skills is usually the most effective course of treatment. The alcoholics most likely to recover completely are those who developed their dependencies after the age of 20, those with intact and supportive family units, and those who have reached a high level of personal disgust coupled with strong motivation to recover.

Summary

- Alcohol is a central nervous system depressant used by 70 percent of all Americans and 85 percent of all college students; 44 percent of college students are binge drinkers. While consumption trends are slowly creeping downward, college students are under extreme pressure to consume alcohol.

- Alcohol's effect on the body is measured by the blood alcohol concentration (BAC), the ratio of alcohol to total blood volume. The higher the BAC, the greater the impaired judgment and coordination and drowsiness. Some negative consequences associated with alcohol use and college students are lower grade point averages, academic problems, dropping out of school, unplanned sex, hangovers, and injury. Long-term effects of alcohol overuse include damage to the nervous system, cardiovascular damage, liver disease, and increased risk for cancer. Use during pregnancy can cause fetal alcohol effects (FAE) or fetal alcohol syndrome (FAS). Alcohol is also a causative factor in traffic accidents.

- Alcohol use becomes alcoholism when it interferes with school, work, or social and family relationships or entails violations of the law. Causes of alcoholism include biological and family factors and social and cultural factors. Alcoholism has far-reaching effects on families, especially on children. Children of alcoholics have problematic childhoods and generally take those problems into adulthood.

- Recovery is problematic for alcoholics. Most alcoholics do not admit to a problem until reaching a major life crisis or having their families intervene. Treatment options include detoxification at private medical facilities, therapy (family, individual, or group), and programs like Alcoholics Anonymous. Most alcoholics relapse (60 percent within three months) because alcoholism is a behavioral addiction as well as a chemical addiction.

Discussion Questions

1. When it comes to drinking alcohol, how much is too much? How can you avoid slipping from having a drink or two in an evening to loosen up to having enough drinks to impinge upon your judgment? When you see a friend having "too many" drinks at a party, what actions do you normally take? What actions could you take?

2. Determine what your BAC would be if you drank four beers in two hours (assume they are spaced at equal intervals). What physiological effects will you feel after each drink? Would a person of similar weight show greater effects after having four gin and tonics instead of beer? Why or why not? At what point in your life

should you start worrying about the long-term effects of alcohol abuse?

3. Describe a social drinker, a problem drinker, and an alcoholic. What factors may cause someone to slip from being a social drinker to being an alcoholic? What effect does alcoholism have on an alcoholic's family?

4. Does anyone recover from alcoholism? Why or why not?

Application Exercise

Reread the What Do You Think? scenarios at the beginning of the chapter and answer the following questions.

1. From what you have learned in this chapter, how might Dave cope with the peer pressure to drink alcohol?

2. How is the perception that "everyone" drinks reinforced on college campuses?

3. What are some alternatives to drinking alcohol that Dave can pursue?

4. If Dave is somewhere that alcohol is being served and he doesn't want to drink, what can he do?

5. What responsibility does the restaurant have in protecting the fetus from a known teratogen?

6. What responsibility does the mother have for protecting the fetus?

7. If you were the waiter/waitress, what would you do?

Further Reading

Michael Dorris, *The Broken Cord* (New York: HarperCollins, 1992).

A personal story about and a current source of information on fetal alcohol syndrome.

G. Leaton and J. Kinney, *Loosening the Grip* (St. Louis: Times Mirror/Mosby, 1990).

A handbook of alcohol information. Covers the basic information that an alcohol counselor or other professional confronted with alcohol problems needs to know. Synthesizes and organizes information from the fields of medicine, psychology, psychiatry, anthropology, sociology, and counseling as it applies to alcohol use and treatment.

National Institute on Alcohol Abuse and Alcoholism (NIAAA), *Research Monographs* (Washington DC: U.S. Department of Health and Human Services).

A series of publications containing the results of a number of studies conducted by research scientists under the auspices of NIAAA during the late 1970s and 1980s. Addresses such issues as alcohol use among the elderly, occupational alcoholism, social drinking, and the relationship between heredity and alcoholism.

S. Peele and A. Brodsky, *The Truth about Addiction and Recovery* (New York: Simon and Schuster, 1991).

A powerful, well-documented challenge to the concept of addiction as disease and to the 12-step ideology of recovery.

M. Sandmaier, *The Invisible Alcoholics: Women and Alcohol Abuse,* 2nd ed. (Blue Ridge Summit, PA: Tab Books, 1992).

Explores why women drink, social attitudes toward their drinking, their treatment needs, and how and where they can get help. Includes in-depth interviews with diverse women.

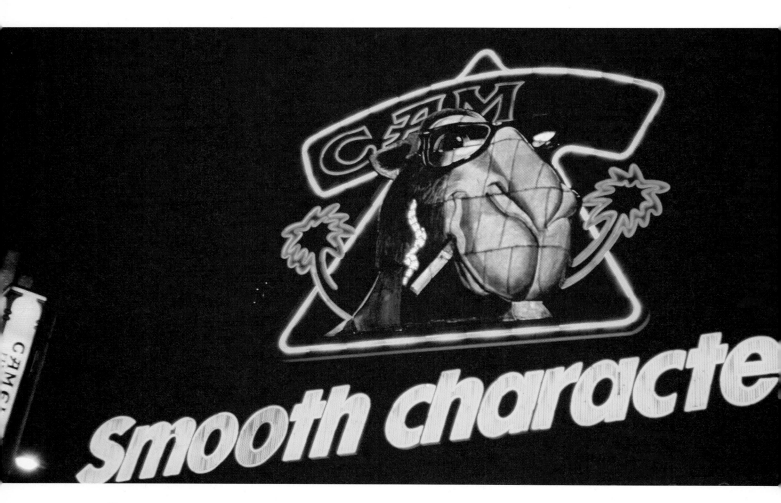

CHAPTER OBJECTIVES

◆ Discuss the social issues involved in tobacco use, including advertising and the medical costs associated with tobacco use.

◆ Discuss how the chemicals in tobacco products affect a smoker's body.

◆ Review how smoking affects a smoker's risk for cancer, cardiovascular disease, and respiratory diseases, and how it adversely affects a fetus's health.

◆ Discuss the risks associated with using smokeless tobacco.

◆ Evaluate the risks to nonsmokers associated with environmental tobacco smoke.

◆ Describe strategies people adopt to quit using tobacco products, including strategies aimed at breaking the nicotine addiction as well as habit.

◆ Compare the benefits and risks associated with caffeine, and summarize the health consequences of long-term caffeine use.

$\mathcal{T}$obacco and Caffeine

Legal Addictions

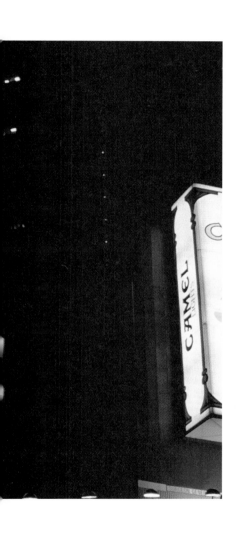

Mike's roommate John uses chewing tobacco. He has chewed tobacco for years without noticing any ill effects. Other than the annoying habit chewers have of spitting into bottles or cans, Mike really doesn't see what is so bad about chewing tobacco. After all, chewing tobacco doesn't seem as harmful as cigarettes because John doesn't inhale any smoke. John has offered Mike a chew on several occasions. Mike likes the pleasant lift he gets from using the chewing tobacco.

■ What health problems should both Mike and John be concerned about? What are the major health risks associated with smokeless tobacco use? Is using smokeless tobacco safer than smoking? Why would Mike want to begin a habit that is difficult to break and has so many health risks associated with it?

Tracy's vacation is finally here! She has been looking forward for months to going on vacation with Jodi and her friends. But when they arrive to pick Tracy up, Tracy finds out that one of Jodi's friends who is going with them smokes two packs of cigarettes a day, practically one right after the other. Tracy cannot stand breathing cigarette smoke, especially in cars or other enclosed places. The smoke makes her eyes water, her throat sore, and her nose run. She cannot bear the thought of an eight-hour car ride under these smoky conditions.

■ What should Tracy do in this situation? What do you think most people would do under these circumstances? What issues are involved for both the smokers and the nonsmokers?

obacco use is the single most preventable cause of death in the United States.[1] Each year, smoking claims more lives than alcohol and drug abuse combined. More Americans die annually from tobacco-related health problems than died in World War I, World War II, and the Vietnam War combined (see Figure 14.1). While tobacco companies continue to publish full-page advertisements refuting the dangers of smoking, over 418,000 Americans die each year of tobacco-related diseases.[2]

OUR SMOKING SOCIETY

In 1990, more than 55 million Americans—approximately 26.5 percent of the population aged 17 or older—smoked cigarettes, consuming more than 533 billion cigarettes per year. This translates to 10,000 cigarettes per smoker. The average age at which Americans begin smoking is 11.6 years, and those who begin smoking this early have only a 15 percent chance of ever quitting.

Children in homes where the parents smoke are not only exposed to harmful second-hand smoke, but they are 90 percent more likely to take up smoking than children raised in nonsmoking households.

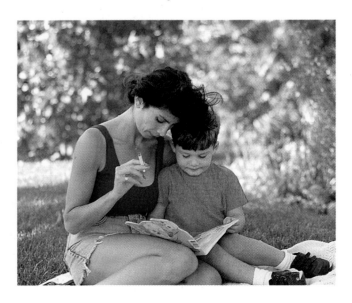

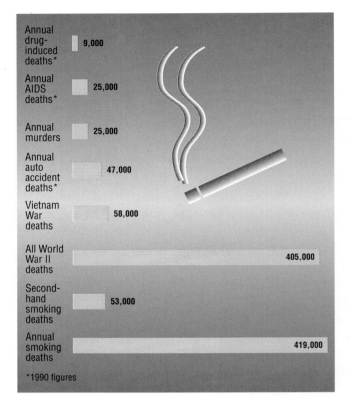

Annual drug-induced deaths* 9,000
Annual AIDS deaths* 25,000
Annual murders 25,000
Annual auto accident deaths* 47,000
Vietnam War deaths 58,000
All World War II deaths 405,000
Second-hand smoking deaths 53,000
Annual smoking deaths 419,000

*1990 figures

FIGURE 14.1

Smoking's Toll

Source: Data from National Center for Health Statistics, U.S. Department of Defense, as they appeared in a graph in the *Boston Globe,* 11 April 1994, 25.

The desire to model adult behavior plays a major role in teenagers' smoking. In households where one parent smokes, children are 90 percent more likely to take up smoking than are children from households where neither parent smokes.[3] In addition, children whose peers smoke were found to have an 80 percent chance of adopting the habit.

How many teenagers smoke? A 1987 survey of American teens indicated 10 percent. An identical survey conducted one year later found the proportion of teen smokers had increased to 13 percent, with more girls smoking than boys.[4] By 1993, almost 19 percent of high school seniors were smoking. This increase is partly attributed to the ready availability of tobacco products through vending machines and the aggressive drive by tobacco companies to entice young people to smoke.

Cigarette smoking in the United States results in untold loss of human potential. In 1991, it caused over 400,000 premature deaths.[5] According to the Department of Health and Human Services, 29.5 percent of males and 23.8 percent of females smoke. The age group with the highest percentage of smokers is the 35-to-44-year-old group. This makes sense, as most of these people developed their habit as adolescents 20 to 30 years ago, when the practice of smoking was commonplace.

The percentage of Americans who smoke dropped throughout the 1980s. In fact, the 26.5 percent figure quoted above for 1990 is the lowest percentage recorded since the 1950s. But because the population has grown, there are 1.5 million more smokers today than there were 20 years ago.[6] See Table 14.1 for a group profile of American smokers.

Tobacco and Social Issues

The production and distribution of tobacco products in the United States and abroad involve many political and economic issues. During the 1980s, tobacco products were one of the United States' top five exports. Tobacco-growing states derive substantial income from tobacco production, and federal, state, and local governments benefit enormously from cigarette taxes.

More recently, nationwide health awareness has led to a decrease in the use of tobacco products among U.S. adults. To compensate for revenue losses, many major tobacco companies have merged with or purchased other corporations that market food or beverage products.

Advertising. Tobacco companies spend billions of dollars advertising their products to keep them in the public eye. With the number of U.S. smokers declining by about 1 million each year, the industry must actively recruit new smokers. Campaigns are directed at all age, social, and ethnic groups, but because children and teenagers constitute 90 percent of all new smokers, much of the advertising has been directed at them.

Tobacco companies' campaigns aimed at young people suggest that smoking is a mature, elegant, sophisticated activity. Cartoon characters such as Old Joe have been used on campuses, in magazines, and even to promote a line of clothing. A recent study indicated that over 95 percent of school-age children can identify this character.[7] After Camel, Marlboro and Newport were the most heavily advertised brands during 1990. A survey found that 84 percent of adolescents who smoke purchased one of these three brands.[8] Millions of young people are persuaded to light up by magazine and billboard ads depicting the strength and independence of the Marlboro man, the suave character of Joe Camel, and the vibrancy of young, successful, physically fit people enjoying Newport cigarettes.

Advertisements in women's magazines imply that cigarette smoking is a liberating thing to do. These ads have apparently been working. From 1975 through 1988, cigarette sales to women increased dramatically. Recently, the Reynolds company targeted 18-to-20-year-old women—the only age group of Americans whose rate of smoking continues to rise. By 1987, statistics indicated that cigarette-induced lung cancer had surpassed breast cancer as the leading form of cancer death among women.

Women are not the only targets of gender-based cigarette advertisements. Males are depicted changing clothes in a locker room, charging over rugged terrain in off-road vehicles, or riding bay stallions into the sunset in blatant appeals to a need to feel and appear masculine. In addition, minorities are often targeted, as discussed in the Multicultural Perspectives box.

Financial Costs to Society. The use of tobacco products is costly to all of us in terms of lost productivity and lost lives. Health care for smoking-related illnesses (in smokers and passive smokers alike) and lost productivity costs the nation an estimated $68 billion annually (see Figure 14.2). Employers must bear another $13 billion a year in expenses related to smoking (absenteeism, added cost of fire insurance, training costs to replace employees who die prematurely, disability payments, and so on).[9] These expenses increase the costs of goods and services for us all. In 1995, the state of Florida took action against the tobacco industry to recover money spent treating Medicaid

TABLE 14.1 ■ Percentage of Population that Smokes (Age 18 and Older) among Select Groups in the United States

	Percentage
Males	
Overall	27.5
White	27.0
Black	32.9
Hispanic	25.6
Females	
Overall	23.0
White	23.3
Black	23.2
Hispanic	13.4
Occupation	
White-collar	25.9
Service workers	30.2
Blue-collar	41.1

Source: Reprinted from U.S. Department of Health and Human Services, *Strategies to Control Tobacco Use in the U.S.*, NIH Publication No. 92–3316, (October 1991), iii.

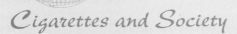
Cigarettes and Society

- Billboards advertising tobacco products are placed in African-American communities four to five times more often than in white communities. In 1985, tobacco companies spent $5.8 million for advertisements on 8-foot billboards in African-American communities, accounting for 37 percent of total advertising in this medium.

- Not only do cigarette companies advertise heavily in popular black magazines, they also successfully target the African-American community by sponsoring entertainment, sporting, and cultural events and political and literacy campaigns.

- Developing nations often lack the legislative controls necessary to regulate tobacco use. In many of these countries, cigarettes are sold without the warning label required in the countries where they are manufactured. American cigarettes sold in the Philippines contain more tar and nicotine and produce more carbon monoxide than do the

same brands sold in the United States. Cigarettes sold in Asia have a higher tar content than do cigarettes sold in Western countries.

- In order to increase sales in developing countries, promotional ads are often aimed at women. The reason for this is simple: Half the men in developing countries already smoke, while only 5 percent of the women do. In contrast, about 30 percent of both men and women in most industrialized countries are smokers.

- As the smoking of tobacco has become a popular habit around the world, it has taken a tremendous toll. Worldwide, tobacco use is responsible for 90 percent of all lung cancer deaths, 75 percent of bronchitis deaths, and 25 percent of cardiovascular deaths. The World Health Organization (WHO) estimates that every year over 2.5 million people die prematurely as a result of smoking cigarettes.

patients with smoking-related illnesses. The Health Headlines box details the lawsuit.

Because of their work environments, some industrial workers face increased risks for lung disease. Workers who smoke and are also exposed to toxic chemicals or fumes from rubber, chlorine, asbestos, or coal or cotton dust are up to 60 times more likely to develop lung cancer as are nonsmokers who work in the same environments.

WHAT DO YOU THINK?

What would it be like if the United States were smoke-free? What types of repercussions would there be? Who would be affected? What do you think needs to be done to reduce the number of smokers in the United States?

TOBACCO AND ITS EFFECTS

Tobacco is available in several forms: Cigarettes, cigars, and pipes are used for burning and inhaling tobacco. **Snuff** is a finely ground form of tobacco that can be inhaled, chewed, or placed against the gums. **Chewing tobacco,** also known as "smokeless tobacco," is placed between the gums and teeth for sucking or chewing.

The chemical stimulant **nicotine** is the major psychoactive substance in all these tobacco products. In its natural form, nicotine is a colorless liquid that turns

brown upon oxidation (exposure to oxygen). When tobacco leaves are burned in a cigarette, pipe, or cigar, nicotine is released and inhaled into the lungs. Sucking or chewing a quid of tobacco releases nicotine into the saliva, and the nicotine is then absorbed through the mucous membranes in the mouth.

Smoking is the most common form of tobacco use. Smoking delivers a strong dose of nicotine to the user, along with an additional 4,000 chemical substances. Among these chemicals are various gases and vapors that carry particulate matter in concentrations that are 500,000 times greater than the most air-polluted cities in the world.[10]

Particulate matter condenses in the lungs to form a thick, brownish sludge called **tar.** Tar contains various carcinogenic (cancer-causing) agents such as benzopyrene and chemical irritants such as phenol. Phenol has the potential to combine with other chemicals to contribute to the development of lung cancer.

In healthy lungs, millions of tiny hairlike tissues called cilia sweep away foreign matter. Once the foreign material is swept up and collected by the cilia, it can be expelled from the lungs by coughing. Nicotine impairs the cleansing function of the cilia by paralyzing them for up to one hour following the smoking of a single cigarette. Tars and other solids in tobacco smoke are thus allowed to accumulate and irritate sensitive lung tissue.

Tar and nicotine are not the only harmful chemicals in cigarettes. In fact, tars account for only 8 percent of the components of tobacco smoke. The remaining 92 percent

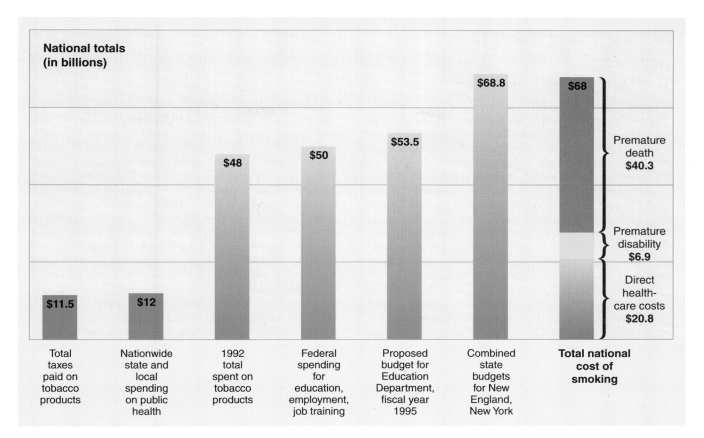

National totals (in billions)

- Total taxes paid on tobacco products — $11.5
- Nationwide state and local spending on public health — $12
- 1992 total spent on tobacco products — $48
- Federal spending for education, employment, job training — $50
- Proposed budget for Education Department, fiscal year 1995 — $53.5
- Combined state budgets for New England, New York — $68.8
- Total national cost of smoking — $68
  - Premature death $40.3
  - Premature disability $6.9
  - Direct health-care costs $20.8

FIGURE 14.2

Costs of Smoking to Society

Source: Data from National Center for Health Statistics, U.S. Department of Defense, as they appeared in a graph in the *Boston Globe,* 11 April 1994, 26.

is made up of various gases, the most dangerous of which is **carbon monoxide.** In tobacco smoke, the concentration of carbon monoxide is 800 times higher than the level considered safe by the U.S. Environmental Protection Agency (EPA). In the human body, carbon monoxide reduces the oxygen-carrying capacity of the red blood cells by binding with the receptor sites for oxygen. Smoking thus diminishes the capacity of the circulatory system to carry oxygen, causing oxygen deprivation in many body tissues.

The heat from tobacco smoke, which can reach 1,616 degrees Fahrenheit, is also harmful to the smoker. Inhaling hot gases and vapors exposes sensitive mucous membranes to irritating chemicals that weaken the tissues and contribute to the development of cancers of the mouth, larynx, and throat.

Filtered cigarettes designed to reduce levels of gases such as hydrogen cyanide and hydrocarbons may actually deliver more hazardous carbon monoxide to the user than do nonfiltered brands. Some smokers use low-tar and nicotine products as an excuse to smoke more cigarettes.

This practice is self-defeating, because such smokers wind up exposing themselves to more harmful substances than they would if they smoked regular-strength cigarettes.

Clove cigarettes contain about 40 percent ground cloves (a spice) and about 60 percent tobacco. Many users mis-

Snuff: A powdered form of tobacco that is sniffed and absorbed through the mucous membranes in the nose or placed inside the cheek and sucked.

Chewing tobacco: A stringy type of tobacco that is placed in the mouth and then sucked or chewed.

Nicotine: The stimulant chemical in tobacco products.

Tar: A thick, brownish substance condensed from particulate matter in smoked tobacco.

Carbon monoxide: A gas found in cigarette smoke that binds at oxygen receptor sites in the blood.

Florida Sues the Tobacco Industry

Ira Stark, a retired cabbie, has a smoking habit that cost taxpayers more than $20,000 last year, and the meter is still running. The 53-year-old Miami resident smoked three packs a day for almost four decades; now he has emphysema and needs bottled oxygen to breathe. Medicaid—i.e., taxpayers—foots the bill for his respiratory problems ($400 a month for oxygen, $18,000 for a nine-day hospital stay last year). Despite the tab he's already rung up, Stark still puffs his way through half a pack a day: "I just have this unbelievable craving," he says. Stark admits nobody made him start smoking, but since tobacco companies make the product he just can't seem to quit, he figures they're at least partly responsible for his costly state of misery.

The state of Florida agrees. Last week it filed a $1.43 billion suit against the tobacco industry to recoup money spent treating Medicaid patients with smoking-related ailments. West Virginia, Minnesota, and Mississippi have filed similar suits. Meanwhile, a U.S. district judge in New Orleans just cleared the way for a class action by three current smokers and the wife of a deceased smoker who claim that tobacco manufacturers hid the addictive properties of nicotine. If the suit proceeds, almost anyone who is "nicotine dependent" could join and seek up to $50,000 each from cigarette makers. Says Florida Governor Lawton Chiles: "It's time for the tobacco industry to take responsibility for the damage it does."

So far, that's something the industry has avoided. More than 800 antismoking lawsuits have been filed since 1954, but not a single cigarette maker has been forced to pay a single penny in damages. Says Maura Ellis, a spokeswoman for R. J. Reynolds Tobacco Co.: "Juries have consistently found that smokers should be held responsible for their own actions." But public sentiment began to shift during last year's congressional hearings, in which tobacco executives stubbornly refused to admit that smoking was addictive, even as internal company memos revealed that cigarette makers have long understood—and hidden—nicotine's addictive properties. Says Sheldon Schlesinger, a lawyer working on Florida's case: "For years we said to smokers, 'If you want to quit, why don't you quit?' But now people understand that nicotine is addictive, just like a lot of other substances that are outlawed."

Lawyers also understand that if juries begin to turn on tobacco manufacturers, the potential for making money is mind-boggling. There are 46 million smokers in this country and 400,000 smoking-related deaths each year. In the Florida Medicaid case alone, the attorneys who succeed in winning the legally mandated triple damages and collecting their 25 percent contingency fee would divvy up a $350 million pot. So it's hardly surprising that some of the country's best product-liability lawyers have been eager to join Chiles' Dream Team. Meanwhile, 60 U.S. law firms have pledged $100,000 each to support the New Orleans class action, attracted, no doubt, by speculation that the damage award could run as high as $100 billion if the antismoking forces prevail. "It's no longer David vs. Goliath," says John Banzhaf, executive director of the antismoking group Action on Smoking and Health. "The big law firms are willing to put up lots of money because they think there's a big payoff."

In the Florida case, the state also tried to even out the odds by amending its product-liability laws last year. Now it can claim damages based on general health statistics, and cigarette makers can be assessed financial penalties based on their market share, rather than having to prove that an individual patient's illness was caused by smoking a particular brand. The tobacco companies have already tried to have this new statute declared unconstitutional, and makers of other products such as alcoholic beverages have expressed concern that the law could be used against them as well. But in a move that should help soothe such corporate fears, the House Judiciary Committee passed a measure that would severely limit punitive damage awards. The measure, which is part of the G.O.P.'s "Contract with America," must still pass the full House and Senate, and would not apply retroactively to Florida's antitobacco efforts.

Whatever that bill's ultimate fate, the tobacco wars are sure to drag on like a bad habit. This week several major health organizations and a bipartisan group of governors will publicly rededicate themselves to the fight, waged with sin taxes, lawsuits, and no-smoking areas. Yet some legal experts doubt that the Medicaid-reimbursement suits will be the decisive new weapon. Says Stephen Sugerman, a law professor at the University of California, Berkeley: "My feeling is that a lot of these untried methods have a dubious likelihood of success." But as any nicotine addict knows, when people want to try to stop smoking, they're willing to try almost anything.

Source: Reprinted from Christopher John Farley, "Cough Up That Cash," *Time,* March 6, 1995, 47. © 1995 Time Inc. Reprinted by permission.

takenly believe that these products are made entirely of ground cloves and that smoking them eliminates the risks associated with tobacco. In fact, clove cigarettes contain higher levels of tar, nicotine, and carbon monoxide than do regular cigarettes. In addition, the numbing effect of eugenol, the active ingredient in cloves, allows smokers to inhale the smoke more deeply. Most users of clove cigarettes are teenagers and young adults who are smoking

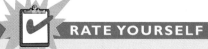
Are You Addicted to Nicotine?

Answer the following questions as honestly as you can.

1. Do you smoke every day?

2. Do you smoke because of shyness and to build up self-confidence?

3. Do you smoke to escape from boredom and worries or while under pressure?

4. Have you ever burned a hole in your clothes, carpet, furniture, or car?

5. Have you ever had to go to the store late at night or at another inconvenient time because you were out of cigarettes?

6. Do you feel defensive or angry when people tell you that your cigarette smoke is bothering them?

7. Has a doctor or dentist suggested that you stop smoking?

8. Have you promised someone that you would stop smoking, then broken your promise?

9. Have you felt physical or emotional discomfort when trying to quit?

10. Have you successfully stopped smoking for a period of time, only to start again?

11. Do you buy extra supplies of tobacco to make sure you won't run out?

12. Do you find it difficult to imagine life without smoking?

13. Do you choose only activities and entertainment during which you can smoke?

14. Do you prefer, seek out, or feel more comfortable in the company of smokers?

15. Do you inwardly despise or feel ashamed of yourself because of your smoking?

16. Do you ever find yourself lighting up without having consciously decided to?

17. Has your smoking caused trouble at home or in a relationship?

18. Do you ever tell yourself that you can stop smoking whenever you want to?

19. Have you ever felt that your life would be better if you didn't smoke?

20. Do you continue to smoke even though you are aware of the health hazards posed by smoking?

If you answered yes to one or two of these questions, there is a chance that you are addicted or are becoming addicted to nicotine. If you answered yes to three or more, you are probably already addicted to nicotine.

Source: © Copyright 1988 Nicotine Anonymous World Services, Inc. For additional information, write: Nicotine Anonymous World Services, 2118 Greenwich Street, San Francisco, CA 94123, or call 415/922–8575.

---

them under the mistaken assumption that these products are safe. Annual imports of clove cigarettes have reached 150 million cigarettes.[11]

Physiological Effects of Nicotine

Nicotine is a powerful central nervous system stimulant that produces a variety of physiological effects. Its stimulant action in the cerebral cortex produces an aroused, alert mental state. Nicotine also stimulates the adrenal glands, increasing the production of adrenaline. The physical effects of nicotine stimulation include increased heart and respiratory rate, constriction of blood vessels, and subsequent increased blood pressure because the heart must work harder to pump blood through the narrowed vessels.

Nicotine decreases the stomach contractions that signal hunger. It also decreases blood sugar levels. These factors, along with decreased sensation in the taste buds, reduce appetite. For this reason, many smokers eat less than nonsmokers do and weigh, on average, 7 pounds less than nonsmokers. Beginning smokers usually feel the effects of nicotine with their first puff. These symptoms, called **nicotine poisoning**, include dizziness, lightheadedness, rapid, erratic pulse, clammy skin, nausea, vomiting, and diarrhea. The effects of nicotine poisoning cease as soon as tolerance to the chemical develops. Medical research indicates that tolerance develops almost immediately in new users, perhaps after the second or third cigarette. In contrast, tolerance to most other drugs, such as alcohol, develops over a period of months or years. See the Rate Yourself box to find out if you are addicted to nicotine.

Nicotine poisoning: Symptoms often experienced by beginning smokers; they include dizziness; diarrhea; lightheadedness; rapid, erratic pulse; clammy skin; nausea; and vomiting.

HEALTH HAZARDS OF SMOKING

Cigarette smoking adversely affects the health of every person who smokes. Each pack of cigarettes has a warning label alerting smokers to some of the dangers. Smoking has been estimated to be responsible for almost 19 percent of all U.S. deaths each year—that's almost one out of every five deaths. Each day cigarettes contribute to over 1,000 deaths from cancer, heart disease, and respiratory diseases.

Cancer

The American Cancer Society estimates that tobacco smoking is the cause of approximately 30 percent of all deaths from cancer and of more than 85 to 90 percent of all cases of lung cancer. Lung cancer, the leading cause of cancer deaths in the United States, kills more than 153,000 Americans each year: 94,000 men and 59,000 women. Less than 10 percent of lung cancers occur among nonsmokers.[12] Figure 14.3 illustrates how tobacco smoke damages the lungs.

Lung cancer can take from 10 to 30 years to develop. The outlook for victims of this disease is poor. Most lung cancer is not diagnosed until it is fairly widespread in the body; at that point, the five-year survival rate is only 13 percent. When a malignancy is diagnosed and recognized while still localized, the five-year survival rate rises to 46 percent.

If you are a smoker, your risk of developing lung cancer is dependent on several factors. First, the number of cigarettes you smoke per day is important. Someone who smokes two packs a day is 15 to 25 times more likely to develop lung cancer than a nonsmoker. If you started smoking in your teens, you have a greater chance of developing lung cancer than people who started later. If you inhale deeply when you smoke, you also increase your chances of developing the disease. Occupational or domestic exposure to other irritants, such as asbestos and radon, will also increase your likelihood of developing lung cancer.[13]

Tobacco is linked to other cancers as well. Cigarette smoking increases the risk of pancreatic cancer by 70 percent. Smokers can reduce those odds by 30 percent if they quit for 11 years or more.[14] Cancers of the lip, tongue, salivary glands, and esophagus are five times more likely to occur in smokers than in nonsmokers. Smokers are also more likely to develop kidney, bladder, and larynx cancers.

Cardiovascular Disease

Half of all tobacco-related deaths occur as a result of some form of heart disease.[15] Smokers have a 70 percent higher death rate from heart disease than nonsmokers do, and heavy smokers have a 200 percent higher death rate than moderate smokers do. In fact, smoking cigarettes poses as great a risk for developing heart disease as high blood pressure and high cholesterol levels do.

The likelihood of developing cancer and other smoking-related illnesses increases for smokers who start in their teens.

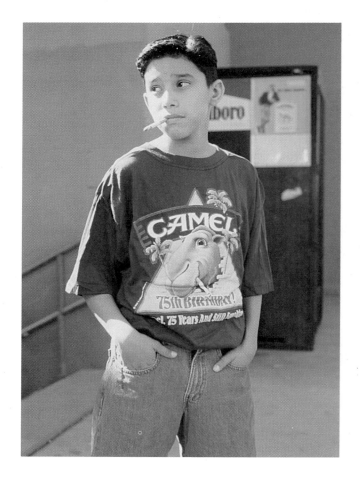

Platelet adhesiveness: Stickiness of red blood cells associated with blood clots.

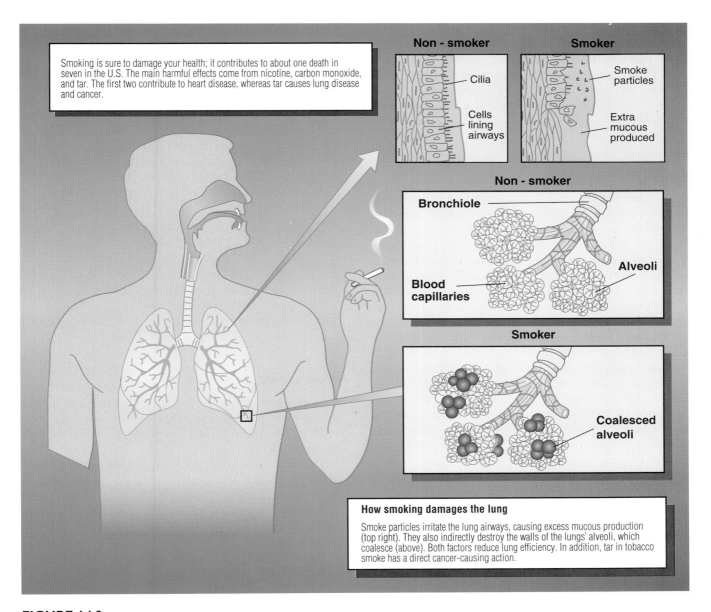

Smoking is sure to damage your health; it contributes to about one death in seven in the U.S. The main harmful effects come from nicotine, carbon monoxide, and tar. The first two contribute to heart disease, whereas tar causes lung disease and cancer.

Non - smoker

Cilia

Cells lining airways

Smoker

Smoke particles

Extra mucous produced

Non - smoker

Bronchiole

Blood capillaries

Alveoli

Smoker

Coalesced alveoli

How smoking damages the lung

Smoke particles irritate the lung airways, causing excess mucous production (top right). They also indirectly destroy the walls of the lungs' alveoli, which coalesce (above). Both factors reduce lung efficiency. In addition, tar in tobacco smoke has a direct cancer-causing action.

FIGURE 14.3

How Cigarette Smoking Damages the Lungs

Smoking contributes to heart disease by adding the equivalent of 10 years of aging to the arteries.[16] One possible explanation for this is that smoking increases the development of atherosclerosis, the buildup of fatty deposits in the heart and major blood vessels. For unknown reasons, smoking decreases blood levels of HDLs (high-density lipoproteins), which help protect against heart attacks. Smoking also contributes to **platelet adhesiveness,** or the sticking together of red blood cells that is associated with blood clots. The oxygen deprivation associated with smoking decreases the oxygen levels supplied to the heart and can weaken tissues. Smoking also contributes to irregular heart rhythms, which can lead to a sudden heart attack.

The number of years a person has smoked does not seem to bear much relation to his or her risk for cardiovascular disease. If a person quits smoking, the risk of dying from a heart attack is reduced by half after only one year of not smoking and declines gradually thereafter. After 15 years of not smoking, the ex-smoker's risk of cardiovascular disease is similar to that of people who have never smoked.

Stroke. Smokers are twice as likely to suffer strokes as nonsmokers. A stroke occurs when a small blood vessel in the brain bursts or is blocked by a blood clot, denying oxygen and nourishment to vital portions of the brain. Depending on the area of the brain supplied by the vessel, the stroke can result in paralysis, loss of mental functioning, or death. Smoking contributes to strokes by raising blood pressure, thereby increasing the stress on vessel walls. Platelet adhesiveness contributes to clotting. Five to 15 years after they have stopped smoking, the risk of stroke for ex-smokers is the same as that for people who have never smoked.

Respiratory Diseases

The respiratory system is quickly impaired by smoking. Smokers can feel the impact of their smoking in a relatively short period of time—they are more prone to breathlessness, chronic cough, and excess phlegm production than nonsmokers their age. Smokers tend to miss work one-third more often than nonsmokers do, primarily because of respiratory diseases. Cigarette smokers are up to 18 times more likely than nonsmokers to die of diseases of the lungs.

Chronic bronchitis is the presence of a productive cough that persists or reoccurs frequently. It may develop in smokers because their inflamed lungs produce more mucus and constantly try to rid themselves of this mucus and foreign particles. The effort to do so results in the "smoker's hack," the persistent cough experienced by most smokers. Smokers are more prone than nonsmokers to respiratory ailments such as influenza, pneumonia, and colds.

Emphysema is a chronic disease in which the alveoli (the tiny air sacs in the lungs) are destroyed, impairing the lungs' ability to obtain oxygen and remove carbon dioxide. As a result, breathing becomes difficult. Whereas healthy people expend only about 5 percent of their energy breathing, people with advanced emphysema expend nearly 80 percent of their energy breathing. A simple movement such as rising from a seated position may be painful and difficult for the emphysema patient. Since the heart has to work harder to do even the simplest tasks, it may become enlarged and the person may die from heart damage. There is no known cure for emphysema. Approximately 80 percent of all cases of emphysema are related to cigarette smoking.

Emphysema: A chronic lung disease in which the tiny air sacs in the lungs are destroyed, making breathing difficult.

Sudden infant death syndrome (SIDS): Death that occurs without apparent cause in babies under two years of age; some cases may be associated with tobacco use by the mother during pregnancy.

Other Health Effects of Smoking

Gum disease is three times more common in smokers than in nonsmokers. Smokers also lose significantly more teeth than do nonsmokers, despite any efforts to practice good oral hygiene.[17] Smokers are also likely to use more medications than are nonsmokers. Nicotine and the other ingredients in cigarettes interfere with the metabolism of drugs: nicotine speeds up the process by which the body uses and eliminates drugs, so that medications become less effective. The smoker may therefore have to take a higher dosage of a drug or take it more frequently.

---

*W*HAT DO YOU THINK?

Given all the dramatic health hazards related to cigarette smoking, why is it difficult for people to stop smoking? Do you think tobacco companies should be held liable for damages resulting from tobacco use?

Women and Smoking

A study released in 1989 indicated that smokers have a greater risk of developing cervical cancer than do nonsmokers. The risk seemed to be higher for women under the age of 30.[18]

The risk of heart disease for women smokers who smoke more than 25 cigarettes per day is 500 percent higher than it is for nonsmokers. Even smoking one to four cigarettes per day doubles a woman's risk for heart attack. It makes no difference if she smokes low- or high-nicotine cigarettes.

Women who smoke and use oral contraceptives run a higher risk of stroke and heart attack, though just how much higher is difficult to estimate. Current birth control pills have lower—and theoretically safer—levels of hormones, so it is hard to tell if earlier research on the risks of heart disease and stroke still holds true.

Smoking appears to cause women to begin menopause one to two years early. But former smokers start their menopause at about the same age as do women who have never smoked. Smoking also contributes to osteoporosis, a condition involving bone loss that particularly afflicts women.

Smoking and Pregnancy

Although cigarette smoking is dangerous for all women, it presents special risks for pregnant women and their fetuses. Each year in the United States, approximately 50,000 miscarriages are attributed to smoking during pregnancy. On average, babies born to mothers who

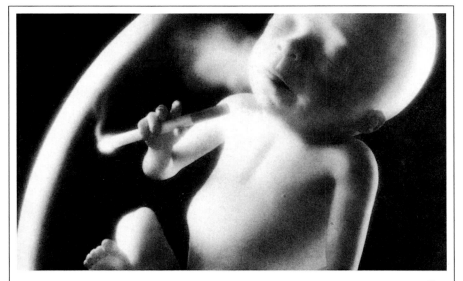

PREGNANT MOTHERS: PLEASE DON'T SMOKE!

If you are pregnant or planning a family, here are three good reasons to quit smoking now:

1. Smoking retards the growth of your baby in your womb.
2. Smoking increases the incidence of infant mortality.
3. Your family needs a healthy mother.

Please don't smoke for your baby's sake. And yours.

AMERICAN CANCER SOCIETY ®

Expectant mothers have been the focus of numerous public service campaigns designed to make people aware of the hazards of smoking.

smoke weigh less than those born to nonsmokers, and low birth weight is correlated with many developmental problems. Pregnant women who stop smoking in the first three or four months of their pregnancies give birth to higher-birth-weight babies than do women who smoke throughout their pregnancies. Infant mortality rates are also higher among babies born to smokers. Moreover, research indicates that babies born to women who smoke during pregnancy are more likely to die of **sudden infant death syndrome (SIDS)** than are babies born to mothers who do not smoke. SIDS, or "crib death," occurs when an infant, usually under one year of age, dies during its sleep for no apparent reason.

WHAT DO YOU THINK?

Do you think it should be illegal for pregnant women to purchase and smoke cigarettes? What do you think is the cause of the dramatic increase over the past 20 years in the number of women smokers?

SMOKELESS TOBACCO

In the wake of strong antismoking campaigns, tobacco companies have increased their advertising for, and production of, chewing tobacco products. Cigarette advertising was banned from television in 1970, but television advertising for chewing tobacco products continues despite campaigns to ban it.

Smokeless tobacco is used by approximately 12 million Americans, 3 million of whom are under the age of 21. Most users are teenage and young adult males, who are often emulating a professional sports figure or a family member. There are two types of smokeless tobacco—chewing tobacco and snuff. Chewing tobacco comes in the form of loose leaf, plug, or twist. Chewing tobacco contains tobacco leaves treated with molasses and other flavorings. The user places a "quid" of tobacco in the mouth between the teeth and gums and then sucks or chews the quid to release the nicotine. Once the quid becomes ineffective, the user spits it out and inserts another.

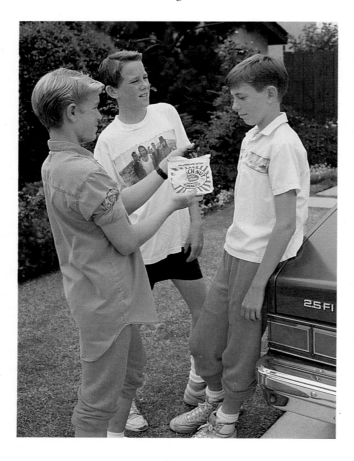

Dipping is another method of using chewing tobacco. The dipper takes a small amount of tobacco and places it between the lower lip and teeth to stimulate the flow of saliva and release the nicotine. Dipping rapidly releases the nicotine into the bloodstream.

Snuff can come in either a dry or moist powdered form or sachets (tea bag-like pouches) of tobacco. The most common placement of snuff is inside the cheek. In European countries, inhaling dry snuff is more common than in the United States.[19] Consumption of moist snuff and other smokeless tobacco products has almost tripled in the United States from 1972 to 1991.

Risks of Smokeless Tobacco

Smokeless tobacco is just as addictive as cigarettes due to its nicotine content. There is nicotine in all tobacco products, but smokeless tobacco contains more nicotine than do cigarettes. Holding an average-sized dip or chew in your mouth for 30 minutes gives you as much nicotine as smoking four cigarettes. A two-can-a-week snuff dipper gets as much nicotine as a one-and-a-half-pack-a-day smoker.

One of the major risks of chewing tobacco is **leukoplakia,** a condition characterized by leathery white patches inside the mouth produced by contact with irritants in tobacco juice. Smokeless tobacco contains 10 times the amount of cancer-producing substances found in cigarettes and 100 times more than the Food and Drug Administration allows in foods and other substances used by the public.[20] Between 3 and 17 percent of diagnosed leukoplakia cases develop into oral cancer. It is estimated that 75 percent of the 30,000 oral cancer cases in 1992 resulted from either smokeless tobacco or cigarettes. Users of smokeless tobacco are 50 times more likely to develop oral cancers than are nonusers. Warning signs of oral cancers include: lumps in the jaw or neck area; color changes or lumps inside the lips; white, smooth, or scaly patches in the mouth or on the neck, lips, or tongue; a red spot or sore on the lips or gums or inside the mouth that does not heal in two weeks; repeated bleeding in the mouth; difficulty or abnormality in speaking or swallowing.

The lag time between first use and contracting cancer is shorter for smokeless tobacco users than for smokers because absorption through the gums is the most efficient route of nicotine administration. A growing body of evidence suggests that long-term use of smokeless tobacco also increases the risk of cancer of the larynx, esophagus, nasal cavity, pancreas, kidney, and bladder. Moreover, many smokeless tobacco users eventually "graduate" to cigarettes.

Chewers and dippers do not face the specific hazards associated with heat and smoke, but they do run other tobacco-related risks. The stimulant effects of nicotine may create the same circulatory and respiratory problems for chewers as for smokers. Chronic smokeless tobacco use also results in delayed wound healing, peptic ulcer disease, and reproductive disturbances.

Smokeless tobacco also impairs the senses of taste and smell, causing the user to add salt and sugar to food, which may contribute to high blood pressure and obesity. Some smokeless tobacco products contain high levels of sodium (salt), which also contributes to high blood pressure. In addition, dental problems are common among users of smokeless tobacco. Contact with tobacco juice causes receding gums, tooth decay, bad breath, and discolored teeth. Damage to both the teeth and jawbone can contribute to early loss of teeth. Users of all tobacco products may not be able to use the vitamins and other nutrients in food effectively. In some cases, vitamin supplements may be recommended by a physician.

Smokeless tobacco users have the same problems that smokers do when trying to quit. Withdrawal symptoms are almost universal; relapse is common. Some or many of the following symptoms often accompany nicotine withdrawal: headache, gastrointestinal discomfort, sleeping problems, irritability, anxiety, aggressiveness, craving for tobacco, and a reduction in heart rate, blood pressure, and hormone secretions.

*W*HAT DO YOU THINK?

Why do you think chewing tobacco has been such a large part of sports in the United States? What is it that has attracted athletes to chewing tobacco? Do you think the use of smokeless tobacco should be banned in high school and college athletics? Should its use be forbidden in residence halls and classrooms just as cigarettes are banned?

*E*NVIRONMENTAL TOBACCO SMOKE

As the population of nonsmokers rises, so does the demand for the right to breathe clean air. Although fewer than 30 percent of Americans are smokers, air pollution from smoking in public places continues to be a problem.

Environmental tobacco smoke (ETS) is divided into two categories: mainstream smoke and sidestream smoke (also called secondhand smoke). **Mainstream smoke** refers to smoke drawn through tobacco while inhaling; **sidestream smoke** refers to smoke from the burning end of a cigarette or to smoke exhaled by a smoker. People who breathe smoke from someone else's smoking product are said to be *involuntary* or *passive* smokers. Approximately 30 percent of the American population is exposed to secondhand smoke on a regular basis.[21]

Although involuntary smokers breathe less tobacco than active smokers do, they still face risks from exposure to tobacco smoke. Sidestream smoke actually contains more carcinogenic substances than the smoke that a smoker inhales. According to the American Lung Association, sidestream smoke has about 2 times more tar and nicotine, 5 times more carbon monoxide, and 50 times more ammonia than mainstream smoke. An Environmental Protection Agency (EPA) report released in January 1993, following a four-year study of sidestream cigarette smoke, stated that lung cancer caused by cigarette smoke kills about 3,000 nonsmokers a year.[22] On the basis of this study, the EPA has designated secondhand tobacco smoke a *group A cancer-causing agent* that is even worse than other group A threats such as benzene, arsenic, and radon.[23] The EPA has no power to regulate levels of indoor tobacco smoke, but officials believe that the agency's recommendations carry weight with employers and local governments. There is also recent evidence that sidestream smoke poses an even greater risk for death due to heart disease than for death due to lung cancer.[24]

Sidestream smoke is estimated to cause more deaths per year than any other environmental pollutant. The risk of dying because of exposure to passive smoking is 100 times greater than the risk that requires the EPA to label a pollutant as carcinogenic and 10,000 times greater than the risk that requires the labeling of a food as carcinogenic.[25]

Lung cancer and heart disease are not the only risks involuntary smokers face. The 1993 EPA report also concluded that sidestream smoke increases the risk of pneumonia and bronchitis in children.[26] Children exposed to sidestream smoke have a greater chance of developing other respiratory problems, such as cough, wheezing, asthma, and chest colds, along with a decrease in pulmonary performance. The greatest effects of sidestream smoke are seen in children under the age of five.

Cigarette, cigar, and pipe smoke in enclosed areas present other hazards to nonsmokers. An estimated 10 to 15 percent of nonsmokers are extremely sensitive (hypersensitive) to cigarette smoke.[27] These people experience itchy eyes, difficulty in breathing, painful headaches, nausea, and dizziness in response to minute amounts of smoke. The level of carbon monoxide in cigarette smoke contained in enclosed places is 4,000 times higher than the standard recommended by the EPA for a definition of clean air.

Efforts to reduce the hazards associated with passive smoking have been gaining momentum in recent years. Groups such as GASP (Group Against Smokers' Pollution) and ASH (Action on Smoking and Health) have been working since the early 1970s to reduce smoking in public places. In response to their efforts, some 44 states have enacted laws limiting or restricting smoking in public places such as restaurants, theaters, bowling alleys, public schools, airports, and bus depots.[28] The federal government has restricted smoking in all government buildings. Hotels and motels now set aside rooms for nonsmokers, and car rental agencies designate certain vehicles for nonsmokers. Since 1990, smoking has been banned on all domestic airline flights. During 1994, McDonald's banned smoking in 1,400 of its company-owned fast food restaurants and 20 major-league baseball parks went smokeless.[29] The Gap airbrushed cigarettes from the fingers of John Wayne and Miles Davis in its advertise-

Leukoplakia: A condition characterized by leathery white patches inside the mouth produced by contact with irritants in tobacco juice.

Environmental tobacco smoke (ETS): Smoke from tobacco products, including sidestream and mainstream smoke.

Mainstream smoke: Smoke that is drawn through tobacco while inhaling.

Sidestream smoke: The cigarette, pipe, or cigar smoke breathed by nonsmokers; also called secondhand smoke.

Saying No to Environmental Smoke

As long as people continue to smoke tobacco, second-hand smoke will threaten the health of nonsmokers. Still, you can take steps to protect yourself from other people's smoke at home, at school, and in public places. How can you share air space with smokers without risking your health? Here are some ideas to help you clear the air.

If You Live with a Smoker

- Ask him or her not to smoke inside your home.
- If he/she is unwilling to go outside, suggest ways to limit the exposure to smoke. Maybe a room could be set aside for smoking—one that is seldom used by other members of the household. Some smokers protect others by keeping a window open or by smoking only when no one is around.
- Keep rooms well ventilated. Open windows.
- Support smokers who decide to quit.

When Visitors Come

- Ask all smokers who visit not to smoke in your house or apartment. It's your right to keep your home free of this health risk.
- Don't keep ashtrays around.

In Other's Homes

- Tell friends and relatives politely that you'd appreciate it if they do not smoke while you're there.
- Let people know when their smoke is causing immediate problems. If it is making your allergies worse, making you cough or wheeze, or making your eyes sting, say so. Some smokers may put their cigarettes away when they see the discomfort it causes.

In Public Places

- Always take the nonsmoking options that are available. Today, many restaurants have nonsmoking sections and hotels offer nonsmoking rooms and floors. You can even get a nonsmoking rental car. If one place doesn't offer a nonsmoking area, choose another that does. The strongest statement against smoking in public places is made by taking your business elsewhere.
- Don't accept what you can change. If a restaurant puts you at a table near smokers (even if you're in a nonsmoking section), ask to move. If smokers don't obey nonsmoking rules, ask those in charge to enforce the rules. When people near you are smoking, ask them politely either to stop or to move the ashtray or to hold their cigarettes away from you.

Increased awareness of the hazards of second-hand smoke and nonsmokers' demands for the right to clean air have prompted many restrictions on smoking in public places in recent years.

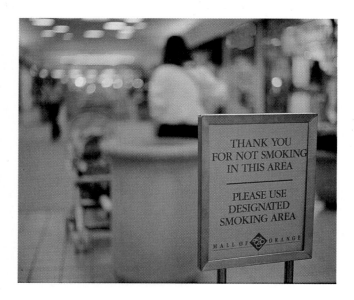

ments, and the Post Office lifted a cigarette from a stamp honoring blues great Robert Johnson.

Learning to express your right to smoke-free air is an important part of attaining good health. The Building Communication Skills box gives practical suggestions about how to avoid inhaling sidestream smoke.

The Tobacco Industry Strikes Back

In July 1994, a U.S. District court judge paved the way for tobacco giants Philip Morris and R. J. Reynolds to sue the EPA for its highly publicized report that sidestream smoke causes cancer. The tobacco industry contends that the EPA report is flawed and asked the court to order the agency to withdraw it. The lawsuit said that the EPA reviewed 30 studies on sidestream smoke and found that 24 did not support its conclusion that cancer was a risk. Three other studies in which animals inhaled sidestream smoke showed no increase in cancer, according to the lawsuit. The tobacco industry is hoping that if the report is withdrawn, smokers will no longer be restricted to smoking areas.

Even if the EPA study regarding sidestream smoke is found to be flawed in regard to cancer, would you support continued restricted smoking areas? What other concerns are there about sidestream smoke that are not addressed in the tobacco industry's lawsuit?

QUITTING

Quitting smoking isn't easy. To stop smoking requires breaking an addiction and a habit. Smokers must break the physical addiction to nicotine. And they must break the habit of lighting up at certain times of the day.

From what we know about successful quitters, quitting is often a lengthy process involving several unsuccessful attempts before success is finally achieved. Even successful quitters suffer occasional slips, emphasizing the fact that quitting smoking is a dynamic process that occurs over time.

Approximately one-third of smokers attempt to quit each year. Unfortunately, 90 percent or more of those attempts fail. The person who wishes to quit smoking has several options. Most smokers try to quit "cold turkey"— that is, they decide simply not to smoke again. Others resort to short-term quitting programs, such as that offered by the American Cancer Society, that are based on behavior modification and a system of self-rewards. Still others turn to treatment centers that are part of large franchises or of a local medical clinic's community outreach plan. Finally, some people work privately with their physicians to reach their goal.

Prospective quitters must decide which method or combination of methods will work best for them. Programs that combine several approaches have shown the most promise. Financial considerations, personality characteristics, and level of addiction should all be analyzed when choosing a plan for quitting. What's the best way to quit? Have a heart attack! Doctors seem to have the most influence with cardiac patients, with an almost 43 percent success rate.

Breaking the Nicotine Addiction

Nicotine addiction may be one of the toughest addictions to overcome. Smokers' attempts to quit lead to withdrawal symptoms. Symptoms of **nicotine withdrawal** include irritability, restlessness, nausea, vomiting, and intense cravings for tobacco.

Nicotine Replacement Products. Nontobacco products that replace depleted levels of nicotine in the bloodstream have helped some people stop using tobacco. The two most common nicotine-replacement products are nicotine chewing gum and the nicotine patch, both available by prescription.

Some patients use a prescription chewing gum containing nicotine, called Nicorette, to help them reduce their nicotine consumption over time. Under the guidance of a physician, the user chews between 12 and 24 pieces of gum per day for up to six months. Nicorette delivers about as much nicotine as a cigarette does, but because it is absorbed through the mucous membrane of the mouth, it doesn't produce the same rush as inhaling a cigarette does. Users experience no withdrawal symptoms and fewer cravings for nicotine as the dosage is reduced until they are completely weaned.

There is some controversy surrounding the use of nicotine replacement gum. Opponents believe that it substitutes one addiction for another. Successful users counter that it is a valid way to help break a deadly habit without suffering the unpleasant withdrawal symptoms and cravings that often lead ex-smokers to resume smoking.

The nicotine patch, first marketed in 1991, is the hottest new method for those attempting to quit smoking. It is generally used in conjunction with a comprehensive smoking-behavior cessation program. A small, thin 24-hour patch placed on the smoker's upper body delivers a continuous flow of nicotine through the skin, helping to relieve the body's cravings. The patch is worn for 8 to 12 weeks under the guidance of a physician. During this time, the dose of nicotine is gradually reduced until the smoker is fully weaned from nicotine. Occasional side effects include mild skin irritation, insomnia, dry mouth, and nervousness. The patch costs the equivalent of two packs of cigarettes a day—about four dollars—and some insurance plans will pay for it.

How effective is the nicotine patch? In 1994 analysis of 17 studies involving 5,098 people, the nicotine patch was at least twice as effective as placebo (fake) patches. At the end of treatment periods lasting at least four weeks, 27 percent of the nicotine patch wearers were free of cigarettes versus 13 percent of placebo patch users. Six months later, 22 percent of the nicotine patch users were absti-nent compared to only 9 percent of the placebo users. The study also showed that the patch was effective with or without intensive counseling.[30]

Nicotine withdrawal: Symptoms including nausea, headaches, and irritability, suffered by smokers who cease using tobacco.

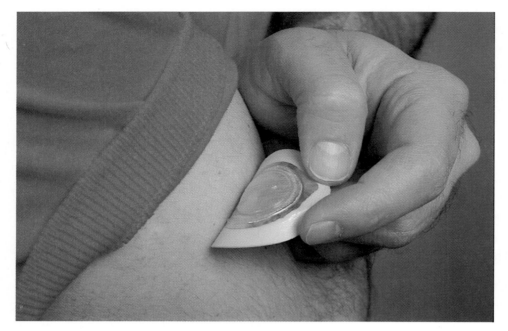

Many smokers find that the unpleasant symptoms of nicotine withdrawal can be mitigated by a nicotine patch that delivers nicotine through the skin, but the success rates for quitting are highest when the patch is combined with counseling or a behavior modification program.

Breaking the Habit

For many smokers, the road to quitting includes some type of antismoking therapy. Among the more common therapy techniques are aversion therapy, operant conditioning, and self-control therapy. One of the American Cancer Society's approaches is shown in the Choices for Change box.

Aversion Therapy. Aversion techniques attempt to reduce smoking by pairing the act of smoking with some sort of noxious stimulus so that smoking itself is perceived as unpleasant. For example, the technique of rapid smoking instructs patients to smoke rapidly and continuously until they exceed their tolerance for cigarette smoke, producing unpleasant sensations. Short-term rates of success are high, but many patients relapse over time.

Operant Strategies. Pairing the act of smoking with an external stimulus is a typical example of this method. For example, one technique requires smokers to carry a timer that sounds a buzzer at different intervals. When the buzzer sounds, the patient is required to smoke a cigarette. Once the smoker is conditioned to associate the buzzer with smoking, the buzzer is eliminated, and, one hopes, so is the smoking.

Self-Control. Self-control strategies view smoking as a learned habit associated with specific situations. Therapy is aimed at identifying these situations and teaching smokers the skills necessary to resist smoking. The Skills for Behavioral Change box offers self-control strategies to overcome the smoking habit.

Benefits of Quitting

According to the American Cancer Society, many tissues damaged by smoking can repair themselves. As soon as smokers stop, their bodies begin the repair process. Within eight hours, carbon monoxide and oxygen levels return to normal, and "smoker's breath" disappears. Within a few days of quitting, the mucus clogging airways is broken up and eliminated. Circulation and the senses of taste and smell improve within weeks. Many ex-smokers who have kicked the cigarette habit say they have more energy, sleep better, and feel more alert. By the end of one year, the risk for lung cancer and stroke decreases. Within two years, the risk for heart attack drops to near normal. At the end of 10 smoke-free years, the ex-smoker can expect to live out his or her normal life span. Figure 14.4 shows the health benefits of quitting smoking.

Caffeine: A stimulant found in coffee, tea, chocolate, and some soft drinks.

Xanthines: The chemical family of stimulants to which caffeine belongs.

*W*HAT DO YOU THINK?

What could you personally do to help someone quit smoking? What are the most common barriers to quitting tobacco use? When trying to stop smoking, why do people often interpret a relapse as a total failure?

Developing a Plan to Kick the Habit

There is no magic cure that can help you stop. Take the first step to quitting. Answer this question: Why do I want to stop smoking?

Write your reasons in the space below. Once you have prepared your list, cut it out and carry it with you. Memorize it. Every time you are tempted to smoke, go over your reasons for stopping.

My Reasons for Stopping

1. _____
2. _____
3. _____
4. _____
5. _____

Develop a Plan; Change Some Habits

Over time, smoking becomes a strong habit. Often, daily events such as finishing a meal, talking on the phone, drinking coffee, and chatting with friends trigger your urge to smoke. Breaking the link between the trigger and your smoking will help you stop. Think about the times and places you usually smoke. What could you do instead of smoking at those times?

Things to Do Instead of Smoking

1. _____
2. _____
3. _____

The Bottom Line: Commit Yourself

There comes a time when you have to say good-bye to your cigarettes.

- Pick a day to stop smoking.
- Fill out a "Stop Smoking Contract."
- Have a family member or friend sign the contract.

THEN

- Throw away all your cigarettes, lighters, and ashtrays at home and at work. You will not need them again.

- Be prepared to feel the urge to smoke. The urge will pass whether or not you smoke. Use the FOUR Ds to fight the urge:
  Delay
  Deep breathing
  Drink water
  Do something else
- Keep "mouth toys" handy: lifesavers, gum, straws, and carrot sticks can help.
- If you've had trouble stopping before, ask your doctor about nicotine chewing gum.
- Tell your family and friends that you've stopped smoking.
- Put "NO SMOKING" signs in your car, work area, and house.
- Give yourself a treat for stopping. Go to a movie, go out to dinner, or buy yourself a gift.

Focus on the Positives

Now that you have stopped smoking, your mind and your body will begin to feel better. Think of the good things that have happened since you stopped. Can you breathe easier? Do you have more energy? Do you feel good about what you've done?

Use the space below to list the good things about not smoking. Carry them with you. Look at them when you have the urge to smoke.

_____
_____
_____
_____
_____
_____

Source: Reprinted by permission from *Smart Move! A Stop Smoking Guide.* © 1988, American Cancer Society, Inc.

CAFFEINE

Caffeine is the most popular and widely consumed drug in the United States. Almost half of all Americans drink coffee every day, and many others use caffeine in some other form, mainly for its well-known "wake-up" effect. Drinking coffee is legal, even socially encouraged. Many people believe caffeine is a nondrug item and not really addictive. Besides, it tastes good. Coffee and other caffeine-containing products seem harmless; with no cream or sugar added, they are calorie-free and therefore a good way to fill yourself up if you are dieting. If you share these attitudes, you should think again, because research in the last decade has linked caffeine to certain health problems.

Caffeine is a drug derived from the chemical family called **xanthines.** Two related chemicals, *theophylline* and

Breaking the Habit

Beating the nicotine addiction is only half the battle when you want to stop smoking. You also have to break the behavioral habit of reaching for a cigarette. When you encounter cues that normally result in your lighting up a cigarette, try the suggested strategy instead. Although it is hard to break the habit, with persistence you can.

Cues and High-Risk Situations	Suggested Strategies
Awakening in morning	Brush your teeth as soon as you wake up.
	Stay busy and try not to think about smoking.
Drinking coffee	Do something else with your hands.
	Drink tea or another beverage instead.
Eating meals	Eat in a different location.
	Sit in nonsmoking sections in restaurants.
	Get up from the table right away after eating and start another activity.
	Brush your teeth right away after eating.
Driving a car	Have the car cleaned when you quit smoking.
	Chew sugarless gum or eat a low-calorie snack.
	Take public transportation or ride your bike.
	Remove the cigarette lighter from your car.
Socializing with friends who smoke	Suggest nonsmoking events (movies, theater, shopping).
	Tell them you've quit and ask them not to smoke around you, offer you cigarettes, or give you cigarettes if you ask for them.
	Start an exercise program with a friend.
Drinking at a bar, restaurant, or party	Try to take a nonsmoker with you or associate with nonsmokers.
	Let friends know you've just quit.
	Moderate your intake of alcohol (it can weaken your resolve).
	Keep something in your hand.
	Try to go to a smoke-free bar or restaurant.
Encountering stressful situations	Practice relaxation techniques.
	Get out of your room or house. Go somewhere that doesn't allow smoking.
	Take a shower, chew gum, or call a friend.
	Go for a walk.

Source: Adapted by permission from *Postgraduate Medicine* 90, no. 1 (July 1991).

---

theobromine, are found in tea and chocolate, respectively. The xanthines are mild central nervous system stimulants. They enhance mental alertness and reduce feelings of fatigue. Other stimulant effects include increases in heart muscle contractions, oxygen consumption, metabolism, and urinary output. These effects are felt within 15 to 45 minutes of ingesting a caffeine-containing product.

Side effects of the xanthines include wakefulness, insomnia, irregular heartbeat, dizziness, nausea, indigestion, and sometimes mild delirium. Some people also experience heartburn. As with some other drugs, the user's psychological outlook and expectations will influence the stimulant effects of xanthine-containing products.

Different products contain different concentrations of caffeine. A 5-ounce cup of coffee contains between 60 and 180 milligrams of caffeine. Caffeine concentrations vary with the brand of the beverage and the strength of the brew. Small chocolate bars contain up to 15 milligrams of caffeine and theobromine. A comparison of various caffeine-containing products can be found in Table 14.2.

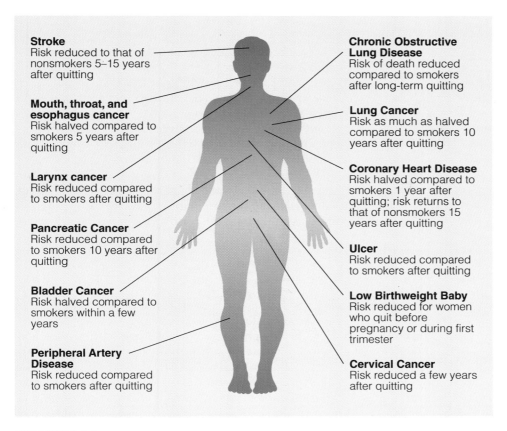

FIGURE 14.4

Benefits of Quitting Smoking

Source: Reprinted from U.S. Department of Health and Human Services, "The Health Benefits of Smoking Cessation: A Report of the Surgeon General 1990, at a Glance."

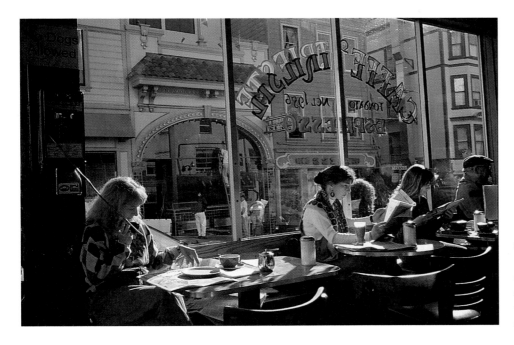

Though caffeine products, especially coffees, colas, and chocolate, are widely consumed, it is important to remember that caffeine is an addictive drug.

TABLE 14.2 ■ Caffeine Content of
Various Products

Product	Caffeine Content (average mg per serving)
Coffee (5-oz. cup)	
Regular brewed	65–115
Decaffeinated brewed	3
Decaffeinated instant	2
Tea (6-oz. cup)	
Hot steeped	36
Iced	31
Soft Drinks (12-oz. servings)	
Jolt Cola	100
Dr. Pepper	61
Mountain Dew	54
Coca-Cola	46
Pepsi-Cola	36–38
Chocolate	
1 oz. baking chocolate	25
1 oz. chocolate candy bar	15
½ cup chocolate pudding	4–12
Over-the-Counter Drugs	
No Doz (2 tablets)	200
Excedrin (2 tablets)	130
Midol (2 tablets)	65
Anacin (2 tablets)	64

Caffeine Addiction

As the effects of caffeine begin to wear off, users may feel let down, mentally or physically depressed, exhausted, and weak. To counteract these effects, people commonly choose to drink another cup of coffee. Habitually engaging in this practice leads to tolerance and psychological dependence. Until the mid-1970s, caffeine was not medically recognized as addictive. Chronic caffeine use and its attendant behaviors were called "coffee nerves." This syndrome is now recognized as *caffeine intoxication,* or **caffeinism.** Symptoms of caffeinism include chronic insomnia, jitters, irritability, nervousness, anxiety, and involuntary muscle twitches. Withdrawing the caffeine may compound the effects and produce severe headaches. (Some physicians ask their patients to take a simple test for caffeine addiction:

Caffeinism: Caffeine intoxication brought on by excessive caffeine use; symptoms include chronic insomnia, irritability, anxiety, muscle twitches, and headaches.

Don't consume anything containing caffeine, and if you get a severe headache within four hours, you are addicted.) Because caffeinism meets the requirements for addiction—tolerance, psychological dependence, and withdrawal symptoms—it can be classified as addictive.

Although you would have to drink between 67 and 100 cups of coffee in a day to produce a fatal overdose of caffeine, you may experience sensory disturbances after consuming only 10 cups of coffee within a 24-hour period. These symptoms include tinnitus (ringing in the ears), spots before the eyes, numbness in arms and legs, poor circulation, and visual hallucinations. Because 10 cups of coffee is not an extraordinary amount for many people to drink within a 24-hour period, caffeine use clearly poses health threats.

The Health Consequences of Long-Term Caffeine Use

Long-term caffeine use has been linked to a number of serious health problems ranging from heart disease and cancer to mental dysfunction and birth defects. Reexamination of these findings in 1989, however, indicated that moderate caffeine use (less than 500 milligrams daily, which is approximately five cups of coffee) produces very few harmful effects in healthy, nonpregnant people.

The links between caffeine consumption and heart and circulatory disorders are still disputed, but it seems that caffeine does not cause long-term high blood pressure and it has not been linked to strokes.[31] Researchers associated with the Framingham Heart Study have concluded that there is no evidence of a relationship between coffee and heart disease. However, people who suffer from irregular heartbeat are cautioned against the use of caffeine because the resultant increase in heart rate can be life-threatening.

A debate about the relationship between caffeine and cholesterol has been raging for more than 30 years. In the early 1960s, some research indicated that caffeine consumption significantly raised cholesterol levels. More recent research suggests that caffeine-containing products in and of themselves do not raise cholesterol but that people who have high cholesterol levels and who consume large amounts of caffeine also tend to engage in other behaviors (such as eating high-fat foods) that contribute to their cholesterol problems. Another possibility is that some as-yet-unidentified substance (not caffeine) in caffeine-containing substances is the real culprit behind the high blood cholesterol levels found in heavy users of these substances.

For years, caffeine consumption was linked with fibrocystic breast disease, a condition characterized by painful, noncancerous lumps in the breast. Then a 1986 study, substantiated in 1988 by a National Cancer Institute study, found no link between caffeine consumption and fibrocystic breast disease.[32]

Managing Tobacco and Caffeine

Acommon mistake people make when they are trying to stop smoking is picking a stressful time to quit. It is best to wait until you have a month that is relatively free of stress. Follow these guidelines to prepare yourself to stop smoking or share them with someone you know who smokes.

Making Decisions for You

Making healthy behavior changes is never easy but always beneficial. In the case of choosing to be tobacco-free, breaking the habit is even more difficult because of the chemical addiction caused by nicotine. The behavior change techniques described throughout this book will help give you the willpower needed to overcome your tobacco habit. After you have decided to quit, outline the steps you will take to quit. The Choices for Change box gave an example of one outline. What reinforcers or rewards can you give yourself along the way? Who might you call upon to help keep you motivated? Can any of the behavior change techniques described in Chapter 1 help you (such as modeling, changing self-talk, etc.)?

Checklist for Change: Making Personal Choices

✓ Identify your smoking habits. Keep a daily journal and record when and where you smoked and whom you were with at the time. Write down how you felt and note how important that cigarette was to you at the time on a scale of one to five. Maintain your diary for one or two weeks.

✓ Get support. It can be extremely difficult to go it alone when you are trying to quit smoking. Friends who have never smoked probably don't realize the enormous problems smokers face when trying to stop. Phone your local chapter of the American Cancer Society or community hospital to find out what programs are being offered and what support groups you can join.

✓ Begin by tapering off. For a period of one to two weeks, either aim at cutting down or change to a lower-nicotine brand (in the latter case, be careful not to increase the number of cigarettes you smoke). Stop carrying matches. Don't buy a new pack until you finish the one you're smoking, and never buy a carton. Cut back on those cigarettes you smoke automatically (e.g., when you get into your car or every time you have a cup of coffee).

✓ Set a quit date. At some point when you are tapering off, announce to family, friends, and roommates when you are going to stop.

✓ Stop. A week before you quit, cut your cigarette consumption down to five cigarettes per day. Smoke these cigarettes in the late day or evening. By this time, you may be able to notice some of the negative effects of smoking every time you do light up, such as the harshness of the smoke in your lungs and throat. On the day

you quit, treat yourself to something nice—dinner out with a friend, new clothes, or a movie.

✓ Follow up by continuing to seek support from your support-group members. Increase your physical activity. Avoid situations you most closely associate with smoking. Find a substitute for cigarettes. Do deep breathing exercises when you get the urge to smoke.

✓ If you fail to stop despite your best efforts, do not hit on yourself. Try again soon.

Checklist for Change: Making Personal Choices to Reduce Caffeine Consumption

✓ For some people, caffeine consumption has unpleasant side effects, such as headaches, nervousness, diarrhea, frequent urination, and insomnia. If you feel that your caffeine consumption is interfering with your life, you should consider cutting back.

✓ Cut back gradually, though, because going cold turkey can result in severe headaches and other unpleasant symptoms, such as irritability and insomnia. Cut down by one serving a day every few days until you have reached your goal.

✓ Another alternative is to mix caffeinated products with decaffeinated products, gradually increasing the proportion of the latter until the former is eliminated.

✓ Smokers should be aware that nicotine affects the way the body uses caffeine. Caffeine is metabolized faster in smokers than in nonsmokers, so smokers need more caffeine to feel its effects. If you try to quit smoking, the caffeine you ingest will have very potent effects, producing greater degrees of irritability and nervousness. Therefore, you may want to cut down on caffeine before you give up the nicotine habit.

✓ If you are a confirmed coffee drinker, you may require some medical assistance and support from friends and family when taking the first step toward reducing your caffeine intake. Because caffeinated products play a central role in social customs ("Let's get together over a cup of coffee"), quitting or cutting down may be very difficult. Finding satisfying alternatives to coffee-associated behaviors will help you in this process.

Checklist for Change: Making Community Choices

✓ Have you become familiar with the policies and issues surrounding smoke-free environments on your campus and in your community?

✓ Are you aware of the influence that the media have on society? Have you thought of ways to counter the advertisements aimed at yourself and those you associate with?

(continued)

✓ Are you cognizant of the powerful influence you may have now or in the future as a role model? Is being a role model a responsibility you feel comfortable assuming?

✓ Do you take an active part in community organizations that are designed to help youth reduce their risky behaviors?

✓ Are you an active participant in community or nation-wide activities, such as the Great American Smokeout, that encourage the adoption or maintenance of healthy behaviors?

✓ When you vote in local, state, or national elections, do you vote in support of legislation that supports healthy lifestyles (such as laws that ban the sale of cigarettes to those under age)?

✓ Do you support organizations in your community that are working to protect nonsmokers?

✓ Do you write to public officials, newspapers, and businesses to promote policies protecting nonsmokers?

Critical Thinking

The health department at your school is holding its annual health fair, and you are chairing the organizing committee. The fair is a popular event, and a large percentage of students turn out to participate. You are particularly interested, because as a first-year student you learned from the free screenings offered that you had elevated blood pressure and high cholesterol. But you have run into a major glitch this year: The major corporate sponsors have withdrawn support due to economic conditions. Without corporate support, you can't hold the event. However, a major tobacco company has offered to fund the entire event. All they ask in return is the right to hand out free T-shirts to people leaving the fair. On the one hand, you feel that the event is valuable to students; certainly it alerted you to health problems. On the other hand, you think it is hypocritical for a tobacco company to be sponsoring a health event.

Using the DECIDE model described in Chapter 1, decide what you will recommend to your organizing committee. Remember to be creative in thinking about your options.

Coffee is still considered a gastric irritant that can contribute to ulcers. Decaffeinated coffee products contain some of the same irritants as caffeine-containing products and thus can also be harmful to people with stomach ulcers.

The link between caffeine and birth defects is still unclear. Most studies have shown evidence of fetal deformities in rats whose mothers consumed the equivalent of 18 cups of coffee per day. Although the majority of people do not consume this much caffeine, pregnant women are nevertheless advised to eliminate caffeine from their diets because any drug ingested during pregnancy, particularly during the first three months, may be hazardous to the fetus. The relationship between caffeine and low-birthweight babies is also unclear. Again, however, because in pregnancy it is better to be safe than sorry, pregnant women should probably eliminate or restrict caffeine intake.

Studies conducted in 1989 indicated an association between caffeine consumption and infertility in women. Based on these results, women who were having difficulty conceiving were told to stop using caffeine-containing products. But later studies found no correlation between caffeine consumption and infertility. It may be several years before we have any conclusive evidence regarding a link between caffeine and infertility.[33]

*W*HAT DO YOU THINK?

Do you consider caffeine a drug? Is the amount of caffeine you consume a concern, or has it ever been a concern? On an average day, how much caffeine do you think you consume? Do you think you could decrease the amount of caffeine you consume and not feel any ill effects?

Summary

◆ The use of tobacco involves many social issues, including advertising targeted at youth and women, the largest growing populations of smokers. Health care and lost productivity resulting from smoking cost the nation about $68 billion.

◆ Tobacco is available in smoking and smokeless forms, both containing addictive nicotine (a psychoactive substance). Smoking also delivers 4,000 other chemicals to the lungs of smokers.

◆ The health hazards of smoking include markedly higher rates of cancer, heart and circulatory disorders, respiratory diseases, and gum diseases. Smoking while pregnant presents risks for the fetus, including miscarriage or low birth weight.

◆ Smokeless tobacco contains more nicotine than do cigarettes and dramatically increases risks for oral cancer and other oral problems.

- Environmental tobacco smoke (sidestream smoke) puts nonsmokers at risk for elevated rates of cancer and heart disease according to an EPA study. While many businesses and local governments have responded by banning smoking, the tobacco industry contends that flaws in the study make it invalid.

- Quitting is complicated by the dual nature of smoking: Smokers must kick a chemical addiction as well as a habit. Nicotine replacement products (gum and the patch) are available to help wean smokers off nicotine. Several therapy methods can help smokers break the habit of lighting up.

- Caffeine is a widely used central nervous system stimulant. No long-term ill-health effects have been proven, although caffeine may produce withdrawal symptoms for chronic users who try to quit.

Discussion Questions

1. Given that you have a 90 percent greater chance of smoking if your parents smoke, and an 80 percent greater chance of smoking if your peers smoke, how effective are tobacco ads at luring young people to smoke?

2. Discuss the varied forms in which you can ingest tobacco. In each form, how do chemicals enter your system? What are the physiological effects of nicotine?

3. List the health hazards of smoking. Given all the health problems associated with smoking, why don't more people quit?

4. Discuss the varied risks of smokeless tobacco. Do you think that smokeless tobacco should be banned from major league baseball, as it was from the minor leagues?

5. Smokers often claim they have the right to smoke in public places. From what you have learned about sidestream smoke, how would you argue against a smoker's right to smoke in public?

6. Describe varied methods of quitting tobacco products. Which do you think would be most effective for you? Explain why.

7. After learning about the potential problems associated with caffeine use, have you considered altering the amount you consume?

Application Exercise

Reread the What Do You Think? scenarios at the beginning of the chapter and answer the following questions.

1. From what you have learned in this chapter, what steps would you suggest each of the tobacco users in the scenarios take to quit their tobacco use?

2. How could people who do not use tobacco best assert themselves so as not to be exposed to tobacco?

3. Given that each individual in the scenarios has some knowledge that using tobacco is an unhealthy behavior, what do you think it will take to get each to stop using tobacco?

4. In each of the scenarios, the tobacco users are young adults. What is so alluring about the use of tobacco? Why are some people so quick to start using tobacco? What benefits do they perceive? When most people start using tobacco, do you think they intend to use it for the rest of their lives?

Further Reading

U.S. Department of Health and Human Services, *Strategies to Control Tobacco Use in the United States: A Blueprint for Public Health Action in the 1990s* (NIH Publication No. 92–3316, December 1991).

An extensive overview of current and suggested strategies for smoking cessation programs. Includes extensive coverage of the impact of smoking on lung cancer death rates. Overall emphasis is on getting public health officials to recognize the importance of smoking as a public health issue.

G. Boyd and C. M. Darbey, eds., *Smokeless Tobacco Use in the United States* (National Cancer Institute Monograph, 1990).

A comprehensive examination of the role of smokeless tobacco in causing cancer.

Smoking and Health: A Report to the Congress, 2nd ed. (Rockville, MD: U.S. Department of Health and Human Services, 1990).

A summary of statistics, trends, and research on smoking and its impact on Americans.

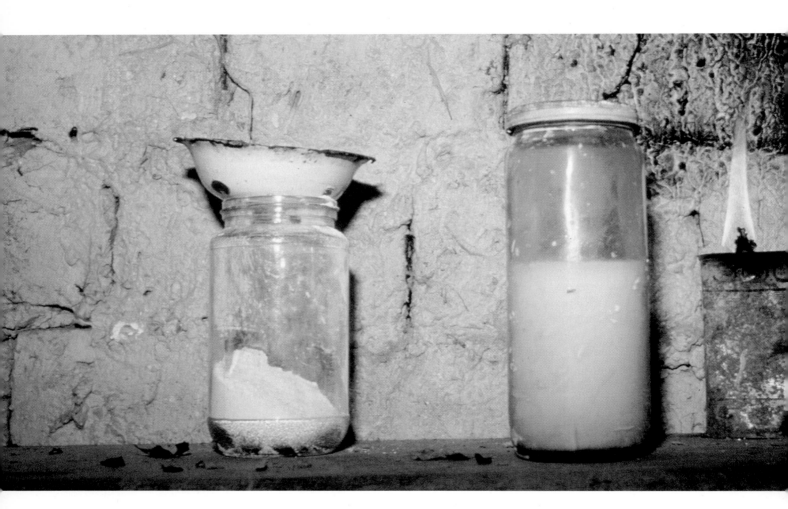

CHAPTER OBJECTIVES

◆ Discuss patterns of illicit drug use, including who uses illicit drugs and why they use them.

◆ Describe the use and abuse of controlled substances, including cocaine, amphetamines, marijuana, opiates, psychedelics, deliriants, designer drugs, and inhalants.

◆ Profile overall illegal drug use in the United States, including frequency, financial impact, arrests for drug offenses, and impact on the workplace.

Illicit Drugs

Use, Misuse, and Abuse

WHAT DO YOU THINK?

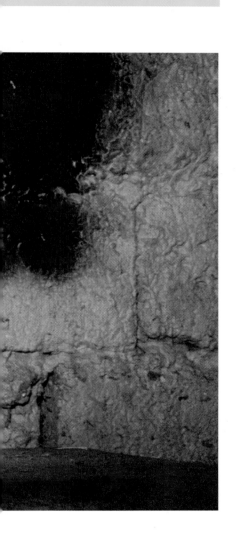

The company for which Richard works as a machine operator recently introduced random drug testing for all employees. At a party last weekend, Richard smoked a little marijuana, unaware that the drug would remain in his body for a few days. On Monday, he tested positive for drug use and was suspended from work without pay for a week. He was informed that he would receive a dismissal warning if he tested positive again. Richard argues that his personal life is his own business as long as he can perform his job.

- Is Richard justified in maintaining that his use of drugs off the job is his own business? Is his attitude toward drug use a potential danger to co-workers? Is random drug testing in the workplace a viable deterrent?

Susan is a pharmacy major attending a large university. She is a junior and is a live-in at her sorority. When she was living in the residence halls, Susan was asked to move out because she was caught smoking marijuana. Recently, she has begun experimenting with LSD. She believes the drug presents a low risk for her developing a dependency and that the adverse health effects are negligible. Susan and her friends have found this drug easy to access and find that it has much less effect on their school work than using alcohol or other drugs.

- Does Susan's history of other drug use suggest a problem? Does Susan's background in pharmacy suggest that she knows how to use drugs at a level that offers greater safety for herself and others? What are the ethical concerns surrounding Susan's chosen profession and her drug use? How do you feel about medical professionals who use or abuse alcohol and other drugs? Is the use or abuse of one more acceptable than the other? Why?

Illicit drug abuse is a problem of staggering proportions in our society. We need to understand how these drugs work and why people use them. Human beings appear to have a need to alter their consciousness, or mental state. We like to feel good. Sometimes we like to change our awareness of things and to feel different. Consciousness can be altered in many ways. Children spinning until they become dizzy and adults enjoying thrilling high-speed activities are altering their consciousness. Many of us listen to music, skydive, ski, skate, read, daydream, meditate, pray, or have sexual relations to change our awareness or to alter our consciousness. For others, illicit drugs offer an easy way to alter consciousness. For example, smoking a marijuana cigarette requires less time and effort than climbing a mountain. The high achieved is not necessarily the same, but both actions produce altered awareness.

ILLICIT DRUGS

The drug problem touches us all. While some people become addicted to prescription drugs and painkillers, we focus our attention here on **illicit drugs**—those drugs that are illegal to possess, produce, or sell. We may choose to use illicit drugs ourselves, be forced to watch someone we love struggle with drug abuse, or become the victim of a drug-related crime. At the very least, we are forced to pay increasing taxes for law enforcement and drug rehabilitation. An estimated 10 to 23 percent of the U.S. workforce is under the influence of illicit drugs or alcohol on any given day. When our co-workers use drugs, the effectiveness of our own work is diminished. If the car we drive was assembled by drug-using workers at the plant, we are in danger. Our safety is jeopardized by a drug-using bus driver, train engineer, or pilot who is transporting us.[1]

The good news is that there has been a significant decline in the use of illicit drugs in recent years. Use of most drugs increased from the early 1970s to the late 1970s, peaked between 1979 and 1986, and has been declining

---

Illicit drugs: Drugs that are illegal to possess, produce, or sell.

---

ever since[2] (see Table 15.1). The bad news is that drug use is still so prevalent.

Who Uses Illicit Drugs?

Illicit drug users come from all walks of life. Not all illicit drug use occurs in dilapidated crack houses and not all users fit the stereotype of the crazed junkie. A 1993 survey conducted by the National Institute on Drug Abuse (NIDA) noted that 11.8 percent of the population age 12 and older reported using an illicit drug during the past year.[3]

The reasons for using drugs vary from one situation to another and from one person to another. A person's age, gender, genetic background, physiology, personality, experiences, and expectations are all factors.

Patterns of drug use vary considerably by age. For example, a recent nationwide study of college campuses reported that approximately 28 percent of students had tried marijuana during the previous year.[4] In contrast, only 9 percent of all Americans took marijuana in the past year. Approximately 3 percent of college students sur-

---

Numerous anti-drug programs in recent years have focused on prevention of drug use in school, including middle schools, which in some areas have been forced to fence in students to protect them from easy-to-find drug sales.

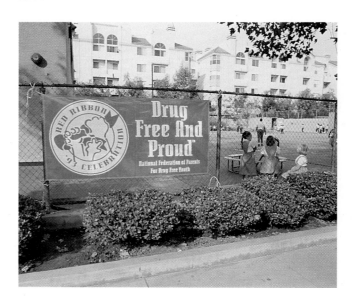

TABLE 15.1 ▪ Trends in the Percentage of Persons Reporting any Illicit Drug Use: 1979–1993

Age of Respondent and Recency of Drug Use	Year					
	1979	1982	1985	1988	1990	1993
12–17						
Ever	34.3%	27.6%	29.5%	24.7%	22.7%	17.9%
Past year	26.0	22.0	23.7	16.8	15.9	13.6
Past 30 days	17.6	12.7	14.9	9.2	8.1	6.6
18–25						
Ever	69.9%	65.3%	64.3%	58.9%	55.8%	50.9%
Past year	49.4	43.4	42.6	32.0	28.7	26.6
Past 30 days	37.1	30.4	25.7	17.8	14.9	13.5
26 and older						
Ever	23.0%	24.7%	31.5%	33.7%	35.3%	29.9%
Past year	10.0	11.8	13.3	10.2	10.0	6.3
Past 30 days	6.5	7.5	8.5	4.9	4.6	2.8

Note: Prior to 1979, data were not totaled for overall drug use and instead were published by specific drug type only.

Source: Reprinted from Substance Abuse and Mental Health Services Administration, Office of Applied Studies, 1993 National Household Survey on Drug Abuse.

veyed reported using cocaine in the past year (see Figure 15.1), while only 2.2 percent of all Americans said they had used cocaine during the previous year.

Antidrug programs have been developed to deal with the problems of illegal drug use. The major drawback of most of these programs is their failure to take a multidimensional approach. The tendency has been to focus on only one aspect of drug abuse rather than to examine all factors that contribute to the problem. For example, many programs consider the drugs themselves the culprits. Others oversimplify the problem by exhorting potential users to "just say no," ignoring the fact that drugs are an integral part of many people's social or cultural lives. The pressures to take drugs are often tremendous, and the reasons for using them are complex.

People who develop drug problems generally begin with the belief that they can control their drug use. Initially, they often view drug taking as a fun and controllable pastime. Peer influence is a strong motivator, especially among adolescents, who greatly fear not being accepted as part of the group. Other people use drugs to cope with feelings of worthlessness and despair or to battle depression and anxiety. Drugs are seen as the quick answer to life's difficulties in our society. Since the majority of illegal drugs produces physical and psychological dependence, the idea that a person can use these substances regularly without becoming addicted is foolish. To find out if you are controlled by drugs, see the Rate Yourself box.

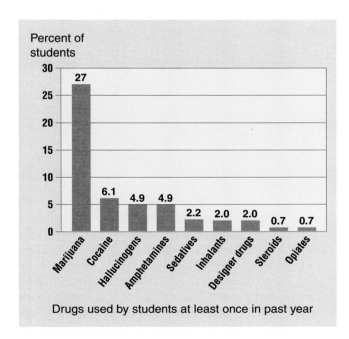

FIGURE 15.1

College Students' Use of Illicit Drugs

𝒲HAT DO YOU THINK?

Would you change any of the current laws governing drugs? If so, what would you consider legitimate and illegitimate use of a drug? What types of changes do you think are needed to help reduce the level of substance abuse in the United States?

Recognizing a Drug Problem

Are You Controlled by Drugs?

How do you know whether you are chemically dependent? A dependent person can't stop using drugs. This abuse hurts the user and everyone around him or her. Take the following assessment. The more "yes" checks you make, the more likely you have a problem.

Yes No

☐ ☐ Do you use drugs to handle stress or escape from life's problems?

☐ ☐ Have you unsuccessfully tried to cut down or quit using your drug?

☐ ☐ Have you ever been in trouble with the law or been arrested because of your drug use?

☐ ☐ Do you think a party or social gathering isn't fun unless drugs are available?

☐ ☐ Do you avoid people or places that do not support your usage?

☐ ☐ Do you neglect your responsibilities because you'd rather use your drug?

☐ ☐ Have your friends, family, or employer expressed concern about your drug use?

☐ ☐ Do you do things under the influence of drugs that you would not normally do?

☐ ☐ Have you seriously thought that you might have a chemical dependency problem?

Are You Controlled by a Drug User?

Is your life controlled by a chemical abuser? Your love and care (codependency) may actually be enabling the chemical abuser to continue the abuse, hurting you and others. Try this assessment; the more "yes" checks you make, the more likely there's a problem.

Yes No

☐ ☐ Do you often have to lie or cover up for the chemical abuser?

☐ ☐ Do you spend time counseling the person about the problem?

☐ ☐ Have you taken on additional financial or family responsibilities?

☐ ☐ Do you feel that you have to control the chemical abuser's behavior?

☐ ☐ At the office, have you done work or attended meetings for the abuser?

☐ ☐ Do you often put your own needs and desires after the user's?

☐ ☐ Do you spend time each day worrying about your situation?

☐ ☐ Do you analyze your behavior to find clues to how it might affect the chemical abuser?

☐ ☐ Do you feel powerless and at your wit's end about the abuser's problem?

Source: Reprinted by permission of Krames Communications, 1100 Grundy Lane, San Bruno, CA 94066–3030.

CONTROLLED SUBSTANCES

In order to counteract the increased use of illegal drugs and the overuse of certain prescription drugs, Congress passed the Controlled Substances Act of 1970 (Public Law 91-513). This law created categories for both prescription and illegal substances that the federal government felt required strict regulation. The Drug Enforcement Agency (DEA) was founded within the Department of Justice to administer the law.

The law established these control measures for drugs defined as "controlled substances": registration of handlers; record-keeping requirements; quotas on manufacturing; restrictions on distribution and dispensation; limitation of imports and exports; conditions for storage of drugs; requirements for reporting drug transactions to the government; and criminal, civil, and administrative directives for actions involving illegal drugs or the illegal use of prescription drugs.

The law divided drugs into five "schedules," or categories, based on their potential for abuse, their medical uses, and accepted standards for their safe use (see Table 15.2). Schedule I drugs were those with the highest potential for abuse; they are considered to have no valid

Cocaine: A powerful stimulant drug made from the leaves of the South American coca shrub.

medical uses. Although Schedule II, III, IV, and V drugs have known and accepted medical applications, many of them present serious threats to health when abused or misused. Penalties for illegal use were also tied to the schedule level of various drugs. Despite the 1970 law, however, trafficking and manufacturing of illegal drugs in the United States have not diminished.

In 1986, the Drug Free America Act superseded the Controlled Substances Act and expanded penalties for the sale, manufacture, possession, and trafficking of illicit drugs. The goal of the new act was to eliminate drug abuse in schools and communities and to focus efforts on drug rehabilitation, medical treatment, and education.

Hundreds of illegal drugs exist. For general purposes, they can be divided into five representative categories: stimulants, like cocaine; marijuana and its derivatives; depressants, like the opiates; psychedelics and deliriants; and so-called designer drugs. All are Schedule I or Schedule II drugs. These categories include the drugs that are illegal to grow, manufacture, sell, or distribute in any form in the United States.

Cocaine

The rise of **cocaine,** or "coke," as the drug of choice among upper- and middle-class Americans in the 1980s was well chronicled in the media. Professional athletes were frequently banned from competition for cocaine use. National toll-free cocaine hotlines were established. The country became more aware of cocaine abuse with the spread of the relatively inexpensive and smokeable cocaine derivative called crack. Crack use turned into a national epidemic in the mid-1980s.

Between 1987 and 1990, there was a dramatic reversal in patterns of cocaine use. The number of people actively using cocaine fell from 2.9 million to 1.6 million.[5] Decreases occurred in every age group evaluated[6] (see Figure 15.2). Recent studies have revealed that, in general, cocaine is not as acceptable among high school and college students as it was previously, which undoubtedly has contributed to the decline in its use. The amount of money spent on the purchase of cocaine also decreased, from $22.5 billion in 1989 to $17.5 billion in 1990.[7] Cocaine is no longer viewed as a glamorous drug

TABLE 15.2 ■ How Drugs Are Scheduled

Schedule	Characteristics	Examples
Schedule I	High potential for abuse and addiction; no accepted medical use.	Amphetamine (DMA, STP) Heroin Phencyclidine (PCP) LSD Marijuana Methaqualone
Schedule II	High potential for abuse and addiction; restricted medical use.	Cocaine Codeine* Methadone Morphine Opium Secobarbital (Seconal) Pentobarbital (Nembutal)
Schedule III	Some potential for abuse and addiction; currently accepted medical use.	Butalbital combinations (Fiorinal) Nalorphine Noludar
Schedule IV	Low potential for abuse and addiction; currently accepted medical use.	Chlorpromazine (Thorazine) Phenobarbital Minor tranquilizers
Schedule V	Lowest potential for abuse; accepted medical use.	Robitussin A-C OTC preparations

*Can also be Schedule III or Schedule IV, depending on use.

Source: Information from *Drug Enforcement,* July 1979; National Institute on Drug Abuse, Statistical Series, *Annual Data Report, 1989* (Rockville, MD: U.S. OHHS, 1989), 228–236.

of the rich and famous but rather as a potentially dangerous substance.

NIDA describes cocaine as "the most powerful naturally occurring stimulant."[8] Despite a few chemical similarities to less potent stimulants, such as those found in coffee and tea, cocaine is very dangerous and cannot be compared with these substances.

Cocaine is a crystalline white alkaloid powder derived from the leaves of the South American coca shrub (not related to cocoa plants). Coca grows only in the Andes Mountains at elevations between 1,500 and 5,000 feet. Coca leaves have been chewed for their stimulant effects for thousands of years by the Incas and their descendants. Then, in 1860, a German pharmacology graduate student named Albert Niemann "invented" cocaine. He was the first person to extract cocaine from the coca leaf, making possible a pure, stable substance (coca leaves lose their potency over time). Within three years, a wine called Vin Mariani, billed as a tonic and restorative, became popular in Paris. It contained 6 milligrams of cocaine per ounce. The public hailed cocaine's curative properties. Thomas Edison, Robert Louis Stevenson, Jules Verne, and Sigmund Freud were satisfied customers.

With the discovery that cocaine was a potent local anesthetic, the drug's popularity skyrocketed in the late nineteenth and early twentieth centuries. Manufacturers began producing it in larger quantities to answer demand. Patent-medicine men sold bottles of tonic that contained high concentrations of cocaine. Cocaine was used as an ingredient in Coca-Cola when it first appeared on the market. (It is reported that this popular beverage may still contain a drug-free extract of coca leaves.)

The medical establishment grew concerned about the drug when it became apparent that many users suffered from both dependence and unpleasant side effects. In 1914, the Harrison Act outlawed the use of cocaine in the United States.

Methods of Cocaine Use. Cocaine can be taken in several ways. The powdered form of the drug is "snorted" through the nose. Smoking (freebasing) and intravenous injections are more dangerous means of ingesting cocaine.

When cocaine is snorted, it can cause both damage to the mucous membranes in the nose and sinusitis. It can destroy the user's sense of smell, and occasionally it even creates a hole in the septum. Smoking cocaine can cause lung and liver damage. Freebasing has become more popular than injecting in recent years because people fear contracting diseases such as AIDS and hepatitis by sharing contaminated needles. But freebasing involves other dangers. Because the volatile mixes it requires are very explosive, some people have been killed or seriously burned.

Many cocaine users still occasionally "shoot up." Injecting allows the user to introduce large amounts of cocaine into the body rapidly. Within seconds, there is an incredible sense of euphoria. This intense high lasts only 15 to 20 minutes, and then the user heads into a "crash." To prevent the unpleasant effects of the crash, users must shoot up frequently, which can severely damage their veins. Besides AIDS and hepatitis, injecting users place themselves at risk for skin infections, inflammation of the arteries, and infection of the lining of the heart.

Physical Effects of Cocaine. The effects of cocaine are felt rapidly. Snorted cocaine enters the bloodstream through the lungs in less than one minute and reaches the brain in less than three minutes. When cocaine binds at its receptor sites in the central nervous system, it produces intense pleasure. The euphoria quickly abates, however, and the desire to regain the pleasurable feelings makes the user want more cocaine.

Cocaine is both an anesthetic and a central nervous system stimulant. In tiny doses, it can slow heart rate. In larger doses, the physical effects are dramatic: increased heart rate and blood pressure, loss of appetite that can lead to dramatic weight loss, convulsions, muscle twitching, irregular heartbeat, even eventual death due to overdose. Other effects of cocaine include temporary relief of depression, decreased fatigue, talkativeness, increased alertness, and heightened self-confidence. Again, however, as the dose increases, users become irritable and apprehensive and their behavior may turn paranoid or violent. The Skills for Behavior Change box lists further symp-

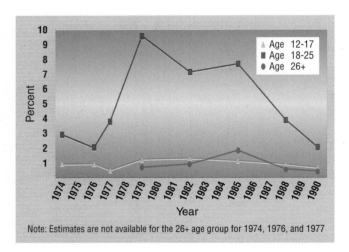

FIGURE 15.2

Trends in Americans' Cocaine Use by Age Group, 1974–1990

These data represent the percentages of those surveyed who reported using cocaine 30 days before the survey.

NIDA's 1990 National Household Survey had a sample of 9,259 Americans age 12 and over, living in the contiguous 48 states.

Source: Reprinted from *NIDA Notes* 5 (Winter 1991): 22.

Detecting and Helping Drug Users

The National Institute on Drug Abuse lists the following behaviors as indications of a drug problem:

- An abrupt change in attitude, including a lack of interest in activities once enjoyed.
- Frequent vague, withdrawn moods.
- A sudden decline in work or school performance or the regular skipping of classes.
- A sudden resistance to discipline or criticism.
- Secret telephone calls and meetings and a demand for greater privacy in terms of personal possessions.
- Increased frustration levels.
- Changes in sleeping or eating habits.
- A sudden weight loss.
- Evidence of drug use (smell of marijuana, drug paraphernalia).
- Frequent borrowing of money.
- Stealing.
- Disregard for personal appearance.
- Impaired relationships with family and friends.
- Disregard for deadlines, curfews, or other regulations.
- Unusual flare-ups of temper.

- New friends, especially known drug users, and strong allegiance to these friends.

Bear in mind that some of these behaviors may just be the result of college stress. But if you note several fairly sudden behavior changes in your friend, you may need to get your friend help. To help your friend, try the following:

- Get as much information as you can so you can understand what you and your friend are up against.
- Get some intervention training. Talk to a counselor with special training in chemical dependency; some offer advice by telephone.
- Confront the user—with other loved ones and a counselor if possible.
- Don't expect the drug abuser to quit without help.
- Offer your support, but make it clear that you expect your friend to undergo therapy.
- Don't believe abusers who say they have learned to control their drug use. Abstinence is the key to any good treatment program.
- Encourage the user to attend support groups such as Narcotics Anonymous or Cocaine Anonymous.

---

toms of drug use that you may recognize in yourself or friends along with some practical advice on how to help.

Cocaine-Affected Babies. In the mid-1980s, a problem began to emerge that may have devastating long-term effects on society: the use of cocaine by pregnant women. Because cocaine rapidly crosses the placenta (as virtually all drugs do), the fetus is vulnerable when a pregnant women snorts or shoots up. It is estimated that between 2.4 and 3.5 percent of pregnant women between the ages of 12 and 34 abuse cocaine. It is difficult to gauge how many newborns have been exposed to cocaine because pregnant women who are users are often reluctant to discuss their drug habit with their health-care providers for fear of prosecution. The most threatening problem during pregnancy is the increased risk of a miscarriage.

Many cocaine-exposed babies are born with brain damage, heart defects, kidney problems, and malformed heads, arms, and fingers. They tend to show signs of withdrawal at birth, including irritability, jitteriness, and the inability to eat or sleep properly. They seem to be unable to respond or to relate to people the way normal babies do, and they are difficult to console and comfort. Because

it is so difficult for adults to interact with them, their social and emotional development is negatively affected. There is also a significant increase in the risk of crib death—approximately 15 percent of cocaine-exposed babies die this way.

Since these babies often require extensive medical attention for their birth defects or abnormalities, many are abandoned by their mothers in the hospital. There they remain until foster care can be arranged. The cost for hospital and foster care is enormous—an estimated $500 million a year nationwide. In addition, preparing cocaine-affected babies for school is estimated to cost $1.5 billion annually. For both financial and humane reasons, developing prenatal care and education programs for mothers at risk should be a state and local government priority.

Freebase Cocaine. Freebase is a form of cocaine that is more powerful and costly than the powder or chip (crack)

Freebase: The most powerful distillate of cocaine.

form. Street cocaine (cocaine hydrochloride) is converted to pure base by removing the hydrochloride salt and many of the "cutting agents." The end product, freebase, is smoked through a water pipe.

Because freebase cocaine reaches the brain within seconds, it is more dangerous than cocaine that is snorted. It produces a quick, intense high that disappears quickly, leaving an intense craving for more. Freebasers typically increase the amount and frequency of the dose. They often become severely addicted and experience serious health problems and financial ruin.[9]

Side effects of freebasing cocaine include weight loss, increased heart rate and blood pressure, depression, paranoia, and hallucinations. Freebase is an extremely dangerous drug and is responsible for a large number of cocaine-related hospital emergency-room visits and deaths.

Crack. Crack is the street name given to freebase cocaine that has been processed from cocaine hydrochloride using ammonia or sodium bicarbonate (baking soda) and water and heating the substance to remove the hydrochloride. Crack can also be processed with ether, but this is much riskier because ether is a flammable solvent.

The mixture (90 percent pure cocaine) is then dried. The soapy-looking substance that results can be broken up into "rocks" and smoked. These rocks are approximately five times as strong as cocaine. Crack gets its name from the popping noises it makes when burned. Crack is also sometimes called "rock," an alias that should not be confused with rock cocaine. Rock cocaine is a cocaine hydrochloride substance that is primarily sold in California. White in color, it is about the shape of a pencil eraser and is typically snorted.

Because crack is such a pure drug, it takes much less time to achieve the desired high. One puff of a pebble-sized rock produces an intense high that lasts for approximately 20 minutes. The user can usually get three or four hits off a rock before it is used up. Crack is typically sold in small vials, folding papers, or heavy tinfoil containing two or three rocks, and costing between $10 and $20.

A crack user may quickly become addicted to the drug. Addiction is accelerated by the speed at which crack is absorbed through the lungs (it hits the brain within seconds after use) and by the intensity of the high. It is not uncommon for crack addicts to spend over $1,000 a day on their habits.

There is no definitive way of estimating the extent of crack use in the United States, but most authorities agree that it is highly popular. According to NIDA estimates, 4 to 5 million people use crack at least once a month.[10] Media attention to the large numbers of crack houses, crack-addicted babies, crack-related crimes, and other problems has drawn national attention to the enormity of the crack problem since the drug first gained notice around 1986.

Cocaine Addiction and Society. Cocaine addicts often suffer both physiological damage and serious disruptions of their lifestyle, including loss of employment and self-esteem. It is estimated that the annual cost of cocaine addiction in the United States exceeds $100 million. However, there is no way to measure the cost in wasted lives. An estimated 5 million Americans from all socioeconomic groups are addicted to cocaine. In the early 1980s, 1 person in 7 in the $50,000 income bracket was a regular user of crack or cocaine.[11] Today 5,000 new users try cocaine or crack every day. Federal agencies estimate that 5 to 6 million people use the drug at least once a month.[12]

The DEA has to date found no successful method to fight the cocaine and crack epidemic in the United States. Cocaine has been called unpredictable by drug experts, deadly by coroners, dangerous by former users, and disastrous by the media. Apparently, the risks associated with the use of the drug do not override users' desire to experience its euphoria.

Because cocaine is illegal, a complex network has developed to manufacture and sell the drug. Buyers may not always get the product they think they are purchasing. Cocaine marketed for snorting may be only 60 percent pure. Usually, it is mixed, or "cut," with other white powdery substances such as mannitol or sugar, though occasionally, it is cut with arsenic or other cocaine-like powders that may themselves be highly dangerous.

Amphetamines

The amphetamines include a large and varied group of synthetic agents that stimulate the central nervous system. Small doses of amphetamines improve alertness, lessen fatigue, and generally elevate mood. With repeated use, however, physical and psychological dependence develops. Sleep patterns are affected (insomnia); heart rate, breathing rate, and blood pressure increase; restlessness, anxiety, appetite suppression, and vision problems are common. High doses over long time periods can produce hallucinations, delusions, and disorganized behavior. Abusers become paranoid, fearing everything and everyone. Some become very aggressive or antisocial.

Amphetamines for recreational use are sold under a variety of names. "Bennies" (amphetamine/Benzedrine), "dex" (dextroamphetamine/Dexedrine), and "meth" or "speed" (methamphetamine/Methedrine) are some of the most common. Other street terms for amphetamines are "cross tops," "crank," "uppers," "wake-ups," "lid poppers," "cartwheels," and "blackies." Amphetamines do have therapeutic uses (see Chapter 2) in the treatment of attention deficit-hyperactivity disorder in children (Ritalin, Cylert) and of obesity (Pondimin).

Newer-Generation Stimulants

Illicit stimulants such as **crank** and **ice** have created further concerns because their effects last considerably longer than those produced by crack and cocaine. The elevated mood and excitability caused by crank, an amphetamine-like stimulant, last from two to four hours. For this reason, crank is becoming more and more popular among people whose occupations require long periods of wakefulness, such as truck drivers.

Ice is an even more potent stimulant that has begun to gain popularity in the United States, particularly in Hawaii. In just over four years after its introduction into the state, ice had reportedly surpassed marijuana and cocaine as Hawaii's leading problem drug.[13] Called *shabu* by the Japanese and *hiroppon* by the Koreans, ice can be manufactured in the laboratory using easily obtained chemicals. Purer and more crystalline than the crank manufactured in many large U.S. cities, most ice comes from Asia, particularly South Korea and Taiwan. Because it is odorless, public use of ice often goes unnoticed.

Typically, ice quickly becomes addictive. Some users have reported severe cravings after using the drug only once. The effects of ice are long-lasting. They include wakefulness, mood elevation, and excitability, all of which appeal to work-addicted young adults, particularly those who must put in long hours in high-stress jobs. Because the drug is very inexpensive and produces such an intense high (lasting from 4 to 14 hours), it has become popular among young people looking for a quick high. A pennysized plastic bag, called a "paper," may cost $50, but when smoked, it can keep a person high for a few days or for as long as a week. In contrast, an ounce of cocaine causes a high that lasts only about 20 minutes.

Addicts call the sensation from smoking ice *amping*, for the amplified euphoria it gives them. However, as is true of other *methamphetamines* (sympathetic nervous system stimulants), the "down" side of this drug can be devastating. Prolonged use can cause fatal lung and kidney damage as well as long-lasting psychological damage. In some instances, major psychological dysfunction has lasted as long as two and a half years after last use. Aggressive behavior is also associated with the drug's use, as evidenced by the dramatic increase in the number of ice-related violent crimes.[14] The number of babies born severely addicted to the drug is also increasing at an alarming rate.

Marijuana

Although archaeological evidence documents **marijuana** ("grass," "weed," "pot") use as far back as 6,000 years ago, the drug did not become popular in the United States until the 1960s. Marijuana receives less media attention today than it did then, but it is still the most extensively used illicit drug by far. NIDA reports that nearly 62 million Americans over the age of 12—about 1 in 3—have tried marijuana at least once.[15] About 19 million used the drug during 1991, according to the Department of Justice.[16] Although marijuana use has declined since 1982, 18 percent of all 18- to 34-year-olds surveyed in 1993 reported trying marijuana at least once in the previous month.[17] Among college students, marijuana is still the most popular illicit drug. (See Figure 15.1.)

Physical Effects of Marijuana. Marijuana is derived from either the cannabis sativa or cannabis indica (hemp) plants. The American-grown marijuana of the 1990s is a turbo-charged version of the hippie weed of the late 1960s. Developed using crossbreeding, genetic engineering, and American farming ingenuity, today's top-grade cannabis packs a punch very similar to hashish. **Tetrahydrocannabinol (THC)** is the psychoactive substance in marijuana, and the key to determining how powerful a high the marijuana will produce. Whereas marijuana from two decades ago ranged in potency from 1 to 5 percent THC, today's crop averages 8 percent, although concentrations as high as 15 percent may be found.

Hashish, a potent cannabis preparation derived mainly from the thick, sticky resin of the plant, contains high concentrations of THC. Hash oil, a substance produced by percolating a solvent such as ether through dried marijuana to extract the THC, is a tarry liquid that may contain up to 70 percent THC.

Crack: A distillate of powdered cocaine that comes in small, hard "chips" or "rocks."

Crank: An amphetamine-like stimulant having effects that last longer than those of crack or cocaine.

Ice: A potent, inexpensive stimulant that has long-lasting effects.

Marijuana: Chopped leaves and flowers of the cannabis indica or cannabis sativa plant (hemp); a psychoactive stimulant that intensifies reactions to environmental stimuli.

Tetrahydrocannabinol (THC): The chemical name for the active ingredient in marijuana.

Hashish: The sticky resin of the cannabis plant, which is high in THC.

Marijuana can be brewed and drunk in tea. It may also be baked into quick breads or brownies. THC concentrations in such products are impossible to estimate. Most of the time, however, marijuana is rolled into cigarettes (joints) or packed firmly into a pipe. Some people smoke marijuana through water pipes called bongs. Effects are generally felt within 10 to 30 minutes and usually wear off within three hours.

The most noticeable effect of THC is the dilation of the eyes' blood vessels, which produces the characteristic bloodshot eyes. Smokers of the drug also exhibit coughing, dry mouth and throat ("cotton mouth"), increased thirst and appetite, lowered blood pressure, and mild muscular weakness, primarily exhibited in drooping eyelids. Those users who take a high dose in an unfamiliar or uncomfortable setting are more likely to experience anxiety and the paranoid belief that their companions are ridiculing or threatening them.

Users may experience intensified reactions to various stimuli. For example, normal laugh responses may stretch into prolonged giggling and silliness. Colors and sounds, as well as the speed at which things move, may be magnified greatly. High doses of hashish may produce vivid visual hallucinations.

Effects of Chronic Marijuana Use. Because the use of marijuana is illegal in most parts of the United States, and because the drug has only been widely used since the 1960s, long-term studies of its effects are difficult to conduct. Also, studies conducted in the 1960s involved marijuana with THC levels that were only a fraction of the levels found in plants today. Thus the results of these studies may not be relevant to the more toxic forms of the drug presently in use. Most of the current information gathered about chronic marijuana use has been obtained from countries such as Jamaica and Costa Rica, where the drug is not illegal. These studies of chronic users (people who have used the drug for 10 or more years) indicate that long-term use of marijuana causes lung damage comparable to that caused by tobacco smoking. Smoking a single joint may be as damaging to the lungs as smoking five tobacco cigarettes. The chemicals do not damage the heart, but the effects of inhaling burning material do. Inhalation of marijuana transfers carbon monoxide to the bloodstream. Because the blood has a greater affinity for carbon monoxide than it does for oxygen, the oxygen-carrying capacity of the blood is diminished. The heart must then work harder to pump the vital element to oxygen-starved tissues.

Other suspected risks associated with marijuana include suppression of the immune system, blood pressure changes, and impaired memory function. Recent studies suggest that pregnant women who smoke marijuana are at a higher risk for stillbirth or miscarriage and for delivering low-birthweight babies and babies with abnormalities of the nervous system. Babies born to women who use marijuana during pregnancy are five times more likely to have features similar to those exhibited by children with fetal alcohol syndrome.

Debates concerning the effects of marijuana on the reproductive system have yet to be resolved. Studies conducted in the mid-1970s suggested that marijuana inhibited testosterone (and thus sperm) production in males and caused chromosomal breakage in both ova and sperm. Subsequent research in these areas is inconclusive. The question of whether the high-level THC plants currently available will increase the risks associated with this drug is, as yet, unanswered.

Marijuana and Medicine. Although recognized as a dangerous drug by the U.S. government, marijuana has at least two medical purposes. It has been used to help control the side effects, such as severe nausea, produced by chemotherapy (chemical treatment for cancer). Some reports claim that marijuana also reduces the pressure in the eyeball caused by glaucoma (a progressive disease characterized by increased fluid pressure in the eyeball).

In past years, the federal government has provided marijuana cigarettes to certain AIDS, cancer, and glaucoma patients for therapeutic use. But recently, the Public Health Service decided to halt supplies to new cancer and AIDS patients because of concern that marijuana may further compromise their immune systems.[18]

Marijuana and Driving. Marijuana use presents clear hazards for drivers of motor vehicles as well as for others on the road. The drug substantially reduces a driver's ability to react and to make quick decisions. A recent study revealed that one-third of the most seriously injured accident victims admitted to a hospital had levels of THC in their blood that indicated use of marijuana two to four hours prior to admission. The same study found that 4 out of every 10 drivers under 30 who were involved in car accidents were under the influence of marijuana at the time of their accidents.[19] Perceptual and other performance deficits resulting from using marijuana may persist for some time after the high subsides, though users who

Narcotics: Drugs that induce sleep and relieve pain; primarily the opiates.

Opium: The parent drug of the opiates; made from the seedpod resin of the opium poppy.

Morphine: A derivative of opium; sometimes used by medical practitioners to relieve pain.

Codeine: A drug derived from morphine; used in cough syrups and certain painkillers.

Heroin: An illegally manufactured derivative of morphine, usually injected into the bloodstream.

Black tar heroin: A dark brown, sticky substance made from morphine.

attempt to drive, fly, or operate heavy machinery often fail to recognize their impairment.

Opiates

The opiates are among the oldest analgesics known to humans. These drugs cause drowsiness, relieve pain, and induce euphoria. Also called **narcotics,** they are derived from the parent drug **opium,** a dark, resinous substance made from the milky juice of the opium poppy. Other opiates include *morphine, codeine, heroin,* and *black tar heroin.*

The word *narcotic* comes from the Greek word for "stupor" and is generally used to describe sleep-inducing substances. For many years, opiates were widely used by the medical community to relieve pain, induce sleep, curb nausea and vomiting, stop diarrhea, and sedate psychiatric patients. During the late nineteenth and early twentieth centuries, many patent medicines contained opiates. Suppliers advertised these concoctions as cures for everything from menstrual cramps to teething pains.

Among the opiates once widely used by medical practitioners was **morphine.** First manufactured in the early nineteenth century, morphine was named after Morpheus, the Greek god of sleep. More powerful than opium, morphine was first widely used as a painkiller during the Civil War. **Codeine,** a less powerful analgesic derived from morphine, also became popular.

As opiate use became more common, physicians noted that patients tended to become dependent on these substances. Contrary to earlier belief, all of the opiates are highly addictive. Growing concern about addiction led to government controls of narcotic use. The Harrison Act of 1914 prohibited the production, dispensation, and sale of opiate products unless prescribed by a physician. Subsequent legislation required physicians prescribing opiates to keep careful records. Physicians are still subject to audits of their prescriptions of these agents.

Some of the opiates are still used today for medical purposes. Morphine is sometimes prescribed by doctors in hospital settings for relief of severe pain. Codeine is found in prescription cough syrups and in other painkillers. Several prescription drugs, including Percodan, Demerol, and Dilaudid, contain synthetic opiates. All opiate use is strictly regulated.

Physical Effects of Opiates. Opiates are powerful central nervous system depressants. In addition to relieving pain, these drugs lower heart rate, respiration, and blood pressure. Side effects include weakness, dizziness, nausea, vomiting, euphoria, decreased sex drive, visual disturbances, and lack of coordination. Of all the opiates, heroin is the most notorious. Because all opiate addiction follows a similar progression, we will use heroin as a model for narcotic abuse.

Heroin Addiction. Heroin and **black tar heroin** are illegal opiates. Heroin is a white powder derived from morphine. Black tar heroin is a sticky, dark brown, foul-smelling substance. It is estimated that 750,000 Americans use heroin and that one-half of them live in New York City.[20] Authorities believe that the United States is at the beginning of a new heroin epidemic, which may result in increased crime and further spread of AIDS. There is concern that this epidemic will be worse than previous ones because the drug is now two to three times more available than ever before. The contemporary version of heroin is so potent that users can get high by snorting or smoking the drug rather than by injecting it and putting themselves at risk for AIDS (see Chapter 18). Once primarily an inner-city drug, heroin use is now becoming more widespread among middle-class people who tend to try whatever drug is new and trendy. Many people have switched from cocaine to heroin because the heroin high is not so stimulating and the drug is less expensive than cocaine.

Once considered a cure for morphine dependency, heroin was later discovered to be even more addictive and potent than morphine. Today, heroin has no medical use.

Heroin is a depressant. It produces a dreamy, mentally slow feeling and drowsiness in the user. In addition to its depressant effects, it can cause drastic mood swings in some users, with euphoric highs followed by depressive lows. Heroin also slows respiration and urinary output and constricts the pupils of the eyes. In fact, pupil constriction is a classic sign of narcotic intoxication; hence the image of the stereotypical drug user hiding his eyes

Cultivation of the opium poppy—from which opium, morphine, codeine, and heroin are produced—has been a staple of the economy of many underdeveloped countries.

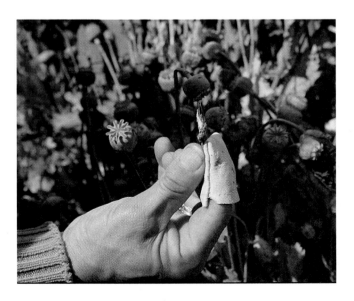

behind a pair of dark sunglasses. Symptoms of tolerance and withdrawal can appear within three weeks of the first use of the drug.

The most common route of administration for heroin addicts is "mainlining"—intravenous injection of powdered heroin mixed in a solution—though fear of AIDS has induced some people to change to nonneedle methods. Many users describe the "rush" they feel when injecting themselves as intensely pleasurable, whereas others report unpredictable and unpleasant side effects. The temporary nature of the rush contributes to the drug's high potential for addiction—many addicts shoot up four or five times a day. Mainlining can cause veins to become scarred, and if this practice is frequent enough, the veins collapse. Once a vein has collapsed, it can no longer be used to introduce heroin into the bloodstream. Addicts become expert at locating new veins to use: in the feet, the legs, even the temples. When they do not want their needle tracks (scars) to show, they inject themselves under the tongue or in the groin.

The physiology of the human body could be said to encourage opiate addiction. Opiate-like substances called **endorphins** are manufactured in the body and have multiple receptor sites, particularly in the central nervous system. When endorphins attach themselves at these points, they create feelings of painless well-being (see Chapter 12). Medical researchers have referred to endorphins as "the body's own opiates." When endorphin levels are high, people feel euphoric. The same euphoria occurs when opiates or related chemicals are active at the endorphin receptor sites.

Treatment for Heroin Addiction. Programs to help heroin addicts kick their habits have not been very successful. The rate of recidivism (tendency to return to previous behaviors) is high. Some addicts resume their drug use even after years of drug-free living because the craving for the injection rush is very strong. It takes a great deal of discipline to seek alternative, nondrug highs.

Heroin addicts experience a distinct pattern of withdrawal. They begin to crave another dose four to six hours after their last dose. Symptoms of withdrawal include intense desire for the drug, yawning, a runny nose, sweating, and crying. About 12 hours after the last dose, addicts experience sleep disturbance, dilated pupils, loss of appetite, irritability, goose bumps, and muscle tremors. The most difficult time in the withdrawal process occurs 24 to 72 hours following last use. All of the preceding symptoms continue, along with nausea, abdominal cramps, restlessness, insomnia, vomiting, diarrhea, extreme anxiety, hot and cold flashes, elevated blood pressure, and rapid heartbeat and respiration. Once the peak of withdrawal has been passed, all these symptoms begin to subside. Still, the recovering addict has many hurdles to jump; one of these is explored in the Building Communication Skills box.

Methadone maintenance is one type of treatment available for people addicted to heroin or other opiates.

Methadone is a synthetic narcotic that blocks the effects of opiate withdrawal. It is chemically similar enough to the opiates to control the tremors, chills, vomiting, diarrhea, and severe abdominal pains of withdrawal. Methadone dosage is decreased over a period of time until the addict is weaned off the drug.

Methadone maintenance is controversial because of the drug's own potential for addiction. Critics contend that the program merely substitutes one addiction for another. Proponents argue that people on methadone maintenance are less likely to engage in criminal activities to support their habits than heroin addicts are. For this reason, many methadone maintenance programs are state or federally financed and are available to clients free of charge or at reduced costs.

Psychedelics

The term **psychedelic** was adapted from a Greek phrase meaning "mind manifesting." Psychedelics are a group of drugs whose primary pharmacological effect is to alter feelings, perceptions, and thoughts in the user. The major receptor sites for most of these drugs are in the part of the brain that is responsible for interpreting outside stimuli before allowing these signals to travel to other parts of the brain. This area is called the **reticular formation** and is located in the brain stem at the upper end of the spinal cord (see Figure 15.3). When a psychedelic drug is present at a reticular formation receptor site, messages become

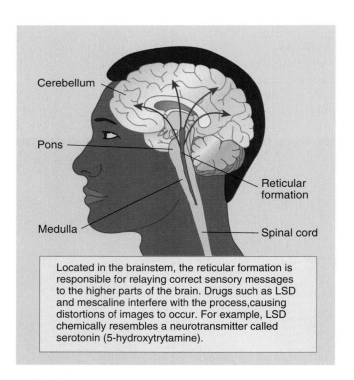

Cerebellum

Pons

Medulla

Reticular formation

Spinal cord

Located in the brainstem, the reticular formation is responsible for relaying correct sensory messages to the higher parts of the brain. Drugs such as LSD and mescaline interfere with the process, causing distortions of images to occur. For example, LSD chemically resembles a neurotransmitter called serotonin (5-hydroxytrytamine).

FIGURE 15.3

The Reticular Formation

Recovering Addicts Need Communication Skills, Too

An often overlooked area in drug rehabilitation is the teaching of communication skills to recovering addicts. At the DeKalb Medical Center in DeKalb, Georgia, addicts begin with a week of detoxification. Then they have nightly education programs with two main goals: staying off their drug and reentering a society filled with people not on drugs. People whose lives have been immersed in drugs have been seeing themselves and others in an altered state. As they start to move back to mainstream society, they need to learn basic communication skills and relationship development skills.

So much of our self-esteem is based on our ability to communicate with others, and these addicts generally tend to lack skills. Without training, addicts may feel tremendous stress in dealing with others, and stress is considered the "big kicker" for developing relapse.

Addicts learn to change their negative self-talk to positive self-talk, whereby they can help themselves to beat the habit and reestablish their lives. [One of the self-talk techniques you learned in Chapter 1 was the Rational-Emotive Theory.] Addicts may be taught that when they feel an urge to relapse, they should not say to themselves, "I'm a useless drug addict"; instead, they could say, "I am learning to cope without drugs and will not return to their use."

Relationship training is also important. Addicts need to be reminded of what relationships are about and how to form them. Many women addicts are abused, and need to learn to assert themselves in relationships so that they do not have another abusive relationship.

How could you help a recovering addict? As friends or family members come out of rehab programs, give them some extra time and attention. Realize that as they adjust to a drug-free life, their communications behavior might not always be appropriate; allow them to make errors. Help them by letting them know that you care. And most of all, let them know that they can reestablish the relationship that was ruined by the disease of drug addiction.

Source: Reprinted by permission from "Traditional Treatment," CNN News Segment, 23 February 1994; Andrew Holtz reporting. © 1994 Cable News Network, Inc. All rights reserved. Published by arrangement with Turner Educational Services, Inc.

---

scrambled, and the user may see wavy walls instead of straight ones or may smell colors or hear tastes. This mixing of sensory messages is known as **synesthesia.**

In addition to synesthetic effects, users may recall events long buried in the subconscious mind or become less inhibited than they are in a nondrug state. Some psychedelic drugs are erroneously labeled "hallucinogens." Hallucinogens are substances that are capable of creating auditory or visual **hallucinations,** or images that are perceived but are not real. Not all of the psychedelic drugs are capable of producing hallucinations. The most widely recognized psychedelics are LSD, mescaline, psilocybin, and psilocin. All are illegal and carry severe penalties for manufacture, possession, transportation, or sale.

LSD. Of all the psychedelics, **lysergic acid diethylamide** (LSD) has achieved the most notoriety. This chemical was first synthesized in the late 1930s by the Swiss chemist Albert Hoffman. It resulted from experiments aimed at deriving medically useful drugs from the ergot fungus found on rye and other cereal grains. Because LSD seemed capable of unlocking the secrets of the mind, psychiatrists initially felt it could be beneficial to patients unable to remember and recognize suppressed traumas. From 1950 through 1968, the drug was used for such purposes.

Media attention was drawn to LSD in the late 1960s. Young people were using the drug to "turn on" and "tune out" the world that gave them the war in Vietnam, race riots, and political assassinations. In 1970, federal author-ities, under intense pressure from the public, placed LSD on the list of controlled substances (Schedule I). This ruling did not curtail the use of the drug, however. Its popularity peaked in 1972, then tapered off, primarily because of users' inability to control dosages accurately.

Because of the recent wave of nostalgia for the 1960s, this dangerous psychedelic drug has been making a come-

Endorphins: Opiate-like hormones that are manufactured in the human body and contribute to natural feelings of well-being.

Methadone maintenance: A treatment for people addicted to opiates that substitutes methadone, a synthetic narcotic, for the opiate of addiction.

Psychedelics: Drugs that distort the processing of sensory information in the brain.

Reticular formation: An area in the brain stem that is responsible for relaying messages to other areas in the brain.

Synesthesia: A (usually) drug-created effect in which sensory messages are incorrectly assigned—for example, hearing a taste or smelling a sound.

Hallucination: An image (auditory or visual) that is perceived but is not real.

Lysergic acid diethylamide (LSD): Psychedelic drug causing sensory disruptions; also called acid.

back. Known on the street as "acid," LSD is now available in virtually every state, and its availability is increasing. Over 10 million Americans, most of them under 35 years of age, have tried LSD at least once. LSD especially attracts younger users.[21] Although a national survey of college students showed that only 3.6 percent had tried LSD in 1991,[22] it is the fastest-growing illicit drug among the under-20 age group. In 1990, nearly 50 percent of LSD-related emergency room visits involved people who were younger than 20; of these, 80 percent were white and 76 percent were male.[23]

An odorless, tasteless, white crystalline powder, LSD is most frequently dissolved in water to make a solution that can then be used to manufacture the street forms of the drug: tablets, blotter acid, and windowpane. What the LSD consumer usually buys is blotter acid—small squares of blotterlike paper that have been impregnated with the liquid. The blotter is swallowed or chewed briefly. LSD also comes in tiny thin squares of gelatin called windowpane and in tablets called microdots, which are less than an eighth of an inch across (it would take 10 or more of these to add up to the size of an aspirin tablet). Microdots and windowpane are just a sideshow; blotter is the medium of choice. It comes decorated with a mind-boggling array of designs, some of them copied from characters created by Disney and other cartoon studios.

LSD is one of the most powerful drugs known to science and can produce strong effects in doses as low as 20 micrograms. (To give you an idea of how small a dose this is, the average-sized postage stamp weighs approximately 60,000 micrograms.) The potency of the typical dose of LSD currently ranges from 20 to 80 micrograms, com-pared to 150 to 300 micrograms commonly used in the 1960s.

Despite its reputation for being primarily a psychedelic, LSD produces a large number of physical effects, including slightly increased heart rate, elevated blood pressure and temperature, goose flesh (roughened skin), increased reflex speeds, muscle tremors and twitches, perspiration, increased salivation, chills, headaches, and mild nausea. Since the drug also stimulates uterine muscle contractions, it can lead to premature labor and miscarriage in pregnant women.

Research into the effects of long-term LSD use has been inconclusive. As with any illegally purchased drug, users run the risk of purchasing an impure product.

The psychological effects of LSD vary from person to person. The set and setting in which the drug is used are very influential factors. Euphoria is the common psychological state produced by the drug, but *dysphoria* (a sense of evil and foreboding) may also be experienced. The drug also shortens attention span, causing the mind to wander. Thoughts may be interposed and juxtaposed as well. The user may thus be able to experience several different thoughts simultaneously. Synesthesia occurs occasionally. Users become introspective, and suppressed memories may surface, often taking on bizarre symbolism. Many more effects are possible, including decreased aggressiveness and enhanced sensory experiences.

Although LSD rarely produces hallucinations, it can create illusions. These distortions of ordinary perceptions may include movement of stationary objects. "Bad trips" are the most publicized risk of LSD. These negative experiences are commonly related to set or setting. The user,

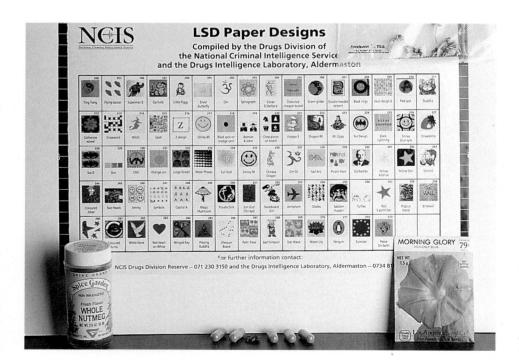

The dangerous psychedelic drug, LSD, which was heavily used by the "consciousness-raising" generation of the 1960s, is making a comeback despite its many risks.

Separation of Church and Drugs

The peyote cactus is a sacred plant to many Native Americans. It has been used as an integral part of many of their religious ceremonies dating back to the pre-Columbian period of American history. These cacti are still used today in religious practices by Northern Mexican tribes and the Southwestern Plains Indian tribes. In addition, the Native American Church of North America, with a membership of over 250,000, also uses peyote as a sacrament.

Mescaline is the active component of peyote and San Pedro cacti. Its effects include kaleidoscope-like displays of vivid colors, auditory and tactile hallucinations, and synesthetic experiences. Seen in the context of a religious service as a "communion with the gods," peyote was regarded as a sacred substance. A peyote ceremony might consist of ingesting the peyote buttons, then singing, drumming, chanting hymns, and trying to understand the psychedelic changes in order to have spiritual experiences.

Until a 1990 U.S. Supreme Court ruling, Native American Church members believed that their right to use peyote in religious ceremonies was protected under the U.S. Constitution. The Supreme Court, however, upheld an Oregon state law that declared the use of the hallucinogen for any purpose illegal in that state (the federal government and 23 states make exceptions for the use of peyote by the Native American Church). The Court, by a six to three majority, ruled in favor of Oregon and against Native-American traditions, stating that an individual's religious beliefs do not excuse him or her from compliance with an otherwise valid law prohibiting conduct that the state is free to regulate. Native Americans have pointed out that their practice predates the U.S. Constitution.

Source: Adapted by permission from Robert R. Pinger et al., *Drugs: Issues for Today,* 2nd ed. (St. Louis, MO: Mosby-Year Book, 1995), 333–334.

---

for example, may interpret increased heart rate as a heart attack (a "bad body trip"). Often bad trips result when a user confronts a suppressed emotional experience or memory (a "bad head trip") while using the drug.

While there is no evidence that LSD creates a physical dependence, it may well create a psychological dependence. Many LSD users become depressed for one or two days following a trip and turn to the drug to relieve this depression. The result is a cycle of LSD use to relieve post-LSD depression, which often leads to psychological addiction.

WHAT DO YOU THINK?

Discuss the reasons for use of LSD in the United States during the 1960s. Discuss the prevalence of LSD's use in the 1990s. What are the similarities and differences between the two periods and the use of this drug during them?

Mescaline. Mescaline is one of the hundreds of chemicals derived from the **peyote** cactus. The small, buttonlike cactus grows in the southwestern United States and parts of Latin America. Natives of these regions have long used the dried peyote buttons during religious ceremonies. In fact, members of the Native American Church (a religion practiced by thousands of North American Indians) have been granted special permission to use the drug during religious ceremonies in some states, as discussed in the Multicultural Perspectives box.

Users normally swallow 10 to 12 dried peyote buttons. These buttons taste bitter and generally induce immediate nausea or vomiting. Long-time users claim that the nausea becomes less noticeable with frequent use.

Those who are able to keep the drug down begin to feel the effects within 30 to 90 minutes, when mescaline reaches maximum concentration in the brain. (It may persist for up to 9 or 10 hours.) Unlike LSD, mescaline is a powerful hallucinogen. It is also a central nervous system stimulant.

Products sold on the street as mescaline are likely to be synthetic chemical relatives of the true drug. Street names of these products include DOM, STP, TMA, and MMDA. Any of these can be toxic in small quantities.

Psilocybin. Psilocybin and *psilocin* are the active chemicals in a group of mushrooms sometimes called "magic

Mescaline: A hallucinogenic drug derived from the peyote cactus.

Peyote: A cactus with small "buttons" that, when ingested, produce hallucinogenic effects.

Psilocybin: The active chemical found in psilocybe mushrooms; it produces hallucinations.

mushrooms." Psilocybe mushrooms, which grow throughout the world, can be cultivated from spores or can be harvested wild. Because many mushrooms resemble the psilocybe variety, people who use wild mushrooms for any purpose should be certain of what they are doing. Mushroom varieties can easily be misidentified, and mistakes can be fatal. Psilocybin is similar to LSD in physical effects. These effects generally wear off within 4 to 6 hours.

The Deliriants

Delirium is an agitated mental state characterized by confusion and disorientation. Almost all of the psychoactive drugs will produce delirium at high doses, but the **deliriants** produce this condition at relatively low (subtoxic) levels.

PCP. **Phencyclidine,** or **PCP,** is one of the best-known deliriants. It is a synthetic substance that became a black-market drug in the early 1970s. PCP was originally developed as a "disassociative anesthetic," which means that patients administered this drug could keep their eyes open, apparently remain conscious, and feel no pain during a medical procedure. Patients would afterward experience amnesia for the time the drug was in their system. Such a drug had obvious advantages as an anesthetic during surgery, but its unpredictability and drastic effects (postoperative delirium, confusion, and agitation) made doctors abandon it and it was withdrawn from the legal market.

On the illegal market, PCP is a white, crystalline powder that users often sprinkle onto marijuana cigarettes. It is dangerous and unpredictable regardless of the method of administration. Common street names for PCP are "angel dust" for the crystalline powdered form and "peace pill" and "horse tranquilizer" for the tablet form.

The effects of PCP depend on the dosage. A dose as small as 5 mg will produce effects similar to those of strong central nervous system depressants. These effects include slurred speech, impaired coordination, reduced sensitivity to pain, and reduced heart and respiratory rate. Doses between 5 and 10 mg cause fever, salivation, nausea, vomiting, and total loss of sensitivity to pain. Doses greater than 10 mg result in a drastic drop in blood pressure, coma, muscular rigidity, violent outbursts, and possible convulsions and death.

Psychologically, PCP may produce either euphoria or dysphoria. It is also known to produce hallucinations as well as delusions and overall delirium. Some users experience a prolonged state of "nothingness." The long-term effects of PCP use are unknown.

Designer Drugs

Designer drugs are structural analogs (drugs that produce similar effects) of drugs already included under the Con-

trolled Substances Act. These illegal drugs are manufactured by underground chemists to mimic the psychoactive effects of controlled drugs. At present, at least three types of synthetic drugs are available on the illegal drug market: analogs of phencyclidine (PCP), analogs of *fentanyl* and *meperidine* (both synthetic narcotic analgesics), and analogs of amphetamine and methamphetamine, which have hallucinogenic and stimulant properties.[24]

Although PCP analogs have been identified in street samples of drugs, they are less frequently used today than are other forms of designer drugs. Analogs of fentanyl are much more common. The pharmacological properties of most fentanyl analogs are similar to those of heroin or morphine. These analogs are known as "synthetic heroin," "china white," or "new heroin." These designer drugs may be addictive and carry the risk for overdose.

Meperidine, commonly known by its trade name Demerol, is a narcotic with several designer analogs. When heroin becomes difficult to obtain, street analogs of meperidine, known as MPPP and PEPAP, often surface. Both of these drugs pose significant risk for overdose. An impure form of MPPP, known as MPTP, has been known to cause an irreversible brain syndrome similar to Parkinson's disease in some users.[25]

Amphetamine and methamphetamine analogs are the most common forms of designer drugs on college campuses today. These analogs often cause hallucinations and euphoria. *Ecstasy,* which was dubbed the "LSD of the 80s," is one such analog that became popular on many college campuses in the 1980s. It is actually a chemical called methylenedioxymethylamphetamine, or MDMA, and it is similar to the hallucinogen MMDA.

Users claim that Ecstasy provides the rush of cocaine combined with the mind-expanding characteristics of the hallucinogens. Psychological effects of MDMA include confusion, depression, anxiety, and paranoia. Physical symptoms may include muscle tension, nausea, blurred vision, faintness, chills, and sweating. MDMA also increases heart rate and blood pressure and may destroy neurons that regulate aggression, mood, sexual activity, and sensitivity to pain.[26]

A number of deaths were initially attributed to MDMA, but subsequent research indicated that these deaths were actually related to other factors. Researchers are continuing to explore the effects of this and other designer drugs.

In the 1980s, states began regulating the manufacture of drug analogs, and by 1989, 47 states had enacted "look-alike" laws. Illinois, for example, imposes penalties that include five years in prison and up to a $20,000 fine for possessing, advertising, producing, or selling look-alike, or designer, drugs.[27]

An analog of phencyclidine, Special K or ketamine, is an anesthetic drug used in many hospital and veterinary clinics around the country. Over the past few years, it has become more available and popular. The appeal of ketamine stems from its low cost and hallucinogenic effects. Called the "yuppie LSD," it produces a rush of energy but also mental confusion. Ketamine's effects are not as severe as Ecstasy's, so it appeals to people who have to go to work or school after a night of partying.[28]

Inhalants

Inhalants are chemicals that produce vapors that, when inhaled, can cause hallucinations as well as create intoxicating and euphoric effects. They are not commonly recognized as drugs. They are legal to purchase and universally available but are potentially dangerous. These drugs are generally used by young people who can't afford illicit substances.

Some of these agents are organic solvents representing the chemical by-products of the distillation of petroleum products. Rubber cement, model glue, paint thinner, lighter fluid, varnish, wax, spot removers, and gasoline belong to this group. Most of these substances are sniffed by users in search of a quick, cheap high.

Because they are inhaled, the volatile chemicals in these products reach the bloodstream within seconds. An inhaled substance is not diluted or buffered by stomach acids or other body fluids and thus is more potent and dangerous than the same substance would be if swallowed. This characteristic, along with the fact that dosages are extremely difficult to control because everyone has unique lung and breathing capacities, makes inhalants particularly dangerous.

The effects of inhalants usually last for less than 15 minutes. Users may experience dizziness, disorientation, impaired coordination, reduced judgment, and slowed reaction times. Signs of inhalant use include: unjustifiable collection of glues, paints, lacquer thinner, cleaning fluid, and ether; sniffles similar to those produced by a cold; and a smell on the breath similar to the inhalable substance. The effects of inhalants are similar to those of central nervous system depressants. Combining inhalants with alcohol produces a synergistic effect. In addition, these substances in combination can cause severe liver damage that may lead to death.

An overdose of fumes from inhalants can cause unconsciousness. If the user's oxygen intake is reduced during the inhaling process, death can result within five minutes.

Amyl Nitrite. Sometimes called "poppers" or "rush," **amyl nitrite** is often prescribed to alleviate chest pain in heart patients. It is packaged in small, cloth-covered glass capsules that can be crushed to release the active chemical. The drug relieves chest pains because it causes rapid dilation of the small blood vessels and reduces blood pressure. That same dilation of blood vessels in the genital area is thought to enhance sensations or perceptions of orgasm. It also produces fainting, dizziness, warmth, and skin flushing.

Nitrous Oxide. "Laughing gas" is the popular term for **nitrous oxide.** It is sometimes used as an adjunct to dental anesthesia or minor surgical anesthesia. It is also used as a propellant chemical in aerosol products such as whipped toppings. Users experience a state of euphoria, floating sensations, and illusions. Effects also include pain relief and a "silly" feeling, demonstrated by laughing and giggling (hence the term *laughing gas*). Regulating dosages of this drug can be difficult. Sustained inhalation can lead to unconsciousness, coma, and death.

Steroids

Public awareness of **anabolic steroids** has recently been heightened by media stories about their use by amateur and professional athletes, including Arnold Schwarzenegger during his competitive bodybuilding days. Anabolic steroids are artificial forms of the male hormone testosterone that promote muscle growth and strength. These **ergogenic drugs** are used primarily by young men to increase their strength, power, bulk (weight), and speed. These attributes are sought either to enhance athletic performance or to develop the physique that users perceive will make them more attractive and increase their sex appeal.

Most steroids are obtained through black market sources. It is estimated that approximately 17 to 20 percent of college athletes use steroids. Overall, it is estimated that there are 1 million steroid abusers in the

Delirium: An agitated mental state characterized by confusion and disorientation that can be produced by psychoactive drugs.

Deliriant: Any substance that produces delirium at relatively low doses, including PCP and some herbal substances.

Phencyclidine (PCP): A deliriant commonly called "angel dust."

Designer drug: A synthetic analog (a drug that produces similar effects) of an existing illicit drug.

Inhalants: Products that are sniffed or inhaled in order to produce highs.

Amyl nitrite: A drug that dilates blood vessels and is properly used to relieve chest pain.

Nitrous oxide: The chemical name for "laughing gas," a substance properly used for surgical or dental anesthesia.

Anabolic steroids: Artificial forms of the hormone testosterone that promote muscle growth and strength.

Ergogenic drug: Substance that enhances athletic performance.

United States, many of whom take steroids for noncompetitive bodybuilding.[29] Steroids are available in two forms: injectable solution and pills.[30] Anabolic steroids produce a state of euphoria, diminished fatigue, and increased bulk and power in both sexes. These qualities give steroids an addictive quality. When users stop, they appear to undergo psychological withdrawal, mainly caused by the disappearance of the physique they have become accustomed to.

Several adverse effects occur in both men and women who use steroids. These drugs cause mood swings (aggression and violence), sometimes known as "roid rage"; acne; liver tumors; elevated cholesterol levels; hypertension; kidney disease; and immune system disturbances. There is also a danger of AIDS transmission through shared needles. In women, large doses of anabolic steroids trigger masculine changes, including lowered voice, increased facial and body hair, male pattern baldness, enlarged clitoris, decreased breast size, and changes in or absence of menstruation. When taken by healthy males, anabolic steroids shut down the body's production of

The use of steroids to increase bulk and power carries many health risks, including disturbance of the immune system from the drug itself, plus the risk of AIDS transmission through the use of shared needles.

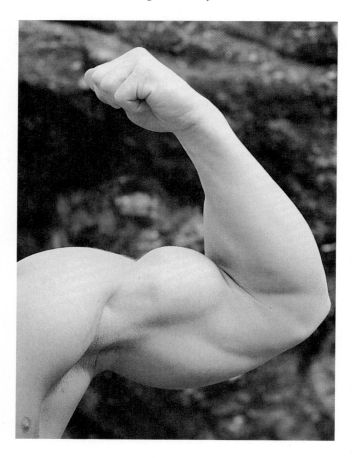

testosterone, causing men's breasts to grow and testicles to atrophy.

To combat the growing problem of steroid use, Congress passed the Anabolic Steroids Control Act (ASCA) of 1990. This law makes it a crime to possess, prescribe, or distribute anabolic steroids for any use other than for the treatment of specific diseases. Anabolic steroids are now classified as a Schedule III drug. Penalties for their illegal use include up to five years' imprisonment and a $250,000 fine for the first offense, and up to 10 years' imprisonment and a $500,000 fine for subsequent offenses.

A new and alarming trend is the use of other drugs to achieve the "performance-enhancing" effects of steroids. These steroid alternatives are sought in order to avoid the stiff penalties now in effect against those who possess anabolic steroids without a valid prescription.

The two most common steroid alternatives are gamma hysroxybutyrate (GHB) and clenbuterol. GHB is a deadly, illegal drug that is a primary ingredient in many of these "performance-enhancing" formulas. GHB does not produce a high. It does, however, cause headaches, nausea, vomiting, diarrhea, seizures and other central nervous system disorders, and possibly death. Clenbuterol, another steroid alternative, has become an extremely popular item on the black market. The drug is used in some countries for certain veterinary treatments, but is not approved for any use—in animals or humans—in the United States.

WHAT DO YOU THINK?

How do you think reports in the media about the use of stimulants and/or steroids by athletes affect the popularity of these drugs? Would you consider using such a drug to improve your appearance?

ILLEGAL DRUG USE IN THE UNITED STATES

Stories of people who have tried illegal drugs, enjoyed them, and suffered no consequences may tempt you to try them yourself. You may tell yourself it's "just this once," convincing yourself that one-time use is harmless. Given the dangers surrounding these substances, however, you should carefully consider nondrug alternatives. Many such alternatives, although often time-consuming, are more rewarding and usually contribute more to personal growth than chemically induced experiences do. The Choices for Change box gives some alternatives to drug use that you may wish to consider.

The risks associated with drug use extend beyond the personal level. The decision to try any illicit substance encourages illicit drug manufacture and transportation and

Alternatives to Drug Use

People use drugs for a variety of reasons—to achieve altered states of consciousness or to cope with the stresses of everyday life. Fortunately, nondrug alternatives are available that can accomplish the same results. If you feel tempted to experiment with drugs, try some of these activities in preference to risking your health and stability by taking drugs.

- If you need physical relaxation, try exercise or outdoor hobbies.
- If you feel a need for excitement or risk taking, try hiking, biking, or other outdoor activities.
- Look for challenges and satisfaction in your work or studies.
- Participate in social or political activities that provide meaning and a sense of accomplishment in your life.

Assume responsibility for someone or something outside yourself.

- Learn to practice meditation or biofeedback to help yourself relax.
- Turn to religious or spiritual sources for comfort and guidance. If you want to expand your personal awareness, explore various philosophical theories through classes, seminars, and discussion groups.
- If you feel pressure from your peers, look for new friends or roommates. Take a class or join an organization that attracts health-conscious people.
- If you're anxious, depressed, or uptight and want relief from stress or emotional pains, turn to friends, support groups, or counselors.

---

contributes to the national drug problem. The DEA estimates that illegal drug sales in the United States in 1990 totaled $40 billion, an amount that exceeded the annual sales volume of all but the largest U.S. corporations. Expenditures for cocaine alone were $17.5 billion. Retail sales of heroin surpassed $12 billion, and for marijuana the figure was $9 billion.[31] Thus illegal drugs are not only big business, they are one of the largest businesses in the United States.[32] The financial burden of illegal drug use on the U.S. economy is staggering. Health-care costs attributable to it total $60 billion annually.

Roughly one-half of all expenditures to combat crime are related to illegal drugs. The same laws that restrict drug use and warn us of potential dangers also contribute to the mystique surrounding illicit drug use. For this reason, some people have proposed legalizing—or at least decriminalizing—the use of presently illicit drugs, as discussed in the Health Headlines box.

Women and Drug Abuse

More than 4 million U.S. women of all ages, races, and cultures use drugs. It is estimated that 9 million women have used illicit drugs during the past year and almost half of all women between the ages of 15 and 44 have used drugs at least once in their lifetimes. Today, more than 28,000 (70 percent) of AIDS cases among women are related either to injecting drugs or to having sex with a man who injects drugs; AIDS is now the fourth leading cause of death among women.

Many women who use drugs have had troubled lives. Studies have found that at least 70 percent of women drug users have been sexually abused by the age of 16. Most of these women had at least one parent who abused alcohol or drugs. Furthermore, these women often have low self-esteem, little self-confidence, and feel powerless. They often feel lonely and are isolated from support networks.

Unfortunately, many of these women have good reasons not to seek help. Some may not be able to find or afford child care. Others fear that the courts may take away their children. Many fear violence from their husbands, boyfriends, or partners.

Research has shown that women drug abusers get better when treatment takes care of all their basic needs. Some women need the basic services of food, shelter, and clothing. Other women also need transportation, child care, and parenting training. Good treatment also teaches reading, basic education, and the skills needed to find a job. As a woman's self-esteem increases, her chances of remaining drug-free increase.

What Do You Think?

What are the societal factors that make getting treatment so difficult for women? Do you think women begin using drugs for reasons that are different from men's? Does society perceive women who abuse substances differently from men? If so, why?

Drugs in the Workplace

NIDA estimates that between 10 and 23 percent of all U.S. workers use dangerous drugs on the job—that's one in every five workers aged 18 to 25 and one in every eight workers aged 26 to 34. Employees caught up in substance

Should Illicit Drugs Be Legalized?

Recently, there has been an increase in public debate on the issue of legalizing illicit drugs. The rationale for legalization rests on the assumption that it is drug laws, rather than drugs themselves, that are damaging to society. However, people do not control drugs; drugs control people.

Myth: Legalization would eliminate the profitable black market and its accompanying violence.

Fact: Unless we are willing to make every drug available in unlimited quantities and combinations on demand of the user/addict, regardless of age or occupation, there will always be a thriving black market for drugs. If we are not willing to provide the most potent marijuana and the strongest, purest heroin, cocaine, crack, and methamphetamine to anyone who requests these substances, the black market will continue to flourish as drug users and abusers search for an ever-higher high.

Myth: Drug use is a victimless crime. What a person does with his or her own body is no one else's business.

Fact: Illicit drugs are illegal because they are dangerous not only to users/addicts but to everyone else around them: family, employers, fellow employees, and all those who share the roads and highways with drug-impaired drivers.

If drug users work, other citizens pay in lost productivity, increased on-the-job accidents, and higher absenteeism and medical costs. If drug users don't work, they and their families become a financial burden on the taxpayer or they become involved in criminal activities that are not only costly but often vicious as well.

Myth: Legalizing drugs for adults will not increase drug use by minors.

Fact: Research studies show that adults' use of drugs in the home results in substantially increased usage by their children. No education or prevention program could counter the lure of illicit drugs if they become legal, more readily available, and socially acceptable.

Myth: The drug laws are hypocritical. Alcohol and tobacco, the two major legal drugs, kill more people than all illegal drugs put together.

Fact: Tobacco addiction and alcoholism kill more people because they are legal and more people use them. In time, if legalized, other dangerous drugs would become just as common and even more deadly. Because we now have two legal drugs that destroy many lives is no reason to add more dangerous drugs to the legal list.

Myth: Legalization will eliminate most crimes.

Fact: It is true that many drug-linked crimes are money related, but an equal number of crimes committed by drug users do not involve quick-cash schemes. These are violent and destructive crimes that result from the effects of psychoactive drugs on the individual. If dangerous drugs were legalized, the number of crimes committed by users would certainly increase rather than decrease, both in the community and on the job.

Myth: We're wasting money on law enforcement; if people want drugs, they will find ways to get them.

Fact: This argument loses sight of the moral implications of legalization. Who are we willing to sacrifice so we can save money and protect our personal property? With lower prices and greater availability, drug use would go up among those who are presently most vulnerable: our youth, the working poor, and the chronically unemployed.

Source: Adapted from Citizens for a Drug Free Oregon (1988), NE Sandy Blvd, Suite 320-I, Portland, OR 97220.

---

abuse tend to be absent from the job up to 16 times as often, claim three times as many sickness benefits, and file five times as many workers' compensation claims as nonusers.[33] Costs are seen in reduced work performance and efficiency, lost productivity, absenteeism and turnover costs, increased health benefits utilization, accidents, and losses stemming from impaired judgment.

Many employers have instituted drug testing for their employees to counteract the drug epidemic. The use of mandatory drug urinalysis is controversial. Critics argue that such testing violates Fourth Amendment rights of protection from unreasonable search and seizure. Proponents believe the personal inconvenience entailed in testing pales in comparison to the problems caused by drug use in the workplace. Some court decisions have affirmed the right of employers to test their employees for drug use. They contend that Fourth Amendment rights pertain only to employees of government agencies, not to those of private businesses. Most Americans apparently support some type of drug testing for certain types of job categories.[34]

Drug testing is expensive, with costs running as high as $100 per individual test. Moreover, some critics question the accuracy and the reliability of these tests. Both false positives and false negatives can occur. As drug testing becomes more common in the work environment, it is gaining greater acceptance by employees, who see testing as a step to improving safety and productivity.

WHAT DO YOU THINK?

What do you believe are the moral and ethical issues surrounding drug testing? Are you in favor of drug testing? Should all employees be subjected to drug tests or just those employees in high-risk jobs? Is it the employer's right to conduct drug testing at the worksite?

Solutions to the Problem

Americans are alarmed by the increasing use of illegal drugs, particularly crack and other forms of cocaine. In recent years, we have been constantly warned through the media about this "chemical menace" to our society. Respondents in a poll felt that the most important strategy for fighting drug abuse was educating young people. Other strategies endorsed were working with foreign governments to stop drug trafficking, making a concerted effort to arrest dealers, providing treatment assistance, and arresting drug users.

The most popular antidrug strategies for many years were total prohibition and "scare tactics." Both approaches proved ineffective. Prohibition of alcohol during the 1920s created more problems than it solved, as did prohibition of opiates in 1914. Likewise, prohibition of other illicit drugs has neither eliminated them nor curtailed their trafficking across U.S. borders.

In general, researchers in the field of drug education agree that a multimodal approach to drug education is best. Students should be taught the difference between drug use and abuse. Factual information that is free from scare tactics must be presented; moralizing about drug use and abuse does not work. Programs that teach people to control drugs, as opposed to allowing drugs to control them, are needed, as are programs that teach about the influences of set and setting. Reinforcement of self-esteem is mandatory. It is not adequate to urge people to "just say no." Alternatives to drugs should be taught.

At-risk groups must be targeted for study so that we can better understand the circumstances that make each group more or less prone to drug use. Time, money, and effort by educators, parents, and policymakers are needed to ensure that today's youths are given the love and security essential for building productive and meaningful lives.[35]

Among the various strategies suggested for combating drug abuse are stricter border surveillance to reduce drug trafficking, longer prison sentences for drug pushers, increased government spending on prevention and enforcement of antidrug laws, and greater cooperation between government agencies and private groups and individuals. All of these approaches will probably help up to a point, but neither alone nor in combination do they offer a total solution to the problem. Drug abuse has been a part of human behavior for thousands of years, and it is not likely to disappear in the near future. For this reason, it is necessary to educate ourselves and to develop the self-discipline necessary to avoid dangerous drug dependencies.

WHAT DO YOU THINK?

What is the cost society pays for drug use? Have you ever personally known someone who has suffered because of addiction to drugs? How did you respond?

Many people believe that the most effective strategy for fighting illicit drug use is educating young people, particularly if they can learn about its dangers and consequences from someone who has "been there."

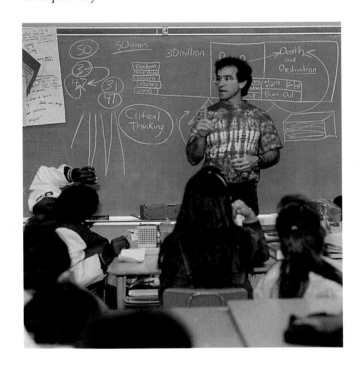

Summary

◆ People from all walks of life use illicit drugs, although college students report higher usage rates than does the general population. Drug use has declined since the mid-1980s.

◆ Controlled substances include cocaine and its derivatives, amphetamines, newer-generation stimulants, marijuana, the opiates, the psychedelics, the deliriants, designer

Managing Drug Use Behavior

As long as illicit drugs have existed, people have been weighing the costs and benefits of using them. It may be useful for you to explore your own attitudes about illicit drug use.

Making Decisions for You

Drug use often comes from the desire to change your state of consciousness or perhaps to experience something new. Before you try a new drug, take a moment to think. Begin by writing down what you want to experience or why you want to change your mental state. Then think about whether or not your chosen drug will really achieve that. Are there alternatives? For example, the natural endorphins generated by exercise may bring you out of a bad mood in a more predictable manner than will taking a drug. What are the potential side effects to your body—and your social life? Are you willing to risk those side effects? Are you willing to risk potential addiction?

Checklist for Change: Making Personal Choices

✓ What illicit drugs are you familiar with? How did you become familiar with them? What drugs are most popular among your peers? What is it about these drugs that makes them popular?

✓ How do you and your peers feel about illicit drug use? Is it condoned or condemned? Has that changed in the last few years? What has led to these feelings?

✓ Have you thought of recreational activities that you can do in place of using drugs?

✓ Are you prepared for the challenge of refusing to use illicit drugs that you may be offered and for dealing with the consequences associated with that decision?

✓ Do you practice assertiveness? Do you practice speaking up and voicing your opinion regardless of the subject?

✓ Are you someone who takes pride in your accomplishments? Do you view setbacks as times for growth?

✓ Do you have strategies for coping with stress? Do you use exercise, meditation, or some other healthy activity as a method of stress reduction?

Checklist for Change: Making Community Choices

✓ Do you take the time to find out what the current drug problems on your campus and in your community are?

✓ Would you be willing to assist a friend in combating his or her substance abuse problem? Would you take him or her or accompany him or her to support groups?

✓ Would you be willing to be a role model in community programs such as Big Brothers or Big Sisters?

✓ Do you volunteer your time for any campus or community organizations that provide opportunities for high-risk youth?

✓ Would you be willing to volunteer to help out at an addiction hotline or community center?

Critical Thinking

You have a major term paper due in three days, and you've just completed the reading for it. You're worried about how you'll get it done, and realize you may have to pull an all-nighter. If you don't get at least a B, you'll lose your academic scholarship and will be forced to leave your college. A friend tells you that, last semester, she took a few lines of coke; it not only helped her stay awake, but also stimulated her thinking. She got an A– on the paper and experienced no side effects. She suggests you try it, too.

Using the DECIDE model described in Chapter 1, decide how you will keep yourself awake to finish your paper. What stimulant, if any, are you willing to take to stay awake?

---

drugs, inhalants, and steroids. Users tend to become addicted quickly to such drugs.

◆ The drug problem reaches everyone through crime and elevated health-care costs. Women addicts have special

problems associated with seeking treatment. Drugs are a major problem in the workplace; workplace drug testing is one proposed solution to this problem.

Discussion Questions

1. Create an antidrug program aimed at grade-school children. Think about what antidrug message would have reached you.

2. List the varied types of drugs. Then discuss their physiological and psychological effects. Why is it that newer, purer forms of drugs (like crack cocaine) are developed?

3. Debate the issue of workplace drug testing. Would you apply for a job that had drug testing as an interview requirement? As a continuing requirement?

4. List nondrug alternative behaviors to drug use. Are these realistic? What could make them more enticing?

Application Exercise

Reread the What Do You Think? scenarios at the beginning of the chapter and answer the following questions.

1. Do you think employers have the right to require drug screenings? How about potential employers? Would you want airline pilots or train engineers to be tested regularly? How about cafeteria workers?

2. Do you think that the NCAA should be able to test college athletes for drugs? Why or why not? Which drugs would you test for?

3. If you were Susan's roommate, what would you do, if anything, to help her? If she was resistant to your offers for help, what options might you have?

4. Where on your campus could Susan (or other students with drug problems) go for help? Are there resources available for students who are seeking help for their drug-abusing friends? Are there any student assistance programs on your campus where students can go for self-referrals?

Further Reading

National Institute on Drug Abuse, *Statistical Series, Annual Data Report* (Rockville, MD: U.S. Department of Health and Human Services, 1992).

Data are presented on the use of drugs in the United States. A detailed description of drug categories, including use, symptoms of use and abuse, and schedule classification, is provided.

R. G. Schlaadt and P. T. Shannon, *Drugs,* 4th ed. (Englewood Cliffs, NJ: Prentice Hall, 1994).

A very useful book about the widening use of drugs in our society. Includes a unique chapter on the consumer and drug legislation. Provides an overview of the history and social impact of drug use in the United States.

R. Tricker and D. L. Cook, *Athletes at Risk: Drugs and Sport* (Dubuque, IA: Wm. C. Brown, 1990).

Written with the intention of teaching athletes, coaches, and others interested in sports how to achieve athletic excellence without using drugs. Presents the thoughts of those who are professionally and personally committed to the health and well-being of athletes.

G. Winger, F. Hoffman, and J. Woods, *A Handbook on Drug and Alcohol Abuse: The Biomedical Aspects,* 3rd ed. (New York: Oxford University Press, 1992).

Excellent resource book that covers the essential theories and principles of drug use and abuse.

16

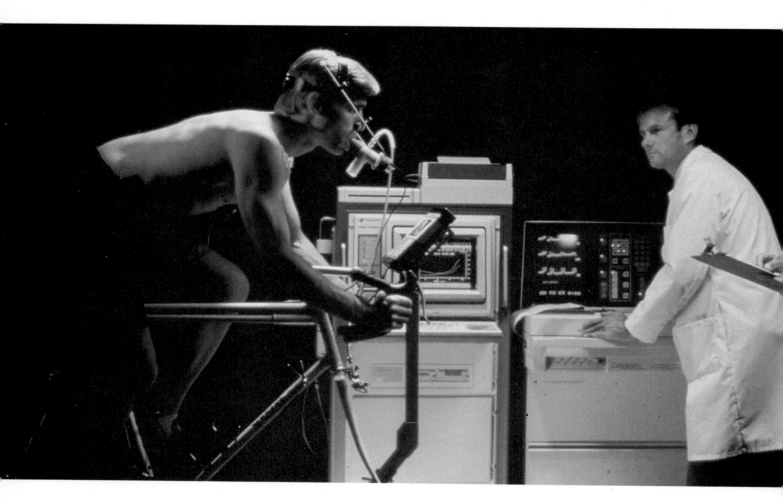

CHAPTER OBJECTIVES

◆ Describe the anatomy and physiology of the heart and the circulatory system.

◆ Review the various types of heart disease and their diagnoses and treatments.

◆ Discuss the controllable risk factors for cardiovascular disease, including smoking, blood fat and cholesterol

levels, hypertension, exercise, diet and obesity, diabetes, and stress. Examine the risk factors you cannot control.

◆ Discuss the issues uniquely concerning women in relationship to cardiovascular disease.

◆ Discuss some of the new methods of diagnosis and treatment of cardiovascular disease.

Cardiovascular Disease

Helping the Beat Go On

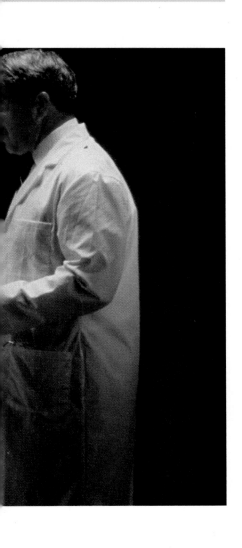

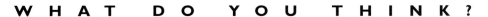

WHAT DO YOU THINK?

Thirty-two-year-old Clay is an avid exerciser. He runs 40 miles a week, lifts weights, and keeps his weight under control. His father died of a heart attack at the age of 43, and Clay does not intend to follow in his footsteps. Believing that a sedentary lifestyle and a high-fat diet are the major risk factors for heart disease, he has reduced his consumption of red meats and exercises aerobically every day. He tells his friends that he is "lean and mean" and extremely healthy. He has never had his blood pressure or cholesterol level checked and has never been to a doctor for any reason.

■ Is Clay correct in assuming that exercising and avoiding red meats will protect him from heart disease? Are there other things that he is doing that may put him at risk for a heart attack? Is heredity a risk factor in heart disease? As a responsible health consumer, what actions should Clay take to insure that his risk is as low as he believes it is?

Jan, aged 54, has noticed that she is becoming short of breath after performing light physical activities and feels dizzy when getting out of bed in the morning. She worries that her cancer—in remission for over 10 years—may have recurred. At a routine physical examination, she tells her doctor about her symptoms. The doctor says that she should exercise more and try to lose a few pounds; otherwise, her mammogram and pap smears look fine and she appears to be in good health. Her doctor listens to her heart and checks her blood pressure but orders no additional tests. Two weeks after her visit, Jan suffers a heart attack.

■ Given her age and her medical history, what risk factors for heart disease is Jan likely to have? Why do you think her doctor failed to test further for possible cardiac symptoms? What advice about her interactions with her doctor would you give to someone like Jan? How can consumers protect themselves from similar incidents?

During the last century, "the American way of life" became synonymous with abundant food, the best medical treatment, and astonishing technological progress. Slowly but surely, we consumed more and more protein-rich, high-fat, high-sugar, high-sodium, and high-calorie foods to the point that, today, over 35 percent of us are obese and a large percentage of the rest of us is so out of shape that a simple trip up the stairs leaves us gasping for breath. Escalators and elevators, automobiles, and numerous other laborsaving devices have released us from much physical exertion. We sit on plump couches and flip through the TV channels by remote control rather than exert ourselves to get up and change them by hand. We buy blowers to whisk our leaves away rather than get out the old rake. To compound the problem, millions of us continue to smoke and drink. It is no wonder that **cardiovascular diseases (CVDs)** are the leading cause of death in the United States today, accounting for more than 42 percent of all deaths. That is nearly three times the number of deaths caused by the second leading killer, cancer, and more than the number of deaths caused by all other diseases combined. In fact, the number-one killer in the United States in every year but one (1918) since 1900 has been CVD.[1]

Every 34 seconds, an American dies of CVD. That's more than 925,000 deaths annually.[2] But these deaths don't tell the whole story. Many people live with their CVD problems: of the current U.S. population of about 255 million, nearly 60 million people have some form of CVD.[3] They, and often their relatives, suffer disruptions of work, fear and anxiety, pain, disability, and diminished quality of life. For additional information concerning CVD statistics, see the Health Headlines box.

It is important to put these figures into perspective in terms of their overall impact on American society. According to the most recent computations done by the National Center for Health Statistics, if all forms of major cardiovascular disease were eliminated, total life expectancy would rise by nearly 10 years.[4] For comparison, if all forms of cancer were eliminated, the gain would be three years.

Although it is impossible to place a monetary value on human life, the economic burden of cardiovascular disease on our society is overwhelming. In 1995, cardiovascular diseases will cost us in excess of $137.7 billion.[5] This figure includes the cost of physician and nursing services, hospital and nursing home services, medications, and lost productivity of the victim resulting from disability. Fig-

ure 16.1 shows the relative distribution of these costs. If all direct and indirect costs for care, family productivity losses, rehabilitation, and other services and losses were included, these numbers would be even higher.

Despite all these gloomy statistics, there is reason for optimism. Medical scientists have made tremendous progress in fighting cardiovascular diseases. The death

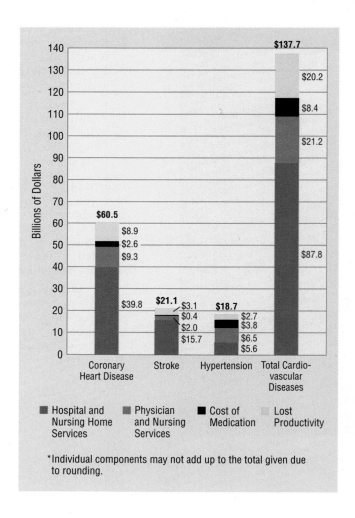

FIGURE 16.1

Estimated Cost of Major Cardiovascular Diseases in the United States in Billions of Dollars (1990)

Source: Reproduced with permission from *Heart and Stroke Facts, 1990,* 11. Copyright American Heart Association.

CVD Facts

- People who survive a heart attack have a two to nine times higher chance of illness and death than does the general population. Within six years after suffering a heart attack,

  23 percent of men and 31 percent of women survivors will have another heart attack.

  41 percent of men and 34 percent of women survivors will develop angina.

  about 20 percent of survivors will be disabled.

  9 percent of men and 18 percent of women survivors will have a stroke.

  13 percent of men and 6 percent of women survivors will experience sudden death.

- 66 percent of survivors don't make a complete recovery, but 88 percent of those under age 65 are able to return to work.

- More than 2,500 Americans die each day from CVDs.

- More than one-sixth of all people killed by CVD are under age 65.

- CVD accounts for 48.2 percent of all male deaths and 51.8 percent of all female deaths.

- In 1950, the CVD death rate was 424.2 per 100,000; in 1991, it had dropped to 186 per 100,000.

- One in six men and one in eight women aged 45 or over has had a heart attack or stroke.

- About 80 percent of coronary mortality in people under age 65 occurs during the initial attack.

- In 48 percent of men and 63 percent of women who have died suddenly of coronary heart disease, there was no previous evidence of disease.

- At older ages, women who have heart attacks are twice as likely as men to die from them within a few weeks.

- 27 percent of men and 44 percent of women will die within one year after having a heart attack.

Source: American Heart Association.

rate (numbers per 100,000 persons) from cardiovascular disease has declined by more than 25 percent during the last decade, even though numbers of deaths have held fairly constant.[6] How do health experts account for this decline in CVD death rates?

There are no simple answers. Advances in medical techniques, earlier and better diagnostic procedures and treatments, better emergency medical assistance programs, and training of ordinary citizens in *cardiopulmonary resuscitation (CPR)* have greatly aided victims of cardiovascular disease. Refinements in surgical techniques and improvements in heart transplants and artificial heart devices have enabled many to live longer lives. Educational programs have promoted public awareness of the role individual efforts, including diet and exercise, can play in risk reduction. Although recent studies show conflicting data on self-reported improvements in diet, obesity, exercise, and smoking behaviors, it is generally assumed that many Americans are making some positive changes in many areas. All these factors have contributed to increasing optimism about treating and preventing CVD.

Although there are many forms of cardiovascular disease and many of them are interrelated, it is important that you know how the cardiovascular system functions, what these different diseases are, what your personal risk factors are, and the steps that you can take to prevent CVD or to protect yourself from additional injury.

You can reduce your risk for CVD by taking steps to change certain behaviors. For example, controlling high blood pressure and reducing your intake of saturated fats and cholesterol are two things you can do to lower your chances of heart attack. By maintaining your weight, decreasing your intake of sodium, exercising, and changing your lifestyle to reduce stress, you can lower your blood pressure. You can also monitor the levels of fat and cholesterol in your blood and adjust your diet to prevent your arteries from becoming clogged. By understanding how your cardiovascular system works, you will have a better chance of understanding your risks and of changing your behaviors to reduce them.

UNDERSTANDING YOUR CARDIOVASCULAR SYSTEM

The **cardiovascular system** is the network of elastic tubes through which blood flows as it carries oxygen and nutri-

Cardiovascular diseases (CVDs): Diseases of the heart and blood vessels.

Cardiovascular system: A complex system consisting of the heart and blood vessels that transports nutrients, oxygen, hormones, and enzymes throughout the body and regulates temperature, the water levels of cells, and the acidity levels of body components.

ents to all parts of the body. It includes the *heart, lungs, arteries, arterioles* (small arteries), and *capillaries* (minute blood vessels). It also includes *venules* (small veins) and *veins,* the blood vessels though which blood flows as it returns to the heart and lungs.[7]

The heart is a muscular, four-chambered pump, roughly the size of a man's fist. It is a highly efficient, extremely flexible organ that manages to contract 100,000 times each day, pumping the equivalent of 2,000 gallons of blood to all areas of the body. In a 70-year lifetime, an average human heart beats 2.5 billion times. This number may be significantly higher when our hearts fight to keep those of us who are out of shape and overweight functioning.

Under normal circumstances, the human body contains approximately 6 quarts of blood. This blood transports nutrients, oxygen, waste products, hormones, and enzymes throughout the body. It also regulates body temperature, cellular water levels, and acidity levels of body components, and aids in bodily defense against toxins and harmful microorganisms. An adequate blood supply is essential to health and well-being.

How does the heart ensure that blood is constantly recirculated to body parts? The four chambers of the heart work together to achieve this (see Figure 16.2). The two upper chambers of the heart, called **atria,** or auricles, are large collecting chambers that receive blood from the rest of the body. The two lower chambers, known as **ventricles,** pump the blood out again. Small valves regulate the steady, rhythmic flow of blood between chambers and prevent inappropriate backwash. The *tricuspid valve,* located between the right atrium and the right ventricle; the *pulmonary (pulmonic) valve,* between the right ventricle and the pulmonary artery; the *mitral valve,* between the left atrium and left ventricle; and the *aortic valve,* between the left ventricle and the aorta, permit blood to flow in only one direction.[8]

Heart activity depends on a complex interaction of biochemical, physical, and neurological signals. The following is a simplified version of the steps involved in heart function:

1. Deoxygenated blood enters the right atrium after having been circulated through the body.

2. From the right atrium, blood moves to the right ventricle and is pumped through the pulmonary artery to the lungs, where it receives oxygen.

3. Oxygenated blood from the lungs then returns to the left atrium of the heart.

4. Blood from the left atrium is forced into the left ventricle.

5. The left ventricle pumps blood through the aorta to all body parts.

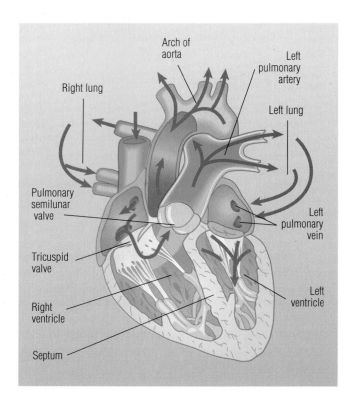

FIGURE 16.2

Anatomy of the Heart

Different types of blood vessels are required for different parts of this process. **Arteries** carry blood away from the heart—except for pulmonary arteries, which carry deoxygenated blood to the lungs, where it picks up oxygen and gives off carbon dioxide. As they branch off from the heart, the arteries divide into smaller blood vessels called **arterioles,** and then into even smaller blood vessels called **capillaries.** Capillaries have thin walls that permit the exchange of oxygen, carbon dioxide, nutrients, and waste products with body cells. The carbon dioxide and waste products are transported to the lungs and kidneys through **veins** and venules (small veins).

For the heart to function properly, the four chambers must beat in an organized manner. This is governed by an electrical impulse that directs the heart muscle to move when the impulse moves across it, which results in a sequential contraction of the four chambers. This signal starts in a small bundle of highly specialized cells, the **sinoatrial node (SA node),** located in the right atrium. The SA node serves as a form of natural pacemaker for the heart.[9] People with damaged or nonfunctional natural pacemaker activity must often have a mechanical pacemaker inserted to insure the smooth passage of blood through the sequential phases of the heart beat.

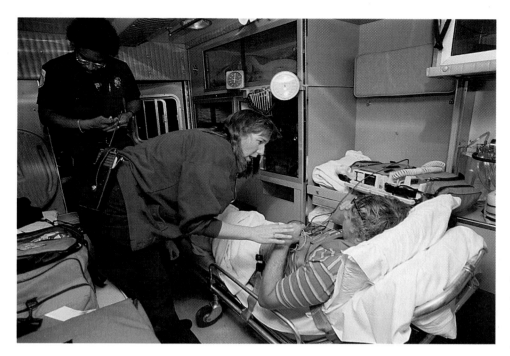

Because 40 percent of heart attack victims die within the first hour, immediate attention is vital to the patient's survival.

The average adult heart at rest beats 70 to 80 times per minute, although a well-conditioned heart may beat only 50 to 60 times per minute to achieve the same results. When overly stressed, a heart may beat over 200 times per minute, particularly in an individual who is overweight or out of shape. A healthy heart functions more efficiently and is less likely to suffer damage from overwork than is an unhealthy one.

$\mathcal{W}$HAT DO YOU THINK?

What risk factors for heart disease do you currently have? What is your current resting heart rate? Do you know what your current cholesterol level is? Have you taken any action to reduce your fat intake or to improve your cardiovascular function? If not, why not? What actions can you take to improve your overall cardiovascular condition?

$\mathcal{T}$YPES OF CARDIOVASCULAR DISEASES

Although most of us associate cardiovascular disease with heart attacks, there are actually a number of different types of cardiovascular system diseases. Current efforts are aimed at preventing and treating the most common forms of cardiovascular diseases:

- Atherosclerosis (fatty plaque buildup in arteries).
- Heart attack (myocardial infarction).
- Chest pain (angina pectoris).
- Irregular heartbeat (arrhythmia).
- Congestive heart failure.
- Congenital and rheumatic heart disease.
- Stroke (cerebrovascular accident).

Prevention and treatment of these diseases range from changes in diet and lifestyle to use of medications and surgery.

Atria: The two upper chambers of the heart, which receive blood.

Ventricles: The two lower chambers of the heart, which pump blood through the blood vessels.

Arteries: Vessels that carry blood away from the heart to other regions of the body.

Arterioles: Branches of the arteries.

Capillaries: Minute blood vessels that branch out from the arterioles; their thin walls allow for the exchange of oxygen, carbon dioxide, nutrients, and waste products with body cells.

Veins: Vessels that carry blood back to the heart from other regions of the body.

Sinoatrial node (SA node): Node serving as a form of natural pacemaker for the heart.

Atherosclerosis: A Major Culprit

Atherosclerosis is a general term for thickening and hardening of the arteries. Atherosclerosis is actually a type of **arteriosclerosis** and is characterized by deposits of fatty substances, cholesterol, cellular waste products, calcium, and *fibrin* (a clotting material in the blood) in the inner lining of an artery. The resulting buildup is referred to as **plaque**.[10]

Plaque may partially or totally block the blood's flow through an artery. Two things that can happen where plaque occurs are (1) bleeding (hemorrhage) into the plaque, or (2) formation of a blood clot (thrombus) on the plaque's surface. If either of these occurs and an artery is blocked, the chances of a heart attack or stroke occurring are great.[11]

Atherosclerosis does not suddenly occur after a few months spent eating chocolate cheesecake and lounging on the couch. Evidence suggests that atherosclerotic plaque may actually begin to form while a person is still in the womb, and it becomes progressively worse as the years pass. Some individuals seem to be "plaque formers," while others exhibiting the same behavior have much less buildup. In some people, their 20s seem to be a significant plaque-forming period; in others, plaque doesn't become a problem until their 50s or 60s.[12]

WHAT DO YOU THINK?

Did you realize that you may lay down significant deposits of atherosclerotic plaque during your 20s? What risk factors for plaque formation do you have right now? What is your cholesterol level? Have your parents been diagnosed with high cholesterol? What actions can you take now that may keep your risks for atherosclerosis low?

Exactly why some people are "atherosclerotic prone" and others are not remains in question. There are several theories. Many scientists believe that the process of plaque buildup begins because the protective inner lining of the artery (*endothelium*) becomes damaged and that fats, cholesterol, and other substances in the blood are deposited in the damaged area, eventually obstructing blood flow. The three major causes of such damage are (1) dramatic fluctuations in blood pressure, (2) elevated levels of cholesterol and triglycerides in the blood, and (3) cigarette smoking. Cigarette smoke aggravates and speeds up the development of atherosclerosis particularly in the coronary arteries, the aorta, and the arteries of the legs.[13] We discuss each of these factors in detail in other sections of this chapter dealing with risk factors for CVD.

Atherosclerosis: A general term for thickening and hardening of the arteries.

Arteriosclerosis: Characterized by deposits of fatty substances, cholesterol, cellular waste products, calcium, and fibrin in the inner lining of an artery.

Plaque: Buildup of deposits in the arteries.

Myocardial infarction (MI): Heart attack.

Heart attack: A blockage of normal blood supply to an area in the heart.

Coronary thrombosis: A blood clot occurring in the coronary artery.

Collateral circulation: Adaptation of the heart to partial damage accomplished by rerouting needed blood through unused or underused blood vessels while the damaged heart muscle heals.

Ischemia: Reduced oxygen supply to the heart.

Angina pectoris: Severe chest pain occurring as a result of reduced oxygen flow to the heart.

Beta blockers: Major type of drug used to treat angina, they control potential overactivity of the heart muscle.

Arrhythmia: An irregularity in heartbeat.

Fibrillation: A sporadic, quivering pattern of heartbeat resulting in extreme inefficiency in moving blood through the cardiovascular system.

Heart Attack

Those of you raised on a weekly dose of TV doctor programs will recognize *Code Blue* as the term for a **myocardial infarction (MI)**, or heart attack. However, you may not know exactly what a heart attack is. A **heart attack** involves a blockage of normal blood supply to an area of the heart. This condition is often brought on by a **coronary thrombosis**, or blood clot in the coronary artery. Coronary heart disease (CHD) and coronary artery disease (CAD) are general names for heart attack (and angina).

When blood does not flow readily, there is a corresponding decrease in oxygen flow. If the heart blockage is extremely minor, the otherwise healthy heart will adapt over time by utilizing small unused or underused blood vessels to reroute needed blood through other areas. This system, known as **collateral circulation**, is a form of self-preservation that allows a damaged heart muscle to heal.

When heart blockage is more severe, however, the body is unable to adapt on its own and outside lifesaving support is critical. The hour following a heart attack is believed to be the most critical period because over 40 percent of heart attack victims die within this time. For information on how to assist a heart attack victim, see the Skills for Behavioral Change box.

It is believed that normal nonatherosclerotic arteries can also go into spasm and cause circulatory impairment. Excessive calcium and potassium are among the suspected causes of these spasms.

Angina Pectoris

As a result of atherosclerosis and other circulatory impairments, the heart's oxygen supply is often reduced, a condition known as **ischemia.** Individuals with ischemia often suffer from varying degrees of **angina pectoris,** or chest pains. Many people experience short episodes of angina whenever they exert themselves physically. Symptoms may range from a slight feeling of indigestion to a feeling that the heart is being crushed. Generally, the more serious the oxygen deprivation, the more severe the pain. Although angina pectoris is not a heart attack, it does indicate underlying heart disease.

Currently, there are several methods of treating angina. In mild cases, rest is critical. The most common treatments for more severe cases involve using drugs that affect (1) the supply of blood to the heart muscle or (2) the heart's demand for oxygen. Pain and discomfort are often relieved with *nitroglycerin,* a drug used to relax (dilate) veins, thereby reducing the amount of blood returning to the heart and thus lessening its workload. Patients whose angina is caused by spasms of the coronary arteries are often given drugs called *calcium channel blockers.* These drugs prevent calcium atoms from passing through coronary arteries and causing heart contractions. They also appear to reduce blood pressure and to slow heart rates. **Beta blockers** are the other major type of drugs used to treat angina. The chemical action of beta blockers serves to control potential overactivity of the heart muscle.

Arrhythmias

An **arrhythmia** is an irregularity in heartbeat. It may be suspected, for instance, when a person complains of a racing heart in the absence of exercise or anxiety; *tachycardia* is the medical term for this abnormally fast heartbeat. On the other end of the continuum is *bradycardia,* or abnormally slow heartbeat. When a heart goes into **fibrillation,** it exhibits a totally sporadic, quivering pattern of beating resulting in extreme inefficiency in moving blood through the cardiovascular system. If untreated, this condition may be fatal. Not all arrhythmias are life-threatening. In many instances, excessive caffeine or nicotine consumption can trigger an arrhythmia episode. For the most part, in the absence of other symptoms, arrhythmias are not serious. However, severe cases may require drug therapy or external electrical stimulus to prevent serious complications.

Congestive Heart Failure

When the heart muscle is damaged or overworked and lacks the strength to keep blood circulating normally through the body, its chambers are often taxed to the limit. Patients who have been afflicted with rheumatic fever, pneumonia, or other cardiovascular problems in the past often have weakened heart muscles. In addition, the walls of the heart and the blood vessels may be damaged from previous radiation or chemotherapy treatments for cancer. These weakened muscles respond poorly when stressed, blood flow out of the heart through the arteries is diminished, and the return flow of blood through the veins begins to back up, causing congestion in the tissues.[14] This pooling of blood causes enlargement of the heart and decreases the amount of blood that can be circulated. Blood begins to accumulate in other body areas, such as in the vessels in the legs and ankles or the lungs, causing swelling or difficulty in breathing. If untreated, congestive heart failure will result in death. Most cases respond well to treatment that includes *diuretics* (water pills) for relief of fluid accumulation; drugs, such as *digitalis,* that increase the pumping action of the heart; and drugs called *vasodilators* that expand blood vessels and decrease resistance, allowing blood to flow more easily and making the heart's work easier.

Congenital and Rheumatic Heart Disease

Approximately 1 out of every 125 children is born with some form of **congenital heart disease** (disease present at birth). These forms may range from slight murmurs caused by valve irregularities, which some children outgrow, to serious complications in heart function that can be corrected only with surgery. Their underlying causes are unknown but are believed to be related to hereditary factors; maternal diseases, such as German measles (rubella), occurring during fetal development; or chemical intake (particularly alcohol) by the mother during pregnancy. Because of advances in pediatric cardiology, the prognosis for children with congenital heart defects is better than ever before.

Rheumatic heart disease can cause similar heart problems in children. It is attributed to rheumatic fever, an inflammatory disease that may affect many connective tissues of the body, especially those of the heart, the joints, the brain, or the skin, and which is caused by an unresolved *streptococcal infection* of the throat (strep throat). In a small number of cases, this infection can lead to an immune response in which antibodies attack the heart as well as the bacteria.

Stroke

Like heart muscle, brain cells must have a continuous adequate supply of oxygen in order to survive. A **stroke** (also called a cerebrovascular accident) occurs when the blood supply to the brain is cut off. Strokes may be caused by a **thrombus** (blood clot), an **embolus** (a wandering clot), or an **aneurysm** (a weakening in a blood vessel that causes it to bulge and, in severe cases, burst). Figure 16.3 illustrates these blood vessel disorders.

When any of these events occurs, the result is the death of brain cells, which do not have the capacity to heal or regenerate. Strokes may cause speech impairments, mem-

Congenital heart disease: Heart disease that is present at birth.

Rheumatic heart disease: A heart disease caused by untreated streptococcal infection of the throat.

Stroke: A condition occurring when the brain is damaged by disrupted blood supply.

Thrombus: Blood clot.

Embolus: Blood clot that is forced through the circulatory system.

Aneurysm: A weakened blood vessel that may bulge under pressure and, in severe cases, burst.

Transient ischemic attacks (TIAs): Mild form of stroke; often an indicator of impending major stroke.

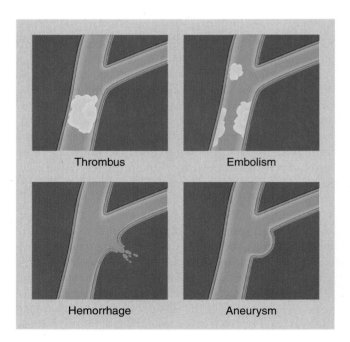

Thrombus Embolism

Hemorrhage Aneurysm

FIGURE 16.3

Common Blood Vessel Disorders

ory loss, and loss of motor control. Although some strokes affect parts of the brain that regulate heart and lung function and kill within minutes, others are mild and cause only temporary dizziness or slight weakness or numbness. These mild forms of strokes are called **transient ischemic attacks (TIAs)** and are often indications of an impending major stroke. Knowing the warning signs or symptoms of stroke may help you or a loved one get medical attention earlier, when treatment may be more effective. Among the most common symptoms are:

- Sudden weakness or numbness of the face, arm, or leg on one side of the body.

- Sudden dimness or loss of vision, particularly in only one eye.

- Loss of speech, or trouble talking or understanding speech.

- Sudden, severe headaches with no known cause.

- Unexplained dizziness, unsteadiness, or sudden falls, especially along with any of the previous symptoms.

The prognosis for stroke victims today is much better than it was a decade ago. Surgery, drugs, acute hospital care and rehabilitation are all effective ways of improving a stroke victim's chances of survival. Improvements in physical therapy and a recognition of the importance of early involvement by patients in their own rehabilitation have allowed many stroke victims to resume nearly normal activity levels. The best way to prevent a stroke from occurring is to reduce the risk factors that predispose you to suffer one.

CONTROLLING YOUR RISKS FOR CARDIOVASCULAR DISEASES

Our understanding of the role of stress management, sodium reduction, low-fat diets, and other preventive actions, coupled with better diagnostic aids, has allowed many people to avoid major CVD episodes. Figure 16.5 summarizes known ways to reduce your risk for heart attack.

A knowledge of the factors that contribute to cardiovascular disease can lead to health-promoting lifestyle changes. Different risks can have a compounded effect when combined. For example, if you have high blood pressure, smoke cigarettes, have a high cholesterol level, and have a family history of heart disease, you run a much greater risk of having a heart attack than does someone with only one of these risks. To assess your own risks for heart disease, see the Rate Yourself box.

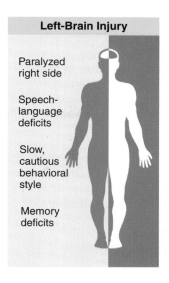
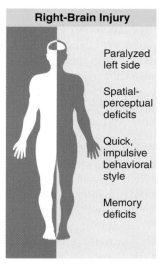

FIGURE 16.4

Effects of Stroke on the Body

Risks You Can Control

Factors that increase the risk for cardiovascular disease fall into two categories: those that can be controlled and those that cannot. The following risk factors can be controlled. As you read about each factor, ask yourself whether it applies to you and note the steps you can take to reduce its influence.

Cigarette Smoking. As early as 1984, the surgeon general of the United States asserted that smoking was the greatest risk factor for heart disease. Generally, the more a person smokes, the greater the risk for heart attack or stroke. The risk for cardiovascular disease is 70 percent greater for smokers than for nonsmokers. Smokers who have a heart attack are more likely to die suddenly (within one hour) than are nonsmokers. Available evidence also indicates that chronic exposure to environmental tobacco smoke (*passive smoking*) increases the risk of heart disease by as much as 30 percent.[15] When the effects of smoking are combined with the effects of other risk factors, the danger is greater than the sum of the added effects.

Although we do not fully understand how cigarette smoking damages the heart, there are two plausible explanations. One theory states that nicotine increases heart rate, heart output, blood pressure, and oxygen use by heart muscles. Because the carbon monoxide in cigarette smoke displaces oxygen in heart tissue, the heart is forced to work harder to obtain sufficient oxygen. The other theory states that chemicals in smoke damage the lining of the coronary arteries, allowing cholesterol and plaque to accumulate more easily. This additional buildup constricts the vessels, increasing blood pressure and causing the heart to work harder.

When people stop smoking, regardless of how long or how much they've smoked, their risk of heart disease declines rapidly.[16] Three years after quitting, the risk of death from heart disease and stroke for people who smoked a pack a day or less is almost the same as for people who never smoked. It's important to stop smoking before the signs of heart disease appear. If you smoke, quit now. And if you don't smoke, don't start.

Blood Fat and Cholesterol Levels. Excess fats in the body can contribute to CVD. In fact, researchers are now discovering that high-fat diets are even more dangerous than previously thought. Fatty diets not only raise cholesterol levels slowly over time, but also can send the body's blood-clotting system into high gear and make the blood sludgy in just a few hours, increasing the risk for heart attack. Recent studies indicate that fatty foods apparently trigger production of factor VII, a blood-clotting substance. Switching to a low-fat diet promptly eliminates the risk of clotting.[17]

A fatty diet also increases the amount of cholesterol in the blood, contributing to atherosclerosis. In past years, cholesterol levels of between 200 and 250 milligrams per 100 milliliters of blood (mg/dl) were considered normal. Recent research indicates that levels between 180 and 200 mg/dl are more desirable for reducing the risk for CVD. Cholesterol comes in two varieties: **low-density lipoproteins (LDLs)** and **high-density lipoproteins (HDLs)**. Scientists used to think that the critical question was whether a person had more of the "good" HDLs than the "bad" LDLs. But now according to scientists, what may really count is the HDL component *LpA-I*. The more of this protective protein a person has, it seems, the lower the risk for heart disease.[18] A study published in 1994 in the *Journal of the American Medical Association* has raised questions about the role of cholesterol in increased risk for CVD among the elderly. Researchers studied 997 people whose cholesterol was measured as part of a longitudinal (covering several years) study of older Americans. Results indicated that there was no association between elevated total serum cholesterol and any outcome, including myocardial infarction.[19] Although it should be noted that this was just one study, it does challenge the screening for cholesterol and treatment of high cholesterol levels in the elderly as possible unnecessary.

Low-density lipoproteins (LDLs): Compounds that facilitate the transport of cholesterol in the blood to the body's cells.

High-density lipoproteins (HDLs): Compounds that facilitate the transport of cholesterol in the blood to the liver for metabolism and elimination from the body.

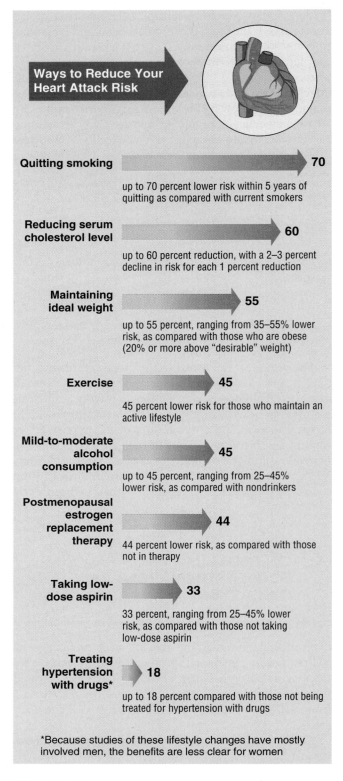

FIGURE 16.5

Estimated Average Reduction in Risk for Heart Attack*

*Estimated risk reductions refer to the independent contribution of each risk factor to heart attack and do not address the wide range of known or hypothesized reactions among them.

Source: Adapted from information appearing in J. E. Mason, "Medical Progress: The Primary Prevention of Myocardial Infarction," *The New England Journal of Medicine* 326 (21 May 1992): 1406–1416.

Cardiac Risk Factor Index

You can estimate your chance of suffering a heart attack or stroke by using this risk index. Remember, it's an estimate, not a diagnosis. Study each risk factor and its entire row. Choose the most appropriate description and circle the point number. For example, if your age is 25, circle 2 points. After checking out all 13 risk factors, total your score. Your score is an estimate of your risk.

Age	10–20 years	21–30 years	31–40 years	41–50 years	51–60 years	61 and over
	1	2	3	4	6	8
Heredity (Parents' and siblings' cardiac health)	No family history of heart disease	One with heart disease after age 60	Two with heart disease after age 60	One with heart disease before age 60	Two with heart disease before age 60	Three with heart disease before age 60
	1	2	3	4	6	8
Weight	More than 5 lbs. below standard	-5 to +5 lbs. of standard weight	5 to 20 lbs. overweight	21 to 35 lbs. overweight	36 to 50 lbs. overweight	51 to 65 lbs. overweight
	0	1	2	3	5	7
Smoking	Nonsmoker	Occasional cigar or pipe; live or work with someone who smokes	10 cigarettes or fewer per day	11–20 cigarettes per day	21–30 cigarettes per day	31 cigarettes or more per day
	0	1	2	4	6	10
Exercise	Intensive job and recreational exertion	Moderate job and recreational exertion	Sedentary job and intensive recreation	Sedentary job and moderate recreation	Sedentary job and occasional recreation	Sedentary job; no special exercise
	0	1	2	4	6	8
Cholesterol level or fat % in diet	Cholesterol below 180 mg. Diet contains no animal or solid fat	Cholesterol 181–205 mg. Diet contains 10% animal or solid fat	Cholesterol 206–230 mg. Diet contains 20% animal or solid fat	Cholesterol 231–255 mg. Diet contains 30% animal or solid fat	Cholesterol 256–280 mg. Diet contains 40% animal or solid fat	Cholesterol 281–300 mg. Diet contains 50% animal or solid fat
	1	2	3	4	5	7
Gender	Female under age 40	Female age 40–50	Female under 50, male under 20	Male between 20–35	Male between 35–55	Male over 50
	1	2	4	5	6	7
Systolic blood pressure	Below 110	111–130	131–140	141–160	161–180	Above 180
	0	1	2	3	5	7

(continued)

Diastolic blood pressure	Below 80	80–85	86–90	91–95	96–100	Above 100
	0	1	2	4	7	9
Stress	No mental-emotional stress	Occasional mild stress	Frequent mild stress	Frequent moderate stress	Frequent high stress	Constant high stress
	0	1	2	3	4	5
Present heart disease symptoms	None	Occasional fast pulse and/or irregular rhythm	Frequent fast pulse and/or irregular rhythm	Dizziness on exertion	Occasional angina (chest pain)	Frequent angina (chest pain)
	0	2	4	6	8	10
Past personal history of heart disease	Completely benign	Heart disease symptoms; not physician confirmed	History of heart disease symptoms; examined by physician	Mild heart disease; no present treatment	Heart disease under treatment	Hospitalized for heart disease
	0	2	4	6	8	10
Diabetes	No symptoms; negative family history	Positive family history of diabetes	Impaired glucose tolerance	Dietary control	Oral medication control	Insulin control
	0	1	3	5	7	9

If your total score is:

  6–14 = Risk well below average

15–19 = Risk below average

20–25 = Risk generally average

26–32 = Risk moderately high

33–40 = Risk dangerous

41–56 = Risk very dangerous

57+   = Risk extreme

If your total score is "above average," work with your physician to reduce your risk factors.

_____

Source: Used by permission of St. Vincent Hospital & Medical Center, The Heart Institute, Portland, OR 97225.

Triglycerides, the type of fat we normally consume, are also manufactured by our own bodies. As people get older or fatter or both, their triglyceride and cholesterol levels tend to rise. Although some CVD patients have elevated triglyceride levels, a causal link between high triglyceride levels and CVD has yet to be established. It may be that high triglyceride levels do not directly cause atherosclerosis but rather are among the abnormalities that speed its development.

Monitoring Your Cholesterol Levels. If a blood test reveals that you have a high level of total cholesterol (more than 240 mg/dl), the first thing you should do is to have the test retaken to make sure that the reading is accurate. (Remember that prior to having your blood drawn, you must not eat or drink anything for 12 hours.) If your total cholesterol level is still high, you should request that a lipoprotein analysis be done to determine the level of LDLs and HDLs in your blood.

Lipoprotein analysis, which also requires that you fast for 12 hours, measures the level of three substances: total cholesterol, HDL, and triglycerides. The level of LDL is derived using a standard formula: LDL = Total cholesterol – HDL – (Triglycerides ÷ 5). For example, if the level

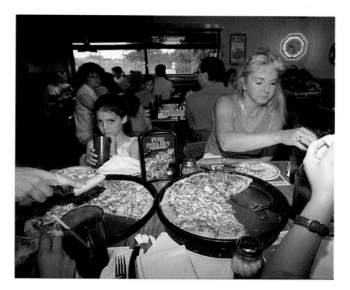

Controlling the amount and type of fat you eat is something you can do to lower your risk for cardiovascular disease.

of total cholesterol is 200, the level of HDL 45, and the level of triglycerides 150, the LDL level would be 125 (200 − 45 − 30).

In general, LDL is more closely associated with cardiovascular risks than is total cholesterol. However, most authorities agree that by looking only at LDL, we ignore the positive effects of HDL. Perhaps the best method of evaluating risk is to examine the ratio of HDL to total cholesterol or the percentage of HDL in total cholesterol. If the percentage of HDL is less than 35, the risk increases dramatically.

The ratio of HDL to total cholesterol can be controlled either by lowering LDL levels or by raising HDL levels. The best way to lower LDL levels is to reduce your dietary intake of the major sources of saturated fat. However, medications can also be used.

Hypertension. **Hypertension** refers to sustained high blood pressure. If it cannot be attributed to any specific cause, it is known as **essential hypertension.** Approximately 90 percent of all cases of hypertension fit this category. **Secondary hypertension** refers to hypertension caused by specific factors, such as kidney disease, obesity, or tumors of the adrenal glands. In general, the higher your blood pressure, the greater your risk for CVD. Hypertension is known as the "silent killer," because it usually has no symptoms. Although hypertension affects nearly 61 million Americans, 20 percent of them don't know they have the condition, and only one-third of those who are aware of it have it under control.[20] Common forms of treatment are dietary changes (reducing salt and

calorie intake), weight loss (when appropriate), the use of diuretics and other medications (only when prescribed by a physician), regular exercise, and the practice of relaxation techniques and effective coping and communication skills.

Blood pressure is measured in two parts and is expressed as a fraction—for example, 110/80, or 110 over 80. Both values are measured in *millimeters of mercury* (mm Hg). The first number refers to **systolic pressure,** or the pressure being applied to the walls of the arteries when the heart contracts, pumping blood to the rest of the body. The second value is **diastolic pressure,** or the pressure applied to the walls of the arteries during the heart's relaxation phase. During this phase, blood is reentering the chambers of the heart, preparing for the next heartbeat.

Normal blood pressure varies for different individuals depending on weight and physical condition and for different groups of people, such as women and minorities. As a rule, men have a greater risk for high blood pressure than women have until age 55, when their risks become about equal. At age 75 and over, women are more likely victims of high blood pressure than are men.[21] For the average person, 110 over 80 is a normal blood pressure level. If your blood pressure exceeds 140 over 90, you probably need to take steps to lower it. See Table 16.1 for a summary of blood pressure values and what they mean.

Exercise. According to the American Heart Association, inactivity is a definite risk factor for CVD.[22] Moreover, physically inactive people also tend to be overweight and are more likely to smoke and to pay less attention to their overall health than are active people. The good news is that you don't have to be an exercise fanatic to reduce your

Triglycerides: The most common form of fat in the body; excess calories are converted into triglycerides and stored as body fat.

Hypertension: Sustained elevated blood pressure.

Essential hypertension: Hypertension that cannot be attributed to any cause.

Secondary hypertension: Hypertension caused by specific factors, such as kidney disease, obesity, or tumors of the adrenal glands.

Systolic pressure: The upper number in the fraction that measures blood pressure, indicating pressure on the walls of the arteries when the heart contracts.

Diastolic pressure: The lower number in the fraction that measures blood pressure, indicating pressure on the walls of the arteries during the relaxation phase of heart activity.

TABLE 16.1 ■ Blood Pressure Values and What They Mean to You

Classification	Systolic Reading	Diastolic Reading	Actions
Normal	Below 130	Below 85	Recheck in two years.
High normal	130–139	85–89	Recheck in one year.
Mild hypertension	140–159	90–99	Check in two months.
Moderate hypertension	160–179	100–109	See physician within a month.
Severe hypertension	180 or above	110 or above	See physician immediately.

Note: Systolic and diastolic values are based on an average of two or more readings taken at different times.

Source: Adapted from "Fifth Report of the Joint National Committee on Detection, Evaluation, and Treatment of High Blood Pressure," *Archives of Internal Medicine* 153 (25 January 1993): 154–183 (published by the American Medical Association); and American Heart Association.

risk. Even modest levels of low-intensity physical activity are beneficial if done regularly and long term. Such activities include walking for pleasure, gardening, housework, and dancing.

Diet and Obesity. Like exercise, diet and obesity are believed to play a role in CVD. Researchers are not certain whether high-fat, high-sugar, high-calorie diets are a direct risk for CVD or whether they invite risk by causing obesity, which forces the heart to strain to push blood through the many miles of capillaries that supply each pound of fat. A heart that continuously has to move blood through an overabundance of vessels may become damaged. In fact, people who are overweight or obese are more likely to develop heart disease and stroke even if they have no other risk factors. Moreover, recent evidence indicates that how fat is distributed on the body may affect a person's risk. A waist/hip ratio greater than 1.0 for men or 0.8 for women indicates a significant increase in risk. This means that a man's waist measurement should not exceed his hip measurement, and a woman's waist measurement should not be more than 80 percent of her hip measurement.[23]

Diabetes. Diabetics, particularly those who have taken insulin for a number of years, appear to run an increased risk for the development of CVD. In fact, CVD is the leading cause of death among diabetic patients. Because overweight people have a higher risk for diabetes, distinguishing between the effects of the two conditions is difficult. Diabetics also tend to have elevated blood fat levels, increased atherosclerosis, and a tendency toward deterioration of small blood vessels, particularly in the eyes and extremities. Through a prescribed regimen of diet, exercise, and medication, diabetics can control much of their increased risk for CVD.

Individual Response to Stress. During the 1960s and 1970s, stress was considered a leading cause of CVD. Some scientists have noted a relationship between CVD risk and a person's stress level, behavior habits, and socioeconomic status. These factors may affect established risk factors. For example, people under stress may start smoking or smoke more than they otherwise would.[24] Other studies have challenged the apparent link between emotional stress and heart disease. Although it was once widely assumed that the Type A personality who suffered from high stress levels was a time bomb ticking toward a heart attack, this theory has not been proven clinically.

Recently, researcher-physician Robert S. Eliot demonstrated that approximately one out of five people has an extreme cardiovascular reaction to stressful stimulation. These people experience alarm and resistance so strongly that, when under stress, their bodies produce large amounts of stress chemicals, which in turn cause tremendous changes in the cardiovascular system, including remarkable increases in blood pressure. These people are called hot reactors. Although their blood pressure may be normal when they are not under stress—for example, in a doctor's office—it increases dramatically in response to even small amounts of everyday stress.

Cold reactors are those who are able to experience stress (even to live as Type As) without reacting with harmful cardiovascular responses. Cold reactors may internalize stress, but their self-talk and perceptions about the stressful events lead them to a nonresponse state in which their cardiovascular system remains virtually unaffected.[25] New research indicates that people who have an

Should You Drink to Improve Your Cardiovascular Health?

The choices we make about our health are often based on what the mass media choose to cover. One medical issue that got great media attention during the 1980s was the hypothesis that red wine might prevent heart disease. After all, France has the lowest rate of heart disease of any industrialized nation other than Japan. Just 174 of every 100,000 middle-aged French men die of heart disease, compared to 315 of every 100,000 middle-aged American men. During the 1980s, some researchers suggested that wine consumption was responsible for this difference. The French consume 10 times more red wine per capita than we do. But other researchers believe that the critical factor is the ethyl alcohol found in many types of alcoholic beverages, not only red wine. They base their belief on several studies indicating that alcohol consumed in moderation raises HDL (good cholesterol) levels. Take a look at some of the evidence:

- The Honolulu Heart Study followed 7,705 Japanese men living in Hawaii. Subjects who said they never drank had a heart disease rate of 5 percent, while men who had three to six drinks a week had a heart disease rate of only 3 percent.

- A study by the American Cancer Society followed more than 275,000 middle-aged men for 12 years. Subjects who reported having one or two drinks a day were 20 percent less likely to die of heart disease than were those who did not drink.

- An ongoing study of 128,934 Californians who participate in the Kaiser Permanente medical plan found fewer cardiac deaths and nonfatal heart attacks among light to moderate drinkers.

- A 1994 Harvard study indicated that the death rate from heart disease was 11 percent lower for someone who has one drink per week than for someone who does not drink; 20 percent lower for someone who has two to four drinks per week; 46 percent lower for someone who has five to six drinks per week; 4 percent lower for someone who has one drink a day; but 62 percent *higher* for someone who has two or more drinks a day.

We must be cautious in interpreting these findings. It is conceivable (though not likely) that it was not alcohol consumption but lifestyle that was responsible for the lower risk found in these studies—perhaps moderate drinkers lead less stressful lives. In the Kaiser Permanente study, Arthur Klatsky, chief of cardiology at Kaiser Permanente Medical Center in Oakland, California, found that "wine drinkers did a little better than beer drinkers, and the beer drinkers did a little better than the liquor drinkers." But among the northern Californians studied, wine drinkers were more likely than beer or liquor drinkers to be female, to be nonsmokers, and to be better educated. In other words, they were people at low risk for heart disease to begin with.

The French may be reaping benefits of antioxidant vegetables and fruits or of leaner cuts of meat. In addition, the manner in which the French eat may also have protective effects. The French eat heavier meals at midday than at night. In addition, they tend to consume alcohol with meals, rather than at bars or parties with little or no caloric intake to help moderate the alcohol.

There is no direct proof that alcohol protects against CVD, so before you start drinking for your heart's sake, you would be wise to consider the negative effects of alcohol consumption on other areas of health. You should not drink if you are pregnant; if you are planning to drive; if you are taking antihistamines, sedatives, or other medications that can magnify alcohol's effects; if you are a recovering alcoholic; if you are under age 21; or if you have medical conditions that may be exacerbated by the use of alcohol (e.g., ulcers or diabetes). People with a family history of alcoholism should be wary, too.

Sources: Information from *Nutrition Action Health Letter,* November 1992, 5–7; E. N. Frankel, J. Kanner, J. B. German, E. Parks, and J. E. Kinsella, "Inhibition of Oxidation of Human Low-Density Lipoprotein by Phenolic Substances in Red Wine," *Lancet* 341 (1993): 454–457; Patricia Thomas, "A Toast to the Heart," *Harvard Health Letter,* March 1994, 4–5; and H. Wechsler, "Health and Behavioral Consequences of Binge Drinking in College," *Journal of the American Medical Association* 272 (1994): 1672–1677.

---

underlying predisposition toward a toxic core personality (in other words, who are chronically hostile and hateful) may be at greatest risk for a CVD event.

Risks You Cannot Control

There are, unfortunately, some risk factors for CVD that you cannot prevent or control. The most important are:

- *Heredity:* Having a family history of heart disease appears to increase risks significantly. Whether this is because of genetics or environment is an unresolved question.

- *Age:* Seventy-five percent of all heart attacks occur in people over age 65. The risk for CVD increases with age for both sexes.

- *Gender:* Men are at much greater risk for CVD until old age. Women under 35 have a fairly low risk unless they have high blood pressure, kidney problems, or diabetes. Using oral contraceptives while smoking also increases risk. Hormonal factors appear to reduce risk for women, although after menopause or after estrogen levels are otherwise reduced (e.g., hysterectomy), women's LDL levels tend to go up, increasing their risk for CVD. (For a more detailed discussion of the gender factor, see the next section.

- *Race:* Blacks are at 45 percent greater risk for hypertension and thus a greater risk for CVD than are whites. In addition, African Americans have a worse chance of surviving heart attacks, as discussed in the Multicultural Perspectives box.

*W*HAT DO YOU THINK?

Which do you think is your biggest CVD risk factor right now? What is your second biggest risk factor? List four actions that you can take this week to reduce these two risk factors. Who can you get to help you in your attempt to change your health behaviors?

*W*OMEN AND CARDIOVASCULAR DISEASE

Heart disease is the number one killer of both men and women. In the United States, heart attacks kill about 240,000 women a year; stroke takes another 88,000 women's lives. That compares with about 43,000 women who die annually from breast cancer. In fact, nearly twice as many women die of CVD than all cancers combined.[26]

While men do have more heart attacks and have them earlier in life, women have a much lower chance of surviving a heart attack. We understand the mechanisms that cause CVD in men from years of male-oriented research. But only within the last decade have we moved toward a better understanding of how CVD manifests itself in women.

Risk Factors for Heart Disease in Women

Premenopausal women are unlikely candidates for heart attacks, except for those who suffer from diabetes, high blood pressure, or kidney disease, or who have a genetic predisposition to high cholesterol levels. Family history and smoking can also increase the risk for premenopausal women.

The Estrogen Element. Once her estrogen production drops with menopause, a woman's chances of developing CVD rise rapidly. A 60-year-old woman has the same

heart attack risk as a 50-year-old man. By her late 70s, a woman has the same heart attack risk as a man her age. To date, much of this changing risk has been attributed to the aging process, but some preliminary evidence indicates that hormones may play a bigger role than once thought. Recent results from the *Postmenopausal Estrogen/Progestin Interventions (PEPI)* study, a longitudinal study of how various **hormone replacement therapies** (HRT) affect cardiovascular risks, indicate that HRT may reduce CVD by as much as 12 to 25 percent. In this study, HRT seemed to reduce a woman's risk for CVD by raising HDL cholesterol levels and lowering LDL cholesterol levels. Even when their total blood cholesterol levels are higher than men's, women may be at less risk because they typically have a higher percentage of HDL.[27]

But that's only part of the story. It's true that women aged 25 and over tend to have lower cholesterol levels than do men of the same age. But when they reach 45, things change. Most men's cholesterol levels become more stable, while both LDL and total cholesterol levels in women start to rise. And the gap widens further beyond age 55.[28]

Before age 45, women's total blood cholesterol levels average below 220 mg/dl. By the time she is 45 to 55, the average woman's blood cholesterol rises to between 223 and 246 mg/dl. Studies of men have shown that for every 1 percent drop in cholesterol, there is a 2 percent decrease in CVD risk.[29] If this holds true for women, prevention efforts focusing on dietary interventions and exercise may significantly help postmenopausal women.

Symptoms of Heart Disease in Postmenopausal Women

Postmenopausal women often do not display the same extreme symptoms of heart disease that men do. The first sign of heart disease in men is generally a myocardial infarction. In women, the first sign is usually uncomplicated angina pectoris. Because chest discomfort rather than pain is the common manifestation of angina in women, and because angina has a much more favorable prognosis in women than in men, many physicians ignore the condition in their female patients or treat it too casually.

A heart attack also shows different signs in women than in men. In men, a heart attack usually manifests itself as crushing chest pain radiating to the arm. But in women, a heart attack can feel like severe abdominal pain or indigestion. If these symptoms are neglected, the outcome can be dire.

Neglect of Heart Disease Symptoms in Women

Research has suggested three main reasons for the widespread neglect of the signs of heart disease in women: (1) physicians may often be gender-biased in their delivery of health care, tending to concentrate on women's reproductive organs rather than on the whole woman;

Racial Inequality in Heart Attack Treatment

Do all our citizens receive equally good health care? As you have probably already guessed, the answer is no.

For instance, researchers at the University of Chicago studied 6,000 cardiac arrest victims. They found that blacks were twice as likely to suffer sudden cardiac arrest and twice as likely to die as whites. At every link in what doctors call the "chain of survival," blacks fared worse than whites. They had more unwitnessed cardiac arrests, which kept them from getting treatment. They were more likely to die in the emergency room. And when it came to cardiopulmonary resuscitation (CPR), there was a lower rate of bystander CPR in blacks than in whites.

Further studies suggest that once blacks make it to a hospital, they receive inferior care. A study of more than 400,000 men admitted to veterans hospitals across the United States showed that blacks are less likely to get sophisticated heart procedures—such as cardiac catheterization and angioplasty—and far less likely to get heart bypass surgery. The study echoes similar results found in private hospitals.

Dr. Paul Crawford, a black inner-city doctor in Chicago, believes that the roots of these problems include a "lack of education. We're dealing with no money to purchase medications we want and . . . we're dealing with a really major educational job in the communities."

Dr. Crawford's point is well-taken: Education is key to promoting health. If you know the early symptoms of a heart attack, you are more likely to seek help earlier. If more inner-city neighbors knew CPR, blacks would not experience as many delays in getting critical treatment.

But the problem reaches beyond such education for blacks: An editorial in the *New England Journal of Medicine* concluded that a patient's race influences physicians' decisions about medical treatment and that there are deep-seated racial inequities in the U.S. health-care system.

Source: Reprinted by permission from Jeff Flock, "Medical Master 318, story #16," CNN News, 25 August 1993. © 1993 Cable New Network, Inc. All rights reserved. Published by arrangement with Turner Educational Services, Inc.

---

(2) physicians tend to view male heart disease as a more severe problem because men have traditionally had a higher incidence of the disease; and (3) women decline major procedures more often than men do. Other possible explanations for the diagnostic and therapeutic difficulties women with heart disease encounter include:[30]

- Delay in diagnosing a possible heart attack.

- The complexity involved in interpreting chest pain in women.

- Typically less aggressive treatment of women heart attack victims.

- Their older age, on average, and more frequent comorbidities (other diseases/problems).

- Their coronary arteries are often smaller than men's, making surgical or diagnostic procedures more difficult technically.

- Their increased incidence of postinfarction angina and heart failure.

Although there is much debate about whether women have actually been ignored by past research concerning cardiovascular diseases, at least one study points out that the differences in treatment of suspected acute cardiac ischemia in men cannot be applied directly to women. More importantly, at least one study suggests that these differences may reflect overtreatment of men rather than undertreatment of women.[31]

Gender Bias in CVD Research

The traditional view that heart disease is primarily a male problem has carried over into research as well. A well-publicized example was research suggesting that aspirin could help prevent heart attacks—based entirely on a study of 22,000 male doctors. To address such concerns, the National Institutes of Health has launched a 15-year, $625 million study of 140,000 postmenopausal women, focusing on the leading causes of death and disease. Researchers hope to determine how a healthy lifestyle and increased medical attention can help prevent women's heart disease, as well as cancer and osteoporosis.

WHAT DO YOU THINK?

How do men and women differ in their CVD experiences? Why do you think women's risks were largely ignored until fairly recently? What actions do you think individuals can take to help improve these situations for both men and women? What actions can communities and members of the medical community take?

Hormone replacement therapies (HRT): Therapies that replace estrogen in postmenopausal women.

NEW WEAPONS AGAINST HEART DISEASE

The victim of a heart attack today has a variety of options that were not available a generation ago. Medications designed to strengthen heartbeat, control irregularities in rhythm, and relieve pain are widely prescribed. Triple and quadruple bypasses and angioplasty have become relatively commonplace procedures in hospitals throughout the nation.

Techniques of Diagnosing Heart Disease

Several techniques are used to diagnose heart disease, including electrocardiogram, angiography, and positron emission tomography scans. An **electrocardiogram (ECG)** is a record of the electrical activity of the heart measured during a stress test. Patients walk or run on treadmills while their hearts are monitored. A more accurate method of testing for heart disease is **angiography,** (often referred to as *cardiac catheterization*) in which a needle-thin tube called a *catheter* is threaded through blocked heart arteries, a dye is injected, and an X-ray is taken to discover which areas are blocked. A more recent and even more effective method of measuring heart activity is **positron emission tomography,** also called a **PET scan,** which pro-

duces three-dimensional images of the heart as blood flows through it. During a PET scan, a patient receives an intravenous injection of a radioactive tracer. As the tracer decays, it emits positrons that are picked up by the scanner and transformed by a computer into color images of the heart.

Newer tests that are now performed at many medical centers include:[32]

- *Radionuclide imaging* (includes such tests as thallium test, MUGA scan, and acute infarct scintigraphy). These tests involve injecting substances called radionuclides into the bloodstream. Computer-generated pictures can then show them in the heart. These tests can show how well the heart muscle is supplied with blood, how well the heart's chambers are functioning, and which part of the heart has been damaged by a heart attack.

- *Magnetic resonance imaging* (also called MRI or NMR). This test uses powerful magnets to look inside the body. Computer-generated pictures can show the heart muscle, identify damage from a heart attack, diagnose certain congenital heart defects, and evaluate disease of larger blood vessels such as the aorta.

- *Digital cardiac angiography* (also called DCA or DSA). This modified form of computer-aided imaging records pictures of the heart and its blood vessels.

Angioplasty versus Bypass Surgery

During the 1980s, **coronary bypass surgery** seemed to be the ultimate technique for treating patients who had coronary blockages or who had suffered heart attacks. In coronary bypass surgery, a blood vessel taken from another site in the patient's body (usually the saphenous vein in the leg or the internal mammary artery) is implanted to transport blood by bypassing blocked arteries. Recently, experts have begun to question the effectiveness of bypass operations, particularly for elderly people. Bypass patients typically spend 10 days or more in the hospital to recuperate from the surgery. The average cost of the procedure itself is well over $25,000 and the additional intensive care treatments and follow-ups often result in total medical bills that are closer to $100,000. The death rate is generally 2 percent at medical centers where surgical teams do large numbers of these operations. At hospitals where the procedure is performed infrequently, death rates can be much higher.

A procedure called **angioplasty** (sometimes called balloon angioplasty) is associated with fewer risks and is believed by many experts to be more effective than bypass surgery in selected cardiovascular cases. This procedure is similar to angiography. A needle-thin catheter is threaded through blocked heart arteries. The catheter has a balloon at the tip, which is inflated to flatten fatty

---

Electrocardiogram (ECG): A record of the electrical activity of the heart measured during a stress test.

Angiography: A technique for examining blockages in heart arteries. A catheter is inserted into the arteries, a dye is injected, and an X-ray is taken to find the blocked areas. Also called cardiac catheterization.

Positron emission tomography (PET scan): Method for measuring heart activity by injecting a patient with a radioactive tracer that is scanned electronically to produce a three-dimensional image of the heart and arteries.

Coronary bypass surgery: A surgical technique whereby a blood vessel is implanted to bypass a clogged coronary artery.

Angioplasty: A technique in which a catheter with a balloon at the tip is inserted into a clogged artery; the balloon is inflated to flatten fatty deposits against artery walls, allowing blood to flow more freely.

Thrombolysis: Injection of an agent to dissolve clots and restore some blood flow, thereby reducing the amount of tissue that dies from ischemia.

---

deposits against the artery walls, allowing blood to flow more freely. Angioplasty patients are generally awake but sedated during the procedure and spend only one or two days in the hospital after treatment. Most people can return to work within five days. Only about 1 percent of all angioplasty patients die during or soon after the procedure. Compared to bypass operations, angioplasty is far less expensive, costing about $12,000. However, there are some hazards in this procedure. In 3 to 7 percent of cases, the blood vessel that is stretched open by the balloon collapses spontaneously, and a bypass has to be done anyway. In addition, in about 30 percent of all angioplasty patients, the treated arteries become clogged again within six months. Some patients may undergo the procedure as many as three times within a five-year period. Some surgeons argue that given angioplasty's high rate of recurrence, bypass may be a more effective method of treatment.

New research suggests that in many instances, drug treatments may be just as effective in prolonging life as the invasive surgical techniques, but it is critical that doctors follow an aggressive drug treatment program and that patients comply with the doctors' drug orders.[33] How do you make a decision about your own treatment? The Building Communication Skills box can help.

Aspirin for Heart Disease: Can It Help?

Research has indicated that the use of low-dose aspirin (325 milligrams daily or every other day) is beneficial to heart patients. Aspirin has also proved helpful for patients undergoing certain cardiovascular surgery. It has even been advised as a preventive strategy for individuals with no current heart disease symptoms. However, a major problem associated with aspirin use is gastrointestinal intolerance, and this factor may outweigh its benefits for some people. Although the findings concerning the overall benefits of using aspirin to treat or prevent heart disease are inconclusive, the research seems promising thus far.[34]

Thrombolysis

Whenever a heart attack occurs, prompt action is the key factor in the patient's eventual prognosis. When a coronary artery gets blocked, the heart muscle doesn't die immediately, but time determines how much damage occurs. If a victim gets to an emergency room and is diagnosed fast enough, a form of reperfusion therapy called **thrombolysis** can sometimes be performed. Thrombolysis involves injecting an agent such as TPA (tissue plasminogen activator) to dissolve the clot and restore some blood flow, thereby reducing the amount of tissue that dies from ischemia.[35] These drugs must be used within one to three hours of a heart attack for best results.

Extensive CVD research in many areas has resulted in numerous strategies and techniques for prevention, diagnosis, and treatment that were not available a generation ago.

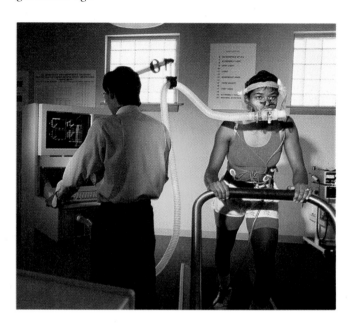

Knowledge about signs and symptoms of CVD and a readiness to take prompt action can do much to save your or a loved one's life. However, the ideal situation is to prevent a heart attack or other CVD crisis from happening in the first place. The choices that you make in your dietary habits, your exercise patterns, your management of stress, your prompt attention to suspicious symptoms, and other behaviors can greatly enhance your overall chances of remaining CVD-free. How much emphasis our health-care systems place on access to health care for all underserved populations, education about risks, and other community-based interventions for those at high risk is another factor that will influence your relative risk. You cannot totally reduce your risk of CVD: if you live long enough, chances are that some part of your cardiovascular system will begin to fail. However, the actions you take today may have a substantial and significant impact on the future health of your body systems.

*W*HAT DO YOU THINK?

With all the new diagnostic procedures, treatments, and differing philosophies about various prevention and intervention techniques, how can the typical health consumer insure that he or she will get the best treatment when entering the health-care system? Where can one go for information? Why might women, members of certain minority groups, and the elderly need a "health advocate" who can help them get through the system?

Be a Heart-Wise Consumer

The typical person who suspects that he or she may have a cardiovascular disease is often overwhelmed and frightened. Where should one go for diagnosis? What are the risks? Who has the best record of treatment success? What actions may reduce or enhance risks? Is this procedure my only option? Answering these and other questions becomes even more difficult if you are emotionally upset, scared, or tend to listen unquestioningly to doctors' orders.

If you or a loved one must face a CVD crisis, it is important to act with knowledge, strength, and assertiveness. Following these suggestions may help insure that you feel comfortable with your choices.

1. *Know your rights as a patient.* Ask about the relative risks and costs of various diagnostic tests. Some procedures, particularly angiography, may pose significant risks for the elderly, those who have had a history of TIAs, or those who have had chemotherapy or other treatments which may have damaged blood vessels. Ask for test results and an explanation of any abnormalities.

2. *Find out about informed consent procedures, living wills, durable power of attorney, organ donation, and other legal issues before you are sick.* Having someone shove a clipboard in your face and ask you if life support can be terminated in case of a problem is one of the great horrors of many people's hospital experiences. If you aren't prepared, this can be an unnecessary emotional burden.

3. *Ask about alternative procedures.* If possible, seek a second opinion at a health-care facility that is unrelated to your present one (in other words, get at least two opinions from doctors who are not in the same group and who cannot read each other's diagnoses). New research indicates that doctors may not use drug treatments as aggressively as they could and that drug treatments may be as effective as major bypass or open heart surgeries. Ask, ask, and ask again. Remember, it is your life, and there is always the possibility that another treatment may be better for you.

4. *Remain with your loved one as his or her "personal advocate."* If your loved one is weak and unable to ask ques-

tions, ask questions for him or her. Ask questions about new medications that are being given, new tests that are being run, and other potentially risky procedures that may be undertaken during the course of treatment or recovery. If your loved one is being removed from intensive care or other closely monitored areas prematurely, ask if the hospital is taking this action to comply with DRGs (established limits of treatment for certain conditions) and if this action is warranted. Most hospitals have waiting areas or special rooms that family members can use to stay close to a patient. Exercise your rights to this option.

5. *Monitor the actions of health-care providers.* In an attempt to control costs by means of managed care, some hospitals are hiring nursing aides and other untrained personnel to perform duties previously performed by registered nurses. Ask about the patient-to-nurse ratio, and make sure that people monitoring you or your loved ones have appropriate credentials.

6. *Be kind to and considerate of your care provider.* One of the most stressful jobs any person can be entrusted with is care of a critically ill person after a major cardiac event. Although questions are appropriate, be as tactful and considerate as possible, even though your emotions may be running high. Nurses often carry a disproportionate responsibility for the care of patients during critical times. They are often forced to carry a higher than necessary patient load. Try to remain out of their way, ask questions as necessary, and report any irregularities in care to the supervisor in charge.

7. *Be patient with the patient.* The pain, suffering, and fears associated with a cardiac event often cause otherwise nice people to act in not-so-nice ways. Be patient, helpful, and allow time for the patient to get his or her rest. Talk with the patient about how he or she is feeling, and about his or her concerns, fears, etc. Do not ignore his or her concerns in an attempt to ease your own anxieties.

Summary

◆ The cardiovascular system consists of the heart and circulatory system and is a carefully regulated, integrated network of vessels that supply the body with the nutrients and oxygen necessary to perform daily functions.

◆ Cardiovascular diseases include atherosclerosis (hardening of the arteries), heart attack, angina

pectoris, arrhythmias, congestive heart failure, congenital and rheumatic heart disease, and stroke. These combine to be the leading cause of death in the United States today.

◆ Risk factors for cardiovascular disease include cigarette smoking, high blood fat and cholesterol levels, hypertension, lack of exercise, high-fat diet, obesity, diabetes,

Managing Your Cardiovascular Health

Although it is easy to read through a chapter like this and learn what we should be doing to keep our hearts and circulatory systems healthy, few of us every really make a healthy heart one of our priorities. Relationships, financial worries, grades, time for fun, and other issues often take precedence over our long-term commitments to cardiovascular wellness.

Making Decisions for You

List the five things that matter to you most right now. Is appearance part of your list? Is being able to get through a day without feeling tired or unusually fatigued important? Are you motivated to change your health behaviors and take action to reduce your cardiovascular risks by exercising more, reducing stress, and cutting down on fat consumption? Was there anything about this chapter that got to you—that helped you become more concerned about making a change now? Why is this important? Are you really worried about your health, or are you more motivated by how you look to friends, by how your swimsuit may fit, or by other social reasons? Are you really ready to change right now? What actions do you plan to take?

Checklist for Change: Making Personal Choices

✓ Determine your hereditary risk. If it is high, outline the steps that you can take to reduce your overall risk.

✓ Regardless of your sex, take actions to reduce your risk factors.

✓ Know about the normal CVD risk changes that occur with age. Take the extra steps needed to minimize your risks as you age.

✓ If you smoke, quit. If you don't smoke, don't start.

✓ Find out what your cholesterol level is, including your HDL and LDL levels.

✓ Reduce saturated fat in your diet and take steps to reduce your triglyceride and cholesterol levels.

✓ Get out and exercise. Even a relaxing walk every day is a good CVD risk reducer. Nobody says you have to run and exercise until you drop. Take it easy, but keep it up.

✓ Control your blood pressure. Monitor it regularly and see your doctor if you are hypertensive.

✓ Lose weight if you are overweight. Obesity is a significant risk factor for both men and women.

✓ Control your stress levels.

Checklist for Change: Making Community Choices

✓ Take a class in CPR. Your local Red Cross likely offers them; even your college may. Be prepared to offer bystander CPR.

✓ Consider becoming an Emergency Medical Technician (EMT). You don't have to make a career of it. But you could be prepared to save people in your dorm, your office building, and your community.

✓ Volunteer for the local chapter of the American Heart Association. Give a few hours of your time answering phone calls and mailing information.

Critical Thinking

Your mother, now in her 50s, has recently begun complaining about indigestion. It seems to come and go, accompanying the pressure she is under at work. She saw her long-time doctor recently, who told her that she didn't appear to have a major indigestion problem. He suggested an improved diet and exercise. One day, when you are home for spring break, you find your mother sitting on the sofa in obvious pain, clutching her stomach. She tells you not to worry, it's just a particularly bad bout of indigestion. She adamantly denies that there is a problem beyond indigestion, and she does *not* want you to call the doctor.

It's now been 15 minutes since you discovered your mother, and she is in worsening pain. Using the DECIDE model described in Chapter 1, what should you do to help your mother?

---

and emotional stress. Some factors, such as age, gender, and heredity, are risk factors that are not under your control. Many of these factors have a compounded effect when combined. Dietary changes, exercise, weight reduction, and attention to lifestyle risks can reduce your susceptibility to cardiovascular disease.

◆ Women have a unique challenge in controlling their risk for CVD, particularly after menopause, when estrogen

levels are no longer sufficient to be protective.

◆ New methods developed for treating heart blockages include coronary bypass surgery and angioplasty. Also, beta blockers and calcium channel blockers are being used to reduce high blood pressure and to treat other symptoms.

Discussion Questions

1. Trace a drop of blood from the time it enters the heart until it reaches your extremities.

2. List the different types of CVDs. Compare and contrast their symptoms, risk factors, prevention, and treatment.

3. What are the major indicators that CVD poses a particularly significant risk to people your age? To the elderly? To people from selected minority groups?

4. Discuss the role exercise, stress management, dietary changes, checkups, sodium reduction, and other factors can play in reducing your risk for CVD.

5. Discuss why age is such an important factor in women's risk for CVD. What can be done to improve women's risks in later life?

6. Describe some of the diagnostic and treatment alternatives for CVD. If you had a heart attack today, which treatment would you prefer? Explain why.

Application Exercise

Reread the What Do You Think? scenarios at the beginning of the chapter and answer the following questions:

1. Consider Clay's case in the chapter opener. Why do you think so many young Americans deny their risk for CVD?

2. As a friend of either Clay or Jan, what advice might you give?

3. Think about people in your family who have significant CVD risks. What could you do to help them become aware of their risks without preaching to them about their behaviors and turning them off?

4. What kinds of community support could people like Jan and Clay use?

Further Reading

American Heart Association, *Heart and Stroke Facts* (Dallas, TX: American Heart Association)

An overview providing facts and figures concerning cardiovascular disease in the United States. Supplement provides key statistics about current trends and future directions in treatment and prevention.

Institute of Medicine, *Women and Health Research,* vol. 1 (National Academy Press, 1994).

Provides an outstanding overview of key issues surrounding research on women's health.

C H A P T E R   *17*

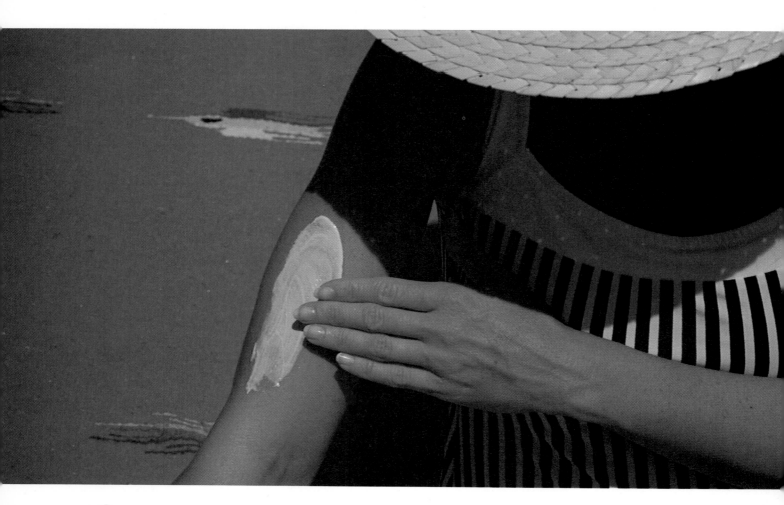

𝒞HAPTER OBJECTIVES

◆ Define *cancer* and discuss how cancer develops.

◆ Discuss the probable causes of cancer, including biological causes, occupational and environmental causes, social and psychological causes, chemicals in foods, viral causes, medical causes, and combined causes.

◆ Understand and act in response to self-exams, medical exams, and symptoms related to different types of cancers.

◆ Discuss cancer detection and treatment, including radiation therapy, chemotherapy, and immunotherapy.

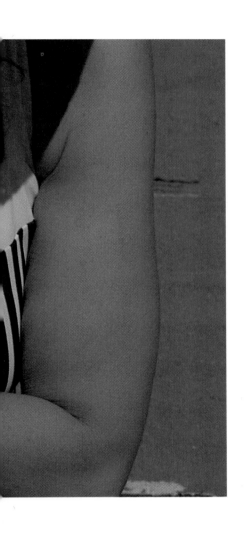

Cancer

Reducing Your Risks

Last year, Nasira's 28-year-old sister died of a rapidly growing form of inflammatory breast cancer. Although Nasira is only 21, she decides to have a mammogram, which reveals a very small malignant mass in one of the ducts of her right breast. Although her doctor recommends that she schedule a lumpectomy and begin radiation treatment, Nasira insists that she have both breasts removed and also her ovaries be removed to further reduce her risk.

- Before making such a decision, what factors should Nasira consider? Where should she go for the most current and reliable information about her best options? In situations like Nasira's, are such drastic surgical procedures typically warranted? If you were Nasira's friend, what advice might you give her?

Nick is an avid sunbather and lives in Phoenix. He routinely sits by the pool or on the deck sunning for one to two hours a day. When the weather is bad, he goes to the health spa for tanning sessions to help maintain his rugged, dark tan. When his girlfriend tells him that all that sun isn't good for him, he says that it helps his complexion and that the tanning booths filter out all the bad ultraviolet light, so there is nothing to worry about. He believes that because he has naturally dark hair and skin he isn't at risk for any form of skin cancer. Anyway, he says, it's no big deal. Even if he does get skin cancer, he'll just go in and get it taken care of.

- Is Nick's information about skin cancer correct? What are the risks associated with sunbathing in artificial and natural environments? If Nick insists on getting his tan, what actions can he take to reduce his risks?

As few as 50 years ago, a diagnosis of cancer was usually a death sentence. To make matters even worse, having a case of cancer in the family often led to ostracism, whispers about the possibility of infecting others with the disease, and an accompanying need for secrecy. Patients and their families thus often lacked any outside support. Moreover, even health professionals played guessing games about cancer's probable causes, laying a fertile ground for mystery, myth, and tremendous amounts of bigotry.

Fortunately, we've come a long way since then. Today, we know that there are multiple causes of cancer and that very few are linked to any type of infectious agent. In short, your chances of catching cancer from others are very slight. We also know that those who develop cancer do not face an inevitable death sentence. Early detection and vast improvements in technology have dramatically improved the prognosis for the majority of cancer patients. Finally, we know that a whole array of possibilities exists for actions that we can take individually or as a society to prevent cancer. Promising research puts us closer and closer to better solutions. Knowing the facts about cancer, recognizing your personal risks and risks to others, and taking action to reduce these risks are important steps in the battle to reduce cancer rates. Let's start by taking a look at just what this menace called cancer is.

AN OVERVIEW OF CANCER

Approximately 547,000 people will have died of cancer in 1995, which amounts to 1,500 cancer deaths each day.[1] To put this into perspective, about 170,000 lives will be lost to cancer caused by tobacco use, and another 18,000 cancer deaths will be related to excessive alcohol use, frequently undertaken in combination with cigarette smoking.[2] Thus, over one-third of today's cancer deaths could be prevented by sharp reductions in smoking and excessive alcohol use.

Although over 4.5 million people in the United States died of cancer during the 1980s, over 8 million people diagnosed with cancer during the 1980s are still alive, and 5 million of the 8 million are considered to be cured. Cured means that a patient has had no evidence of disease since treatment and now has the same life expectancy as a person who has never had cancer. Some cancers that only a few decades ago presented a very poor outlook are often cured today: acute lymphocytic leukemia in children, Hodgkin's disease, Burkitt's lymphoma, Ewing's sarcoma (a form of bone cancer), Wilms' tumor (a kidney cancer in children), testicular cancer, and osteogenic (bone) sarcoma are among the most remarkable indicators of progress in treatment techniques.

Not everyone is equally at risk for all types of cancers. Cancer incidence and mortality vary greatly by age, sex, race, and socioeconomic status. For instance, the National Cancer Institute (NCI) estimates that black Americans have greater incidence and mortality rates than white Americans do for most cancers. In 1991, the incidence rates were 439 per 100,000 for blacks and 406 for whites, about an 8 percent difference. In addition, blacks have a lower five-year survival rate than whites have—40 percent versus 56 percent. Cancer sites for which blacks have significantly higher incidence and mortality rates include the esophagus, uterus, cervix, stomach, liver, prostate, and larynx. Blacks also have greater rates for multiple myeloma, a bone marrow cancer. Rates for esophageal cancer are over three times higher among blacks than among whites. Researchers at the NCI believe that these differences are due more to blacks' lower average socioeconomic status and generally more limited access to health care than to any inherent physical characteristics.[3] In addition, it is possible that because large numbers of black Americans live in heavily industrialized areas and heavily populated inner cities, they may be exposed to more toxic chemicals in their home and work environments. However, recent findings indicate that some cancers may simply manifest themselves in different races, as the Multicultural Perspectives box discusses.

Cancer incidence and mortality rates within other minority groups, such as Hispanics, are often lower (sometimes by as much as 25 percent or more) than those of white or black Americans. Due to Hispanics' low average socioeconomic status, we might expect that they would have cancer rates similar to blacks' rates. But Hispanics seem to be "protected" from high rates. Why is this so? No one knows for sure, but the answer may lie in differences in various groups' diets, exercise patterns, or other culturally influenced behaviors. Because cancer risk is strongly associated with lifestyle and behavior, differences in ethnic and cultural groups can provide clues to factors involved

Deadliness of Breast Cancer in Blacks Defies Easy Answer

In the two decades that the National Cancer Institute has been gathering data on breast cancer, one thing has been clear: although white women are more likely than black women to get breast cancer, black women are much more likely to die from it. But the question is, why?

Now, several recent studies indicate that breast cancer might appear in a more deadly form among black woman. The tumors tend to be more malignant, as measured by cellular indicators of a poor prognosis.

Cancer experts said it was too soon to say whether this indicated that more aggressive treatment was warranted for black women or whether mammography was more—or less—likely to make a difference in the prognosis. But they said it was becoming clear that the high breast cancer death rates among black women were not solely the result of poverty or lack of access to medical care.

"There's a difference and I don't think we can ignore it," said Dr. Brenda K. Edwards, associate director of the surveillance program at the National Cancer Institute. She added, "The jury is still out on whether these differences alter our conclusions on the effectiveness of screening."

One study, by Dr. Richard M. Elledge, Dr. C. Kent Osborne and colleagues at the University of Texas Health Science Center in San Antonio, examined more than 6,000 tumors sent to them from hospitals throughout the United States. They found that tumors from black women had more actively dividing cells than those from white women and had tumor cells that lacked hormone receptors, another indicator of a poor prognosis.

Signs of Poor Prognosis

A study by Dr. Vivien W. Chen of the Louisiana State Medical Center and colleagues examined 963 newly diagnosed tumors and found that tumors from black women were more likely to have several histological features associated with a poor prognosis, including the features found by Dr. Elledge and his colleagues.

A third study, by Dr. Robert S. Siegel of George Washington University Medical Center in Washington, examined laboratory data on 708 tumors from women treated at his hospital and found that the tumors from the black women were more actively growing, were less likely to have hormone receptors and appeared more deranged.

Dr. Larry Kessler, chief of the cancer institute's applied research branch, said the racial differences in breast cancer incidence and mortality had long puzzled investigators. Breast cancer seems to strike black women under the age of 45 at a particularly high rate and to be especially deadly.

No one knows why breast cancer should be more common among young black women, but many cancer specialists have looked for sociological factors to explain why breast cancer is so deadly among blacks when it does occur.

One theory is that the high death rate reflects poor access to medical care among black women. But, Dr. Edwards said, a study she directed found that this can account for only about half of the increased death rate for blacks.

The study included 1,222 women in Atlanta, New Orleans, and the San Francisco-Oakland area. The black women, the investigators found, had about twice the death rate of the white women. But, Dr. Edwards said, a substantial proportion of the increased mortality seems to result from biological differences in the cancers of black women.

Dr. Siegel said that in his study he looked at the subset of women who were members of health maintenance organizations where the black and white members had equal access to mammograms and medical care. Even so, he said, the black women tended to have larger, more advanced tumors when their cancer was diagnosed, which may reflect a faster rate of tumor growth.

And Dr. Osborne said that his study looked at the treatments that women received once the disease was diagnosed and found that this factor also did not account for the dismal survival rates for black women.

Another theory is that black women put off seeing a doctor when they find a lump in their breasts, so by the time they get treatment their cancer is advanced and their mortality rate is higher.

Dr. Edwards said investigators in her study asked women who had symptoms, like a lump they could feel or bleeding, pain, or discharge from the breast, how long they had waited to see a doctor. Black women waited no longer than whites, she said. "The bottom line is that there was very little difference," she said.

Some investigators said the new findings confirmed a widespread suspicion among cancer doctors that black women really do have more intransigent cancers. . . .

Dr. Howard Ozer, director of the Winship Cancer Center at Emory University in Atlanta, said there might be too much blaming the victim for high breast cancer death rates. When black women go to a doctor with already advanced cancer, "it is always said that they don't come to the doctor soon enough," Dr. Ozer said. But, he said, with the evidence that the cancers might also be much more aggressive, "it may not be their fault at all."

in the development of cancer. Culturally influenced values and belief systems can also affect whether or not a person seeks care, participates in screenings, or follows recommended treatment options. Socioeconomic factors such as lack of health insurance or lack of transportation to major treatment centers can lead to late diagnosis and poor survival prospects.

Statistics from the American Cancer Society and the National Cancer Institute point to an increase in overall cancer mortality rates during the last 50 years despite the fact that mortality rates for many cancers are leveling off or declining. The overall increase is due mainly to a dramatic rise in lung cancer deaths.

What Is Cancer?

Cancer is the name given to a large group of diseases characterized by the uncontrolled growth and spread of abnormal cells. It may seem hard to understand how normal, healthy cells become cancerous, but if you think of a cell as a small computer, programmed to operate in a particular fashion, the process will become clearer. Under normal conditions, healthy cells are protected by a powerful overseer, the immune system, as they perform their daily functions of growing, replicating, and repairing body organs. When something interrupts normal cell pro-

---

Cancer: A large group of diseases characterized by the uncontrolled growth and spread of abnormal cells.

Neoplasm: A new growth of tissue that serves no physiological function resulting from uncontrolled, abnormal cellular development.

Tumor: A neoplasmic mass that grows more rapidly than surrounding tissues.

Malignant: Very dangerous or harmful; refers to a cancerous tumor.

Benign: Harmless; refers to a noncancerous tumor.

Biopsy: Microscopic examination of tissue to determine if a cancer is present.

Metastasis: Process by which cancer spreads from one area to different areas of the body.

Mutant cells: Cells that differ in form, quality, or function from normal cells.

Carcinogens: Cancer-causing agents.

Oncogenes: Suspected cancer-causing genes present on chromosomes.

Protooncogenes: Genes that can become oncogenes under certain conditions.

Oncologists: Physicians who specialize in the treatment of malignancies.

---

gramming, however, uncontrolled growth and abnormal cellular development results in a new growth of tissue serving no physiologic function called a **neoplasm.** This neoplasmic mass often forms a clumping of cells known as a **tumor.**

Not all tumors are **malignant** (cancerous); in fact, most are **benign** (noncancerous). Benign tumors are generally harmless unless they grow in such a fashion as to obstruct or crowd out normal tissues or organs. A benign tumor of the brain, for instance, is life-threatening when it grows in a manner that causes blood restriction and results in a stroke. The only way to determine whether a given tumor or mass is benign or malignant is through **biopsy,** or microscopic examination of cell development.

Benign and malignant tumors differ in several key ways. Benign tumors are generally composed of ordinary-looking cells enclosed in a fibrous shell or capsule that prevents their spreading to other body areas. Malignant tumors are usually not enclosed in a protective capsule and can therefore spread to other organs. This process, known as **metastasis,** makes some forms of cancer particularly aggressive in their ability to overcome bodily defenses. By the time they are diagnosed, malignant tumors have frequently metastasized throughout the body, making treatment extremely difficult. Unlike benign tumors, which merely expand to take over a given space, malignant cells invade surrounding tissue, emitting clawlike protrusions that disrupt chemical processes within healthy cells. More specifically, malignant cells disturb the ribonucleic acid (RNA) and deoxyribonucleic acid (DNA) within the normal cells. Tampering with these substances, which control cellular metabolism and reproduction, produces **mutant cells** that differ in form, quality, and function from normal cells.

WHAT CAUSES CANCER?

Although we can describe the process by which malignant cells spread throughout the body, we don't know for sure why this process occurs. We also do not know why some people have malignant cells in their bodies but never develop cancer. Scientists have proposed several theories for the cellular changes that produce cancer.

One theory of cancer development proposes that cancer results from some spontaneous error that occurs during cell reproduction. Perhaps cells that are overworked or aged are more likely to break down, causing genetic errors that result in mutant cells.

Another theory suggests that cancer is caused by some external agent or agents that enter a normal cell and initiate the cancerous process. Numerous environmental factors, such as radiation, chemicals, hormonal drugs, immunosuppressant drugs (drugs that suppress the normal activity of the immune system), and other toxins, are considered possible **carcinogens** (cancer-causing agents); perhaps the most common carcinogen is the tar in cigarettes. This theory of environmental carcinogens obviously has profound implications for our industrialized society. As in most disease-related situations, the greater the dose or the exposure to environmental hazards, the greater the risk of disease. People who are forced to work, live, and pass through areas that have high levels of environmental toxins may, in fact, be at greater risk for several types of cancers.

A third theory came out of research on certain viruses that are believed to cause tumors in animals. This research led to the discovery of **oncogenes,** suspected cancer-causing genes that are present on chromosomes. Although oncogenes are typically dormant, scientists theorize that certain conditions such as age, stress, and exposure to carcinogens, viruses, and radiation may activate these oncogenes. Once activated, they begin to grow and reproduce in an out-of-control manner.

There is still a great deal that remains unanswered about the oncogene theory of cancer development. Scientists are uncertain whether only people who develop cancer have oncogenes or whether we all have **protooncogenes,** genes that can become oncogenes under certain conditions. Many **oncologists** (physicians who specialize in the treatment of malignancies) believe that the oncogene theory may lead to a greater understanding of how individual cells function and may bring us closer to developing an effective treatment for cancerous cells.

The broad, underlying mechanisms for the development of cancer cells have been outlined, but much research needs to be conducted before we understand the exact mechanisms. Scientists have classified many substances as possible carcinogens, but we cannot state with certainty that these substances produce cancer in human beings. Some of the most widely suspected causes of cancer are shown in Figure 17.1 and are discussed in the following section.

Biological Factors

Some early cancer theorists believed that we inherit a genetic predisposition toward certain forms of cancer.[4] Recent research conducted by the University of Utah indicates that a gene for breast cancer exists. To date, however, the research in this area remains inconclusive. Although a rare form of eye cancer does appear to be passed genetically from mother to child, most cancers are not genetically linked. It is possible that we can inherit a tendency toward a cancer-prone, weak immune system or, conversely, that we can inherit a cancer-fighting potential. Both possibilities are considered rather remote at this time. But the complex interaction of hereditary predisposition, lifestyle, and environment on the development of cancer makes the likelihood of determining a single cause fairly remote.

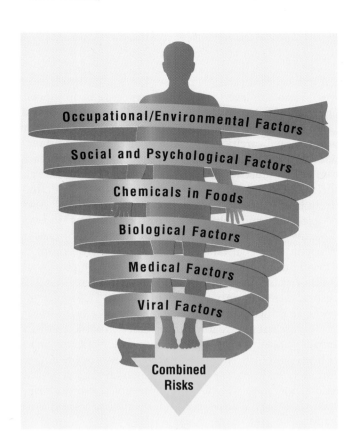

FIGURE 17.1

Suspected Causes of Cancer

Cancers of the breast, stomach, colon, prostate, uterus, ovaries, and lungs do appear to run in families. For example, a woman runs a much higher risk of having breast cancer if her mother or sisters have had the disease. Hodgkin's disease and certain leukemias show similar familial patterns. Whether these familial patterns are attributable to genetic susceptibility or to the fact that people in the same families experience similar environmental risks remains uncertain.

Gender also affects the likelihood of developing certain forms of cancer. For example, breast cancer occurs primarily among females, although men do occasionally get breast cancer. Obviously, factors other than heredity and familial relationships affect which sex develops a particular cancer. In the 1950s and 1960s, for example, women rarely contracted lung cancer. But with increases in the number of women who smoked and the length of time they had smoked, lung cancer became the leading cause of cancer deaths for American women in the 1980s. Lifestyle is clearly a critical factor in the interaction of variables that predispose a person toward cancer. Although gender plays a role in certain cases, other variables are probably more significant.

Occupational / Environmental Factors

Various occupational hazards are known to cause cancer when exposure levels are high or exposure is prolonged. Overall, however, workplace hazards account for only a small percentage of all cancers. One of the most common occupational carcinogens is asbestos, a fibrous substance once widely used in the construction, insulation, and automobile industries. Nickel, chromate, and chemicals such as benzene, arsenic, and vinyl chloride have definitively been shown to be carcinogens for humans. Also, people who routinely work with certain dyes and radioactive substances may have increased risks for cancer. Working with coal tars, as in the mining profession, or working near inhalants, as in the auto-painting business, is also hazardous. Those who work with herbicides and pesticides also appear to be at higher risk, although the evidence is inconclusive to date for low-dose exposures.

Because people are sometimes forced to work near hazardous substances, it is imperative that worksites enact policies and procedures designed to minimize and/or eliminate toxic exposure to the above substances. Several federal and state agencies are responsible for monitoring such exposures and insuring that businesses comply with standards designed to protect workers.
Radiation: Ionizing and Nonionizing. Ionizing radiation—radiation from X-rays, radon, cosmic rays, and ultraviolet radiation (primarily UV-B radiation)—is the only form of radiation proven to cause human cancer. (See the section on skin cancer.)

Incidents such as the Chernobyl accident have focused attention on the potentially disastrous effects of ionizing radiation emissions from nuclear power facilities and from medical radioactive wastes. Such facilities and wastes are closely monitored for safety in the United States. While reports about cancer case clusters in communities around nuclear power facilities have raised public concerns, studies show that clusters do not occur more often near nuclear power plants than they do by chance in wider geographical areas.[5]

Although nonionizing radiation produced by radio waves, microwaves, computer screens, televisions, electric blankets, and other products has been a topic of great concern in recent years, this form of radiation has not been shown to cause cancer. While some epidemiological studies suggest associations with cancer, others do not, and experimental studies have not yielded conclusive evidence of carcinogenic mechanisms.[6]

Social and Psychological Factors

Many researchers claim that social and psychological factors play a major role in determining whether a person gets cancer. Stress has been implicated in increased susceptibility to several types of cancers. By reducing stress levels in your daily life, you may, in fact, be reducing your risk for cancer. A number of therapists have even established preventive treatment centers where the primary focus is on "being happy" and "thinking positive thoughts." Is it possible to laugh away cancer?

Although orthodox medical personnel are skeptical of overly simplistic prevention centers that focus on humor and laughter as the way to prevent cancer, we cannot rule out the possibility that negative emotional states contribute to disease development. People who are lonely, depressed, and lack social support have been shown to be more susceptible to cancer than are their mentally healthy counterparts. Similarly, people who are under chronic stress and have poor nutrition or sleep habits develop cancer at a slightly higher rate than does the general population. Experts believe that severe depression or prolonged stress may reduce the activity of the body's immune system, thereby wearing down bodily resistance to cancer.

Although psychological factors may play a part in cancer development, exposure to substances such as tobacco and alcohol in our social environment are far more important. The American Cancer Society states that cigarette smoking is responsible for 30 percent of all cancer deaths—87 percent of all lung cancer deaths. Heavy consumption of alcohol has been related to cancers of the mouth, larynx, throat, esophagus, and liver. These cancers show up even more frequently in people whose heavy drinking is accompanied by smoking. The negative effects of smoking are not just concerns for the active smoker. Environmental (passive) tobacco smoke causes an estimated 4,000 deaths from lung cancer in the United States annually among family members and co-workers exposed to smokers' smoke.[7]

Chemicals in Foods

Among the food additives suspected of causing cancer is *sodium nitrate,* a chemical used to preserve and give color to red meat. Research indicates that the actual carcinogen is not sodium nitrate but nitrosamines, substances formed when the body digests the sodium nitrates. Sodium nitrate has not been banned, primarily because it kills the bacterium botulism, which is the cause of the highly virulent food-borne disease known as botulism. It should also be noted that the bacteria found in the human intestinal tract may contain more nitrates than a person could ever take in from eating cured meats or other nitrate-containing food products. Nonetheless, concern about the carcinogenic properties of nitrates has led to the introduction of meats that are nitrate-free or that contain reduced levels of the substance. See the Skills for Behavior Change box for guidelines on how to eat to reduce your risk of cancer.

Much of the concern about chemicals in foods today centers on the possible harm caused by pesticide and herbicide residue left on foods by agricultural practices. While some of these chemicals cause cancer at high doses in experimental animals, the very low concentrations

Diet and Cancer: Reducing Your Risk

If you've tuned in to the talk shows in recent months, you're almost certain to have heard claims and counterclaims about the mysterious health and protective benefits of some common nutrients. Although the debate about any role these foods may play in preventing cancer continues, many health professionals believe that there is at least some truth to the claims that eating certain foods may actually reduce your risks.

Folic Acid: The Good Vitamin?

Studies at the University of Alabama at Birmingham and the Harvard Medical School have repeatedly shown a positive link between the B vitamin known as folic acid and risks for cervical, colon, and rectal cancer. Increased amounts of folic acid appeared to play a role in preventing *precancerous polyps* (small growths) and to reduce the incidence of all *dysplasia* (abnormal cell development).

Antioxidants: The Debate Goes On

Perhaps no other group of nutrients has attracted so much attention in recent months as the antioxidants—vitamins A, C, E, and betacarotene; the *retinoids,* which are related to vitamin A; and the mineral selenium. Do these substances offer the promise of a cancer-free world, do they increase your risk for selected cancers, or are they just another example of cancer-prevention quackery?

Fortunately, amid the clamor of pro and con claims, a reputable body of research is beginning to provide useful information for consumers. Much of this research focuses on the idea that antioxidants offset a normal body process

in which healthy cells produce a destructive by-product—a highly reactive, unstable form of oxygen molecules known as free radicals.

While some free radicals serve useful purposes in the body's defenses, others appear to steal electrons from other molecules, thereby causing irreversible damage to a cell's membrane and DNA. According to John Bertram, professor of genetics and molecular biology at the University of Hawaii Cancer Research Center, "We know without a doubt that oxidative damage harms cells. An affected cell, for example, may fail to activate its natural cancer fighting defenses, shirk some of its other chemical functions, or even copy damaged DNA into new cells." Researchers believe that antioxidants have the ability to control "out of control" free radicals and perhaps repair their damage, deactivate them, or transform them into less toxic substances.

Even though some studies have found no association between antioxidants and reduced cancer risks, the antioxidant theory gained respectability in the early 1990s. So, does this mean that you should rush out and buy a heavy dose of the antioxidants and try to beat the cancer odds? Probably not. An April 1994 study of over 29,000 Finnish male smokers threw a monkey wrench into the antioxidant debate by reporting that among those male smokers who ate diets high in antioxidant-rich fruits and vegetables, risks for lung cancer and hemorrhagic stroke actually appeared to increase. Experts caution that the Finnish study provides interesting information, but that smokers represent a much different health profile than do nonsmokers and thus may not be similar in level of risk. Much more research must be

(continued)

---

found in some foods are well within established government safety levels. Continued research regarding pesticide and herbicide use is essential for maximum food safety and the continuous monitoring of agricultural practices is necessary to insure a safe food supply. Scientists and consumer groups stress the importance of a balance between chemical use and the production of quality food products.[8] Policies protecting consumer health and insuring the continued improvement in food production through development of alternative, low-chemical pest and herbicide control and reduced environmental pollution should be the goal of prevention efforts.

Viral Factors

The chances of becoming infected with a "cancer virus" are very remote. Over the years, several forms of virus-induced cancers have been observed in laboratory animals and there is some indication that human beings display a similar tendency toward virally transmitted cancers. Evidence that the *herpes-related viruses* may be

involved in the development of some forms of leukemia, Hodgkin's disease, cervical cancer, and Burkitt's lymphoma has surfaced in recent years. The *Epstein-Barr virus,* associated with mononucleosis, may also contribute to cancer development. Cervical cancer has also been linked to the *human papillomavirus,* the virus that causes genital warts.[9]

Although research is inconclusive, many scientists believe that selected viruses may help to provide an *opportunistic* environment for subsequent cancer development. It is likely that a combination of immunological bombardment by viral or chemical invaders and other risk factors substantially increases the risk of cancer.

Medical Factors

In some cases, medical treatment increases a person's risk for cancer. One famous example is the widespread use of the prescription drug *diethylstilbestrol (DES)* during the years 1940 to 1960 to control problems with bleeding during pregnancy and to reduce the risk of miscarriage. It was

conducted before we have a true picture of the antioxidant risk/benefit quotient.

Meanwhile, it is clear that chugging down megadoses of antioxidants can be harmful. Although toxic effects from overdosing on vitamin E or betacarotene have not yet been noted, vitamin A and selenium do have toxic effects. Too much vitamin C increases the risk of urinary stones. Instead of popping pills to get sufficient antioxidants, eating more green, red, and yellow vegetables and fruits in a normal diet will put you in line with the best advice to date. Supplements are not a substitute for a healthy diet. Until we know more about the actions of these and other dietary substances, the guidelines established by the American Cancer Society offer the most sensible framework for a diet that reduces the risk of cancer.

- Maintain desirable weight. Sensible eating habits and regular exercise will help you avoid excessive weight gain. Being 40 percent overweight significantly increases your risk for colon, breast, gallbladder, prostate, ovarian, and uterine cancers.

- Eat a varied diet. A varied diet consumed in moderate quantities seems to lower the risk for cancer.

- Eat vegetables and fruits every day. Five servings daily of fruits and vegetables can help reduce your chances of getting lung, prostate, bladder, esophagus, and stomach cancers.

- Include cruciferous vegetables in your diet. Certain vegetables in this family—cabbage, broccoli, brussels sprouts, kohlrabi, and cauliflower—seem to help prevent the development of certain cancers.

- Eat more high-fiber foods. A high-fiber diet—including whole-grain cereals, breads, and pasta—may reduce your risk for colon cancer.

- Cut down on total fat intake. A high-fat diet may be a factor in the development of certain cancers, particularly breast, colon, and prostate cancers.

- Avoid salt-cured, smoked, and nitrate-cured foods. In areas of the world where salt-cured and smoked foods are eaten frequently, there is a higher incidence of cancer of the esophagus and stomach.

- Keep alcohol consumption moderate. The heavy use of alcohol, especially when accompanied by cigarette smoking or chewing tobacco, increases risks for cancers of the mouth, larynx, throat, esophagus, and liver.

Sources: Information from L. Katzenstein, *American Health,* October 1993, 13–14; "Taking a Closer Look at Antioxidants," *American Institute for Cancer Research Newsletter,* August, 1994; "Cancer Protection in Our Food," *American Institute for Cancer Research Newsletter,* Spring 1993, 4; A. Kardinaal, F. Kok, Ringstad et al., "Antioxidants in Adipose Tissue and Risk of Myocardial Infarction: The EURAMIC Study," *Lancet* 342 (4 December 1993): 1379–1382; and O. Heinonen and D. Albanes, "The Effect of Vitamin E and Beta Carotene on the Incidence of Lung Cancer and Other Cancers in Male Smokers," *New England Journal of Medicine* 330 (14 April 1994): 1029–1035.

---

not until the 1970s that the dangers of this drug became apparent. Although DES caused few side effects in the millions of women who took it, their daughters were found to have an increased risk for cancers of the reproductive organs.

Some scientists claim that the use of estrogen replacement therapy among postmenopausal women is dangerous because it increases the risks for uterine cancer. Others believe that because estrogen is critical to the prevention of osteoporosis and heart disease in aging women, its use should not be curtailed. Most medical professionals believe that properly administered estrogen therapy poses no substantially increased risks to most patients.

Numerous drug regimens given to patients in the form of chemotherapy to treat one cancer may also increase the risks of the patient developing other forms of cancer.

Combined Risks

Currently, many factors are believed to contribute to cancer development. How large an effect each risk factor has is unknown. Experts believe, however, that combining risk factors can dramatically increase a person's risk for cancer. For example, a person who smokes heavily and works as an auto-body painter runs a much greater risk for developing lung cancer than a person who has only one of these risks. To assess your personal risk factors, complete the Rate Yourself box.

*W*HAT DO YOU THINK?

Based on what you've read and heard, what do you think causes most people to get cancer? Which risk factors do you think your family has? Which ones do you have, if any, that are different from your family's? What can you do about your personal risks?

*T*YPES OF CANCERS

As we said earlier, the term *cancer* refers not to a single disease but to hundreds of different diseases. However, four

Cancer: Assessing Your Risk

You can reduce your risk of developing some types of cancer, such as lung cancer, by changing your lifestyle behaviors. For other types of cancer, such as breast and colorectal cancers, your chance for cure is greatly increased if the cancer is found at an early stage through periodic screening examinations.

The following has been designed by the American Cancer Society to help you learn about (1) your risk factors for certain types of cancer and (2) the chances that cancer would be found at an early stage when a cure is possible.

Read each question concerning each site and its specific risk factors. Be honest in your responses. Circle the number in parentheses next to your response.

Individual numbers for specific questions are not to be interpreted as a precise measure of relative risk, but the totals for a given site should give a general indication of your risk.

Lung Cancer

1. Sex: a. Male (2)   b. Female (1)

2. Age: a. 39 or less (1)   b. 40–49 (2)   c. 50–59 (5)   d. 60+ (7)

3. Exposure to any of these:
   a. Mining (3)   b. Asbestos (7)   c. Uranium and radioactive products (5)   d. None (0)

4. Habits: a. Smoker: (10)*   b. Nonsmoker (0)*

5. Type of smoking:
   a. Cigarettes or little cigars (10)   b. Pipe and/or cigar, but not cigarettes (3)   c. Nonsmoker (0)

6. Number of cigarettes smoked per day:
   a. 0 (1)   b. less than ½ pack per day (5)   c. ½–1 pack (9)   d. 1–2 packs (15)   e. 2+ packs (20)

7. Type of cigarette:
   a. High tar/nicotine (10)**   b. Medium tar/nicotine (9)**   c. Low tar/nicotine (7)**   d. Nonsmoker (1)

8. Length of time smoking:
   a. Nonsmoker (1)   b. Up to 15 years (5)   c. 15–25 years (10)   d. 25+ years (20)

Subtotal _____

Reducing Your Risk

*If you stopped smoking more than 10 years ago, count yourself as a nonsmoker. If you have stopped smoking in the past 10 years, you are an ex-smoker. Ex-smokers should answer questions 4 through 8 according to how they previously smoked. Then ex-smokers may reduce their point total on questions 5 through 8 by 10% for each year they have not smoked. Current smokers also answer questions 5 through 8.

9. I am stopping smoking today. (If yes, subtract 2 points.)   Yes   No

Total _____

**High Tar/Nicotine: 20 mg. or more tar/1.3 mg. or more nicotine
Medium Tar/Nicotine: 16–19 mg. tar/1.1–1.2 mg. nicotine
Low Tar/Nicotine: 15 mg. or less tar/1.0 mg. or less nicotine

Colon and Rectum Cancer
Risk factors

1. Age: a. 40 or less (2)   b. 40–49 (7)   c. 50 and over (12)

2. Has anyone in your family ever had:
   a. Colon cancer (18)   b. Colon polyps (18)   c. Neither (1)

3. Have you ever had:
   a. Colon cancer (25)   b. Colon polyps (25)   c. Ulcerative colitis for more than seven years (18)
   d. Cancer of the breast, ovary, uterus, or stomach (13)   e. None of the above (1)

Total _____

(continued)

Symptoms

1. Do you have bleeding from the rectum?   Yes   No

2. Have you had a change in bowel habits (such as altered frequency, size, consistency, or color of stool)?   Yes   No

Reducing Your Risks and Detecting Cancer Early

1. I have altered my diet to include less fat and more fruits, fiber, and cruciferous vegetables (broccoli, cabbage, cauliflower, brussel sprouts).   Yes   No

2. I have had a negative test for blood in my stool within the past year.   Yes   No

3. I have had a negative examination for colon cancer and polyps within the past year (porcosigmoidoscopy, colonscopy, barium enema x-rays).   Yes   No

Skin Cancer

1. Live in the southern part of the U.S.:   Yes   No

2. Frequent work or play in the sun: Yes   No

3. Fair complexion or freckles (natural hair color of blonde, red, or light brown, or eye color of grey, green, blue, or hazel):   Yes   No

4. Work in mines, around coal tars or radioactivity: Yes   No

5. Experienced a severe, blistering sunburn before the age of 18:   Yes   No

6. Have any family members with skin cancer or history of melanoma: Yes   No

7. Had skin cancer or melanoma in the past: Yes   No

8. Use or have used tanning beds or sun lamps: Yes   No

9. Have large, many, or changing moles: Yes   No

Reducing Your Risks and Detecting Cancer Early

10. I cover up with a wide-brimmed hat and wear long-sleeved shirts and pants   Yes   No

11. I use sun screens with an SPF rating of 15 or higher when going out in the sun   Yes   No

12. I examine my skin once a month for changes in warts or moles   Yes   No

Breast Cancer

1. Age group: a. under 35 (10)   b. 35–39 (20)   c. 40–49 (50)   d. 50 and over (90)

2. Race: a. Oriental (10)   b. Hispanic (10)   c. Black (20)   d. White (25)

3. Family history   a. None (10)   b. Mother, sister, daughter with breast cancer (30)

4. Your history: a. No breast disease (10)   b. Previous lumps or cysts (15)   c. Previous breast cancer (100)

5. Maternity: a. 1st pregnancy before 30 (10)   b. 1st pregnancy at 30 or older (15)   c. No pregnancies (20)

Detecting Cancer Early

6. I practice breast self-examination monthly. (If yes, subtract 10 points.)   Yes   No

7. I have had a negative mammogram and examination by a physician in accordance with American Cancer Society Breast Health Guidelines. (If yes, subtract 25 points.)   Yes   No

Total _____

Cervical Cancer

(Lower Portion of Uterus)—These questions do not apply to a woman who has had a total hysterectomy.

1. Age group: a. Less than 25 (10)   b. 25–39 (20)   c. 40–54 (30)   d. 55 and over (30)

2. Race: a. Oriental or white (10)   b. Black (20)   c. Hispanic (20)

3. Number of pregnancies: a. 0 (10)   b. 1 to 3 (20)   c. 4 and over (30)

(continued)

4. Viral infections:
   a. Viral infections of the vagina such as venereal warts, herpes, or ulcer formations (10)   b. Never (1)

5. Age at first intercourse:
   a. Before 15 (40)   b. 15–19 (30)   c. 20–24 (20)   d. 25 and over (10)   e. Never had intercourse (5)

6. Bleeding between periods or after intercourse: a. Yes (40)   b. No (1)

7. Smoker: a. Non-smoker (2)   b. Smoker (3)

Subtotal _____

Detecting Cancer Early

8. I have had a negative Pap smear and pelvic examination within the past year.
   (If yes, subtract 50 points.)   Yes   No

Total _____

Endometrial Cancer

(Body of Uterus)—These questions do not apply to a woman who has had a total hysterectomy.

1. Age group: a. 39 or less (5)   b. 40–49 (20)   c. 50 and over (60)

2. Race: a. Oriental (10)   b. Black (10)   c. Hispanic (10)   d. White (20)

3. Births: a. None (15)   b. 1 to 4 (7)   c. 5 or more (5)

4. Weight: a. 50 or more pounds overweight (50)   b. 20–49 pounds overweight (15)
   c. Normal or underweight for height (10)

5. Diabetes (elevated blood sugar):   a. Yes (3)   b. No (1)

6. Estrogen hormone intake*:   a. Yes, regularly (15)   b. Yes, occasionally (12)   c. None (10)

7. Abnormal uterine bleeding: a. Yes (40)   b. No (1)

8. Hypertension (high blood pressure):   a. Yes (3)   b. No (1)

Subtotal _____

Detecting Cancer Early

9. I have had a negative pelvic examination and Pap smear or endometrial tissue sampling
   (endometrial biopsy) performed within the past year. (If yes, subtract 50 points.)   Yes   No

Total _____

NOTE: This excludes birth control pills.

Test Analysis
Lung Answers

If Your Total Is:

24 or less . . .   You have a low risk for lung cancer.

25–49 . . .   You may be a light smoker and would have a good chance of kicking the habit.

50–74 . . .   As a moderate smoker, your risks for lung and upper respiratory tract cancer are increased. The time to stop is now!

75 or over . . .   As a heavy cigarette smoker, your chances of getting lung cancer and cancer of the upper respiratory or digestive tract are greatly increased.

Reducing Your Risk

Make a decision to quit today. Join a smoking cessation program. If you are a heavy drinker of alcohol, your risks for cancer of the head and neck and esophagus are further increased. Use of "spitting" tobacco increases your risks of cancer of the mouth. Your best bet is not to use tobacco in any form. See your doctor if you have a nagging cough, hoarseness, persistent pain or sore in the mouth, or throat or lumps in the neck.

(continued)

Colon and Rectum Answers

I. Risk Factors*—If Your Total Is:

5 or less . . .   You are currently at low risk for colon and rectum cancer. Eat a diet high in fiber and low in fat and follow cancer checkup guidelines.

6–15 . . .   You are currently at moderate risk for colon and rectum cancer. Follow the American Cancer Society guidelines for early detection of colorectal cancer. These are: (1) a digital rectal exam** every year after 40 and (2) a fecal occult blood test every year and a sigmoidoscopic, preferably flexible, exam every 3–5 years after age 50.

16 or greater . . .   You are in the high risk group for colon and rectum cancer. This rating requires a lifetime, on-going screening program that includes periodic evaluation of your entire colon. See your doctor for more information.

*If your answers to any of these questions change, you should reassess your risk.
**This test has an additional advantage in that it is also an early detection method for cancer of the prostate in men.

II. Symptoms

The presence of rectal bleeding or a change in bowel habits may indicate colon/rectum cancer. See your physician right away if you have either of these symptoms.

III. Reducing Your Risks and Detecting Cancer Early

Regular tests for hidden blood in the stool and appropriate examinations of the colon will increase the likelihood that colon polyps are discovered and removed early and that cancers are found in an early, curable state. Modifying your diet to include more fiber, cruciferous vegetables, and foods rich in Vitamin A; and less fat and salt-cured foods may result in a reduction of cancer risks.

Skin Answers

If you answered "yes" to any of the first nine questions, you need to use protective clothing and use a sunscreen with an SPF rating of 15 or greater whenever you are out in the sun and check yourself monthly for any changes in warts or moles. An answer of "yes" to questions 10, 11, and 12 can help reduce your risk of skin cancer or possibly detect skin cancer early.

Reducing Your Risks and Detecting Cancer Early

Numerical risks for skin cancer are difficult to state. For instance, a person with a dark complexion can work longer in the sun and be less likely to develop cancer than a person with a light complexion. Furthermore, a person wearing a long-sleeved shirt and wide-brimmed hat may work in the sun and be less at risk than a person who wears a bathing suit for only a short time. The risk for skin cancer goes up greatly with age.

Melanoma, the most serious type of skin cancer, can be cured when it is detected and treated at a very early stage. Changes in warts and moles are important and should be checked by your doctor.

Breast Answers

If Your Total Is:

Under 100 . . .   Low risk women (and all others). You should practice monthly Breast Self-Examination, have your breasts examined by a doctor as part of a regular cancer-related checkup, and have mammography in accordance with ACS guidelines.

100–199 . . .   Moderate risk women. You should practice monthly BSE and have your breasts examined by a doctor as part of a cancer-related checkup, and have periodic mammography in accordance with American Cancer Society guidelines, or more frequently as your physician advises.

200 or higher . . .   High risk. You should practice monthly BSE and have your breasts examined by a doctor, and have mammography more often. See your doctor for the recommended frequency of breast examinations and mammography.

Detecting Cancer Early

One in 9 American women will get breast cancer in her lifetime. Being a woman is a risk factor! Most women (75 percent) who get breast cancer don't have other risk factors. BSE and mammography may diagnose a breast cancer in its earliest stage with a greatly increased chance of cure. When detected at this stage, cure is more likely and breast-saving surgery may be an option.

(continued)

Cervical Answers

If Your Total Is:

40–69 . . .   This is a low risk group. Ask your doctor for a Pap test and advice about frequency of subsequent testing.

70–99 . . .   In this moderate risk group, more frequent Pap tests may be required.

100 or more . . .   You are in a high risk group and should have a Pap test (and pelvic exam) as advised by your doctor.

Detecting Cancer Early

Early detection of this cancer by the Pap test has markedly improved the chance of cure. When this cancer is found at an early stage, the cure rate is extremely high and uterus-saving surgery and child-bearing potential may be preserved.

Endometrial Answers

If Your Total Is:

45–59 . . .   You are at very low risk for developing endometrial cancer.

60–99 . . .   Your risks are slightly higher. Report any abnormal bleeding immediately to your doctor. Tissue sampling at menopause is recommended.

100 and over . . .   Your risks are much greater. See your doctor for tests as appropriate.

Detecting Cancer Early

Once again, early detection is a key to your chance of a cure for this cancer. Regular pelvic examinations may find other female cancers such as cancer of the ovary.

Source: Reprinted by permission of the American Cancer Society, Texas Division, Inc., from *Cancer: Assessing Your Risk,* © 1981, revised 1990, 1992, 1993.

---

broad classifications of cancer are made according to the type of tissue from which the cancer arises.

Classifications of Cancer

Carcinomas. Epithelial tissues (tissues covering body surfaces and lining most body cavities) are the most common sites for cancers. Carcinoma of the breast, lung, intestines, skin, and mouth are examples. These cancers affect the outer layer of the skin and mouth as well as the mucous membranes. They metastasize through the circulatory or lymphatic system initially and form solid tumors.

Sarcomas. Sarcomas occur in the mesodermal, or middle, layers of tissue—for example, in bones, muscles, and general connective tissue. They metastasize primarily via the blood in the early stages of disease. These cancers are less common but generally more virulent than carcinomas. They also form solid tumors.

Lymphomas. Lymphomas develop in the lymphatic system—the infection-fighting regions of the body—and metastasize through the lymph system. Hodgkin's disease is one type of lymphoma. Lymphomas also form solid tumors.

Leukemia. Cancer of the blood-forming parts of the body, particularly the bone marrow and spleen, is called leukemia. A nonsolid tumor, leukemia is characterized by an abnormal increase in the number of white blood cells.

The seriousness and general prognosis of a particular cancer are determined through careful diagnosis by trained oncologists. Once laboratory results and clinical observations have been made, cancers are rated by level and stage of development. Those diagnosed as "carcinoma in situ" are localized and are often curable. Cancers that are given higher level or stage ratings have spread farther and are less likely to be cured.

Figure 17.2 shows the most common sites of cancer and the number of deaths annually from each type of cancer. We discuss some of these common cancers in this section.

Lung Cancer

Although lung cancer rates have dropped among white males during the last decade, the incidence among white females (particularly young teens) and black males and females continues to rise. Lung cancer caused an estimated 157,400 deaths in 1995. In 1987, for the first time, more women died from lung cancer than from breast cancer, which for over 40 years had been the major cause of cancer deaths in women.[10]

Symptoms of lung cancer include a persistent cough, blood-streaked sputum, chest pain, and recurrent attacks of pneumonia or bronchitis. Treatment depends on the type and stage of the cancer. Surgery, radiation therapy, and chemotherapy are all treatment options. If the cancer is localized, surgery is usually the treatment of choice. If the cancer has spread, surgery is used in combination with radiation and chemotherapy. Unfortunately, despite advances in medical technology, survival rates for lung cancer have improved only slightly over the past decade. Just 13 percent of lung cancer patients live five or more years after diagnosis. These rates improve to 47 percent with early detection, but only 15 percent of lung cancers are discovered in their early stages of development.[11]

Prevention. Smokers, especially those who have smoked for over 20 years, and people who have been exposed to certain industrial substances such as arsenic and asbestos or to radiation from occupational, medical, or environmental sources are at the highest risk for lung cancer. Exposure to sidestream cigarette smoke increases the risk for nonsmokers. Some researchers have theorized that as many as 90 percent of all lung cancers could be avoided if people did not smoke. Substantial improvements in overall prognosis have been noted in smokers who quit at the first signs of precancerous cellular changes and allowed their bronchial linings to return to normal.

Breast Cancer

About 1 out of 10 women will develop breast cancer at some time in her life. Although this oft-repeated ratio has frightened many women, it represents a woman's lifetime risk. Thus, not until the age of 80 does a woman's risk of

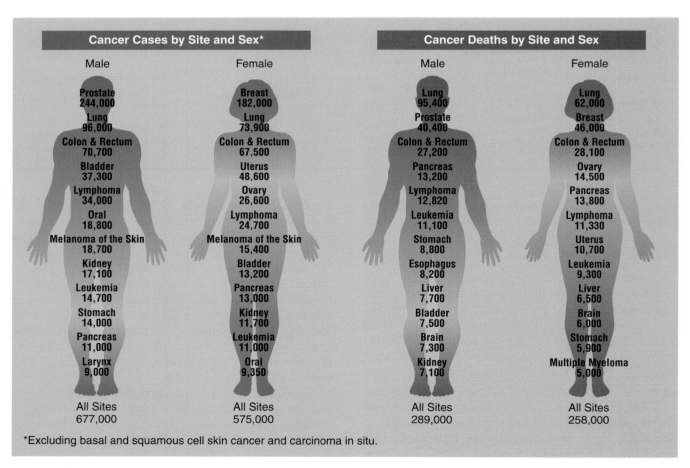

Cancer Cases by Site and Sex*		Cancer Deaths by Site and Sex	
Male	Female	Male	Female
Prostate 244,000	Breast 182,000	Lung 95,400	Lung 62,000
Lung 96,000	Lung 73,900	Prostate 40,400	Breast 46,000
Colon & Rectum 70,700	Colon & Rectum 67,500	Colon & Rectum 27,200	Colon & Rectum 28,100
Bladder 37,300	Uterus 48,600	Pancreas 13,200	Ovary 14,500
Lymphoma 34,000	Ovary 26,600	Lymphoma 12,820	Pancreas 13,800
Oral 18,800	Lymphoma 24,700	Leukemia 11,100	Lymphoma 11,330
Melanoma of the Skin 18,700	Melanoma of the Skin 15,400	Stomach 8,800	Uterus 10,700
Kidney 17,100	Bladder 13,200	Esophagus 8,200	Leukemia 9,300
Leukemia 14,700	Pancreas 13,000	Liver 7,700	Liver 6,500
Stomach 14,000	Kidney 11,700	Bladder 7,500	Brain 6,000
Pancreas 11,000	Leukemia 11,000	Brain 7,300	Stomach 5,900
Larynx 9,000	Oral 9,350	Kidney 7,100	Multiple Myeloma 5,000
All Sites 677,000	All Sites 575,000	All Sites 289,000	All Sites 258,000

*Excluding basal and squamous cell skin cancer and carcinoma in situ.

FIGURE 17.2

Leading Sites of New Cancer Cases and Deaths—1995 Estimates

Source: Reprinted by permission from American Cancer Society, *Cancer Facts and Figures—1995* (Atlanta: ACS, 1995), 11.

breast cancer rise to 1 in 10.[12] Here is the risk at earlier ages:

Age 50: 1 in 50

Age 60: 1 in 24

Age 70: 1 in 14

Age 80: 1 in 10

In 1995, approximately 182,000 women in the United States will have been diagnosed with breast cancer for the first time. About 46,000 women (and 240 men) will die, making breast cancer the second leading cause of cancer death for women.[13]

Warning signals of breast cancer include persistent breast changes such as a lump, thickening, swelling, dimpling, skin irritation, distortion, retraction or scaliness of the nipple, nipple discharge, pain, or tenderness. Risk factors for breast cancer may vary considerably.[14] Typically, risk factors include being over the age of 40, having a primary relative (a grandmother, mother, or sister) who had breast cancer, never having had children or having breast-fed, having your first child after age 30, having had early menarche, having had a late age of menopause, and having a higher education and socioeconomic status. International variability in breast cancer incidence rates correlate with differences in diet, with more affluent societies having significantly higher cancer rates. However, it is important to note that a causal role for dietary factors has not been firmly established.[15]

Although risk factors are useful tools, they do not always adequately predict individual susceptibility. However, because of increased awareness, better diagnostic techniques, and improved treatments, breast cancer victims have a better chance of surviving today than they did in the past. The five-year survival rate for victims of localized breast cancer (which includes all women living five years after diagnosis, whether the patient is in remission, disease-free, or under treatment) has risen from 78 percent in the 1940s to 94 percent today. These statistics vary dramatically, however, based on when the cancer is first detected. For example, if the cancer has spread to surrounding tissue, the five-year survival rate is 73 percent; if it is spread to distant parts of the body, these rates fall to 18 percent; and, if the breast cancer has not spread, the survival rate approaches 100 percent. Thus, it is apparent that a key factor in survival rests with individual recognition of early symptoms.[16]

Prevention. A recent study of the role of exercise in reducing the risk for breast cancer has generated excitement in the scientific community. The study, involving 1,090 women who were 40 or younger (545 with breast cancer and 545 without) analyzed subjects' exercise patterns since they began menstruating. The risk of those who averaged four hours of exercise a week since menstruation

was 58 percent lower than that of women who did no exercise at all. The good news was that subjects did not have to be avid joggers to have reduced risk. Among the activities reported were team sports, individual sports, dance, exercise classes, swimming, walking, and a variety of other activities. Researchers speculated that exercise may protect women by altering the production of the ovarian hormones estrogen and progesterone during menstrual cycles.[17] For more on the role of exercise in preventing cancer, see the Health Headlines box.

Other research has shown that vigorous athletics can delay the onset of menstruation and halt ovulation in some women. A woman's cumulative exposure to the sex hormones is believed to be associated with breast cancer risk. It may also be possible that exercise increases muscle mass and decreases body fat, another potential risk for breast cancer. Although this research is not definitive and other studies have yet to replicate these results, it does

Mammography and other early detection techniques greatly increase a woman's chance of surviving breast cancer.

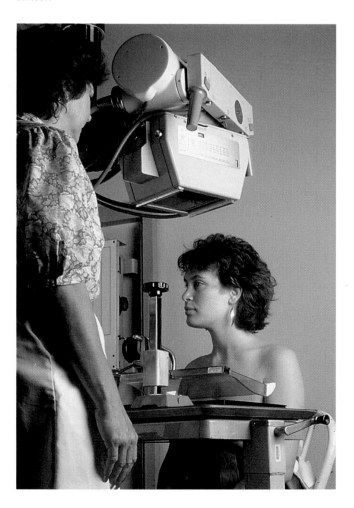

Can Exercise Ward Off Cancer?

Just in case you need another reason to head to the gym, there's a growing body of evidence that regular moderate exercise lowers the risk of colon cancer, as well as cancers of the breast, uterus, ovaries, cervix, and vagina.

Researchers questioned 17,000 male Harvard University alumni about their exercise habits in 1962 or 1966, and then again in 1977. Those who reported at both interviews that they typically burned at least 1,000 calories a week through exercise (equal to walking 10 miles or playing two hours of tennis) had a colon cancer risk half that of those who didn't work out. Experts theorize that exercise speeds the transit of wastes through the intestines, moving along food-borne carcinogens that might otherwise linger in the colon. But since the disease can take years to develop, consistency is key: The men who reported exercising at only one interview did not benefit.

Working out over the long haul may also reduce the body's exposure to estrogen, which is thought to play a role in breast cancer and reproductive-tract cancer. (The hormone seems to stimulate cell division, which increases the chance of a harmful mutation.) Since one-third of a woman's estrogen before menopause is produced by body fat, leaner, fitter women tend to make less of it.

In a study at the Harvard School of Public Health, 5,400 women who had graduated from college between 1925 and 1981 were asked about their diet, their health and their reproductive and exercise histories. Half the subjects were nonathletes; the other half had been college athletes, and 75 percent of this group reported that they had continued to exercise. After eliminating factors such as smoking and family history of cancer, "We found that the former athletes had a significantly lower rate of breast cancer and cancers of the reproductive system," says Dr. Rose Frisch, an associate professor of population sciences emerita, who headed the research.

Exercise may also help fight other forms of cancer because of its ability to boost the performance of two types of immune system cells—natural killer (NK) cells and macrophages. According to Dr. J. Mark Davis, an associate professor of exercise science at the University of South Carolina in Columbia, mice put through both moderate and exhaustive treadmill exercise showed improvement in macrophage assault on breast tumor cells. And in a study at the University of Waterloo in Ontario, mice made to exercise for nine weeks had enhanced NK-cell ability to kill lung tumor cells. Moreover, their heightened immunity was sustained once they stopped.

Animal data can't be directly applied to people, of course. Although intense treadmill running seems to enhance the immunity of laboratory animals, studies show that humans who exercise too intensely may be *more* susceptible to certain infections. Still, Frisch believes that active people do have a greater ability to fight cancer. "With the exception of skin cancer, the athletes had markedly less of *all* types of cancer—including nonreproductive-tract cancers—than sedentary subjects," she says.

Although NK cells and macrophages seem to nip cancers in the bud, Davis emphasizes that once a tumor takes hold, working out won't help the immune system get rid of it. (It may, however, prevent malignant cells from spreading.) Moreover, the jury is still out on exactly how much exercise is needed to lower cancer risk. The best advice? Work up a sweat for 20 to 30 minutes, three times a week—and keep at it.

Source: Reprinted by permission from Michele Wolf, "Can Exercise Ward Off Cancer?" *American Health,* October 1993, 77. © 1993 by Michele Wolf.

---

provide another indicator of actions that may, in fact, be part of the answer to reducing risk.

Regular self-examination (see Figure 17.3) and mammography offer the best hope for early detection of breast cancer. Recommendations for when a woman should obtain her first baseline mammogram are included in the American Cancer Society guidelines, presented in Table 17.1. It is important to note that there is tremendous controversy over the cost effectiveness and usefulness of getting a mammogram before the age of 40. Figure 17.4 shows what a difference a mammogram can make in getting early treatment. However, many health professionals recommend that if you have any of the risk factors listed above, are prone to fibrous breasts, and are excessively worried about your own condition, a mammogram may be warranted. Consult with your physician if you are

in doubt, as it is generally best to be a proactive health consumer.

Treatment. Today, women with breast cancer (and people with nearly any other type of cancer) have many decisions to make in determining the best treatment options available for them. Fortunately, there are services available to help you get the best information, even if you live in a fairly remote area of the country. The important thing to remember is that in most instances, taking the time to thoroughly check out your physician's track record and his or her philosophy on the best treatment is always a good idea. Is his or her treatment recommendation consistent with that of the major cancer centers in the country? (This information can be obtained by calling any of the Help Lines listed in the book's appendix.) Check out

How to Examine Your Breasts

Do you know that 95% of breast cancers are discovered first by women themselves? And that the earlier the breast cancer is detected, the better the chance for a complete cure? Of course, most lumps or changes are not cancer. But you can safeguard your health by making a habit of examining your breasts once a month – a day or two after your period or, if you're no longer menstruating, on any given day. And if you notice anything changed or unusual – a lump, thickening, or discharge – contact your doctor right away.

How to Look for Changes

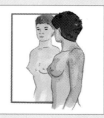

Step 1
Sit or stand in front of a mirror with your arms at your side. Turning slowly from side to side, check your breasts for
• changes in size or shape
• puckering or dimpling of the skin
• changes in size or position of one nipple compared to the other

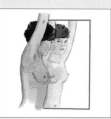

Step 2
Raise your arms above your head and repeat the examination in Step 1.

Step 3
Gently press each nipple with your fingertips to see if there is any discharge.

How to Feel for Changes

Step 1
Lie down and put a pillow or folded bath towel under your left shoulder. Then place your left hand under your head. (From now on you will be feeling for a lump or thickening in your breasts.)

Step 2
Imagine that your breast is divided into quarters.

Step 3
With the fingers of your right hand held together, press firmly but gently, using small circular motions to feel the inner, upper quarter of your left breast. Start at your breastbone and work toward the nipple. Also examine the area around the nipple. Now do the same for the lower, inner portion of your breast.

Step 4
Next, bring your arm to your side and feel under your left armpit for swelling.

Step 5
With your arm still down, feel the upper, outer part of your breast, starting with your nipple and working outwards. Examine the lower, outer quarter in the same way.

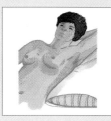

Step 6
Now place the pillow under your right shoulder and repeat all the steps using your left hand to examine your right breast.

FIGURE 17.3

The illustration demonstrates breast self-examination—the 10-minute habit that could save your life.

Average Size of Lumps

| Found by mammography | Found by regular breast self-exam | Found by chance |

FIGURE 17.4

Comparison of Average-size Breast Lumps Found by Various Means of Detection

Source: Adapted by permission from American Cancer Society, *Special Touch: A Personal Plan of Action for Breast Health,* rev. February 1992, document 2095-LE.OR.

the doctors' credentials and the past experiences of patients who have seen this doctor and the surgeon who will perform your biopsy and other surgical techniques. If possible, seek a facility that has a significant number of breast cancer patients, does many surgeries, treats large numbers of patients, and is highly regarded by past patients. Often, cancer support groups can give you invaluable information and advice. Treatments range from the simple lumpectomy to radical mastectomy to various combinations of radiation or chemotherapy. Figure 17.5 reviews these options. Remember that it is always a good idea to seek more than one opinion before making a decision.

WHAT DO YOU THINK?

Why do you think there is such a big difference between mammography screening rates for varied ethnic groups? What actions could be taken to change such disparities? Why do you think so many women fail to be tested for breast cancer? Do you think men are better at seeking recommended screenings for cancers? Why or why not?

Colon and Rectum Cancers

Although colon and rectum cancers are the third leading cause of cancer deaths, with an estimated 47,500 deaths from colon cancer and 7,800 deaths from rectum cancer in 1995, many people are unaware of their potential risk. Bleeding from the rectum, blood in the stool, and changes in bowel habits are the major warning signals. People who are over the age of 40, who have a family history of colon and rectum cancer, a personal or family history of polyps (benign growths) in the colon or rectum, or inflammatory bowel problems such as colitis run an increased risk. Diets high in fats or low in fiber may also increase risk.[18]

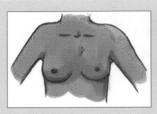

Lumpectomy
Performed when tumor is in earliest localized stages. Prognosis for recovery is better than 95 percent. Only tumor itself is removed. Some physicians may also remove normal tissue in surrounding area.

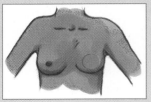

Simple mastectomy
Removal of breast and underlying tissue. Prognosis for full recovery better than 80 percent.

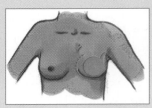

Modified radical mastectomy
Breast and lymph nodes in immediate area removed. Prognosis for full recovery dependent on level of spread.

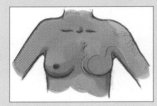

Radical mastectomy
Removal of breast, lymph nodes, pectoral muscles, all fat and underlying tissue. Prognosis for recovery may be as low as 60 percent dependent on level of spread.

FIGURE 17.5

The illustration depicts selected surgical procedures for diagnosed breast cancer. These surgeries are typically followed by radiation treatment and/or chemotherapy.

Because colorectal cancer tends to spread slowly, the prognosis is quite good if it is caught in the early stages. Treatment often consists of radiation or surgery. Chemotherapy, although not used extensively in the past, is today a possibility. A permanent colostomy, the creation of an abdominal opening for the elimination of body wastes, is seldom required for people with colon cancer and even less frequently for those with rectum cancer.[19]

Prostate Cancer

Cancer of the prostate is the second leading cause of cancer deaths in males, killing an estimated 40,400 men in 1995. Most signs and symptoms of prostate cancer are nonspecific—that is, they mimic the signs of infection or enlarged prostate. Symptoms include weak or interrupted urine flow or difficulty starting or stopping the urine flow; the need to urinate frequently; pain or difficulty in urinating; blood in the urine; and pain in the lower back, pelvis, or upper thighs. Many males mistake these symptoms for other nonspecific conditions such as infections and delay treatment.[20]

Incidence of prostate cancer increases with age; over 80 percent of all prostate cancers are diagnosed in men over age 65, although increasing numbers of young men seem to be affected. Incidence is 30 percent higher among black men than it is among whites. The disease is more common in northwestern Europe and North America. It is rare in the Near East, Africa, Central America, and South America. There seems to be a slightly increased risk if a family member has the disease, but it is unclear whether this is due to genetic or environmental factors.[21]

Fortunately, even with so many generalized symptoms, most prostate cancers are detected while they are still localized and tend to progress slowly. Because most men detect cancer in their late 60s and early 70s, it is likely that they will die of other causes before prostate cancer leads to their deaths. For this reason, health-care groups are beginning to question the cost-effectiveness and necessity of prostate surgeries and other costly procedures that may have little real effect on life expectancy. Prostate patients have an average five-year survival rate of 80 percent. Because the incidence of prostate cancer increases with age, every man over the age of 40 should have an annual prostate examination.[22]

Skin Cancer

Skin cancer may be one of the most underrated of all of the cancers, particularly among young people. Although it is true that most people do not die of the common, highly curable *basal* or *squamous cell* skin cancers, over 800,000 people develop this disease each year. What most people do not know is that another, highly virulent form of skin cancer known as **malignant melanoma,** has become the number-one cancer killer of American women ages 25 to 29 and the number-two killer for women ages 30 to 34. The death rate for men over 50 is increasing faster than the rate of any other cancer. Yet few people in this tan-crazed country make the connection between death from melanoma and sunlight overexposure. The perception that health and a well-tanned body go together couldn't be further from the truth. For more information on protecting yourself from skin cancer, see the Choices for Change box.

Symptoms. Many people do not have any idea what to look for when considering skin cancer. Any unusual skin condition, especially a change in the size or color of a mole or other darkly pigmented growth or spot, should be considered suspect. Scaliness, oozing, bleeding, the appearance of a bump or nodule, the spread of pigment beyond the border, change in sensation, itchiness, tenderness, and pain are all warning signs of the basal and squamous cell

In spite of painful sunburns, too often we learn at an early age to yearn for a "healthy tan" and risk overexposure to sunlight, which causes the number-one cancer killer of young American women.

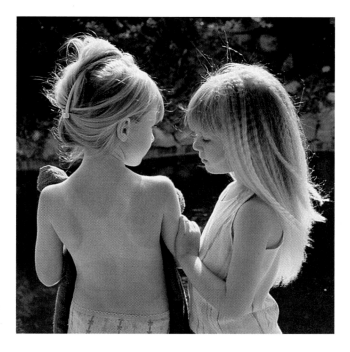

skin cancers. However, melanoma symptoms are slightly different. Often there is a sudden or progressive change in a mole's appearance from a small, mole-like growth to a large, ulcerated, and easily-prone-to-bleeding growth. A simple *ABCD* rule outlines the warning signals of melanoma: *A* is for asymmetry. One half of the mole does not match the other half. *B* is for border irregularity. The edges are ragged, notched, or blurred. *C* is for color. The pigmentation is not uniform. *D* is for diameter greater than 6 millimeters. Any or all of these symptoms should cause you to visit a physician.[23]

Treatment of skin cancer depends on the seriousness of the condition. Surgery is used in 90 percent of all cases. Radiation therapy, *electrodesiccation* (tissue destruction by heat), and *cryosurgery* (tissue destruction by freezing) are also common forms of treatment. For melanoma, treatment may involve surgical removal of the regional lymph nodes, radiation, or chemotherapy.[24]

Testicular Cancer

Testicular cancer is currently one of the most common types of solid tumors found in males entering early adulthood. Those between the ages of 17 and 34 are at greatest risk. There has been a steady increase in tumor frequency over the past several years in this age group.

Although the exact cause of testicular cancer is unknown, several possible risk factors have been identified. Males with undescended testicles appear to be at greatest risk for the disease. In addition, some studies indicate that there may be a genetic influence.

In general, testicular tumors are first noticed as a painless enlargement of the testis or as an apparent thickening in testicular tissue. Because this enlargement is often painless, it is extremely important that all young males practice regular testicular self-examination (see Figure 17.6). If a suspicious lump or thickening is found, medical follow-up should be sought immediately.

Ovarian Cancer

Ovarian cancer is often silent, showing no obvious signs or symptoms until late in its development. The most common sign is enlargement of the abdomen (or a feeling of bloating) in women over the age of 40. Other symptoms include vague digestive disturbances, such as gas and stomach aches that persist and cannot be explained.[25]

The risk for ovarian cancer increases with age, with the highest rates found in women in their 60s. Women who have never had children are twice as likely to develop ovarian cancer as are those who have. This is because the main risk factor appears to be exposure to the reproductive hormone estrogen. Women who have multiple pregnancies or use oral contraceptives, which both inhibit estrogen, are at lower risk. In addition, having one or more primary relatives (mother, sisters, grandmothers) who have had the disease appears to increase individual risk. With the exception of Japan, the highest incidence rates are reported in the industrialized countries of the world.[26]

Prevention. A recent Yale University study indicates that diet may also play a role in ovarian cancer.[27] Researchers found that when comparing 450 Canadian women with newly diagnosed ovarian cancer with 564 demographically similar, healthy women, the women without ovarian cancer had a diet lower in saturated fat. For every 10 grams of saturated fat a woman ate per day, her risk of ovarian cancer rose 20 percent. Conversely, women who lowered their saturated fat consumption by 10 grams a day experienced a 20 percent drop in risk. Every 10 grams of vegetable fiber (but not fruit or cereal fiber) added to a woman's daily menu lowered her risk by 37 percent. The study also found that each full-term pregnancy lowered risk by about 20 percent and each year of oral contraceptive use lowered it by 5 to 10 percent. So, should you go

Malignant melanoma: A virulent cancer of the melanin (pigment-producing portion) of the skin.

Reducing Your Risk for Skin Cancer

One of the best ways to reduce your risks for skin cancer is to become aware of your body. By establishing a personal base line of information and regular self-checks, you will be able to spot changes early.

- Stand in front of a large, well-lit mirror and look at your body from front to back and head to toe. Be careful to pay attention to hidden areas on the backs of your arms, between your fingers and toes, and on your genitals or buttocks. Use a hand-held mirror to examine hard-to-reach areas. Look for unusual growths or moles that bother you or that fit the symptoms of skin cancer.

- If you note potential areas of concern, consult a dermatologist. Many dermatologists will do baseline "mole mapping" to chart locations and sizes of moles for follow-up examinations.

- Check yourself at least once a month to note changes. Pay attention.

- Avoid sun exposure during high UV ray periods—particularly from 10 A.M. to 2 P.M.

- Wear protective hats, sunglasses that block harmful rays, and clothing that protects the arms and legs.

- Wear a sunscreen with an SPF of 17 or more.

- Be cautious in settings where reflective rays may cause considerable harm, such as when at a beach or lake, or when out in the snow.

- If you have sensitive, fair skin, use extra precautions. Cover up and pick the shady spots when outdoors. Remember, the fairer the hair and skin, the higher the SPF sunscreen you normally need—usually 17 to 30 or higher.

---

out and get pregnant or start taking birth control pills to reduce risk? Probably not. Although isolated studies provide useful information that may lead to definitive results when combined with similar findings from other studies, when considered alone, they do not make for scientific certainty. However, such results, particularly when com-

bined with cardiovascular risks and other health risks, may provide yet another reason to hold the fat—or at least cut down on your overall intake.

To protect yourself, annual thorough pelvic examinations are important. Pap tests, although useful in detecting cervical cancer, do not reveal ovarian cancer. Women

Follow the instructions in the diagram carefully and examine your testes immediately after your next hot bath or shower. Heat causes the testicles to descend and the scrotal skin to relax, making it easier to find unusual lumps.

Examine each testicle by placing the index and middle fingers of both hands on the underside of the testicle and the thumbs on the top. Gently roll the testicle between your thumb and fingers, feeling for small lumps.

Changes or anything abnormal will appear at the front or side of your testicle. Did you find any unusual lumps? Are there any unusual signs of any kind? Are there any markings or lumps at any site?

Keep in mind that not all lumps are a sign of testicular cancer. Unusual lumps at any location, however, should be checked by a physician. Early detection greatly increases your chances of a complete cure. Repeat the examination every month and record your findings.

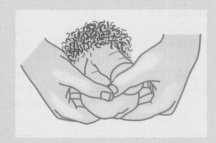

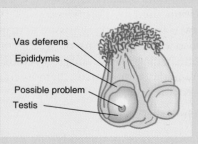

FIGURE 17.6

Testicular Self-exam

over the age of 40 should have a cancer-related checkup every year. If you have any of the symptoms of ovarian cancer and they persist, see your doctor. If they continue to persist, get a second opinion.[28]

Uterine Cancer

In 1995, an estimated 103,600 new cases of uterine cancer will have been diagnosed in the United States. Most uterine cancers develop in the body of the uterus, usually in the endometrium (lining). The rest develop in the cervix, located at the base of the uterus. The overall incidence of early-stage uterine cancer—that is, cervical cancer—has increased slightly in recent years in women under the age of 50. In contrast, invasive, later-stage forms of the disease appear to be decreasing. Much of this apparent trend may be due to more effective regular screenings of younger women using the **Pap test,** a procedure in which cells taken from the cervical region are examined for abnormal cellular activity. Although these tests are very effective for detecting early-stage cervical cancer, they are less effective for detecting cancers of the uterine lining and are not effective at all for detecting cancers of the fallopian tubes or ovaries.[29]

Risk factors for cervical cancer include early age of first intercourse, multiple sex partners, cigarette smoking, and certain sexually transmitted diseases, such as the herpes virus and the human papillomavirus. For endometrial cancer, a history of infertility, failure to ovulate, obesity, and treatment with tamoxifen or unopposed estrogen therapy appear to be major risk factors.[30]

Early warning signs of uterine cancer include bleeding outside the normal menstrual period or after menopause or persistent unusual vaginal discharge. These symptoms should be checked by a physician immediately.[31]

Cancer of the Pancreas

The incidence of cancer of the pancreas, known as a "silent" disease, has increased substantially during the last 30 years. Although chronic inflammation of the pancreas, diabetes, cirrhosis, and a high-fat diet may contribute to the development of pancreatic cancer, the research on causes is inconclusive. Unfortunately, pancreatic cancer is one of the worst cancers to get, with only 3 percent of pancreatic cancer victims living more than five years after diagnosis, usually because the disease is well advanced by the time there are any symptoms. Smokers have double the risk of pancreatic cancer as have nonsmokers, but other factors such as diets high in fat appear to increase risk.[32]

Leukemia

Leukemia is a cancer of the blood-forming tissues that leads to proliferation of millions of immature white blood cells. These abnormal cells crowd out normal white blood cells (which fight infection), platelets (which control hemorrhaging), and red blood cells (which prevent anemia). As a result, symptoms such as fatigue, paleness, weight loss, easy bruising, repeated infections, nosebleeds, and other forms of hemorrhaging occur. In children, these symptoms can appear suddenly.[33]

Leukemia can be acute or chronic in nature and can strike both sexes and all age groups. Chronic leukemia can develop over several months and have few symptoms. Although many people believe that leukemia is a childhood disease, leukemia struck many more adults (23,100) than children (2,600) in 1994.[34] The five-year survival rate for patients with leukemia is 38 percent, due partly to very poor survival for patients with some types of leukemia. Over the last 30 years, however, there has been a dramatic improvement in survival of patients with acute lymphocytic leukemia—from a five-year survival rate of 4 percent for people diagnosed in the early 1960s to 28 percent in the early 1970s to 52 percent in the mid-1980s. In children, the improvement has been from 4 percent to 73 percent.[35]

Oral Cancer

Cancer may develop in any part of the oral cavity. Most often it is found on the lips, the lining of the cheeks, the gums, and the floor of the mouth. The tongue, the pharynx, and the tonsils are other common sites. Tobacco use—smoking, chewing, or dipping—is the most common risk factor for oral cancer.

WHAT DO YOU THINK?

What types of cancers do you think you and your friends are at greatest risk for right now? Do you practice regular breast or testicular self-exam? Do you think it's important for a man to know how to do a breast self-exam or a woman to do a testicular self-exam—or are these individual responsibilities only? Would you be able to help your spouse or intimate partner with his or her exam?

FACING CANCER

While heart disease mortality rates have declined steadily over the past 50 years, cancer mortality rates have in-

Pap test: A procedure in which cells taken from the cervical region are examined for abnormal cellular activity.

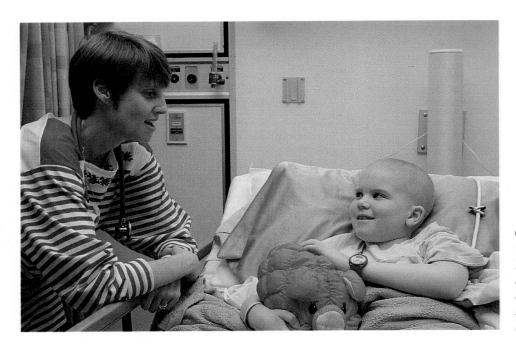

The treatment for childhood leukemia remains a difficult and disturbing experience for both children and parents even though survival rates have risen dramatically in recent years.

creased consistently in the same period. Based on current rates, about 83 million—or one in three of us now living—will eventually develop cancer. Many factors have contributed to the rise in cancer mortality, but the increase in the incidence of lung cancer is probably the most important reason. Despite these gloomy predictions, recent advancements in the diagnosis and treatment of many forms of cancer have reduced much of the fear and mystery that once surrounded this disease.

Detecting Cancer

The earlier a person is diagnosed as having cancer, the better the prospect for survival. Various high-tech diagnostic techniques exist to detect cancer. These medical techniques, along with regular self-examinations and checkups, play an important role in the early detection and secondary prevention of cancer.

Most of the sites that pose the highest risk for cancer have screening tests available for early detection. Other common forms of cancer present with symptoms that are often readily identifiable. The key seems to be whether or not the individual has the financial resources (insurance) to seek medical diagnosis and early treatment. A health-care reform package that focuses on payment for regular checkups, and preventive services would help many poor and middle-class Americans seek medical care earlier when the chances of curing their disease are better.

Accept responsibility for personal cancer detection. Figure 17.7 shows the Seven Warning Signals of cancer. If you notice any of these signals, and they don't appear to be related to anything else, you should see a doctor immediately. For example, difficulty swallowing may be due to a cold or flu. But if you are otherwise symptomless and the difficulty continues, you should see a doctor. You may have a far less serious problem than cancer, but you should get all medical problems treated!

Make sure that appropriate diagnostic tests are completed whenever any warning signals appear. Also make a realistic assessment of your individual risk factors and try to avoid those you have some control over. Even if there is a history of cancer in your immediate family, for instance, you can reduce your risk for cancer by changing your dietary patterns and avoiding known carcinogens and other environmental hazards. Heeding the suggestions for primary prevention may significantly decrease your chances of getting cancer.

Recommended Cancer Checkups

Detecting cancer early is half the battle. The American Cancer Society recommends the following:

- Get a yearly Pap test and pelvic exam if you are sexually active or 18 or older (endometrial and cervical cancer).

- Do a monthly breast self-exam starting at age 20 (breast cancer).

- Get a mammogram every year or two between the ages of 40 and 49 and every year starting at age 50 (breast cancer).

- Have a prostate-specific antigen (PSA) blood test every year starting at age 50 (prostate cancer).

- Have your stool tested for hidden blood once a year after age 50 (colon and rectum cancer).

- Have a sigmoidoscope exam every three to five years after age 50 (colon and rectum cancer).

- Get a dental checkup at least once a year (cancer of the mouth/tongue).[36]

New Hope in Cancer Treatments

Although cancer treatments have changed dramatically over the last 20 years, surgery, in which the tumor and surrounding tissue are removed, is still common. Today's surgeons tend to remove less surrounding tissue than previously and to combine surgery with either **radiotherapy** (the use of radiation) or **chemotherapy** to kill cancerous cells.

Radiation works by destroying malignant cells or stopping cell growth. It is most effective in treating localized cancer masses. Unfortunately, in the process of destroying malignant cells, radiotherapy also destroys some healthy cells. In addition, in recent years, many scientists have come to suspect that radiotherapy may increase the risks for other types of cancers. Despite these qualifications, radiation continues to be one of the most common and effective forms of treatment.

When cancer has spread throughout the body, it is necessary to use some form of chemotherapy. Currently, over 50 different anticancer drugs are in use, some of which have excellent records of success. A chemotherapeutic regimen including four anticancer drugs in combination with radiation therapy has resulted in remarkable survival

Advances in methods for diagnosing and treating cancer have improved the prognosis for many cancer victims and enabled them to live full and productive lives.

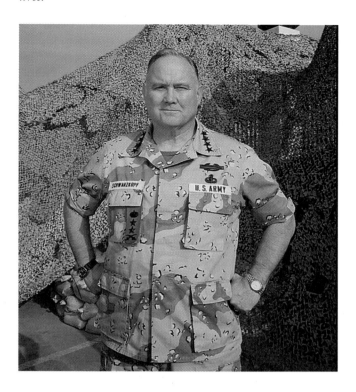

rates for some cancers, including Hodgkin's disease. Ongoing research into new drug development will result in compounds that are less toxic to normal cells and more potent against tumor cells.[37] Current research indicates that some tumors may actually be resistant to certain forms of chemotherapy and that the treatment drugs do not reach the core of the tumor.[38] Scientists are currently working to circumvent resistance to chemotherapeutic drugs and to make tumor cells more vulnerable throughout treatment.

Whether used alone or in combination, radiotherapy and chemotherapy have possible side effects, including extreme nausea, nutritional deficiencies, hair loss, and general fatigue. Long-term damage to the cardiovascular system and many other systems of the body can be significant. It is important that you discuss these matters fully

Cancer's Seven Warning Signals

1 Changes in bowel or bladder habits.

2 A sore that does not heal.

3 Unusual bleeding or discharge.

4 Thickening or lump in breast or elsewhere.

5 Indigestion or difficulty in swallowing.

6 Obvious change in a wart or mole.

7 Nagging cough or hoarseness.

If you have a warning signal, see your doctor.

FIGURE 17.7

Cancer's Seven Warning Signals

Radiotherapy: The use of radiation to kill cancerous cells.

Chemotherapy: The use of drugs to kill cancerous cells.

TABLE 17.1 ■ Summary of American Cancer Society Recommendations for the Early Detection of Cancer in Asymptomatic People

Test or Procedure	Sex	Age	Frequency
Sigmoidoscopy, preferably flexible	M and F	50 and over	Every 3–5 years
Fecal Occult Blood Test	M and F	50 and over	Every year
Digital Rectal Exam	M and F	40 and over	Every year
*Prostate Exam**	M	50 and over	Every year
Pap Test	F	All women who are, or who have been, sexually active, or have reached the age of 18, should have an annual Pap test and pelvic examination. After a woman has had three or more consecutive satisfactory normal annual examinations, the Pap test may be performed less frequently at the discretion of her physician.	
Pelvic Examination	F	18–40	Every 1–3 years with Pap test
		Over 40	Every year
Endometrial Tissue Sample	F	At menopause, if at high risk**	At menopause and thereafter at the discretion of the physician
Breast Self-Examination	F	20 and over	Every month
Breast Clinical Examination	F	20–40	Every 3 years
		Over 40	Every year
*Mammography****	F	40–49	Every 1–2 years
		50 and over	Every year
*Health Counseling and Cancer Checkup*****	M and F	Over 20	Every 3 years
	M and F	Over 40	Every year

*Annual digital rectal examination and prostate-specific antigen should be performed on men 50 years and older. If either is abnormal, further evaluation should be considered.

**History of infertility, obesity, failure to ovulate, abnormal uterine bleeding, or unopposed estrogen or tamoxifen therapy.

***Screening mammography should begin by age 40.

****To include examination for cancers of the thyroid, testicles, ovaries, lymph nodes, oral region, and skin.

Source: Reprinted by permission from American Cancer Society, *Guidelines for the Cancer-Related Checkup: An Update* (Atlanta: *ACS,* 1994), 9.

with your doctors. The Building Communication Skills box offers advice on how to talk to your doctor about your cancer.

Substances found in nature, such as taxol (originally found in Pacific Yew trees), are being synthesized in laboratories and tested on a variety of cancers. Other compounds, including those derived from sea urchins, are rich in resources for anticancer drugs.[39]

Other promising advances in the battle against cancer include:[40]

■ A large clinical trial is underway to evaluate the usefulness of an estrogen-blocking drug called tamoxifen. Used to treat women who have breast cancer that is estrogen positive, or grows more rapidly when estrogen levels are high, this drug is often an alternative to chemotherapy for many women with breast cancer.

Talking with Your Doctor about Cancer

Anytime there is the suspicion of cancer, the person involved is likely to react with great anxiety, fear, and anger. Emotional distress is sometimes so intense that the person involved is unable to serve as his or her own best advocate in making critical health-care decisions. If you find it difficult to know what to ask your doctor on a routine exam, imagine how hard it would be to discuss life or death options for yourself or a loved one. Having a list of important questions to ask when you appear at the doctor's office may help tremendously. Remember, your health-care provider should be your partner in making the best decisions for you. By actively challenging, questioning, and letting the physician know your wishes, difficult decisions may become easier.

If the diagnosis is cancer, you may want to ask these questions:

- What kind of cancer do I have? What stage is it in? Based on my age and stage, what type of prognosis do I have?
- What are my treatment choices? Which do you recommend? Why?
- What are the expected benefits of each kind of treatment?
- What are the long- and short-term risks and possible side effects?
- Would a clinical trial be appropriate for me? (Clinical trials are research studies designed to answer specific questions and to find better ways to prevent or treat cancer. Often new cancer-fighting treatments are used.)

If surgery is recommended, you may want to ask these questions:

- What kind of operation will it be and how long will it take? What form of anesthesia will be used? How many similar procedures has this surgeon done in the last month? What is his or her success rate?
- How will I feel after surgery? If I have pain, how will you help me?

- Where will the scars be? What will they look like? Will they cause disability?
- Will I have any activity limitations after surgery? What kind of physical therapy, if any, will I have? When will I get back to normal activities?

If radiation is recommended, you may want to ask these questions:

- Why do you think this treatment is better than my other options?
- How long will I need to have treatments and what will the side effects be in the short and long term? What body organs/systems may be damaged?
- What can I do to take care of myself during therapy? Are there services available to help me?
- What is the long-term prognosis for people my age with my type of cancer using this treatment?

If chemotherapy is recommended, you may want to ask these questions:

- Why do you think this treatment is better than my other options?
- Which drug combinations pose the least risks and most benefits?
- What are the short- and long-term side effects on my body?
- What are my options?

Before beginning any form of cancer therapy, it is imperative that you be a vigilant and vocal consumer. Read and seek information from cancer support groups. Check the skills of your surgeon, your radiation therapist, and your doctor in terms of clinical work and interpersonal interactions. The time spent asking these questions and seeking information is well worth the effort.

- **Immunotherapy** is a new technique designed to enhance the body's own disease fighting systems to help control cancer. Interferon (a naturally occurring body protein that protects healthy cells and kills cancer cells), interleukin 2 (a growth factor that stimulates cells of the immune system to find cancer), and other biologic response modifiers are under study. Vaccines against several types of cancers are also being studied.

- New high-technology diagnostic imaging techniques have replaced exploratory surgery for some cancer patients. **Magnetic resonance imaging (MRI)** is one example of such technology. In MRI, a huge electro-

magnet is used to detect hidden tumors by mapping the vibrations of the various atoms in the body on a

Immunotherapy: A process that stimulates the body's own immune system to combat cancer cells.

Magnetic resonance imaging (MRI): A device that uses magnetic fields, radio waves, and computers to generate an image of internal tissues of the body for diagnostic purposes without the use of radiation.

computer screen. **Computerized axial tomography scanning** (CAT scan) uses x-rays to examine parts of the body. In both of these painless, noninvasive procedures, cross-section pictures can show a tumor's shape and location more accurately than can conventional x-rays.

- Cell mutations can cause increased production of destructive enzymes that allow them to invade surrounding tissues and penetrate blood vessels to travel to other parts of the body. A powerful enzyme inhibitor, TIMP-2, is showing promise for slowing the metastasis of tumor cells. A metastasis suppressor gene, NM23, has also been identified.

- *Neoadjuvant chemotherapy* (giving chemotherapy to shrink the cancer and then removing it surgically) has been tried against various types of cancers. This is a promising new treatment approach.

- *Prostatic ultrasound* (a rectal probe using ultrasonic waves to produce an image of the prostate) is currently being investigated as a potential means to increase the early detection of prostate cancer. Recently, prostatic ultrasound has been combined with a blood test for **prostate-specific antigen** (PSA), an antigen found in prostate cancer patients. Although the reliability of PSA tests for screening has been questioned, it appears to show promise.

In addition, psychosocial and behavioral research has become increasingly important as health professionals seek the answers to questions concerning complex lifestyle factors that appear to influence risks for cancer as well as the survivability of patients with particular psychological and mental health profiles. Also, health-care practitioners have become more aware of the psychological needs of patients and families and have begun to tailor treatment programs to meet the diverse needs of different people.

Life After Cancer

Heightened public awareness and an improved prognosis for cancer victims have made the cancer experience less threatening and isolating than it once was. While you may hear of some stories of recovering cancer patients experiencing job discrimination and being unable to obtain

health or life insurance, these cases are increasingly fewer. Several states have even enacted legislation to prevent insurance companies from cancelling policies or from instituting other forms of discrimination. Health insurance can be obtained through large employers. Because large employers spread the insurance risk among many employees, insurance companies accept all new employees without underwriting. A young college grad, who had survived a type of bone cancer, secured health insurance through the group policy of the publisher of this text. When she went to another publisher, she again received insurance, through the new company's group policy.

Life insurance, too, is often available to cancer survivors. An insurer will likely charge a higher rate (either for a period of a few years or permanently), but coverage is available. It is true that some companies do not write insurance on cancer survivors; however, other insurers specialize in such coverage. Ask your insurance broker, your local chapter of the American Cancer Society, or people in your support group for suggestions.

On the personal side, assistance for the cancer patient is more readily available than ever before. Cancer support groups, cancer information workshops, and low-cost medical consultation are just a few of the forms of assistance now offered in many communities. Breast cancer

The efforts of lobbyists and activist groups, such as this group of people on a fund-raising hike, have brought about a dramatic increase of funding for cancer research as well as community programs and treatment centers.

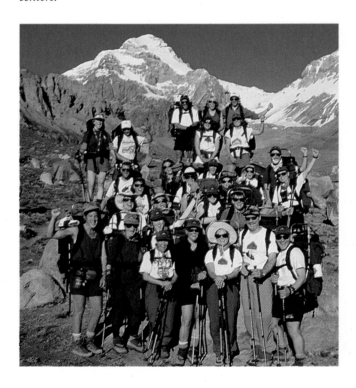

Computerized axial tomography (CAT scan): A machine that uses radiation to view internal organs not normally visible on X-rays.

Prostate-specific antigen (PSA): An antigen found in prostate cancer patients.

Managing Cancer Risks

Cancer is no longer an automatic death sentence. Oncologists continually increase our chances of surviving cancer with new and improved medical care as well as better early detection tests. But we each hold the key to fulfilling our own hopes by doing what we can to prevent cancer. Regular check-ups and monthly self-exams will improve our odds of survival by providing early diagnosis. Proper diet, regular exercise, and attempts to stay clear of carcinogens will help improve our odds of avoiding cancer.

Making Decisions for You

Cancer is caused both by things we do as well as by things that are out of our control. From the self-assessment that you completed earlier in the chapter, which factors appear to put you at risk for certain types of cancers? Which of these things are out of your personal control? Of those things that you can control, which ones should you be most concerned about? What actions can you take today that will reduce these risks? Write a personal plan that you can follow every day for the next seven days to reduce risk.

Checklist for Change: Making Personal Choices

✓ *Stop smoking.* Smoking accounts for about 30 percent of all cancer deaths and 90 percent of all lung cancer deaths. Those who smoke two or more packs of cigarettes a day have lung cancer mortality rates 17 to 25 times greater than nonsmokers. In fact, only 13 percent of patients live more than five years after being diagnosed. Cancers that smokers are most susceptible to include lung, pancreas, stomach, bladder, esophagus, mouth, and throat cancers.

✓ *Avoid excessive sunlight.* Almost all of the more than 600,000 cases of nonmelanoma skin cancer diagnosed each year in the United States are considered to be sun-related.

✓ *Avoid excessive alcohol consumption.* Oral cancer and cancers of the larynx, throat, esophagus, breast, and liver occur more frequently among heavy drinkers of alcohol. If you drink alcoholic beverages, limit them to one a day (for women) or two a day (for men).

✓ *Do not use smokeless tobacco.* Use of chewing tobacco or snuff increases risk for cancer of the mouth, larynx, throat, and esophagus and is highly habit-forming.

✓ *Properly monitor estrogen use.* Estrogen treatment to control menopausal symptoms increases risk for endometrial cancer. While estrogen therapy does seem to lower women's risk for heart disease and osteoporosis, it should not be undertaken without careful discussion between a woman and her physician.

✓ *Avoid occupational exposures to carcinogens.* Exposure to several different industrial agents (nickel, chromate, asbestos, vinyl chloride, etc.) increases risk for various cancers. Risk from asbestos is greatly increased when combined with cigarette smoking.

✓ *Avoid obesity.* Risk for colon, breast, endometrial, and uterine cancers increases in obese people. Following the suggestions listed on dietary choices in this chapter will help you reduce your risk.

✓ *Eat your fruits and vegetables.* Eat at least five servings of fruits and vegetables every day to reduce your risk for lung, colon, pancreatic, stomach, bladder, esophageal, mouth, and throat cancer.

✓ *Cut back on fats.* Reduce fat consumption, especially saturated fats and red meats, to reduce risk for colon, breast, prostate, pancreatic, and ovarian cancers.

Checklist for Change: Making Community Choices

✓ Does your community have any major sources of carcinogens (toxic waste dumps, chemical factories, etc.)? What precautions are taken to ensure that any environmental risks are reduced?

✓ Does the American Cancer Society have a local office at which you could volunteer some time?

✓ Does your community have cancer support groups that you could join if you were found to have cancer? Where would you find out about such support groups?

Critical Thinking

You've been good friends with one of your 30-something neighbors for some time. Recently, after spending a good deal of time working on a community project together, you start to date. After a few terrific dates, during which you really hit it off socially, you find out that your friend had cancer two years ago. In addition, there is a 50 percent chance that the cancer will return within five years. You truly love this person, but wonder what to do. If you commit yourself to this relationship and the cancer returns, then what? In addition, you've always wanted to have children, but are concerned about what would happen if your partner died of cancer while the kids were young. On the other hand, there is a 50 percent chance that the cancer will not return.

Using the DECIDE model described in Chapter 1, decide whether or not you would continue the relationship. Does it make any difference to you whether the cancer survivor described is a male or female? Explain why.

activists learned a great deal from the success of the AIDS activists who pressured Congress to provide funds for AIDS research. The National Breast Cancer Coalition and other grass-roots groups have lobbied to increase cancer research dollars. Their efforts have been paying off. Gov-ernment funding went from $87 million in 1990 to $408 million in 1993. The battle for funds continues. Increasing efforts in cancer research, improvements in diagnostic equipment, and advances in treatment provide hope for the future.

Summary

- Cancer is a group of diseases characterized by uncontrolled growth and spread of abnormal cells. These cells may create tumors. Benign (noncancerous) tumors grow in size but do not spread; malignant (cancerous) tumors spread to other parts of the body.

- Several probable causes of cancer have been identified. Biological factors include inherited genes and gender. Occupational and environmental hazards are carcinogens present in people's home or work environments. Research shows that people who are lonely, depressed, or under chronic stress tend to have a higher incidence of cancer. Chemicals in foods that may act as carcinogens include preservatives and pesticides. Viral diseases

that may lead to cancer include herpes, mononucleosis, and human papillomavirus (which causes vaginal warts). Medical factors include certain drug therapies given for other conditions that may elevate the chance of cancer. Combined risk refers to a combination of the above factors, which tends to compound the risk for cancer.

- Early diagnosis affects your survival rate. Self-exams for breast, testicular, and skin cancer and knowledge of the Seven Warning Signals of cancer aid early diagnosis.

- New types of cancer treatments include various combinations of radiotherapy, chemotherapy, and immunotherapy.

Discussion Questions

1. What is cancer? How does it spread? What is the difference between a benign and a malignant tumor?

2. List the likely causes of cancer. Do any of these causes put you at greater risk? What can you do to reduce this risk?

3. What are the symptoms of lung, breast, prostate, and testicular cancer? What can you do to increase your chances of surviving these cancers?

4. Discuss the Seven Warning Signals of cancer. What could signal that you have cancer instead of a minor illness? How soon should you seek treatment for any of the warning signs?

Application Exercise

Reread the What Do You Think? scenarios at the beginning of this chapter and answer the following questions:

1. From what you learned in the chapter, what are Nasira's chances of getting breast cancer? Is Nasira reacting more from fear or from medical knowledge? What factors besides genetics could have contributed to her sister's onset of cancer? What factors could have contributed to death from a disease with a good cure rate?

2. Aside from the mastectomies and removal of her ovaries, what are Nasira's options? What preventive

measures could Nasira take? If you were Nasira (and, yes, men do get breast cancer), what would you do?

3. From what you learned in the chapter, how much of a risk is Nick's lifestyle? Is the risk for skin cancer serious at his age? Do you think Nick's current lifestyle may affect his chances of getting malignant melanoma later in life?

4. What could Nick do to reduce his risk for skin cancer? What factors beside sitting in the sun might contribute to the risk for skin cancer?

Further Reading

American Cancer Society, *Cancer Facts and Figures,* Atlanta, GA, published annually.

A summary of major facts relating to cancer. Provides information on incidence, prevalence, symptomology, prevention, and treatment. Available through local divisions of the American Cancer Society.

Nutrition and Cancer Journal, published monthly.

Focuses on etiological aspects of various dietary factors and research on risks for cancer development. Also includes current research on dietary factors and prevention.

American Cancer Institute Journal, published monthly.

Focuses on current risk factors, prevention, and treatment research in the area of cancer.

Susan Love, *Dr. Susan Love's Breast Book* (Addison Wesley).

Joan Swirsky and Barbara Balaban, *The Breast Cancer Handbook: Taking Control after You've Found a Lump* (Harper-Perennial).

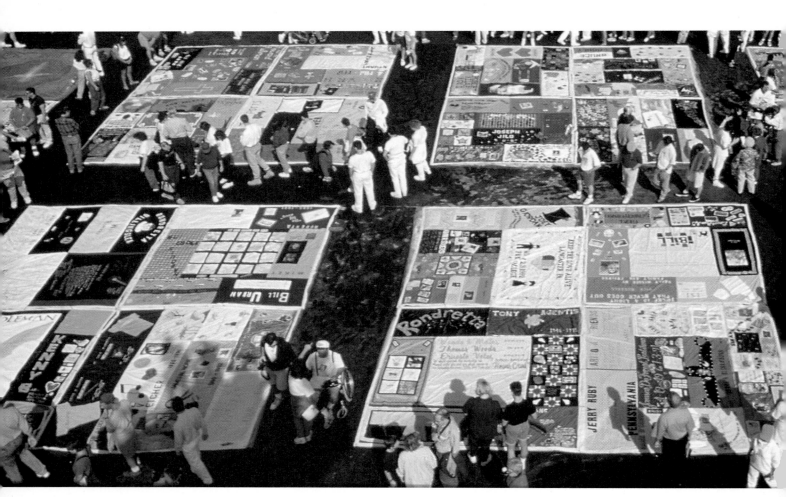

CHAPTER OBJECTIVES

◆ Discuss the risk factors for infectious diseases, including those you can control and those you cannot.

◆ Describe the most common pathogens.

◆ Discuss the immune system and explain the role of vaccinations in fighting disease.

◆ Discuss the various sexually transmitted diseases, their means of transmission, and actions that prevent the spread of STDs.

◆ Discuss the transmission, symptoms, treatment, and prevention of transmission of the HIV virus.

Infectious and Sexually Transmitted Diseases

Risks and Responsibilities

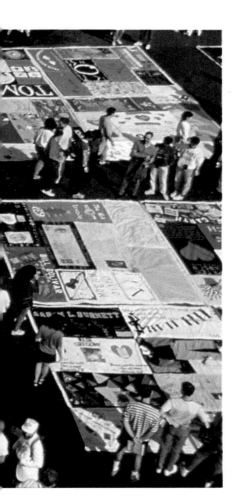

WHAT DO YOU THINK?

Jimmy is a 26-year-old living in a large city in the Pacific Northwest. He was recently charged with attempted murder for knowingly infecting three young women with the AIDS virus. He had been diagnosed with the disease at the age of 21, and, angry about his "fate," had decided to get even by passing the virus on to others.

- Do you believe that someone who knowingly infects another person with a potentially fatal disease should be criminally prosecuted? Is the policy of allowing anonymity in medical records to persons with AIDS a wise one? Why or why not? If you can prosecute someone for giving you a disease such as AIDS, should you also be able to sue or prosecute the person who gives you a cold or a herpes infection? Where would you draw the line? What policies or procedures should be put in place to reduce risk of infection by deadly diseases? To help people who are infected lead relatively normal lives? Who ultimately bears responsibility for establishing such policies and offering such help?

Gayle and Patrick have been in a monogamous marriage for seven years. During a medical checkup, Gayle finds that she is HIV positive. Because she has not been sexually active outside her marriage and has never injected drugs, received a blood transfusion, or been hospitalized, she is quite certain that Patrick must have infected her. When she calls the local health clinic to discover if Patrick has been tested for HIV, they tell her that this information is confidential. She does not want to confront Patrick for fear that he may not be infected and she will have to explain her own infection.

- What do you think Gayle should do? What would you do in a similar situation? What laws does your state have regarding partner notification for HIV, AIDS, and other sexually transmitted diseases?

Every moment of every day you are in constant contact with microscopic organisms that have the ability to make you sick. These disease-causing agents, or **pathogens,** are found in the air you breathe, in the foods you eat, and on nearly every person or object that you come into contact with. Although new varieties of pathogens arise all the time, scientific evidence indicates that pathogens have existed for at least as long as we have. There is fossil evidence that infections, cancer, heart disease, and a host of other ailments afflicted the earliest human beings. At times, infectious diseases wiped out whole groups of people through **epidemics** such as the Black Death, or bubonic plague, that wiped out more than half of the population of Europe and Asia in the 1300s and the influenza, tuberculosis, cholera, and other deadly epidemics of more recent centuries. In modern times, some infectious diseases have been conquered or contained by scientific advances such as vaccinations and pasteurization and by wholesale improvements in sanitation.[1]

Still, we continue to be susceptible to a vast number of potentially threatening organisms. *Endogenous microorganisms* are those that live in peaceful coexistence with their human hosts most of the time. Your intestines, body openings, and skin contain a great variety of these organisms. If you are in good health and your immune system is functioning properly, endogenous organisms are usually harmless. But in sick people, these organisms can cause serious health problems. *Exogenous microorganisms* are organisms that do not normally inhabit the body.

When these pathogens invade the body, they can produce an infection and/or illness. The more **virulent,** or aggressive the organism, the higher the probability that it will overcome your body defenses and cause disease. However, if your immune system is strong and your internal capacity to ward off disease is substantial, you will often be able to fight off even the most virulent attacker. Just because you inhale a flu virus does not mean that you will get the flu. Just because your hands are teeming with bacteria does not mean that you will get a bacterial disease. Several factors influence your susceptibility to diseases.

*I*NFECTIOUS DISEASE RISK FACTORS

At one time, it was believed that most diseases were caused by a single factor, but today we recognize that most diseases are **multifactorial,** or caused by the interaction of several factors from inside and outside the person. For a disease to occur, the *host* must be *susceptible,* meaning that the immune system must be in a weakened condition; an *agent* capable of transmitting a disease must be present; and the *environment* must be hospitable to the pathogen in terms of temperature, light, moisture, and other requirements. Other risk factors also apparently increase or decrease levels of susceptibility. Figure 18.1 summarizes the body's defenses against invasion. Table 18.1 summarizes the disease factors you can and cannot control.

Risk Factors You Can't Control

Uncontrollable risk factors are those that increase your susceptibility and over which you may have little or no control. Some of the most common factors are:

Heredity. Perhaps the single greatest factor influencing your longevity is your parents' longevity. Being born into a family in which heart disease, cancer, or other illnesses are prevalent seems to increase your risk. Some people having a close relative who is a diabetic become diabetic themselves even though they take precautions, watch their weight, and exercise regularly. Still other diseases are caused by direct chromosomal inheritance. **Sickle cell**

Pathogen: A disease-causing agent.

Epidemic: Disease outbreak that affects many people in a community or region at the same time.

Virulent: Said of organisms able to overcome host resistance and cause disease.

Multifactorial disease: Disease caused by interactions of several factors.

Sickle cell anemia: Genetic disease commonly found among African Americans; results in organ damage and premature death.

Immunological competence: Ability of the immune system to defend the body from pathogens.

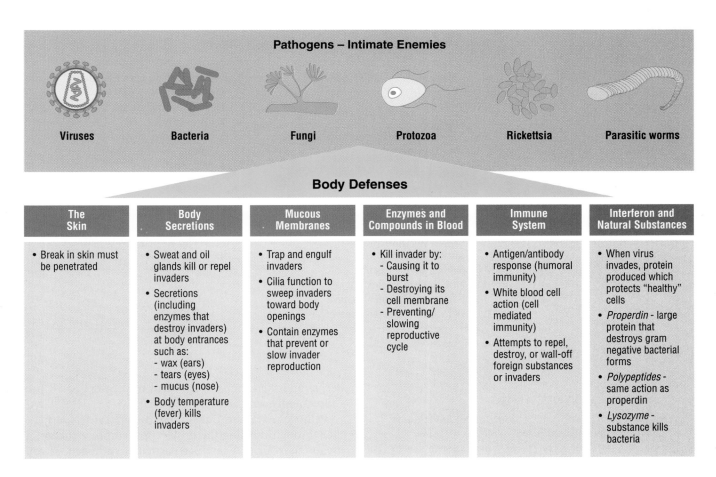

FIGURE 18.1

These are the body's defenses against disease-causing pathogens.

anemia, an inherited blood disease that primarily affects African Americans, is often transmitted to the fetus if both parents carry the sickle cell trait.

It is often unclear whether hereditary diseases occur as a result of inherited chromosomal traits or inherited insufficiencies in the immune system. In either case, if your grandparents, parents, and siblings have developed certain diseases at early ages, you are probably at increased risk for those diseases.

Aging.   Although we can do a great deal to lessen the effects of many negative aspects of the aging process, it is widely documented that after the age of 40 we become more vulnerable to most of the chronic diseases. Moreover, as we age, our immune systems respond less efficiently to invading organisms, increasing our risk for infection and illness. The same flu that produces an afternoon of nausea and diarrhea in a younger person may cause days of illness or even death in an older person. The very young are also at risk for many diseases, particularly if they are not vaccinated against them.

Environmental Conditions.   Unsanitary conditions and the presence of drugs, chemicals, and hazardous pollutants and wastes in our food and water probably have a great effect on our immune systems. That **immunological competence**—the body's ability to defend itself against pathogens—is weakened in such situations has been well documented.[2]

Risk Factors You Can Control

Although our degree of control over risk factors for disease may vary according to our socioeconomic condition, cultural upbringing, geographic location, and a host of other variables, we all have some degree of personal control over certain risk factors for disease. Too much stress, inadequate nutrition, a low physical fitness level, lack of sleep, misuse or abuse of legal and illegal substances, personal hygiene, high-risk behaviors, and other variables significantly increase the risk for a number of diseases. These variables are discussed individually in various chapters of this text.

TABLE 18.1 ■ Risk Factors for Infectious Diseases

Factors You Can't Control	Factors You Can Control
1. Your age	1. Nutritional status
2. Your sex	2. Pregnancy
3. Menstruation/hormonal status*	3. Psychological stressors/emotional status
4. Immunological competence*	
5. Previous risk from other microbial infections	4. Adequate rest
	5. Drug/chemical use
6. Underlying diseases*	6. Personal hygiene/sanitation
7. Heredity	7. Risk-taking behaviors
8. Infection in the community	8. Exposure to many pathogens
9. Community hygiene/ sanitation/pollution*	9. Seeking early treatment
	10. Fitness level
10. Season of the year	
11. Normal body "flora"*	
12. Early access to health care (vaccination, treatment, etc.)*	

*You may have some control.

ᴡHAT DO YOU THINK?

What current risk factors do you have for an infection by some form of invading pathogen? Which of these risk factors can you take actions to avoid? Which ones appear to be unavoidable? Outline a strategy that may help you improve your ability to ward off infectious agents.

ᴛHE PATHOGENS: ROUTES OF INVASION

Pathogens enter the body in several ways. They may be transmitted by direct contact between infected persons, such as during sexual relations, kissing, or touching, or by indirect contact, such as by touching an object the infected person has had contact with. The hands are probably the greatest source of transmission. For example, you may touch the handle of a drinking fountain that was just touched by a person whose hands were contaminated by a recent sneeze or failure to wash after using the toilet. You may also **autoinoculate** yourself, or transmit a pathogen from one part of your body to another. For example, you may touch a sore on your lip that is teeming with viral

Autoinoculation: Transmission of a pathogen from one part of your body to another.

Bacteria: Single-celled organisms that may be disease-causing.

herpes and then transmit the virus to your eye when you subsequently scratch your itchy eyelid.

Pathogens are also transmitted by *airborne contact*, either through inhaling the droplet spray from a sneeze or breathing in air that carries a particular pathogen, or you may become the victim of *food-borne infection* if you eat something contaminated by microorganisms. Recent episodes of food poisoning from *salmonella* bacteria found in certain foods and *E. coli* bacteria found in undercooked beef have raised concerns about the safety of our food supply in the United States and forced many food handlers to make sure that their burgers and chicken are cooked to the proper organism-killing temperatures. Recently introduced labels cautioning consumers to cook meats thoroughly, to wash utensils, and the like have been the direct result of these concerns.

Your best friend may be the source of *animal-borne pathogens*. Dogs as well as cats, livestock, and wild animals can spread numerous diseases through their bites or feces or by carrying infected insects into your living areas. For example, ticks carry Lyme disease. Water-borne diseases are transmitted directly from drinking water and indirectly from foods washed or sprayed with water containing their pathogens. These pathogens can also invade your body if you wade or swim in contaminated streams, lakes, and reservoirs. What are the most common pathogens and how can you best protect yourself against them?

Bacteria

Bacteria are single-celled organisms that are plantlike in nature but lack chlorophyll (the pigment that gives plants their green coloring). There are three major types of bac-

Assessing Your Risks for the New Diseases

Recently, the media has been beseiging the public with sensationalized accounts of powerful—and often fatal—new diseases. In 1994, several young children died after eating a fast-food hamburger tainted with E. Coli; a rare outbreak of a strain of hantavirus—quickly (and incorrectly) dubbed "Navajo disease"—sent waves of panic through the Southwest; and 1995 began with news of an outbreak in Zaire of the dreaded Ebola virus.

These diseases may be real, but just how real is their threat to you? A closer look at a few of these diseases will help put your personal risk into perspective.

Ebola Virus

There is no lack of sensationalism surrounding the scare of the Ebola virus. Richard Preston's best-selling novel *The Hot Zone*, the TV movie *Virus*, and the movie *Outbreak* all hypothesized that a disease such as Ebola could rapidly spread throughout the world and wipe out millions of people.

Scientific evidence paints a different story. The only outbreaks of Ebola—in 1976, 1979, and 1995—were concentrated in Zaire and nearby western Sudan. Ebola can by transferred only by direct contact with infected blood, organs, secretions, semen, or contaminated needles.

Many of the victims of Ebola came in contact with the disease through unsanitary conditions in medical facilities. A medical team that performed surgery without surgical gowns, gloves, or masks on an early victim were stricken with Ebola. Other hospital patients were infected through the reuse of hypodermic needles.

Like many public health epidemics, poor sanitation, poverty, and over-crowded housing units and medical facilities provide ripe breeding grounds for highly contagious diseases such as Ebola. Strict attention to infection-control measures in most U.S. health-care facilities limits our risk of exposure to such diseases. While U.S. sanitation policies are among the best in the world, the Centers for Disease Control and Prevention (CDC) remains vigilant in monitoring potential routes of infection.

Although remote, the chance of a major epidemic remains a possibility. Today, people may cross the globe in a matter of hours by commercial aircraft. They may breathe the same air in aircraft, share body fluids, or come into close physical contact with people who have been exposed to pathogens that are virtually unheard of in the United States. If you travel, exercising common-sense precautions may help reduce your risk for many of these diseases.

Hantavirus

Another scare of 1994 was the outbreak of a strange disease in the Southwest. Victims had flu-like symptoms until suddenly their lungs flooded with fluid, resulting in death. After one such death, an alert medical worker in the Navajo nation realized that a similar death had occurred at another local medical facility. The CDC sent a team of experts, who were able to identify and trace the cause of the disease in 17 days.

The disease was identified as a hantavirus, which was spread through human contact with the feces of contaminated mice. Residents of the reservation were taught how to rid their homes of mice and dispose of the feces. Isolated cases have since been identified in 20 states; transmission in each case was linked to mouse feces.

E. Coli

Another of 1994's outbreaks involved hamburgers at a fast-food restaurant in the Northwest. The hamburger meat had been tainted with the *Escherichia Coli* (better known as E. Coli) bacteria. People who ate undercooked burgers became ill; several young children died.

The best way to protect yourself from E. Coli is to cook ground meat to an internal temperature of at least 155 degrees. In a restaurant, never order a hamburger cooked less than medium. If any meat appears pink, send it back for further cooking. In many communities, local health regulations no longer allow hamburgers to be cooked to anything less than medium.

Flesh-Eating Strep

Although the media might try to convince you that incidents of a form of *Andromeda* strain of flesh-eating bacteria has become common, the facts are really quite different. This strain of Group A Strep is very rare: between 10,000 and 15,000 occurrences annually. Your chances of infection are very slight. One of the strange aspects of this bacterium is that it produces materials that dissolve tissue and once it infects a person, it is difficult to stop with the available array of antibiotics. Death may occur, particularly in persons who are already weakened by another disease. Only by removing the dead tissue and infusing large amounts of antibiotics can the disease be stopped. While this may seem quite drastic, it is important to realize that if the infection is caught early, antibiotics usually do stop it before it progresses. Early diagnosis and infection control measures that stop this bacterial threat in hospitals and other health-care facilities are critical aspects of prevention and intervention.

Disease and You

As you can see, your risks of contracting these "hot" new diseases are negligible. While some diseases such as Tuberculosis are developing antibiotic-resistant strains, medical researchers are constantly searching for new medicines to help eradicate these enemies. And organizations such as the CDC are on the prowl to locate potential epidemics and stop them in their tracks.

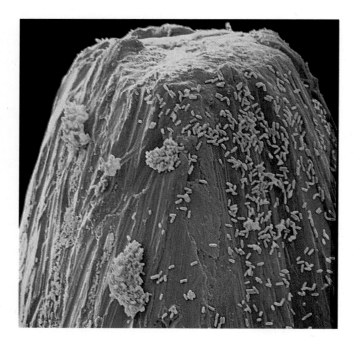

Bacteria (shown here on the head of a pin) are single-celled plantlike organisms that produce infection-causing toxins.

teria: cocci, bacilli, and spirilla. Bacteria may be viewed under a standard light microscope.

Although there are several thousand species of bacteria, only approximately 100 cause diseases in humans. In many cases, it is not the bacteria themselves that cause disease but rather the poisonous substances, called **toxins,** that they produce. Some of these toxins are extremely powerful. Bacterial infections can take many forms. The following are the most common.

Staphylococcal Infections. One of the most common forms of bacterial infection is the staph infection. **Staphylococci** are normally present on our skin at all times and usually cause few problems. But when there is a cut or break in the **epidermis,** or outer layer of the skin, staphylococci may enter and cause a localized infection. If you have ever suffered from acne, boils, styes (infections of the eyelids), or infected wounds, you have probably had a staph infection.

At least one staph-caused disorder, **toxic shock syndrome,** is potentially fatal. Media reports in the early 1980s indicated that the disorder was exclusive to menstruating women, particularly those who used high-absorbency tampons and left them inserted for prolonged periods of time. Although most cases of toxic shock syndrome have occurred in menstruating women, the disease was first reported in 1978 in a group of children and continues to be reported in men, children, and nonmenstruating women. Most cases that are not related to menstruation occur in patients recovering from wounds, surgery, and similar incidents. Although tampons are strongly implicated, the actual mechanisms that produce this disease remain uncertain.

To reduce the likelihood of contracting toxic shock syndrome, take the following precautions: (1) avoid superabsorbent tampons except during the heaviest menstrual flow; (2) change tampons at least every four hours; and (3) use napkins at night instead of tampons. Call your doctor immediately if you have any of the following symptoms during menstruation: high fever, headache, vomiting, diarrhea and the chills, stomach pains, or shocklike symptoms such as faintness, rapid pulse, pallor (which can be caused by a drop in blood pressure), or a sunburnlike rash, particularly on fingers and toes.

Streptococcal Infections. Another common form of bacterial infection is caused by microorganisms called **streptococci.** A "strep throat" (severe sore throat characterized by white or yellow pustules at the back of the throat) is the typical streptococcal problem. Scarlet fever (characterized by acute fever, sore throat, and rash) and rheumatic fever (said to "lick the joints and bite the heart") are serious streptococcal infections.

Pneumonia. In the late nineteenth century and early twentieth century, **pneumonia** was one of the leading causes of death in the United States. This disease is characterized by chronic cough, chest pain, chills, high fever, fluid accumulation, and eventual respiratory failure. One of the most common forms of pneumonia is caused by bacterial infection and responds readily to antibiotic treatment. Other forms are caused by the presence of viruses, chemicals, or other substances in the lungs. In these types of pneumonia, treatment may be more difficult. Although medical advances have reduced the overall incidence and severity of pneumonia, it remains the fifth leading cause of death in the United States. HIV-infected individuals are particularly vulnerable to certain forms of pneumonia, some of which may be fatal.

Legionnaire's Disease. This bacterial disorder gained widespread publicity in 1976, when several Legionnaires at the American Legion convention in Philadelphia contracted the disease and died before the invading organism was isolated and effective treatment devised. The symptoms are similar to those for pneumonia, which sometimes makes identification difficult. In people whose resistance is lowered, particularly the elderly, delayed identification can have serious consequences. If they are misdiagnosed as suffering from pneumonia, they may be given **penicillin,** which is ineffective as a treatment for Legionnaire's disease, instead of the required erythromycin (Ilotycin).

Tuberculosis. One of the leading fatal diseases in the United States in the early 1900s, **tuberculosis (TB)** was largely controlled by the mid-1900s through improved

Although tuberculosis was nearly eradicated in the United States, the incidence of new drug-resistant strains of the disease is on the rise, with the poor—especially those living in homeless shelters—among those at special risk.

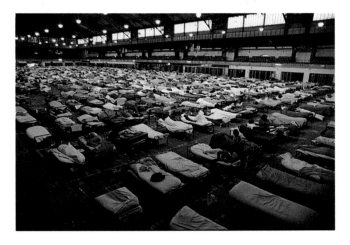

sanitation, isolation of infected persons, and treatment with drugs such as rifampin or Isoniazid. In fact, the number of reported cases in 1985 reached an all-time low of about 22,000 cases. But during the last decade, deteriorating social conditions, including overcrowding and poor sanitation, and the failure to isolate active cases have led to an epidemic of tuberculosis in some U.S. communities; there are nearly 30,000 active cases in the United States today. Newer strains of *drug resistant* tuberculosis make this new epidemic potentially more devastating than previous outbreaks. People residing in overcrowded prisons and homeless shelters having poor ventilation (which means that people continually inhale contaminated air) are at special risk. Early release programs for infected prisoners and the migratory patterns of infected homeless people make the spread of tuberculosis difficult to control. The poor, especially the chronically ill and children, seem to be especially at risk. The influx of large numbers of TB-infected illegal aliens has contributed substantially to our escalating tuberculosis rates. Globally, tuberculosis kills 2.9 million persons a year.[3]

Tuberculosis is caused by bacterial infiltration of the respiratory system. It is transmitted from person to person by the breathing of air infected by coughing or sneezing, but it is normally fairly difficult to catch. In fact, you need, on average, to be in contact with the disease eight hours a day for six straight months, and even then, the chances of getting it are only about 50 percent. Many people infected with TB are contagious without actually showing any symptoms themselves. Fortunately, the average healthy person is not at high risk; however, those who may be fighting other diseases, such as some of the HIV-related diseases, may be at increased risk. Symptoms include persistent coughing, weight loss, fever, and spitting up blood. If you or someone in your household has these symptoms, see your doctor. A quick test can usually detect TB. If you do have it, you can usually be treated and made noncontagious within two weeks. You can often be cured within six months. Although tests for detecting the TB organism are available, those most likely to be infected are often the very people who are least likely to have access to the health-care facilities where such tests are done. The usual test involves a superficial injection of weakened tuberculosis bacteria just under the skin. If the site of the injection becomes red or swells within 48 hours, a positive test result is recorded, indicating that the person may be infected. Confirming tests, including a chest X-ray, are done before a diagnosis is made. Treatment includes rest, careful infection-control procedures, and drugs to combat the infection.

Periodontal Diseases.   Diseases of the tissue around the teeth, called **periodontal diseases,** affect three out of four adults over 35. Improper home tooth care, including lack of flossing and poor brushing habits, and the failure to obtain professional dental care regularly lead to increased bacterial growth, caries (tooth decay), and gum infections. If left untreated, permanent tooth loss may result.

Rickettsia.   Once believed to be closely related to viruses, **rickettsia** are now considered to be a small form of bacteria. They produce toxins and multiply within small blood vessels, causing vascular blockage and tissue death. Rickettsia require an insect vector (carrier) for transmission to humans. Two common forms of human rickettsia disease

Toxins: Poisonous substances produced by certain microorganisms that cause various diseases.

Staphylococci: Round, gram-positive bacteria, usually found in clusters.

Epidermis: The outermost layer of the skin.

Toxic shock syndrome: A potentially life-threatening bacterial infection that is most common in menstruating women.

Streptococci: Round bacteria, usually found in chain formation.

Pneumonia: Bacterially caused disease of the lungs.

Penicillin: Antibiotic used to fight a variety of bacterially caused ailments.

Tuberculosis (TB): A disease caused by bacterial infiltration of the respiratory system.

Periodontal diseases: Diseases of the tissue around the teeth.

Rickettsia: A small form of bacteria that live inside other living cells.

are Rocky Mountain spotted fever, carried by a tick, and typhus, carried by a louse, flea, or tick. Both diseases can be life-threatening. They produce similar symptoms, including high fever, weakness, rash, and coma. You do not actually have to be bitten by a vector to contract these diseases. Because the vectors themselves harbor the developing rickettsia in their intestinal tracts, insect excrement deposited on the skin and entering the body through abrasions and scratches may be a common source of infection.

$\mathcal{W}$HAT DO YOU THINK?

Why do you think we are experiencing increases in many infectious diseases today? Why are some bacterial agents becoming more resistant to current treatment regimens? What can be done to reduce the spread of infectious diseases such as tuberculosis? What can you do to reduce your own risks?

Viruses

Viruses are the smallest of the pathogens, being approximately 1/500th the size of bacteria. Because of their tiny size, they are visible only under an electron microscope and were therefore not identified until this century. By the 1960s, viruses were being effectively grown outside the body in tissue cultures.

At present, over 150 viruses are known to cause diseases in humans. The role of viruses in the development of various cancers and chronic diseases is still unclear. In fact, much remains to be learned about viruses, perhaps the most unusual of all the microorganisms that infect humans.

Viruses: Minute parasitic microbes that live inside another cell.

Incubation period: The time between exposure to a disease and the appearance of the symptoms.

Slow-acting viruses: Viruses having long incubation periods and causing slowly progressive symptoms.

Interferon: A protein substance produced by the body that aids the immune system by protecting healthy cells.

Endemic: Describing a disease that is always present to some degree.

Influenza: A common viral disease of the respiratory tract.

Hepatitis: A virally caused disease in which the liver becomes inflamed, producing such symptoms as fever, headache, and jaundice.

Essentially, a virus consists of a protein structure that contains either *ribonucleic acid (RNA)* or *deoxyribonucleic acid (DNA)*. It is incapable of carrying out the normal cell functions of respiration and metabolism. It cannot reproduce on its own and can only exist in a parasitic relationship with the cell it invades. In fact some scientists question whether viruses should be considered living organisms.

When viruses attach themselves to host cells, they inject their own RNA or DNA, causing the host cells to begin reproducing new viruses. Once they take control of a cell, these new viruses overrun it until, filled to capacity, the cell bursts, putting thousands of new viruses into circulation to begin the process of cell invasion and reproduction all over again.

Because viruses cannot reproduce outside living cells, they are especially difficult to culture in a laboratory, making detection and study of these organisms extremely time-consuming. Treatment of viral diseases is also difficult because many viruses can withstand heat, formaldehyde, and large doses of radiation with little effect on their structure. In addition, some viruses may have **incubation periods** (the length of time required to develop fully and therefore to cause symptoms in their hosts) that are measured in years rather than hours or days. Termed **slow-acting viruses,** these viruses infect the host and remain in a semidormant state for years, causing a slowly developing illness. HIV is the most recent deadly example of a slow-acting virus.

Drug treatment for viral infections is limited. Drugs powerful enough to kill viruses also kill the host cells, although there are some drugs available that block stages in viral reproduction without damaging the host cells.

We have another form of virus protection within our own bodies. When exposed to certain viruses, the body begins to produce a protein substance known as **interferon**. Interferon does not destroy the invading microorganisms but sets up a protective mechanism to aid healthy cells in their struggle against the invaders. Although interferon research is promising, it should be noted that not all viruses stimulate interferon production.

The Common Cold. In everyday life, perhaps no ailment is as bothersome as the common cold, with its irritating symptoms of runny nose, itchy eyes, and generally uncomfortable sensations. Colds are responsible for more days lost from work and more uncomfortable days spent at work than any other ailment.

Caused by any number of viruses (some experts claim there may be over 100 different viruses responsible for the common cold), colds are **endemic** (always present to some degree) among peoples throughout the world. Current research indicates that otherwise healthy people carry cold viruses in their noses and throats most of the time. These viruses are held in check until the host's resistance is lowered. In the true sense of the word, it is possible to "catch" a cold—from the airborne droplets of another person's sneeze or from skin-to-skin or mucous membrane contact—though recent studies indicate that the hands may be the greatest avenue of cold and other viral transmission. Obviously, then, covering your mouth with a tissue or handkerchief when sneezing is better than covering it with your bare hand, particularly if you next use your hand to touch food in a restaurant, shake your friend's hand, or open the door.

Although there are numerous theories about how to "cure" the common cold, including that concerning megadoses of vitamin C, there is little hard evidence to support any of them. The best rule of thumb is to keep your resistance level high. Sound nutrition, adequate rest, stress reduction, and regular exercise appear to be your best bets in helping you fight off infection. Also, avoiding people with newly developed colds (colds appear to be most contagious during the first 24 hours of onset) is advisable. Once you contract a cold, bed rest, plenty of fluids, and aspirin for relief of pain and discomfort are the tried-and-true remedies for adults. Children should not be given aspirin for colds or the flu because of the possibility that this may lead to a potentially fatal disease known as Reye's syndrome. Several over-the-counter preparations have proved effective for alleviating certain cold symptoms.

Influenza. In otherwise healthy people, **influenza,** or flu, is usually not serious. Symptoms, including aches and pains, nausea, diarrhea, fever, and coldlike ailments, generally pass very quickly. (See Figure 18.2 for a comparison of cold and flu symptoms.) However, in combination with other disorders, or among the elderly (people over the age of 65), those with respiratory or heart disease, or the very young (children under the age of 5), the flu can be very serious.

To date, three major varieties of flu virus have been discovered, with many different strains existing within each variety. The "A" form of the virus is generally the most virulent, followed by the "B" and "C" varieties. Although if you contract one form of influenza you may develop immunity to it, you will not necessarily be immune to other forms of the disease. There is little that can be done to treat flu patients once the infection has become established. Some vaccines have proved effective preventives for certain strains of flu virus, but they are totally ineffective against others. In spite of minor risks, it is recommended that people over the age of 65, pregnant women, people with heart disease, and those with certain other illnesses be vaccinated. Because flu shots take anywhere from 2 to 3 weeks to become effective, you should get these shots in the fall, before the flu season begins.

Infectious Mononucleosis. This affliction of college-aged students is often jokingly referred to as the "kissing disease." The symptoms of mononucleosis, or "mono," include sore throat, fever, headache, nausea, chills, and a pervasive weakness or tiredness in the initial stages. As the disease progresses, lymph nodes may become increasingly

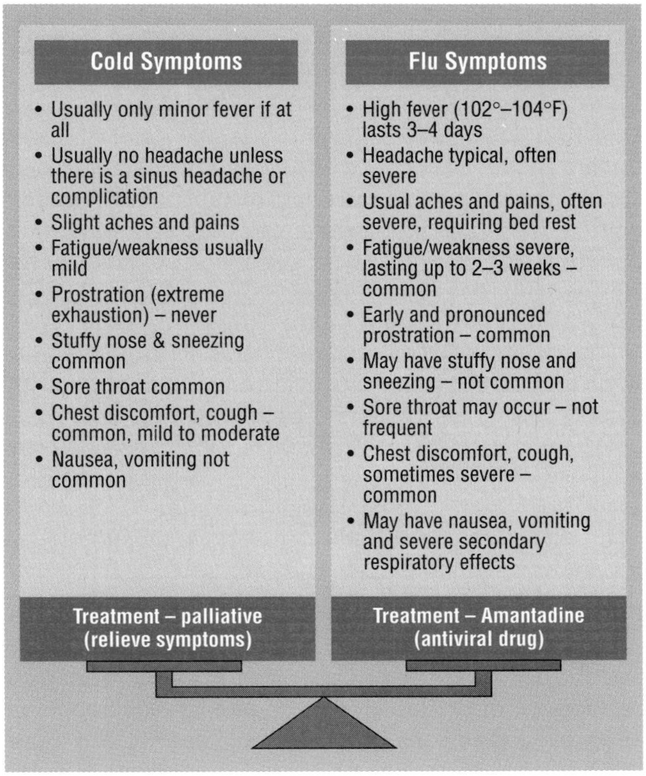

Cold Symptoms	Flu Symptoms
• Usually only minor fever if at all	• High fever (102°–104°F) lasts 3–4 days
• Usually no headache unless there is a sinus headache or complication	• Headache typical, often severe
• Slight aches and pains	• Usual aches and pains, often severe, requiring bed rest
• Fatigue/weakness usually mild	• Fatigue/weakness severe, lasting up to 2–3 weeks – common
• Prostration (extreme exhaustion) – never	• Early and pronounced prostration – common
• Stuffy nose & sneezing common	• May have stuffy nose and sneezing – not common
• Sore throat common	• Sore throat may occur – not frequent
• Chest discomfort, cough – common, mild to moderate	• Chest discomfort, cough, sometimes severe – common
• Nausea, vomiting not common	• May have nausea, vomiting and severe secondary respiratory effects
Treatment – palliative (relieve symptoms)	**Treatment – Amantadine (antiviral drug)**

FIGURE 18.2

Cold or flu? Weighing your symptoms may answer your questions.

Source: Adapted from *National Institutes of Health Bulletin* and H. Sheldon, *Introduction to Human Diseases* (Philadelphia: W. B. Saunders, 1992).

enlarged, and jaundice, spleen enlargement, aching joints, and body rashes may occur.

Theories on the transmission and treatment of mononucleosis are highly controversial. Caused by the *Epstein-Barr virus,* mononucleosis is readily detected through a *monospot test,* a blood test that measures the percentage of specific forms of white blood cells. Because many viruses are caused by transmission of body fluids, many people once believed that young people passed the disease on by kissing. Although this is still considered a possible cause, mononucleosis is not believed to be highly contagious. It does not appear to be easily contracted through normal, everyday personal contact. Multiple cases among family members are rare, as are cases between intimate partners.

Treatment of mononucleosis is often a lengthy process that involves bed rest, balanced nutrition, and medications to control the symptoms of the disease. Gradually, the body develops a form of immunity to the disease and the person returns to normal activity levels.

Hepatitis. One of the most highly publicized viral diseases is **hepatitis.** In some regions of the country and among certain segments of the population, hepatitis has at times reached epidemic proportions. Massive educational programs aimed at prevention of this disease have been initiated in the hope of preventing new outbreaks. Hepatitis is generally defined as a virally caused inflammation of the liver, characterized by symptoms that include fever, headache, nausea, loss of appetite, skin rashes, pain in the upper right abdomen, dark yellow (with a brownish tinge) urine, and the possibility of jaundice (the "disease your friends diagnose" because of the yellowing of the whites of the eyes and the skin).

Treatment of all the forms of viral hepatitis is somewhat limited. A proper diet, bed rest, and antibiotics to combat bacterial invaders that may cause additional problems are recommended. Vaccines for hepatitis are available, although costs are high for the series of injections. Many states are beginning to require vaccinations against hepatitis B for health-care workers and others who may be exposed to blood-borne pathogens.

Mumps. Until 1968, mumps was a common viral disorder among children. That year a vaccine become available and the disease seemed to be largely under control, with reported cases declining from 80 per 100,000 people in 1968 to less than 2 per 100,000 people in 1984. But today the incidence of mumps, as well as of many other childhood diseases, is on the increase nationally.[4] Failure to vaccinate children due to public apathy, misinformation, and social and economic conditions is responsible for the rise. Approximately one-half of all mumps infections are not apparent because they produce only minor symptoms. Typically, there is an incubation period of 16 to 18 days, followed by symptoms caused by the lodging of the virus in the glands of the neck. The most common symptom is the swelling of the parotid (salivary) glands. One of the greatest dangers associated with mumps is the potential for sterility in men who contract the disease in young adulthood. Also, some victims suffer hearing loss.

Chicken Pox. Caused by the herpes zoster varicella virus, chicken pox produces the characteristic symptoms of fever and tiredness 13 to 17 days after exposure, followed by skin eruptions that itch, blister, and produce a clear fluid. The virus is present in these blisters for approximately one week. Symptoms are generally mild, and immunity to subsequent infection appears to be lifelong. Although a vaccine for chicken pox is now available, many believe that it is not necessary and fail to vaccinate their children. Many children still contract the disease. Scientists believe that after the initial infection, the virus goes into permanent hibernation and, for most people, there are no further complications. For a small segment of the population, however, the zoster virus may become reactivated. Blisters will develop, usually on only one side of the body and tending to stop abruptly at the midline. Cases in which the disease covers both sides of the body are far more serious. This disease, known as shingles, affects over 5 percent of the population each year. More than half the sufferers are over 50 years of age.

Measles. Technically referred to as rubeola, **measles** is a viral disorder that often affects young children. Symptoms, appearing about 10 days after exposure, include an itchy rash and a high fever. **German measles (rubella),** is a milder viral infection that is believed to be transmitted by inhalation, after which it multiplies in the upper respiratory tract and passes into the bloodstream. It causes a rash, especially on the upper extremities. It is not generally a serious health threat and usually runs its course in three to four days. The major exceptions to this rule are among newborns and pregnant women. Rubella can damage a fetus, particularly during the first trimester, creating a condition known as congenital rubella, in which the infant may be born blind, deaf, retarded, or with heart defects. Immunization has reduced the incidence of both measles and German measles. Infections in children not immunized against measles can lead to fever-induced problems such as rheumatic heart disease, kidney damage, and neurological disorders.

Rabies. The **rabies** virus infects many warm-blooded animals. Bats are believed to be **asymptomatic** (symptom-free) carriers. Their urine, which they spray when flying, contains the virus, and even the air of densely populated bat caves may be infectious. In most other hosts, the disease is extremely virulent and usually fatal. A characteristic behavior of rabid animals is the frenzied biting of other animals and people. Not only does this behavior cause injury but it also spreads the virus through the infected animal's saliva. The most obvious symptoms of the disease are extreme cerebral excitement and rage, spasms in the pharynx (throat) muscles, especially at the sight of water, and the inability to drink water.

The incubation period for rabies is usually one to three months, yet may range from one week to one year. The disease may be fatal if not treated immediately with the rabies vaccine. Anyone bitten by an animal that may carry rabies should seek medical attention as soon as possible and try to bring the animal along for testing.

Other Pathogens

Fungi. Hundreds of species of **fungi**, multi- or unicellular primitive plants, inhabit our environment and serve useful functions. Moldy breads, cheeses, and mushrooms used for domestic purposes pose no harm to humans. But some species of fungi can produce infections. Candidiasis (a vaginal yeast infection), athlete's foot, ringworm, and jock itch are examples of fungal diseases. Keeping the affected area clean and dry plus treatment with appropriate medications will generally bring prompt relief from these infections.

Protozoa.   Protozoa are microscopic, single-celled organisms that are generally associated with tropical diseases such as African sleeping sickness and malaria. Although these pathogens are prevalent in the developing countries of the world, they are largely controlled in the United States. The most common protozoal disease in the United States is trichomoniasis, an infection discussed further in the sexually transmitted diseases section of this chapter. A common water-borne protozoan disease in many regions of the country is giardiasis. Persons who drink or are exposed to the giardia pathogen may suffer symptoms of intestinal pain and discomfort weeks after infection. Protection of water supplies is the key to prevention.

Parasitic Worms.   Parasitic worms are the largest of the pathogens. Ranging in size from the relatively small pinworms typically found in children to the relatively large tapeworms found in all forms of warm-blooded animals, most parasitic worms are more a nuisance than a threat. Of special note today are the new forms of worm infestations commonly associated with eating raw fish in Japanese sushi restaurants. Cooking fish and other foods to temperatures sufficient to kill the worms or their eggs is an effective means of prevention.

*Y*OUR BODY'S DEFENSES: KEEPING YOU WELL

Although all of the pathogens described in the preceding section pose a threat if they take hold in your body, the chances that they will take hold are actually quite small. To do so, they must overcome a number of effective barriers, many of which were established in your body before you were born.

Physical and Chemical Defenses

Perhaps our single most critical early defense system is the skin. Layered to provide an intricate web of barriers, the skin allows few pathogens to enter. **Enzymes,** complex proteins manufactured by the body that appear in body secretions such as sweat, provide additional protection, destroying microorganisms on skin surfaces by producing inhospitable pH levels. Normal body pH is 7.0, but enzymatic or biochemical changes may cause the body chemistry to become more acidic (pH of less than 7.0), or more alkaline (pH of more than 7.0). In either case, microorganisms that flourish at a selected pH will be weakened or destroyed as these changes occur. A third protection is our frequent slight elevations in body temperature, which create an inhospitable environment for many pathogens. Only when there are cracks or breaks in the skin can pathogens gain easy access to the body.

The linings of the body provide yet another protection against pathogens. Mucous membranes in the respiratory tract and other linings of the body trap and engulf invading organisms. *Cilia*, hairlike projections in the lungs and respiratory tract, sweep unwanted invaders toward body openings, where they are expelled. Tears, nasal secretions, ear wax, and other secretions found at body entrances contain enzymes designed to destroy or neutralize invading pathogens. Finally, any invading organism that manages to breach these initial lines of defense faces a formidable specialized network of defenses thrown up by the immune system.

The Immune System: Your Body Fights Back

Immunity is a condition of being able to resist a particular disease by counteracting the substance that produces the disease. Any substance capable of triggering an immune response is called an **antigen.** An antigen can be a virus, a bacterium, a fungus, a parasite, or a tissue or cell from another individual. When invaded by an antigen, the body responds by forming substances called **antibodies** that are matched to the specific antigen much as a key is matched to a lock. Antibodies belong to a mass of large molecules known as immunoglobulins, a group of nine chemically distinct protein substances, each of which plays a role in neutralizing, setting up for destruction, or actually destroying antigens. Once an antigen breaches the body's initial defenses, the body begins a careful

Measles: A viral disease that produces symptoms including an itchy rash and a high fever.

German measles (rubella): A milder form of measles that causes a rash and mild fever in children and may cause damage to a fetus or a newborn baby.

Rabies: A viral disease of the central nervous system often transmitted through animal bites.

Asymptomatic: Without symptoms, or symptom-free.

Fungi: A group of plants that lack chlorophyll and do not produce flowers or seeds; several microscopic varieties are pathogenic.

Protozoa: Microscopic, single-celled organisms.

Enzymes: Organic substances that cause bodily changes and destruction of microorganisms.

Antigen: Substance capable of triggering an immune response.

Antibodies: Substances produced by the body that are individually matched to specific antigens.

process of antigen analysis. It considers the size and shape of the invader, verifies that the antigen is not part of the body itself, and then begins to produce a specific antibody to destroy or weaken the antigen. This process, which is much more complex than described here, is part of a system called *humoral immune responses*. Humoral immunity is the body's major defense against many bacteria and bacterial toxins.

Cell-mediated immunity is characterized by the formation of a population of lymphocytes that can attack and destroy the foreign invader. These lymphocytes constitute the body's main defense against viruses, fungi, parasites, and some bacteria. Key players in this immune response are specialized groups of white blood cells known as *macrophages* (a type of phagocytic, or cell-eating, cell) and *lymphocytes,* other white blood cells in the blood, lymph nodes, bone marrow, and certain glands.

Two forms of lymphocytes in particular, the *B-lymphocytes* (B-cells) and *T-lymphocytes* (T-cells), are involved in the immune response. There are different types of B-cells, named according to the area of the body in which they develop. Most are manufactured in the soft tissue of the hollow shafts of the long bones. T-cells, in contrast, develop and multiply in the thymus, a multilobed organ that lies behind the breastbone. T-cells assist your immune system in several ways. *Regulatory T-cells* help direct the activities of the immune system and assist other cells, particularly B-cells, to produce antibodies. Dubbed "helper Ts," these cells are essential for activating B-cells, other T-cells, and macrophages. Another form of T-cell, known as the "killer Ts" or "cytotoxic Ts," directly attacks infected or malignant cells. Killer Ts enable the body to rid itself of cells that have been infected by viruses or transformed by cancer; they are also responsible for the rejection of tissue and organ grafts. The third type of T-cells, "suppressor Ts," turns off or suppresses the activity of B-cells, killer Ts, and macrophages. Suppressor Ts circulate in the bloodstream and lymphatic system, neutralizing or destroying antigens, enhancing the effects of the immune response, and helping to return the activated immune system to normal levels. After a successful attack on a pathogen, some of the attacker T- and B-cells are preserved as *memory T- and B-cells,* enabling the body to quickly recognize and respond to subsequent attacks by the same kind of or-

ganism at a later time. Thus macrophages, T- and B-cells, and antibodies are the key factors in mounting an immune response.

Once people have survived certain infectious diseases, they become immune to those diseases, meaning that in all probability they will not develop them again. Upon subsequent attack by the disease-causing microorganism, their memory T- and B-cells are quickly activated to come to their defense. Immunization works on the same principle. Vaccines containing an attenuated (weakened) or killed version of the disease-causing microorganism or containing an antigen that is similar to but not as dangerous as the disease antigen are administered to stimulate the person's immune system to produce antibodies against future attacks—without actually causing the disease.

Autoimmune Diseases. Although white blood cells and the antigen-antibody response generally work in our favor by neutralizing or destroying harmful antigens, the body sometimes makes a mistake and targets its own tissue as the enemy, builds up antibodies against that tissue, and attempts to destroy it. This is known as autoimmune disease (*auto* means "self"). Common examples of this type of disease are rheumatoid arthritis, lupus erythematosus, and myasthenia gravis.

In some cases, the antigen-antibody response completely fails to function. The result is a form of *immune deficiency syndrome.* Perhaps the most dramatic case of this syndrome was the "bubble boy," a youngster who died in 1984 after living his short life inside a sealed-off environment designed to protect him from all antigens. A much more common immune system disorder is *acquired immune deficiency syndrome* (AIDS), which we will discuss later in this chapter.

Fever

If an infection is localized, pus formation, redness, swelling, and irritation often occur. These symptoms indicate that the invading organisms are being fought systematically. Another indication is the development of a fever, or a rise in body temperature above the norm of 98.6°F. Fever is frequently caused by toxins secreted by pathogens that interfere with the control of body temperature. Although this elevated temperature is often harmful to the body, it is also believed to act as a form of protection. Elevations of body temperature by even 1 or 2 degrees provide an environment that destroys some types of disease-causing organisms. Also, as body temperature rises, the body is stimulated to produce more white blood cells which destroy more invaders.

Pain

Although pain is not usually thought of as a defense mechanism, it plays a valuable role in the body's response to invasion. Pain is generally a response to injury. Pain

---

Vaccination: Inoculation with killed or weakened pathogens or similar, less dangerous antigens in order to prevent or lessen the effects of some disease.

Acquired immunity: Immunity developed during life in response to disease, vaccination, or exposure.

Natural immunity: Immunity passed to a fetus by its mother.

---

may be either direct, caused by the stimulation of nerve endings in an affected area, or referred, meaning it is present in one place while the source is elsewhere. An example of referred pain is the pain in the arm or jaw often experienced by someone having a heart attack. Regardless of the cause of pain, most pain responses are accompanied by inflammation. Pain tends to be the earliest sign that an injury has occurred and often causes the person to slow down or stop the activity that was aggravating the injury, thereby protecting against further damage. Because it is often one of the first warnings of disease, persistent pain should not be overlooked or masked with short-term pain relievers.

Vaccines: Bolstering Your Immunity

Our natural defense mechanisms are our strongest allies in the battle against disease, being with us from birth until death. There are periods in our life, however, when either invading organisms are too strong or our own natural immunity is too weak to protect us from catching a given disease. It is at such times that we need outside assistance in developing immunity to an invading organism. Such assistance is generally provided in the form of a **vaccination,** which, as we said earlier, consists of killed or weakened versions of disease microorganisms or of antigens that are similar to but far less dangerous than the disease microorganism. Vaccines are given orally or by injection, and this form of artificial immunity is termed **acquired immunity,** in contrast to **natural immunity,** which a mother passes to her fetus via their shared blood supply.

Today, depending on the virulence of the organism, vaccines containing live, weakened, or dead organisms are given to people for a variety of diseases. In some instances, if a person is already weakened by other diseases, vaccination may provoke an actual case of the disease. This was what happened with the smallpox vaccinations administered routinely in the 1960s. It was believed that the risk of contracting smallpox from the vaccine was actually greater than was the chance of contracting the disease in an environment where it had essentially been eradicated. For this reason, routine smallpox inoculations were eliminated in the late 1960s. The 1995 schedule for childhood vaccinations is in Table 18.2.

Active and Passive Immunity

If you are exposed to an organism, either during your day-to-day life or through vaccination, you will eventually develop an active acquired immunity to that organism. Your body will produce its own antibodies, and, in most cases, you will not have to worry about subsequent exposures to the disease. In some cases, however, the risks associated with contracting a disease are so severe that you may not be able to wait the days or weeks that your own body needs to produce antibodies. Also, in the event that your resistance is terribly weakened as a result of cancer chemotherapy or for other reasons, your body may be unable to produce its own antibodies. In either of these situations, antibodies formed in another person or animal (called the donor) are often given. Termed passive immunity, this type of immunity is often short-lived but provides the necessary boost to get you through a potentially critical period. Antibodies utilized for passive immunity are taken from gammaglobulins, proteins synthesized from a donor's blood. A mother also confers passive immunity on her newborn baby through breastfeeding.

TABLE 18.2 ■ Recommended Childhood Immunization Schedule

		Age								
Vaccine	Birth	2 mos	4 mos	6 mos	12 mos	15 mos	18 mos	4–6 yrs	11–12 yrs	14–16 yrs
Hepatitis B	HB-1	HB-2		HB-3						
Diphtheria, Tetanus, Pertussis		DTP	DTP	DTP	DTP or DTaP at ≥15 months			DTP or DTaP	Td	
H. influenzae type b		Hib	Hib	Hib	Hib					
Polio		OPV	OPV	OPV				OPV		
Measles, Mumps, Rubella						MMR		MMR or	MMR	

Source: "Recommended Childhood Immunization Schedule, United States—January 1995" (Washington, D.C.: American Academy of Pediatrics, 1995).

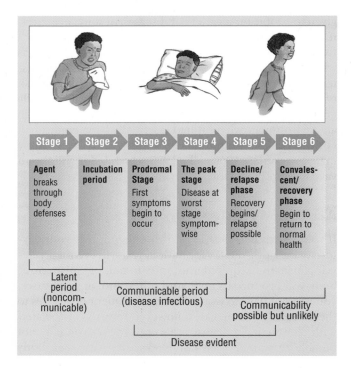

Stage 1	Stage 2	Stage 3	Stage 4	Stage 5	Stage 6
Agent breaks through body defenses	**Incubation period**	**Prodromal Stage** First symptoms begin to occur	**The peak stage** Disease at worst stage symptom-wise	**Decline/ relapse phase** Recovery begins/ relapse possible	**Convales-cent/ recovery phase** Begin to return to normal health

Latent period (noncom-municable)

Communicable period (disease infectious)

Communicability possible but unlikely

Disease evident

FIGURE 18.3

The illustration depicts stages in the course of disease and recovery and periods of likely communicability.

SEXUALLY TRANSMITTED DISEASES

Public health researchers estimate that every year over 10 million people in the United States are afflicted with one or more of the over 20 different types of **sexually transmitted diseases (STDs)**. These diseases were once referred to as venereal diseases, but the newer classification is believed to be broader in scope and more reflective of the numbers and types of these communicable diseases. At the present rate of infection, it is expected that the incidence of STDs will double by the year 2000, with more virulent, antibiotic-resistant, and untreatable strains appearing regularly.

In many victims, the early symptoms of an STD are not serious. They may range from mild discomfort to annoying itching or discharge. (See Figure 18.3 for signs that may indicate the presence of an STD.) Left untreated, however, some of these diseases can have grave consequences, such as sterility, blindness, central nervous system destruction, disfigurement, and even death. Infants born to mothers carrying the organisms for these diseases are at risk for a variety of health problems.

As with many of the communicable diseases, much of the pain, suffering, and anguish associated with STDs could be eliminated or substantially reduced through ed-

ucation, responsible action, and prompt treatment when symptoms first occur. Overcoming the tendency to pass moral judgments on victims would certainly lower the barriers to treatment. Being prepared to deal with the pressure to engage in sexual activity can also be helpful.

Possible Causes: Why Me?

Sexually transmitted diseases affect people of both sexes and of all socioeconomic levels, ages, ethnic groups, and regions of the world. Several reasons have been proposed to explain the present high rates of STDs. The first relates to the moral and social stigma associated with these diseases. Shame and embarrassment often keep infected people from seeking treatment. Unfortunately, these people usually continue to be sexually active, thereby infecting unsuspecting partners. People who are uncomfortable discussing sexual issues may also be less likely to use and/or ask their partners to use condoms as a means of protection against STDs and/or pregnancy.

Another reason proposed for the STD epidemic is our casual attitude about sex. Bombarded by media hype that

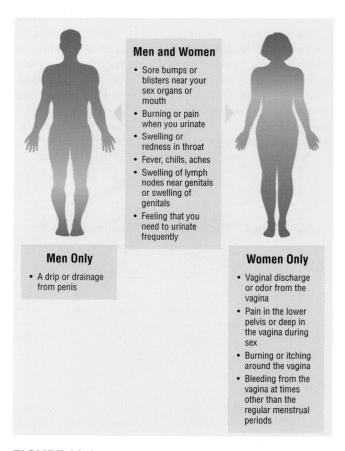

Men and Women
- Sore bumps or blisters near your sex organs or mouth
- Burning or pain when you urinate
- Swelling or redness in throat
- Fever, chills, aches
- Swelling of lymph nodes near genitals or swelling of genitals
- Feeling that you need to urinate frequently

Men Only
- A drip or drainage from penis

Women Only
- Vaginal discharge or odor from the vagina
- Pain in the lower pelvis or deep in the vagina during sex
- Burning or itching around the vagina
- Bleeding from the vagina at times other than the regular menstrual periods

FIGURE 18.4

The illustration lists signs or symptoms that may mean you have an STD.

glamorizes easy sex, many people take sexual partners without considering the consequences. Others are pressured into sexual relationships they don't really want. Generally, the more sexual partners a person has, the greater the risk for contracting an STD. Evaluate your attitude about STDs by taking the Rate Yourself box self-assessment.

Ignorance about the diseases themselves and an inability to recognize actual symptoms or to acknowledge that a person may be asymptomatic yet still have the disease are also factors behind the STD epidemic. A person who is infected but asymptomatic may unknowingly spread an STD to an unsuspecting partner, who may then ignore or misinterpret any symptoms that do appear. By the time either partner seeks medical help, he or she may have infected several others.

Modes of Transmission

Sexually transmitted diseases are generally spread through some form of intimate sexual contact. Sexual intercourse, oral-genital contact, hand-genital contact, and anal intercourse are the most common modes of transmission. More rarely, pathogens for STDs are transmitted mouth to mouth or, even more infrequently, through contact with fluids from body sores. While each STD is a different disease caused by a different pathogen, all STD pathogens prefer dark, moist places, especially the mucous membranes lining the reproductive organs. The majority of these organisms is susceptible to light, excess heat, cold, and dryness, and many die quickly on exposure to air. (The toilet seat is not a likely breeding ground for most bacterial or viral STDs!) Although most STDs are passed on by sexual contact, other kinds of close contact, such as sleeping on the sheets used by someone who has pubic lice, may also cause you to get an STD. One method of preventing the spread of STDs, the use of condoms, is discussed in the Skills for Behavior Change box.

Like other communicable diseases, STDs have both pathogen-specific incubation periods and periods of time during which transmission is most likely, called periods of communicability. Although there are over 20 different types of sexually transmitted diseases, we will discuss only those STDs that are most likely to pose a risk for the average adult.

Chlamydia

Often referred to as the "silent epidemic," **chlamydia** is now the most common STD among heterosexual white Americans. The Centers for Disease Control estimate that over 3 million Americans have chlamydia and that between 3 million and 10 million new cases occur every year.[5] Chlamydia affects 5 times as many people as does gonorrhea and 10 times as many people as does syphilis. Over 10 percent of all college students are infected, and chlamydia is more prevalent than genital herpes and trichomoniasis in this group.

The name of the disease is derived from the Greek verb *chlamys,* meaning to "to cloak," because, unlike most bacteria, chlamydia can only live and grow inside other cells. Although many people classify chlamydia as either *nonspecific* or *nongonococcal urethritis (NGU),* a person may have NGU without having the organism for chlamydia. In over half of the cases of NGU (infections of the urethra and surrounding tissues that are not caused by gonococcal bacteria), however, *Chlamydia trachomatis,* the bacterial organism that causes chlamydia, is present. For this reason, the two disease terms tend to be used interchangeably, even though NGU may be caused by other organisms.

In males, early symptoms may include painful and difficult urination, frequent urination, and a watery, puslike discharge from the penis. Symptoms in females may include a yellowish discharge, spotting between periods, and occasional spotting after intercourse. Unfortunately, many chlamydia victims display no symptoms and therefore do not seek help until the disease has done secondary damage. Females are especially prone to be asymptomatic; over 70 percent do not realize they have the disease until secondary damage occurs.

The secondary damage resulting from chlamydia is serious in both sexes. Male victims can suffer damage to the prostate gland, seminal vesicles, and bulbourethral glands as well as arthritislike symptoms and damage to the blood vessels and heart. In females, secondary damage from chlamydia may include inflammation that damages the cervix or fallopian tubes, causing sterility, and damage to the inner pelvic structure, leading to pelvic inflammatory disease (PID). If an infected woman becomes pregnant, she has a high risk for miscarriages and stillbirths. Chlamydia may also be responsible for one type of **conjunctivitis,** an eye infection that affects not only adults but also infants, who can contract the disease from an infected mother during delivery. Untreated conjunctivitis can cause blindness.

Chlamydia can be controlled through responsible sexual behavior and familiarity with the early symptoms of the disease. If detected early enough, chlamydia is easily treatable with antibiotics such as tetracycline, doxycy-

Sexually transmitted diseases (STDs): Infectious diseases transmitted via some form of intimate, usually sexual, contact.

Chlamydia: Bacterially caused STD of the urogenital tract.

Conjunctivitis: Serious inflammation of the eye caused by any number of pathogens or irritants; can be caused by STDs such as chlamydia.

STD Attitude and Belief Scale

The following quiz will help you evaluate whether your beliefs and attitudes about STDs lead you to take risks that may heighten your risk for contracting an STD.

Directions

Indicate that you believe the following items are true or false by circling the T or the F. Then consult the answer key that follows.

T   F   1.   You can usually tell whether someone is infected with an STD, especially HIV infection.

T   F   2.   Chances are that if you haven't caught an STD by now, you probably have a natural immunity and won't get infected in the future.

T   F   3.   A person who is successfully treated for an STD needn't worry about getting it again.

T   F   4.   So long as you keep yourself fit and healthy, you needn't worry about STDs.

T   F   5.   The best way for sexually active people to protect themselves from STDs is to practice safer sex.

T   F   6.   The only way to catch an STD is to have sex with someone who has one.

T   F   7.   Talking about STDs with a partner is so embarrassing that you're best off not raising the subject and hope the other person will.

T   F   8.   STDs are mostly a problem for people who are promiscuous.

T   F   9.   You don't need to worry about contracting an STD so long as you wash yourself thoroughly with soap and hot water immediately after sex.

T   F   10.   You don't need to worry about AIDS if no one you know has ever come down with it.

T   F   11.   When it comes to STDs, it's all in the cards. Either you're lucky or you're not.

T   F   12.   The time to worry about STDs is when you come down with one.

T   F   13.   As long as you avoid risky sexual practices, such as anal intercourse, you're pretty safe from STDs.

T   F   14.   The time to talk about safer sex is before any sexual contact occurs.

T   F   15.   A person needn't be concerned about an STD if the symptoms clear up on their own in a few weeks.

Scoring Key

1.   *False.* While some STDs have telltale signs, such as the appearance of sores or blisters on the genitals or disagreeable genital odors, others do not. Several STDs, such as chlamydia, gonorrhea (especially in women), internal genital warts, and even HIV infection in its early stages, cause few if any obvious signs or symptoms. You often cannot tell whether your partner is infected with an STD. Many of the nicest looking and well-groomed people carry STDs, often unknowingly. The only way to know whether a person is infected with HIV is by means of an HIV-antibody test.

2.   *False.* If you practice unprotected sex and have not contracted an STD to this point, count your blessings. The thing about good luck is that it eventually runs out.

3.   *False.* Sorry. Successful treatment does not render immunity against reinfection. You still need to take precautions to avoid reinfection, even if you have had an STD in the past and were successfully treated. If you answered true to this item, you're not alone. About one in five college students polled in a recent survey of more than 5,500 college students across Canada believed that a person who gets an STD cannot get it again.

4.   *False.* Even people in prime physical condition can be felled by the tiniest of microbes that cause STDs. Physical fitness is no protection against these microscopic invaders.

5.   *True.* If you are sexually active, practicing safer sex is the best protection against contracting an STD.

6.   *False.* STDs can also be transmitted through nonsexual means, such as by sharing contaminated needles or, in some cases, through contact with disease-causing organisms on towels and bed sheets or even toilet seats.

7.   *False.* Because of the social stigma attached to STDs, it's understandable that you may feel embarrassed raising the subject with your partner. But don't let embarrassment prevent you from taking steps to protect your own and your partner's welfare.

8.   *False.* While it stands to reason that people who are sexually active with numerous partners stand a greater chance that one of their sexual partners carries an STD, all it takes is one infected partner to pass along an STD to you, even if he or she is the only partner you've had or even if the two of you only had sex once. STDs are a potential problem for anyone who is sexually active.

(continued)

cline, or erythromycin. In most cases, treatment is successfully completed in two to three weeks. Unfortunately, when you are tested for STDs, chlamydia checks are not a routine part of many health clinics' testing procedures. You usually have to request a chlamydia check specifically before one is performed on you.

9. *False.* While washing your genitals immediately after sex may have some limited protective value, it is no substitute for practicing safer sex.

10. *False.* You can never know whether you may be the first among your friends and acquaintances to become infected. Moreover, symptoms of HIV infection may not appear for years after initial infection with the virus, so you may have sexual contacts with people who are infected but don't know it and who are capable of passing along the virus to you. You in turn may then pass it along to others, whether or not you are aware of any symptoms.

11. *False.* Nonsense. While luck may play a part in determining whether you have a sexual contact with an infected partner, you can significantly reduce your risk of contracting an STD.

12. *False.* The time to start thinking about STDs (thinking helps, but worrying only makes you more anxious than you need be) is now, not after you have contracted an infection. Some STDs, like herpes and AIDS, cannot be cured. The only real protection you have against them is prevention.

13. *False.* Any sexual contact between the genitals, or between the genitals and the anus, or between the mouth and genitals, is risky if one of the partners is infected with an STD.

14. *True.* Unfortunately, too many couples wait until they have commenced sexual relations to have "a talk." By then it may already be too late to prevent the transmis-

sion of an STD. The time to talk is before any intimate sexual contact occurs.

15. *False.* Several STDs, notably syphilis, HIV infection, and herpes, may produce initial symptoms that clear up in a few weeks. But while the early symptoms may subside, the infection is still at work within the body and requires medical attention. Also, as noted previously, the infected person is capable of passing along the infection to others, regardless of whether noticeable symptoms were ever present.

Interpreting Your Score

First, add up the number of items you got right. The higher your score, the lower your risk. The lower your score, the greater your risk. A score of 13 correct or better may indicate that your attitudes toward STDs would probably decrease your risk of contracting them. Yet even one wrong response on this test may increase your risk of contracting an STD. You should also recognize that attitudes have little effect on behavior unless they are carried into action. Knowledge alone isn't sufficient to protect yourself from STDs. You need to ask yourself how you are going to put knowledge into action by changing your behavior to reduce your chances of contracting an STD.

Source: From Jeffrey S. Nevid with Fern Gotfried, *Choices: Sex in the Age of STDs,* 10–13. © Copyright 1995 by Allyn and Bacon. Reprinted by permission.

$\mathcal{W}$HAT DO YOU THINK?

Why do you think that even though many college students have heard about the risks of STDs and HIV disease, they remain apathetic, fail to use condoms, and in general, act irresponsibly? What actions do you think could be taken to make more of your friends heed warnings about STDs and either use condoms more regularly, abstain from sex, and/or engage in other self-protecting behaviors? What would it take to make you change your behaviors?

Pelvic Inflammatory Disease (PID)

Pelvic inflammatory disease (PID) is actually not one disease but a term used to describe a number of infections of the uterus, fallopian tubes, and ovaries. Although PID is often the result of an untreated sexually transmitted disease, especially chlamydia and gonorrhea, it is not actually

an STD. Nonsexual causes of PID are also common, including excessive vaginal douching, cigarette smoking, and substance abuse.

Women make over 2 million visits to private physicians each year for PID symptoms, which may include acute inflammation of the pelvic cavity, severe pain in the lower abdomen, menstrual irregularities, fever, nausea, painful intercourse, tubal pregnancies, and severe depression.[6] The major consequences of untreated PID are infertility, ectopic pregnancy, chronic pelvic pain, and recurrent upper genital infections. Risk factors include young age at first sexual intercourse, multiple sex partners, high frequency of sexual intercourse, and change of sexual part-

Pelvic inflammatory disease (PID): Term used to describe various infections of the female reproductive tract.

Protect Yourself: Condoms

If you choose to be sexually active, it is crucial that you carefully consider your personal protection options. To date, with the exception of abstinence, the most effective method for reducing the risk of STD infection is use of a condom. But remember, condoms are not 100 percent effective. They do not give absolute assurance that you will not come into contact with your sexual partner's body fluids at some time during the sex act. The most common problems are: failure to put the condom on in time, failure to use it every time, failure to completely unroll it and leave a reservoir at the tip, failure to keep the condom on during sex, and holes in or rupture of the condom due to improper storage.

To protect yourself, stick to the following rules:

- Decide ahead of time that you will not have sex without using a condom. Make sure that you have one with you. (If you are female, you may purchase a female condom that will help you take greater charge of your sexual encounters and decrease your reliance on others for your protection.)
- Never reuse a condom.

- Purchase latex condoms only. The other types are more likely to break or leak.
- Store condoms in a cool, dry place—not in the glove compartment of your car or in your wallet.
- If a condom appears brittle or sticky, get rid of it.
- Put the condom on (correctly) before having any contact between genitals.
- Use condoms for oral sex as well; use a dental dam for oral sex with a female.
- Apply a water-based lubricant containing spermicide to the condom for additional protection.
- If the condom breaks, tears, or becomes dislodged, wash the genitals thoroughly with soap and water, apply a spermicide to the area, and put on another condom before additional contact. It only takes a fraction of a second to become infected with disease-laden body fluids or to infect someone else if you are a carrier.
- Make sure the condom doesn't come off by holding it in place during withdrawal.

---

ners within the last 30 days.[7] Regular gynecological examinations and early treatment for STD symptoms reduce risk.

Gonorrhea

Gonorrhea is one of the most common STDs in the United States, being surpassed only by chlamydia in number of cases. Although over 2 million new cases of gonorrhea are reported annually in the United States, a significant number probably go unreported. Caused by the bacterial pathogen, *Neisseria gonorrhoea,* this disease primarily infects the linings of the urethra, genital tract, pharynx, and rectum. It may be spread to the eyes or other body regions via the hands or body fluids. Most victims are males between the ages of 20 and 24, with sexually active females between the ages of 15 and 19 also at high risk.[8]

In males, a typical symptom is a white milky discharge from the penis accompanied by painful, burning urination two to nine days after contact. This is usually enough to send most men to their physician for treatment. Only about 20 percent of all males with gonorrhea are asymptomatic.

In females, the situation is just the opposite. Only about 20 percent of all females experience any form of discharge, and few develop a burning sensation upon urinating until much later in the course of the disease (if ever). The organism can remain in the woman's vagina,

cervix, uterus, or fallopian tubes for long periods with no apparent symptoms other than an occasional slight fever. Thus a woman can be unaware that she has been infected and that she may be infecting her sexual partners.

Upon diagnosis, an antibiotic regimen using penicillin, tetracycline, spectiomycin, ceftriaxone, or other drugs is begun. A penicillin-resistant form of gonorrhea may require a particularly strong combination of antibiotics. Treatment is generally completely effective within a short period of time if the disease is detected early.

If the disease goes undetected in a woman, it can spread throughout the genital-urinary tract to the fallopian tubes and ovaries, causing sterility, or at the very least, severe inflammation and pelvic inflammatory disease symptoms. If an infected woman becomes pregnant, the disease can cause conjunctivitis in her infant. To prevent this, physicians routinely administer silver nitrate or penicillin preparations to the eyes of newborn babies.

Untreated gonorrhea in the male may spread to the prostate, testicles, urinary tract, kidney, and bladder. Blockage of the vasa deferentia due to scar tissue formation may cause sterility. In some cases, the penis develops a painful curvature during erection.

Syphilis

Syphilis, the other well-known sexually transmitted disease, is also caused by a bacterial organism, the spirochete known as *Treponema pallidum.* Because it is extremely delicate and dies readily upon exposure to air, dryness, or cold, the organism is generally transferred only through direct sexual contact. Typically, this means contact between sexual organs during intercourse, but in rare instances, the organism enters the body through a break in the skin, through deep kissing in which body fluids are exchanged, or through some other transmission of body fluids.

Syphilis peaked in the United States after World War II, then declined through the 1950s and 1960s as penicillin became more widely used. The number of cases increased significantly in the late 1980s and early 1990s. Lack of access to health care and exchanges of sex for drugs are among the social conditions that have contributed to the recent rise.[9]

Syphilis is called the "great imitator" because its symptoms resemble those of several other diseases. Only an astute physician who has reason to suspect the presence of the disease will order the appropriate tests for a diagnosis. What are the symptoms? Unlike most of the other STDs, syphilis generally progresses through several distinct stages.

Primary Syphilis. The first stage of syphilis, particularly for males, is often characterized by the development of a sore known as a **chancre** (pronounced "shank-er"), located most frequently at the site of the initial infection. This chancre is usually about the size of a dime and is painless, but it is oozing with bacteria, ready to spread to an unsuspecting partner. Usually the chancre appears between three to four weeks after contact.

In males, the site of the chancre tends to be the penis or scrotum because this is the site where the organism first makes entry into the body. But, if the disease was contracted through oral sex, the sore can appear in the mouth, throat, or other "first contact" area. In females, the site of infection is often internal, on the vaginal wall or high on the cervix. Because the chancre is not readily apparent, the likelihood of detection is not great. In both males and females, the chancre will completely disappear in three to six weeks.

Secondary Syphilis. From a month to a year after the chancre disappears, secondary symptoms may appear, including a rash or white patches on the skin or on the mucous membranes of the mouth, throat, or genitals. Hair loss may occur, lymph nodes may become enlarged, and the victim may run a slight fever or develop a headache. In rare cases, sores develop around the mouth or genitals. As during the active chancre phase, these sores contain infectious bacteria, and contact with them may spread the disease. In some people, symptoms follow a textbook pattern; in others, there are no symptoms at all. In a few cases, there may be arthritic pain in the joints. Because symptoms vary so much and because the symptoms that do appear are so far removed from previous sexual experience that the victim seldom connects the two, the dis-

ease often goes undetected even at this second stage. Symptoms may persist for a few weeks or months and then disappear, leaving the victim thinking that all is well.

Latent Syphilis. The syphilis spirochetes begin to invade body organs after the secondary stage. There may be periodic reappearance of previous symptoms, including the presence of infectious lesions, for between two and four years after the secondary period. After this period, the disease is rarely transmitted to others, except during pregnancy, when it can be passed on to the fetus. The child will then be born with congenital syphilis, which can cause death or severe birth defects such as blindness, deafness, or disfigurement. Because in most cases the fetus does not become infected until after the first trimester, treatment of the mother during this period will usually prevent infection of the fetus.

In some instances, a child born to an infected mother will show no apparent signs of the disease at birth but, within several weeks, will develop body rashes, a runny nose, and symptoms of paralysis. *Congenital syphilis* is usually detected before it progresses much farther. But sometimes the child's immune system will ward off the invading organism, and further symptoms may not surface until the teenage years. Fortunately, most states protect against congenital syphilis by requiring prospective marriage partners to be tested for syphilis prior to obtaining a marriage license.

In addition to causing congenital syphilis, latent syphilis, if untreated, will continue to progress, infecting more and more organs until the disease reaches its final stage, late syphilis.

Late Syphilis. Most of the horror stories concerning syphilis involve the late stages of the disease. Years after syphilis has entered the body and progressed through the various organs, its net effects become clearly evident. Late-stage syphilis indications may include heart damage, central nervous system damage, blindness, deafness, paralysis, premature senility, and, ultimately, insanity.

Treatment for Syphilis. Treatment for syphilis resembles that for gonorrhea. Because the organism is bacterial, it is treated with antibiotics, usually penicillin, benzathine penicillin G, or doxycycline. Blood tests are administered to determine the exact nature of the invading organism,

---

Gonorrhea: Second most common STD in the United States; if untreated, may cause sterility.

Syphilis: One of the most widespread STDs; characterized by distinct phases and potentially serious results.

Chancre: Sore often found at the site of syphilis infection.

and the doses of antibiotics are much stronger than those taken by the typical gonorrhea patient. The major obstacle to treatment is misdiagnosis of this "imitator" disease.

Pubic Lice

Often called crabs, pubic lice are more annoying than dangerous. **Pubic lice** are small parasites that are usually transmitted during sexual contact. They prefer the dark, moist regions of the body and, during sex, move easily from partner to partner. They have an affinity for pubic hair, attaching themselves to the base of these hairs, where they deposit their eggs (nits). Between one and two weeks later, these nits develop into adults that lay eggs and migrate to other body parts, thus perpetuating the cycle.

Treatment includes washing clothing, furniture, and linens that may harbor the eggs. It usually takes two to three weeks to kill all larval forms. Although sexual contact is the most common mode of transmission, you can become infested with pubic lice from lying on sheets that an infected person has slept on. Sleeping in hotel and dormitory rooms in which blankets and sheets are not washed regularly or sitting on toilet seats where the nits or larvae have been dropped and lie in wait for a new carrier may put you at risk.

Venereal Warts

Venereal warts (also known as genital warts or condylomas) are caused by a small group of viruses known as *human papilloma viruses* (HPVs). A person becomes infected when an HPV penetrates the skin and mucous membranes of the genitals or anus through sexual contact. The virus appears to be relatively easy to catch. The typical incubation period is from six to eight weeks after contact. Many people have no apparent symptoms, particularly if the warts are located inside the reproductive tract. Others may develop a series of itchy bumps on the genitals, which may range in size from a small pinhead to large cauliflowerlike growths that can obstruct normal urinary or reproductive activity. On dry skin (such as on the shaft of the penis), the warts are commonly small, hard, and yellowish-gray, resembling warts that appear on other parts of the body.

Venereal warts are of two different types: (1) *full-blown genital warts* that are noticeable as tiny bumps or growths, and (2) the much more prevalent *flat warts* that are not usually visible to the naked eye. In females, these flat warts are often first detected by a doctor during a routine Pap test. Abnormal Pap results may prompt the physician to perform a procedure in which a vinegarlike solution is applied to the insides of the vaginal walls and cervix to bleach potential warts. The area is then viewed through a special magnifying instrument known as a colposcope. A relatively new photographic procedure known as a cerviscope is being used in some clinics to detect venereal warts. During a cerviscope, vinegar is applied to the vagi-

nal and cervical areas, and an image of the area is projected onto a screen for a specialist to diagnose. This technique is relatively inexpensive and is believed to be five times more sensitive than standard colposcopy. An even newer method that is being used at medical research centers throughout the United States is the *DNA probe,* a technique that identifies the genetic makeup of possible warts.

Whereas women must see a physician for a diagnosis, a male can check for suspicious lesions by wrapping his penis in vinegar-soaked gauze or cloth, waiting for five minutes, and then checking for white bleached areas indicative of flat warts. But venereal warts of the rectum must be diagnosed by a physician.

Risks of Venereal Warts. Many venereal warts will eventually disappear on their own. Others will grow and generate unsightly flaps of irregular flesh on the external genitalia. Although these flaps may be a source of embarrassment, they typically do not cause serious problems. If they grow large enough to obstruct urinary flow or become irritated by clothing or sexual intercourse, they can cause significant problems.

The greatest threat from venereal warts may lie in the apparent relationship between them and a tendency for *dysplasia,* or changes in cells that may lead to a precancerous condition. Exactly how HPV infection leads to cervical cancer is uncertain. What is known is that within five years after infection, 30 percent of all HPV cases will progress to the precancerous stage. Of those cases that become precancerous and are left untreated, 70 percent will eventually result in actual cancer. In addition, venereal warts may pose a threat to a pregnant woman's unborn fetus if the fetus is exposed to the virus during birth. Cesarean deliveries may be considered in serious cases.

Treatment for Venereal Warts. Treatment for venereal warts may take several forms:

1. Warts are painted with a medication called podophyllin during a visit to the doctor's office. The podophyllin is washed off after about four hours, and a few days later the warts begin to dry up and fall off. Sometimes more than one trip to the doctor is necessary. This procedure is relatively painless, but there are potential side effects. Because podophyllin may be absorbed through the skin, pregnant women should not use it. Some patients may experience skin reactions.

2. Warts may be removed by *cryosurgery,* a procedure in which an instrument treated with liquid nitrogen is held to the affected area, "freezing" the tissue. Within a few days, the warts fall off.

3. Depending on size and location, some warts are removed by *simple excision.*

4. For larger warts, *laser surgery* is often used. This is a major procedure that generally requires general anesthesia. The frequency of laser use for wart removal is currently being questioned by many health experts.

(Precautions must also be taken during this procedure to shield medical staff from infection by viral spray.)

5. Creams containing 5-Fluoracil (an anticancer drug) are being used to prevent further precancerous cell development.

6. For warts located externally, injections of interferon are sometimes given to keep the virus from spreading to healthy tissue. This treatment shows promise, but it is expensive and, in large doses, may cause flulike symptoms.

Prevention is clearly a better approach. What is true about protecting yourself from AIDS is also true about protecting yourself from genital warts and other STDs (see the section on AIDS prevention later in this chapter).

Candidiasis (Moniliasis)

Unlike many of the other sexually transmitted diseases, which are caused by pathogens that come from outside the body, the yeastlike fungus caused by the *Candida albicans* organism normally inhabits the vaginal tract in most women. Only under certain conditions will these organisms multiply to abnormal quantities and begin to cause problems.

The likelihood of **candidiasis** (also known as moniliasis) is greatest if a woman has diabetes, if her immune system is overtaxed or malfunctioning, if she is taking birth control pills or other hormones, or if she is taking broadspectrum antibiotics. All of the above factors decrease the acidity of the vagina, making conditions more favorable for the development of a yeastlike infection.

Symptoms of candidiasis include severe vaginal itching, a white cheesy discharge, swelling of the vaginal tissue due to irritation, and a burning sensation. These symptoms are often collectively called **vaginitis**. When this microbe infects the mouth, whitish patches form, and the condition is referred to as thrush. This monilial infection also occurs in males and is easily transmitted between sexual partners.

Candidiasis strikes at least half a million American women a year. Antifungal drugs applied on the surface or by suppository usually cure the disease in just a few days. For approximately 1 out of 10 women, however, nothing seems to work, and the organism returns again and again. In patients with this chronically recurring infection, symptoms are often aggravated by contact of the vagina with soaps, douches, perfumed toilet paper, chlorinated water, and spermicides. Tight-fitting jeans and pantyhose can provide the combination of moisture and irritant the organism thrives on.

Trichomoniasis

Unlike many of the other STDs, **trichomoniasis** is caused by a protozoan. Although as many as half of the men and women in the United States may have this organism present, most remain free of symptoms until their bodily defenses are weakened. Both men and women may transmit the disease, but women are the more likely candidates for infection. The "trich" infection may cause a foamy, yellowish discharge with an unpleasant odor that may be accompanied by a burning sensation, itching, and painful urination. These symptoms are most likely to occur during or shortly after menstruation, but they can appear at any time or be absent altogether in an infected woman. Although usually transmitted by sexual contact, the "trich" organism may be easily spread by toilet seats, wet towels, or other items that have discharged fluids on them. You can also contract trichomoniasis by sitting naked on the bench of the dressing room of your local health spa or locker room. Treatment includes oral metronidazole, usually given to both sexual partners to avoid the possible "ping-pong" effect of repeated cross-infection so typical of the STDs.

General Urinary Tract Infections

Although *general urinary tract infections (UTIs)* can be caused by various factors, some forms are sexually transmitted. Any time invading organisms enter the genital area, there is a risk that they may travel up the urethra and enter the bladder. Similarly, organisms normally living in the rectum, urethra, or bladder may travel to the sexual organs and eventually be transmitted to another person.

You can also get a UTI through autoinoculation (transmission to yourself by yourself). This frequently occurs during the simple task of wiping yourself after defecating. Wiping from the anus forward may transmit organisms found in feces to the vaginal opening or to the urethra. Contact between the hands and the urethra and between the urethra and other objects are also common means of autoinoculation of bacterial and viral pathogens. Women, with their shorter urethras, are more likely to contract UTIs.

Treatment depends on the nature and type of pathogen. For minor infections, some practitioners recom-

---

Pubic lice: Parasites that can inhabit various body areas, especially the genitals; also called "crabs."

Venereal warts: Warts that appear in the genital area or the anus; caused by the human papilloma viruses (HPVs).

Candidiasis: Yeastlike fungal disease often transmitted sexually.

Vaginitis: Set of symptoms characterized by vaginal itching, swelling, and burning.

Trichomoniasis: Protozoan infection characterized by foamy, yellowish discharge and unpleasant odor.

mend drinking 8 to 10 glasses of fluids per day, particularly those high in acid, such as cranberry juice, to alter the acidity of the vagina in order to kill the pathogen. This treatment is considered worthless by some authorities, however, since it has been estimated that a person would have to drink over 4 quarts of cranberry juice a day over a period of several days to even begin to alter vaginal acidity. Considering the caloric intake, cost of the juice, and minimal effectiveness of this home treatment, you would probably be better off visiting a doctor and obtaining proven medications from a pharmacy.

Herpes

Herpes is a general term for a family of diseases characterized by sores or eruptions on the skin. Herpes infections range from mildly uncomfortable to extremely serious. One subcategory, *herpes simplex,* is caused by a virus. Herpes simplex virus type 1 (HSV-1) causes the cold sores and fever blisters that most of us have been afflicted with at one time or another. Although figures are difficult to come by, it is believed that four out of five adult Americans have herpes simplex type I (also called orofacial herpes) and that one out of six has genital herpes.[10]

Genital herpes, caused by *herpes simplex virus type 2,* is one of the most widespread STDs in the world. Typically, genital herpes is characterized by distinct phases. First, the herpes virus must gain entrance to the body, which it usually does through the mucous membranes of the genital area. Once these organisms invade, the victim will experience the *prodromal* (precursor) phase of the disease, which is characterized by a burning sensation and redness at the site of the infection. This phase is typically followed by the formation of a small blister filled with a clear fluid containing the virus. If you pick at this blister or otherwise spread this clear fluid by your hands, you can autoinoculate other body parts. Particularly dangerous is the possibility of spreading the infection to your eyes this way because a herpes lesion on the eye may cause blindness.

Over a period of days, this unsightly blister will crust, dry, disappear, and the virus will travel to the base of an affected nerve supplying the area and become dormant. Only when the victim becomes overly stressed, when diet is inadequate, when the immune system is overworked, or when there is excessive exposure to sunlight or other stressors will the virus reactivate (at the same site every

time) and begin the blistering cycle all over again. This cyclical recurrence can be painful, unsightly, and, most importantly, highly contagious. Fluids from these blisters may readily be transmitted to sexual partners. Through oral sex, herpes simplex type 2 may be transmitted to the mouth. Symptoms are similar to those of herpes simplex type 1. Figure 18.5 summarizes the herpes cycle.

Genital herpes is especially serious in pregnant women because of the danger of infecting the baby as it passes through the vagina during birth. For that reason, many physicians recommend cesarean deliveries for infected women. Additionally, women who have a history of genital herpes also appear to have a greater risk of developing cervical cancer.

The many myths and misconceptions surrounding this disease have greatly contributed to the stigma associated with it. Herpes is not only embarrassing, painful, and ugly, but it may also cause social ostracism based on a misunderstanding of the disease.

First, herpes is not a form of plague. It is a communicable disease for which no cure presently exists, but it is not transmissible all of the time. In fact, the only time

Genital herpes, a highly contagious sexually transmitted disease—for which no cure is currently available—is characterized by recurring cycles of painful blisters on the genitalia.

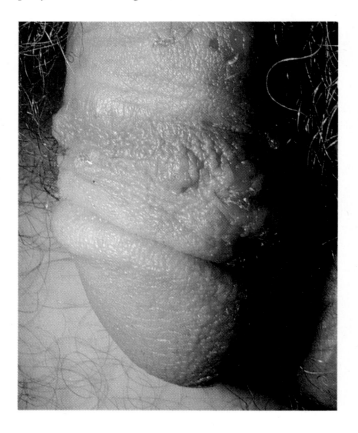

Genital herpes: STD caused by herpes simplex virus type 2.

Acquired immune deficiency syndrome (AIDS): Extremely virulent sexually transmitted disease that renders the immune system inoperative.

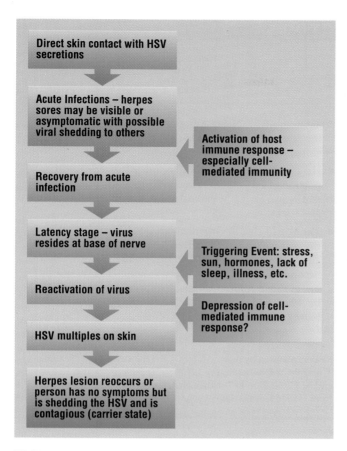

FIGURE 18.5

The Herpes Cycle

Source: Adapted by permission of J. B. Lippincott from "Sexually Transmitted Diseases in the 1990's," *STD Bulletin* 11 (1992): 4.

that sexual partners should refrain from contact is when active lesions are present. At other times, the risk of infection appears to be quite small, although viral shedding is possible.

Second, it is often just as necessary to treat the psychological problems of the herpes victim as it is to treat the physical symptoms. People with this disease often experience fear, frustration, depression, and a feeling that they have been dealt a "dirty blow" by someone. Counseling and support groups for herpes victims and their intimate partners have proved very effective.

Finally, although there is no cure for herpes at present, certain drugs have shown some success in reducing symptoms. Unfortunately, they only seem to work if the disease is confirmed during the first few hours after contact. As you may guess, this is rather rare. The effectiveness of other treatments, such as L-lysine, is largely unsubstantiated to date. Although lip balms and cold-sore medications may provide temporary anesthetic relief, it is useful to remember that rubbing anything on a herpes blister

may spread herpes-laden fluids to other tissues or, via the hands, to other body parts.

Preventing Herpes. If you are worried about contracting herpes, there are several precautions that you should take:

- Avoid any form of kissing if you notice a sore or blister on your partner's mouth. Kiss no one, not even a peck on the cheek, if you know that you have a herpes lesion. Allow a bit of time after the sores go away before you start kissing again.

- Be extremely cautious if you have casual sexual affairs. Not every partner will feel obligated to tell you that he or she may have a problem. Protecting against risk is up to you.

- Wash your hands immediately with soap and water after any form of sexual contact.

- If you have herpes, reduce the risk of a herpes episode by avoiding excessive stress, sunlight, or whatever else appears to trigger a herpes outbreak in you.

- If you have questionable sores or lesions, seek medical help at once. Do not be afraid to name your contacts.

- Since the herpes organism dies quickly upon exposure to air, toilet seats, soap, and similar sources are not likely means of transmission.

- If you have herpes, be responsible in your sexual contacts with others. If you have herpes lesions that might put your partner at risk, let that person know. Although it is not necessary to announce openly a herpes problem, use common sense in determining the appropriate time and place for a candid herpes discussion with your partner.

ACQUIRED IMMUNE DEFICIENCY SYNDROME (AIDS)

Acquired immune deficiency syndrome (AIDS) became the leading killer among Americans aged 25 to 44 as of January, 1995.[11] In 1994, 80,691 new AIDS cases were reported, for a total of over 440,000 U.S. AIDS cases since 1981.[12] To date, over 250,000 people have died of AIDS in the United States, and despite massive efforts aimed at prevention and treatment, the number of cases continues to rise.[13] AIDS is now the leading killer of young adults in 79 of the 169 U.S. cities with populations greater than 100,000, including such places as Bridgeport, Connecticut, Providence, Rhode Island, and Miami, Florida.[14] Overall, new AIDS cases being reported to the Centers for Disease Control and Prevention average about 20,000 every three months. Statistics show that rising incidence

The Global AIDS Picture: Grim and Worsening

AIDS has reached overwhelming proportions in some of the poorest countries of the world, far outstripping their governments' resources to deal with the situation. For example:

- Between 20 and 30 percent of all adults in eastern and central Africa are infected by HIV.

- HIV is now the major cause of loss of health and productivity in the average Third World city—surpassing the traditionally debilitating diseases such as malaria, gastroenteritis, and pneumonia.

- In Rwanda, half of all midwives trained in the last 10 years have died of AIDS.

- In one district in Uganda, one in three households is without parents because they have died of AIDS.

- In Kenya, half of the women seeking treatment for some other STD are HIV-positive.

- Worldwide, 75 percent of the 16 million people infected with HIV are heterosexual. Nearly 65 percent live in sub-Saharan Africa. North America (1.7 million), Latin America (1.4 million), and Africa account for 96 percent of global infections.

- Heterosexual transmission accounts for a growing proportion of HIV/AIDS cases in Europe and Latin America, and is increasing at explosive rates in parts of Thailand and India.

- The World Health Organization (WHO) projects that by the year 2000, up to 90 percent of all HIV infections globally will be transmitted heterosexually. Two women are becoming HIV infected every minute. The WHO estimates that 6 million women had been infected with HIV by 1994, and over 1 million of these women had full-blown AIDS.

Source: Adapted by permission of J. B. Lippincott from "Sexually Transmitted Diseases in the 1990s," *STD Bulletin* 11 (1992): 3–6; and by permission of Prentice Hall, Inc., Englewood Cliffs, N.J., from Gerald J. Stine, *AIDS Update, 1994–1995,* © 1995, 196–197.

of the disease has shifted from the gay male population to heterosexuals, women, African Americans, Hispanic Americans, and those living in the South and Northeast.[15]

Global estimates of the epidemic also present a rapidly worsening picture. Few regions of the world have been spared, and it is estimated that over 16 million people around the world have been infected.[16] The Multicultural Perspectives box gives some of the statistics concerning the global AIDS problem. Where did the disease originate? How is it contracted? What is the prognosis once a person is infected? What are the major risk factors? Can AIDS be prevented?

The Onset of AIDS

Researchers believe that the AIDS virus may actually have been present in the United States ever since the early 1950s, although medical and government officials did not note problems related to the disease until the spring of 1981. Suddenly, federal officials began to receive an increasing number of requests for an experimental drug used to treat a rare disease called *pneumocystis carinii*

Human immunodeficiency virus (HIV): The slow-acting virus that causes AIDS.

pneumonia (PCP). Caused by a protozoan, PCP appeared to be affecting significant numbers of previously healthy young homosexual males in New York and California.

At about the same time, increasing numbers of homosexual men in California were being diagnosed with a rare form of cancer known as *Kaposi's sarcoma.* These two groups of patients—those with PCP and those with Kaposi's sarcoma—tended to share many characteristics. They were typically white, homosexual, came from similar geographical regions, used specific types of drugs, and had generalized lymphadenopathy (chronic swelling of the lymph nodes) and general malfunctioning of the immune system. Because of the last problem, many of these people developed several diseases at the same time, making diagnosis of one underlying cause extremely difficult.

For many months, epidemiologists investigated possible causes of this apparent "gay plague," including the types of drugs used by many gay men and the water supplies in their communities. In 1984, two researchers, Robert C. Gallo at the National Cancer Institute in the United States and Luc Montagnier at the Pasteur Institute in Paris, independently isolated the retrovirus (a type of slow-acting virus) that causes AIDS. Initially called the human T-cell lymphotropic virus type III (HTLV-III) by most American researchers, this virus is today generally referred to as the **human immunodeficiency virus (HIV).**

Although during the early days of the epidemic it appeared that HIV infected only homosexuals, it quickly became apparent that the disease was not confined to groups of people but rather was related to high-risk behaviors such as promiscuous sex and sharing of intravenous needles.

New Definition, Increasing Numbers

Since 1981, when HIV infections were first noticed and the earliest victims began to die, the numbers of HIV-infected persons and AIDS-diagnosed individuals have skyrocketed. Recent expansions in the definition of AIDS will certainly cause these overall numbers to shoot up.

Under old definitions, people with HIV were diagnosed as having AIDS only when they developed blood infections, the blood vessel cancer known as Kaposi's sarcoma, or any of 21 other indicator diseases, most of which were common in male victims only. The Centers for Disease Control expanded the definition under pressure from AIDS activists and women's groups, who charged that the CDC was ignoring AIDS symptoms peculiar to drug-injecting individuals and women, thereby making it difficult for these people to obtain health insurance payments and federally funded health benefits. Thus, the new definition adds pulmonary tuberculosis, recurrent pneumonia, and invasive cervical cancer to the indicator list. Perhaps the most significant new indicator, however, is a dip in the level of the body's master immune cells, called CD4s, to 200 per cubic millimeter (that's one-fifth the level in a healthy person). It is estimated that 190,000 Americans have this low CD4 count and don't know it.[17] The average CD4 test runs $200, making it hard to afford for many people.

The true number of infected people may never be established. Currently, only 25 states require that HIV-positive individuals be reported to state health divisions by name; 10 other states require anonymous reporting; and 15 states do not require any reporting to state health officials. All states require reporting of AIDS cases by name at the local and state level.[18]

Women and AIDS: The Newest Epidemic

Homosexuals, drug-injecting individuals, prostitutes, children, promiscuous heterosexual males, Haitians, and other groups all had their turn in discussions of HIV and the AIDS epidemic during the 1980s. Now there is increasing realization that HIV is not an infection that certain groups get because of inherent group characteristics but rather an equal-opportunity pathogen that can attack anyone who engages in certain high-risk behaviors. If you engage in these high-risk behaviors, it doesn't matter who you are, what your race or socioeconomic status group may be, or what your sexual orientation is.

With this realization, the focus has finally fallen on the 50 percent of the population that was long ignored: women. These are a few of the facts that have emerged:

- Women are the fastest growing segment of the HIV population in the United States today.

- Women now make up over 13 percent of the total number of people with HIV infection in the United States.

- Worldwide, an estimated 3 million women will die of AIDS during the 1990s.

- In the United States, African-American women are at greatest risk, followed by white and then Latino women.[19]

- HIV/AIDS contracted by heterosexual transmission is increasing faster in rural America than in any other part of the country. Women most at risk are ethnic minorities and the poor.

- By the end of 1993, over 11 percent, or nearly 45,000 cases, of the total adult AIDS cases were among women. This number is expected to increase by nearly 18,000 cases by the end of 1994.

- Among sexually active teenagers, college students, and health-care workers nationwide, nearly 60 percent of the heterosexual spread of HIV is among women, usually as a result of contact with an injecting drug partner or with a partner whose HIV infection is unknown or unreported.[20]

- Contrary to popular beliefs, non-drug-using prostitutes in the United States play a small role in HIV transmission.

Compounding the problems of women with HIV are serious deficiencies in our health and social service systems, including inadequate treatment for women addicts and lack of access to child care, health care, and social services for families headed by single women.[21] Women with HIV/AIDS are of special interest because they are the major source of infection in infants. In 1993, about 95 percent of children up to four years of age infected with HIV got the virus from their mothers.[22]

Special Concerns of Women with HIV/AIDS. Although contracting HIV/AIDS is a serious problem for both males and females, women often have an even more difficult time protecting themselves from infection and taking care of themselves once they become ill. Traditionally, women have played a relatively passive role in taking responsibility for protection during sexual intercourse and in general sexual decision making, particularly in Third World countries. Efforts must be initiated to help women take more control of their sexual health and to participate actively in sexual decisions made with their sexual partners.[23]

Women, the fastest growing segment of the HIV population in the United States, not only carry the burden of their own health, but frequently that of a child infected before birth or at the time of delivery.

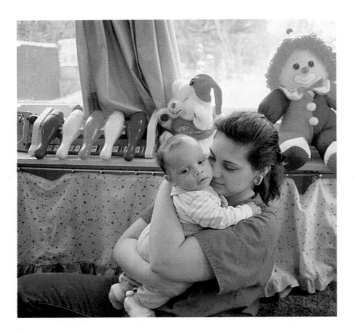

In addition, women often carry the responsibility for caring for their children or caring for others who may be infected with HIV or suffering from AIDS. If the mother's role as caretaker must be abandoned due to illness, family members often suffer. As a result, the mother may add a feeling of guilt to her already heavy burden. If the mother transmits HIV to her fetus, she will almost certainly feel even more guilt.[24]

Although increasing numbers of women are contracting HIV and developing AIDS worldwide, much of what we know about the clinical course of the disease, treatment modalities, and other AIDS-related topics has been determined from studies conducted on men. However, research following HIV progression in women and the effectiveness of certain treatments has been initiated. As more and more women become infected with HIV, national efforts aimed at prevention, intervention, and treatment will undoubtedly increase.

*W*HAT DO YOU THINK?

Why do you think HIV/AIDS is increasing among women and minority groups in America? Why are some women particularly vulnerable to diseases such as AIDS? What actions can we take as a nation to reduce the spread of HIV/AIDS among women and other minority groups? Why is the global HIV/AIDS epidemic of concern to Americans?

How HIV Is Transmitted

The HIV virus typically enters one person's body when another person's infected body fluids (semen, vaginal secretions, blood, etc.) gain entry through a breach in body defenses. Mucous membranes of the genital organs and the anus provide the easiest route of entry. If there is a break in the mucous membranes (as can occur during sexual intercourse, particularly anal intercourse), the virus enters and begins to multiply.

After initial infection, the HIV typically begins to multiply rapidly in the body, invading the bloodstream and cerebrospinal fluid. It progressively destroys helper T-lymphocytes, weakening the body's resistance to disease. The virus also changes the genetic structure of the cells it attacks. In response to this invasion, the body quickly begins to produce antibodies.

Despite some rather hysterical myths, HIV is not a highly contagious virus. Countless studies of people living in households with a person with HIV/AIDS have turned up no documented cases of HIV infection due to casual contact. Other investigations provide overwhelming evidence that insect bites do not transmit the HIV virus. The virus is actually quite selective in the way it transmits itself from person to person.

Engaging in High-Risk Behaviors. AIDS is not a disease of certain groups. People are not predestined to get the disease because they belong to a group or associate with a

The AIDS-causing HIV virus multiply rapidly after infection, weakening the body's resistance and changing the genetic structure of the cells it attacks.

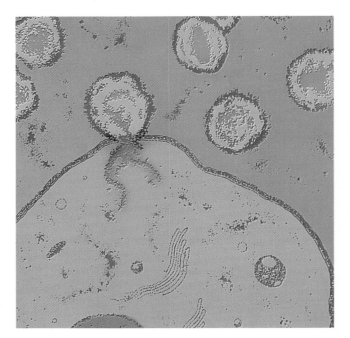

group. Thus, AIDS is not a gay disease, or a disease of minority groups, or Haitians, or any other class of people. It is a disease of certain high-risk behaviors. If you engage in the behavior, you increase your risk for the disease. If you don't engage in the behavior, your risk is minimal. Seems pretty simple, doesn't it? Unfortunately, the message has not gotten through to many Americans. They assume that because they are not homosexual, or do not do illegal drugs via injections, or do not have sex with prostitutes they are not at risk. They couldn't be more wrong. Anyone at any time who engages in unprotected sex with a person who has engaged in high-risk behaviors is at risk. It could be that handsome, clean-cut guy on the football team, or that wholesome-looking girl from a small rural city in the Midwest. If they've had sex with others, they may carry HIV. Promiscuous sex—in males and females of all ages, races, ethnic groups, sexual orientations, and socioeconomic conditions—is the greatest threat. A celibate or monogamous gay man or a drug-injecting woman who never shares her needles is at very low risk for HIV. But if they've had sex with anyone who's ever had sex with an injecting drug user, they could be infected. You can't tell by looking at them; you can't tell by questioning them, unless they've been tested recently and are HIV negative. So, what should you do? The Building Communication Skills box offers some direct advice.

Of course, the most simple answer is abstinence. If you don't exchange body fluids, you won't get the disease. As a second line of defense, if you decide to be intimate, the next best option is to use a condom. In spite of the message, in spite of all the educational campaigns, surveys consistently indicate that the vast majority of college-age people throw caution to the wind if they think they "know" someone—they have unprotected sex. Even when they do not know the individual involved, the majority have unprotected sex. Why do so many people act so irresponsibly when the outcome is potentially deadly? The answers to this question are unclear. It is probably a combination of ignorance, denial that it could be you who is HIV positive, a certain degree of apathy, and a bit of very real fear. People who are afraid often avoid testing. If they have symptoms, they may still avoid testing out of fear that they may be diagnosed positive and not have any real options for a cure. You must recognize what the risk factors are. The important thing to realize is that if you do not engage in activities that are known to spread the virus, your chances of becoming infected are extremely small. The following activities are high-risk behaviors.

Exchange of Body Fluids.   The exchange of HIV-infected body fluids during sexual intercourse is the greatest risk factor. Substantial research evidence indicates that blood, semen, and vaginal, cervical, and anal secretions are the major fluids of concern. Although the virus was found in 1 person's saliva (out of 71 people in a study population), most health officials state that saliva is not a

high-risk body fluid. But the fact that the virus has been found in saliva does provide a good rationale for using caution when engaging in deep, wet kissing.

Initially, public health officials also included breast milk in the list of high-risk fluids because a small number of infants apparently contracted HIV while breast-feeding. Subsequent research has indicated that HIV transmission could have been caused by bleeding nipples as well as by actual consumption of breast milk and other fluids. Infection through contact with feces and urine is believed to be highly unlikely though technically possible.

Receiving a Blood Transfusion prior to 1985.   A small group of people became infected with HIV as a result of having received a blood transfusion before 1985, when the Red Cross and other blood donation programs implemented a stringent testing program for all donated blood. Today, because of these massive screening efforts, the risk of receiving HIV-infected blood is almost nonexistent.

Injecting Drugs.   A significant percentage of cases of AIDS in the United States are believed to be the result of sharing or using HIV-contaminated needles. While illegal drug users are the people we usually think of as being in this category, it is important to remember that others may also share needles—for example, diabetics who inject insulin. People who share needles and also engage in sexual activities with members of high-risk groups, such as those who exchange sex for drugs, increase their risks dramatically.

Mother-to-Infant Transmission (Perinatal).   Approximately one in three of the children who have contracted AIDS received the virus from their infected mothers while in the womb or while passing through the vaginal tract during delivery.

Symptoms of AIDS

A person may go for months or years after infection by HIV before any significant symptoms appear. The incubation time varies greatly from person to person. Children have shorter incubation periods than do adults. Newborns and infants are particularly vulnerable to AIDS because human beings do not become fully immunocompetent (that is, their immune system is not fully developed) until they are 6 to 15 months old. New information suggests that some very young children show the "adult" progression of AIDS. In adults, the average length of time it takes the virus to cause the slow, degenerative changes in the immune system that are characteristic of AIDS is 8 to 10 years. During this time, the person may experience a large number of opportunistic infections (infections that gain a foothold when the immune system is not functioning effectively). Colds, sore throats, fever, tiredness, nausea, night sweats, and other generally non-life-threatening conditions commonly appear. People who show these

Communicating with Your Partner about HIV Infection

In the decade and a half since the identification of the first known cases of AIDS, what is and is not known about HIV disease has changed a great deal. As the scientific knowledge has grown, so has public understanding. Over the years, we've come to understand the destructive actions of the virus inside the human body, how the virus is transmitted from one person to another, and the importance of knowledge in fighting the disease. The more people learned about the disease, the more they realized that everyone was susceptible if they practiced unsafe behaviors.

Today we recognize that the more people know about how the virus is transmitted and the more they internalize personal susceptibility, the greater the chance that they will adopt safer behaviors. Yet, despite the millions of dollars spent on public awareness campaigns and AIDS education programs, the rate of infection continues to rise, particularly among women, members of minority groups, and young people. Many medical, education, and youth officials feel that the major obstacle to preventing HIV infection among young people is the discomfort most feel about discussing personal needs and feelings regarding HIV infection, AIDS, and practicing safer sex behaviors. For many young people, discussing HIV status and safer sex practices, such as condom use, can be uncomfortable. Some fear that raising the issue suggests lack of trust in the partner; others worry that safer behaviors will ruin their sexual enjoyment; and still others fail to recognize their personal vulnerability. As a result, a great many put themselves at risk for infection rather than hurt the other person's feelings. Therefore, a major goal in the fight against HIV infection is to improve the one-on-one communication between young people considering sexual intimacy. The following tips can help open the lines of communication about HIV infection.

- *Remember that you have a responsibility to your partner to disclose your status.* You also have a responsibility to yourself to do what needs to be done to stay healthy. Do not be afraid to ask your partner's HIV status. If either person's status is unknown, suggest going through the testing together as a means of sharing something important with each other.

- *Be direct, honest, and determined in talking about sex before you become involved.* Do not act silly or evasive. Get to the point, ask clear questions, and do not be put off re-

ceiving a response. Remember, a person who does not care enough to talk about sex probably does not care enough to take responsibility for his or her actions.

- *Discuss the issues without sounding defensive or accusatory.* Develop a personal comfort level with the subject prior to raising the issue with your partner. Be prepared with complete information and articulate your feelings clearly. Reassure your partner that your reasons for desiring abstinence or safer sex arise from respect and not distrust. Sharing feelings is easier in a calm, suspicion-free environment in which both people feel comfortable.

- *Encourage your partner to be honest and to share feelings.* This will not happen overnight. If you have never had a serious conversation with this person before you get into an intimate situation, you cannot expect honesty and openness when the lights go out.

- *Analyze your own beliefs and values ahead of time.* The worst thing you can do is to get yourself into an awkward situation before you have had time to think about what is important to you and what you believe in. Know where you will draw the line on certain actions, and be very clear with your partner about what you expect. If you believe that using a condom is necessary, make sure you communicate this to your partner.

- *Decide what you will do if your partner does not agree with you.* Anticipate your partner's potential objections or excuses and prepare your responses accordingly.

- *Ask questions about past history.* Although it may seem as though you are prying into another person's business, your own health future depends upon you knowing basic information about your partner's past. An idea of your partner's past sexual practices and use of drug injecting works is very valuable. Again, it is important to let your partner know why you are concerned and that you are not inquiring due to jealousy or other ulterior motives.

- *Ask about the significance of monogamy in your partner's relationships.* A basic question to ask before becoming involved in a regular sexual relationship is: "How important is a committed relationship to you?" You will need to decide early how important this relationship is to you and how much you are willing to work at arriving at an acceptable compromise on lifestyle.

combinations of symptoms have been described as having pre-AIDS symptoms.

Testing for HIV Antibodies

Once antibodies have begun to form in reaction to the presence of the HIV virus, a blood test known as the **ELISA** test may detect their presence. If sufficient antibodies are present, the ELISA test will be positive. When a

person who previously tested *negative* (no HIV antibodies present) has a subsequent test that is *positive,* seroconversion is said to have occurred. In such a situation, the person would typically take another ELISA test, followed by a more expensive, more precise test known as the **Western blot** to confirm the presence of HIV antibodies.

Although the ELISA is viewed as quite accurate, it is a conservative test in that it errs on the side of caution, meaning it produces a large number of *false positive re-*

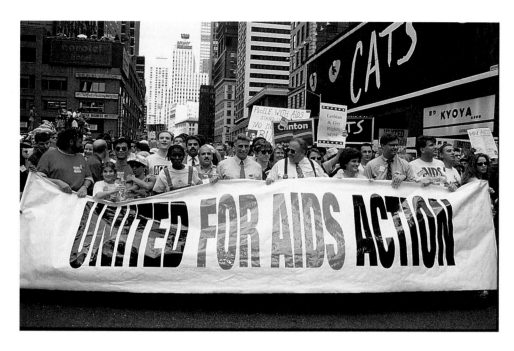

Numerous demonstrations by gay activists have successfully called attention to the need for AIDS research and treatment programs.

sults. It was deliberately designed to do this because it was intended as a test for screening the nation's blood supply. There have also been instances of *false negative results.* Some health professionals believe that there are chronic carriers of HIV who, for unknown reasons, continually show false negative results on both the ELISA and Western blot tests. This, of course, raises serious concerns about risks for these people's sexual partners. It should be noted that these tests are not AIDS tests per se. Rather, they detect antibodies for the disease, indicating the presence of the HIV in the person's system. Whether or not the person will develop AIDS depends to some extent on the strength of the immune system. However, the vast majority of all infected people does develop some form of the disease.

Treatment in the 1990s: New Hope

Although the list of possible anti-HIV agents has grown considerably in the last five years, many would-be cures remain on the unapproved list for human testing. Of those that have gained approval, *Zidovudine (AZT),* an anticancer drug known to delay the progress of the immunodeficiency that leads to AIDS, has had promising results. AZT also decreases the frequency of opportunistic infections and mental dysfunction. Clinical benefits may be apparent within six weeks of therapy, and continued treatment appears to prolong survival. But not all HIV-infected individuals can tolerate AZT treatments. Extreme nausea, headache, anemia, insomnia, and other side effects have forced many patients to seek alternative treatments.[25] Moreover, the cost of AZT treatment (about $6,400 per year) makes it prohibitively expensive for some patients.[26]

Newer forms of treatment include *ddI (29,39-dideoxyinosine),* a drug that blocks HIV reproduction with fewer side effects than seen with AZT; and *ddA (29,39-dideoxyadenosine)* and *ddC (29,39-dideoxycytidine),* chemicals that also fight HIV reproduction. *Pentamidine,* in both the injectable and aerosol forms, has been used to treat *pneumocystis carinii* pneumonia, the type of pneumonia that frequently attacks HIV-infected persons. The injected form of Pentamidine causes severe pain and other adverse effects, while the newer aerosol version is said to be less toxic.[27] In addition to these antiviral treatments, scientists are experimenting with immunomodulators, which regenerate or revitalize a failing immune system.[28]

Present methods of treatment have extended life in some patients, but these treatments are often tremendously costly, prompting close scrutiny by insurance companies. Consequently, testing for AIDS has become a fairly common requirement for applicants for life and health insurance policies in the United States.

Preventing HIV Infection

Although scientists have been searching for over a decade for a vaccine to protect people from HIV infection, they have had no success so far. The only effective prevention strategies known all closely relate to the means by which people contract AIDS. As we said earlier, it is not the mere

---

ELISA: Blood test that detects presence of antibodies to HIV virus.

Western blot: More precise test than the ELISA to confirm presence of HIV antibodies.

Reducing Your Risks for HIV Disease

HIV disease is not uncontrollable. HIV cannot, like cold or flu viruses, be caught casually. The transmission of HIV depends upon specific behaviors. Therefore, HIV infection can be prevented by following safe practices. The following list offers ways to reduce your risk for infection and limit the impact of the disease.

- Avoid casual sexual partners. Ideally, only have sex if you are in a long-term mutually monogamous relationship with someone who is equally committed to the relationship and whose HIV status is negative.

- Avoid unprotected intimate sexual activity involving the exchange of blood, semen, or vaginal secretions with people whose present or past behaviors put them at risk for infection. Do not be afraid to ask intimate questions about your partner's sexual past. You expose yourself to your partner's history whenever you choose to have sexual relations. Postpone sexual involvement until you are assured that he or she is not infected.

- All sexually active adults who are not in a lifelong monogamous relationship should practice safer sex by using latex condoms. Remember, however, that condoms still do not provide 100 percent safety.

- Never share injecting needles with anyone for any reason.

- Never share any devices through which the exchange of blood could occur, including needles, razors, tattoo instruments, any body-piercing instruments, and any other sharp objects.

- Avoid injury to body tissue during sexual activity. HIV can enter the bloodstream through microscopic tears in anal or vaginal tissues.

- Avoid unprotected oral sex or any sexual activity in which semen, blood, or vaginal secretions could penetrate mucous membranes through breaks in the membrane. Always use a condom or a dental dam during oral sex.

- Avoid using drugs that may dull your senses and affect your ability to make decisions about responsible precautions with potential sex partners.

- Wash your hands before and after sexual encounters. Urinate after sexual relations and, if possible, wash your genitals.

- Although total abstinence is the only absolute means of preventing the sexual transmission of HIV, abstinence can be a difficult choice to make. If you are in doubt about the potential risks of having sex, consider other means of intimacy, at least until you can assure your safety. Enjoyable and safer alternatives include massage, dry kissing, hugging, holding and touching, and masturbation (alone or with a partner).

- When receiving care from medical professionals such as dentists or doctors, make sure they take appropriate precautions to prevent potential transmission, including washing their hands and wearing gloves and masks. Be sure that all equipment used for treatment is properly sterilized.

- If you are worried about your own HIV status, have yourself tested rather than risk infecting others inadvertently.

- If you are a woman and HIV positive, you should take the steps necessary to ensure that you do not become pregnant.

- If you suspect that you may be infected or if you test positive for HIV antibodies, DO NOT donate blood, semen, or body organs.

---

fact of membership in a so-called high-risk group (homosexuals, prostitutes, intravenous drug users, etc.) that increases the probability of HIV infection but instead risky behaviors.

HIV infection and AIDS are not uncontrollable conditions. You can reduce your risks by the choices you make in sexual behaviors and the responsibilities you take for your health and for that of your loved ones. The Choices for Change box presents ways to reduce your risk for contracting HIV.

Because the status of your immune system is an important factor in whether or not you are susceptible to any of the STDs, it is important that you do everything possible to protect yourself. Adequate nutrition, sleep, stress management, vaccinations, and other preventive mainte-

nance activities can do a great deal to ensure your long-term health.

Where to Go for Help. If you are concerned about your possible risk or the risk of a close friend, arrange a confidential meeting with the health educator or other health professional at your college health service. He or she will provide you with the information that you need to decide whether you should be tested for HIV antibodies. If the student health service is not an option for you, seek assistance through your local public health department or community STD clinic. Local physicians, clergy members, counselors, professors, and other responsible people can often help you discover the answers you are looking for.

Managing Your Disease Risks

Infectious diseases pose serious challenges in the United States as well as throughout the world. In particular, sexually transmitted diseases, including HIV infection, present an increasing health risk to our nation's youth. All infectious diseases can be prevented by practicing safe and responsible behaviors. These are sensible steps you can take to avoid infectious diseases.

Making Decisions for You

Protecting yourself from infectious diseases is not always easy. Because most pathogens are microscopic, exposure to one can occur without your knowledge. Therefore, you need to be aware of your risks. What can you do to improve your own awareness of your potential exposure to disease-causing pathogens?

What are some actions you can take to reduce your risk of contracting a sexually transmitted disease, including HIV infection? What steps could you take right now to ensure the sexual health of your partners? Finally, if you thought you had been exposed to HIV, would you seek testing?

Checklist for Change: Making Personal Choices

✓ Be aware of factors that can threaten your health status.

✓ Know your disease and immunization history.

✓ Take the proper precautions to protect yourself from exposure to infectious pathogens.

✓ Know the health status of your intimate partners.

✓ Communicate openly and honestly with your partners about your feelings regarding sexual intimacy.

✓ If you have an infectious disease that can be spread through casual contact, remember to wash your hands frequently.

✓ Avoid traveling to places where outbreaks of infectious diseases have not been controlled.

✓ Maintain a healthy routine of sleep, nutrition, and exercise.

✓ Follow safe measures when around someone with an infectious disease.

✓ Cook foods at their appropriate temperatures.

✓ Respect the symptoms that indicate a possible infection and seek treatment immediately.

✓ Recognize your responsibility for the health of others.

✓ Behave in sexually responsible ways.

✓ Limit your sexual partners.

✓ Avoid using alcohol or other drugs during intimate sexual encounters.

✓ Assess your level of risk for acquiring an STD, including HIV infection.

✓ Respect the rights and needs of individuals affected by an infectious disease.

✓ Follow your physician's instructions completely when seeking help.

Checklist for Change: Making Community Choices

✓ Does your student health service offer testing for STDs? How about HIV?

✓ Is there a local free clinic where you could be tested for STDs or HIV?

✓ Do you support government spending for HIV research and health promotion (education)?

✓ Do you write your congressional representatives regarding your support of funding?

✓ Does your local school system offer a sex education curriculum including discussion about how to stop the spread of the HIV virus?

Critical Thinking

You have been in a relationship for several months that has grown from a nice friendship to a state of passionate sexual intimacy. During this time, a close and trusting bond has also developed. You have remained monogamous and believe that your partner has as well, although you have never discussed it. Nor has any discussion arisen about each other's sexual history or HIV status. You have been involved in sexual relationships in the past and have never been tested for HIV antibodies, and you're quite certain your partner is experienced as well. You trust your partner but recognize that, without complete information, you are both at risk for HIV infection. You want to take some precautionary steps but worry about insulting your partner's feelings.

Use the DECIDE model described in Chapter 1 to decide what you would do in this situation. Develop several different strategies and approaches for reaching the desired result.

Summary

◆ The major uncontrollable risk factors for contracting infectious diseases are heredity, age, and environmental conditions. The major controllable risk factors are stress, nutrition, fitness level, sleep, hygiene, avoidance of high-risk behaviors, and drug use.

◆ The major pathogens are bacteria, viruses, fungi, protozoa, and parasitic worms. Bacterial infections include staphylococcal infections, streptococcal infections, pneumonia, Legionnaire's disease, tuberculosis, periodontal diseases, and rickettsia. Major viruses include the common cold, influenza, infectious mononucleosis, hepatitis, mumps, chicken pox, measles, and rabies.

◆ Your body uses a number of defense systems to keep pathogens from invading. The skin is our major protection, helped by enzymes. The immune system creates antibodies to destroy antigens. In addition, fever and pain play a role in defending the body. Vaccines bolster the body's immune system against specific diseases.

◆ Sexually transmitted diseases are spread through intercourse, oral sex, anal sex, hand-genital contact, and sometimes through mouth-to-mouth contact. Major STDs include chlamydia, pelvic inflammatory disease, gonorrhea, syphilis, pubic lice, venereal warts, candidiasis, trichomoniasis, and herpes.

◆ Acquired immune deficiency syndrome (AIDS) is caused by the human immunodeficiency virus (HIV). HIV is not confined to certain high-risk groups. Anyone can get HIV by engaging in high-risk sexual activities that include exchange of body fluids, by having received a blood transfusion before 1985, and by injecting drugs (or having sex with someone who does). Your risk for AIDS can be cut by deciding not to engage in risky sexual activities.

Discussion Questions

1. What is a pathogen? What are the similarities and differences between pathogens and antigens? What are the uncontrollable risk factors that can threaten your health? What factors are controllable? What can be done to limit the effects of either type of risk factor?

2. What are the five types of pathogens? What are the various means by which they can be transmitted? How have social conditions among the poor and homeless increased the risks for certain diseases, such as tuberculosis, influenza, and hepatitis? Why are these conditions challenges to the efforts of public health officials?

3. What is the difference between active and passive immunity? How do they compare to natural and acquired immunity? Explain why it is important to wash your hands often when you have a cold.

4. Identify five sexually transmitted diseases. What are their symptoms? How do they develop? What are their potential long-term risks?

5. Why might it be inappropriate to identify groups as at high risk for HIV infection? Why might HIV infection be better referred to as a sexually transmissible disease than as a sexually transmitted disease?

Application Exercise

Reread the What Do You Think? scenarios at the beginning of this chapter and answer the following questions:

1. What was your initial reaction to each of the scenarios presented in the chapter opener?

2. What are some other legal issues that could arise or that already exist regarding all infectious diseases, including STDs? Why do the rights of all the individuals involved in these relationships need to be considered?

3. What services exist on your campus for people living with HIV infection or AIDS? What services focus on informing people about sexually transmitted diseases?

Jeffrey S. Nevid with Fern Gotfried, *Choices: Sex in the Age of STDs* (Boston: Allyn and Bacon, 1995).

Straightforward discussion of STDs. Geared toward college students.

Jeffrey S. Nevid with Fern Gotfried, *201 Things You Should Know about AIDS and Other Sexually Transmitted Diseases* (Boston: Allyn and Bacon, 1993).

Easy, enjoyable book gives you all the facts about STDs you need to be safe.

G. Stine, *Acquired Immune Deficiency Syndrome* (Englewood Cliffs, NJ: Prentice Hall, 1993).

Excellent text describing the biological, medical, social, and legal issues relating to HIV infection and the AIDS epidemic.

S. Rathus and S. Boughn, *AIDS: What Every Student Needs to Know* (New York: Harcourt Brace Jovanovich, 1993).

Readable college-level text designed to answer students' basic questions about HIV infection and other STDs.

J. Mann, D. Tarantola, and T. Netter, eds., *AIDS in the World: A Global Report* (Cambridge, MA: Harvard University Press, 1993).

A global consideration of the policies and issues surrounding the AIDS epidemic, including regional differences, cultural factors, and various methods of prevention, intervention, and control.

19

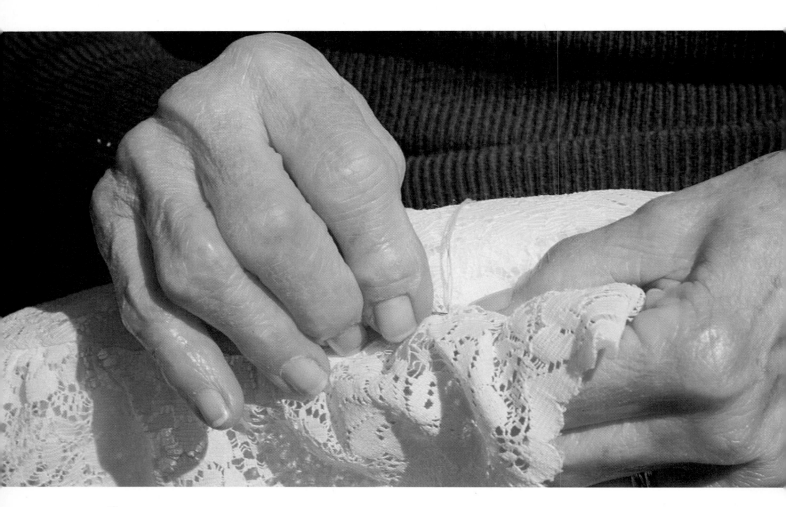

CHAPTER OBJECTIVES

◆ Discuss the respiratory disorders, including allergies, hay fever, asthma, emphysema, and chronic bronchitis.

◆ Explain the common neurological disorders, including the varied types of headaches and seizure disorders.

◆ Describe the common gender disorders, risk factors for these conditions, their symptoms, and methods of their control or prevention.

◆ Discuss diseases of the digestive system, including their symptoms, prevention, and control.

◆ Discuss the varied musculoskeletal diseases and their effects on the body.

◆ Describe chronic fatigue syndrome and job-related disorders.

Noninfectious Conditions

The Modern Maladies

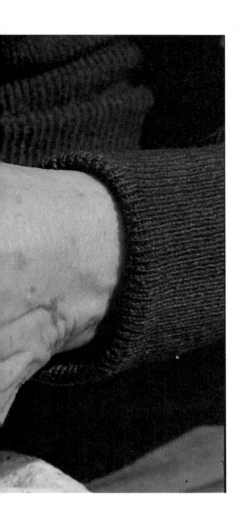

W H A T   D O   Y O U   T H I N K ?

Tom is an overweight, out-of-shape, 24-year-old. His father has type II diabetes and has been dependent on insulin for 10 years. His grandmother and grandfather are also diabetics. Tom realizes that he is at risk but finds it extremely difficult to maintain his weight and to exercise. He says that he is sure he'll become diabetic anyway, so he refuses to bother with trying to prevent the disease.

■ Why is Tom's rationale for not taking action to reduce the likelihood of getting diabetes justified or unjustified? As a friend, what actions could you take to help him? From a community health perspective, what actions can be taken to help him? If he gets sick, should the rest of society be forced to pay his medical bills? Why or why not? Where could Tom go on your campus to get help?

Bev, aged 65, suffers from self-diagnosed chronic fatigue syndrome. She complains that she is tired all the time, can't get through the day without a nap, and is ornery and nasty to her family. She nabs anyone who will listen to talk about her CFS problem.

■ What actions should Bev take to help herself? As a friend, what advice would you give her? Have any of your close friends been diagnosed by a physician with CFS? What do you know about this disease?

ypically, when we think of the major ailments and diseases affecting Americans today, we think of "killer" diseases such as cancer and heart disease. Clearly, these diseases make up the major portion of our life-threatening diseases—accounting for nearly two-thirds of all deaths. They're the ones we think of when we think of what Grandpa Joe or Aunt Martha died of, and the ones that strike fear in the hearts of those who are diagnosed. But although these diseases capture much of the media attention, other forms of chronic disease often cause substantial pain, suffering, and disability. Fortunately, the majority of these diseases can be prevented or their onset delayed.

To prevent the development of certain noninfectious and chronic diseases, we must identify the major common characteristics of these diseases. They are not transmitted by any pathogen or by any form of personal contact. They usually develop over a long period of time, and they cause progressive damage to human tissues. Although these conditions normally do not result in death, they do lead to illness and suffering for many people. Lifestyle and personal health habits appear to be major contributing factors to the general increase observed in the incidence of chronic diseases in the United States in recent years. Education, reasonable changes in lifestyle behaviors, and public health efforts aimed at prevention and control could minimize the effects of many of these diseases. In this chapter, we will discuss some of the more common forms of these diseases and the factors that contribute to them.

Allergy: Hypersensitive reaction to a specific antigen or allergen in the environment in which the body produces excessive antibodies to that antigen or allergen.

Histamines: Chemical substances that dilate blood vessels, increase mucous secretions, and produce other allergy-like symptoms.

Hay fever: A chronic respiratory disorder that is most prevalent when ragweed and flowers bloom.

Asthma: A chronic respiratory disease characterized by attacks of wheezing, shortness of breath, and coughing spasms.

RESPIRATORY DISORDERS

Allergy-Induced Problems

An **allergy** occurs as a part of the body's attempt to defend itself against a specific *antigen* or *allergen* by producing specific *antibodies*. When foreign pathogens such as bacteria or viruses invade the body, the body responds by producing antibodies to destroy these invading antigens. Under normal conditions, the production of antibodies is a positive element in the body's defense system. However, for unknown reasons, in some people the body overreacts by developing an overly elaborate protective mechanism against relatively harmless allergens or antigens. The resultant *hypersensitivity reaction* to specific allergens or antigens in the environment is fairly common, as anyone who has awakened with a runny nose or itchy eyes will testify. Most commonly, these hypersensitivity, or allergic, responses occur as a reaction to environmental antigens such as molds, animal dander (hair and dead skin), pollen, ragweed, or dust. Once excessive antibodies to these antigens are produced, they trigger the release of **histamines,** chemical substances that dilate blood vessels, increase mucous secretions, cause tissues to swell, and produce other allergylike symptoms (see Figure 19.1).

Although many people think of allergies as childhood diseases, in reality allergies tend to become progressively worse with time and with increased exposure to allergens. In these circumstances, allergic responses become chronic in nature, and treatment becomes difficult. Many people take allergy shots to reduce the severity of their symptoms with some success. In most cases, once the offending antigen has disappeared, allergy-prone people suffer few symptoms. Although allergies can cause numerous problems, one of the most significant effects is on the immune system. The Health Headlines box describes allergic reactions to some well-known plants.

Hay Fever

Perhaps the best example of a chronic respiratory disease is **hay fever.** Usually considered to be a seasonally related disease (most prevalent when ragweed and flowers are blooming), hay fever is common throughout the world. Hay fever attacks, which are characterized by sneezing and

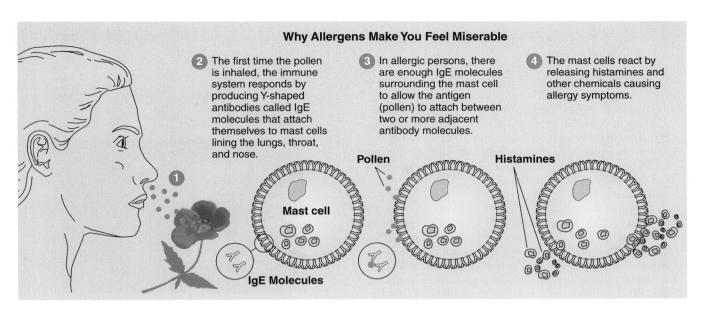

Why Allergens Make You Feel Miserable

2. The first time the pollen is inhaled, the immune system responds by producing Y-shaped antibodies called IgE molecules that attach themselves to mast cells lining the lungs, throat, and nose.

3. In allergic persons, there are enough IgE molecules surrounding the mast cell to allow the antigen (pollen) to attach between two or more adjacent antibody molecules.

4. The mast cells react by releasing histamines and other chemicals causing allergy symptoms.

Mast cell

Pollen

Histamines

IgE Molecules

FIGURE 19.1

Steps of an Allergy Response

itchy, watery eyes and nose, cause a great deal of misery for countless people. Hay fever appears to run in families, and research indicates that lifestyle is not as great a factor in developing hay fever as it is in other chronic diseases. Instead, an overzealous immune system and an exposure to environmental allergens including pet dander, dust, pollen from various plants, and other substances appear to be the critical factors that determine vulnerability. Moving from a rural area into a city or to an area of the country where spring flowers and pollen are less plentiful may provide relief from hay fever. For those people who are unable to get away from the cause of their hay fever response, medical assistance in the form of injections or antihistamines may provide the only possibility of relief.

Asthma

Unfortunately for many hay fever sufferers, their condition is often complicated by the development of another chronic respiratory disease, **asthma.** Asthma is characterized by attacks of wheezing, difficulty in breathing, shortness of breath, and coughing spasms. Although most asthma attacks are mild, they can trigger bronchospasms (contractions of the bronchial tubes in the lungs) of such a severe nature that, unless treatment is rapid, death may occur. Between attacks, most people have few symptoms.

In the majority of cases, asthma occurs in children under the age of 10, afflicting males nearly twice as often as females. Although many children outgrow the condition, a number of them suffer recurrences as adults.

Although exposure to allergens such as dust, pollen, and animal dander may trigger many asthmatic episodes,

emotional factors and excessive anxiety or stress can also trigger an attack. *Exercise-induced asthma (EIA)* is a type of asthma that has gained increasing attention. Friends who bow out of a long run or a tennis game by claiming to be allergic to exercise may not be joking. Track dynamo Jackie Joyner-Kersee, for example, is one of several Olym-

Prescription drugs, including inhalants, are more effective and safer in bringing relief to asthma sufferers than over-the-counter inhalers, which contain medicines that raise the pulse and stress the heart.

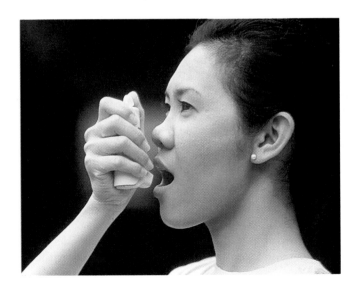

Poison Ivy and Poison Oak Alert

A common case of "poison ivy" may be a response to allergens produced by several different but related plants. If you live in the central or eastern part of the United States, you are more likely to come into contact with true poison ivy. In western states, you are more likely to come into contact with poison oak. In the South, the culprit may be poison sumac.

In each of these cases, your body comes into contact with the resin (an oily substance) from the leaves of the plant and has an allergic reaction. The more resin you are exposed to, the more likely it is that you will have a reaction. Thus exposed areas of the skin—ankles and wrists, for example—are more vulnerable than covered areas. Also, if you have been exposed before, your next reaction is likely to be more severe.

Can you get poison ivy through contact with anything other than the plants themselves? Yes. You can come into contact with the resin if you touch a dog after it has been exposed to the plant or if you touch clothing that has resin on it. Also, resin can be carried in the air, particularly by smoke from forest fires.

What to Do If You Are Exposed

- If you are exposed to any of these plants, wash the affected area with cool water. Avoid spreading the resin to other parts of your body.

- Using soap is not advised because it may spread the oil to other areas.

- Applying rubbing alcohol to the affected area after washing with water may help remove any remaining resin.

- If you know that you have been exposed to one of these plants, you can receive oral or injected steroid treatments before blisters develop.

- Once blisters form, the best treatment is calamine lotion, which helps to dry the blisters and to prevent any further spread of the resin.

Prescription pills that contain resinlike substances designed to help immunize you against future outbreaks are available. However, these pills often have side effects or are ineffective.

The best method of prevention is to avoid areas known to have poison ivy plants and to wear appropriate clothing when in these areas to avoid contact with the resin.

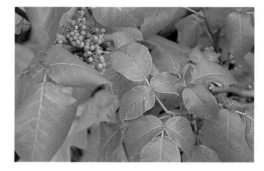

Poison Ivy

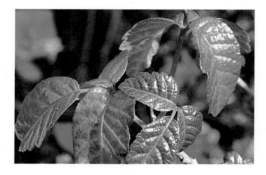

Poison Oak

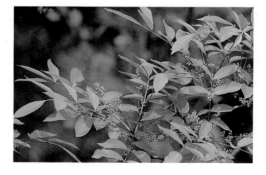

Poison Sumac

pians who have racked up gold medals despite allergies to exercise.

Doctors do not know what causes EIA or understand its exact connection with allergies. Some athletes without other allergies have EIA, and 35 percent of people with allergies and 90 percent of people with both allergies and asthma suffer from it.[1] It is known that histamines are a factor in EIA.

Those who suspect that they have exercise allergies can find out easily by describing the symptoms to an allergist or sports-medicine doctor, who may perform some simple lung-function tests. Once EIA is diagnosed, breathing easy is no sweat. Cold, dry air is a major cause of EIA, so keeping the air in your lungs moist could stave off an attack. Warming up for at least 10 minutes before working out and breathing through your nose also help. Runners, cross-country skiers, and other outdoor athletes can wear a scarf or light mask or consider changing sports. The warm, moist air around swimming pools is one of the best environments for asthmatics.

Relaxation techniques appear to help some asthma sufferers. Drugs may be necessary for serious cases. Doctors warn against using over-the-counter inhalers because the medication in them wears off quickly, raises the pulse rate, and stresses the heart. New prescription drugs such as Seldane, inhalers containing albuterol, and Cromolyn, appear to work better than OTC products and without serious side effects. Determining the specific allergen that provokes asthma attacks and taking steps to reduce your exposure, avoiding triggers such as exercise or stress, and finding the most effective medications are big steps in asthma prevention and control.

Emphysema

If you have ever seen someone hooked up to an oxygen tank and struggling to breathe while climbing a flight of stairs or listened to someone gasping for air for no apparent reason, you have probably witnessed an emphysemic episode. **Emphysema** involves the gradual destruction of the **alveoli** (tiny air sacs) of the lungs. As the alveoli are destroyed, the affected person finds it more and more difficult to exhale. The victim typically struggles to take in a fresh supply of air before the air held in the lungs has been expended. The chest cavity gradually begins to expand, producing the barrel-shaped chest characteristic of the chronic emphysema victim.

The exact cause of emphysema is uncertain. There is, however, a strong relationship between the development of emphysema and long-term cigarette smoking and exposure to air pollution. Victims of emphysema often suffer discomfort over a period of many years. What we all take for granted—the easy, rhythmic flow of air in and out of our lungs—becomes a continuous struggle for people with emphysema. Inadequate oxygen supply, combined with the stress of overexertion on the heart, eventually takes its toll on the cardiovascular system and leads to premature death. Unfortunately, there is little that can be done to reverse the effects of the disease. Emphysema and other chronic respiratory diseases are often classified as chronic obstructive pulmonary diseases (COPDs) by health officials. Collectively, the COPDs are the fifth leading cause of death in the United States.

Chronic Bronchitis

Although often dismissed as "smoker's cough" or a bad case of the common cold, **chronic bronchitis** may be a serious, if not life-threatening, respiratory disorder. In this ailment, the bronchial tubes become so inflamed and swollen that normal respiratory function is impaired. Symptoms of chronic bronchitis include a productive cough and shortness of breath that persist for several weeks over the course of the year. Cigarette smoking is the major risk factor for this disease, although fumes, dust, and particulate matter in the air are also contributing factors. Victims of chronic bronchitis must often use respiratory devices similar to those used by emphysema patients. They must also avoid those factors, such as cigarettes, that contributed to the development of bronchitis. Bronchitis coupled with a severe cold may be serious enough to warrant obtaining immediate medical attention.

---

*W*HAT DO YOU THINK?

Which of the respiratory diseases described in this section do you or your family have problems with? Do you have risk factors for any of these problems? Why do you think that COPDs tend to be among the leading causes of death in the United States? What actions can you and/or the people in your community take to reduce risks/problems from these diseases?

---

*N*EUROLOGICAL DISORDERS

Headaches

Almost all of us have experienced the agony of at least one major headache in our lives, whether it be of the mild, throbbing variety or the severe, pounding ache that makes us nauseated or dizzy. Not all headaches are equal; more important, it's possible that not all headaches have the same cause, although some headache experts suggest that all serious headaches share the same basic causes but fall

---

Emphysema: A respiratory disease in which the alveoli become distended or ruptured and are no longer functional.

Alveoli: Tiny air sacs of the lungs.

Chronic bronchitis: A serious respiratory disorder in which the bronchial tubes become so inflamed and swollen that respiratory function is impaired.

along a spectrum, with ordinary tension headaches at one end and full-blown migraines at the other.[2] Headaches may result from dilated blood vessels within the brain, underlying organic problems, or excessive stress and anxiety. The following are the most common forms of headaches and the most effective methods of treatment.

Tension Headache. Tension headaches are generally caused by muscle contractions or tension in the neck or head. This tension may be caused by actual strain placed on neck or head muscles due to overuse, static positions held for long periods of time, or tension triggered by stress. Recent research indicates that tension headaches may be a product of a more "generic mechanism" in which chemicals deep inside the brain may cause the muscular tension, pain, and suffering often associated with an attack. Triggers for this chemical assault may be red wine, lack of sleep, fasting, menstruation, or other factors, and the same symptoms (sensitivity to light and sound, nausea, and/or throbbing pain) may be characteristic of different types of headaches. Symptoms may vary in intensity and duration. Relaxation, hot water treatment, and massage have surfaced as the new "holistic treatments," while aspirin, Tylenol, Aleve, and Advil are the old standby forms of pain relief. Although such painkillers may bring temporary relief of symptoms, it is believed that, over

Tension headaches are triggered by many factors, including lack of sleep, stress, and strain on head and neck muscles.

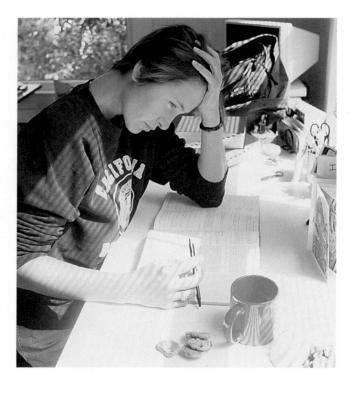

time, the drugs may dull the brain's own pain-killing weapons and result in more headaches rather than fewer.

Migraine Headache. If you've ever experienced pulsating pain on one side of the head in combination with dizzy spells, nausea, and a severe intolerance for light and noise, you are probably one of the more than 20 percent of Americans (mostly females) who suffer from **migraine.** Many of these migraine sufferers experience the appearance of an "aura" in their visual field, a red flag that a bad headache will soon follow. Some aura victims become disoriented, but for most the aura affects only their vision, and they may see stars, sparks, or zigzag lines and experience blind spots.[3] Many migraine victims suffer excruciatingly painful, recurring headaches that last for minutes, hours, or even days. The pain often tends to worsen over time. In some cases, migraine headaches are so severe that the person is unable to work or to continue normal activity.

While past research has focused on an unusual alternating dilation and constriction of blood vessels in the brain as a possible cause of migraine attacks, more recent thinking questions this theory. If the dilation causes vessels to press against nerves and inflict pain, why aren't joggers, people who take lots of hot baths, and other people prone to vessel dilation more susceptible to such headaches? Many believe that the answer to this question is that the key to the origin of migraines lies in the cortex of the brain. According to Harvard University neurology professor Michael Moskowitz, triggers, such as caffeine or wine, set off an electrical ripple on the surface of the cortex. Waves of nerve cells fire and then go quiet, creating an aura. This spurs a reaction in the meninges, the membranes above the cortex. The meninges contain endings of the brain's major nerve, the *trigeminus,* which release chemicals that inflame nearby tissues. The result is pain.[4]

Other doctors believe that pain signals start deep in the brain in areas normally rich in the painkilling chemical serotonin. Migraines are started by disturbances that keep the pain-regulating chemicals from doing their jobs. Susceptibility to these disturbances may be hereditary. This theory would explain why drugs that interact with serotonin work to reduce headaches. (It must be said that there is no proof that serotonin irregularities cause headaches, only that serotonin drugs work.)[5]

When true migraines occur, relaxation is only minimally effective as a treatment. Often, strong pain-relieving drugs prescribed by a physician are necessary. In 1994, the FDA approved Imitrex, a new drug tailor-made for migraines that works for about 80 percent of those who try it. But the cost of a single dose is a stunning $35 and second doses are often needed. In addition, its side effects make Imitrex inappropriate for anyone having uncontrolled high blood pressure or heart disease.

Secondary Headaches. Secondary headaches arise as a result of some other underlying condition. A good example is a person with a severe sinus blockage that causes pressure in the sinus cavity. This pressure may induce a headache. Hypertension, allergies, low blood sugar, diseases of the spine, the common cold, poorly fitted dentures, problems with eyesight, and other types of pain or injury can trigger this condition. Relaxation and pain relievers such as aspirin are of little help in treating secondary headaches. Rather, medications or other therapies designed to relieve the underlying organic cause of the headache must be included in the treatment regimen.

Psychological Headaches. With this type of headache, the "it's all in your head" diagnosis may, in fact, be correct. Rather than having a physical cause, psychological headaches stem from anxiety states, depression, and other emotional factors.

How do these headaches differ from tension headaches? Although it can be difficult to distinguish between the two, psychological headaches result from the stress of severe emotional disturbances, particularly depression. Unlike tension headaches, no muscles or blood vessels appear to be involved, thereby making relaxation and painkillers virtually worthless as treatment.

Victims of depression-related headaches tend to suffer from sleep disturbances and to experience symptoms over a period of years. Only therapy designed to treat the underlying depression or emotional problem appears to be effective in reducing the headache. Depression-related headaches, like all headaches, may indicate a more serious underlying condition. If severe headaches do not improve with aspirin or relaxation techniques, persist for more than three days, or are accompanied by visual disturbances, nausea, speech difficulties, numbness or tingling in the face or limbs, you should see your doctor.

Seizure Disorders

The word **epilepsy** is derived from the Greek *epilepsia,* meaning "seizure." Reports of epilepsy appeared in Greek medical records as early as in 300 B.C. Ancient peoples interpreted seizures as invasions of the body by evil spirits or as punishments by the gods. Although much of the mystery surrounding epileptic seizures has been solved in recent years, the stigma and lack of understanding remain. Approximately 1 percent of all Americans suffer from some form of seizure-related disorder.

These disorders are generally caused by abnormal electrical activity in the brain and are characterized by loss of control of muscular activity and unconsciousness. Symptoms vary widely from person to person.

There are several forms of seizure disorders, the most common of which are:

1. *Grand mal, or major motor seizure:* These seizures are often preceded by a shrill cry or a seizure aura (body sensations such as ringing in the ears or a specific smell or taste that occurs prior to a seizure). Convulsions and loss of consciousness generally occur and may last from 30 seconds to several minutes or more. Keeping track of the length of time elapsed is one aspect of first aid.

2. *Petit mal, or minor seizure:* These seizures involve no convulsions. Rather, a minor loss of consciousness that may go unnoticed occurs. Minor twitching of muscles may take place, usually for a shorter time than the duration of grand mal convulsions.

3. *Psychomotor seizure:* These seizures involve both mental processes and muscular activity. Symptoms may include mental confusion and a listless state characterized by such activities as lip smacking, chewing, and repetitive movements.

4. *Jacksonian seizure:* This is a progressive seizure that often begins in one part of the body, such as the fingers, and moves to other parts, such as the hand or arm. Usually only one side of the body is affected.

Theories concerning the factors that predispose a person to seizure disorders are varied. About half of all cases are of unknown origin. Head injury or trauma is one possible cause; other causes include congenital abnormalities, injury or illness resulting in inflammation of the brain or spinal column, drug or chemical poisoning, tumors, nutritional deficiency, and heredity.

In the majority of cases, people afflicted with seizure disorders can lead normal, seizure-free lives when under medical supervision. Epilepsy is seldom fatal. The greatest risk for epileptics whose seizures are uncontrolled is motor vehicle or other accidents. Anticonvulsant drugs such as phenobarbital, phenytoin (Dilantin), and primidone (Mysoline) have helped victims to lead normal lives in the absence of a definitive cure. Driving automobiles and other activities are usually not restricted for people whose seizures are medically controlled. In spite of massive campaigns to educate the public about the facts that epileptics are not psychologically unstable, lacking in intelligence, or otherwise abnormal, many people are still afraid to hire those with seizure disorders and discriminate against them in numerous other ways. Public ignorance about these disorders is one of the most serious obstacles confronting victims of seizure disorders. Improvements in medication and surgical interventions to

---

Migraine: A condition characterized by localized headaches that result from alternating dilation and constriction of blood vessels.

Epilepsy: A neurological disorder caused by abnormal electrical brain activity; can be accompanied by altered consciousness or convulsions.

reduce some causes of seizures are among the most promising treatments today.

Giving First Aid for Seizures. There are several things you can do to help seizure victims during their seizures and as they recover.

1. *Note the length of the attack.* Seizures in which a person remains unconscious for long periods of time should be monitored closely. If medical help arrives, be sure to tell the medical personnel how long it has been since the person became unconscious.

2. *Remove obstacles that may harm the victim.* Because seizure victims may lose motor control during a convulsion, they inadvertently thrash around, hitting objects in their way. To reduce the chances of serious injury, clear away any objects that may pose a threat to the victim.

3. *Loosen clothing and turn the victim's head to the side.* To ensure adequate ventilation, loosen clothing around the victim's neck and turn the head to the side to ensure that any fluids or vomit will drain from the mouth.

4. *Do not force objects into the victim's mouth.* Although seizure victims may bite their tongues, causing possible damage, they will not swallow them. If the victim's mouth has been clamped shut, forcing objects into the mouth may break teeth or cause more serious damage than would have occurred if you had done nothing.

5. *Get help.* After you have completed the above steps, get help or send someone for help. This is particularly important if the victim does not regain consciousness within a few minutes.

6. *Reassure the victim.* In too many instances, the seizure victim regains consciousness only to face a crowd of staring people. When administering first aid, try to dissuade curious bystanders from hanging around. Reassure the victim that you are not shocked or otherwise upset by the seizure episode.

7. *Allow the victim to rest.* After a seizure, many victims will be exhausted and may want to sleep. Allow them to do so if possible.

WHAT DO YOU THINK?

Do you suffer from recurrent headaches or other neurological problems? What do you think are the major causes of your problems? What actions might you take to reduce your risks and/or symptoms?

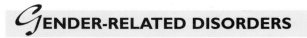

GENDER-RELATED DISORDERS

Fibrocystic Breast Condition

Fibrocystic breast condition is a common, noncancerous problem among women in the United States. Symptoms range in severity from a small palpable lump to large masses of irregular tissue found in both breasts. The underlying causes of the condition are unknown. Although some experts believe it to be related to hormonal changes that occur during the normal menstrual cycle, many women report that their conditions neither worsen nor improve during their cycles. In fact, in most cases, the condition appears to run in families and to become progressively worse with age, irrespective of pregnancy or other hormonal disruptions. Although the majority of these cyst formations consists of fibrous tissue, some are filled with fluid. Treatment often involves removal of fluid from the affected area or surgical removal of the cyst itself.

Does fibrocystic breast condition predispose a woman to later cancer development? Experts believe that the risks for breast cancer among women with certain types of fibrocystic disease may be slightly higher than among the general populace, but it is likely that a host of other factors, discussed in detail in Chapter 17, present much greater risks.

Premenstrual Syndrome (PMS)

Premenstrual syndrome (PMS), a syndrome describing a series of characteristic symptoms that occur prior to menstruation in some women, has generated a great deal of controversy in recent years. Although the monthly problems experienced by many women have been discussed for decades, they were largely dismissed as insignificant until the 1980s. Psychiatrists and other mental health professionals who convened for a major conference in 1986 refused, after much debate, to classify PMS as a psychiatric disorder, although they did agree that it was a problem that merited consideration. PMS is currently "provided for further study" as a psychiatric disorder in the American Psychiatric Association's *Diagnostic and Statistical Manual of Mental Disorders, Fourth Edition* (DSM-IV).

Why the sudden interest in PMS? What are its typical signs and symptoms? Why has a women been acquitted of murder by claiming PMS as her defense? How legitimate are these claims? As psychologist Carol Tavris points out in her book *The Mismeasure of Woman,* PMS as a diagnosis has been around for most of the century. During times when women have been needed in the work force, such as during the world wars, PMS was never considered a factor. But whenever women began to make inroads into the

Speaking Out on PMS

Psychologist Carol Tavris provides an excellent discussion of PMS in her book The Mismeasure of Woman. *In the following passage, she suggests why the concept of PMS is so widely accepted:*

Many institutions and individuals now benefit from the concept of PMS. Biomedical researchers, medical schools, and drug companies profit financially. Gynecologists, many of whom have closed their obstetrical services because of malpractice insurance costs, have lost a traditional source of income and are turning to new patient groups and new diagnoses for replenishment. Many psychiatrists have shifted from conducting long-term psychotherapy to prescribing short-term (repeatable) drug treatments. Indeed, obstetricians and psychiatrists are already engaging in turf wars over who is best suited to diagnose and treat all those women with premenstrual symptoms.

But the success of PMS is not entirely a conspiracy of big institutions, although, as [psychologist Mary Brown] Parlee says, if PMS didn't exist as a "psychologically disturbing, socially disruptive, biologically caused disease" they would have needed to invent it. (They did.) We must also ask why so many women have responded so favorably to the term and use it so freely. Parlee suggests that "the language of 'PMS' is a means by which many women can have their experiences of psychological distress, or actions they do not understand, validated as 'real' and taken seriously." In that sense the language of PMS is empowering for women, she believes, because it gives a medical and social reality to experiences that were previously ignored, trivialized, or misunderstood.

Like all good psychological diagnoses, then, PMS cuts two ways: It validates women, but it also stigmatizes them. Psychiatrist Leslie Hartley Gise directs a PMS program at Mt. Sinai Hospital in New York, yet she too is worried about the stigmatizing effects of making PMS a psychiatric diagnosis. "If even the rumor that [presidential candidate] Michael Dukakis had undergone treatment for depression could be held against him," Gise told an interviewer, "think of what a PMS diagnosis would mean for a woman seeking public office."

Source: Reprinted by permission of Simon & Schuster, Inc., and Lescher & Lescher from *The Mismeasure of Woman,* p. 143, by Carol Tavris. Copyright © 1992 by Carol Tavris. (Footnotes omitted.)

work force (after the world wars and during the 1970s), the effect of PMS on female work performance has become an issue. Tavris points out that in 1964, only one medical journal article was written on PMS; in 1976 the number was 146; in 1988 the number was 305. As women make further gains in the work force, Tavris predicts we will continue to hear more about PMS.[6] The Building Communication Skills box has more on Tavris's view of PMS.

So just what is PMS? Premenstrual syndrome is characterized by as many as 150 possible physical and emotional symptoms that vary from person to person and from month to month. These symptoms usually appear a week to 10 days preceding the menstrual period and affect between 20 and 40 percent of U.S. women of menstruating age to some degree. They include depression, tension, irritability, headaches, tender breasts, bloated abdomen, backache, abdominal cramps, acne, fluid retention, diarrhea, and fatigue. It is believed that women who have PMS develop a predictable pattern of symptoms during the menstrual cycle and that the severity of their symptoms may be influenced by external factors, such as stress.

Women usually experience PMS for the first time after the age of 20, and it may remain a regular part of their re-

productive life unless they seek treatment. For many women, the first day of their period brings immediate relief. For others, the depressive symptoms persist all month and are only heightened prior to the menstrual period.

Most authorities believe that the most plausible cause of PMS is a hormonal imbalance related to the rise in estrogen levels preceding the menstrual period. This theory is substantiated by the fact that women with PMS who are given prescriptions for progesterone often experience relief of symptoms. Critics of this theory argue that controlled research has not yet been conducted on the effects of progesterone on PMS.

Common treatments for PMS include hormonal therapy in addition to drugs and behaviors designed to relieve

Fibrocystic breast condition: A common, noncancerous condition in which a woman's breasts contain fibrous or fluid-filled cysts.

Premenstrual syndrome (PMS): A series of physical and emotional symptoms that may occur in women prior to their menstrual periods.

the symptoms. These include aspirin for pain, diuretics for fluid buildup, decreases in caffeine and salt intake, increases in complex carbohydrate intake, stress reduction techniques, and exercise.

Endometriosis

Whether the incidence of **endometriosis** is on the rise in the United States or whether the disorder is simply attracting more attention is difficult to determine. Victims of endometriosis tend to be women between the ages of 20 and 40. Symptoms include severe cramping during and between menstrual cycles, irregular periods, unusually heavy or light menstrual flow, abdominal bloating, fatigue, painful bowel movements with periods, painful intercourse, constipation, diarrhea, menstrual pain, infertility, and low back pain. What is this disease? What causes it? What are the common methods of treatment?

Although much remains unknown about the causes of endometriosis, we do know that the disease is characterized by the abnormal growth and development of endometrial tissue (the tissue lining the uterus) in regions of the body other than the uterus. Among the most widely accepted theories concerning the causes of endometriosis are the transmission of endometrial tissue to other regions of the body during surgery or through the birthing process; the movement of menstrual fluid backward through the fallopian tubes during menstruation; and abnormal cell migration through body-fluid movement. Women with cycles shorter than 27 days and those with flows lasting over a week are at increased risk. The more aerobic exercise a woman engages in and the earlier she starts, the less likely she is to develop endometriosis.

Treatment of endometriosis ranges from bed rest and reduction in stressful activities to **hysterectomy** (the removal of the uterus) and/or the removal of one or both ovaries and the fallopian tubes. Recently, physicians have been criticized by some segments of the public for being too quick to select hysterectomy as the treatment of choice. More conservative treatments that involve dilation and curettage, surgically scraping endometrial tissue off the fallopian tubes and other reproductive organs, and combinations of hormone therapy have become more acceptable in most regions of the country. Hormonal treatments include gonadotropin-releasing hormone (GnRH) analogs, various synthetic progesterone-like drugs (Provera), and oral contraceptives. The drugs most commonly used by specialists—danazol and the GnRH analogs—are very expensive. Once the patient stops using them, the condition recurs.

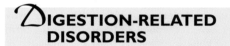

WHAT DO YOU THINK?

Which of the preceding health problems do you think causes the most problems for women in the United States? Are these problems related to stigma associated with the condition, the condition's physiological effects, or psychological in nature? What actions should be taken to increase awareness and understanding of these conditions?

DIGESTION-RELATED DISORDERS

Diabetes

In healthy people, the *pancreas,* a powerful enzyme-producing organ, produces the hormone **insulin** in sufficient quantities to allow the body to use or store glucose (blood sugar). When this organ fails to produce enough insulin to regulate sugar metabolism or when the body fails to use insulin effectively, a disease known as **diabetes** occurs. Diabetics exhibit **hyperglycemia,** or elevated blood sugar levels, and high glucose levels in their urine. Other symptoms include excessive thirst, frequent urination, hunger, tendency to tire easily, wounds that heal slowly, numbness or tingling in the extremities, changes in vision, skin eruptions, and, in women, a tendency toward vaginal yeast infections.

Of the estimated 15 million diabetics in the United States today, nearly 6 million are unaware that they have a problem. Many diabetics remain ignorant of their condition until they begin to show overt symptoms. How does a person become diabetic? The more serious form, known as type 1 (insulin-dependent) diabetes or diabetes mellitus, usually begins early in life. Type 1 diabetics typically must depend on insulin injections or oral medications for the rest of their lives because insulin is not present in their bodies. Adult-onset (noninsulin-dependent), or type 2 diabetes, in which insulin production is deficient, tends to develop in later life. These diabetics can often control the symptoms of their disease, with minimal medical inter-

---

Endometriosis: Abnormal development of endometrial tissue outside the uterus resulting in serious side effects.

Hysterectomy: Surgical removal of the uterus.

Insulin: A hormone produced by the pancreas; required by the body for the metabolism of carbohydrates.

Diabetes: A disease in which the pancreas fails to produce enough insulin or the body fails to use insulin effectively.

Hyperglycemia: Elevated blood sugar levels.

Ulcerative colitis: An inflammatory disorder that affects the mucous membranes of the large intestine, producing bloody diarrhea.

Are You at Risk for Diabetes?

Certain characteristics tend to place people at greater risk for the development of diabetes. Nevertheless, many people remain unaware of the symptoms of diabetes until after the disease has begun to progress. If you answer yes to several of the following questions, you should consider seeking medical advice about your symptoms and degree of risk. Talk to health professionals at your student health center, or make an appointment with your family physician.

1. Do you have a history of diabetes in your family?

2. Do any of your primary relatives (mother, father, sister, brother, grandparents) have diabetes?

3. Are you overweight or obese?

4. Are you typically sedentary (seldom, if ever, engage in vigorous aerobic exercise)?

5. Have you noticed an increase in your craving for water or other beverages?

6. Have you noticed that you have to urinate more frequently than you used to during a typical day?

7. Have you noticed any tingling or numbness in your hands and feet, which might indicate circulatory problems?

8. Do you often feel a gnawing hunger during the day, even though you usually eat regular meals?

9. Have you noticed that you are losing weight but don't seem to be doing anything in particular to make this happen?

10. Are you often so tired that you find it difficult to stay awake to study, watch television, or engage in other activities?

11. Have you noticed that you have skin irritations more frequently and that minor infections don't heal as quickly as they used to?

12. Have you noticed any unusual changes in your vision (blurring, difficulty in focusing, etc.)?

13. Have you noticed unusual pain or swelling in your joints?

14. If you are a woman, have you had several vaginal (yeast) infections during the past year?

15. Do you often feel weak or nauseated if you have to wait too long to eat a meal?

---

vention, through a regimen of proper diet, weight control, and exercise. They may be able to avoid oral medications or insulin indefinitely.

Diabetes tends to run in families, and a tendency toward being overweight, coupled with inactivity, dramatically increases a person's risk. Older persons and mothers of babies weighing over 9 pounds also run an increased risk. Approximately 80 percent of all patients are overweight at the time of diagnosis. Weight loss and exercise are important factors in lowering blood sugar and improving the efficiency of cellular use of insulin. Both can help to prevent overwork of the pancreas and the development of diabetes. People who develop diabetes today have a much better prognosis than did those who developed diabetes just 20 years ago. Our present understanding of the role that stress, illness, alcohol, smoking, and other lifestyle characteristics may play in the development of diabetes can aid in prevention and earlier diagnosis. Recognizing your risks and taking steps to reduce the likelihood of developing this problem is a good start. The Rate Yourself box contains a self-assessment that will help you find out if you are at risk for diabetes.

Most physicians attempt to control diabetes with a variety of insulin-related drugs. Most of these drugs are taken orally, although self-administered hypodermic injections are prescribed when other treatments are inadequate. Recent breakthroughs in individual monitoring and the implanting of insulin monitors and insulin infusion pumps that regulate insulin intake "on demand" have provided many diabetics with the opportunity to lead normal lives. Other diabetics have found that they can help to control their diabetes by eating foods that are rich in complex carbohydrates, low in sodium, and high in fiber; by losing weight; and by getting regular exercise.

Colitis and Irritable Bowel Syndrome (IBS)

Ulcerative colitis is a disease of the large intestine in which the mucous membranes of the intestinal walls become inflamed. Victims with severe cases may have as many as 20 bouts of bloody diarrhea a day. Colitis can also produce severe stomach cramps, weight loss, nausea, sweating, and fever. What causes colitis? Although some experts believe that it occurs more frequently in people with high stress levels, this theory is controversial. Hypersensitivity reactions, particularly to milk and certain foods, have also been considered as a possible cause. It is difficult to determine the cause of colitis because the disease goes into unexplained remission and then recurs without apparent reason. This pattern often continues over periods of years and may be related to the later development of colorectal cancer. Because the cause of colitis remains unknown, treatment focuses exclusively on relieving the symptoms. Increasing fiber intake and taking anti-inflammatory drugs, steroids, and other medications designed to reduce inflammation and soothe irritated intestinal walls have been effective in relieving symptoms.

Many people develop a condition related to colitis known as **irritable bowel syndrome (IBS),** in which nausea, pain, gas, diarrhea attacks, or cramps occur after eating certain foods or when a person is under unusual stress. IBS symptoms commonly begin in early adulthood. Symptoms may vary from week to week and can fade for long periods of time only to return. The cause of IBS is unknown, but researchers suspect that people with IBS have digestive systems that are overly sensitive to what they eat and drink, to stress, and to certain hormonal changes. They may also be more sensitive to pain signals from the stomach. Stress management, relaxation techniques, regular activity, and diet can bring IBS under control in the vast majority of cases. If diarrhea is a problem, cut down on fat in your diet; avoid caffeine and excessive amounts of sorbitol, a sweetener found in dietetic foods and chewing gum. Many IBS patients are lactose intolerant. To relieve constipation, gradually increase fiber in your diet. Some sufferers benefit from anticholinergic drugs, which relax the intestinal muscle, or from antidepressant drugs and psychological counseling. Medical advice should be sought whenever such conditions persist. The Choices for Change box gives advice on when you need to see a doctor.

Diverticulosis

Diverticulosis occurs when the walls of the intestine become weakened for undetermined reasons and small pea-sized bulges develop. These bulges often fill with feces and, over time, become irritated and infected, causing pain and discomfort. If this irritation persists, bleeding and chronic obstruction may occur, either of which can be life-threatening.

Although diverticulosis may appear in any part of the intestinal wall, it most commonly occurs in the small intestine. Often the person affected may be unaware that the problem exists. However, in some cases, a person may actually have an attack similar to the pain of appendicitis except that the pain is on the left side of the body instead of the right, where the appendix is located. Although diverticulosis most frequently occurs during and after middle age, it can appear at any age. If you have a persistent pain in the lower abdominal region, seek medical attention at once.

Peptic Ulcers

An ulcer is a lesion or wound that forms in body tissue as a result of some form of irritant. A **peptic ulcer** is a chronic ulcer that occurs in the lining of the stomach or the section of the small intestine known as the *duodenum*. It has been thought to be caused by the erosive effect of digestive juices on these tissues. The lining of these organs becomes irritated, the protective covering of mucus is reduced, and the gastric acid begins to digest the dying tissue, just as it would a piece of food. Typically, this irritation causes pain that disappears when the person eats, but returns about an hour later.

In 1994, the National Institutes of Health (NIH) announced that a common bacteria, *Helicobacter pylori,* may be the cause of most ulcers, and called for the use of powerful antibiotics to treat the disorder, which affects over 4 million Americans every year. This is a dramatic departure from the typical treatment using acid-reducing drugs known as H2 blockers, such as cimetidine (Tagamet) or ranitidine (Zantec). The new treatment recommends a two-week course of antibiotics. H2 blockers will still be used in ulcer cases in which excess stomach acid or overuse of drugs such as aspirin and ibuprofen have caused an irritation. The good news is that by treating ulcers with germ-killing drugs, the ulcers appear less likely to recur.

Ulcers appear to run in families and to be more prevalent in people who are highly stressed over long periods of time and who consume high-fat foods or excessive amounts of alcohol. People with ulcers should avoid high-fat foods, alcohol, and substances such as aspirin that may irritate organ linings or cause increased secretion of stomach acids and thereby exacerbate this condition. In some cases, surgery has been necessary to relieve persistent symptoms.

Heartburn

Anyone who's ever experienced the fiery pain of post-pepperoni pizza will know what *heartburn* feels like. This pain is often a symptom of *gastroesophageal reflux,* the backup of stomach contents, including acids, into the lower esophagus that occurs when a valve-like ring of muscle at the entrance to the stomach becomes too relaxed. This disease has nothing to do with a heart problem, but the pain is often experienced in the region of the chest near the heart; hence the name.

Simple cases of heartburn are readily relieved by antacids; however, excessive antacid intake can lead to diarrhea or constipation. Current thinking is that diet and other lifestyle variables may increase risk. Fried and fatty foods, chocolate, coffee, bananas, alcohol, and cigarettes can trigger heartburn. Being overweight, eating large meals, or lying down soon after a meal can cause prob-

Seeking Care for Digestive Problems

Digestive problems are common afflictions that most of us face at some time or another. We tend not to want to discuss our bowel habits with others and often ignore very real problems for too long. There are many actions that you can take to reduce your symptoms and your risk, including making dietary changes, reducing stress levels, exercising, and losing weight. However, there are some symptoms that should not be ignored and should be checked by your doctor:

- Severe stomach cramps or pain.
- Blood in stools or vomit or dark, tarry-looking stools.
- A sudden change in bowel habits or consistency of stools lasting for more than a few days.

- Pain or difficulty when swallowing foods.
- Unexpected feeling of "fullness" after eating only small amounts.
- Loss of appetite or unexpected weight loss.
- Persistent diarrhea or constipation.

Source: Information from National Digestive Diseases Information Clearinghouse, Box NDDIC, 9000 Rockville Pike, Bethesda, MD 20892; and Crohn's and Colitis Foundation of America, 386 Park Avenue South, New York, NY 10016 (phone 800/343–3636).

lems by increasing pressure on the stomach and its sphincter muscles. Waterbeds are particularly troublesome for heartburn sufferers, as they do not allow you to raise your head enough to reduce gastric reflux. By reducing risks and avoiding foods that cause problems, heartburn problems often go away. If these actions don't work, drugs that alter gastric secretions or surgery to repair weakened muscles may provide relief.

Gallbladder Disease

Gallbladder disease, also known as *cholecystitis,* occurs when the gallbladder has been repeatedly irritated by chemicals, infection, or overuse, thus reducing its ability to release bile used for the digestion of fats. Usually, gallstones, consisting of calcium, cholesterol, and other minerals, form in the gallbladder itself. When the patient eats foods that are high in fats, the gallbladder contracts to release bile; these contractions cause pressure on the stone formations. One of the characteristic symptoms of gallbladder disease is acute pain in the upper right portion of the abdomen after eating fatty foods. This pain, which can last several hours, may feel like a heart attack or an ulcer attack and is often accompanied by nausea.

Who gets gallbladder disease? The old adage about the "five f's" of risk factors frequently holds true. Anyone who is "female, fat, fair, forty, and flatulent" (prone to passing gas) appears to be at increased risk. However, people who don't fit this picture also get the disease.

Not all gallstones cause acute pain. In fact, small stones that pass through one of the bile ducts and become lodged may be more painful than gallstones that are the size of golf balls. Many people find out that they have gallstones only after undergoing ultrasound and diagnostic X-rays

to rule out other conditions. The absence of symptoms is significant because gallstones are considered to be a predisposing factor for gallbladder cancer. In fact, gallstones were present in 75 percent of all gallbladder cancers in 1989.[7]

Current treatment of gallbladder disease usually involves medication to reduce irritation, restriction of fat consumption, and surgery to remove the gallstones. New medications designed to dissolve small gallstones are currently being used in some patients. In addition, some doctors are using a new technique known as lithotripsy, in which a series of noninvasive shock waves break up small stones. Experiments are being done with lasers and various forms of laparoscopy to eliminate the risks associated with large surgical incisions.

What Do You Think?

What role does improved diet have in reducing your risks for and symptoms of the above diseases? Are you or any of your family members at risk for these problems? What actions can you take today that will begin to reduce your risks?

Irritable bowel syndrome (IBS): Nausea, pain, gas, or diarrhea caused by certain foods or stress.

Diverticulosis: A condition in which bulges form in the walls of the intestine; results in irritation and infection of the intestine.

Peptic ulcer: Damage to the stomach or intestinal lining, usually caused by digestive juices.

Western Problems, Eastern Cures

Certainly the best "cure" for backache and other chronic musculoskeletal disorders is prevention. But for those suffering already, Western and Eastern science offer very different views of how to solve the problem. In the United States, you may take pain relievers for temporary relief, visit an M.D. or chiropractor, and do physical therapy. If your back hurts in China, you may visit an acupuncturist.

Originating in China over 2,000 years ago, acupuncture is based on the idea that the body has 14 well-defined pathways (called meridians) of energy. These pathways convey the body's life force, known as *qi* (pronounced *chee*). According to Chinese medical theory, pain and illness occur when *qi* builds up or diminishes. To adjust its flow, acupuncturists insert stainless-steel needles into one or more of the nearly 2,000 acupuncture points on the skin. The needles, which cause little if any sensation, stay in place for 10 to 45 minutes.

Recently, acupuncture has gained more acceptance in the United States. Although the FDA estimates that 9 to 12 million acupuncture treatments are performed each year in the United States, the medical uses of acupuncture remain limited. Many patients suffer from untraceable or intractable pain in the back, head, neck, and other areas. They report milder symptoms and often lasting relief after acupuncture.

At the Boston Veterans Affairs Medical Center and the neurology department of the Boston University School of Medicine, Margaret Naeser has used acupuncture needles and low-energy lasers to stimulate acupuncture points on stroke patients, helping them regain partial mobility and strength in their hands, arms, and legs. For the 60 percent of patients who benefited, the progress was significant; many were long-time stroke survivors who had plateaued in their recoveries and were no longer expected to gain motor improvement.

In Asia, acupuncture is used for a wide spectrum of problems: pain, menstrual disorders, digestive problems, infertility, even schizophrenia and depression. Here, acupuncture needles are still considered "investigational" by the FDA, and thus ineligible for reimbursement by many insurance companies.

Source: Adapted by permission of the author from Madeline Drexler, "Healing Needles," *Boston Globe Magazine*, 11 September 1994, 10–11.

MUSCULOSKELETAL DISEASES

Most of us will encounter some form of chronic musculoskeletal disease during our lifetime. Some form of arthritis will afflict half of those over 65; low back pain hits 80 percent of us at some point in our life. While these diseases are found throughout the world, the cures differ in different places. The Multicultural Perspectives box looks at one alternative cure.

Arthritis

Called the "nation's primary crippler," **arthritis** strikes one in seven Americans, or over 38 million people. Symptoms range from the occasional tendinitis of the weekend athlete to the horrific pain of rheumatoid arthritis. Arthritis accounts for over 30 million lost workdays annually and costs the U.S. economy over $10 billion per year, including $4.5 billion in hospital and nursing home services. In addition, arthritis sufferers spend more than $1 billion a year on dubious cures.

Osteoarthritis is a progressive deterioration of bones and joints that has been associated with the "wear and tear" theory of aging. More recent research indicates that as joints are used, they release enzymes that digest cartilage while other cells in the cartilage try to repair the damage. When the enzymatic breakdown overpowers cellular repair, the pain and swelling characteristic of arthritis may occur. Weather extremes, excessive strain, and injury often lead to osteoarthritis flare-ups. But a specific precipitating event does not seem to be necessary.

Arthritis: Painful inflammatory disease of the joints.

Osteoarthritis: A progressive deterioration of bones and joints that has been associated with the "wear and tear" theory of aging.

Rheumatoid arthritis: A serious inflammatory joint disease.

Lupus: A disease in which the immune system attacks the body, producing antibodies that destroy or injure organs such as the kidneys, brain, and heart.

Although age and injury are undoubtedly factors in the development of osteoarthritis, heredity, abnormal use of the joint, diet, abnormalities in joint structure, and impaired blood supply to the joint may also contribute. Osteoarthritis of the hands seems to have a particularly strong genetic component. Extreme disability as a result of osteoarthritis is rare. However, when joints become so distorted that they impair activity, surgical intervention is often necessary. Joint replacement and bone fusion are common surgical repair techniques. For most people, anti-inflammatory drugs and pain relievers such as aspirin and cortisone-related agents ease discomfort. In some sufferers, applications of heat, mild exercise, and massage may also relieve the pain.

Rheumatoid arthritis is similar to, but far more serious than, osteoarthritis. Rheumatoid arthritis is an inflammatory joint disease that can occur at any age, but most commonly appears between the ages of 20 and 45. It is three times more common among women than among men during early adulthood but equally common among men and women in the over-70 age group. Symptoms may be gradually progressive or sporadic, with occasional unexplained remissions.

Rheumatoid arthritis typically attacks the synovial membrane, which produces the lubricating fluids for the joints. Advanced rheumatoid arthritis often involves destruction of the bony ends of joints. The remedy for this condition is typically bone fusion, which leaves the joint immobile. In some instances, joint replacement may be a viable alternative. Figure 19.2 illustrates the bone destruction that typically occurs in a joint affected by rheumatoid arthritis.

Although the exact cause of this form of arthritis is unknown, some experts theorize that it is an autoimmune disorder, in which the body responds as if its own cells were the enemy, eventually destroying the affected body parts. Other theorists believe that rheumatoid arthritis is caused by some form of invading microorganism that takes over the joint. Certain toxic chemicals and stress have also been mentioned as possible causes.

Regardless of the cause, treatment of rheumatoid arthritis is similar to that for osteoarthritis. Emphasis is placed on pain relief and attempts to improve the functional mobility of the patient. In some instances, immunosuppressant drugs are given to reduce the inflammatory response.

Fibromyalgia is a chronic, painful rheumatological-like disorder that affects approximately 6 million Americans. Symptoms include widespread pain; stiffness and numerous tender points; weakness; swelling; and neurovascular complaints including coldness, numbness, tingling, mottled skin, headaches, auditory sensitivity, irritable bowel syndrome, sleep disorders, depression, and dysmenorrhea. The cause of fibromyalgia remains a mystery, with many theories under investigation. Acute sleep disturbances, muscular irregularities, and forms of psychopathological disturbance have been considered as possible culprits. What is known is that the disease primarily affects women (particularly in their 30s and 40s), that the disease causes

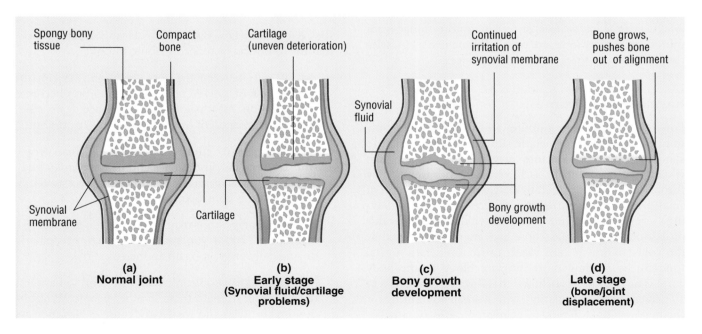

FIGURE 19.2

The Stages of Rheumatoid Arthritis

more chronic pain and debilitation than other muscloskeletal disorders, and that significant research must be conducted before an effective, long-term treatment will be available.

Systemic Lupus Erythematosus (SLE)

Lupus is a disease in which the immune system attacks the body, producing antibodies that destroy or injure organs such as the kidneys, brain, and heart. The symptoms vary from mild to severe and may disappear for periods of time. A butterfly-shaped rash covering the bridge of the nose and both cheeks is common. Nearly all SLE sufferers have aching joints and muscles, and 60 percent of them develop redness and swelling that moves from joint to joint. The disease affects 1 in 700 Caucasians but 1 in 250 African Americans; 90 percent of all victims are females. Extensive research has not yet found a cure for this sometimes fatal disease.

Scleroderma

Scleroderma (hardening of the skin) is a disease characterized by an increasing fibrous growth of connective tissue underlying the skin and body organs. These areas may form hard skin patches or form a more generalized "evertightening case of steel," making movement difficult. Some cases of scleroderma are related to certain occupations, such as working with vibrating machines and exposure to chemicals in plastics or in mining. Others have an abrupt, unknown etiology. Scleroderma may cause swelling of the hands, face, or feet. Symptoms range from minor discomfort to severe pain. In some instances, scleroderma has life-threatening consequences.

Raynaud's Syndrome

For most of us, a few minutes in the cold causes only minor discomfort. For people suffering from **Raynaud's syndrome,** fingers and toes may go numb, then turn white, then deep purple; as fingers and toes warm, they throb. Raynaud's is caused by exaggerated constriction of small arteries in the extremities that results in blood moving away from them and toward the vital organs. Why this disease occurs in people whose lives are not threatened by the cold (in which case vasoconstriction serves a vital function by sending more, warmer blood to the body core) is unknown. It is believed that Raynaud's affects 5 to 10 percent of the population, with women accounting for the majority of sufferers. In women, onset is usually between the ages of 15 and 40; men tend to develop Raynaud's later in life. Treatment for Raynaud's consists of trying to control body temperature by wearing warm gloves and boots, avoiding drugs that may alter blood flow (e.g., nicotine), taking drugs to regulate blood flow, and surgery to improve circulation and/or repair damaged areas.

Low Back Pain

Approximately 80 percent of all Americans will experience low back pain at some point during their lifetimes. Although some of these low back pain (LBP) episodes may result from muscular damage and be short-lived and acute, others may involve dislocations, fractures, or other problems with spinal vertebrae or discs and be chronic or require surgery. Low back pain is epidemic throughout the world. It is the major cause of disability for people aged 20 to 45 in the United States,[8] who suffer more frequently and severely from this problem than older people do.

In 1993, LBP caused more lost work time in the United States than did any other illness except upper respiratory infections. In fact, costs associated with back injury exceeded those associated with all other industrial injuries combined. Back injuries are the most frequently mentioned complaints in injury-related lawsuits, and the average cost of medical bills and compensation claims cited in these suits is $8,500.[9] Low back injuries cost business and industry in the United States over $20 billion annually in direct costs. As a result, employers throughout the country have become increasingly interested in preventing these injuries. Note that these figures do not include the costs of human suffering, self-worth, and other emotional problems that occur when a person becomes disabled.

Risk Factors for Low Back Pain. Health experts believe that the following factors contribute to LBP:

- *Age.* People between the ages of 20 and 45 run the greatest risk of LBP. At age 50, the condition becomes less common. After age 65, the incidence again rises, apparently because of bone and joint deterioration.

- *Body types.* Many studies have indicated that people who are very tall, are overweight, or have lanky body types run an increased risk of LBP. However, much of this research is controversial.

- *Posture.* Poor posture may be one of the greatest risk factors for LBP. If you routinely slouch, particularly during daily tasks, you run an increased risk.

- *Strength and fitness.* People with LBP tend to have less overall trunk strength than do other people. Weak abdominal muscles and weak back muscles also increase your risk. In addition, your total level of fitness and conditioning is a factor. The more fit you are, the lower your risk.

- *Psychological factors.* Numerous psychological factors appear to increase risk for LBP. Depression, apathy, inattentiveness, boredom, emotional upsets, drug abuse, and family and financial problems all heighten risk.

- *Occupational risks.* Evidence indicates that employees who are new to a particular job run the greatest risk of LBP problems. In addition, the type of work that you do and the conditions under which you work greatly affect your risk. For example, truck drivers, who must endure the bumps and jolts of the road while in a sitting position, frequently suffer from back pain.

Preventing Back Pain and Injury. What can you do to protect yourself from possible back injury? First, to prevent back pain, you must be knowledgeable about what area of the spinal column is most at risk and attempt to protect that area as much as possible. Almost 90 percent of all back problems occur in the lumbar spine region

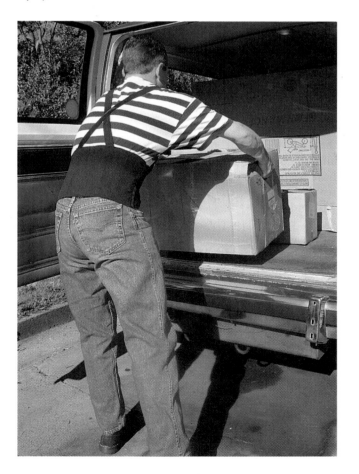

Taking precautions, such as wearing a protective belt when moving heavy objects, can help you avoid back injury.

(lower back). Consciously protecting this region of the body from blows, excessive strain, or sharp twists when muscles are not warmed up is essential. You can avoid many problems by consciously attempting to maintain good posture.

In addition, exercise, particularly exercises that strengthen the abdominal muscles and stretch the back muscles, is important. New research indicates that many traditional surgical and medicinal treatments for back injury may be less effective than most practitioners currently think.[10] If you injure your back, be sure to consult with at least two different experts in rehabilitation and therapy to determine your best options. Consult an exercise physiologist, biomechanist, physical therapist, or physician specializing in bone and joint injuries for recommended exercises. The Skills for Behavior Change box offers suggestions for protecting your back.

OTHER MALADIES

During the last decade, numerous afflictions have surfaced that seem to be products of our times. Some of these health problems relate to specific groups of people, some are due to technological advances, and some are unexplainable. Still other diseases have been present for many years and continue to cause severe disability (see Table 19.1). Among the conditions that have received the most attention in recent years are chronic fatigue syndrome and disorders related to the use of video display terminals.

Chronic Fatigue Syndrome (CFS)

Fatigue is a subjective condition in which people feel tired before they begin activities, lack the energy to accomplish tasks that require sustained effort and attention, or become abnormally exhausted after normal activities. Does this sound familiar? To many Americans, such symptoms are all too common. In the late 1980s, however, a characteristic set of symptoms including chronic fatigue,

Scleroderma: A disease in which fibrous growth of connective tissue underlying the skin and body organs hardens and makes movement difficult.

Raynaud's syndrome: A disease in which exposure to cold temperatures produces exaggerated constriction of the small arteries in the extremities, causing fingers and toes to go numb, turn white, and then turn deep purple.

Protecting Your Back

These guidelines will help you protect your spine from undue stress during work, recreation, and sleep:

- Purchase a firm mattress. Avoid sleeping on your stomach. Some experts recommend that you sleep in a fetal position (on your side, with your knees drawn up slightly) to ease spinal pressure. Try to determine what works best for your back.

- Avoid high-heeled shoes. These shoes often tilt the pelvis forward, causing excessive curvature of the spine and LBP.

- Control your weight. Excessive weight puts an added burden on the back muscles and may lead to LBP.

- Practice proper lifting techniques. Bend your knees and keep your back straight, taking the load on your legs rather than on your back. Try to hold the object you are lifting as close to your body as possible.

- Purchase a car with the right seat. The structure of the driver's seat and the amount of support that the seat gives to the low back should be major considerations when you are buying a car. If possible, choose a car that has adjustable lumbar spine supports (common in newer models).

- Adjust your auto seat for comfort. If you are driving long distances, move the car seat forward, which elevates your knees slightly, increases circulation, and reduces pressure on the low back.

- Don't skimp on chairs. We often spend tremendous amounts on fancy desks, tables, and other flashy items, yet go the cheap route on chairs and other items that we spend large amounts of time sitting on. Buy a good chair for doing your work, preferably one with lumbar support and adjustments for height and angle of the seat.

- Warm up before exercising. This is critical for preventing injury to muscles supporting the back. Stretching back muscles and warming up abdominal and leg muscles will probably reduce your chances of causing LBP.

If you are plagued with periodic aches and pains in the low back area, heat, massage, or whirlpool baths may help ease your pain by relaxing muscles in the affected area. Rest is a key factor in recovery. In addition, pain relievers such as aspirin may be effective for minor problems. However, if your low back pain persists, if you have difficulty moving, or if you experience numbness or pain radiating to the extremities, consult a physician. These could be early signs of a disk alignment problem, a ruptured disk, or another condition requiring immediate attention.

---

headaches, fever, sore throat, enlarged lymph nodes, depression, poor memory, general weakness, nausea, and symptoms remarkably similar to mononucleosis were noted in several U.S. clinics. Researchers initially believed that they were really talking about a series of symptoms caused by the same virus as mononucleosis, the Epstein-Barr virus. The disease was initially called *chronic Epstein-Barr disease,* or the "yuppie flu," because the pattern of symptoms appeared most commonly in baby boomers in their early 30s. In some instances, the symptoms were so severe that patients required hospitalization. Since those initial studies, however, researchers have all but ruled out the possibility of a mystery form of the Epstein-Barr virus. Despite extensive testing, no viral cause has been found to date.

Today, in the absence of a known pathogen, many researchers believe that the illness, now commonly referred to as chronic fatigue syndrome (CFS), may have strong psychosocial roots. According to Harvard psychiatrist Arthur Barsky, our heightened awareness of health makes some of us scrutinize our bodies so carefully that the slightest deviation becomes amplified. The more we focus on our body and on our perception of our health, the worse we feel.[11] In addition, the growing number of people who suffer from depression seem to be good candidates for chronic fatigue syndrome. Chronic fatigue among college students seems to correlate not with too little sleep or too much work but rather with indicators of psychopathology: emotional instability, introversion, anxiety, and depression.[12]

The diagnosis of chronic fatigue syndrome depends on two major criteria and eight or more minor criteria. The major criteria are debilitating fatigue that persists for at least six months and the absence of diagnoses of other illnesses that could cause the symptoms. Minor criteria include headaches, fever, sore throat, painful lymph nodes, weakness, fatigue after exercise, sleep problems, and rapid onset of these symptoms. Because an exact cause is not apparent, treatment of CFS focuses on improved nutrition, rest, counseling for depression, judicious exercise, and development of a strong support network.

Job-Related Disorders

During the last decade, a new potential health risk for computer users has been the topic of growing debate.

TABLE 19.1 ▪ Other Modern Afflictions

Disease	Victims	Symptoms	Risks	Prevention and Treatment
Parkinson's disease	Affects 1.5 million Americans; rare before age 40; typically begins after age 55.	Gradual, insidious development of 5 major symptoms: **1.** *Tremors*—typically of hand, leg, foot, chin, thumbs, or fingers when not being used. **2.** *Rigidity*—Tightness caused by muscle contractions; cramplike pain. **3.** *Slowed movement* (bradykinesia). **4.** *Loss of autonomic movements*—diminished control of blinking, smiling, frowning, and other facial expressions. **5.** *Walking difficulties*—shuffling of feet.	Affects men and women equally. No occupational, ethnic, geographic, or social group is at greater risk. Not contagious; no links to a specific dietary or environmental cause; not hereditary.	Emotional upsets cause symptom flare-ups. Because the cause is not known, prevention is difficult. Major tranquilizers are useful in controlling nerve responses from affected region of brain.
Multiple sclerosis	Affects approximately 250,000 Americans per year.	Variable; often sudden onset of unexplained blurred vision or blindness; tingling and numbness in extremities; sporadic urinary control problems; chronic fatigue; neurological problems characterized by remission and relapse.	Cause unknown; viral cause suspected; affects more women than men; most common in adults in their 30s.	Stress management may be helpful. Disease is often progressive. Medications can be used to control symptoms.
Cystic fibrosis	Occurs in 1 out of every 1,600 births.	Large amounts of mucus cause lung complications and infections; digestive disturbances; large greasy stools; excessive sodium excretion.	Inherited disease. If both parents have the gene for cystic fibrosis, there is a 25 percent chance that the child will have the disease.	Treatment is geared toward relief of symptoms. Antibiotics are administered for infection.
Sickle cell disease	Between 8 and 10 percent of all African Americans carry genes for this disease.	Abnormality in body's hemoglobin; sickle-shaped red blood cells form that interfere with body's ability to supply oxygen to tissues; causes anemia, crippling, severe pain, and premature death.	Inherited disease.	People at risk should seek genetic counseling.
Cerebral palsy	Believed to occur in people who suffer from a lack of oxygen at birth; a brain disorder or accident before or after birth; poisoning; or brain infections.	Loss of voluntary control over motor functioning.	(See "Victims")	Avoidance of risks is best method of prevention. Improved neonatal and birthing techniques.
Graves' disease	Can occur at any age.	Thyroid disorder characterized by swelling of the eyes, staring gaze, retraction of the eyelid; in severe cases, blindness may result.	Cause unknown. Autoimmune dysfunction suspected as cause.	Medication may help to control symptoms. Radioactive iodine supplements can also be administered.

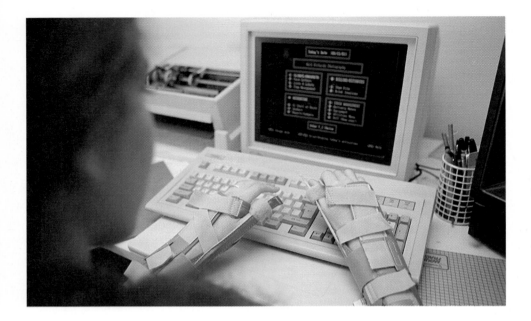

Carpal tunnel syndrome, which causes numbness, tingling, and pain in the fingers and hands, is a common occupational injury for people who work at a computer for long hours every day.

Adverse health effects have been noted in people who work at computer video display terminals (VDTs) for several hours per day. More than 15 million Americans, including many college students, are regular high-volume users of VDTs and therefore at risk.

Most of these problems relate to eyestrain and discomfort in the low back, neck, shoulders, and wrists. Questions about the danger posed by radiation from the electrical fields produced within the circuits of the VDT and about the potential effects on pregnant women and their fetuses remain unanswered. **Carpal tunnel syndrome** is a common occupational injury in which the median nerve in the wrist becomes irritated, causing numbness, tingling, and pain in the fingers and hands. This condition is worsened by the repetitive typing motions made by computer users and is often classified as one of the common repetitive motion injuries. To prevent problems, experts recommend that if you must work on a computer for hours at a time, day after day, you should take regular breaks and remove your hands from the keyboard to exercise them about every 20 minutes. You should also stretch other body parts, such as the neck and shoulders, periodically. Attention to the design, height, and support of your chair and placement of the keyboard at a comfortable angle and height can save you countless hours of suffering.

Carpal tunnel syndrome: A common occupational injury in which the median nerve in the wrist becomes irritated, causing numbness, tingling, and pain in the fingers and hands.

Summary

◆ Respiratory disorders include allergies, hay fever, asthma, emphysema, and chronic bronchitis. Allergies are part of the body's natural defense system. Chronic obstructive pulmonary diseases are the fifth leading cause of death in the United States.

◆ Neurological conditions include headaches and seizure disorders. Headaches may be caused by a variety of factors, the most common of which are tension, dilation and/or contraction of blood vessels in the brain, chemical influences on muscles and vessels that cause inflammation and pain, and underlying physiological and psychological disorders.

◆ Several modern maladies affect only women. Fibrocystic breast condition is a common, noncancerous buildup of irregular tissue. Premenstrual syndrome (PMS) is the name given to a wide variety of symptoms that appear

Managing Chronic Ailments

The majority of chronic noninfectious diseases can be prevented, delayed in their onset, or treated, meaning that patients may experience substantially reduced symptoms, improved quality of life, and longer life span. Lifestyle and personal health habits appear to be major contributing factors to the rise in the incidence of chronic diseases in the United States in recent years. What is important is that all of us learn to recognize our own risks, identify early potential symptoms, act responsibly in reducing risks, and act to support promotion policies and procedures designed to help people cope more effectively with their health problems. By carefully thinking about the following questions, you may be able to determine those actions most prudent for you and your family and loved ones.

Making Decisions for You

Think about the varied maladies from which you have suffered or may be genetically predisposed to suffer. What can you do now to ease current suffering or to postpone suffering from chronic disorders? Make a list of these actions. Are you willing to take such steps? Why or why not?

Checklist for Change: Making Personal Choices

✓ How much individual responsibility should we each accept for chronic diseases we could have prevented? What will it take for people to accept more responsibility for their own personal health habits?

✓ Do you have any lifestyle or personal health habits that could cause a chronic disease? For instance, do you smoke? Do you exercise regularly? Do you have healthy eating habits? Are you overweight?

✓ If you have any of these habits, why did you choose them? Have you tried to change your habits? If so, what approaches have worked best? What approaches have not worked at all?

✓ What actions can you take today to reduce your own risks for the diseases and disorders discussed in this chapter? Which concern you most?

Checklist for Change: Making Community Choices

✓ If you worked for a government agency charged with helping people improve their personal health habits, what approaches would you take? For instance, would you try to use information to convince people that their habits were harmful? Would you use rewards (such as tax credits) to persuade people to improve their personal health habits?

✓ Should the cost of harmful substances, such as cigarettes, be raised to discourage their use?

✓ What role should businesses play in improving employee health? Should businesses be held liable for situations in which employees get carpal tunnel syndrome or experience low back problems? Should the federal government provide tax credits to help businesses buy proper equipment?

Critical Thinking

Last summer, you started working at a data-entry company, entering banking transactions into a computer. The task is repetitious and boring, but it pays more than twice what you'd make elsewhere. During the summer you worked full time; during the school year you work Saturdays and Sundays. You've begun to notice that sitting in front of the computer screen is starting to have physical effects: your back and shoulders seem to hurt half the week. And your wrists and fingers (particularly on the hand that you use for your computer mouse) seem to have chronic pain. You mention this to your supervisor and take the actions suggested in this chapter, which include using adjustable equipment and taking breaks every 20 minutes to exercise your hands. Your boss suggests that you do your job or quit.

Using the DECIDE model in Chapter 1, decide what you will do. Balance the short-term high pay against the chronic effects of repetitive motion injury. Consider whether there is a better way to approach your supervisor.

---

to be related to the menstrual cycle. Endometriosis is the buildup of endometrial tissue in regions of the body other than the uterus.

◆ Diabetes occurs when the pancreas fails to produce enough insulin to regulate sugar metabolism. Other conditions, such as colitis, irritable bowel syndrome, gallbladder disease, and ulcers are the direct result of functional problems in various digestion-related organs or systems. Pathogens, problems in enzyme or hormone production, anxiety or stress, functional abnormalities, and other problems are often listed as probable causes.

◆ Musculoskeletal diseases such as arthritis, lower back pain, repetitive motion injuries, and other problems cause significant pain and disability in millions of people. Age, occupation, gender, posture, abdominal strength, and psychological factors contribute to the development of lower back problems.

◆ Chronic fatigue syndrome (CFS) and job-related disorders (such as carpal tunnel syndrome) have emerged in the last decade as major chronic maladies. CFS is associated with depression. Many job-related disorders are preventable by proper equipment placement and usage.

Discussion Questions

1. What are some of the major noninfectious chronic diseases affecting Americans today? Do you think there is a pattern in the types of diseases that we get? What are the common risk factors?

2. List the common respiratory diseases affecting Americans. Which of these diseases has a genetic basis? An environmental basis? An individual basis? What, if anything, is being done to prevent, treat, and/or control each of these conditions?

3. Compare and contrast the different types of headaches, including their symptoms and treatments.

4. Do you believe that PMS is a disorder or disease or simply a catch-all name for many naturally occurring events in the menstrual cycle?

5. What are the medical risks of fibrocystic breast condition and endometriosis? How can they be treated?

6. Describe the symptoms and treatment of diabetes.

7. Compare the symptoms of colitis, diverticulosis, peptic ulcers, heartburn, and gallbladder disease. How can you tell whether your stomach is reacting to final exams or telling you you have a serious medical condition?

8. What are the major disorders of the musculoskeletal system? Why do you think there aren't any cures?

9. Chronic fatigue syndrome (CFS) is often associated with depression. Experts argue about whether depression precedes CFS or CFS causes depression. What do you think?

Application Exercise

Reread the What Do You Think? scenarios at the beginning of the chapter and answer the following questions:

1. Given that Tom has a hereditary predisposition toward diabetes, is he to blame if his diabetic onset comes at an earlier than expected date? Do you think there is a tendency to blame the victim when people get diseases such as diabetes? Is this victim-blaming ever justified? Explain.

2. Do you think that chronic fatigue syndrome is a real physical disease? Or is it the physical manifestation of a mental disorder? Explain your answer.

Further Reading

Boston Women's Health Book Collective, *The New Our Bodies, Ourselves* (New York: Simon and Schuster, New York, 1992).

Discusses the many concerns related to women and their health. Covers specific health problems in the area of modern maladies and concerns of all age groups.

Carol Tavris, *The Mismeasure of Woman* (New York: Touchstone, 1992).

Subtitled "Why women are not the better sex, the inferior sex, or the opposite sex." Looks at the nature and development of so-called women's disorders. Very well written, often humorous, always thought-provoking.

National Center for Health Statistics, *Monthly Vital Statistics Report* and *Advance Data from Vital and Health Statistics*, Public Health Service, Hyattsville, MD.

Detailed government reports, usually published monthly. Provide mortality and morbidity data for the United States. Focus on changes occurring in the rates of particular diseases and in health practices so patterns and trends can be analyzed.

Public Health Services, Centers for Disease Control, *Chronic Disease News and Notes*, U.S. Department of Health and Human Services, Washington, DC.

Quarterly publication focusing on relevant chronic disease topics and issues.

Brownson, Remington, and Davis, *Chronic Disease Epidemiology and Control* (American Public Health Association, 1993).

An excellent book covering the epidemiology of major human illnesses. Provides historical, pathological, and epidemiological perspectives on illness and infirmity.

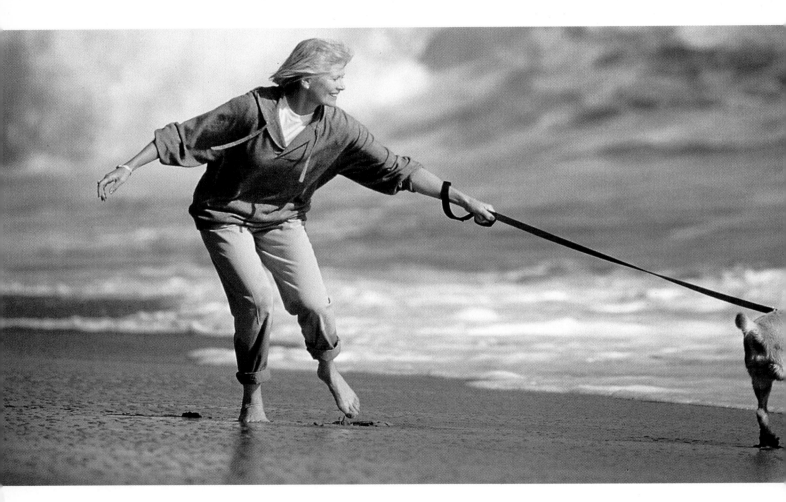

CHAPTER OBJECTIVES

◆ Review the definition of aging, and explain the related concepts of biological age, psychological age, social age, legal age, and functional age.

◆ Explain the impact on society of the growing population of the elderly, including considerations of economics, health care, housing and living arrangements, and ethical and moral issues.

◆ Discuss the biological and psychosocial theories of aging and examine how knowledge of these theories may have an impact on your own aging process.

◆ Identify the major physiological changes that occur as a result of the aging process.

◆ Discuss the unique health challenges faced by the elderly, such as alcohol abuse, prescription medication and over-the-counter drug use, osteoporosis, urinary incontinence, depression, senility, and Alzheimer's disease.

◆ Examine the differences between males and females in terms of their numbers among the elderly population and of their roles as caregivers for others.

Healthy Aging

A Lifelong Process

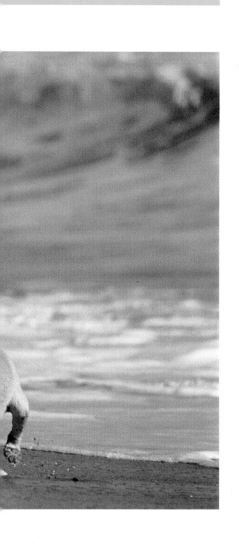

Jovier's widowed grandmother has just begun to date an elderly man from her church. When Jovier shows up at his grandmother's door early one morning, he finds her friend sitting at the kitchen table in his pajamas having a cup of coffee. Jovier is shocked and a bit disgusted by his grandmother's behavior. He quickly says hello, makes some idle conversation, and leaves, feeling embarrassed.

- Is Jovier's reaction typical? Why do you think he feels the way he does? Do you have difficulty thinking about your parents or grandparents having sexual relations? Why do you feel the way you do? What can Jovier do to change his feelings about this situation?

Bonnie, aged 82, is a springboard diver. Every morning, she walks 10 blocks to the city pool, where she practices her diving and swims to stay in shape. Erin, aged 79, is an internationally recognized expert in family dysfunction. She travels extensively, giving several lectures a week, volunteering her services to community groups, and maintaining an active social life with many close friends. Stewart, aged 83, is a master's level marathoner. He lifts weights regularly, rides a bike, and hikes the hills and valleys around his home when he is not training for his next race. He is a professional writer and has just learned how to run the software programs Word for Windows and Excel on his computer. Ben, aged 87, recently appeared on the *Love Connection* on TV looking for a woman to enjoy an active social, emotional, and sexual relationship with him.

- What do all these people have in common? Do you know any elderly people like them? How do they compare to your own grandparents? What factors do you think have contributed to their healthy aging? Why do you think these people seem atypical? Are they really that unusual?

Grow old along with me!
The best is yet to be,
The last of life, for which the first was
made. . . .
—Robert Browning, *Rabbi Ben Ezra*

In a society that seems to worship youth, researchers have finally begun to offer some good—even revolutionary—news about the aging process: Growing old doesn't have to mean a slow slide to disability, loneliness, and declining physical and mental health. Health promotion, disease prevention, and wellness-oriented activities can prolong vigor and productivity, even among those who haven't always had model lifestyles or given healthful habits priority. In fact, getting older may actually mean getting better in many ways—particularly socially, psychologically, and intellectually.

Every moment of every day, we are involved in a steady aging process. Everything in the universe—animals, plants, mountain peaks, rivers, planets, even atoms—changes over time. This process is commonly referred to as aging. Aging is something that cannot be avoided, despite the perennial human quest for a fountain of youth. Since you can't stop the process, why not resolve to have a positive aging experience by improving your understanding of the various aspects of aging, taking steps toward maximizing your potential, and learning to adapt and develop strengths you can draw upon over a lifetime?

Who you are as you age and the manner in which you view aging (either as a natural part of living or as an inevitable move toward disease and death) are important factors in how successfully you will adapt to life's transitions. If you view these transitions as periods of growth, as changes that will lead to improved mental, emotional, spiritual, and physical phases in your development as a human being, your journey through even the most difficult times may be easier. No doubt you have encountered active, vigorous, positive 80-year-olds who wake up every morning looking forward to whatever challenges the day may bring. Such persons are socially active and have a zest for life. Many of them seem much younger than their

chronological age, even though their physical casing may be weathered and gray. In contrast, you have probably met 50-year-olds who lack energy and enthusiasm, who seem resigned to tread water for the rest of their lives. These people often appear much older than their chronological age. In short, people experience the aging process in different ways. Explore your own notions about aging in the Rate Yourself box. See how they change after you have read this chapter.

From the moment of conception, we have genetic predispositions that influence our vulnerabilities to many diseases, our physical characteristics, and many other traits that make us unique. Maternal nutrition and health habits influence our health while we are in the womb and during the early months after birth. From the time we are born, we begin to take on characteristics that distinguish us from everyone else. We grow, we change, and we pass through many physical and psychological phases. **Aging** has traditionally been described as the patterns of life changes that occur in members of all species as they grow older. Some believe that it begins at the moment of conception. Others contend that it starts at birth. Still others believe that true aging does not begin until we reach our 40s.

Typically, experts and laypersons alike have used chronological age to assign a person to a particular life-cycle stage. However, people of different chronological ages view age very differently. To the 4-year-old, a college freshman seems quite old. To the 20-year-old, parents in their 40s are over the hill. Have you ever heard your 65-year-old grandparents talking about "those old people down the street"? Views of aging are also colored by occupation. For example, a professional linebacker may find himself too old to play football in his mid-30s. Although some baseball players have continued to demonstrate high levels of skills into their 40s, most players are considering other careers by the time they reach 40. Airline pilots and policemen are often retired in their 50s, while college professors, U.S. senators, and even U.S. presidents may work well into their 70s. Perhaps our traditional definitions of aging need careful reexamination.

REDEFINING AGING

Discrimination against people based on age is known as **ageism.** When directed against the elderly, this type of dis-

Aging: The patterns of life changes that occur in members of all species as they grow older.

Ageism: Discrimination based on age.

What's Your Aging IQ?

Test your knowledge of healthy aging by taking the following test. Answer true or false to each question. Then improve your aging IQ by reading the answers below.

1. Families don't bother with their older relatives.

2. All people become confused or forgetful if they live long enough.

3. You can become too old to exercise.

4. Heart disease is a much bigger problem for older men than for older women.

5. The older you get, the less you sleep.

6. Most older people are depressed. Why shouldn't they be?

7. Older people take more medications than do younger people.

8. People begin to lose interest in sex around age 55.

9. Older people may as well accept urinary accidents as a fact of life.

10. Suicide is mainly a problem for teenagers, not for older people.

11. Falls and injuries just happen to older people.

12. Extremes of heat and cold can be especially dangerous for older people.

Answers

1. False. Most older people live close to their children and see them often. Many live with their spouses. An estimated 80 percent of men and 60 percent of women live in family settings. Only 5 percent of the elderly live in nursing homes.

2. False. Although the confusion and forgetfulness caused by Alzheimer's disease is irreversible, there are at least 100 other problems (head injury, high fever, poor nutrition, adverse drug effects, depression, etc.) that can cause the same symptoms.

3. False. Exercise at any age is beneficial, though the elderly should see a physician for specific guidelines.

4. False. The risk of heart disease after menopause increases dramatically for women. By age 65, both men and women have a one in three chance of showing symptoms of heart disease.

5. False. In later life, it's the quality of sleep that declines, not total sleep time. As people age, their night sleeping becomes more fragmented and they tend to take more naps during the day.

6. False. Most older people are not depressed. When depression does occur in older people, it is treatable with the same approaches used earlier in the life cycle: family support, psychotherapy, and antidepressant medications.

7. True. Older people often have a combination of conditions that require drugs. They consume 25 percent of all medications sold in the United States. Since the chance of adverse reactions to drugs rises with age, careful monitoring is necessary.

8. False. Most older people can lead active, satisfying sex lives.

9. False. Urinary incontinence is a symptom, not a disease. It may be caused by infection, diseases, or the use of certain drugs, and there are many options for treatment.

10. False. Suicide is most prevalent among people age 65 and older. Also, suicide attempts in this group have a higher success rate.

11. False. Falls are the most common cause of injuries among people over 65. Many falls can be avoided by regular vision checks, hearing tests, and improved safety habits in the home. Also important is monitoring the effects of certain medications on balance and coordination.

12. True. The body's thermostat tends to function less efficiently with age, making the older person's body less able to adapt to extreme temperature changes.

Source: Adapted from U.S. Department of Health and Human Services, National Institutes of Health, National Institute on Aging, *What's Your Aging IQ?* (Washington, D.C.: Government Printing Office, 1991).

---

crimination carries with it social ostracism and negative portrayals of older people. A developmental task approach to life-span changes tends to reduce the potential for ageist or negatively biased perceptions about what occurs as a person ages chronologically.

Researchers such as Erik Erikson, Abraham H. Maslow, and R. J. Havighurst believe that people experience considerable change during their lives. Some of these changes occur fairly predictably as rites of passage, such as gradu-

ating from high school, securing a first job, voting, moving away from home, and retirement. As people pass through critical periods in their lives, they are either successful or unsuccessful in their attempts to achieve specified goals. Those who are successful usually develop positive coping skills that carry over into other areas of their lives. They tend to think confidently and independently and are more prepared to "experience" life. Those who fail in these rites of passage either develop a sense of

Learning to cope with challenges and changes early in life develops attitudes and skills that contribute to a full and satisfying old age.

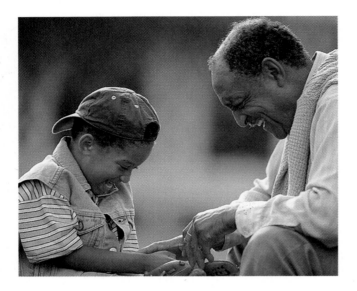

learned helplessness and lose confidence in their ability to succeed or learn to cope by compensating for their failures in productive ways.

The study of individual and collective aging processes, known as **gerontology,** explores the reasons for aging and the ways in which people cope with and adapt to this process. Gerontologists have identified several types of age-related characteristics that should be used to determine where a person is in terms of biological, psychological, social, legal, and functional life-stage development:[1]

- *Biological age* refers to the relative age or condition of the person's organs and body systems. Does the person who is 70 years old have the level of physiological functioning that might be expected of someone in that age group? You have heard of the 70-year-old runner who has the cardiovascular system of a 40-year-old. In contrast, a 20-year-old suffering from progeria (symptoms resembling accelerated aging) may be physiologically closer to a 60-year-old. Arthritis and other chronic conditions often accelerate the aging process.

- *Psychological age* refers to a person's adaptive capacities, such as coping abilities and intelligence, and to the

---

Gerontology: The study of our individual and collective aging processes.
Young-old: People aged 65 to 74.
Middle-old: People aged 75 to 84.
Old-old: People 85 and over.

---

person's awareness of his or her individual capabilities, self-efficacy, and general ability to adapt to a given situation. A lifetime of experiences helps people cope with adversity and with life's challenges. Although chronic illness may render someone physically handicapped, that person may possess tremendous psychological reserves and remain alert and fully capable of making decisions. Psychological age is typically assessed on the basis of everyday behavior, personal interviews, or tests.

- *Social age* refers to a person's habits and roles relative to society's expectations. People in a particular life stage usually share similar tastes in music, television shows, and politics. Whereas rap music and/or heavy metal often appeal to teenagers and people in their 20s, they may repel middle-aged and older people. Cartoons and children's shows probably don't offer the same attraction for you in college that they did when you were a child.

- *Legal age* is probably the most common definition of age in the United States. Legal age is based on chronological years and is used to determine such things as voting rights, driving privileges, drinking age, eligibility for Social Security payments, and a host of other rights and obligations.

- *Functional age* refers to the ways in which people compare to others of a similar age. Heart rate, skin thickness, hearing, and other individual characteristics are analyzed and compared. A person's ability to perform a given job-related task is also part of this assessment. It is difficult to separate functional aging from many of the other types of aging, particularly chronological and biological aging.

What Is Normal Aging?

Contemporary gerontologists have begun to analyze the vast majority of people who continue to live full and productive lives throughout their later years. In the past, our youth-oriented society has viewed the onset of the physiological changes that occur with aging as something to be dreaded. The aging process was seen primarily from a pathological (disease) perspective, and therefore as a time of decline; the focus was not on the gains and positive aspects of normal adult development throughout the life span. Many of these positive developments occur in the areas of emotional and social life as older adults learn to cope with and adapt to the many changes and crises that life may hold in store for them.

Gerontologists have devised several categories for specific age-related characteristics. For example, people who reach the age of 65 are considered to fit the general category of old age. They receive special consideration in the form of government assistance programs such as Social

Security and Medicare. People aged 65 to 74 are viewed as the **young-old**; those aged 75 to 84 are the **middle-old** group; those 85 and over are classified as the **old-old**.

You should note that chronological age is not the only component to be considered when objectively defining *aging*. The question is not how many years a person has lived, but how much life the person has packed into those years. This quality-of-life index, combined with the inevitable chronological process, appears to be the best indicator of the "aging gracefully" phenomenon. The eternal question then becomes "How can I age gracefully?" Most experts today agree that the best way to experience a productive, full, and satisfying old age is to take appropriate action to lead a productive, full, and satisfying life prior to old age. Essentially, older people are the product of their lifelong experiences, molded over years of happiness, heartbreak, and day-to-day existence.

*W*HAT DO YOU THINK?

What factors influence the aging process? Which of these factors do you have the power to change through the behaviors that you engage in right now?

*W*HO ARE THE ELDERLY?

Contrary to popular belief, the elderly in the United States are not and never will be the "forgotten minority." The 65-and-over age group will unquestionably be a major force in the future social, political, and economic plans of the nation because of their sheer numbers and buying power. By the year 2010, a whole generation of 1960s "flower children," who once proclaimed that no one over 30 could be trusted, will begin turning 65. The baby-boomer generation, over 77 million strong and making up over one-third of today's U.S. population, will undoubtedly have a profound impact on the way America looks, thinks, and behaves after the year 2000. Whereas people aged 65 and older made up 13 percent of the U.S. population in 1992, they are projected to make up 21.8 percent of the population by 2030 (see Figure 20.1). The Multicultural Perspectives box looks at worldwide aging demographics in more detail.

A Profile of Today's Elderly

Whereas the average American could expect to live until age 47 in 1900, the typical American today has an average life expectancy of well over 75 years. Where will these elderly people live? Who will pay for their increasing medical costs? How will they support themselves? These questions become more urgent when we consider the factors discussed below.

According to the most recent, 1990 census data, about one in eight Americans today is age 65 years or older. The percentage of the population in this age group more than tripled between 1900 and 1990 (from 4.1 percent to 13 percent) and its number increased 10-fold (from 3.1 million to over 31 million).[2]

In 1990, there were 18.7 million older women and 12.7 million older men, for a gender ratio of 146 women to every 100 men. The sex ratio increases with age, ranging from 120 women for every 100 men in the 65-to-69-year-old group to a high of 258 women for every 100 men in the 85-and-older age group.[3] In 1988, Americans who reached age 65 had an average life expectancy of an additional 16.9 years (18.6 years for females and 14.8 for males). About 2.2 million people celebrated their 65th birthday that year (5,960 birthdays per day). In the same year, about 1.6 million people 65 or older died.[4]

Impact on Society

Economic Considerations. The median income for older persons in 1990 was slightly over $13,500 for males and $7,800 for females. In addition, about 3.5 million elderly Americans lived at or below the poverty level. One of every ten elderly whites was poor compared to about

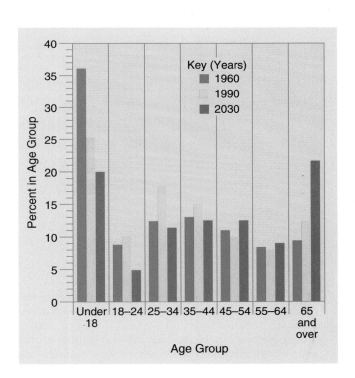

FIGURE 20.1

The Changing Age Distribution of the U.S. Population

Source: Reprinted from *Profile of Older Americans* (Washington, D.C.: American Association on Aging and U.S. Department of Health and Human Services, Administration on Aging, 1992); and National Center for Health Statistics.

Aging: Worldwide Comparative Indicators and Future Trends

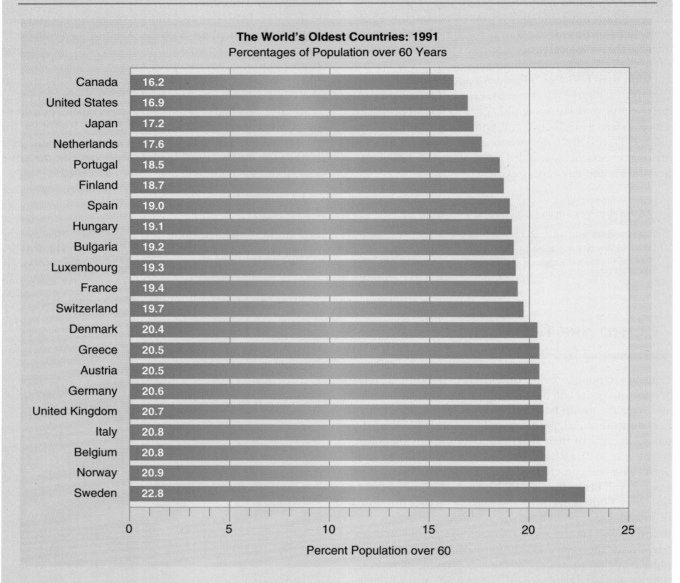

The World's Oldest Countries: 1991
Percentages of Population over 60 Years

Country	Percent
Canada	16.2
United States	16.9
Japan	17.2
Netherlands	17.6
Portugal	18.5
Finland	18.7
Spain	19.0
Hungary	19.1
Bulgaria	19.2
Luxembourg	19.3
France	19.4
Switzerland	19.7
Denmark	20.4
Greece	20.5
Austria	20.5
Germany	20.6
United Kingdom	20.7
Italy	20.8
Belgium	20.8
Norway	20.9
Sweden	22.8

Percent Population over 60

The numerical and proportional growth of older populations around the world is a result of major achievements—reliable birth control that has decreased fertility rates, improvements in medical care and sanitation that have reduced infant and maternal mortality and infectious and parasitic diseases, and improvements in nutrition and education. Every month, the net increase in the world's population aged 60 and over is more than 1 million; 70 percent of this increase occurs in developing countries and 30 percent in developed countries. Based on projected estimates, the percent increase in world population over the age of 60

(continued)

one of every three elderly blacks and one of every five elderly Hispanics.[5]

Health-Care Costs. Although the elderly represented only 13 percent of the U.S. population in 1990, they accounted for over 36 percent of total national health-care costs. Although exact figures are unavailable, it is likely that these numbers have increased substantially in the last five years. Annual health-care expenditures for the elderly total $180 billion—an average of $5,800 per person,

will be 59 percent for the developed countries of the world and 159 percent for the less developed countries between 1991 and 2020.

The world's elderly population—defined here as persons aged 60 and over—numbers 495 million today and is expected to exceed 1 billion by the year 2020. Almost half of today's elderly population lives in just four nations: the People's Republic of China, India, the Commonwealth of Soviet States, and the United States. There is intense debate over issues—social security costs, health care, educational investments, and so on—that are directly linked to this changing age structure of societies.

How could these changes in demographics affect you? Your parents? What do you think the nations of the world could do to plan effectively for the large increases in their elderly populations? What do you think the United States government could do? What do all the "world's oldest countries" have in common?

Source: U.S. Department of Commerce, Bureau of the Census, Economics and Statistics Administration, *Global Aging: Comparative Indicators and Future Trends* (Washington, D.C.: Government Printing Office, 1991).

---

which is more than four times the $1,500 per person spent for the health care of younger Americans.[6] To a large extent, these figures reflect the intense use of expensive medical procedures in treating people with diseases such as cancer, heart disease, and respiratory ailments. With projected future increases in life expectancy, many analysts fear that health-care costs will skyrocket even more. Will working Americans be willing to pay an increased share of the health-care costs for people on fixed incomes who cannot pay for themselves?

Housing and Living Arrangements. With the costs of owning and maintaining a home slowly moving beyond the reach of the average American, housing problems for low-income elderly people are becoming more acute. Where will the generation of baby-boom elderly find suit-able housing? Who will provide the necessary social services, and who will pay the bill? Will the family of the future be forced to coexist with several generations under one roof?

Contrary to popular opinion, most older people do not live in nursing homes. In fact, only about 1 percent of all people between the ages of 65 and 74, 6 percent of those between 75 and 84, and 22 percent of those over 85 are forced to seek nursing-home care. The great majority of all older males (82 percent) and more than half (57 percent) of all older females live in family settings until their final days. For an overview of the living arrangements of these noninstitutionalized elderly, see Figure 20.2.

Ethical and Moral Considerations. As we have already noted, the "senior boom" of the 1990s and beyond may

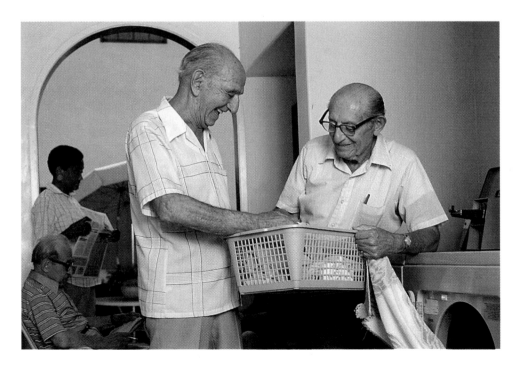

Older people in good health can maintain their independence and find companionship in community housing for the elderly.

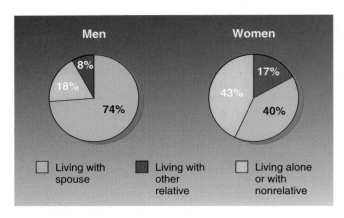

FIGURE 20.2

The chart measures living arrangements of elderly people (65 and over) in the United States in 1992. Note that many more women than men live alone.

force us to reexamine many of our present attitudes and practices. At the present time, the implications for an already overburdened health-care delivery system are staggering. For example, with our current shortage of donor organs, will we be continually forced to decide whether a 75-year-old should receive a heart transplant instead of a 50-year-old? Questions have already surfaced regarding the efficacy of hooking a terminally ill older person up to costly machines that may prolong life for a few weeks or months but overtax our health-care resources. Is the prolongation of life at all costs a moral imperative, or will future generations be forced to devise a set of criteria for deciding who will be helped and who will not? These questions represent potential concerns and problems for all of us.

𝒲HAT DO YOU THINK?

Why are so many people concerned about the graying of America? What impact will the boom of elderly people have on society? What actions can we take now to minimize problems in the future?

𝒯HEORIES ON AGING

Biological Theories

Of the various theories about the biological causes of aging, the following are among the most commonly accepted.

■ *The wear-and-tear theory* states that, like everything else in the universe, the human body wears out. Inher-

ent in this theory is the idea that the more you abuse your body, the faster it will wear out. A great deal of controversy exists today regarding the relative benefits and disadvantages of various exercise programs for middle-aged and elderly people. Proponents of the wear-and-tear theory argue that activities such as jogging may actually predispose people to premature bone and joint injuries in later years, particularly in the lower back, hip, and knee areas.

■ *The cellular theory* states that at birth we have only a certain number of usable cells, and these cells are genetically programmed to divide or reproduce only a limited number of times. Once these cells reach the end of their reproductive cycle, they begin to die and the organs they make up begin to show signs of deterioration. The rate of deterioration varies from person to person, and the impact of the deterioration depends on the system involved.

■ *The autoimmune theory* attributes aging to the decline of the body's immunological system. Studies indicate that as we age, our immune systems become less effective in fighting disease. Eventually, bodies that are subjected to too much stress, especially if this is coupled with poor nutrition, begin to show signs of disease and infirmity. In some instances, the immune system appears to lose control and to turn its protective mechanisms inward, actually attacking the person's own body. Although this type of disorder may occur in all

Some people seem to defy many of the theories of aging by remaining fit and even able to participate in competitive sports well into their seventies.

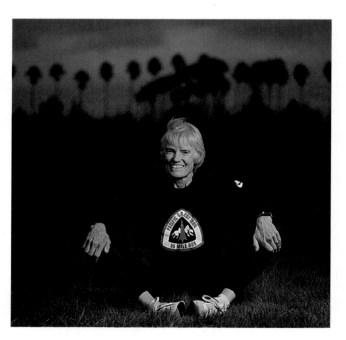

age groups, some gerontologists believe that the condition increases in frequency and severity with age.

- *The genetic mutation theory* proposes that the number of cells exhibiting unusual or different characteristics increases with age. Proponents of this theory believe that aging is related to the amount of mutational damage within the genes. The greater the mutation, the greater the chance that cells will not function properly, leading to eventual dysfunction of body organs and systems.

Psychosocial Theories

Numerous psychological and sociological factors also have a strong influence on the manner in which people age. Psychologists Erik Erikson and Robert Peck have formulated theories of personality development that encompass the human life span. Their theories emphasize adaptation and adjustment as related to self-development. In his developmental model, Erikson states that people must progress through eight critical stages during their lifetimes. If a person does not receive the proper stimulus or develop effective methods of coping with life's turmoil from infancy onward, problems are likely to develop later in life. According to this theory, attitudes, behaviors, and beliefs related to maladjustments in old age are often a result of problems encountered in earlier stages of a person's life.

Peck focuses much of his developmental theory on the crucial issues of middle and old age. He argues that during these periods people face a series of increasingly stressful tasks. Those who are poorly adjusted psychologically or who have not developed appropriate coping skills are likely to undergo a painful aging process.

A key element in the theories of both Erikson and Peck is the incorporation of age-related factors into lifelong behavior patterns. Both models stress that successful aging involves maintaining emotional as well as physical well-being. Most probably, a combination of psychosocial and biological factors and environmental "trigger mechanisms" causes each of us to age in a unique manner. The question then arises as to what is considered normal in the aging process. How much change is inevitable and how much can be avoided? Which factors slow down the aging process and which ones actually cause us to age prematurely?

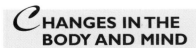

CHANGES IN THE BODY AND MIND

Answers to the question of what is "typical" or "normal" when applied to aging are highly speculative. In order to assess the typical aging process, we should probably ask ourselves what we can reasonably expect to happen to our bodies as we grow older.

Physical Changes

Although the physiological consequences of aging differ in their severity and timing from person to person, there are standard changes that occur as a result of the aging process.

The Skin. As a normal consequence of aging, the skin becomes thinner and loses elasticity, particularly in the outer surfaces. Fat deposits, which add to the soft lines and shape of the skin, begin to diminish. Starting at about age 30, lines develop on the forehead as a result of smiling, squinting, and other facial expressions. These lines become more pronounced, with added "crow's-feet" around the eyes, during the 40s. During a person's 50s and 60s, the skin begins to sag and lose color, leading to pallor in the 70s. Body fat in underlying layers of skin continues to be redistributed away from the limbs and extremities into the trunk region of the body. Age spots become more numerous because of excessive pigment accumulation under the skin. The sun tends to increase pigment production, leading to more age spots.

Bones and Joints. Throughout the life span, your bones are continually changing because of the accumulation and loss of minerals. By the third or fourth decade of life, mineral loss from bones becomes more prevalent than mineral accumulation, resulting in a weakening and porosity (diminishing density) of bony tissue. This loss of minerals (particularly calcium) occurs in both sexes, although it is much more common in females. Loss of calcium can contribute to **osteoporosis,** a condition characterized by weakened, porous, and fractured bones.

Although many people consider osteoporosis a disease of the elderly, it is actually a progressive disorder that may already have begun to affect you. When you hear of osteoporosis, you may envision a slumped over individual with a characteristic "dowager's hump" in the upper back, but this is the rare extreme of the condition. Bone loss occurs over many years and may be without symptoms until actual fractures occur or are diagnosed via X rays. The spine, hips, and wrists are the most common sites of fractures, though other bones of the body may be involved.[7]

In the United States, osteoporosis affects over 25 million Americans and causes 1.5 million fractures annually. Of these fractures, about 250,000 occur at the hip. An estimated 12 to 20 percent of patients with hip fractures die

Osteoporosis: A degenerative bone disorder characterized by increasingly porous bones.

within one year.[8] Osteoporosis affects one in three post-menopausal women and a majority of people of both sexes over the age of 70.[9] Although more common in women than in men, osteoporosis in men is a significant problem.[10] About 14 percent of all vertebral fractures and 25 percent of all hip fractures occur in men.[11] Several risk factors for developing osteoporosis have been identified:

- *Gender:* Women have a four times greater risk than men have. Their peak bone mass is lower than men's, and they experience an accelerated rate of bone loss after menopause.

- *Age:* After the third and fourth decade of life, all individuals lose bone mass and are more susceptible.

- *Low bone mass:* Low bone mass is one of the strongest predictors of osteoporosis. Measurement of bone density is an important aspect of risk assessment.

- *Early menopause:* The early occurrence of menopause, whether natural or caused by surgery, means that the positive effects of estrogen are lost for a longer period of time. (Decreases in sex hormones—estrogen in females and testosterone in males—appear to increase risk for the disease.) Menstrual disturbances, such as those caused by anorexia or bulimia or excessive exercise, may similarly result in an early loss of bone mass.

- *Thin, small-framed body:* Petite, thin women usually have a relatively low peak bone mass and are therefore at greater risk for osteoporosis. (This is one of the few health areas in which being larger and even slightly overweight is an advantage.)

- *Race:* Whites and Asians are at higher risk of developing osteoporosis than are blacks because blacks have heavier bone density on average. Black women have about one-half the incidence of hip fractures as white women have.

- *Lack of calcium:* A lifetime of low calcium intake (well below the RDA and below the natural loss of calcium of 300 to 400 milligrams per day) may result in low peak bone mass and above-average loss of bone mass throughout adulthood.

- *Lack of physical activity:* Immobilized, bedridden, or very inactive people usually have less muscle and bone mass.

- *Cigarette smoking:* Though the mechanism is not clear, smoking is linked to the development of osteoporosis.

- *Alcohol and/or caffeine:* Abuse of these substances is also linked to the development of osteoporosis.

- *Heredity:* Unidentified hereditary factors may play a role in the development of osteoporosis.[12]

Although all these factors have been implicated in osteoporosis, there are people who have few of these risk factors and yet develop osteoporosis and people who have many of these risk factors who never develop the condition. The many unknowns about the disease make prevention and treatment difficult. Currently, there are several options open to you for reducing your own risks. In general, prevention focuses on building the largest possible bone mass (within genetic limits), particularly at skeletal maturity, and maintaining these levels with minimal bone loss, especially after menopause.[13] Both of these strategies help prevent bone fractures.

The goal of both treatment and prevention of osteoporosis is to decrease the likelihood and severity of bone fractures. Currently accepted treatments of established osteoporosis include adequate calcium intake, daily weight-bearing exercises approved by a physician, fall-prevention measures, and use of the hormones estrogen (in those not at high risk for certain forms of cancer) and calcitonin.[14] A recent study has shown that increasing calcium intake to 1,380 milligrams per day—an amount that exceeds the current RDA for calcium—both reduces bone loss and increases bone mineralization in women aged 58 to 77.[15] Other therapies for osteoporosis, such as sodium fluoride, various metabolites of vitamin D, and bisphosphonates, are under investigation.[16]

Of these treatments, increasing calcium intake during childhood and young adulthood appears to be quite effective in reducing lifelong risk by promoting denser bone mass.[17] By 1989, the large numbers of studies documenting this relationship led the Food and Nutrition Board of the National Research Council to raise the RDA for calcium from 800 to 1200 milligrams per day for people between 19 and 24 years of age. Many experts suggest that these numbers should be even higher and recommend a standard of 1500 milligrams per day for postmenopausal women.

Although the vitamin industry would like all of us to take megadoses of calcium every day, the preferred source of calcium is a nutritionally balanced diet.[18] Dairy products, including milk, yogurt, and cheese, are the best sources of dietary calcium; canned fish, certain dark green leafy vegetables (such as kale and broccoli), legumes, calcium-enriched grain products, and fortified fruit juices may also be good sources.

Regular exercise of weight-bearing joints, maintenance of muscular strength and flexibility, and an adequate intake of calcium are probably your best routes of prevention during early adulthood. As you approach menopause or if you have other ailments that could increase your risk, consult an endocrinologist or orthopedic specialist to determine what forms of medical treatment may be most effective for minimizing your risk for osteoporosis.

The Head. With age, features of the head enlarge and become more noticeable. Increased cartilage and fatty tissue cause the nose to grow a half-inch wider and another half-inch longer. Earlobes get fatter and grow longer, while overall head circumference increases one-quarter of an inch per decade, even though the brain itself shrinks. The skull becomes thicker with age.

The Urinary Tract. At age 70, the kidneys can filter waste from the blood only half as fast as they could at age 30. The need to urinate more frequently occurs because the bladder's capacity declines from 2 cups of urine at age 30 to 1 cup at age 70.

One problem often associated with aging is **urinary incontinence,** which ranges from passing a few drops of urine while laughing or sneezing to having no control over when and where urination takes place. Although exact estimates vary, as many as 19 percent of older men and 38 percent of older women have some degree of urinary incontinence.[19]

However, incontinence is not an inevitable part of the aging process. Most cases are caused by highly treatable underlying neurological problems that affect the central nervous system, medications, infections of the pelvic muscles, weakness in the pelvic walls, or other problems. When the problem is treated, the incontinence usually vanishes.[20]

Incontinence poses major social, physical, and emotional problems for the elderly. Embarrassment and fear of wetting oneself may cause an older person to become isolated and to avoid social functions. Caregivers may become frustrated and angry with their incontinent elderly patients. Prolonged wetness and the inability to properly care for oneself can lead to irritation, infections, or other problems. Fortunately, there are many treatments for this problem. Drug therapy can slow bladder contractions, increase bladder capacity, contract or relax the bladder sphincter, and increase fluid output. Surgery to repair the pelvic floor is often successful in stress incontinence. Artificial devices that slow urine flow, improvements in access to toilet facilities, rigid schedules for urination, and many newer treatments have also shown promise.[21] In addition, women can learn exercises to strengthen the pelvic floor to reduce their susceptibility to this problem later in life. Biofeedback to control urine flow and improve mind/body responses is another approach to prevention.

The Heart and Lungs. Resting heart rate stays about the same during a person's life, but the stroke volume (the amount of blood the muscle pushes out per beat) diminishes as heart muscles deteriorate. Vital capacity, or the amount of air that moves when you inhale and exhale at maximum effort, also declines with age. Exercise can do a great deal to reduce potential deterioration in heart and lung function.

Eyesight. By the age of 30, the lens of the eye begins to harden, causing specific problems by the early 40s. The lens begins to yellow and loses transparency, while the pupil of the eye begins to shrink, allowing less light to penetrate. Activities such as reading become more difficult, particularly in dim light. By age 60, depth perception declines and farsightedness often develops. A need for glasses usually develops in the 40s that evolves into a need for bifocals in the 50s and trifocals in the 60s. **Cataracts** (clouding of the lens) and **glaucoma** (elevation of pressure within the eyeball) become more likely. There may eventually be a tendency toward color blindness, especially for shades of blue and green.

Hearing. The ability to hear high-frequency consonants (for example, *s, t,* and *z*) diminishes with age. Much of the actual hearing loss is in the ability to distinguish not normal conversational tones but extreme ranges of sound. The Building Communication Skills box offers tips on communicating with those who are hearing impaired.

Taste. The sense of taste begins to decline as a person gets older. At age 30, each tiny elevation on the tongue (called papilla) has 245 taste buds. By the age of 70, each has only 88 left. The mouth gets drier as salivary glands secrete less fluid. The ability to distinguish sweet, sour, bitter, and salty tastes diminishes. Elderly people often compensate for their diminished sense of taste by adding excessive amounts of salt, sugar, and other flavor enhancers to their food.

Smell and Touch. The sense of smell also diminishes with age. As a result of this loss, coupled with the loss of the sense of taste, food is often less appealing to older people. Pain receptors also become less effective. The tactile senses decline.

Sexual Changes. As men age, they experience notable changes in sexual functioning. Whereas the degree and rate of change vary greatly from person to person, the following changes generally occur:

1. The ability to obtain an erection is slowed.

2. The ability to maintain an erection is diminished.

3. The length of the refractory period between orgasms increases.

4. The angle of the erection declines with age.

5. The orgasm itself grows shorter in duration.

Urinary incontinence: The inability to control urination.

Cataracts: Clouding of the lens that interrupts the focusing of light on the retina, resulting in blurred vision or eventual blindness.

Glaucoma: Elevation of pressure within the eyeball, leading to hardening of the eyeball, impaired vision, and possible blindness.

Tips on Communicating with Hearing-Impaired Individuals

- Speak clearly, distinctly, and slowly: do not shout or exaggerate your mouth movements.

- Face the person when talking and look him or her in the eye. If the person to whom you are speaking is in a wheelchair, lower yourself to eye level.

- Be sure that there is enough light for the person to see you speaking but also that there is no glare.

- Try to avoid conversing with the person in noisy areas.

- Use visual cues such as hand movements and facial expressions in addition to your verbal message.

- If you are asked to repeat what you said, find other words to say the same thing.

- In a group situation, sit in a circle so everyone can see one another's lip movements and expressions. Clue the hearing-impaired into the conversation by summarizing occasionally.

- Be patient. Don't create the feeling that you are in a hurry.

- Learn to read the individual's reactions to be certain you are heard and understood.

- Keep hands, scarves, and tobacco away from your mouth. Don't chew gum, eat, or smoke while talking.

- Get the person's attention before you start to speak.

- Don't talk from too far away.

- Make an attempt to discuss topics other than what is absolutely necessary, even though these may be harder to communicate. Don't resort to curt, necessary exchanges and avoid everything else.

Source: From Armeda F. Ferrini with Rebecca L. Ferrini, *Health in the Later Years,* 2nd edition. Copyright © 1993 Wm. C. Brown Communications, Inc., Dubuque, Iowa. Reprinted by permission of Times Mirror Higher Education Group, Inc., Dubuque, Iowa.

Women also experience several changes:

1. Menopause usually occurs between the ages of 45 and 55. Women may experience such symptoms as hot flashes, mood swings, weight gain, development of facial hair, and other hormone-related problems.

2. The walls of the vagina become less elastic, and the epithelium thins, making painful intercourse more likely.

3. Vaginal secretions during sexual activity diminish.

4. The breasts decrease in firmness. Loss of fat in various areas leads to fewer curves, with a decrease in the soft lines of the body contours.

Body Comfort. Because of the loss of body fat, thinning of the epithelium, and diminished glandular activity, elderly people experience greater difficulty in regulating body temperature. This change means that their ability to withstand extreme cold or heat may be very limited, thus increasing the risks of hypothermia, heatstroke, and heat exhaustion.

Senility: A term associated with loss of memory and judgment and orientation problems occurring in a small percentage of the elderly.

Alzheimer's disease: A chronic condition involving changes in nerve fibers of the brain that results in mental deterioration

WHAT DO YOU THINK?

Of the health conditions listed in this section, which ones can you prevent? Which ones can you delay? What actions can you take now to protect yourself from these problems?

Mental Changes

Intelligence. Stereotypes concerning inevitable intellectual decline among the elderly have been largely refuted. Recent research has demonstrated that much of our previous knowledge about elderly intelligence was based on inappropriate testing procedures. Given an appropriate length of time, elderly people may learn and develop skills in a similar manner to younger people. Researchers have also determined that what many elderly people lack in speed of learning they make up for in practical knowledge—that is, the "wisdom of age."

Memory. Have you ever wondered why your grandfather seems unable to remember what he did last weekend even though he can graphically depict the details of a social event that occurred 40 years earlier? This phenomenon is not unusual among the elderly. Research indicates that although short-term memory may fluctuate on a daily basis, the ability to remember events from past decades seems to remain largely unchanged in many elderly people. The Skills for Behavior Change box offers suggestions on improving your memory.

Many elderly retain their intellectual and artistic abilities into old age, despite the inevitable physical declines and progressive diminishment of the sensory functions of sight, sound, taste, smell, and touch.

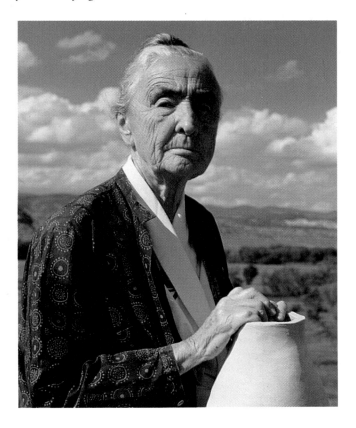

Flexibility versus Rigidity. Although it is widely believed that people become more like one another as they age, nothing could be farther from the truth. Having lived through a multitude of experiences and having faced diverse joys, sorrows, and obstacles, the typical elderly person has developed unique methods of coping with life. These unique adaptive variations make for interesting differences in how the elderly confront the many changes brought on by the aging process. As a group, the elderly are extremely heterogeneous.

Depression. Most adults continue to lead healthy, fulfilling lives as they grow older. However, some elderly people do suffer from mental and emotional disturbances. Some research indicates that depression may be the most common psychological problem facing older adults. However, the rate of major depression is 4 percent lower among older people than among younger adults.[22]

Regardless of age, those who have a poor perception of their health, who have multiple chronic illnesses, who take a lot of medications, and who do not exercise have greater rates of depression.[23] Strong coping skills and support systems will often lessen the duration and severity of the

depression. However, those who are ill-equipped to deal with life's changes or who lack close ties may consider suicide as a means of solving their problems.

Senility: Getting Rid of Ageist Attitudes. Over the years, the elderly have often been the victims of ageist attitudes. People who were chronologically old were often labeled "senile" whenever they displayed memory failure, errors in judgment, disorientation, or erratic behaviors. Today scientists recognize that these same symptoms can occur at any age and for various reasons, including disease or the use of OTC and prescription drugs. When the underlying problems are corrected, the memory loss and disorientation also improve. Currently, the term **senility** is seldom used except to describe a very small group of organic disorders.

Alzheimer's Disease. Dementias are progressive brain impairments that interfere with memory and normal intellectual functioning. Although there are many types of dementia, one of the most common forms is **Alzheimer's disease.** In November 1994, the announcement that former president Ronald Reagan has Alzheimer's disease dramatized the Alzheimer patient's struggle for those who had not yet experienced its effects on a relative or friend. Attacking over 4 million Americans, and killing over 100,000 of them every year, this disease is one of the most painful and devastating conditions that families can endure. It kills its victims twice: First through a slow loss of their personhood (memory loss, disorientation, personality changes, and eventual loss of the ability to function as a person), and then as their bodily systems

Alzheimer's disease, a progressive impairment of the brain, strikes over 4 million older Americans in all walks of life every year.

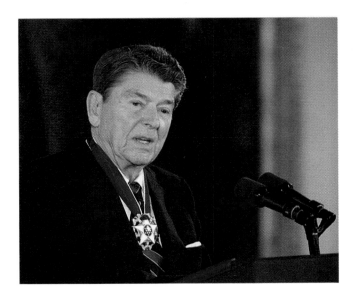

Exercising Your Memory

Mnemonics, the art of improving short-term recall and ferreting out stored facts, depends on strong visual images and meaningful associations: it's a system for cross-indexing stored information in arresting ways. These methods only take a little time to master. They work because they seize the attention and demand concentration. The more outrageous the connections you set up, the better. [For example:] . . .

Make up rhymes. Nobody ever forgets the useful "I before E, except after C." But to remember home chores, make up your own rhymes: "Skitty, skat, let in the cat," for instance. The cornier the better.

Compose mental pictures, particularly when you're trying to remember a name: Helen Decker, say, might conjure up a vision of Helen of Troy on shipboard.

Repeat or rehearse new facts. "How do you do, Helen," you say when introduced at a party. A few minutes later you say to yourself, "That's Helen Decker." And a minute or so after that, "Can I get you anything to drink, Helen?" You probably won't forget Helen's name.

Make up acronyms or sentences. "Maple" could help an out-of-towner remember the order of Madison, Park, and Lexington Avenues. "The postman at Sutter's Mill was bushed from pining for California" could help a visitor remember the order of five San Francisco streets, Post, Sutter, Bush, Pine, and California.

Chunk or regroup clusters of data to give them a pattern. Telephone numbers are already partially grouped, but you can give them further meaning. Helen's three-digit exchange, 744, is easy to remember, but you won't forget the rest of the number either, 4591, when you reflect that she looks to be about 45, almost halfway to 91.

Write things down. Writing notes and making lists will often fix things in your mind. You may not even have to refer to your notes or lists.

Structure your life. Even the hook for the house keys by the back door is a mnemonic device: you'll always look there first. Similarly, keep your checkbook in the drawer of your desk, or park your reading glasses on the night table.

Ease your mind. If you feel you are forgetting too much, consider the following:

- Give yourself time. The sky won't fall in if you forget a name or a number, and if you employ a few delaying tactics (don't rush right up to the friend whose name you've forgotten), the missing data may surface. If they don't, don't make a big fuss over it. Just admit you've forgotten.

- Don't expect too much. If you're nervous about forgetting, you usually do.

- Play games. Crossword puzzles, Scrabble, and card games are all good exercises for improving memory.

- Improve your mind. Going to lectures, taking classes, and joining groups will introduce new stimuli and keep your neurons transmitting.

Source: Excerpted by permission from "Exercising Your Memory," *University of California at Berkeley Wellness Letter,* October 1988, p. 5. © Health Letter Associates, 1988.

---

gradually succumb to the powerful impact of neurological problems.

Currently, Alzheimer's afflicts an estimated 1 in 20 people between the ages of 65 and 75 and 1 in 5 people over the age of 80. These numbers are certain to increase. It is estimated to cost society over $100 billion a year currently. With the U.S. population gradually aging, the economic burden of the future seems even more dismal. While the disease is associated in most people's minds strictly with the elderly, it has been diagnosed in people as young as in their late 40s. In fact, about 5 percent of all cases occur before age 65.

What is Alzheimer's? Actually, contrary to what many people think, Alzheimer's is not a new disease. Named after Alois Alzheimer, a German neuropathologist who recorded it as early as 1906, Alzheimer's refers to a degenerative disease of the brain in which nerve cells stop communicating with one another. Ordinarily, brain cells communicate by releasing chemicals that allow the cells to receive and transmit messages for various types of behavior. In Alzheimer's patients, the brain doesn't produce enough of these chemicals, cells can't communicate, and eventually the cells die.

This degeneration happens in the sections of the brain that affect memory, speech, and personality, leaving the parts that control other bodily functions, such as heartbeat and breathing, working just fine. Thus, the mind begins to go as the body lives on. It all happens in a slow, progressive manner, and it may be as long as 20 years before you notice symptoms.

The only known detection test for Alzheimer's was announced in November 1994. Researchers at Harvard Medical School found that people with Alzheimer's appear to be very sensitive to eye drops similar to those used by doctors to dilate the pupils before performing an eye exam. Although many people feel a sensitivity to such eye drops, people with Alzheimer's show reaction with just 1 percent of the normal dose. The test should be available clinically by the end of 1996. Experts hope to use the test to detect Alzheimer's early enough that experimental drugs that may slow progress of the disease will be most effective.[24]

Alzheimer's is generally detected first by families, who note changes, particularly unusual memory losses and personality changes, in their loved ones. Medical tests rule out underlying causes, and certain neurological tests help confirm the likelihood of this disease.

What are the symptoms of Alzheimer's? Alzheimer's disease is characteristically diagnosed in three stages. During the first stage, symptoms include forgetfulness, memory loss, impaired judgment, increasing inability to handle routine tasks, disorientation, lack of interest in one's surroundings, and depression. These symptoms accelerate in the second stage, which also includes agitation and restlessness (especially at night), loss of sensory perceptions, muscle twitching, and repetitive actions. Many patients become depressed and there is a tendency to be combative and aggressive. In the final stage, disorientation is often complete. The person becomes completely dependent on others for eating, dressing, and other activities. Identity loss and speech problems are common symptoms. Eventually, control of bodily functions may be lost.

Once Alzheimer's disease strikes, the victim's life expectancy is cut in half. Tragically, there is little that can be done at present to treat the disorder. Scientists are experimenting with various drug regimens, but it is unlikely that a drug will be discovered in the immediate future that will undo the damage associated with Alzheimer's disease.

The results of research into the causes of Alzheimer's disease are inconclusive. Current research is looking into genetic predisposition, malfunction of the immune system, a slow-acting virus, chromosomal or genetic defects, and neurotransmitter imbalance, among other possibilities.

Preliminary research indicates that a defect in the chromosomes may be the most likely cause, partly because virtually everyone with Down's syndrome eventually develops Alzheimer's.[25] Treatments for Alzheimer's tend to focus on the only medication that has been approved by the Food and Drug Administration, Cognex, which slows the loss of memory by preventing the destruction of neurotransmitters. Unfortunately, this drug seems to be effective in only about 20 percent of the patients who receive it.

Some researchers are looking at anti-inflammatory drugs, theorizing that Alzheimer's may develop in response to an inflammatory ailment. Others are focusing on estrogen as a possible preventive measure, noting that women who take estrogen during menopause have been found to develop Alzheimer's much later on average than women who don't. Still others are focusing on stimulating the brains of Alzheimer's-prone individuals, believing that as people learn, more connections between cells are formed that may offset those that are lost. All such research is very preliminary.

Much attention has also been focused on the family, as the family is often another victim when Alzheimer's occurs. Having to decide between trying to tend to the needs of a loved one at home or seeking the assistance of a long-term-care facility can be difficult for relatives of Alzheimer's victims. Caring for such patients is a challenge for even the most dedicated family members. And even the best preparation for the final days of a loved one with this disease does not make the process an easy one.

Knowing what the options are and being able to recognize the differences between normal physiological aging and the ravages of certain diseases can help make age-related problems easier to cope with for both the elderly themselves and their families. Although we have focused on some negative aspects of aging in this chapter, we must emphasize again that elderly people who have developed self-confidence, self-reliance, healthy attitudes about themselves and others, and effective coping mechanisms typically lead active, healthy lives. In fact, older people who have a support network and are socially adept are happier and more satisfied in many ways than are younger people who do not have these social skills or networks.

HEALTH CHALLENGES OF THE ELDERLY

The elderly are disproportionately victimized by a number of societally induced problems. Other problems result when people do not develop the ability to cope properly with life's hurdles. Still other problems come from a perceived loss of control over the circumstances of their lives by the elderly—who watch loved ones die, are forced to retire, face problems with personal health, and confront an uncertain economy on a fixed income. If you develop certain skills in your earlier years and acquire strong social supports, you may significantly reduce your risk for problems in old age

Alcohol Use and Abuse: Myth or Reality?

Although the elderly are often believed to be at high risk for alcoholism, exact numbers in this area are difficult to obtain. Some early studies reported incidence rates of 2 to 10 percent, but more recent studies indicate that fewer than 2 percent of the elderly are alcoholics.[26] However, if you are prone to alcoholism in your younger and middle years, the chances are great that you will continue with these patterns of abuse in your older years. The old alcoholic is probably no more common in American society than the young alcoholic, even though the stereotype is an old, lost soul, hiding his or her sorrows in a bottle. Often, when many people think they see a drunken older person they are really seeing a confused older person who has taken too many different prescription medications and is experiencing a form of drug interaction.

Men tend to have higher risks for alcoholism at all ages. Alcohol abuse is five times more common among elderly men than among elderly women. Yet as many as half of all elderly men and an even higher proportion of elderly women don't drink at all. Those who do drink do so less than younger persons, consuming only five to six drinks weekly.[27]

If the more recent studies are accurate, the reason there aren't many heavy drinkers among the elderly may be that very heavy drinkers tend either to die of alcoholic complications before they reach old age or to reform their drinking habits. Some older people reduce their consumption of alcohol because they find they cannot process it as readily as they did when they were younger or because they are afraid of combining alcohol with the prescription drugs they must take. If the older reports are accurate, alcoholism in the elderly may be disguised by a tendency among health professionals and family members to associate forgetfulness, incontinence, poor grooming, dementia-like reactions, injuries, and so on with old age rather than with an alcohol problem.[28] It is important to note that most of the elderly who consume alcohol are neither alcoholics nor people who drink to cope with their losses.[29] Most drinking among the elderly is social drinking, and may, in fact, be much less of a problem than previously thought.[30]

Prescription Drug Use: Unique Problems for the Elderly

It is extremely rare for elderly people to use illicit drugs, but some do overuse, and grow dependent upon, prescription drugs. Beset with numerous aches, pains, and inexplicable as well as diagnosable maladies, some elderly people take between four and six prescription drugs a day. Reported numbers of drugs taken are substantially higher for residents of health-care institutions, but this may be because drugs that many of us purchase over the counter, such as aspirin, are counted in the total numbers.

Anyone who combines different drugs runs the risk of dangerous drug interactions. The risks of adverse effects are even greater for people with circulation impairments and declining kidney and liver functions. Elderly people displaying symptoms of these drug-induced effects, which may include bizarre behavior patterns or an appearance of being out of touch, are often misdiagnosed as being senile rather than examined for underlying causes and treated. As the Health Headlines box points out, doctors often misprescribe for the elderly.

Over-the-Counter Remedies

Although today's elderly appear to be more receptive to medical treatment than the elderly of previous generations, a substantial segment of the over-60 population avoid orthodox medical treatment, viewing it as only a last resort. This is becoming increasingly true as Medicare coverage becomes less and less adequate and the elderly are forced to pay greater amounts of their medical bills out of their own resources. The poor are particularly prone to turn to folk medicine and over-the-counter preparations as cheaper, less intimidating alternatives. As might be expected, aspirin and laxatives head the list of commonly used OTC medications for relief of arthritic pain and the irregular bowel activity sometimes experienced by the elderly.

Vitamins and Mineral Supplements

As with many bodily processes, the digestion of food begins to slow with age. Nevertheless, the body can still use almost all nutrients if they are consumed in moderate quantities and in the right combination. There is a great deal of concern among gerontologists and other health professionals that the elderly may be particularly vulnerable to nutritional hucksters who promote the magical qualities of their brands of vitamin and mineral concoctions. Following is a description of some of the more common vitamin and mineral products promoted as being especially important to the elderly:

- *Calcium:* Many elderly people do not believe that they need as much milk and other dairy products as they did when they were young. As a result, they may not consume adequate amounts of calcium, or they may take it as an individual supplement without vitamin D, which is necessary for calcium absorption in the body. Calcium deficiencies contribute to osteoporosis, "dowager's hump," shrinking height, and other bone disorders that are common among the elderly. Fear of these ailments has led to soaring sales of calcium supplements. However, research has begun to refute much of the previous thinking about the benefits of calcium supplements versus other treatments after bone and joint deterioration occurs.[31] Adequate calcium intake should be a part of a lifelong regimen of preventive health care.

- *Vitamin E:* Although some gerontologists believe that we should take extra vitamin E because it stops the formation of substances believed to cause aging, this theory is largely unsubstantiated. In fact, evidence suggests that megadoses of any of the fat-soluble vitamins may damage already deteriorating kidneys and livers.

- *Vitamin C:* Although Linus Pauling, a Nobel prize-winning scientist, actively promoted the intake of megadoses of vitamin C as a preventive measure for a host of health-related problems, the likelihood that this vitamin has any appreciable effect on life expectancy is minimal.

- *Vitamin B_6:* Promoted as a kind of "energizer" for deteriorating nervous systems, vitamin B_6 was a key element in the "vitamin mania" of the 1980s. Recent research suggests, however, that megadoses of vitamin B_6 may cause symptoms similar to multiple sclerosis in some people, making it especially hazardous for the elderly.

Wrong Drugs Given to 1 in 4 of Elderly

Close to a quarter of all Americans 65 or older were given prescriptions for drugs that they should almost never take, a study has found.

Some of the drugs can produce amnesia and confusion, others can cause serious side effects like heart problems or respiratory failure. And, the investigators said, there is no need to prescribe these drugs to older people, either because safer alternatives are available or because the drugs are simply not needed.

The study, by Dr. Steffi Woolhandler of Harvard Medical School and colleagues, examined data from a national survey that included more than 6,000 older people who were not in nursing homes and that determined what medicines they were taking. The researchers used a list of 20 drugs that a panel of experts had said should not be prescribed for older people. The survey was conducted in 1987, but the data were only recently made available for analysis, the researchers said, and no similar studies have been conducted since then.

In their paper, being published today in the *Journal of the American Medical Association*, the investigators found, for example, that 1.8 million older people had prescriptions for dipyridamole, a blood thinner that, the researchers say, is useless for all except people with artificial heart valves. Yet only 36,000 Americans, half of them over 65, had heart valves put in in 1987.

More than 1.3 million older Americans had prescriptions for propoxyphene, an addictive narcotic that, the author say, is no better than aspirin in relieving pain. More than 1.2 million were taking diazepam or chlordiapoxide, which are long-acting sedatives and sleeping pills that can make people groggy, forgetful and prone to falls. . . .

[G]eriatrics specialists, including Dr. Woolhandler, said they were disturbed, but not surprised, by the study's findings.

"Based on my own clinical practice, I knew it was a problem," Woolhandler said. "I have had elderly people call up who had taken a Valium and started falling or who had gotten home at night and not known where they were in the day because of amnesia. I have seen patients after a heart attack who were so drugged that they couldn't function at all. I had a lady who almost died from a fainting spell after she took a muscle relaxer that she shouldn't have been given.

"A lot of the problem is that doctors frequently ascribe side effects of drugs to old age," she said. "If a patient loses memory or loses balance, they say it's old age."

Dr. Robert Butler, chairman of the department of "geriatrics at the Mount Sinai School of Medicine, said older people also attributed severe side effects to old age.

Dr. Butler said he often conducted what he called a brown bag test with elderly patients, asking them to bring in every medication they had in a brown bag. "You'd be shocked," he said. "Sometimes Mrs. Jones next door got a good result with her arthritis medication so our patient will take Mrs. Jones's drug. Some are taking medications that are five or six years old." And, he added, many older people do not take their medicines at the right time or in the right doses.

Dr. Robert Kane, a researcher at the University of Minnesota School of Public health, said pressures on doctors might lead to inappropriate prescriptions.

"As physicians feel under pressure to spend less and less time with their patients, they often don't spend the time needed to take a thorough drug history," Dr. Kane said. "And one of the most common ways to terminate an interaction with a patient is to write a prescription. There is a tendency to substitute the use of drugs for time and attention." . . .

Dr. Kane suggested that older people take lists of their medications to their doctors and ask about interactions and side effects. "There are things that older people can do to help themselves and I think they should do them," Dr. Kane said.

Source: Excerpted from Gina Kolata, "Wrong Drugs Given to 1 in 4 of Elderly," *New York Times,* 27 July 1994, 68. © 1994 by The New York Times Company. Reprinted by permission.

Although the list of food additives, beauty aids, and youth enhancers for the elderly is seemingly limitless, the best rule of thumb is "If something in the health area seems too good to be true, it probably is."

Gender Issues:
Caring for the Elderly

According to the most recent census data, elderly women fill a disproportionate place in American society. In 1990, for example, there were 19 million women and 13 million men aged 65 and over. This difference in the number of older women and older men increases with age. Because women live seven years longer then men on average, elderly women are more likely than elderly men to be living alone. Further, they are more likely to experience poverty and multiple chronic health problems, a situation referred to as **comorbidity.** Consequently, more elderly women than men are likely to need assistance from children, other relatives, friends, and neighbors.

Comorbidity: The presence of a number of diseases at the same time.

Women have usually been the primary caregivers for elderly Americans. A national survey found that 72 percent of primary caregivers were women, and 60 percent of these were wives of the person who was receiving care.[32] Research also indicates that women spend more hours than do men (38 hours versus 27 hours per week) in caregiving activities and that women perform a wider range of activities than do men. Regardless of the time spent, caregiving is a difficult and stressful experience for both women and men. **Respite care,** or care that is given by someone who relieves the primary caregiver, should be available to ease the burden of the primary caregiver. As the population ages and more elderly people are in need of care, the importance of the caregiver in maintaining health and well-being will become even more important.

$\mathcal{W}$HAT DO YOU THINK?

Why are women so often the primary caregivers for their aging spouses and other family members? What potential problems can such caregiving cause for women? How can women best learn to cope with the stresses and strains of caregiving?

Respite care: The care provided by substitute caregivers to relieve the principle caregiver from his or her continuous responsibility.

Clubs, hobbies, and organized groups that stimulate social activity, physical exercise, and mental alertness are an effective strategy for helping the elderly adapt to the many challenges of old age.

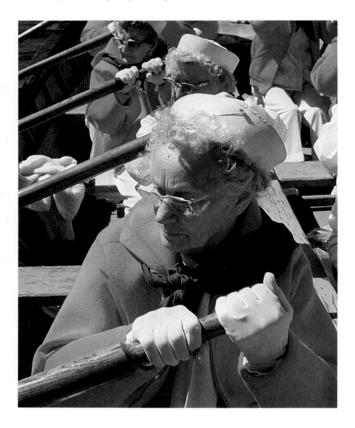

Summary

◆ Aging can be defined in terms of biological age, referring to a person's physical condition; psychological age, referring to a person's coping abilities and intelligence; social age, referring to a person's habits and roles relative to society's expectations; legal age, based on chronological years; or functional age, relative to how other people function at varied ages.

◆ The growing numbers of elderly (people age 65 and older) will have a growing impact on our society in terms of economy, health care, housing, and ethical considerations.

◆ Two broad groups of theories—biological and psychosocial—purport to explain the physiological and psychological changes that occur with aging. The biological theories include the wear-and-tear theory, the

cellular theory, the autoimmune theory, and the genetic mutation theory. Psychosocial theories center on adaptation and adjustments related to self-development.

◆ Aging changes the body and mind in many ways. Physical changes occur in the skin, bones and joints, head, urinary tract, heart and lungs, senses, sexual functioning, and temperature regulation. Major physical concerns are osteoporosis and urinary incontinence. The elderly maintain a high level of intelligence and memory. Potential mental problems include depression and Alzheimer's disease.

◆ Special challenges for the elderly include alcohol abuse, prescription drug and OTC interactions, questions about vitamin and mineral supplementation, and issues regarding caregiving.

Affirmations for Healthy Aging

Who you are today is a good indication of who you may become as an older adult. Your beliefs, attitudes, habits, genetics, the environment you live in, and your health-related behaviors will significantly affect the degree of satisfaction and sense of well-being you experience later in life. Although there is no way to predict individual differences accurately, the following affirmations may help assure that your own aging will be healthy.

1. I am about average in weight and body fat—neither overweight nor underweight.
2. I exercise regularly and consider myself to be in pretty good shape.
3. Although I experience plenty of stress in my life, I seem to be able to cope with it without letting it get to me.
4. I try to eat healthfully most of the time.
5. I am interested in many different activities and find that I am seldom bored.
6. I value my friends and consider them very important in my everyday life.
7. I enjoy other people and usually prefer being around others rather than being alone.
8. I get excited about learning new things.
9. I place a high value on the spiritual side of life.
10. I take time out for myself every day.
11. I generally believe that most people are good and are interested in helping me to succeed.
12. I take care of my body, have regular medical checkups, and make sure that I practice self-care.
13. I set a high priority on having money for health insurance, saving money for health insurance, or trying to get a job with health insurance benefits.
14. I avoid excessive intake of all drugs, including alcohol and cigarettes.
15. I am very independent and do not like to ask people for help; however, if I really need help, I will ask.
16. I like older people and really enjoy interacting and spending time with them.
17. I look forward to getting older and to all of the fun things I can do when I retire.
18. I believe that saving money for retirement is very important, and I plan to start saving as soon as I graduate and get a full-time job.

Discussion Questions

1. Discuss the various definitions of aging. At what age would you place your parents for each category?

2. As the elderly population grows, what implications are there for you? Would you be willing to pay higher taxes to support government social programs for the elderly? For example, do you believe that Social Security should continue its yearly increases in payments, which are pegged to inflation? Explain why or why not.

3. Which of the biological theories of aging do you think is most correct? Why?

4. List the major physiological changes that occur with aging. Which of these, if any, can you change?

5. Explain the major health challenges that the elderly may face. What advice would you give to your grandparents before they took a prescription or OTC drug?

Application Exercise

Reread the What Do You Think? scenarios at the beginning of the chapter and answer the following questions:

1. Do your grandparents ever talk or joke about sex in front of you? Does it make you feel uncomfortable? Explain why.

2. Do you expect to have a fulfilling sex life when you are in your 60s? Why or why not?

3. Do you think the individuals in the second scenario are normal for their age? What is normal for a particular age?

4. What changes have made it easier for elderly people to lead healthy lives? What changes have made it more difficult?

Reducing Age-Related Risks

The question of how to best take responsible action to promote your potential for a full, productive life is not an easy one to answer. There are many obstacles to overcome, some of which may be totally beyond your control. There is no one right way to age. Most people who do age successfully, however, pay attention to their physical, spiritual, emotional, mental, and social well-being.

Making Decisions for You

Think about your own life right now. Are you happy with the way things are going for you? Are your relationships satisfying? Do you feel good about yourself and your social interactions? What would you like to be like when you are 70 years old? What actions should you be taking now to help ensure that you will be able to achieve your own ideal aging profile?

Checklist for Change: Making Personal Choices

✓ Keep physically fit. If you are in good physical shape, exercise regularly, and have good muscle strength and agility, the likelihood that you will be able to perform optimally as you age will be greatly enhanced. Many studies indicate that regular exercisers outlive their sedentary peers and that exercise reduces the risks of cardiovascular disease. Eating properly throughout life will do much to ensure that you maintain strong bones, healthy organs, and optimal weight for your height and frame.

✓ Maintain a variety of support networks. We all need friends we can call on for help or when we want to talk about our sorrows, joys, and frustrations. Although it may be easy to find a friend, it takes care and attention to keep that friend over time. How many of you are still in close contact with your best friends from high school? Why have some of your friends drifted away? What things do you do to let your friends know that they matter to you?

✓ Keep mentally active. For some people, mentally active equals socially active. Gardening, painting, dancing, listening to music, and taking courses are all means of staying mentally active. Take time for quiet reflection, concentrated thought, and idle musing.

✓ Have regular medical checkups. Regardless of your age, you should know what your risk factors are and have periodic medical examinations. One of the best ways to protect yourself against major health problems at any age is to take care of seemingly minor problems early. Whether you are 20 or 45, if you notice a small lump in your breast, have it checked immediately. If your arm aches excessively after playing tennis, make sure it is not the first warning sign of arthritis.

✓ Develop a sense of self. Self-esteem, self-efficacy, and internal locus of control are important in youth and will continue to be important all your life. Maintaining a sense of yourself as a worthwhile, productive member of society can be a challenge in the face of changes that appear to diminish individual prestige.

✓ Learn to accept help when you need it. Just as a healthy level of independence and personal control are important aspects of human development so is the ability to ask questions and to seek advice or assistance without feeling foolish or intimidated. These are important skills at every age and stage of development. If you acquire them early in life, they will help carry you through your later years.

✓ Make optimal use of your time and energy. It would be foolish to assume that, as you age, your energy levels and reserves of strength will continue to be the same. Learn to maximize your energy potential. If you develop a pattern of reducing unnecessary stressors in your life now, you will be better able to expend energy on high-priority activities throughout your life.

✓ Make an honest evaluation of your personal weaknesses and strengths. Once you have made this evaluation, make a conscious effort to improve in weak areas wherever possible and, where not, to give those areas less importance in your life.

✓ Take positive steps now to plan for your secure retirement. Although living for the moment seems like a good idea now, it can result in financial problems that cause undue strain and seriously limit your mobility and options later in life.

✓ Become familiar with services that are available to assist the elderly in need of help. Many communities offer services that help people remain independent for as long as possible.

✓ Do not allow yourself to stagnate. Although the 84-year-old woman who takes up springboard diving and the 82-year-old man who learns to navigate a ship by the stars are unusual, the willingness to encounter change and undertake new activities can add pleasure to life at any age. Similarly, stagnation can occur at any age. How many of us have had whole months go by in which we cannot remember one significant event or one really enjoyable activity? For many of us, this type of stultifying life becomes so ingrained that we grow old inside long before our time. Aging is unavoidable, but the reaction to it is largely in your own hands.

(continued)

Checklist for Change: Making Community Choices

✓ What community services are available to promote health at each of the different levels and stages of life? What services are available for children? For young adults? For people in their middle years? Older years?

✓ What services do you think are needed to help people achieve optimal health through the years?

✓ Do you keep up with the federal government's plans for Social Security and Medicare? Have you taken the time to learn how these programs will affect you in the future?

Critical Thinking

Your grandfather, aged 74, had a heart attack last week. Complications in the hospital have left him unconscious. As his only child, your mother must make an immediate decision about his care. He can have open-heart surgery, but the prognosis is uncertain for someone his age and in his physical condition, according to his doctor. In addition, the operation would deplete your grandfather's savings, which is paying for your college education. Without your grandfather's support, you would have to drop out of college.

Using the DECIDE model described in Chapter 1, what advice would you give your mother? First, think about the moral and ethical obligations of the medical community to keep people alive. Would it make a difference if your grandfather were 85?

Further Reading

A. Ferrini and R. Ferrini, *Health in the Later Years* (Madison, WI: Brown and Benchmark, 1993).

Provides an overview of the physiological, psychological, and sociological dimensions of the aging process. Discusses key factors involved in the successful development of health promotion programs for the elderly. Comprehensive coverage of major aging issues in an easy-to-read format.

For more information about Alzheimer's disease, contact the National Alzheimer's Association at 1-800-272-3900 for the newest readings and research studies focusing on this problem.

M. L. Teague, *Health Promotion: Achieving High-Level Wellness in the Later Years* (Indianapolis: Benchmark Press, 1992).

Comprehensive reference guide for people interested in developing health-promotion programs specifically designed for older people. Provides major components of programs, the unique needs of the elderly, and resources for information.

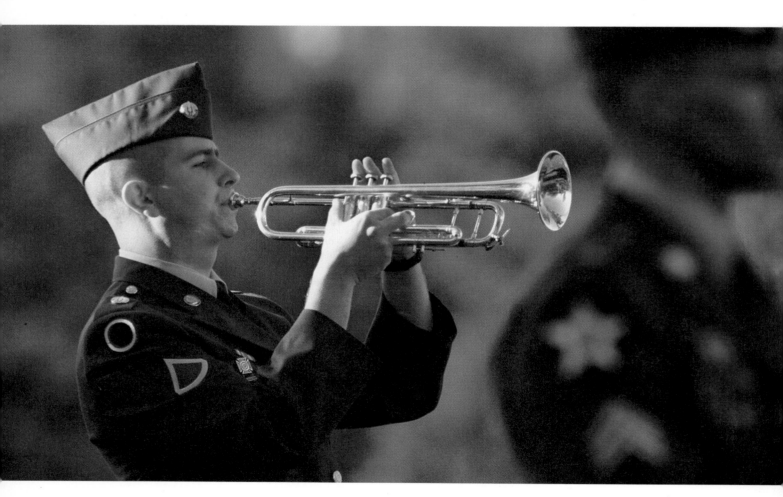

CHAPTER OBJECTIVES

◆ Define *death* using different criteria and evaluate why people deny death.

◆ Discuss the stages of the grieving process and describe several strategies for coping more effectively with death.

◆ Review the decisions that are necessary when someone is dying or has died, including hospice care, funeral arrangements, wills, and organ donations.

◆ Describe the ethical concerns that arise from the concepts of the right to die and rational suicide.

Dying and Death
The Final Transition

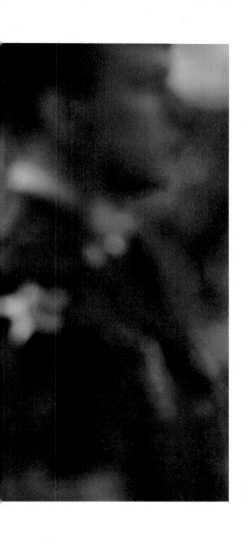

W H A T   D O   Y O U   T H I N K ?

Ed was diagnosed with amyotrophic lateral sclerosis (Lou Gehrig's disease) three years ago. The condition leads to progressive paralysis of the arms, legs, and trunk, finally resulting in the inability to walk, breathe, or swallow. For the past 18 months, he has required 24-hour care. Ed has been progressively losing control of all his muscles, and he now anticipates being put on a respirator when his lungs are unable to expand and contract on their own. It is not certain how long he will live in this condition but Ed knows he will only get worse. Ed does not want to go through any more suffering and asks his doctor to help him end his life.

- Do you think Ed has the right to end his own life? What arguments can you think of that would support his decision? What arguments would refute his decision? What would you do if you were in Ed's situation? Why?

Paulo has just attended the funeral of one of his good friends. This is the third funeral he has gone to in less than two years, and he anticipates attending several more soon. Paulo's friends died of AIDS, and several more are HIV-positive. All three died slow, agonizing deaths, and, despite being there for all of them, Paulo felt helpless. The thought of watching more of his friends die is inconceivable to him, although he knows he must not let his friends die alone.

- How can Paulo cope with the loss of his friends? How can he prepare himself to deal with the upcoming deaths of his other sick friends? What can Paulo do to help his friends as they are dying?

Death eventually comes to everyone. This is a depressing thought, but each of us must eventually accept the inevitable. Distractions and denial may postpone the reality of death, but they cannot eliminate it. The acceptance of death helps us shape our attitudes about the importance of life. Throughout history, humans have attempted to determine the nature and meaning of death. The questioning continues today. Although we will touch on moral and philosophical questions about death in this chapter, we will not explore such issues in depth. Rather, our primary focus is to present dying and death as normal components of life and to discuss how we can cope with these events.

Confrontations with death elicit different feelings depending on many factors, including age, religious beliefs, family orientation, health, personal experience with death, and the circumstances of the death itself. To cope effectively with dying, we must address the individual needs of those involved. We will identify some of these needs and offer information and suggestions that have been helpful to many people as they face the final transition in life.

*U*NDERSTANDING DEATH

Large-scale and impersonal death seems to surround us. Often sensationalized by the news media, it is regularly woven into our entertainment. Nowhere is this more evident than in the public fascination with the 1994 murders of Nicole Simpson and Ron Goldman. In the context of this routine exposure, it seems almost paradoxical that twentieth-century Western society has been characterized as "death-denying." Why is it that we wish to deny, or even postpone, death? Let's begin by investigating what death means, at least in medical terms.

Defining Death

Dying is the process of decline in body functions resulting in the death of an organism. **Death** can be defined as the "final cessation of the vital functions" and also refers to a state in which these functions are "incapable of being restored."[1] This definition has become more significant as medical and scientific advances have made it increasingly possible to postpone death.

In response to legal and ethical questions related to death and dying, a presidential commission developed the Uniform Determination of Death Act in 1981, which was endorsed by the American Medical Association, the American Bar Association, and the National Conference for Commissioners on Uniform State Laws. This act, which has been adopted by several states, reads as follows: "An individual who has sustained either (1) irreversible cessation of circulatory and respiratory functions, or (2) irreversible cessation of all functions of the entire brain, including the brainstem, is dead. A determination of death must be made in accordance with accepted medical standards."[2]

The following definitions have subsequently evolved to facilitate classification of various phases of biological death:

- *Cell death:* The gradual death of a cell after all metabolic activity has ceased. The rate of cellular death varies according to the type of tissue involved. For example, higher brain cells die five to eight minutes after respiration stops; striated muscle cells die after two to four hours; kidney cells die after about seven hours; and epithelial cells (hair and nails) die after several days. Rigor mortis, the temporary stiffening of muscles, is associated with cell death.

- *Local death:* The death of a body part or portion of an organ without the death of the entire organism. For example, a kidney may fail, part of the heart muscle may die, or a limb or section of intestine may die as a result of loss of circulation.

- *Somatic death:* The death of the entire organism, as opposed to death of a part of an organ or an extremity.

- *Apparent death:* The cessation of vital physiologic functions, particularly spontaneous cardiac and respiratory activities, which produces a state simulating actual death but from which recovery is possible through the use of resuscitative efforts.

- *Functional death:* Extensive and irreversible damage to the central nervous system, with respiration and circulatory function maintained only by artificial means.

- *Brain death:* The termination of brain function, as evidenced by loss of all reflexes and electric activity of the brain or by irreversible coma. Brain death is confirmed by an **electroencephalogram** (EEG) reading of electrical activity of brain cells.

As the Ad Hoc Committee of the Harvard Medical School defined it in 1968, brain death occurs when the following criteria are met:

- Unreceptivity and unresponsiveness—that is, no response even to painful stimuli.

- No movement for a continuous hour after observation by a physician and no breathing after three minutes off a respirator.

- No reflexes, including brainstem reflexes; pupils are fixed and dilated.

- A "flat" EEG for at least 10 minutes.

- All of these tests repeated at least 24 hours later with no change.

- Certainty that hypothermia (extreme loss of body heat) and depression of the central nervous system caused by use of drugs such as barbiturates are not responsible for these conditions.[3]

Most of these criteria are relatively easy to understand, but the general public often incorrectly interprets the term *flat (isographic) EEG.* Part of our misconception may stem from exposure to dramatic medical crises on television, in which frantic attempts to save a victim are suddenly discontinued when the EEG tracing drags across the graph paper in an unerring straight line. The patient is declared "dead" at this point, and we logically conclude that a "flat EEG" can be equated with total brain death—that is, a complete absence of electrical activity anywhere in the brain.

This conclusion is inaccurate. In actuality, an EEG records electrical activity only in the outermost layers of the brain. These layers, the cortex and neocortex, are composed of highly differentiated cells that integrate sensory input in an individually characteristic manner, thereby producing a unique personality. Most experts accept that the loss of function of these outer layers of the brain results in death of the person but not necessarily in death of the physical body. Lower brain centers may still retain some degree of electrical activity, thus preserving some vital functions such as breathing, cardiac function, digestion, elimination of wastes, and reflex action. Although a flat EEG is valuable when used with other criteria for brain death, it cannot be considered by itself an adequate indicator of death.

Despite the development of these specific death indicators, the issue of death determination remains problematic and surrounded by ethical dilemmas. In the 1980s, experts modified the standards for death determination in response to ethical questions resulting from organ-transplant technology. The new rules stated that the signs of death for an organ donor must be affirmed by two physicians, neither of whom is on the transplant team. We can expect continued controversy and further modification of policy as medical technology progresses.

𝒲HAT DO YOU THINK?

How long do you think you will live? Do you have concerns about the quality of your life up until you die? What can you do now and in the future to help guarantee not only a long life but a healthy quality of life?

Denying Death

We can look at our attitudes toward death as falling on a continuum. At one end of the continuum, death is viewed as the mortal enemy of humankind. Both medical science and religion have promoted this idea of death. At the other end of the continuum, death is accepted and even welcomed.[4] For people whose attitudes fall at this end, death is a passage to a better state of being. But most of us perceive ourselves to be in the middle of this continuum. From this perspective, death is a bewildering mystery that elicits fear and apprehension as well as profoundly influences our attitudes, beliefs, and actions throughout our lives.

In the United States, there is a high level of discomfort associated with death and dying. As a result, we may avoid speaking about death in an effort to limit our own discomfort. You may wish to deny death if you

- avoid people who are grieving after the death of a loved one so you won't have to talk about it

- fail to validate a dying person's frightening situation by talking to the person as if nothing were wrong

- substitute euphemisms for the word *death* (a few examples are "passing away," "kicking the bucket," "no longer with us," "going to heaven," or "going to a better place")

Dying: The process of decline in body functions resulting in the death of an organism.

Death: The "final cessation of the vital functions" and the state in which these functions are "incapable of being restored."

Electroencephalogram (EEG): A device that measures the electrical activity of brain cells.

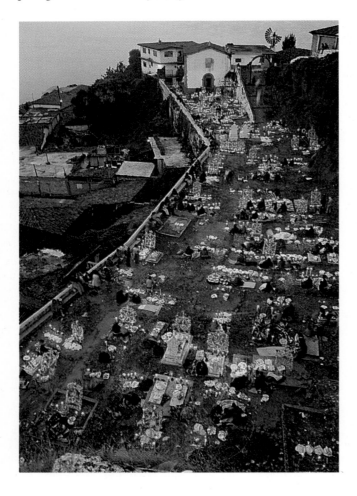

In some cultures death is not feared but viewed as a passage to a better state of being that is to be celebrated.

Throughout the twentieth century, the United States experienced a decrease in the size of households and in the amount of contact between generations. Elders often faced death in relative solitude, with few family members present to conduct traditional funerary (burial) customs such as the "laying out of the dead." The tendency to remove death from the home accelerated after World War II. People who were critically ill or near death were removed to hospitals and nursing homes. Disposal of the body of the deceased became the duty of professionals. Funerals became increasingly efficient, public mourning practically disappeared, and children were often shielded from the unpleasantness of dying and death. Many children sheltered during America's death-denial era eventually became parents and grandparents, still harboring discomfort about death.

As a result of medical breakthroughs during the first half of this century, childhood disease was largely brought under control, "wonder drugs" were developed to combat previously debilitating infections, surgical techniques were refined, and a comprehensive body of knowledge was established with which to begin to unravel the mysteries of human life and health. The miraculous feats of science and medicine during this period created an attitude closer to death-defying than to death-denying.

However, the pendulum appears to be swinging back. Today, a growing number of Americans are rejecting "high-tech" death—death postponed through the use of life-support technology—in favor of more personal, and perhaps more humane, alternatives. The concept of death as an enemy may be giving way to acceptance of dying as a natural part of life.

College Students' Attitudes toward Death

In 1991, researchers asked a group of college students questions that measured their attitudes toward death. They then compared these answers to the answers of college students who were asked the same questions in 1935. Compared to students in 1935, students in 1991[5]

- thought of their own deaths more often
- were more likely to picture themselves as dying or dead
- were more likely to think of dying as a result of some specific disease or accident
- were more likely to dream of being dead or dying
- went to funerals more often
- were more fascinated by newspaper stories about death
- had a stronger fear of death
- were more curious about the existence of life after death

- give false reassurances to people who are dying by saying things like "everything is going to be okay"
- shut off conversation about death by silencing people who are trying to talk about it
- do not touch people who are dying

Although some experts indicate that death denial has always been a predominant characteristic of our society, we must keep in mind that social attitudes change over time. It is therefore important to understand the climate in which our parents and grandparents developed their perceptions so we can understand their reactions to death as well as our own.

Thanatology: The study of death and dying.

THE PROCESS OF DYING

Dying is a complex process that includes physical, intellectual, social, spiritual, and emotional dimensions. Accordingly, we must consider the process of dying from several perspectives. Although the preceding section primarily examined the physical indicators of death, consideration of the emotional aspects of dying and "social death" is essential in establishing an appreciation for the multifaceted nature of life and health.

Coping Emotionally with Death

Science and medicine have enabled us to understand changes associated with growth, development, aging, and social roles throughout the life span, but they have not revealed the nature of death. This may partially explain why the transition from life to death evokes so much mystery and emotion. Although emotional reactions to dying vary, there seem to be many similarities in this process.

Much of our knowledge about reactions to dying stems from the work of Elisabeth Kübler-Ross, a major figure in modern **thanatology**, the study of death and dying. In 1969, Kübler-Ross published *On Death and Dying*, a sensitive analysis of the reactions of terminally ill patients. This pioneering work encouraged the development of death education as a discipline and prompted efforts to improve the care of dying patients. In her book, Kübler-Ross identified five psychological stages that terminally ill patients often experience as they approach death: denial, anger, bargaining, depression, and acceptance (see Figure 21.1). The health-care profession immediately embraced this "stage theory" and hastily applied it in clinical settings. However, research evidence supporting the concept of stages of grief is neither extensive nor convincing. Although it is normal to grieve when a severe loss has been sustained, some people never go through this process and instead remain emotionally calm. Others may pass back and forth between the stages.

A summation of the five stages follows.

- *Denial:* ("Not me, there must be a mistake.") This is usually the first stage, experienced as a sensation of shock and disbelief. A person intellectually accepts the impending death but rejects it emotionally. The patient is too confused and stunned to comprehend "not

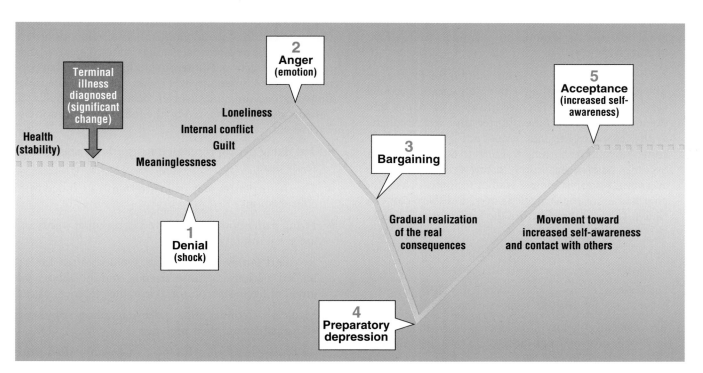

FIGURE 21.1

Kübler-Ross's Stages of Dying

being" and thus rejects the idea. Within a relatively short time, the anxiety level may diminish, enabling the patient to sort through the powerful web of emotions.

- *Anger:* ("Why me?") Anger is another common reaction to the realization of imminent death. The person becomes angry at having to face death when others, including loved ones, are healthy and not threatened. The dying person perceives the situation as "unfair" or "senseless" and may be hostile to friends, family, physicians, or the world in general.

- *Bargaining:* ("If I'm allowed to live, I promise . . .") This stage generally occurs at about the middle of the progression toward acceptance of death. During this stage, the dying person may resolve to be a better person in return for an extension of life or may secretly pray for a short reprieve from death in order to experience a special event, such as a family wedding or birth.

- *Depression:* ("It's really going to happen to me and I can't do anything about it.") Depression eventually sets in as vitality diminishes and the patient begins to experience distressing symptoms with increasing frequency. The patient's deteriorating condition becomes impossible for him or her to deny, and feelings of doom and tremendous loss may become unbearably pervasive. Feelings of worthlessness and guilt are also common in this depressed state because the dying person may feel responsible for the emotional suffering of loved ones and the arduous but seemingly futile efforts of caregivers.

- *Acceptance:* ("I'm ready.") This is often the final stage. The patient stops battling with emotions and becomes very tired and weak. The need to sleep increases, and wakeful periods become shorter and less frequent. With acceptance, the patient does not "give up" and become sullen or resentfully resigned to death, but rather becomes passive. According to one dying patient, the acceptance stage is "almost void of feelings . . . as if the pain had gone, the struggle is over, and there comes a time for the final rest before the long journey."[6] As he

---

Social death: An irreversible situation in which a person is not treated like an active member of society.

Bereavement: The loss or deprivation experienced by a survivor when a loved one dies.

Disenfranchised grief: Grief concerning a loss that cannot be openly acknowledged, publicly mourned, or socially supported.

---

or she lets go, the dying person may no longer welcome visitors and may not wish to engage in conversation. Death usually occurs quietly and painlessly while the victim is unconscious.

Some of Kübler-Ross's contemporaries consider her stage theory to be too neat and orderly. Subsequent research has indicated that the experiences of dying people do not fit easily into specific stages and that patterns vary from person to person. Even if it is not accurate in all its particulars, however, Kübler-Ross's theory offers valuable insights for those seeking to understand or deal with the process of dying.

---

*W*HAT DO YOU THINK?

Do you agree with Elisabeth Kübler-Ross's stages of dying? Have you ever lost someone close to you and then experienced any of these stages?

Social Death

The need for recognition and appreciation within a social group is nearly universal. Although the size and nature of the social group may vary widely, the need to belong exists in all of us. Loss of value or of appreciation by others can lead to **social death,** an irreversible situation in which a person is not treated like an active member of society. Dramatic examples of social death include the exile of nonconformists from their native countries or the excommunication of dissident members of religious orders. More often, however, social death is inflicted by avoidance of social interaction. Numerous studies indicate that people are treated differently when they are dying. The isolation that accompanies social death in terminally ill patients may be promoted by the following common behaviors:

- The dying person is referred to as if he or she were already dead.

- The dying person may be inadvertently excluded from conversations.

- Dying patients are often moved to terminal wards and are given minimal care.

- Bereaved family members are avoided, often for extended periods, because friends and neighbors are afraid of feeling uncomfortable in the presence of grief.

- Medical personnel may make degrading comments about patients in their presence.[7]

A decrease in meaningful social interaction often strips dying and bereaved people of recognition as valued members of society at a time when belonging is critical. Some dying people choose not to speak of their inevitable fate in an attempt to make others feel more comfortable

What You Can Do to Help Dying Friends or Relatives

We may feel uncomfortable and uneasy around a dying friend or relative. We worry about what to say and do. The following points may make your visits more comfortable for both you and the dying person.

- Help the person complete unfinished business that he or she really wants done.

- In the case of family members, help them heal broken family relationships, for this will create peace of mind.

- If they wish, let dying people participate in making funeral and other arrangements.

- Be a good listener. Dying people often need to talk about their feelings.

- Be comfortable with silence when visiting. Your presence is sometimes more important than words.

- Try to anticipate the person's real interests. Don't rattle on about the trivial events of your life when the person appears uninterested. If he or she asks questions, be sensitive, open, and honest in your replies.

- When it's apparent that a person has come to terms with or accepted death, don't deny it. Acknowledge his or her suffering.

- Talk about your own feelings. Let the person know how much you love him or her. It may be your last chance.

- Be sincere. Follow your feelings.

and thus preserve vital relationships. The Skills for Behavior Change box discusses ways that you can help your dying friends or relatives.

Near-Death Experiences

We cannot speak of the process of dying without mentioning near-death experiences. Thousands of similar reports have been given by people who have almost died or who were actually pronounced dead but subsequently recovered. The descriptions of feelings, perceptions, and visions associated with being near death have many common features. Three phases have been identified in a large number of near-death accounts: resistance, life review, and transcendence. During the initial phase, resistance, the dying person is aware of extreme danger and struggles desperately to escape from the unseen threat. Many people have reported a sensation of expanding fear. The second phase, life review, has been described as a feeling of being outside one's body and beyond danger. During this period, the dying person feels a sensation of security while observing his or her physical body from an emotionally detached perspective. The dying person's life experiences may also seem to pass by in rapid review. The last phase, transcendence, is characterized by a reported feeling of euphoria, contentment, and even ecstasy. Some people have recalled a sensation of being unified with nature and of having an awareness of infinity.

Subsequent investigations indicate that many people who are not dying experience sensations similar to these, suggesting that they are not uncommon. Various explanations have been proposed for these hallucinations, including the release of beta-endorphin, a morphine-like chemical produced in the brain that is known to block or reduce the sensation of pain.

Coping with Loss

The losses resulting from the death of a loved one may be extremely difficult to cope with. The dying person, as well as close family and friends, frequently suffers emotionally and physically from the impending loss of critical relationships and roles. Words used to describe feelings and behavior related to losses resulting from death include *bereavement, grief, grief work,* and *mourning.* These terms are related but not identical. An understanding of them may help you to comprehend the emotional processes associated with loss and the cultural constraints that often inhibit normal coping behavior (see Figures 21.2 and 21.3).

Bereavement is generally defined as the loss or deprivation experienced by a survivor when a loved one dies. Because relationships vary in type and intensity, reactions to losses also vary. The death of a parent, a spouse, a sibling, a child, a friend, or a pet will result in different kinds of feelings. In the lives of the bereaved or of close survivors, "holes" will be left by the loss of loved ones. We can think of bereavement as the awareness of these holes. Time and courage are necessary to fill these spaces.

When a person experiences a loss that cannot be openly acknowledged, publicly mourned, or socially supported, coping may be much more difficult. This type of grief is referred to as **disenfranchised grief.**[8] Some examples of loss that may lead to disenfranchised grief include the following:

- *Death of a divorced spouse:* Unresolved anger and hurt along with fond memories are conflicting feelings that may prevent the satisfactory resolution of feelings surrounding the spouse's death.

- *Death of a secret lover:* When a lover dies and no one but the partner knew of the relationship, grief is often

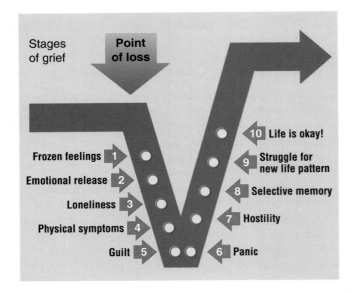

FIGURE 21.2

The diagram shows the stages of grief. People react differently to losses, but most eventually adjust. The common stages of grief and relief are depicted. Generally, the stronger the social support system, the smoother the progression through the stages of grief.

hidden. Examples would include a partner in an extra-marital relationship or a lover of a gay person who is not openly gay.

- *Death of a gay lover:* Homosexuals may find it difficult to mourn the deaths of their lovers when they themselves are not accepted by their own families or the families of their lovers. The situation can be even more difficult if the lover has died of AIDS because of the unjust stigma and discrimination associated with this disease.

A special case of bereavement occurs in old age. Loss is an intrinsic part of growing old. The longer we live, the more losses we are likely to experience. These losses include physical, social, and emotional losses as our bodies deteriorate and more and more of our loved ones die. The theory of *bereavement overload* has been proposed to explain the effects of multiple losses and the accumulation of sorrow in the lives of some elderly people. This theory suggests that the gloomy outlook, disturbing behavior patterns, and apparent apathy that characterize these people may be related more to bereavement overload than to intrinsic physiological degeneration in old age.[9]

Grief is a mental state of distress that occurs in reaction to significant loss, including one's own impending death, the death of a loved one, or a quasi-death experience. Grief reactions include any adjustments needed for one to

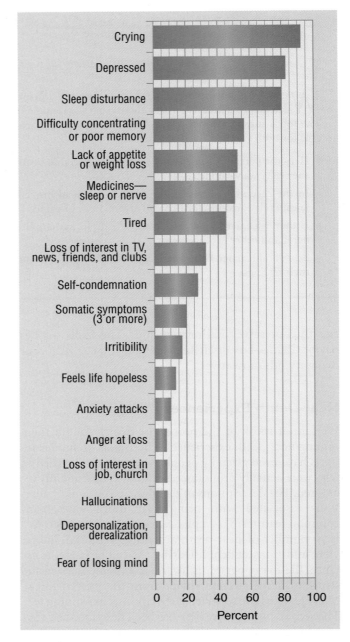

FIGURE 21.3

The graph measures common grief responses of bereaved people. These responses are normal and can be expected to occur as people cope with the death of a loved one. The percentages of specific responses shown in this graph represent expressions of recently widowed people.

"make it through the day" and may include changes in patterns of eating, sleeping, working, and even thinking.

The term **mourning** is often incorrectly equated with the term *grief*. As we have noted, *grief* refers to a wide variety of feelings and actions that occur in response to bereavement. *Mourning,* in contrast, refers to culturally prescribed and accepted time periods and behavior patterns for the expression of grief. In Judaism, for example, "sitting *shivah*" is a designated mourning period of seven days that involves prescribed rituals and prayers. Depending on a person's relationship with the deceased, various other rituals may continue for up to a year.

We have discussed normal grief reactions and have indicated the usual duration of the grieving process. In some cases, however, people are so overwhelmed by grief that they do not return to normal daily living. Support and counseling should be sought when this occurs. Doctors, nurses, psychologists, psychiatrists, and clergy may be helpful in solving problems associated with the loss of a loved one.

Symptoms of grief vary in severity and duration depending on the situation and the individual. However, the bereaved person can benefit from emotional and social support from family, friends, clergy, employers, and the traditional support organizations, including the medical community and the funeral industry. The larger and stronger the support system, the easier readjustment is likely to be.

Religion provides comfort to many dying and grieving people. Although some people question the existence of an afterlife, others gain support from religious beliefs that provide a purpose and meaning to life. By accepting dying as a part of the continuum of life, many people are able to make necessary readjustments after the death of a loved one. This holistic concept, which accepts dying as a part of the total life experience, is shared by both believers and nonbelievers.

What Is "Normal" Grief?

This is a difficult question to answer. Grief responses vary widely from person to person. Despite these differences, a classic acute grief syndrome often occurs when a person acknowledges a loss. This common grief reaction can include the following symptoms:

- Periodic waves of physical distress lasting from 20 minutes to an hour.

- A feeling of tightness in the throat.

- Choking and shortness of breath.

- A frequent need to sigh.

- A feeling of emptiness in the abdomen.

- A feeling of muscular weakness.

- An intense feeling of anxiety that is described as actually painful.

Other common symptoms of grief include insomnia, memory lapse, loss of appetite, difficulty in concentrating, a tendency to engage in repetitive or purposeless behavior, an "observer" sensation or feeling of unreality, difficulty in making decisions, lack of organization, excessive speech, social withdrawal or hostility, guilt feelings, and preoccupation with the image of the deceased. Susceptibility to disease increases with grief and may even be life-threatening in severe and enduring cases.

A bereaved person may suffer emotional pain and may exhibit a variety of grief responses for many months after the death of a loved one. The rate of the healing process depends on the amount and quality of grief work that a person does. **Grief work** is the process of integrating the reality of the loss with everyday life and learning to feel better. Often, the bereaved person must deliberately and systematically work at reducing denial and coping with the pain that results from memories of the deceased. This process takes time and requires emotional effort.

While mourning customs and behaviors are comforting, they can also restrict us from expressing intense grief in a beneficial way.

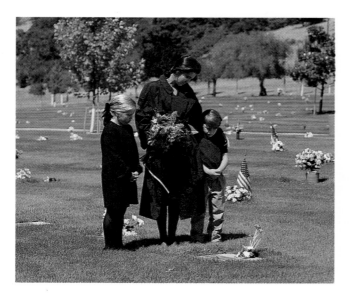

Grief: The mental state of distress that occurs in reaction to significant loss, including one's own impending death, the death of a loved one, or a quasi-death experience.

Mourning: The culturally prescribed behavior patterns for the expression of grief.

Grief work: The process of accepting the reality of a person's death and coping with memories of the deceased.

Gender Differences in Bereavement

While men and women suffer through many of the same stages of bereavement, the Harvard Bereavement Study conducted in the 1970s pointed out some interesting differences. Researchers saw a difference in how men and women interpreted their feelings of loss immediately after the death of a spouse occurred. While women emphasized a sense of abandonment, men reported feeling a sort of dismemberment. The women would speak of being alone, deprived of a comforting and protecting person. The men were more likely to feel "like both my arms and legs were being cut off."[10]

At the funeral, women tended to regard the funeral directors as supporting and caring people rather than as businesspeople. Men, on the other hand, expressed less gratitude toward the funeral directors, and usually felt that the funeral was too expensive. The funeral process was important for women in reaching the realization that their spouses were gone forever. But men tended to feel that the funeral was something to "get through."[11]

As you might expect, widowers showed fewer emotions to other people than did widows. Interestingly, those who came to help the widower emphasized practical help over emotional support. Women were most often the providers of help.[12]

While widowers usually made a more rapid social recovery, the emotional recovery was slower for men. Widowers began dating and remarrying sooner than did widows. But this did not mean that the widowers had worked through their emotional attachment to their late spouses.[13]

𝒲HAT DO YOU THINK?

The Harvard Bereavement Study was done during the early 1970s. Do you think that the gender differences it found still hold true? For example, do you think men are still given practical support rather than social support?

When an Infant or a Child Dies

At the beginning of the twentieth century, children under the age of 15 made up 34 percent of the U.S. population but accounted for 53 percent of the total deaths. Eighty years later, children made up only 22 percent of the population and merely 3 percent of total deaths.[14] Children are highly valued in our society, and their deaths are considered major tragedies. No matter what the cause of premature death—miscarriage, fatal birth defects, childhood illness, accident, suicide, homicide, or war injuries—the grief experienced when a child dies may be overwhelming.

The death of a child is terribly painful for the whole family. However, for several reasons, the siblings of the deceased child have a particularly hard time with grief work. Bereaved children usually have limited experience with death and therefore have not yet learned how to deal with major loss. Children may feel uncomfortable talking about death, and they may also receive less social support and sympathy than do the parents of the deceased child. Because so much attention and energy are devoted to the deceased child, the surviving children may also feel emotionally abandoned by their parents. The Building Communication Skills box discusses helping children through the time following a death.

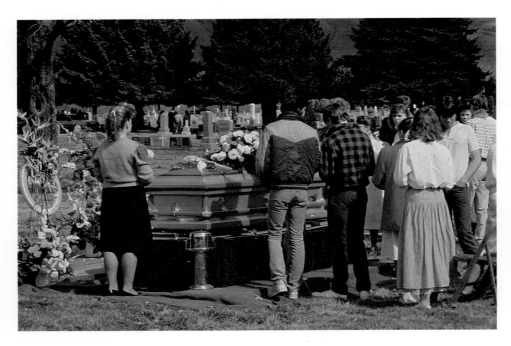

Teenage suicide, a tragically growing cause of death for young people, impacts many people, but siblings and friends—who generally have little experience with death—are especially unable to cope with their grief.

Helping Children Cope with Bereavement

1. *Develop and maintain an open communication pattern with children.* It is difficult and perhaps unrealistic to wait until a crisis situation has developed before including children in the discussion of significant issues. The child who is shunted aside whenever there are "important things" to talk about will have had little opportunity to learn the communication skills that are required to deal with difficult situations. Although limited by their levels of maturation and experience, children observe, think, and make choices. The family in which children feel that they can communicate about anything and everything with their parents and receive a careful and sympathetic hearing is the family that will be able to cope more resourcefully together when faced with bereavement or other stressful life events.

2. *Give children the opportunity to choose attending the funeral.* Adults often assume that children would either not understand funerals or be harmed by the experience. These assumptions may be based on an underestimation of children's cognitive ability as well as their need to be a part of what happens. One set of findings from the Harvard Child Bereavement Study has confirmed that parents tend to give only the illusion of choice: "You don't want to go, do you? No, I know that you don't." As the study also found, children appreciate the opportunity to make their own decisions. In some cases, families encouraged children to make specific recommendations about the funeral, such as, "outside, with lots of flowers, and with bright colors so we can remember all the good things." Furthermore, those who attended the funeral were better able to cope with the loss of the parent. Nevertheless, the child who has decided against attending the funeral should not be forced to do so against his or her wishes.

3. *Encourage the expression of feelings.* . . . The grieving child's thoughts and feelings are a part of reality that cannot be wished away or kept under wraps without adding to the already existing emotional burden. Young children are likely to find valuable means of expression through play and drawings, often accompanied by storytelling. Feelings can also be expressed through a variety of physical activities, including vigorous games through which tension and anger can be discharged. Children of all ages can benefit from open communication with their surviving parent and other empathic adults. An especially valuable way for children to express their feelings is to help comfort others. Even very young children can do this. For example, one child attending a funeral later reported that "at the end while I was crying, my little cousin came up to me and gave me a hug and said it was okay. She was only three." Comforting and altruistic behavior can begin very early in life.

4. *Provide convincing assurance that there will always be somebody to love and look after the child.* The death of a parent arouses or intensifies fears that the surviving parent and other important people may also abandon the child. Verbal assurances are useful, but not likely to be sufficient. Children may become anxious when the surviving parent is out of sight or has not come home at the expected time. Sending the children away for a while is a practice that often intensifies the anxiety of abandonment. Adult relatives and friends who spend time with the children after their bereavement are helping the surviving parent to provide reassurance that there will always be somebody there for them.

5. *Professional counseling should be considered if the bereaved children are at special risk.* The death of both parents, for example, constitutes a special risk, as does a death for which the children might feel that they are somehow [to] blame. There is one special risk that each year rises for thousands of children:

> Mom told us to sit down and she said, "Girls, your Dad died." We both cried right away. We went down to the garage where everybody was. People began holding us and trying to make us feel better. No one knew what to say. We felt like everyone was just staring at us. It was like a big, bad dream. And to make matters worse, we found out from our Mom that Dad had killed himself. . . . It is still hard for us to understand. We were only five and nine years old.

. . . Two girls had to contend—suddenly—with the death of their father and the puzzle and possible stigma of his suicide. Their consuming question was: "If Daddy loved me, why did he leave me?" This became the title of a little book that the girls wrote together over a period of time. In addition to their supportive mother, [they] had the skilled services of a professional counselor, David Dahlke. Every page of the girls' book reflects their personal growth experience as they explored their thoughts, feelings, values, and choices with the counselor's assistance.

Dahlke offers a detailed account of the counseling process along with the girls' own thoughts and comments by the mother. We learn, for example, that the children became afraid that if their mother married again her new husband would also commit suicide. . . .

Other children who suffer parental bereavement under especially traumatic and stressful conditions can also receive valuable assistance from qualified counselors.

Source: Excerpted from Robert J. Kastenbaum, *Death, Society, and Human Experience,* 5th ed., 211–212. © Copyright 1995 by Allyn and Bacon. Reprinted by permission.

Quasi-Death Experiences

Social and emotional support for the bereaved in the aftermath of death is supported by many cultures. Typically, however, there is little support for many other significant losses in life. Losses that in many ways resemble death and that may carry with them a heavy burden of grief include a child running away from home, an abduction or kidnapping, a divorce, a move to a distant place, a move to a nursing home, the loss of a romance or an intimate friendship, retirement, job termination, finishing a "terminal" academic degree, or ending an athletic career.

These **quasi-death experiences**[15] resemble death in that they involve separation, termination, loss, and a change in identity or self-perception. If grief results from these losses, the pattern of the grief response will probably follow the same course as responses to death. Factors that may complicate the grieving process associated with quasi-death include uncomfortable contact with the object of loss (for example, an ex-spouse) and a lack of adequate social and institutional support.

Living with Death and Loss

The reality of death and loss touches everyone. Although the accompanying grief causes painful emotions, it can also bring strength. C. M. Parkes, a British researcher in the psychiatric aspects of bereavement, observed that

> the experience of grieving can strengthen and bring maturity to those who have previously been protected from misfortune. The pain of grief is just as much a part of life as the joy of love; it is, perhaps, the price we pay for love, the cost of commitment. To ignore this fact, or to pretend that it is not so [would] leave us unprepared for the losses that will inevitably occur in our lives and unprepared to help others cope with the losses in theirs.[16]

Different cultures deal with death in varied ways. The Multicultural Perspectives box takes a look at how one small town in northern Greece balances the needs of the living and the dead.

WHAT DO YOU THINK?

Can you remember an experience of grief when you lost a loved one or pet? Try to remember the emotional and physical symptoms that you experienced. Do you think this experience helped you grow as a person and contribute to your personal well-being and philosophy of life?

TAKING CARE OF BUSINESS

Caring for dying people and dealing with the practical and legal questions surrounding death can be difficult and painful. The problems of the dying person and the bereaved loved ones involve a wide variety of psychological, legal, social, spiritual, economic, and interpersonal issues. We will now examine some practical problems associated with death and will present a humanitarian alternative that has been offered as a possible solution to many of these problems.

Hospice: An Alternative for the Dying Person

An increasing number of people now consider the hospice philosophy an acceptable alternative to modern "high-tech" death. The objective of **hospice** programs is to maximize the quality of life when doctors determine that death is inevitable. "The Dying Person's Bill of Rights," reprinted in the Choices for Change box, reflects the sort of humanitarian philosophy on which the hospice idea is based.

The primary goals of the hospice program are to relieve the dying person's pain, to offer emotional support to the dying person and loved ones, and to restore a sense of control to the dying person, the family, and friends. Although home care with maximum involvement by loved ones is emphasized, hospice programs are under the di-

Many terminally ill people choose to spend their last days in a hospice where maximum involvement of loved ones is emphasized.

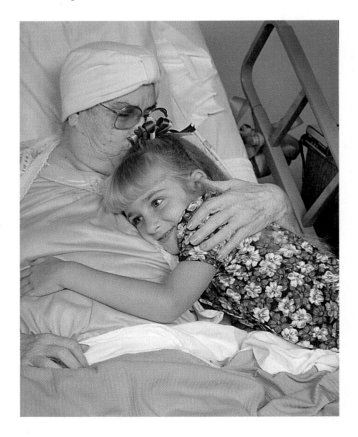

The Graveyard of Potamia

Potamia is a village in northern Greece not far from Mount Olympus. The 600 people who live there remain in close physical and symbolic contact with the dead. The small cemetery is crowded with twenty or more grave markers that memorialize villagers who have died in the past few years. . . .

By local custom, bodies remain in the graveyard for five years and then are removed to the bone house. During this temporary burial the survivors have ample time to visit their lost loved ones. The survivors' feelings often become expressed with great intensity as the time nears to exhume and transfer the body. Tsiaras recorded a mother's lament:

Eleni, Eleni, you died far from home with no one near you. I've shouted and cried for five years, Eleni, my unlucky one, but you haven't heard me. I don't have the courage to shout any more. Eleni, Eleni, my lost soul. You were a young plant, but they didn't let you blossom. You've been here for five years. Soon you'll leave. Then where will I go? What will I do? Five years ago I put a beautiful bird into the ground, a beautiful partridge. But now what will I take out? What will I find?

In contrast to many cemeteries in the United States, the little graveyard in Potamia is often filled with mourners, usually women. They come not only to express their sorrows through song, speech, and prayer but also to tend the graves. Candles are kept burning at the foot of each grave, and the grounds are tended with scrupulous care. When the gravetending activities have been completed for the day, the women sit and talk to their dead and to each other. The conversation may center on death, and one mourner may seek to comfort another. But the conversation may also include other events and concerns. An important aspect of the village's communal life is mediated through their role as survivors of the dead. For the women especially, the graveyard provides an opportunity to express their *ponos* (the pain of grief). The men find a variety of outlets, but the women are usually expected to be at home and to keep their feelings to themselves. "A woman performs the necessary rites of passage and cares for the graves of the dead 'in order to get everything out of her system.'"

Through their graveside laments and rituals the Greek women attempt to achieve a balance between the dead and the living. The custom of temporary burial has an important role in this process. The deceased can still be treated as an individual and as a member of the community, somebody who retains the right of love, respect, and comfort. In effect, the deceased suffers a second and final death when the grave is destroyed and the physical remains are deposited with the bones of the anonymous dead. It is easier to cope with the symbolic claims of the dead when a definite time limit has been set—in this case a rather generous five-year period. Although the memory of the deceased will continue to be honored, removal of the remains to the bone house represents the reemergence of the life-oriented needs of the survivors.

The survivors are *obliged* to tend the graves and carry out other responsibilities to the deceased. As Tsiaras points out, this process involves a symbolic interaction and continuation between the living and the dead. *The dead have the right to expect it, just as those who are now among the living can expect their survivors to honor their postmortem rights when the time comes.* In Potamia and in many other communities where traditional value systems remain in place, the obligations of the living to the dead are clear, specific, and well known.

Source: Excerpted from Robert J. Kastenbaum, *Death, Society, and Human Experience,* 5th ed., 295–296. © Copyright 1995 by Allyn and Bacon. Reprinted by permission.

rection of cooperating physicians, coordinated by specially trained nurses, and fortified with the services of counselors, clergy, and trained volunteers. Hospital inpatient beds are available if necessary. Hospice programs usually include the following characteristics:

1. The patient and family constitute the unit of care, because the physical, psychological, social, and spiritual problems of dying confront the family as well as the patient.

2. Emphasis is placed on symptom control, primarily the alleviation of pain. Curative treatments are curtailed as requested by the patient, but sound judgment must be applied to avoid a feeling of abandonment.

3. There is overall medical direction of the program, with all health care being provided under the direction of a qualified physician.

Quasi-death experiences: Losses or experiences that resemble death in that they involve separation, termination, significant loss, a change of personal identity, and grief.

Hospice: A concept of care for terminally ill patients designed to maximize the quality of life.

The Dying Person's Bill of Rights

As we face death, what are our rights as human beings? This bill of rights was created at a workshop on "The Terminally Ill Patient and the Helping Person" sponsored by the Southwestern Michigan Insurance Education Council and conducted by Amelia J. Barbus. Its affirmations may help you or a loved one to maintain dignity during the dying process. As a survivor, it may help you understand the patient's needs.

- I have the right to be treated as a living human being until I die.

- I have the right to maintain a sense of hopefulness, however changing its focus may be.

- I have the right to be cared for by those who can maintain a sense of hopefulness, however changing this might be.

- I have the right to express my feelings and emotions about my approaching death in my own way.

- I have the right to participate in decisions concerning my care.

- I have the right to expect continuing medical and nursing attention even though "cure" goals must be changed to "comfort" goals.

- I have the right not to die alone.

- I have the right to be free from pain.

- I have the right to have my questions answered honestly.

- I have the right not to be deceived.

- I have the right to have help from and for my family in accepting my death.

- I have the right to die in peace and dignity.

- I have the right to retain my individuality and not be judged for my decisions, which may be contrary to the beliefs of others.

- I have the right to discuss and enlarge my religious and/or spiritual experiences, whatever these may mean to others.

- I have the right to expect that the sanctity of the human body will be respected after death.

- I have the right to be cared for by caring, sensitive, knowledgeable people who will attempt to understand my needs and will be able to gain some satisfaction in helping me face my death.

Source: Copyright 1975 The American Journal of Nursing Company. Reprinted from H. Whitman, "The Dying Person's Bill of Rights," *American Journal of Nursing,* January 1975, vol. 75, no. 1, p. 99. Used with permission. All rights reserved.

---

4. Services are provided by an interdisciplinary team because no one person can provide all the needed care.

5. Coverage is provided 24 hours a day, 7 days a week, with emphasis on the availability of medical and nursing skills.

6. Carefully selected and extensively trained volunteers are an integral part of the health-care team, augmenting staff service but not replacing it.

7. Care of the family extends through the bereavement period.

8. Patients are accepted on the basis of their health needs, not their ability to pay.

Despite the growing number of people considering the hospice option, many people prefer to go to a hospital to die. Others choose to die at home, without the intervention of medical staff or life-prolonging equipment. Each dying person and his or her family should decide as early as possible what type of terminal care is most desirable and feasible. This will allow time for necessary emotional, physical, and financial preparations. Hospice care may also help the survivors cope better with the death experience.

Making Funeral Arrangements

Anthropological evidence indicates that all cultures throughout history have developed some sort of funeral ritual. For this reason, social scientists agree that funerals somehow assist survivors of the deceased in coping with their loss.

In the United States, with its diversity of religious, regional, and ethnic customs, funeral patterns vary. Prior to body disposal, the deceased may be displayed to formalize last respects and increase social support to the bereaved. This part of the funeral ritual is referred to as a wake or viewing. The body of the deceased is usually embalmed prior to viewing to retard decomposition and minimize offensive odors. The funeral service may be held in a church, in a funeral chapel, or at the burial site. Some people choose to replace the funeral service with a simple memorial service held within a few days of the burial. Social interaction associated with funeral and memorial services is valuable in helping survivors cope with their losses. The Rate Yourself box may help you assess your own feelings about funerals.

Common methods of body disposal include burial in the ground, entombment above ground in a mausoleum,

Feelings about Funerals

1. Funerals are a waste of time.
   Agree ____   Tend to agree ____
   Tend to disagree ____   Disagree ____

2. Bodies should be donated for scientific use.
   Agree ____   Tend to agree ____
   Tend to disagree ____   Disagree ____

3. Funerals are a comfort to the next of kin.
   Agree ____   Tend to agree ____
   Tend to disagree ____   Disagree ____

4. People often are too emotional at funerals.
   Agree ____   Tend to agree ____
   Tend to disagree ____   Disagree ____

5. The death of a family member should be published as a notice in the newspaper.
   Agree ____   Tend to agree ____
   Tend to disagree ____   Disagree ____

6. All things considered, most funerals are not excessively costly.
   Agree ____   Tend to agree ____
   Tend to disagree ____   Disagree ____

7. People often do not show enough emotion at funerals.
   Agree ____   Tend to agree ____
   Tend to disagree ____   Disagree ____

8. The size, length, and expense of a funeral should depend on the importance of the deceased person.
   Agree ____   Tend to agree ____
   Tend to disagree ____   Disagree ____

9. Allowing for some exceptions, cemeteries waste valuable space and should be diverted to other uses.
   Agree ____   Tend to agree ____
   Tend to disagree ____   Disagree ____

10. It would be preferable to be cremated.
    Agree ____   Tend to agree ____
    Tend to disagree ____   Disagree ____

11. It would be preferable to be buried in a cemetery.
    Agree ____   Tend to agree ____
    Tend to disagree ____   Disagree ____

12. A funeral director should be required to give a summary of laws stating what is and what is not required before the bereaved purchase a funeral.
    Agree ____   Tend to agree ____
    Tend to disagree ____   Disagree ____

13. The average cost of a funeral in the United States is between $ _____ and $ _____.

14. Embalming the body is required:
    Always ____
    Under certain specified circumstances ____
    Never ____

15. An open-casket funeral can be held after body organs are donated:
    Always ____   Usually ____
    Seldom ____   Never ____

16. My idea of the perfect funeral process is the following:
    _____
    _____
    _____

17. For me the best or most useful aspects of a funeral are:
    _____
    _____
    _____

18. For me the worst or most distressing aspects of a funeral are:
    _____
    _____
    _____

_____

Source: Excerpted from Robert J. Kastenbaum, *Death, Society, and Human Experience,* 5th ed., 279. © copyright 1995 by Allyn and Bacon. Reprinted by permission.

cremation, and anatomical donation. Expenses involved in body disposal vary according to the method chosen and the available options. Examples of options and their costs are listed in Table 21.1. It should be noted that if burial is selected, an additional charge may be assessed for a burial vault. Burial vaults—concrete or metal containers that hold the casket—are required by most cemeteries to limit settling of the gravesite as the casket disintegrates and collapses. The actual container for the body or remains of the dead person is only one of many things that must be dealt with when a person dies. There are many other decisions concerning the funeral ritual that can be burdensome for survivors.

Pressures on Survivors

Stress related to funeral ritual varies culturally as well as individually. In traditional societies, funeral rites and preparation of the body were quite specific. These practices limited the stress on survivors because few decisions

TABLE 21.1 ■ Burial Cost Information

This is a list of the 12 most commonly selected items in an average adult funeral and their average prices in Pennsylvania, New York, and New Jersey.

- Non-declinable professional service charges: $768.75
- Transfer of body to funeral home: $115.65
- Embalming: $366.64
- Other preparation (cosmetology, hairdressing, placing body in the casket): $116.59
- Use of viewing facilities: $290.17
- Use of facilities for service: $227.96
- Other use of facilities: $220.08
- Hearse (local): $140.81
- Limousine (local): $139.48
- Other automotive: $89.94
- Acknowledgment cards: $25.95
- Casket, 18-gauge steel, sealer, velvet interior: $1,883.87

Source: Reprinted by permission of the National Funeral Directors Association, Milwaukee, Wisconsin. (The prices represent averages for funeral homes in Pennsylvania, New York, and New Jersey on 1 January 1994.)

had to be made. Bereaved people fully understood their individual roles in funeral customs and even anticipated carrying out expected duties. In contrast, funeral practices in the United States today are extremely varied. A great number of decisions have to be made, usually within 24 hours. These decisions relate to the method and details of body disposal, the type of memorial service, display of the body, the site of burial or body disposition, the cost of funeral options, organ donation decisions, ordering of floral displays, contacting friends and relatives, planning for the arrival of guests, choosing markers, gathering and submitting obituary information to newspapers, printing of memorial folders, as well as numerous other details. Even though funeral directors are available to facilitate decision making, the bereaved may experience undue stress, especially in the event of a sudden death. In our society, people who make their own funeral arrangements can save their loved ones from having to deal with unnec-

Intestate: The situation in which a person dies without having made a will.

Holographic will: A will written in the testator's own handwriting and unwitnessed.

Testator: A person who leaves a will or testament at death.

essary problems. Even making the decision regarding the method of body disposal can greatly reduce the stress on survivors.

Wills

The issue of inheritance is a controversial one in some families and should be resolved before the person dies in order to reduce both conflict and needless expense. Unfortunately, many people are so intimidated by the thought of making a will that they never do so and die **intestate** (without a will). This is tragic, especially because the procedure involved in establishing a legal will is relatively simple and inexpensive. In addition, if you don't make up a will before you die, the courts (as directed by state laws) will make up a will for you. Legal issues, rather than your wishes, will preside.

For example, let's explore what happens if you die in Massachusetts without a will. If you are married with no children, everything goes to your spouse. If you have children, one-third of your estate goes to your spouse and two-thirds go to the children. If you're not married, it all goes to your parents. Think about the problems this poses for those who choose to live together or are homosexual: Without a will, their partners get *nothing*. Or think of the problems posed when stepchildren who choose not to support the surviving spouse are involved. Clearly, we all need wills, updated regularly.

In some cases, other types of wills may substitute for the traditional legal will. One of these alternative forms is the **holographic will**, written in the handwriting of the **testator** (person who leaves a will) and unwitnessed. Caution should be taken concerning alternatives to legally written and witnessed wills because they are not honored in all states. And holographic wills are contestable in court. Think of the parents who never approved of their child living with someone outside a marriage: They can successfully challenge the holographic will in court.

Organ Donation

Another decision concerns organ donation. Organ transplant techniques have become so refined, and the demand for transplant tissues and organs has become so great, that many people are being encouraged to donate these "gifts of life" upon their death. Uniform donor cards are available through the National Kidney Foundation, donor information is printed on the backs of drivers' licenses, and many hospitals have included the opportunity for organ donor registration as a part of their admission procedures. Although some people are opposed to organ transplants and tissue donation, others experience a feeling of personal fulfillment from knowing that their organs may extend and improve someone else's life after their own deaths (see Figure 21.4).

NATIONAL KIDNEY FOUNDATION
Please detach and give this portion of the card to your family.

This is to inform you that, should the occasion ever arise, I would like to be an organ and tissue donor. Please see that my wishes are carried out by informing the attending medical personnel that I have indicated my wishes to become a donor.

Thank you.

SIGNATURE _____ DATE _____

For further information write or call:
NATIONAL KIDNEY FOUNDATION
30 East 33rd Street, New York, NY 10016
(800) 622-9010

- -

UNIFORM DONOR CARD

Of _____
(print or type name of donor)

In the hope that I may help others, I hereby make this anatomical gift, if medically acceptable, to take effect upon my death. The words and marks below indicate my wishes.

I give: ☐ any needed organs or parts
☐ only the following organs or parts

_____
(specify the organ(s), tissue(s) or part(s)

for the purposes of transplantation, therapy, medical research or education;
☐ my body for anatomical study if needed.

Limitations or special wishes, if any: _____

FIGURE 21.4

Organ Donor Card Provided by the National Kidney Foundation

Source: Reprinted with permission from the National Kidney Foundation, © copyright 1994. New York, NY.

𝒲HAT DO YOU THINK?

If you died suddenly, would you get the kind of end-of-life treatment that you want? What can you do to assure that your wishes will be carried out at the time of your death?

𝓛IFE-AND-DEATH DECISION MAKING

Life-and-death decisions are serious, complex, and often expensive. We will not attempt to present the "answers" to death-related moral and philosophical questions. Instead, we offer topics for your consideration. We hope that discussion of the needs of the dying person and the bereaved will help you to make difficult decisions in the future. A few issues that are problematic or controversial are the

questions concerning the right to die, the concept of rational suicide, and euthanasia.

The Right to Die

Few people would object to a proposal for the right to a dignified death. Going beyond that concept, however, many people today believe that they should be allowed to die if their condition is inevitably terminal and their existence is dependent on mechanical life support devices or artificial feeding or hydration systems. Artificial life support techniques that may be legally refused by competent patients in some states include the following:

- Electrical or mechanical resuscitation of the heart.
- Mechanical respiration by machine.
- Nasogastric tube feedings.
- Intravenous nutrition.
- Gastrostomy (tube feeding directly into the stomach).
- Medications to treat life-threatening infections.

As long as a person is conscious and competent, he or she has the legal right to refuse treatment, even if this decision will hasten death. However, when a person is in a coma or is otherwise incapable of speaking on his or her own behalf, medical personnel and administrative policy will dictate treatment. This issue has evolved into a battle involving personal freedom, legal rulings, health-care administration policy, and physician responsibility. The liv-

Organ donor programs provide registered donors with the satisfaction of knowing they may save another's life and also expedite the transfer of viable organs when the donor dies.

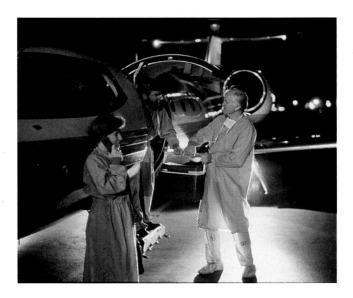

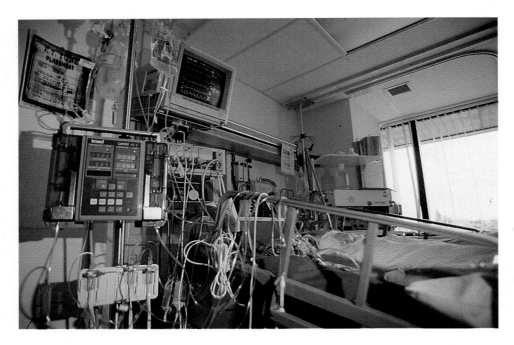

With the advances in modern medicine, the right to die without artificial life support techniques has become a legal and moral issue for patients, their families, and health care professionals.

ing will was developed to assist in solving conflicts among these people and agencies.

Cases have been reported in which the wishes of people who have signed a living will (or advanced directive) indicating their desire not to receive artificial life support were not honored by their physician or medical institution. This problem can be avoided by choosing both a physician and a hospital that will carry out the directives of the living will. Taking this precaution and discussing your personal philosophy and wishes with your family should eliminate anxiety about how you will be treated at the end of your life.

Many legal experts suggest that you take the following steps to assure that your wishes are carried out:

1. *Get specific:* Rather than signing an advanced directive (that only speaks in generalities, fill out a directive like that shown in Figure 21.5. This directive permits you to make specific choices about a variety of procedures under six different circumstances. It is also essential to attach that document to a completed copy of the standard advance directive for your state.

2. *Get an agent:* Even the most detailed directive cannot possibly anticipate every situation that may arise. You may want to also appoint a family member or friend to act as your agent, or *proxy,* by making out a form known as either a durable power of attorney for health care or a health-care proxy.

> **Self-deliverance:** A positive action taken to provide a permanent solution to the long-term pain and suffering for the individual and his or her loved ones faced with terminal illness.

3. *Discuss your wishes:* Discuss your wishes in detail with your proxy and your doctor. Your doctor or proxy may misinterpret or ignore your wishes. Going over the situations described in the form will give them a clear idea of just how much you are willing to endure to preserve your life.

4. *Deliver the directive:* Distribute several copies, not only to your doctor and your agent but also to your lawyer and to immediate family members or a close friend. Make sure *someone* knows to bring a copy to the hospital in the event you are hospitalized.[17]

Rational Suicide

We have discussed suicide in earlier chapters. The concept of *rational suicide* as an alternative to an extended dying process, however, deserves mention here. Although exact numbers are not known, medical ethicists, experts in rational suicide, and specialists in forensic medicine (the study of legal issues in medicine) estimate that thousands of terminally ill people decide to kill themselves rather than endure constant pain and slow decay every year. To these people, the prospect of an undignified death is unacceptable. But does anyone have the right to end his or her life? This issue has been complicated by advances in death prevention techniques that allow terminally ill patients to exist in an irreversible disease state for extended periods of time. Medical personnel, clergy, lawyers, and patients all must struggle with this ethical dilemma.

The Hemlock Society assists terminally ill individuals in the act of **self-deliverance.** *Self-deliverance* has been defined as a positive action taken to provide a permanent solution to the long-term pain and suffering for the individual and his or her loved ones faced with terminal illness.[18] Simply, it is suicide or mercy killing. The Hemlock

Society has sought to eliminate the stigma attached to self-killing and encourages all individuals to have the right to active, rational, and voluntary euthanasia. It supports the Directive to Physicians, a document that can be filled out upon admittance to a hospital that instructs the physician about the desires of the patient (see Figure 21.5).

Still, questions remain. If terminally ill patients wish to die, should they be allowed to commit suicide? Is a person in this situation capable of making a rational decision about suicide? If terminally ill patients are allowed to commit suicide legally, what other groups will demand this option? Should the courts be involved in private de-

---

This directive is made this _____ day of _____ (month) _____ (year).

I, _____ being of sound mind, willfully and voluntarily make known my desire

(a) ☐ **That my life shall not be artificially prolonged** and

(b) ☐ **That my life shall be ended with the aid of a physician under circumstances set forth below, and do hereby declare:**
     (You must initial (a) or (b), or both.)

1. If at any time I should have a terminal condition or illness certified to be terminal by two physicians, and they determine that my death will occur within six months,

   (a) ☐ **I direct that life-sustaining procedures be withheld or withdrawn** and

   (b) ☐ **I direct that my physician administer aid-in-dying in a humane and dignified manner.** (You must initial (a) or (b), or both.)

   (c) ☐ **I have attached Special Instructions on a separate page to the directive.** (Initial if you have attached a separate page.)

   The action taken under this paragraph shall be at the time of my own choosing if I am competent.

2. In the absence of my ability to give directions regarding the termination of my life, it is my intention that this directive shall be honored by my family, agent (described in paragraph 5), and physician(s) as the final expression of my legal right to

   (a) ☐ **Refuse medical or surgical treatment,** and

   (b) ☐ **To choose to die in a humane and dignified manner.** (You must initial (a) or (b), or both and you must initial one box below.)

   ☐ If I am unable to give directions, I *do not* want my attorney-in-fact to request aid-in-dying.

   ☐ If I am unable to give directions, I *do* want my attorney-in-fact to ask my physician for aid-in-dying.

3. I understand that a terminal condition is one in which I am not likely to live for more than six months.

4. a. I, _____
      do hereby designate and appoint _____
      as my attorney-in-fact (agent) to make health-care decisions for me if I am in a coma or otherwise unable to decide for myself as authorized in this document. For the purpose of this document, "health-care decision" means consent, refusal of consent, or withdrawal of consent to any care, treatment, service, or procedure to maintain, diagnose, or treat an individual's physical or mental condition, or to administer aid-in-dying.

   b. By this document I intend to create a Durable Power of Attorney for Health Care under The Oregon Death With Dignity Act and ORS Section 126.407. This power of attorney shall not be affected by my subsequent incapacity, except by revocation.

   c. Subject to any limitations in this document, I hereby grant to my agent full power and authority to make health-care decisions for me to the same extent that I could make these decisions for myself if I had the capacity to do so. In exercising this authority, my agent shall make health-care decisions that are consistent with my desires as stated in this document or otherwise made known to my agent, including, but not limited to, my desires concerning obtaining, refusing, or withdrawing life-prolonging care, treatment, services, and procedures, and administration of aid-in-dying.

5. This directive shall have no force or effect seven years from the date filled in above, unless I am competent to act on my own behalf and then it shall remain valid until my competency is restored.

6. I recognize that a physician's judgment is not always certain, and that medical science continues to make progress in extending life, but in spite of these facts, I nevertheless wish aid-in-dying rather than letting my terminal condition take its natural course.

7. My family has been informed of my request to die, their opinions have been taken into consideration, but the final decision remains mine, so long as I am competent.

8. The exact time of my death will be determined by me and my physician with my desire or my attorney-in-fact's instructions paramount.

FIGURE 21.5

Directive to Physicians
Source: The Oregon Death with Dignity Act, Oregon Revised Statutes, Chapter 97, 1990.

I have given full consideration and understand the full import of this directive, and I am emotionally and mentally competent to make this directive. I accept the moral and legal responsibility for receiving aid-in-dying.

This directive will not be valid unless it is signed by two qualified witnesses who are present when you sign or acknowledge your signature. The witnesses must not be related to you by blood, marriage, or adoption; they must not be entitled to any part of your estate; and they must not include a physician or other person responsible for, or employed by anyone responsible for, your health care. If you have attached any additional pages to this form, you must date and sign each of the additional pages at the same time you date and sign this power of attorney.

Signed: _____

_____
City, County, and State of Residence

(This document must be witnessed by two qualified adult witnesses. None of the following may be used as witnesses: (1) a health-care provider who is involved in any way with the treatment of the declarant, (2) an employee of a health-care provider who is involved in any way with the treatment of the declarant, (3) the operator of a community care facility where the declarant resides, (4) an employee of an operator of a community care facility who is involved in any way with the treatment of the declarant.

FIGURE 21.5

(continued)

cisions? Should any organization be allowed to distribute information that may encourage suicide? Should loved ones or medical caregivers be allowed to assist the person who wants to die by providing the means?

Dyathanasia is a form of "mercy killing" in which someone plays a passive role in the death of a terminally ill person. This passive role may include the withholding of life-prolonging treatments or withdrawal of life-sustaining medical support, thereby allowing the person to die. A recent study, reported in the Health Headlines box, shows that withholding food and water from terminally ill patients may actually ease their suffering. **Euthanasia** is the active form of "mercy killing." An example of euthanasia is direct administration of a lethal drug overdose with the objective of hastening the death of a suffering person. Euthanasia is illegal and is viewed as murder. Nevertheless, euthanasia continues to occur. In fact, some experts believe that some doctors induce euthanasia upon the request of the patient. This type of euthanasia is accomplished by ad-

Euthanasia is illegal, but some doctors do respond to the wishes of terminally ill patients to put an end to their pain and suffering.

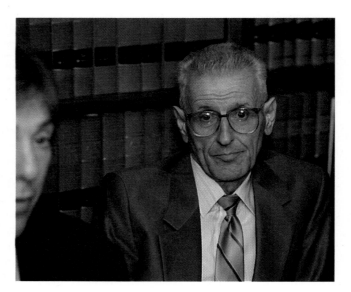

Dyathanasia: The passive form of "mercy killing" in which life-prolonging treatments or interventions are not offered or are withheld, thereby allowing a terminally ill person to die naturally.

Euthanasia: The active form of "mercy killing" in which a person or organization knowingly acts to hasten the death of a terminally ill person.

ministering large doses of painkillers that depress the central nervous system to the extent that basic life-sustaining regulatory centers cease to function. The heart stops beating, breathing ceases, and total brain death follows shortly.

Dr. Jack Kevorkian, a physician in Michigan who is sometimes referred to as Dr. Death, has assisted a number

Study Backs Terminally Ill Refusing Food

Terminally ill people should not be given food or water artificially if they do not want it, because it may only heighten their discomfort, researchers say.

Starving, the researchers report, seems to ease the death of such patients because dehydration lessens consciousness, promotes sleepiness and diminishes pain.

Such patients usually want very little nourishment in their final months.

"Patients terminally ill with cancer generally did not experience hunger, and those who did needed only small amounts of food for alleviation," the researchers say in [the October 1994] issue of The Journal of the American Medical Association.

Similar findings have been reported in previous studies. But they run counter to the behavior of many doctors and families, said the lead author of the new study, Dr. Robert M. McCann.

"There's that whole thing of food as love," said Dr. McCann, head of geriatrics at Rochester General Hospital in Rochester. "That type of emphasis is really misplaced in people who are dying. Families of the dying, they don't know what to do sometimes. So artificial feeding is what they do."

The study involved 32 patients. All expressed a desire not to be fed or given liquids through tubes. They were allowed anything they wanted to eat and drink, including food brought by families.

"They lost their appetite," said Dr. Annmarie Groth-Juncker, a co-author of the study who has cared for the terminally ill. "They didn't want to eat anymore."

People dying of diseases other than cancer, Alzheimer's among them, have the same experience, said Dr. Groth-Juncker, medical director at St. John's Home, a nursing home in Rochester where the research was done.

Almost everyone studied consumed less than 25 percent of the food or fluids needed for basic nutritional requirements. Those who reported thirst or dry mouths sucked ice chips or hard candy and sipped liquids in far smaller quantities than needed to prevent dehydration, the researchers said.

"This is, of course, how people have always died, before there were hospitals with IV's and feeding tubes," Dr. Groth-Juncker said.

Richard Doerflinger, a spokesman for the National Conference of Catholic Bishops, said the bishops agreed with the view of the researchers, as long as no food or fluid was withheld to hasten a death.

"It can be good medicine and good morality to forgo artificial feeding," he said, "when it can only impose additional burdens on a patient who is imminently dying from a progressive terminal illness."

Source: Reprinted by permission of Associated Press from "Study Backs Terminally Ill Refusing Food," *New York Times,* 26 October 1994, A20.

---

of people taking their own lives. Despite a court injunction forbidding him from aiding in any more suicides, in early 1993 he was found at the side of yet another seriously ill woman when she killed herself by inhaling a canister of carbon monoxide that he had provided.

What Do You Think?

Are there any end-of-life situations in which you would ask a physician to help you die? Why or why not?

Summary

◆ *Death* can be defined biologically in terms of the final cessation of vital functions. Various classes of death include cell death, local death, somatic death, apparent death, functional death, and brain death. Death denial results in limited communication about death, which can lead to further death denial.

◆ Death is a multifaceted process and individuals may experience emotional stages of dying including denial,

anger, bargaining, depression, and acceptance. Social death results when a person is no longer treated as living. Grief is the state of distress felt after loss. Men and women differ in their responses to grief. Children, too, need to be helped through the process of grieving.

◆ Practical and legal issues surround dying and death. Choices of care for the terminally ill include hospice

Managing Life-and-Death Decisions

As you have seen in this chapter, your attitudes toward death and dying will affect not only you but also those around you. Many of the decisions we make about how we live our lives will have an impact on how and when we die. Conversely, our attitudes and beliefs about death help to shape the way we live. Where do your beliefs fit on the continuum of death, and what will you change in order to be more accepting of death in the experience of life?

Making Decisions for You

If you find that the subject of managing death still makes you uneasy, consider the following:

1. Talk to someone who has recently lost a loved one and is successfully coping with the loss and try to understand or even compare your feelings with his or hers. Share your thoughts and fears and be open for suggestions.

2. Do some research on the cost of the kind of funeral you want.

3. Visit a funeral home and find out how things operate. It is a fascinating experience!

4. Walk through an old cemetery and read the headstones. Much can be learned from what is said about loved ones who have died.

5. Finally, remember that you have the ability to control much of your life by making decisions that will ultimately affect the nature of your death. Learning all you can that may influence the dying process can make death a much more pleasant event for you and for others.

Checklist for Change: Making Personal Choices

✓ What can you do to decrease your risks for dying an untimely death?

✓ Do you have a will prepared? Do you update it regularly?

✓ Have you completed a directive to physicians?

✓ If you had died yesterday, would your loved ones have known what plans you had for your funeral, body dis-

posal, and asset distribution? What steps can you take to make sure such information is known?

✓ Do you have trouble talking to people about death? If so, what steps can you take to improve your communication skills?

✓ What coping techniques will you turn to if someone you know dies? Do you think you would be able to help someone else who is dealing with a loss?

Checklist for Change: Making Community Choices

✓ What community support is available to help you cope with the death of a loved one? For example, are there widow or widower support groups?

✓ What are your state's laws regarding directives to physicians?

✓ Is physician-assisted suicide legal in your state? Are any laws pending regarding rational suicide?

Critical Thinking

Your child was born 13 weeks prematurely. For the past two weeks, he has been on life-support systems in a neonatal intensive care unit (NICU). Although things were going well, complications have resulted, including bleeding from the lungs. The doctors tell you that your child will eventually die. You must make the decision about whether or not to take him off the life-support systems. If you do, he will die within hours; if not, he may linger for weeks, but will not live. You also need to consider that there is limited space in intensive care units, and your baby is keeping another infant from getting needed care. On the other hand, a pro-life group is threatening to take you to court in order to keep the baby on life support.

Using the DECIDE model described in Chapter 1, what decision would you make? What factors are of greatest concern in making the decision? What factors are of least concern?

---

care. After death, funeral arrangements must be made almost immediately, adding to pressures on survivors. Decisions should be made in advance of death through wills and organ donation cards.

◇ The right to die by rational suicide involves ethical, moral, and legal issues. Dyathanasia involves passive help in suicide for a terminally ill patient; euthanasia involves direct help.

Discussion Questions

1. List the varied definitions of *death*. How do they relate to one another?

2. Discuss why so many of us deny death. How could death become a more acceptable topic to discuss?

3. What are the stages that terminally ill patients theoretically experience? Do you agree with the five-stage theory? Explain why or why not.

4. Define *social death*, *near-death experiences*, and *quasi-death*.

5. Discuss coping with grief, the different grief experiences of men and women, and how to help children overcome their fears of death.

6. Compare and contrast the hospital experience with hospice care. What must one consider before arranging for hospice care?

7. Discuss the legal matters surrounding death, including wills, physician directives, organ donations, and funeral arrangements.

8. Debate whether or not rational suicide should be legalized for the terminally ill. What restrictions would you include in a law?

Application Exercise

Reread the What Do You Think? scenarios at the beginning of the chapter and answer the following questions.

1. Should Ed be able to request rational suicide? If so, when should the suicide occur? As soon as his symptoms start to get intolerable? As soon as Ed feels regular pain?

2. If Ed had made out a directive to physicians asking for assisted suicide 10 years ago, before he had married and had three children, should that document still be used?

Or should his children's or wife's request to keep him alive longer be considered? In other words, is the patient the only person who should have a say in the matter?

3. What kind of help should Paulo receive in order to cope better with the dying experiences of his friends?

4. If helping friends die is a negative experience for Paulo, should he continue helping his friends? Should he think of his own mental and emotional needs and not concern himself with each friend who dies?

Further Reading

Lewis R. Aiken, *Dying, Death, and Bereavement,* 3rd ed. (Boston: Allyn and Bacon, 1994).

An overview of death topics with an emphasis on demographics, cultural diversity, and psychological reactions to death.

Robert J. Kastenbaum, *Death, Society, and Human Experience,* 5th ed. (Boston: Allyn and Bacon, 1995).

Discussion of the experience of death in terms of its psychological and social aspects.

S. L. Bertman, *Facing Death: Images, Insights, and Interventions* (Hemisphere, 1991).

A look at the interpretation of death by the arts.

D. Cundiff, *Euthanasia Is Not the Answer: A Hospice Physician's View* (Clifton, NJ: Humana Press, 1992).

Supports palliative care as a humane alternative to euthanasia.

L. L. Emanuel et al., "Advance Directives for Medical Care: A Case for Greater Use," *New England Journal of Medicine* 324, 889–895.

Advance directives discussed as a way to eliminate the need for euthanasia.

M. R. Leming and G. E. Dickinson, *Understanding Dying, Death and Bereavement,* 2nd ed. (Fort Worth: Holt, Rinehart, and Winston, 1990).

Covers the social and psychological aspects of death as well as topics concerning bereavement and coping strategies for different ages.

J. P. Moreland and N. L. Geisler, *The Life and Death Debate: Moral Issues of Our Time* (New York: Greenwood Press, 1990).

Discusses moral and ethical issues that concern our society today. Discusses who has the power to make such decisions. Presents arguments for the right to die and the right to life.

CHAPTER OBJECTIVES

◆ Discuss violence in the United States, including homicide, bias and hate crimes, gang violence, and campus violence.

◆ Discuss domestic violence (abuse against men, women, and children committed by their family members) and its causes.

◆ Describe sexual victimization, including sexual assault, rape, date rape, and sexual harassment, and why it happens.

◆ Identify the steps you can take to prevent personal assaults at home, on the street, or in your car.

Violence and Abuse

An Epidemic of Fear

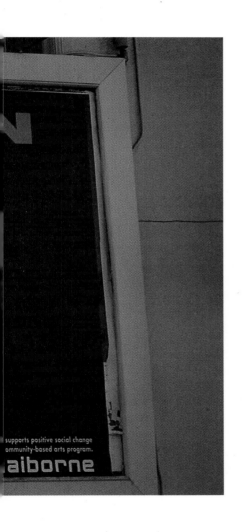

WHAT DO YOU THINK?

In 1991, a group of Navy pilots at a convention verbally abused and then mauled and fondled several Navy and civilian women at the hotel where the pilots were partying. This incident later became known as the Navy Tailhook scandal.

In 1992, a Japanese exchange student was shot to death when he arrived at the wrong address for a Halloween party. Because of communication difficulties and the homeowner's fear of crime and ready access to a gun, the mistake ended in the student's shooting death. The homeowner later explained his behavior as a natural reaction to someone he believed was an intruder on his property. He was acquitted of any crime.

■ What factors in American society have contributed to the seemingly rising incidence of these kinds of violent occurrences? Are there certain values, beliefs, and attitudes pervasive in the United States that make such behaviors more acceptable today than they used to be? In each of the situations described above, who was responsible for the violent action? What can people do to help prevent incidents like these? What types of community action would help reduce violence and abuse? Do you think certain national policies or laws would be useful?

In the 1940s and 50s, life appeared to be much simpler and safer. Kids could play in their neighborhoods, go to school, walk in the park, run to the grocery store or movie, go for a bike ride, and just be kids without the constant fear of muggings, shootings, gang attacks, or other threats.

■ What impact do you think changes in the environments that kids live in will have upon their development as healthy, well-adjusted individuals? What actions should be taken to prevent violence?

*'A*cross the land, waves of violence seem to crest and break, terrorizing Americans in cities and suburbs, in prairie towns and mountain hollow."

"To millions of Americans few things are more pervasive, more frightening, more real today than violent crime. . . . The fear of being victimized by criminal attack has touched us all in some new way."

"Among urban children ages 10–14, homicides are up 150 percent, robberies are up 192 percent, assaults are up 290 percent."

When you read the above quotations, did you think they were headlines from today's newspaper or TV news? They're not. The first comes from President Herbert Hoover's 1929 inauguration speech. The next comes from an 1860 Senate report on crime. And the final quotation comes from a 1967 report on children's violence.[1] Clearly, violence is not a new phenomenon.

However, never before has there been such a universal acknowledgment of the problem of violence in the United States. Chances are that if you go home from class today and flip on the television, you will see graphic footage of violent acts and their outcomes. We are a nation in deep trouble, caught in an epidemic of violence, as evidenced by the Health Headlines box. The term **violence** is used to indicate a set of behaviors that produce injuries, as well as the outcomes of these behaviors (the injuries themselves). In this chapter, we will focus on those violent acts that have particular relevance to you.

*V*IOLENCE IN THE UNITED STATES

In 1985, for the first time in history, the U.S. Public Health Service identified violence as a leading public health problem that was contributing to significant death and disability rates among Americans. In response to the spiraling increase in reported episodes of violence, the Centers for Disease Control and Prevention (CDC) created an entire section devoted to the prevention of violence. Even more significantly, it listed violence as a form of chronic disease that was pervasive in all levels of American society. Younger people's lives were being snuffed out by violent accidents, suicides, and homicides. Young black males seemed to be particularly at risk for violent death.

But is violence in the United States getting worse? Not if you look at the numbers. Since 1991, FBI statistics show that overall crime and certain types of violent crime have actually decreased slightly each year. Still, the odds of being a crime victim are twice what they were in 1963, when the FBI crime index counted 2,180 crimes per 100,000 people. Thirty years later, the number was 5,483 crimes per 100,000 people.[2]

Violence in a society directly or indirectly affects everyone who lives in that society. The direct victims of vio-

Violence in the form of drive-by shootings, fatal stabbings, domestic beatings, brutalizations of the elderly, and mass bombings are not only a major cause of death and disability in the United States, but also a source of fear and anxiety for all who watch the nightly news or read the morning headlines.

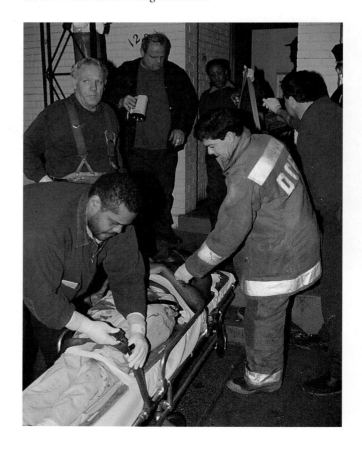

A Violent Nation?

At least 2.2 million Americans are victims of violent injury each year.

Homicide

- In the next 24 hours, 65 men, women, and children will die as a result of handgun fire.

- The United States ranks first among industrialized nations in violent death rates.

- Homicide is the leading cause of death for African Americans aged 15 to 34. In fact, black youths are six times more likely to be homicide victims than are white youths.

- Killers and killed alike are younger than ever, and more people are dying because guns are being used more often.

- The number of teenagers and younger children killed annually by firearms rose from 3373 in 1986 to 6795 in 1994.

- Fourteen percent of 8th-graders and 15 percent of 10th-graders carried a knife to school in 1992. Nearly 1 million teenagers are victims of violent crimes each year.

- In Louisiana and Texas, more people die from firearm-related injuries than from motor vehicle crashes.

Suicide

- Suicide is the third leading cause of death among people aged 15 to 24.

- Alcohol and/or drug use is the most common characteristic among youths who attempt suicide.

Sexual Assault

- According to one study, more than half of convicted rapists were drinking at the time of their offense.

- Over 100,000 rapes were reported in 1992. It is believed that many more rapes are committed than reported.

- According to one survey of high school students, 18 percent of female and 39 percent of male students believe that it is acceptable for a boy to force sex on a girl whose judgment is impaired by drugs or alcohol.

Domestic Violence

- Between 2 million and 4 million people are physically battered each year by their partners.

- More than 1 million women seek medical help every year for injuries caused by battering.

- Most domestic homicides are preceded by episodes of lesser violence.

Source: Adapted from U.S. Department of Health and Human Services, Public Health Service, Office for Substance Abuse Prevention, "Alcohol-Related Injuries and Violence," *OSAP Prevention Pipeline* 5 (May–June 1992): 3–6; and *National Center for Health Statistics Report,* November 1994.

lence and those close to them obviously suffer the most, but others also suffer in various ways because of the climate of fear that such violence generates. Women are afraid to walk the streets at night. Old people are often afraid to go out even in the daytime. Tourists are afraid of being brutalized in many of our nation's cities. Children playing out-of-doors find themselves dodging bullets in many of our major cities. Even people who live in "safe" areas often become victims of violence within their own homes at the hands of family members. At the very least, everyone pays higher tax bills for law enforcement and prisons and higher insurance premiums for damage done to others' or their own property.

Although the underlying causes of violence and abuse are as varied as the individual crimes and people involved, several social, cultural, and individual factors seem to increase the likelihood of violent acts. Poverty, unemployment, hopelessness, lack of education, inadequate housing, poor parental role models, cultural beliefs that objectify women and empower men to act as aggressors, lack of so-

cial support systems, discrimination, ignorance about people who are different, religious self-righteousness, breakdowns in the criminal justice system, stress, economic uncertainty, and a host of other factors may precipitate violent acts (see Table 22.1).

In today's environment, you have to take account of the effects of a climate of fear on your personal health status. By learning more about the etiology of homicide, suicide, and other violent acts that have become all too common in our society, you will reduce your own risk of becoming a victim and help ensure your own level of health. By taking steps to help prevent violence against others, you will help safeguard the health of society.

Violence: Refers to a set of behaviors that produce injuries, as well as the outcomes of these behaviors (the injuries themselves).

TABLE 22.1 ■ Factors That Increase the Risk for Violence

Social/Structural	Cultural	Biological	Interactionist	Personal Factors
Poverty and/or unemployment	Male admiration of physical prowess, toughness, "thrill," action	Male sex	Drug and alcohol consumption	Low self-esteem
Ideology that promotes dominant male social role	Media focus on and glamorization of violence	Youth (20–29 yrs.)	Weapons possession (especially handguns)	Learned helplessness
Dense population area	Peer support for violence and criminal activities	Early parenthood	Lack of support facilities	Ignorance/lack of understanding
Racial segregation and discrimination	Belief in absolutist parental powers and practice of using physical punishment to socialize children		Use of force to compensate for poor communication skills	Attitudes/values/beliefs that accept/condone violence
Breakup of nuclear family			Lack of safe refuge for women from domestic violence	Attitudes/beliefs that denigrate others
Lack of education	"Hands off" policy of criminal justice system concerning domestic violence		Lack of criminal justice and prosecution	History of violent abuse
Prolonged stress	Materialistic values promoting selfishness and acquisitiveness			Disrespect for rights of others
Social isolation	Objectification of women			Unhealthy parental models
Poor housing/unsafe living conditions	Religious oppression/moral self-righteousness			Learned sex roles
				Unhealthy styles for coping with stress

Source: Adapted by permission from Mark Rosenberg and Mary Fenley, *Violence in America* (New York: Oxford University Press, 1991), 30–33.

𝒲HAT DO YOU THINK?

Why do you think there is so much violent behavior in the United States today? What actions can you personally take to prevent violent events from occurring? What actions could be taken on your college campus? In your community?

Homicide

Homicide—death that results from intent to injure or kill—accounts for nearly 25,000 premature deaths every year in the United States. It was the 10th leading cause of death for all age groups in 1992, and the second leading cause of death for those between 15 and 22 years of age. Homicide is now the leading cause of death among black males aged 15 to 22 and 25 to 34.[3] Their homicide rates are 5 to 10 times higher than those for young white men. In fact, young American black men experience the highest homicide rates in the world. Young Hispanic Americans, both male and female, also experience disproportionately high homicide rates.[4]

For the average American, the lifetime probability of being murdered is 1 in 153. For white women, the risk is 1 in 450; for black men, it is 1 in 28. For a black man in the 20 to 22 age group, the risk is 1 in 3.[5]

Most murders are not committed by crazy strangers lurking in the shadows. Over half of all homicides occur among people who know one another. In two-thirds of these cases, the perpetrator and victim are friends or acquaintances; in one-third, they belong to the same family. Over 60 percent of these murders involve firearms. The Choices for Change box discusses some community ac-

Community Strategies for Preventing Violence

Since the causes of homicide and assaultive violence are complex, community strategies for prevention must be multidimensional.

Typical strategies for individual prevention include:

- Developing and implementing educational programs to teach people communication, conflict-resolution, and coping skills.

- Working with individuals to help them develop a sense of personal self-esteem and respect for others.

- Rewarding youngsters for good behavior. Never spanking a child when angry. Children need to know that anger is sometimes acceptable, but violence never is. Use family meetings to resolve conflicts.

- Establishing and enforcing policies that forbid discrimination on the basis of gender, religious affiliation, race, sexual orientation, marital status, and age.

- Increasing and enriching educational programs for family planning.

- Increasing identification by health-care and social service programs of violence victims.

- Improving treatment and support for victims.

- Treating the psychological as well as the physical consequences of violence.

Strategies for stopping violence in communities include:

- Giving judges more power to supervise and incarcerate the most serious offenders. Take into account previous offenses so that older teenagers who have repeatedly committed armed felonies can be identified and sentenced accordingly. Provide enough bed space, security, and anti-suicide assistance to detention centers. Require offenders to do hard work and to learn skills.

- Think of guns as a consumer product. Make them "child-proof." Personalize guns so that only the authorized user can shoot them. Don't leave handguns in the home where children can use them.

- Make it a felony to carry a concealed weapon (including brass knuckles).

- Discipline children swiftly and effectively, but appropriately, so that they realize that actions have real consequences for which they are accountable. Require them to make restitution or to clean up their messes.

- Get young people involved in volunteer service in their neighborhoods.

- Enforce laws forbidding liquor sales to juveniles. In one year, almost 60 percent of males arrested for violent offenses reported using alcohol within 72 hours before committing the crime.

- Get the police into neighborhoods. Establish rapid-response units for domestic violence. Treat family violence as seriously as murder. Provide a safe haven for battered people.

- Establish mandatory training courses for parents who are neglectful. Hold them accountable for their children's delinquency and problems.

- Build prevention and control of violence into the fabric of the community. Organize crime prevention meetings. Get to know your neighbors and establish neighborhood watches. Provide safe places for kids at night and safe corridors on their way to school.

- Improve identification, punishment, and treatment of perpetrators.

- Improve communication between criminal, law enforcement, and social service programs.

- Enact policies to improve social conditions (especially poverty and social injustice).

Source: Adapted by permission from Bill Moyers, "What Can We Do about Violence?" Public Broadcasting Service, January 1995.

---

tions aimed at preventing homicide and other types of violent assault.

Bias and Hate Crimes

As the population of the United States becomes more diverse, and people of color and differing cultures and lifestyles become more visible, there has been a corresponding rise in intolerance. Continuing anti-Semitic acts, Japanese bashing, gay bashing, and racially motivated hate crimes indicate that intolerance is still smoldering in our nation. Neo-Nazi activities, Ku Klux Klan and skin-

head demonstrations, and the growth of extremist religious and cult activity are signs that bigotry and hatred are still present. Cross burnings, religious desecrations, death threats, and actual murders indicate the seriousness of these social problems. Hatred and bigotry divide communities and shatter the social, educational, legal, political,

Homicide: Death that results from intent to injure or kill.

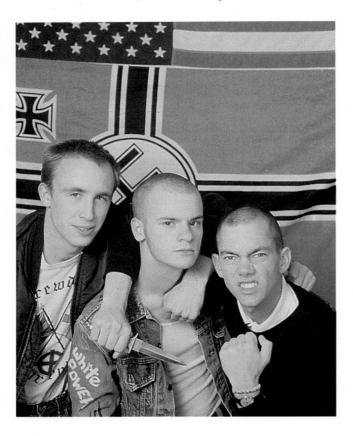

An increase in the number of bias and hate crimes and the growth of extremists groups provide evidence that intolerance smolders in American society.

and economic bonds between people. Such actions lead to deterioration in our spiritual, social, and psychological health.

Preventing Hate and Bias Crimes.   Although the causes of intolerance remain in question, it is believed that much of it stems from a fear of change and a desire to blame others when forces such as the economy and crime seem to be out of control. What can you do to be part of the solution to the problem rather than part of the problem?

- Support educational programs designed to foster understanding and appreciation for differences in people. Many colleges now require diversity classes as part of their academic curriculum.

- Examine your own attitudes and behaviors. Are you intolerant of others? Do you engage in racist, sexist, ethnic, or similar behaviors meant to demean any group of individuals? Have you thought about the reasons why you have problems with a particular group?

- Do you discourage jokes and other forms of social or ethnic bigotry? Do not participate in such behaviors and express your dissatisfaction with others who do.

- Vote for community leaders who respect the rights of others, who value diversity, and who do not have racially or ethnically motivated hidden agendas. Vote against intolerant candidates who are attempting to control our school boards and local government through planned infiltration.

- Educate yourself. Read, interact with, and attempt to understand people who may appear to be different from you. Remember that you do not have to like everything about another person or group. Other people may not like everything about you, either. However, respecting people's right to be different is a part of being a healthy, integrated individual.

- Examine your own values in determining the relative worth of your friends and the others in your life. Are you judgmental? Are you somewhat intolerant of other's differences? How do you resolve your own tendencies to be judgmental and bigoted? Do you judge people on appearances? Do you take time to get to know who they are as individuals?

*W*HAT DO YOU THINK?

Think about the bias or hate crimes that you have heard about in the last six months. Who were the victims? Did you know any of the victims? Why do you think people are motivated to initiate such crimes against people they do not know? What can you do to reduce the risk of such crimes in your area? What should be done nationally?

Gang Violence

The growing influence of street gangs has had a harmful impact on the health of our country. Drug abuse, gang shootings, beatings, thefts, carjackings, and the possibility of being caught in the middle between gangs at war have led to whole neighborhoods being held hostage by gang members. Once thought to be a phenomenon that occurred only in inner-city areas, gang violence now also occurs in both rural and suburban communities, particularly in the southeast, southwest, and western regions of the country.

What causes young people to join gangs? Although these causes are complex, gangs apparently meet the needs of many of today's young people. They provide a sense of belonging to a "family" that gives them self-worth, companionship, security, and excitement. In other cases, they provide a means of attaining economic security through criminal activity, drug sales, or prostitution. Once young people become involved in the gang subculture, it is difficult for them to get out. Threats of violence or fear of not making it on their own dissuade even those people who are most seriously trying to get out.

Who is at risk for gang membership? Gang membership varies considerably from region to region. The age range of gang members is typically 12 to 22 years. Risk factors include low self-esteem, academic problems, low socioeconomic status, alienation from family and society, a history of family violence, and living in gang-controlled neighborhoods.

Protecting against Gang Power.　The best means of preventing a person from joining a gang is trying to keep that person connected to positive influences and programs. From a child's early years, the focus should be on reducing alienation from friends, family, and school and on trying to make sure that any student who has learning disabilities or other problems that make it hard for him or her to keep up has alternative activities at which he or she can be successful.

Prevention programs that are community-based and that involve families, social service organizations, and law enforcement, school, and city officials in a coordinated and visible effort have been shown to be most effective. The staff in such programs, as well as in social service organizations and schools serving at-risk students, must be well-trained, empathic, competent in dealing with emotionally charged issues, and understanding of the underlying factors that make youths choose the gang way of life. Rather than thinking of such youths only as gang members, community members must begin to think of them as people whose circumstances made them susceptible to the gang lifestyle.

In part because the number of gangs and gang-related crimes grows daily, Congress passed a crime bill in 1994

Street gangs, long seen as a source of illegal drug trade and violent crimes in the inner city, have spread to suburban and rural areas, attracting increasing numbers of young people who often become victims of their own gangs if they try to get out.

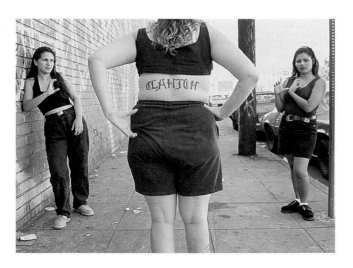

that encompassed the hiring of 100,000 additional police officers, a ban on assault weapons, reform of the welfare system, the creation of a national network of neighborhood banks to boost communities' economic development, and the establishment of "boot camps" for young nonviolent offenders. These boot camps would keep offenders out of prison yet instill discipline, self-esteem, and respect for the law. Although all these proposals have merit, they also cost considerable amounts of money. At the same time, the United States is staggering under the burden of enormous debt. Deciding the place of gang violence prevention in a list of national priorities will be difficult. The Multicultural Perspectives box discusses how China uses its prison system to change attitudes as well as to punish offenders.

Violence on Campus

"Don't walk on campus alone after dark." "Call the escort or shuttle service if you're alone and need a ride." "Lock your room when you go to the shower." These kinds of warnings reverberate across U.S. campuses today.

Students on campus are concerned for their safety for good reason. In the early 1970s, campus "crime" consisted mainly of plagiarism, cheating on an exam, and occasional "streaking." Today there are murders, rapes, vicious assaults, and robberies on campus. Students' "home away from home" has undergone a shocking change. Much of the violent crime on campus seems to be fueled by alcohol abuse and other personal problems. Student victims tend to drink and to use drugs more than do other students, to have lower GPAs, and to be members of fraternities and sororities. Perpetrators also tend to have low GPAs, to drink heavily, and disproportionately to be athletes.[6]

Traditionally, most campus crimes were handled internally. This has changed as more states have passed legislation requiring that colleges and universities warn their students about crime and danger both on campus property and in off-campus housing that they recommend.[7]

In July 1992, Congress passed the Campus Sexual Assault Victim's Bill of Rights, known as the Ramstad Act (for Representative Jim Ramstad of Minnesota, who introduced it). Among other things, the act gives victims the right to call in off-campus authorities to investigate serious campus crimes. In addition, universities must set up educational programs and notify students of available counseling.

Under a recent clarification of the Buckley Privacy Amendment, victims of campus violence have easier access to the previous criminal records of student perpetrators of crime. The Students' Right-to-Know and Campus Security Act requires all colleges and universities receiving federal funds to provide yearly reports of crimes on their campuses and of the actions they are taking to stop them.

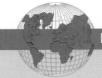

Justice in China

The emphasis . . . throughout the [Chinese] justice system is a "change in attitude." This orientation manifests itself at every stage of the legal process. In the courts, the first change of attitude is expected to take place prior to a trial; it is a confession of guilt. While the confession does confirm the findings of the investigative panel, it is required for "deeper reasons." As in the past, the confession serves to reestablish the "harmony of the social order . . . after the discord created by the crime. From the accused's point of view the process of confession signals his or her capacity to see the facts from society's standpoint and to engage in self-criticism, and thus in time to be changed in order to fit once more into society". . . . Those who do confess tend to receive lighter sentences, while those who resist this resocialization are labeled as having "bad attitudes" and commonly are given much harsher punishments for the same offense.

The lawyer plays an interesting role in the courtroom process. The profession of lawyer was reestablished only in 1979 and its character is still evolving in today's changing Chinese society. In general, though, in criminal proceedings, rather than taking the adversarial position with which we are familiar, the Chinese lawyer, a governmental official, is an active agent in the resocialization process, assisting the accused in making the right choices. This is not to say that the attorney does not try to defend the client, but rather that the lawyer conducts the defense with the interest of society in mind.

Like the Chinese legal system, the correctional system also stresses change. At the juvenile level, the "gong du" or work study schools attempt to reintegrate youthful offenders into the mainstream of Chinese society. The most distinctive feature of the juvenile system is that the gong du operations are administered by the educational branch of local government and only the most severe juvenile offenders are placed in more traditional correctional facilities. At the gong du school, students are constantly reminded of their responsibility to society both in the classroom and on the job that they are required to have. The adult prisons also place considerable emphasis on changing attitudes. Slogans are displayed throughout the prisons urging the offender to "Get to the bottom of your crimes," "Remold yourself quickly," "Make a start towards a new life," or "Criticize your crimes."

Thus, while crime is considered a violation of the social order as it is in numerous other countries, in China it is also viewed as a break that can be mended.

Source: Excerpted from Daniel J. Curran and Claire M. Renzetti, *Social Problems*, 3rd ed., 546. © copyright 1993 by Allyn and Bacon. Reprinted by permission.

DOMESTIC VIOLENCE

During the last decade, the subject of domestic violence has finally grabbed our attention. The Lorena Bobbitt, O. J. Simpson, and Susan Smith cases—as well as many less prominent ones—have brought the truth about domestic violence into the open.

Spousal Abuse

Contrary to common perception, domestic violence does not only happen to people of lower socioeconomic status

> **Domestic violence:** The use of force to control and maintain power over another person in the home environment; it includes both actual harm and the threat of harm.

and to women. It is a widespread social problem affecting all races, ethnic groups, economic classes, and both sexes. By most estimates, it is the most common and least reported crime in the United States today. **Domestic violence** refers to the use of force to control and maintain power over another person in the home environment; it includes both actual harm and the threat of harm.[8] It can involve emotional abuse, verbal abuse, threats of physical abuse, and actual physical violence ranging from slapping and shoving to bone-breaking beatings, rape, and homicide.

Women as Victims

While young men are more apt to become victims of violent acts perpetrated by strangers, women are much more likely to become victims of violent acts perpetrated by spouses, lovers, ex-spouses, and ex-lovers. In fact, 6 of every 10 women in the United States will be assaulted at some time in their lives by someone they know.[9] Every year, approximately 12 percent of married women are the victims of physical aggression perpetrated by their husbands, according to a national survey.[10] These acts of ag-

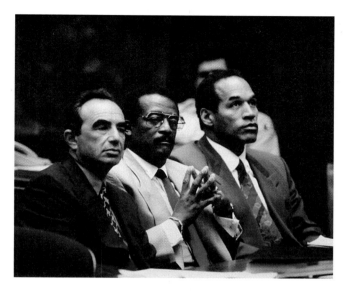

Several highly publicized trials in recent years have heightened our awareness of the widespread domestic violence that pervades our society.

gression are committed in anger and often include pushing, slapping, and shoving.

Some women experience much more severe acts of aggression. About 4 percent of married women each year are the victims of violence that takes the form of beating and/or threats of or actual harm caused by use of a knife or a gun.[11] In fact, acts of aggression by a husband or boyfriend are one of the most common causes of death for young women, and roughly 2,000 women in the United States are killed each year by their partners or ex-partners.[12] Over a recent 10-year period, according to the National Crime Survey, on average, more than 2 million assaults on women occurred each year. More than two-thirds of these assaults were committed by someone the woman knew.[13]

The following United States statistics indicate the seriousness of this long-hidden problem:[14]

- Every 15 seconds, someone batters a woman.

- Only 1 in every 250 such assaults is reported to the police.

- More than a third of women victims of domestic violence are severely abused on a regular basis.

- About five women are killed every day in domestic violence incidents.

- Three of every four women murdered are killed by their husbands.

- Domestic violence is the single greatest cause of injury to women, surpassing rape, mugging, and auto accidents combined.

- About 25 to 45 percent of all women who are battered are battered during pregnancy.

- One-quarter of suicide attempts by women occur as a result of domestic violence.

How many times have you heard of a woman who is repeatedly beaten by her partner or spouse and asked, "Why doesn't she just leave him?" There are many reasons why some women find it difficult, if not impossible, to break their ties with their abusers. Many women, particularly those having small children, are financially dependent on their partners. Others fear retaliation against themselves or their children. There are women who hope that the situation will change with time (it rarely does), and others who stay because their cultural or religious beliefs forbid divorce. Finally, there are women who still love the abusive partner and are concerned about what will happen to him if they leave.[15]

Cycle of Violence Theory. Psychologist Lenore Walker has developed a theory known as the "cycle of violence" to explain how women can get caught in a downward spiral without knowing what is happening to them.[16] The cycle has several phases:

- *Phase One: Tension Building.* In this phase, minor battering occurs, and the woman may become more nurturant, more pleasing, and more intent on anticipating the spouse's needs in order to forestall another violent scene. She assumes guilt for doing something to provoke him and tries hard to avoid doing it again.

Many battered and abused women become trapped in a cycle of violence that also puts their children at risk for physical and psychological abuse.

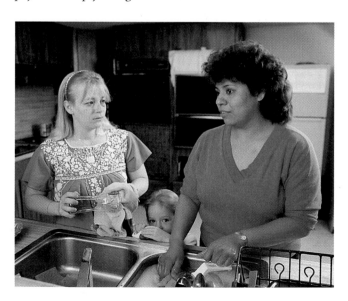

- *Phase Two: Acute Battering.* At this stage, pleasing her man doesn't help and she can no longer control or predict the abuse. Usually, the spouse is trying to "teach her a lesson," and when he feels he has inflicted enough pain, he'll stop. When the acute attack is over, he may respond with shock and denial about his own behavior. Both batterer and victim may soft-peddle the seriousness of the attacks.

- *Phase Three: Remorse/Reconciliation.* During this "honeymoon" period, the batterer may be kind, loving, and apologetic, swearing he will never act violently toward the woman again. He may "behave" for several weeks or months, and the woman may come to question whether she overrated the seriousness of past abuse. Then the kind of tension that precipitated abusive incidents in the past resurfaces, he loses control again, and he once more beats the woman. Unless some form of intervention breaks this downward cycle of abuse, contrition, further abuse, denial, and contrition, it will repeat again and again—perhaps ending only in the woman's, or rarely, the man's death.

It is very hard for most women who get caught in this cycle of violence (which may include forced sexual relations and psychological and economic abuse as well as beatings) to summon up the courage and resolution to extricate themselves. Most need effective outside intervention.

*W*HAT DO YOU THINK?

Can you think of a woman whom you consider a likely victim of domestic violence? What about her has contributed to her current situation? Can you think of a man whom you consider a likely victimizer? What about him has contributed to his current situation?

Men as Victims

Are men also victims of domestic violence? The answer is yes. Clearly, some women do abuse and even kill their partners. Approximately 12 percent of men reported that their wives engaged in physically aggressive behaviors against them in the past year—nearly the same percent-

Child abuse: The systematic harming of a child by a caregiver, generally a parent.

Sexual abuse of children: Sexually suggestive conversations; inappropriate kissing; touching; petting; oral, anal, or vaginal intercourse; and/or other kinds of sexual interaction between a child and an adult or an older child.

age as women. The difference between male and female batterers is twofold. First, although the frequency of physical aggression may be the same, the impact of physical aggression by men against women is drastically different: women are typically injured in such incidents two to three times more often than are men.[17] Women do engage in moderate aggression, such as pushing and shoving, at rates almost equal to men. But the severe form of aggression that is likely to land the victim in the hospital is almost always a male-against-female form of aggression. Second, a woman who is physically abused by a man is generally intimidated by him: she fears that he will use his power and control over her in some fashion. Men, however, generally report that they do not live in fear of their wives.

Causes of Domestic Violence

There is no single explanation for why people tend to be abusive in relationships. Although alcohol abuse is often associated with such violence, marital dissatisfaction seems to predict physical abuse better than does any other variable.[18] Numerous studies also point to differences in the communication patterns between abusive relationships and nonabusive relationships.[19] While some argue that the hormone testosterone is the cause of male aggression, recent studies have failed to show a strong association between physical abuse in relationships and this hormone.[20] Many experts believe that men who engage in severe violence are more likely than other men to suffer from personality disorders.[21]

Regardless of the cause, or of who should shoulder the greatest amount of blame, it is important to remember that it is the dynamics that both people bring to a relationship that result in violence and allow it to continue. Obtaining help from community support and counseling services may help determine the underlying basis of the problem and may help the victim and the batterer come to a better understanding of the actions necessary to stop the cycle of abuse. The Rate Yourself box may help you determine if you are a victim of abuse.

Child Abuse

Children raised in families in which domestic violence and/or sexual abuse occur are at great risk for damage to their personal health and well-being. The effects of such violent acts are powerful and can be very long-lasting. **Child abuse** refers to the systematic harm of a child by a caregiver, generally a parent.[22] The abuse may be sexual, psychological, physical, or any combination of these. Although exact figures are lacking, many experts believe that there are over 2 million cases of child abuse every year in the United States involving severe injury, permanent disability, and/or death. Child abusers exist in all gender, social, ethnic, religious, and racial groups.

Are You a Victim of Abuse?

Although we often think of abuse as physical, much of the abuse that takes place in intimate relationships is more psychological in nature. If you feel constantly put down or controlled by your partner, ask yourself the following questions.

	Never	Sometimes	Usually	Always
1. Are you blamed by your partner whenever things go wrong?	___	___	___	___
2. Does your partner yell at you, curse you, or call you names?	___	___	___	___
3. Is your partner a "nasty" drunk or drug user?	___	___	___	___
4. Does your partner control your money?	___	___	___	___
5. Are you discouraged from enjoying outside friendships?	___	___	___	___
6. Is your free time restricted by your partner?	___	___	___	___
7. Do you "cover" or make excuses for your partner's behavior?	___	___	___	___
8. Do you do more than your fair share of work around the house?	___	___	___	___
9. Are you forced or coerced into having unwanted sex after you've said no?	___	___	___	___
10. Do you feel you must ask permission to do things?	___	___	___	___
11. Are you sometimes "punished" overtly or more subtly for misbehaving?	___	___	___	___
12. Was your mother or your partner's mother abused or was your partner abused in the past?	___	___	___	___
13. If you express opinions opposed to those of your partner, does it cause a scene?	___	___	___	___
14. Are you afraid of your partner?	___	___	___	___
15. Does your partner repeatedly point out things that are wrong with you?	___	___	___	___

Scoring

If you answered Usually or Always to

1 or 2 items	Take notice. Work together to improve troubled areas in the relationship.
3 or 4 items	Seriously examine the relationship. Seek joint counseling from a qualified professional.
5 to 7 items	Abuse is definitely a problem. Counseling is necessary (joint counseling may be appropriate).
8 to 15 items	Crisis intervention is needed. Joint therapy is not appropriate.

Certain personal characteristics tend to be common among child abusers: the experience of being abused as a child, poor self-image, feelings of isolation, extreme frustration with life, higher stress or anxiety levels than normal, a tendency to abuse drugs and/or alcohol, and unrealistic expectations of the child. It is also estimated that half to three-quarters of men who batter their female partners also batter children. In fact, spouse abuse is the single most identifiable risk factor for predicting child abuse. Finally, children with handicaps or other "differences" are more likely to be abused.[23]

Child Sexual Abuse

Sexual abuse of children by adults or older children includes sexually suggestive conversations; inappropriate kissing; touching; petting; oral, anal, or vaginal intercourse; and other kinds of sexual interaction. The most frequent abusers are a child's parents or companions or spouses of the child's parents. Next most frequent are grandfathers and siblings. Girls are more commonly abused than boys, although young boys are also frequent victims, usually of male family members. Between 20 and 30 percent of all adult women report having had an unwanted childhood sexual encounter with an adult male, usually a father, uncle, brother, or grandfather. It is a myth that male deviance or mental illness accounts for most incidents of sexual abuse of children: "Stories of retrospective incest patients typically involved perpetrators who are 'Everyman'—attorneys, mental health practitioners, businessmen, farmers, teachers, doctors, and clergy."[24]

Most sexual abuse occurs in the child's home.[25] Risky situations include:[26]

1. When the child lives without one of his or her biological parents.

2. When the mother is unavailable to the child either because she is working outside the home or because she is disabled or ill.

3. When the parents' marriage is unhappy or rife with conflict.

4. When the child has a poor relationship with his or her parents or is subjected to extremely punitive discipline.

5. When the child lives with a stepfather.

Two points are worth making about the impact of child abuse in later life: 99 percent of the inmates in the maximum security prison at San Quentin were either abused or raised in abusive households; and 300,000 children be-

Sympathetic and sensitive therapy can help abused children cope with the mental and physical pain inflicted on them, most commonly by parents or other family members.

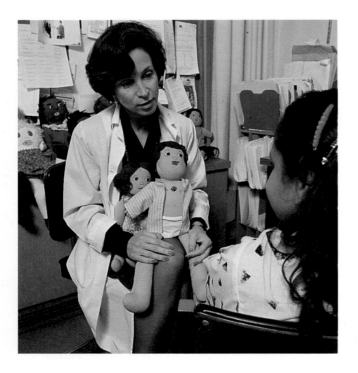

tween the ages of 8 and 15 are living on the nation's streets, willing to prostitute themselves to survive rather than to return to abusive households they ran away from.[27]

Most people who were abused as children, of course, do not end up as convicts or prostitutes. But most do bear spiritual, psychological, and/or physical scars. Clinical psychologist Marjorie Whittaker has found that "of all forms of violence, incest and childhood sexual abuse are considered among the most 'toxic' because of their violations of trust, the confusion of affection and coercion, the splitting of family alignments, and serious psychological and physical consequences."[28]

Not all child violence is physical. Your health can be severely affected by psychological violence—assaults on your personality, character, competence, independence, or general dignity as a human being. The negative consequences of this kind of victimization in close relationships can be harder to discern and therefore harder to combat. They include depression, lowered self-esteem, and a pervasive fear of doing something that will offend the abuser.

> ### ✏️ WHAT DO YOU THINK?
>
> What factors in society lead to child abuse and neglect? What are common characteristics of children's abusers? Why are family members often the perpetrators of child abuse and child sexual abuse? What actions can be taken to prevent such behaviors?

𝒮EXUAL VICTIMIZATION

Sexual Assault and Rape

Sexual violence against women is of epidemic proportions in this country. **Sexual assault** is any act in which one person is sexually intimate with another person without that other person's consent. According to counselor Alan Berkowitz, "sexually assaultive behaviors can be placed on a continuum according to the degree of force or coercion involved."[29] These behaviors include ignoring indications that intimacy is not wanted, threatening force or other negative consequences, and actually using force to obtain sexual intimacy.

Rape is the most extreme form of sexual assault and is defined as "penetration without the victim's consent."[30] Whether committed by an acquaintance, a date, or a stranger, rape is a criminal activity that usually has serious emotional, psychological, social, and physical consequences for the victim. Most victims are young, with 29 percent of rape victims being under 11 years old, 32 percent between the ages of 11 and 17, and another 22 percent between ages 18 and 24.[31]

Most studies of the frequency of sexual assault among college students indicate that from 25 percent to 60 percent of college men have engaged in some form of sexually coercive behavior.[32] This is consistent with the 27.5 percent of college women who have reported experiencing rape or attempted rape since they were 14 years old, and the 54 percent who claim to have been sexually victimized (forced to endure unwanted petting, kisses, and other advances).[33] In one survey, only 39 percent of the men sampled denied coercive involvement, 28 percent admitted to having used a coercive method at least once, and 15 percent admitted that they had forced a woman to have intercourse at least once.[34] And according to a large, nationally representative sample of college and university students, 25 percent of the male respondents had been involved in some form of sexual assault since age 14.[35]

Why Some Males Sexually Assault Women

Over the years, psychologists and others have proposed many theories to explain why so many males sexually victimize women. In a recent study, almost two-thirds of the male respondents had engaged in intercourse unwanted by the woman, primarily because of male peer pressure.[36] Peer pressure is certainly a strong factor in such behavior, but a growing body of research suggests that sexual assault is encouraged by the normal socialization processes that males experience daily.[37]

Male Socialization. Throughout our lives, we are exposed to social norms that "objectify" women. Media portrayals of half-dressed and undressed women in seductive poses promoting products, for instance, contribute to sex-role stereotyping. These portrayals often show males as aggressors and females as targets of aggression. In addition, men are exposed from an early age to anti-female jokes and vulgar and obscene terms for women. These reinforce the idea that females are lesser beings who may be pushed around with impunity.[38] Males are also discouraged from acting in ways that society views as feminine. They are told to strive for power, status, and control; are encouraged to act tough and unemotional; and are expected to be aggressive and to take risks. The inculcation of "tough guy" attitudes during boys' formative years seems to have a significant influence on their attitudes later in life.[39]

Male Attitudes. Several studies have confirmed a greater tolerance of rape in men who accept the myth that rape is something women secretly desire, who believe in adversarial relationships between men and women, who condone violence against women, or who hold traditional attitudes toward sex roles. Such men are more apt to blame the victim and are more likely to commit rape themselves if they think they will get away with it.[40]

Male Sexual History and Hostility. Most rapists are not abnormal or psychologically disturbed. Rather, they tend to be people whose childhoods involved early, multiple sexual experiences (both forced and voluntary) and who feel hostility toward women.[41]

Male Misperceptions. Men who are convinced that women really want sex even if they say they don't are more likely than other men to perpetrate sexual assaults. They more readily misinterpret women's words and behavior and act on their misinterpretations—only to be surprised later when women claim that they have been assaulted.[42]

Situational Factors. Several situations increase the likelihood that men will engage in coercive or aggressive sexual behaviors. Dates in which the male makes all the decisions, pays, drives, and in general controls what happens are more likely to end in sexual aggression. Alcohol and drug use increases the likelihood and severity of sexual assault. Length of relationship is another important situational factor: the more long-standing the relationship, the greater the chance of an assault. Finally, males who belong to a close-knit social group involving intense interaction are more prone to engage in a peer-pleasing assault.

Date Rape

Although acquaintance or date rape occurs among people of all ages, races, and socioeconomic backgrounds, college students are particularly vulnerable—partly because they are in the age group that has the highest rate of rape. While most acquaintance rape victims are females aged 16 to 22 years, surveys indicate that males are victims (usually of other males) in 10 percent of acquaintance rape cases.[43]

In a study of 6,000 college students from 32 different universities, researchers found:

- More than 50 percent of the college women surveyed had endured some form of sexual abuse.

Sexual assault: Any act in which one person is sexually intimate with another person without that other person's consent.

Rape: Sexual penetration without the victim's consent.

- More than 25 percent had been the victims of rape or attempted rape.

- 84 percent of the assault victims knew their assailants.

- 57 percent of the assaults occurred on dates.

- 41 percent of the women raped were virgins at the time of the assault.

- 73 percent of the assailants and 55 percent of the victims had used alcohol or drugs prior to the assault.

- 42 percent of the victims indicated that they had sex with the offender again (it is unknown whether the subsequent sex was voluntary).

- 25 percent of the men in the survey admitted to some degree of aggressive sexual behavior.

- Men were most likely to commit sexual assaults during their senior year in high school or first year in college.[44]

Date rape is not simply miscommunication; it is an act of violence. Susan Jacoby puts it this way:

> Some women (especially the young) initially resist sex not out of real conviction but as part of the elaborate persuasion and seduction rituals accompanying what was once called courtship. And it is true that many men (again, especially the young) take pride in the ability to coax a woman a step further than she intended to go. But these mating rituals do not justify or even explain date rape. Even the most callow youth is capable of understanding the difference between resistance and genuine fear; between a halfhearted 'no, we shouldn't' and tears or screams.[45]

The Skills for Behavior Change box discusses prevention of date rape.

Social Assumptions

According to many experts, certain common assumptions in our society prevent the recognition by both the perpetrator and the wider public of the true nature of sexual assault.[46] The most important of these assumptions are the following.[47]

- *Minimization:* It is often assumed that sexual assault of women is rare because official crime statistics, including the Uniform Crime Reports of the FBI, show very few rapes per thousand population; however, this is the most underreported of all serious crimes. Researchers in this area have found that nearly 25 percent of women in the United States have been raped.

> **Sexual harassment:** Any form of unwanted sexual attention.

- *Trivialization:* Incredibly enough, sexual assault of women is still often viewed as a jocular matter. During a gubernatorial election in Texas a few years back, one of the candidates reportedly compared a bad patch of weather to rape: "If there's nothing you can do about it, just lie back and enjoy it." (He lost the election—to a woman.)

- *Blaming the victim:* Many discussions of sexual violence against women display a sometimes unconscious assumption that the woman did something to provoke the attack—that she dressed too revealingly or flirted too outrageously.

- *"Boys will be boys":* This is the assumption that men just can't control themselves once they become aroused. It has been neatly deflated by one commentator:

> [The] myth that men can't stop once they start is millennia old and typically is stated as "males are slaves to their sexual organs," or "great physical harm can befall the unfortunate male who is denied completion of sexual activity." During my presentations to college-aged audiences, I counter these two statements by pointing out: (a) If a woman's parents walked into the room, it's a sure bet that the male could stop; and (b) there is not a single case reported of a male dying of coitus interruptus.

Sexual Harassment

If we think of violence as including verbal abuse and the threat of coercion, then sexual harassment is a form of violence. **Sexual harassment** is defined as any form of unwanted sexual attention. The issue gained a good deal of attention in the early 1990s with the Anita Hill case and the Navy Tailhook scandal. What had long been dismissed as harmless behavior became a cause for concern in business and schools as well as in government. Many companies established policies against sexual harassment and set up procedures for dealing with it. (The Building Communications Skills box discusses how to avoid and handle sexual harassment situations in the workplace.) Schools—from kindergartens to universities—acted to protect victims and to punish offenders. Across the country, colleges and universities drafted harassment and hate speech codes (though some of the latter ran aground of First Amendment rights) and offered courses designed to sensitize students to the harmful effects of racial and sexual verbal assaults.

How pervasive is sexual harassment in U.S. schools? A nationwide survey sponsored by the Center for Research on Women at Wellesley College and the Legal Defense and Education Fund of the National Organization for Women undertook to answer this question. Of 4,200 girls and young women who responded, 89 percent reported being sexually touched, pinched, or grabbed by other students. About 39 percent said they had been harassed at school on a daily basis during the past year.[48]

Preventing Date Rape

Most date rapes can be prevented by following several general guidelines. To keep yourself from getting into a potentially harmful situation, consider the following:

Women

- Think ahead of time and try to avoid getting into "compromising" situations. Stay out of your date's bedroom, the back seat of the car, or other quiet spots that are away from the rest of the crowd.

- Communicate directly. Don't be wishy-washy in your remarks. If things start to go farther than you would like them to go, say NO loudly and with conviction. Do not worry about hurting feelings or seeming too aggressive. Be firm and stick to your words.

- Be aware that some men, in some situations, will interpret a low cut, sexy dress or other clothing as a come on. Although this is obviously wrong on their part, it is important that you do not naively assume that everyone is enlightened. Be direct and firm with anyone who seems to be assuming too much from your interactions.

- Avoid any substances, alcohol included, that may cause you to think not as clearly as you normally do.

- Pay attention to the nonverbal and verbal cues that your date is giving you. If he is starting to indicate that he is interested in more, make sure you are not caught unawares. Move to stay close to others and quickly let your date know your intentions.

- Decide ahead of time how far you are interested in going. Remember that it is your game, your rules, and no one should be able to pressure or force you into going beyond the line you have drawn.

- Be concerned about any of the following behaviors or expressions exhibited by your date:
  - Continued suggestive or dirty language indicating a disrespect for you and others.
  - Failure to listen to or to value your opinions about where to go, whom to spend time with, etc.
  - Unusual displays of jealousy/rage concerning your interactions with others.
  - Unusual roughness and forceful pushing or shoving to get you to comply with his wishes.

- Wild anger and violent acts toward others.
- Inability to control drinking and to display appropriate behaviors.
- Lack of concern for your feelings; laughter or derisive comments when you say no.

Men

- Take stock of your past behavior in potentially sexual situations. How have you behaved, what have been the outcomes of the encounters, etc.? Have you felt uncomfortable about pushing too hard to have sex with your dates in the past?

- Know your sexual limits. If you feel like you are beginning to lose control in an intimate situation, communicate your feelings and indicate why it is time that you stop.

- Understand that NO means NO—and that it is not a sign of rejection. Respect the woman's right to say no, regardless of how far you've gone or what you thought she might have wanted. Stop NOW and quit trying "another line." Think about how you'd want your sister or close female friend to be treated by another guy in a similar situation.

- Just because you may have been intimate with the woman before, don't assume that it's okay now. When you hear the word NO, or if the woman struggles in any way, STOP.

- Avoid alcohol and other drugs that may cause you to think unclearly.

- Avoid situations likely to get you into trouble. Stay out of bedrooms and avoid dark roads and the back seats of cars. Remember, a rape charge is serious business and could ruin your college and future career aspirations, not to mention the damage you may cause the woman.

- If you encounter a particularly aggressive woman, it is not unmanly to tell her you do not want to have sex and are not interested in being intimate in any way. Say NO and avoid situations that may cause you to be caught in a compromising position. Forget about what she may say or what your friends will say. Remember that sexual activity should be a part of a larger relationship.

*W*HAT DO YOU THINK?

Why do you think women are often reluctant to report sexual harassment cases? Why do you think so many men report that they were unaware of their own sexually harassing behaviors? What can be done to increase awareness in this area?

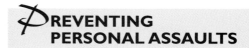

*P*REVENTING PERSONAL ASSAULTS

After a violent act is committed against someone we know, we acknowledge the horror of the event, express sympathy for the victim, and then go on with our lives.

Sexual Harassment in the Workplace

Many of you are currently working to pay for college, and almost all of you will be in the workforce within a few years. Learning what constitutes sexual harassment may save you embarrassment in the future.

Under Title VII of the Civil Rights Act, sexual harassment is "unwelcomed sexual advances, requests for sexual favors, and other verbal or physical contact of a sexual nature." In the real world, though, sexual harassment is anything that the offended person believes is harassment.

You may remember that during the 1991 Senate Judiciary Committee hearings, Anita Hill charged that Supreme Court justice nominee Clarence Thomas had sexually harassed her 10 years earlier when they worked together. The alleged harassment was partly in the form of sexually offensive humor—even though the jokes were not necessarily directed at Hill.

It's always important to watch what you say and how you say it. But nowhere is this more true than at your job. Let's say you want to compliment a colleague on his or her appearance. It's appropriate to say, "You look very nice today." The same compliment may turn into harassment if you say, "That dress looks great on your body," or, "Those jeans look great on your body." Even if the person enjoys your comment, you have to remember that others may overhear your remarks. If you are known as someone who makes such comments, you may be considered a risk the next time a possible promotion comes up.

After you've been in the workforce for a while, you'll notice that there are two subdivisions of people: Those who tell "dirty" jokes and make potentially harassing comments, and those who don't. Those who don't are generally found at the higher-paying positions.

If You Are Harassed

After an incident of sexual harassment, it is generally best to be assertive immediately and to take action to ensure that it will not be repeated. The following suggestions may help you to help yourself:

- *Ask the harasser to stop.* Be clear and direct about what is bothering you and why you are upset: "I don't like this joke/touch/remark/look. It makes me feel uncomfortable and it is hard for me to work/participate/be your friend, etc." This may be the first indication the person has ever had that such behavior is inappropriate. This will usually stop the harassment.

- *Document the harassment.* Make a record of the incident. If the harassment becomes intolerable, having a record of exactly what occurred (and when and where) will be helpful in making your case.

- *Complain to a higher authority.* Talk to your manager about what happened. If the manager or supervisor doesn't take you seriously, find out what the internal grievance procedures are for your organization.

- *Remember that you have not done anything wrong.* You will likely feel awful after being harassed (and especially so if you have to complain to superiors). However, you should feel proud that you are not keeping silent. The person harassing you is wrong, not you. If the situation becomes so uncomfortable that you feel you can't work in the same place as the harasser, why should you be the one to have to leave?

But the person who has been brutalized often takes a long time to recover—and sometimes complete recovery from the assault is not possible (see Table 22.2 for a summary of the most common consequences of victimization). In this section we discuss prevention of violence and abuse rather extensively because it is far better to stop a violent act than to recover from it.

Self-Defense against Rape

Rape can occur no matter what preventive actions you take, but there are some commonsense self-defense tactics that should lower your risk. Self-defense is a process that includes increased awareness, learning self-defense techniques, taking reasonable precautions, and developing the self-confidence and judgment needed to determine appropriate responses to different situations.[49]

Taking Control. Most rapes by assailants unknown to the victim are planned in advance. They are frequently preceded by a casual, friendly conversation. Although many women have said that they started to feel uneasy during such a conversation, they denied the possibility of an attack to themselves until it was too late. Listen to your feelings and trust your intuition. Be assertive and direct to someone who is getting out of line or threatening—this may convince the would-be rapist to back off. Stifle your tendency to be "nice" and don't fear making a scene. Let him know that you mean what you say and are prepared to defend yourself:

- *Speak in a strong voice and use statements like "Leave me alone" rather than questions like "Will you please leave me alone?"* Avoid apologies and excuses.

- *Maintain eye contact with the would-be attacker.*

- *Sound as if you mean what you say.*

- *Stand up straight, act confident, and remain alert.* Walk as if you own the sidewalk.[50]

TABLE 22.2 ■ Common Consequences of Victimization

Psychological	Medical
Recurrent and intrusive recollections, dreams, or flashbacks involving traumatic incidents	Death
Generalized anxiety, mistrust, and/or social isolation	Sexual/reproductive symptoms/consequences Chronic pelvic pain, HIV infection, Urinary tract infections, Premenstrual pain, Fertility problems, Trauma-specific pain, Orgasmic difficulty
Difficulty in forming or maintaining nonexploitive intimate relationships	Battering-related symptoms Bruises, Black eyes, Fractured ribs/broken teeth, Subdural hematomas, Detached retinas, Other head injuries
Chronic depression	Stress-mediated symptoms Headaches, Backaches, TMJ symptoms, High blood pressure, Hyperalertness, Sleep disorders, Gastrointestinal disorders

Dissociative reactions:
  Phobic avoidance, often generalized to apparently unrelated situations
  Feelings of "badness," stigma, and guilt
  Impulsive or self-defeating behavior
	Eating disorders

	Self-mutilation

Source: From Marjorie Whittaker Leidig, "The Continuum of Violence against Women: Psychological and Physical Consequences," *Journal of American College Health* 40 (1992): 151. Reprinted with permission of the Helen Dwight Reid Educational Foundation. Published by Heldref Publications, 1319 Eighteenth Street NW, Washington, D.C. 20036–1802. Copyright © 1992.

Many rapists use certain ploys to initiate their attacks. Among the most common are:

- *Request for help.* This allows him to get close—to enter your house to use the phone, for instance.

- *Offer of help.* This can also help him gain entrance to your home: "Let me help you carry that package."

- *Guilt trip.* "Gee, no one is friendly nowadays. . . . I can't believe you won't talk with me for just a little while."

- *Purposeful accident.* He may bump into the back of your car, and then assault you when you get out to see the extent of the damage. Don't stop unless you have to in these situations, and if you do stop, stay in your car with the doors locked.

- *Authority.* Many women fall for the old "policeman at the door" ruse. If anyone comes to your door dressed in policemen's garb, ask him to show you his ID before you unlock the door. You can also call the police department to get a confirmation on his ID.

If you are attacked, act immediately:

- *Don't worry about causing a scene.* Draw attention to yourself and your assailant. Scream for help.

- *Report the attack* to the appropriate authorities at once.

To prevent an attack from occurring:

- *Always be vigilant.* Even the safest cities and towns have rapes. Don't be fooled by a sleepy-little-town atmosphere.

- *Use campus escort services whenever possible.*

- *Be assertive in demanding a well-lit campus.*

- *Don't use the same routes all the time.* Think about your movement patterns and vary them accordingly.

- *Don't leave a bar alone with a friendly stranger.* Stay with your friends, and let the friendly stranger come along. Don't give your address to anyone you don't know.

- *Let friends/family know where you are going, what route you'll take, and when to expect your return.*

- *Stay close to others.* Avoid shortcuts through dark or unlit paths. Don't be the last one to leave the lab or library late at night.

- *Keep your windows and doors locked.* Don't answer the door to strangers.

What to Do When a Rape Occurs. If you are a rape victim, it should be you who reports the attack. This gives you a sense of control. Calling 911 (if available) is probably the best rule of thumb. Do not bathe, shower, douche, clean up, or touch anything the attacker may have touched. Do not throw away or launder the clothes you were wearing. They will be needed as evidence. Bring a clean change of clothes to the clinic or hospital. Contact the Rape Assistance Hotline in your area and ask for advice on therapists or counseling if you need additional advice or help.

If you want to help a rape victim, the best thing you can do is to believe her. Don't ask questions that may appear to implicate her in the assault. Your hindsight may find some questionable judgment on her behalf, but that doesn't mean she's to blame. Rape is a violent act against someone; the victim was certainly not looking for a violent act. Encourage her to talk, and when she does, listen. Hold back on advice.

Encourage her to see a doctor immediately, as she may have medical needs but be too embarrassed to seek help on her own. Be supportive of her reporting of the crime. And stay her friend. It may take six months to a year for emotional recovery, and you should be understanding during this time. Encourage her to seek counseling if any problems persist.

Preventing Assaults at Home

When at home, there are several precautions you can take to avoid being assaulted:[51]

- *Get deadbolts and peepholes and make sure the entryway to your house is lighted and free of shrubs.*

- *Consider putting a lock, solid-core door, and extension phone with a lighted dial in your bedroom.*

- *Get to know your neighbors and organize a neighborhood watch.*

- *Don't hide your keys under a fake rock or other device.* These are dead giveaways to experienced criminals.

- *Don't open your door to anyone you don't know.*

- *Ask for identification from repairmen and/or call the company to verify that they've sent someone out.*

- *Keep lights on in at least one room other than the one you're in to make it look as if you aren't alone.*

- *Don't put your full name on your mailbox or in the phone book;* use your initials instead.

- *A "Beware of Dog" sign may help deter assailants.* Be careful of "doggy doors." Many an assailant has entered a house through a pet door.

Preventing Assaults on the Street

- *Walk/jog at a steady pace.* Look confident and stay alert to your surroundings.

- *Walk/jog with others.* There is safety in numbers.

- *At night, avoid dark parking lots, wooded areas, and all other good hiding places for assailants.*

- *Listen for footsteps and voices.* Change the pace of your walk if you think you're being followed to see if the person behind you does likewise. If he does, walk down the middle of the street, staying near the streetlights. Run and yell if you feel threatened.

- *Be aware of cars that keep driving around in your vicinity.*

- *Vary your running/walking routes.*[52]

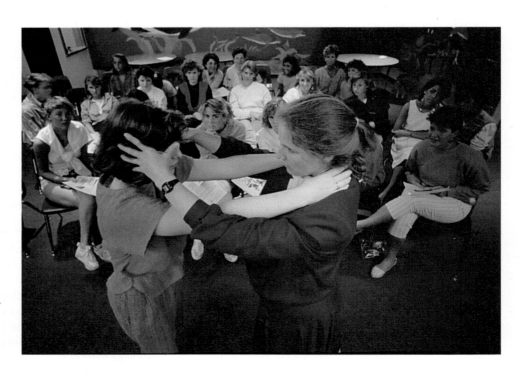

Women who learn self-defense techniques and always remember to take reasonable safety precautions lower their risk for assault and rape.

Managing Campus Safety

College campuses today may be healthy places for student interactions, or they may be settings for violent and aggressive interactions between students. Most campuses have initiated programs, services, and policies designed to protect students from possible violations of their personal health and safety. Answering the following questions may help you determine your college administrators' degree of interest in and commitment to a violence-free setting.

Making Decisions for You

Setting limits on where you go, at what time, and with whom seem to be running themes of this chapter. What types of limits do you set yourself? Think for a moment about your next night out with friends or with your lover. What limits will you set yourself? Will you decide ahead of time to limit your drinking? What time do you want to be home? How far you will go sexually? Will you use condoms? Decide how you will achieve your goals.

Choices for Change: Making Personal Choices

✓ Do you decide before a date to limit your sexual behavior?

✓ Do you travel in groups whenever possible?

✓ Do you avoid being out alone at night?

✓ Do you avoid high-crime areas?

Choices for Change: Making Community Choices

✓ Does your campus have a student health center with a trained staff of health educators?

✓ Does your health center offer workshops on rape prevention and the prevention of other sexual offenses?

✓ Does your campus offer courses focusing on understanding human diversity?

✓ Does your campus offer workshops and/or seminars for men to help them understand their sexuality and refrain from rape and other kinds of assault against women?

✓ Does your campus offer workshops/information for students to help them avoid situations that put them at risk for violent sexual or other interactions?

✓ Does your campus offer confidential counseling and/or assistance to victims of sexual assault?

✓ Does your campus offer workshops/educational sessions dealing with suicide?

✓ Does your campus offer information/workshops/services dealing with partner/domestic violence?

✓ Does your campus offer information/workshops/services dealing with child abuse and/or sexual abuse?

✓ Does your campus offer workshops/seminars that help males learn how to confront peers who express attitudes supportive of "overcoming" women sexually?

✓ Does your campus have strict substance abuse policies designed to reduce the likelihood of possible sexual assaults?

✓ Are sessions designed to negate myths and to increase understanding between the sexes offered in "safe" environments where discussions are open and positive role models encourage positive actions?

✓ Are services such as rides and escort services available to students after hours to prevent rapes/assaults? Do security guards patrol the campus?

✓ Is your campus well-lighted and open in the evenings?

✓ Are campus health educators, counselors, and other professionals trained to spot victimization in clients and recommend appropriate services?

✓ Does your campus have a code of conduct that mandates swift and prudent punishment for alcohol and other drug abuse and acts of campus violence?

Critical Thinking

Your best friend and roommate has been accused of date rape; if the charge is substantiated, he could be dismissed from college. The way your friend tells it, they had a few drinks, started making out, and eventually had intercourse. He claims that she did not try to stop him. Your friend asks you to talk to the girl; after all, she's a friend of yours from high school and you introduced them. He wants you to "find holes in her story" and see if you can get her to "forget about the whole thing." It's hard to believe your best friend is a rapist. But then it's also hard to believe she is lying.

Using the DECIDE model described in Chapter 1, decide what you will do. Reconsider the information about rape in the chapter. Would it make a difference if she came to you to talk?

Preventing Assaults in Your Car

Recent carjackings and murders of individuals driving expensive cars, rental cars, and other vehicles point to the necessity for personal actions to help protect yourself and avoid high risk situations. By taking the following actions, you may avoid a serious assault:

- *Always keep your doors locked and your windows rolled up.*

- *Don't stop for vehicles in distress.* Drive on and call for help.

- *If your car breaks down, lock the doors and wait for help from the police.* Do not accept assistance from strangers, particularly from individuals on isolated roads.

- *If you think someone is following you, do something to attract attention.* Stay in your car with locked windows and doors and drive to a fire station, police station, all-night grocery, restaurant, or other place where there are people. If you are forced to stop on a deserted road, leave your engine running and in gear. Wait until your pursuer gets out of his car, then drive away as fast as you can.

- *Stick to well-traveled routes.* Avoid dark, isolated shortcuts.

- *Fill your car with gas and keep it in good running order.*

- *Don't put your name and address on your key ring.*

- *Before getting into your car, walk around it and check the back seat, floor, and undercarriage.*

- *On long trips, don't make it obvious you're traveling alone.* Never take a map into a restaurant.

- *Don't sleep in your car along the interstate highway.* This is no longer safe in most states.

- *When you stop for a traffic light, leave a car's length so that if you are approached you'll have room to pull out.* Blow your horn and attract attention.

- *Never get out of the car if someone bumps into you until a police officer arrives.* A recent rash of murders and carjackings have involved assailants ramming victims' cars from behind and then shooting or attacking victims who got out to investigate.[53]

Summary

- Violence affects everyone in society—from the direct victims, to those who live in fear, to those who pay higher taxes and insurance premiums. Over half of homicides are committed by people who knew their victims. Bias and hate crimes divide people, but teaching tolerance can reduce risks. Gang violence continues to grow but can be combated by programs aimed at reducing the problems that lead to gang membership. Violence on campus may be increasing, but the victim's rights have also increased as a result of several major pieces of legislation.

- Domestic violence includes spousal and child abuse. Men and women abuse each other physically at about the same rate, but men invoke fear into the women they batter. The cycle of violence theory attempts to explain why many women do not leave abusive relationships. Child abuse includes physical, sexual, and psychological abuse.

- Sexual victimization refers to sexual assault, rape, date rape, and sexual harassment. The possible reasons accounting for why males sexually assault females include male socialization, attitudes, sexual history and hostility, misperceptions, and situational factors. Rape and date rape are not sexual acts; they are violent acts.

- Prevention of violent acts begins with keeping yourself out of situations in which harm may occur.

Discussion Questions

1. What are the major types of crimes in the United States? Who tends to be at risk for becoming victims and for becoming perpetrators of violent crimes?

2. Who tends to be susceptible to the appeal of gang membership? What actions can we take to keep young kids out of gangs?

3. Compare spousal abuse against men and against women: What are the differences? What are the similarities? What are the causes of domestic violence?

4. What puts a child at risk for abuse? Is there anything that can be done to prevent or to decrease the amount of child abuse?

5. What is sexual harassment and what factors contribute to it in the workplace?

6. List the actions you can take to protect yourself from personal assault in your home, car, or on the streets.

7. If your friend was to tell you that she was date-raped last night, what would you do? What would you suggest she do?

Application Exercise

Reread the What Do You Think? scenarios at the beginning of the chapter and answer the following questions:

1. Think about the violent incidents listed. What do you think are the major reasons that these situations occur? What actions could we take as a society to reduce violence?

2. In the Tailhook and the shooting incidents, do you think the participants realized that they were doing anything wrong? If so, why do such incidents happen?

3. Do you believe that violence is really much worse than it was back in the "good old days"? Or are we just made more aware of it due to increased media coverage?

Further Reading

Centers for Disease Control and Prevention, "Firearm Mortality among Children, Youth, and Young Adults 1–34 Years of Age," *Advance Data,* March 1994.

Yearly report on data relating to firearm mortality in the United States.

M. L. Rosenberg and M. A. Fenley, eds., *Violence in America: A Public Health Approach* (New York: Oxford, 1991).

Excellent overview of the epidemiology of violence. Comprehensive approach to concepts of prevention.

"Violence on Campus," *Journal of American College Health* 40 (1992).

Feature issue of this college health journal with articles covering major issues surrounding campus violence. Provides an excellent baseline of data and information.

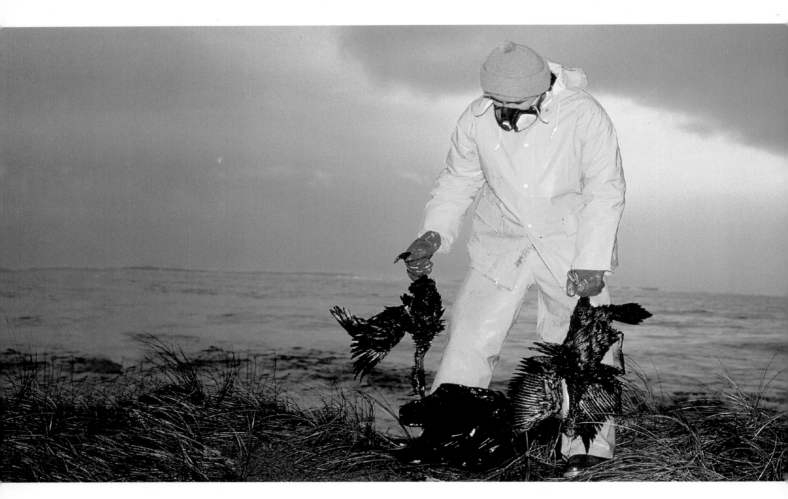

CHAPTER OBJECTIVES

◆ Identify the problems associated with current levels of global population growth.

◆ Discuss the major causes of air pollution, including photochemical smog and acid rain, and the global consequences of the accumulation of greenhouse gases and of ozone depletion.

◆ Identify sources of water pollution and the specific chemical contaminants often found in water.

◆ Describe the physiological consequences of noise pollution.

◆ Distinguish between municipal solid waste and hazardous waste.

◆ Discuss the health concerns associated with ionizing and nonionizing radiation.

Environmental Health

Thinking Globally, Acting Locally

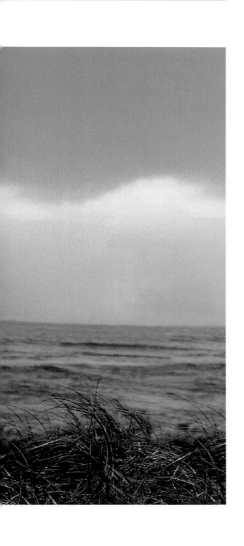

WHAT DO YOU THINK?

The chaotic, unplanned cities of the Third World are often dangerous places. In Calcutta, the Metropolitan Development Authority has been filling in fragile marshlands for new development on the periphery of the city while land in parts of the central city is underused. Many Asian cities have serious housing shortages even though vast tracts of vacant land lie nearby. In Dakar, Senegal, a municipal dump will soon be completely surrounded by housing whose residents will draw their drinking water from nearby wells. The most deadly automobile-caused air pollution and the worst traffic jams are often found in Third World cities even though they have much smaller vehicle fleets than do large cities in the developed world.

- What responsibility do those of us in the developed world have to help reduce population growth and curb pollution in developing nations? Would you be willing to pay 1 percent of your tax dollars to help other nations develop environmental programs?

In 1985, one environmental activist, Pat Bryant, began focusing attention on the poor people living in the lower Mississippi Valley's "Cancer Alley," so-called because one-fourth of the nation's chemicals are produced in this area. Bryant worked with groups to improve housing conditions in the area and then focused on the industrial pollution in the region. Within a year, he had mobilized people from several environmental groups to stage a 10-day demonstration known as the Great Louisiana Toxics March, after which he became the director of the Louisiana Toxics Project. As a result of Bryant's efforts, the Louisiana legislature passed the state's first air quality act in 1989.

- What can we as individuals do to stop pollution and its attendant problems? What factors put environmental groups and big business at odds with each other?

Human health, well-being, and survival are ultimately dependent on the integrity of the planet on which we live. Today the natural world is under attack from the pressure of the enormous numbers of people who live in it, and the wide range of their activities (see the Health Headlines box). Even though the United States has made measurable environmental progress in recent years, our environmental achievements allow no room for complacency. An informed citizenry having a strong commitment to care for the environment is essential to the survival of our planet.

Americans' concern about the environment has intensified since the initial outpouring on the first Earth Day in April 1970. Public opinion polls show that concern for the environment has become a core value for virtually every sector of our society. The number of people who view pollution as a pressing personal concern has tripled in the 1990s. A 1991 study by Environment Opinion Study found that 71 percent of Americans agree that "improving the quality of the environment can create jobs and help the national economy." And a Gallup poll reported that 78 percent of Americans now consider themselves environmentalists.[1]

OVERPOPULATION

Our most challenging environmental problem is population growth. The anthropologist Margaret Mead wrote, "Every human society is faced with not one population problem but two: how to beget and rear enough children and how not to beget and rear too many."[2]

The world population is increasing at unprecedented numbers. In early 1990, it was nearly 5.3 billion and 23 babies were born every 5 seconds: that's 397,440 new people every day, or 145 million every year. This rate gives the planet an annual net population gain of 93 million people. Population experts believe that unless current birth and death rates change radically, 10.4 billion people will be competing for the world's diminishing resources by the year 2029.[3] Table 23.1 shows world population growth by decade, with projections through the year 2029.

The population explosion is not distributed equally around the world. The United States and western Europe have the lowest birth rates. At the same time, these two regions produce more grain and other foodstuffs than their populations consume. Countries that can least afford a high birth rate in economic, social, health, and nutritional terms are the ones with the most rapidly expanding populations.

The vast bulk of population growth in developing countries is occurring in urban areas. Third World cities' populations are doubling every 10 to 15 years, overwhelming their governments' attempts to provide clean water, sewage facilities, adequate transportation, and other basic services. As early as 1964, researcher Ronald Wraith described the Third World giant city plagued by pollution and shantytowns as, "megalopolis—the city running riot with no one able to control it."[4] In 1950, only 3 of the world's 10 largest cities were in the Third World; by 1980, 7 of them were, and this trend is expected to continue into the next century (see Table 23.2).

As the global population expands, so does the competition for the earth's resources. Environmental degradation caused by loss of topsoil, pesticides, toxic residues, deforestation, global warming, air pollution, and acid rain seriously threatens the food supply and undermines world health.

In China, the goal of one child per family is promoted by the government in its effort to reduce the birth rate and gain control of the many problems associated with overpopulation.

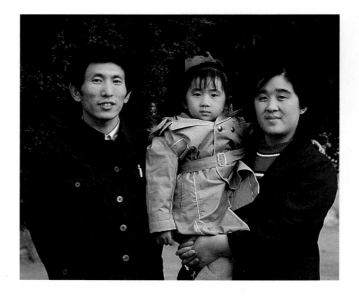

Environmental Facts

- An assessment of urban air quality jointly undertaken by the World Health Organization and the United Nations Environment Programme reports that 625 million people around the globe are exposed to unhealthy levels of sulfur dioxide resulting from fossil fuel burning. More than 1 billion people—a fifth of the planet's population—are exposed to potentially health-damaging levels of air pollutants of all kinds.

- At the end of the International Drinking Water Supply and Sanitation Decade (1981–1990), 1 billion people were without a safe water supply and almost 1.8 billion did not have adequate sanitation facilities.

- The United Nations Conference on Environment and Development—the Earth Summit—met in Rio de Janeiro, Brazil, in June 1992. Perhaps the most remarkable achievement of this conference was Agenda 21, a 900-page action plan for protecting the atmosphere, the oceans, and other global resources. The Earth Summit marked the arrival of environmental concerns as a major new international consideration.

- In the United States, 70 monitoring stations have identified crop-damaging concentrations of ground-level ozone in every part of the country. A joint study by the EPA and the U.S. Department of Agriculture indicates that crops are affected in varying degrees, depending on their sensitivity to air pollutants. Applying these proportions to the annual harvest, which has a market value of around $70 billion, this amounts to a loss of $3 billion to $7 billion caused by air pollution.

- Until cholera broke out in Peru in 1991, there had been no epidemics of that disease in Latin America or the Caribbean for almost a century. Yet, since January 1991, cholera has invaded 19 countries. Over 600,000 cases and more than 6,000 deaths have been reported. The siege of cholera has revealed appalling inadequacies and inequalities in the provision of clean water, sanitation, and health care.

- Lead is a silent hazard in many American homes: 74 percent of all private housing built before 1980 contains some lead paint; one of nine children under the age of six has enough lead in his or her blood to be at risk for serious health problems; children with high lead levels are six times more likely to have reading disabilities.

- An Oregon woman founded Deja, Inc. to manufacture Eco Sneakers from used textiles, rubber products, and other consumer waste. Turtle Plastics in Cleveland, Ohio, turns used swimming pool liners and scrap automobile trim into industrial floor matting and urinal screens. Earth Partners, also based in Oregon, plans to make newsprint into floor paneling material and molded panels for hollow-core doors.

- Refilling bottles, once a common practice in this country, has virtually disappeared. In the early 1960s, 89 percent of all packaged soft drinks and nearly 50 percent of all packaged beer were sold in refillable bottles. Today only about 6 percent of all packaged beer and soft drinks combined is sold in refillables. By comparison, Germany mandates that 72 percent of beverages must be sold in refillable containers.

- Helped by the U.S. Customs Service, the EPA has filed administrative actions, seeking a total of $9.8 million in fines, against 21 companies for illegal import or export of chemicals and hazardous wastes. A number of these cases involve shipments across the Canadian and Mexican borders.

Nowhere are these threats more visible than in Third World countries in Africa, Asia, and Latin America. The combination of falling economic levels and rising grain prices due to grain scarcity has frequently led to famine in these areas. An estimated 40,000 children under the age of five die each day in these countries from severe nutritional deprivation and related infectious diseases.[5] Drought in the late 1980s reduced world grain stocks to their lowest levels since the 1950s. Grain harvests in 1989 were 18 million tons below the projected consumption level, and grain stores were further depleted.[6]

Harvests are directly affected by the state of the environment. Air pollution and acid rain affect crops, as do global warming, deforestation, soil erosion, and toxic waste disposal. The ways in which these environmental issues specifically relate to human health and survival will be discussed throughout this chapter.

At first examination, it may seem that there is little we can do as individuals to alleviate these conditions in Third World countries. We can begin to do our part, however, by recognizing that the United States consumes far more energy and raw materials per person than does any other nation on earth. Many of these resources come from other countries, and our consumption is depleting the resource balances of those countries. Therefore, we must start by living environmentally conscious lives.

Perhaps the simplest course of action we can take is to control our own reproductivity. The concept of zero population growth (ZPG) was born in the 1960s. Proponents of this idea believed that each couple should produce only two offspring. When the parents die, the two offspring are their replacements, and the population stabilizes.

The continued preference for large families in many developing nations is caused by such factors as high infant

It's Not Easy Being Green

Circle the number of each item that describes what you have done or are doing to help the environment.

1. When walking or camping I never leave anything behind.

2. I ride my bike, walk, carpool or use public transportation whenever possible.

3. I have written my representative in the state or federal government about environmental issues.

4. I avoid turning on the air conditioner or heat whenever possible.

5. My shower has a low-flow shower head.

6. I do not run the water while brushing my teeth, shaving, or handwashing clothes.

7. I take showers instead of baths.

8. My sink faucets have aerators installed in them.

9. I have a water displacement device in my toilet.

10. I snip or rip plastic six-pack rings before I throw them out.

11. I choose recycled and recyclable products.

12. I avoid noise pollutants (I sit away from speakers at concerts, select an apartment away from busy streets or airports, and so on.)

13. I make sure my car is tuned and has functional emission control equipment.

14. I try to avoid known carcinogens such as vinyl chloride, asbestos, benzene, mercury, X-rays, and so on.

15. I don't buy products that contain CFCs or methylchloroform.

16. When shopping, I choose products having the least amount of packaging.

17. I dispose of hazardous materials (old car batteries, used oil, or used antifreeze) at gas stations or other appropriate sites.

18. If I have children or when I have children, I will use a diaper service as opposed to disposable diapers.

19. I store food in glass jars and waxed paper rather than in plastic wrap.

20. I use as few paper products as possible.

21. I take my own bag along when I go shopping.

22. I avoid products packaged in plastic and unrecycled aluminum.

23. I recycle newspapers, glass, cans, and other recyclables.

24. I run the clothes dryer only as long as it takes my clothes to dry.

25. I turn off lights and appliances when they are not in use.

Scoring and Interpretation

Count how many items you have circled. Ideally, you can be doing all these things, but if you are trying to do at least some, you can score yourself as follows:

20–25	Good contributions to maintaining the environment.
14–19	Moderate contributions to maintaining the environment.
Below 13	Need to consider the recommendations made in this chapter to help the environment.

mortality rates; the traditional view of children as "social security" (they not only work from a young age to assist families in daily survival but also support parents when they are too old to work); the low educational and economic status of women; and the traditional desire for

sons that keeps parents of several daughters reproducing until they get male offspring. Moreover, some developing nations feel that overpopulation is not as great a problem as the inequitable distribution of wealth and resources, both within their countries and worldwide. For all these reasons, demographers contend that broad-based social and economic changes will be necessary before a stabilization in population growth rates can occur.

Sulfur dioxide: A yellowish-brown gaseous by-product of the burning of fossil fuels.

Particulates: Nongaseous air pollutants.

Carbon monoxide: An odorless, colorless gas that originates primarily from motor vehicle emissions.

Nitrogen dioxide: An amber-colored gas found in smog; can cause eye and respiratory irritations.

What Do You Think?

How would you react to governmentally imposed restriction on family size? Do you favor imposed mandatory limitations in developing nations? What do you think we, as a world community, ought to do about population growth?

TABLE 23.1 ■ World Population Growth by Decade, 1950–1990, with Projections to 2029

Year	Population (billion)	Increase by Decade (million)	Average Annual Increase (million)
1950	2.5		
1960	3.0	504	50
1970	3.7	679	68
1980	4.5	752	75
1990	5.3	842	84
2000	6.3	959	96
2029	10.4	not available	

Source: Information from Lester R. Brown, "The Illusion of Progress," in *State of the World, 1990,* ed. Lester R. Brown (New York: Norton, 1990), 5; Ruth Caplan, *Our Earth, Ourselves* (New York: Bantam, 1990), 248.

*A*IR POLLUTION

As our population has grown, so have the number and volume of the environmental pollutants that we produce. Concern about air quality prompted Congress to pass the Clean Air Act in 1970 and to amend it in 1977 and again in 1990. The object was to develop standards for six of the most widespread air pollutants that seriously affect health: sulfur dioxide, particulates, carbon monoxide, nitrogen dioxide, ozone, and lead.

Sources of Air Pollution

Sulfur Dioxide. **Sulfur dioxide** is a yellowish-brown gas that is a by-product of burning fossil fuels. Electricity generating stations, smelters, refineries, and industrial boilers are the main source points. In humans, sulfur dioxide aggravates symptoms of heart and lung disease, obstructs breathing passages, and increases the incidence of such respiratory diseases as colds, asthma, bronchitis, and emphysema. It is toxic to plants, destroys some paint pigments, corrodes metals, impairs visibility, and is a precursor to acid rain, which we discuss later in this chapter.

Particulates. **Particulates** are tiny solid particles or liquid droplets that are suspended in the air. Cigarette smoke releases particulates. They are also by-products of some industrial processes and the internal combustion engine. Particulates can in and of themselves irritate the lungs and can additionally carry heavy metals and carcinogenic agents deep into the lungs. When combined with sulfur dioxide, they exacerbate respiratory diseases. Particulates can also corrode metals and obscure visibility.

Carbon Monoxide. **Carbon monoxide** is an odorless, colorless gas that originates primarily from motor vehicle emissions. Carbon monoxide interferes with the blood's ability to absorb and carry oxygen and can impair thinking, slow reflexes, and cause drowsiness, unconsciousness, and death. When inhaled by pregnant women, it may threaten the growth and mental development of the fetus. Long-term exposure can increase the severity of circulatory and respiratory diseases.

Nitrogen Dioxide. **Nitrogen dioxide** is an amber-colored gas emitted by coal-powered electrical utility boilers and by motor vehicles. High concentrations of

TABLE 23.2 ■ Population of World's 10 Largest Metropolitan Areas, 1950 and 1980, with Projections for 2000 (in Millions)

City	1950	City	1980	City	2000
New York	12.3	Tokyo	16.9	*Mexico City*	*25.6*
London	8.7	New York	15.6	*São Paulo*	*22.1*
Tokyo	6.7	*Mexico City*	*14.5*	Tokyo	19.0
Paris	5.4	*São Paulo*	*12.1*	*Shangai*	*17.0*
Shangai	*5.3*	*Shangai*	*11.7*	New York	16.8
Buenos Aires	*5.0*	*Buenos Aires*	*9.9*	*Calcutta*	*15.7*
Chicago	4.9	Los Angeles	9.5	*Bombay*	*15.4*
Moscow	4.8	*Calcutta*	*9.0*	*Beijing*	*14.0*
Calcutta	*4.4*	*Beijing*	*9.0*	Los Angeles	13.9
Los Angeles	4.0	*Rio de Janeiro*	*8.8*	*Jakarta*	*13.7*

Source: Information from *World Urbanization Prospects 1990* (New York: United Nations, 1991); Lester R. Brown et al., *State of the World 1992: A Worldwatch Institute Report on Progress toward a Sustainable Society* (New York: Norton, 1992), 122.

Italics indicate city is in the Third World.

nitrogen dioxide can be fatal. Lower concentrations increase susceptibility to colds and flu, bronchitis, and pneumonia. Nitrogen dioxide is also toxic to plant life and causes a brown discoloration of the atmosphere. It is a precursor of ozone, and, along with sulfur dioxide, of acid rain.

Ozone. Ozone is a form of oxygen that is produced when nitrogen dioxide reacts with hydrogen chloride. These gases release oxygen, which is altered by sunlight to produce ozone. In the lower atmosphere, ozone irritates the mucous membranes of the respiratory system, causing coughing and choking. It can impair lung functioning, reduce resistance to colds and pneumonia, and aggravate heart disease, asthma, bronchitis, and pneumonia. This ozone corrodes rubber and paint and can injure or kill vegetation. It is also one of the irritants found in smog. The natural ozone found in the upper atmosphere, however, serves as a protective membrane against heat and radiation from the sun. We will discuss this atmospheric layer, called the ozone layer, later in the chapter.

Lead. Lead is a metal pollutant that is found in the exhaust of motor vehicles powered by fuel containing lead and in the emissions from lead smelters and processing plants. It also often contaminates drinking water systems in homes that have plumbing installed before 1930. Lead affects the circulatory, reproductive, and nervous systems. It can also affect the blood and kidneys and can accumulate in bone and other tissues. Lead is particularly detrimental to children and fetuses. It can cause birth defects, behavioral abnormalities, and decreased learning abilities.

Hydrocarbons. Although not listed as one of the six major air pollutants in the Clean Air Act, hydrocarbons encompass a wide variety of chemical pollutants in the air. Sometimes known as *volatile organic compounds* (VOCs), **hydrocarbons** are chemical compounds containing different combinations of carbon and hydrogen. The principal source of polluting hydrocarbons is the internal combustion engine. Most automobile engines emit hundreds of different types of hydrocarbon compounds. By themselves, hydrocarbons seem to cause few problems, but when they combine with sunlight and other pollutants, they form such poisons as formaldehyde, various ketones, and peroxyacetylnitrate (PAN), all of which are respiratory irritants. Hydrocarbon combinations such as benzene and benzopyrene are carcinogenic. In addition, hydrocarbons play a major part in the formation of smog.

Photochemical Smog

Photochemical smog is a brown, hazy mix of particulates and gases that forms when oxygen-containing compounds of nitrogen and hydrocarbons react in the presence of sunlight. Photochemical smog is sometimes called *ozone pollution* because ozone is created when vehicle exhaust reacts with sunlight. Such smog is most likely to develop on days when there is little wind and high traffic congestion. In most cases, it forms in areas that experience a **temperature inversion,** a weather condition in which a cool layer of air is trapped under a layer of warmer air, preventing the air from circulating. When gases such as the hydrocarbons and nitrogen oxides are released into the cool air layer, they cannot escape, and thus they remain suspended until wind conditions move away the warmer air layer. Sunlight filtering through the air causes chemical changes in the hydrocarbons and nitrogen oxides, which results in smog. Smog is more likely to be produced in valley regions blocked by hills or mountains—for example, the Los Angeles basin, Denver, and Tokyo.

The most noticeable adverse effects of exposure to smog are difficulty in breathing, burning eyes, headaches, and nausea. Long-term exposure to smog poses serious health risks, particularly for children, the elderly, pregnant women, and people with chronic respiratory disorders such as asthma and emphysema. According to the American Lung Association, continued exposure accelerates aging of the lungs and increases susceptibility to infections by hindering the functions of the immune system.

Despite local efforts to reduce the problem, smog and other air pollutants repeatedly surge above federal safe standards. The Clean Air Act Amendments of 1990 are designed to reduce smog levels, as well as those of other air pollutants, significantly.[7] The Air Toxics program established by the Clean Air Act Amendments of 1990 is designed to curb 189 toxic air pollutants produced by industry that are carcinogens, mutagens, or reproductive toxins.[8]

Acid Rain

Acid rain is precipitation that has fallen through acidic air pollutants, particularly those containing sulfur dioxides

---

Ozone: A gas formed when nitrogen dioxide interacts with hydrogen chloride.

Lead: A metal found in the exhaust of motor vehicles powered by fuel containing lead and in emissions from lead smelters and processing plants.

Hydrocarbons: Chemical compounds that contain carbon and hydrogen.

Photochemical smog: The brownish-yellow haze resulting from the combination of hydrocarbons and nitrogen oxides.

Temperature inversion: A weather condition occurring when a layer of cool air is trapped under a layer of warmer air.

Acid rain: Precipitation contaminated with acidic pollutants.

and nitrogen dioxides. This precipitation, in the form of rain, snow, or fog, has a more acidic composition than does unpolluted precipitation. When introduced into lakes and ponds, acid rain gradually acidifies the water. When the acid content of the water reaches a certain level, plant and animal life cannot survive. Ironically, lakes and ponds that are acidified become a crystal-clear deep blue, giving the illusion of beauty and health.

Sources of Acid Rain. More than 95 percent of acid rain originates in human actions, chiefly the burning of fossil fuels. The single greatest source of acid rain in the United States is coal-fired power plants, followed by ore smelters and steel mills.

When these and other industries burn fuels, the sulfur and nitrogen in the emissions combine with the oxygen and sunlight in the air to become sulfur dioxide and nitrogen oxides (precursors of sulfuric acid and nitric acids, respectively). Small acid particles are then carried by the wind and combine with moisture to produce acidic rain or snow. Because of higher concentrations of sunlight in the summer months, rain is more strongly acidic in the summertime. Additionally, the rain or snow that falls at the beginning of a storm is more acidic than that which falls later.

The ability of a lake to cleanse itself and neutralize its acidity depends on several factors, the most critical of which is bedrock geology. Bedrock and topsoil that contain high concentrations of carbonates, bicarbonates, and hydroxides have the greatest neutralizing abilities. Lakes located in areas with low concentrations stand a small chance of remaining unacidified. Figure 23.1 shows those areas in North America that are most vulnerable to acid

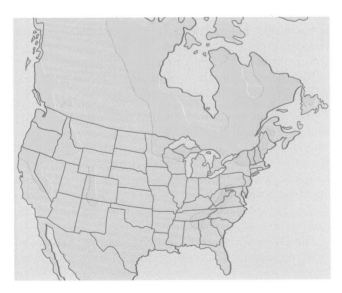

FIGURE 23.1

Areas of North America Most Vulnerable to Acid Rain

Acid rain, the result of airborne acid particles from burning fossil fuels, has many harmful effects on the environment, and it poses numerous health hazards, including the risk of cancer from heavy metals that can make their way into the food chain as a result of acid precipitation.

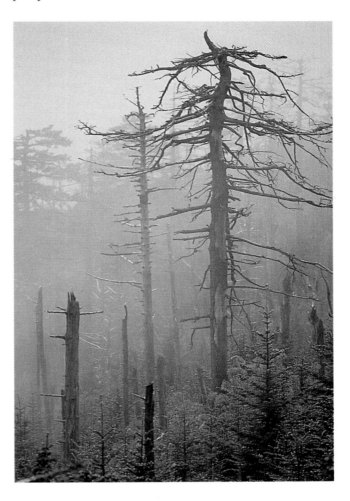

rain because of their bedrock geology and proximity to industries that produce sulfur and nitrogen oxides.

Effects of Acid Rain. The damage caused to lake and pond habitats is not the worst of the problems created by acid rain. Each year, it is responsible for the destruction of millions of trees in forests in Europe and North America. Scientists have concluded that 75 percent of Europe's forests are now experiencing damaging levels of sulfur deposition by acid rain. Forests in every country on the continent are affected.[9]

Doctors believe that acid rain also aggravates and may even cause bronchitis, asthma, and other respiratory problems. People with emphysema and those with a history of heart disease may also suffer from exposure to acid rain. In addition, it may be hazardous to a pregnant woman's unborn child.

Acidic precipitation can cause metals such as aluminum, cadmium, lead, and mercury to **leach** (dissolve and filter) out of the soil. If these metals make their way into water or food supplies (particularly fish), they can cause cancer in humans who consume them.

Acid rain is also responsible for crop damage, which, in turn, contributes to world hunger. Laboratory experiments showed that acid rain can reduce seed yield by up to 23 percent. Actual crop losses are being reported with increasing frequency. In May 1989, China's Hunan Province lost an estimated $260 million worth of crops and seedlings to acid rain. Similar losses have been reported in Chile, Brazil, and Mexico.[10]

A final consequence of acid rain is the destruction of public monuments and structures. Damage to buildings in the United States alone is estimated to cost more than $5 billion annually.[11]

Air pollution is obviously a many-faceted problem. Because we breathe approximately 15,000 to 20,000 liters of air per day (compared to drinking 2 liters of water), we are more likely to be exposed to pollutants by breathing than in any other way.

Indoor Air Pollution

Combating the problems associated with air pollution begins at home. Indoor air can be 10 to 40 times more hazardous than outdoor air. There are between 20 and 100 potentially dangerous chemical compounds in the average American home. Indoor air pollution comes primarily from six sources: woodstoves, furnaces, asbestos, passive smoke, formaldehyde, and radon.

Woodstove Smoke. Woodstoves emit significant levels of particulates and carbon monoxide in addition to other pollutants, such as sulfur dioxide. If you rely on wood for heating, you should make sure that your stove is properly installed, vented, and maintained. Proper adjustments and emission controls taken to recombust potential pol-

---

Leach: A process by which chemicals dissolve and filter through soil.

Asbestos: A substance that separates into stringy fibers and lodges in lungs, where it can cause various diseases.

Formaldehyde: A colorless, strong-smelling gas released through outgassing; causes respiratory and other health problems.

Radon: A naturally occurring radioactive gas resulting from the decay of certain radioactive elements.

Chlorofluorocarbons (CFCs): Chemicals that contribute to the depletion of the ozone layer.

---

lutants can also help to reduce pollution levels from woodstoves. Burning properly seasoned wood reduces the amount of particulates released into the air.

Furnace Emissions. People who rely on oil- or gas-fired furnaces also need to make sure that these appliances are properly installed, ventilated, and maintained. Inadequate cleaning and maintenance can lead to a buildup of carbon monoxide in the home, which can be deadly.

Asbestos. Asbestos is another indoor air pollutant that poses serious threats to human health. Asbestos is a mineral that was commonly used in insulating materials in buildings constructed before 1970. When bonded to other materials, asbestos is relatively harmless, but if its tiny fibers become loosened and airborne, they can embed themselves in the lungs and cannot be expelled. Their presence leads to cancer of the lungs, stomach, and chest lining, and is the cause of a fatal lung disease called mesothelioma.

Formaldehyde. Formaldehyde is a colorless, strong-smelling gas present in some carpets, draperies, furniture, particle board, plywood, wood paneling, countertops, and many adhesives. It is released into the air in a process called outgassing. Outgassing is highest in new products, but the process can continue for many years.

Exposure to formaldehyde can cause respiratory problems, dizziness, fatigue, nausea, and rashes. Long-term exposure can lead to central nervous system disorders and cancer.

To reduce your exposure to formaldehyde, ask about the formaldehyde content of products you purchase and avoid those that contain this gas. If your home has urea-formaldehyde foam insulation, have it removed and replaced with a safer substance. Control the climate of your home. Outgassing is most likely to occur at higher temperatures and in humid areas. Some house-plants, such as philodendrons and spider plants, help clean formaldehyde from the air. If you experience symptoms of formaldehyde exposure, have your home tested by a city, county, or state health agency.

Radon. Radon is one of the most serious forms of indoor air pollution. This odorless, colorless gas is the natural by-product of the decay of uranium and radium in the soil. Radon penetrates homes through cracks, pipes, sump pits and other openings in the foundation. Between 7,000 and 30,000 cancer deaths per year have been attributed to radon, making it second only to smoking as the leading cause of lung cancer.[12]

The EPA estimates that 1 in 15 American homes has an elevated radon level. A home-testing kit from a hardware store will enable you to test your home yourself. "Alpha track" detectors are commonly used for this type of short-term testing. They must remain in your home for 2 to 90 days, depending on the device.

If your home tests high for radon, you should have a professional seal cracks in the floor of the basement or foundation and cover and seal other openings, such as floor drains or sump pumps. Exposed soil should be covered with concrete. Crawl spaces, basements, and attics should be adequately ventilated.

Household Chemicals. When you use cleansers and other cleaning products, do so in a well-ventilated room. Regular cleanings will reduce the need to use potentially harmful substances. Cut down on dry cleaning, as the chemicals used by many cleaners can cause cancer. If your newly cleaned clothes smell of dry-cleaning chemicals, either return them to the cleaner or hang them in the open air until the smell is gone. Avoid the use of household air freshener products containing the carcinogenic agent dichlorobenzene.

*W*HAT DO YOU THINK?

Has the United States government taken strong enough environmental measures to protect citizens? What is the obligation of developing and developed countries regarding the use of fossil fuels? Should the responsibility for curbing their use be equally shared despite disparities in wealth?

Ozone Layer Depletion

We earlier defined *ozone* as a chemical that is produced when oxygen interacts with sunlight. Close to the earth, ozone poses health problems such as respiratory distress. Farther away from the earth, it forms a protective membrane-like layer in the earth's stratosphere—the highest level of the earth's atmosphere, located from 12 to 30 miles above the earth's surface. The ozone layer in the stratosphere protects our planet and its inhabitants from ultraviolet B (UV-B) radiation, a primary cause of skin cancer. Ultraviolet B radiation may also damage DNA and may be linked to weakened immune systems in both humans and animals.

In the early 1970s, scientists began to warn of a depletion of the earth's ozone layer. Special instruments developed to test atmospheric contents indicated that specific chemicals used on earth were contributing to the rapid depletion of this vital protective layer. These chemicals are called **chlorofluorocarbons** (CFCs).

Chlorofluorocarbons were first believed to be miracle chemicals. They were used as refrigerants (Freon), as aerosol propellants in products such as hairsprays and deodorants, as cleaning solvents, and in medical sterilizers, rigid foam insulation, and Styrofoam. But, along with halons (found in many fire extinguishers), methyl chloroform, and carbon tetrachloride (cleaning solvents), CFCs were eventually found to be a major cause of depletion of

the ozone layer. When released into the air through spraying or outgassing, CFCs migrate upward toward the ozone layer, where they decompose and release chlorine atoms. These atoms cause ozone molecules to break apart (see Figure 23.2).

In 1979, a satellite measurement showing a large hole in the ozone layer over Antarctica shocked scientists. Since then, satellite measurements of the ozone layer have regularly shown increases in the size of the hole.

In the early 1970s, the U.S. government banned the use of aerosol sprays containing CFCs in an effort to reduce ozone depletion. But CFCs are still used in various foam products, refrigerators, and air conditioners. In fact, the United States still has the highest per capita use of CFCs in the world, generating approximately 30 percent of all

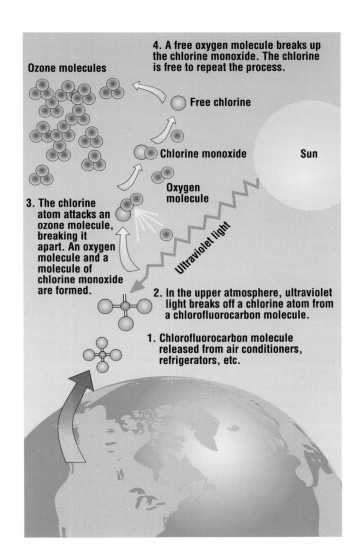

FIGURE 23.2

The diagram shows how the ozone layer is being depleted.

the emissions of ozone-depleting chemicals. Japan is close behind us.

In 1987, after much international negotiation, a group of 24 nations agreed to freeze all production of CFCs immediately and to reduce CFC outputs by 50 percent by the year 2000. This agreement, called the Montreal Protocol, was strengthened in June 1990, when 81 nations signed the Helsinki Declaration, pledging to phase out completely five of the most hazardous CFCs by the year 2000.

Global Warming

More than 100 years ago, scientists theorized that carbon dioxide emissions from fossil-fuel burning would create a buildup of greenhouse gases in the earth's atmosphere and that this accumulation would have a warming effect on the earth's surface. The century-old predictions are now coming true, with alarming effects. Average global temperatures are higher today than at any time since global temperatures were first recorded, and the change in atmospheric temperature may be taking a heavy toll on human beings and crops. Climate researchers predicted in 1975 that the buildup of greenhouse gases would produce life-threatening natural phenomena, including drought in the midwestern United States, more frequent and severe forest fires, flooding in India and Bangladesh, extended heat waves over large areas of the earth, and killer hurricanes. Recently, the planet has experienced all five of these phenomena, although whether they were connected to global warming remains a matter of debate.

Greenhouse gases include carbon dioxide, CFCs, ground-level ozone, nitrous oxide, and methane. They become part of a gaseous layer that encircles the earth, allowing solar heat to pass through and then trapping that heat close to the earth's surface. The most predominant of these gases is carbon dioxide, which accounts for 49 percent of all greenhouse gases. Eastern Europe and North America are responsible for approximately half of all carbon dioxide emissions. Since the late nineteenth century, carbon dioxide concentrations in the atmosphere have increased 25 percent, with half of this increase occurring since the 1950s. Not surprisingly, these greater concentrations coincide with world industrial growth. See Figure 23.3 for more about contributions to global warming.

Rapid deforestation of the tropical rain forests of Central and South America, Africa, and Southeast Asia is also contributing to the rapid rise in the presence of greenhouse gases. Trees take in carbon dioxide, transform it,

> **Greenhouse gases:** Gases that contribute to global warming by trapping heat near the earth's surface.

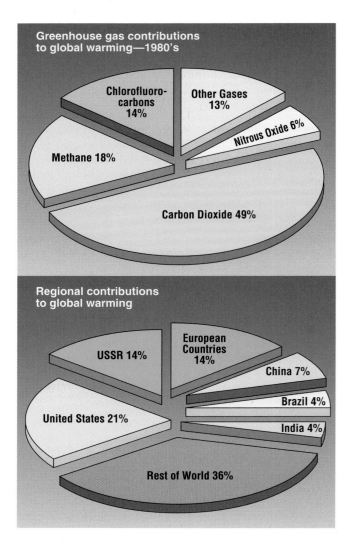

FIGURE 23.3

Greenhouse Gas and Regional Contributions to Global Warming in the 1980s

Source: Reprinted from U.S. Environmental Protection Agency, *Meeting the Environmental Challenge: EPA's Review of Progress and New Directions in Environmental Protection* (EPA Publication No. 21K-2001, 1990).

store the carbon for food, and then release oxygen into the air. As we lose forests, we are losing the capacity to dissipate carbon dioxide.

The potential consequences of global warming are dire. The rising atmospheric concentration of greenhouse gases may be the most economically disruptive and costly change set in motion by our modern industrial society. The cost to the U.S. economy of doubling greenhouse gases, which could occur as early as 2025, would amount to nearly $60 billion, or roughly 1 percent of U.S. gross national product in 1993[13] (see Table 23.3).

Reducing Air Pollution

Our national air pollution problems are rooted in our energy, transportation, and industrial practices. We must develop comprehensive national strategies to address the problem of air pollution in the 1990s in order to clean the air for the coming century. We must support policies that encourage the use of renewable resources such as solar, wind, and water power as the providers of most of the world's energy.[14]

Most experts agree that shifting away from automobiles as the primary source of transportation is the only way to reduce air pollution significantly. Many cities have taken steps in this direction by setting high parking fees, imposing bans on city driving, and establishing high road-usage tolls. Community governments should be encouraged to provide convenient, inexpensive, and easily accessible public transportation for citizens.

Auto makers must be encouraged to manufacture automobiles that provide good fuel economy and low rates of toxic emissions. Incentives given to manufacturers to produce such cars, tax breaks for purchasers who buy them, and gas-guzzler-taxes on inefficient vehicles are three promising measures in this area.

What can you do to help? Find out in the Building Communication Skills box.

TABLE 23.3 ■ Annual U.S. Economic Losses from Global Warming Caused by Doubling of Greenhouse Gases

Source of Loss	Amount of Loss ($ billion)
Agricultural losses due to heat stress and drought	18
Increased electricity for air conditioning	11
Sea level rise	7
Curtailed water supply from reduced runoff	7
Increased urban air pollution	4
Reduced lumber yield from forests	3
Other (includes hurricane and forest fire damage, and increased mortality due to heat stress)	8
Total	58

Source: Adapted with permission from William R. Cline, *Global Warming: The Economic Stakes* (Washington, D.C.: Institute for International Economics, 1992). Copyright © 1992 Institute for International Economics.

𝒲HAT DO YOU THINK?

What products would you be willing to stop using in order to protect the ozone layer? What alternatives are available to replace those products that contain CFCs? What motivations lead to deforestation of the rain forests? What are some measures that might address these problems?

𝒲ATER POLLUTION

Seventy-five percent of the earth is covered with water in the form of oceans, seas, lakes, rivers, streams, and wetlands. Beneath the landmass are reservoirs of groundwater. We draw our drinking water from either this underground source or from surface freshwater sources. The status of our water supply reflects the pollution level of our communities and, ultimately, of the whole earth.

In 1986, the National Wildlife Federation concluded a study revealing that the major environmental concern of Americans was the quality of their drinking water. When the Federation followed up on the original study with an 18-month probe into the quality of drinking water in the United States, it found more than 100,000 violations of federal public health standards. Over 40 million people were affected by these violations. Numerous other studies have found a growing threat to our nation's water supply.

Quality drinking water is a major concern for most Americans; yet we have contaminated our waterways and underground water sources with sewage, industrial waste, pesticides, oil, and other hazardous chemicals.

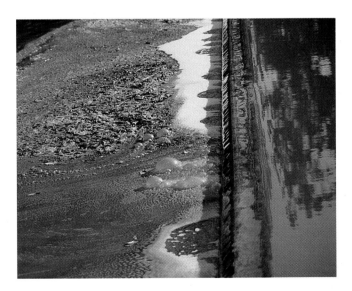

Speaking Out on the Environment

There are many ways for individuals to get involved in the crusade against environmental pollution. Here are eight.

- *Monitor legislation.* All of the key environmental organizations keep tabs on state and national laws being considered in order to offer testimony and to generate letterwriting campaigns on behalf of (or against) proposed laws. [You can ask them for information.] . . .

- *Write letters.* It may not seem like a potent weapon, but letters to state and federal legislators on pending bills *do* influence their opinions. When writing to any public official, keep your letter simple. Focus on one subject and identify a particular piece of legislation. . . . Request a specific action . . . and state your reasons for taking your position. If you live or work in the legislator's district, make sure to say so. . . . Keep the letter to one or two paragraphs, and never write more than one page. [You can send your letters to:

  Hon. _____
  House Office Building
  Washington, D.C. 20515

  Senator _____
  Senate Office Building
  Washington, D.C. 20515

- *Fill out customer comment cards and/or phone toll free numbers on packages* to let companies know your concerns.]

- *Educate others.* You can do this in a variety of ways, from talking to your friends, co-workers, and neighbors to organizing an educational activity. . . .

- *Campaign for environmental candidates.* Don't just be concerned about someone claiming to be an "environmental president." Look at the environmental positions of candidates at all levels of government. . . .

- *Launch a campaign at school or work.* At Rutgers University, for example, members of the law association decided to target the use of plastic foam in the cafeterias. After creating a multistep, long-term strategy, the students first approached the food services department. The director of food services readily agreed to get rid of foam cups in a matter of days, and the foam food containers as soon as current inventory was depleted. . . . Sometimes all you have to do is ask.

- *Invite speakers to your organization.* Most environmental organizations offer speakers on a wide range of topics who will speak at no charge to your civic, school, religious, or social organization. . . . For maximum impact, consider scheduling a debate or panel discussion among representatives of environmental groups, government agencies, and industry.

- *Get involved with government.* Most communities offer a variety of boards, commissions, and committees that deal with environmental issues: planning commissions, zoning and land-use commissions, parks commissions, transit boards, and so on. Each can play a role in setting policies that affect the quality of the environment in your area.

Source: Except for the first paragraph and the bracketed material, from *The Green Consumer Supermarket Guide,* 260–264, by Joel Makower, J. Elkington, and J. Hailes. Copyright © 1991 by John Elkington, Julia Hailes, and Viking Penguin. Used by permission of Viking Penguin, a division of Penguin Books USA Inc.

Water Contamination

Any substance that gets into the soil has the potential to get into the water supply. Contaminants from industrial air pollution and acid rain eventually work their way into the soil and then into the groundwater. Pesticides sprayed on crops wash through the soil into the groundwater. Spills of oil and other hazardous wastes flow into local rivers and streams. Underground storage tanks for gasoline may develop leaks. The list continues.

Pollutants can enter waterways by a number of different routes. Congress has coined two terms, *point source* and *nonpoint source,* to refer to the two general sources of water pollution. Pollutants that enter a waterway at a specific point through a pipe, ditch, culvert, or other such conduit are referred to as **point source pollutants.** The two major sources of this type of pollution are sewage treatment plants and industrial facilities.

Nonpoint source pollutants—commonly known as *runoff* and *sedimentation*—run off or seep into waterways

> **Point source pollutants:** Pollutants that enter waterways at a specific point.
>
> **Nonpoint source pollutants:** Pollutants that run off or seep into waterways from broad areas of land.
>
> **Leachate:** A liquid consisting of soluble chemicals that come from garbage and industrial waste that seeps into the water supply from landfills and dumps.

from broad areas of land rather than through a discrete pipe or conduit. It is currently estimated that 99 percent of the sediment in our waterways, 98 percent of the bacterial contaminants, 84 percent of the phosphorus, and 82 percent of the nitrogen come from nonpoint sources.[15] Nonpoint pollution results from a variety of human land use practices. It includes soil erosion and sedimentation, construction wastes, pesticide and fertilizer runoff, urban street runoff, wastes from engineering projects, acid mine drainage, leakage from septic tanks, and sewage sludge.[16] (See Figure 23.4.)

Septic Systems. Bacteria from human waste can leach into the water supply from improperly installed septic systems. Toxic chemicals that are disposed of by being dumped into septic systems can also get into the groundwater supply.

Landfills. Landfills and dumps generate a liquid called **leachate,** a mixture of soluble chemicals that come from household garbage, office waste, biological waste, and industrial waste. If a landfill has not been properly lined, leachate trickles through its layers of garbage and eventually into the water supply.

Gasoline and Petroleum Products. In the United States, there are more than 2 million underground storage tanks for gasoline and petroleum products, most of which are located at gasoline filling stations. One-quarter of these underground tanks are thought to be leaking.[17]

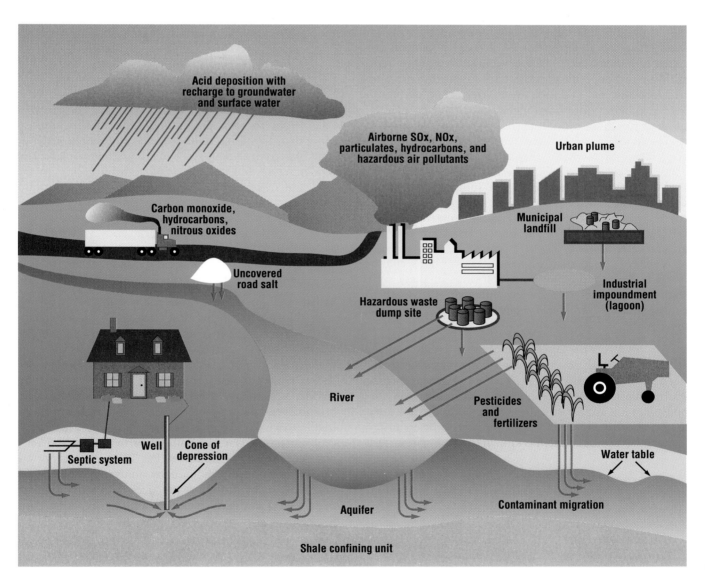

FIGURE 23.4

Sources of Groundwater Contamination

Most of these tanks were installed 25 to 30 years ago. They were made of fabricated steel that was unprotected from corrosion. Over time, pinpoint holes develop in the steel and the petroleum products stored in the tanks leak into the groundwater. The most common way to detect the presence of petroleum products in the water supply is to test for benzene, a component of oil and gasoline. Benzene is highly toxic and is associated with the development of cancer.

Service station owners throughout the country are being informed that their underground storage tanks may be public health hazards because of leakage. In many cases, repairs or reinstallation expenses would bankrupt the businesses, so concerned owners are requesting government aid to solve the problem.

Chemical Contaminants

Most chemicals designed to dissolve grease and oil are called *organic solvents.* These extremely toxic substances, such as carbon tetrachloride, tetrachloroethylene, and trichloroethylene (TCE), are used to clean clothing, painting equipment, plastics, and metal parts. Many household products, such as stain and spot removers, degreasers, drain cleaners, septic system cleaners, and paint removers, also contain these toxic chemicals.

Organic solvents work their way into the water supply in different ways. Consumers often dump leftover products into the toilet. Industries pour leftovers into large barrels, which are then buried. After a while, the chemicals eat their way out of the barrels and leach into the groundwater system.

A related group of toxic substances contains chlorinated hydrocarbons. The most notorious of these substances are the **polychlorinated biphenyls (PCBs)**, their cousins the *polybromated biphenyls (PBBs),* and the *dioxins.*

PCBs. PCBs are fire-resistant and stable at high temperatures and were therefore used for many years as insulating materials in high-voltage electrical equipment such as transformers. PCBs bioaccumulate, meaning that the body does not excrete them but rather stores them in fatty tissues and the liver. PCBs are associated with birth defects, and exposure to them is known to cause cancer. The

Polychlorinated biphenyls (PCBs): Toxic chemicals that were once used as insulating materials in high-voltage electrical equipment.

Dioxins: Highly toxic chlorinated hydrocarbons contained in herbicides and produced during certain industrial processes.

Pesticides: Chemicals that kill pests.

manufacture of PCBs was discontinued in the United States in 1977, but approximately 500 million pounds of PCBs have been dumped into landfills and waterways, where they continue to pose an environmental threat.[18]

Dioxins. Dioxins are chlorinated hydrocarbons that are contained in herbicides (chemicals that are used to kill vegetation) and produced during certain industrial processes. Dioxins have the ability to bioaccumulate and are much more toxic than PCBs.

The long-term effects of bioaccumulation of these toxic substances include possible damage to the immune system, increased risk of infection, and elevated risk for cancer. Exposure to high concentrations of PCBs or dioxins for a short period of time can also have severe consequences, including nausea, vomiting, diarrhea, painful rashes and sores, and chloracne, an ailment in which the skin develops hard, black, painful pimples that may never go away. In 1979, the EPA banned the use of two herbicides that contain dioxin, 2,4,5-T and 2,4-D, after citizen groups organized to publicize the hazards to vegetation, animals, and humans.

Pesticides. Pesticides are chemicals that are designed to kill insects, rodents, plants, and fungi. Americans use more than 1.2 billion pounds of pesticides each year, but only 10 percent actually reach the targeted organisms. The remaining 1.1 billion pounds of pesticides settle on the land and in our water supplies. Pesticide residues also cling to many fresh fruits and vegetables and are ingested when people eat these items.

Most pesticides accumulate in the body. Potential hazards associated with long-term exposure to pesticides include birth defects, cancer, liver and kidney damage, and nervous system disorders.

Trihalomethanes. Most Americans drink water treated with chlorine to kill harmful bacteria. Trihalomethanes (THMs) are synthetic organic chemicals formed at water treatment plants when the added chlorine reacts with natural organic compounds in the water. Any drinking water supply that has been chlorinated is likely to contain THMs, which include such substances as chloroform, bromoform, and dichlorobromomethane. Chloroform in high doses is known to cause liver and kidney disorders, central nervous system problems, birth defects, and cancer. Recent research indicates that THM concentrations can be substantially reduced by adjusting the chlorine dose, improving filtration practices to remove organic material, or adding chlorine after filtration rather than before.[19]

Lead. The Environmental Protection Agency has issued new standards intended to reduce dramatically the levels of lead in U.S. drinking water. These standards are already in place in many municipalities and will eventually reduce lead exposure for approximately 130 million people. The new rules stipulate that tap water lead values must not exceed 15 parts per billion (the previous standard allowed an average lead level of 50 parts per billion). When water suppliers identify problem areas, they will have to lower the water's acidity with chemical treatment because acidity increases water's ability to leach lead from the pipes through which it passes, or they will have to replace old lead plumbing in the service lines.

One way to reduce the possibility of ingesting lead if it does exist in your home's water system is to run the tap water several minutes before taking a drink or cooking with it to flush out water that has been standing overnight in lead-contaminated lines.[20] Although leaded paints and ceramic glazes used to pose health risks, particularly for small children who put painted toys in their mouths, the use of leads in such products has been effectively reduced in recent years (see Figure 23.5).

𝒩OISE POLLUTION

Loud noise has become commonplace. We are often painfully aware of construction crews in our streets, jet air-

planes roaring overhead, stereos blaring next door, and trucks rumbling down nearby freeways. Our bodies have definite physiological responses to noise, and noise can become a source of physical or mental distress.

Prolonged exposure to some noises results in hearing loss. Short-term exposure reduces productivity, concentration levels, and attention spans, and may affect mental and emotional health. Symptoms of noise-related distress include disturbed sleep patterns, headaches, and tension. Physically, our bodies respond to noises in a variety of ways. Blood pressure increases, blood vessels in the brain dilate, and vessels in other parts of the body constrict. The pupils of the eye dilate. Cholesterol levels in the blood rise, and some endocrine glands secrete additional stimulating hormones, such as adrenaline, into the bloodstream.

Sounds are measured in decibels. Table 23.4 shows the decibel levels for various sounds. Hearing can be damaged by varying lengths of exposure to sound. If the duration of allowable daily exposure to different decibel levels is exceeded, hearing loss will result.

At this point, it is necessary to distinguish between sound and noise. Sound is anything that can be heard. Noise is sound that can damage the hearing or cause mental or emotional distress. When sounds become distracting or annoying, they become noise.

Unfortunately, despite gradually increasing awareness that noise pollution is more than just a nuisance, noise

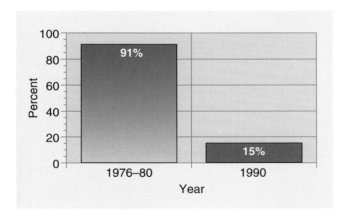

FIGURE 23.5

The graph measures EPA's estimates of the percentage of children with blood lead above 10 micrograms per deciliter of blood, the "level of concern" established by the U.S. Centers for Disease Control. The government's goal is to virtually eliminate the lead problem by the year 2000.

Source: Reprinted from U.S. Environmental Protection Agency, *Securing Our Legacy: An EPA Progress Report, 1989–1991* (EPA Publication No. 175R-92-001, 1992).

TABLE 23.4 ■ Noise Levels of Various Activities (in Decibels)

Decibels (db) measure the volume of sounds. Here are the decibel levels of some common sounds.

Type of Sound	Noise Level (db)
Carrier deck jet operation	150
Jet takeoff from 200 feet	140
Rock concert	120 (painful)
Auto horn (3 feet)	110 (extremely loud)
Motorcycle	100
Garbage truck	100
Pneumatic drill	90
Lawnmower	90
Heavy traffic	80
Alarm clock	80
Shouting, arguing	80 (very loud)
Vacuum cleaner	75 (loud)
Freight train from 50 feet	70
Freeway traffic	65
Normal conversation	60
Light auto traffic	50 (moderate)
Library	40
Soft whisper	30 (faint)

SKILLS FOR BEHAVIOR CHANGE

Reducing the Effects of Noise Pollution

Beyond giving your political support to legislation and enforcement of policies designed to reduce noise pollution, what can you do to lessen the effect of noise pollution on you? The following suggestions are only a few of the recommended approaches:

- Wear ear protectors or ear plugs when working around noisy machinery or when using firearms.

- When listening on a headset with volume settings numbered 1 through 10, keep the volume no louder than 4. Your headset is too loud if you are unable to hear people around you speaking in a normal tone of voice.

- Avoid loud music. Don't sit or stand near speakers or amplifiers at a rock concert and don't play a car radio or stereo above reasonable levels.

- Maintain your automobile, motorcycle, or lawn mower exhaust system in good working order.

- Furnish your room, apartment, home, and office with sound-absorbing materials. Drapes, carpeting, and cork wall tiles are excellent for reducing both interior and exterior noises.

- Avoid any exposure to painfully loud sounds and avoid repeated exposure to any sounds above 80 decibels.

---

control programs at federal, state, and local levels have been given a low budgetary priority. In order to prevent hearing loss, it is important that you take it upon yourself to avoid voluntary and involuntary exposure to excessive noise. Playing stereos in your car and home at reasonable levels, wearing ear plugs when you use power equipment, and establishing barriers (closed windows, etc.) between you and noise will help you keep your hearing intact. The Skills for Behavior Change box discusses more ways to reduce the effects of noise pollution.

WHAT DO YOU THINK?

What do you currently do that places your hearing at risk? What changes can you make in your lifestyle to change these risks?

LAND POLLUTION

Many areas of the United States currently face serious problems concerning safe and effective management of their garbage. As a nation, we are generating more trash than ever before.

Solid Waste

Each day, every person in the United States generates about 4 pounds of **municipal solid waste.** By the year 2000, solid waste generation is projected to reach 216 million tons daily, or 4.2 pounds per person.[21] Approximately 73 percent of this waste is buried in landfills. Cities and smaller communities throughout the country are in danger of exhausting their landfill space. Some cities have already run out of landfill space. Philadelphia, for example,

must ship its garbage to landfills in Ohio, Maryland, and Virginia at an annual cost of more than $44 million.

As communities run out of landfill space, it is becoming more common to haul garbage out to sea to dump it or to ship it to landfills in developing countries for dumping. In mid-1987, a garbage barge from Islip, Long Island, carrying 3,186 tons of waste began a 600-mile odyssey to find a dumping spot. After being rejected by six other states and three foreign countries, the garbage barge returned to the New York harbor to await a solution. Finally, the garbage was incinerated and the ash (some of it toxic) was buried in the Islip landfill.

Figure 23.6 shows the composition of our trash and what happens to our garbage after disposal. Recycling now accounts for only 13 percent of garbage treatment. Experts believe that as much as 90 percent of our trash is ultimately recyclable. Recycling is not a new word or concept in the United States. During World War I, the Depression, and World War II, scrap materials, bottles, clothing, and other goods were recycled regularly because of scarcities. In today's throwaway society, we need to become aware of the amount of waste we generate every day and to look for ways to recycle, reuse, and—most desirable of all—reduce the products we use. The Choices for Change box discusses ways to become a better recycler through better shopping practices.

Hazardous Waste

The community of Love Canal, New York, has come to symbolize **hazardous waste** dump sites. Love Canal was an abandoned canal that was first used as a chemical dump site by the Hooker Chemical Company in the 1920s. Dumping continued for nearly 30 years. Then the area was filled in by land developers and built up with homes and schools.

In 1976, homeowners began noticing strange seepage in their basements and strong, chemical odors. Babies

Become an Environmental Shopper

L earn the 5 R's of recycling:

REDUCE the amount of waste you produce.
REUSE as much as possible.
RECYCLE the recyclables.
REJECT overpackaging and products hazardous to the environment.
REACT by joining with other consumers to let manufacturers and governments know your views.

Reduce

- Buy only what you need.
- Buy products having the least amount of packaging.
- Buy products in recycled or recyclable packaging.
- Avoid disposable products that are not recyclable.
- Buy the larger size or in bulk when possible.

Reuse

- Appliances
- Boxes
- Clothing
- Containers
- Grocery bags
- Wrapping paper

Recycle

Learn what is recyclable in your community:

- Aluminum
- Corrugated cardboard
- Glass
- Motor oil
- Newsprint
- Office paper
- Paperboard
- Plastics
- Steel cans

Reject

- Aerosol containers
- Blister packs
- Mixed material packages
- Nonrecyclable packaging
- Packaging that promises to disappear
- Products harmful to the environment
- Supposedly "biodegradable" plastics
- Overpackaged goods

React

- Write to manufacturers to support environmentally benign packaging and products, and to discourage
  - overpackaging
  - nonrecyclable packaging
  - environmentally harmful products
- Call manufacturers' 800 lines (listed on many packages) to voice your opinion.
- Contact elected officials to request that government at all levels use more recycled products.
- Ask merchants to provide bags made from recycled material or use your own bag.
- Request that your local newspaper use more recycled newsprint.

Source: Johnson County Recycling and Waste Reduction Guide, 4th ed. (1994), 4–6.

---

were born with abnormal hearts and kidneys, two sets of teeth, mental handicaps, epilepsy, liver disease, and abnormal rectal bleeding. The rate of miscarriages was far above normal. Cancer rates were also above normal.

In response to these reports, the New York State Department of Health investigated the area of Love Canal. High concentrations of PCBs were found in the storm sewers near the old canal, but it took the department another two years to order the evacuation of the Love Canal homes. Over 900 families were evacuated, and the state purchased their homes. Finally, in 1978, the expensive process of cleaning up the waste dump began. Many lawsuits for damages are still being litigated.

In 1980, the Comprehensive Environmental Response Compensation and Liability Act (**Superfund**) was enacted to provide funds for cleaning up chemical dump sites that endanger public health and land. This fund is financed through taxes on the chemical and petroleum industries (87 percent) and through general federal tax revenues (13 percent). The 1980 allocation was $1.6 billion. By 1984,

Municipal solid waste: Includes such wastes as durable goods, nondurable goods, containers and packaging, food wastes, yard wastes, and miscellaneous wastes from residential, commercial, institutional, and industrial sources.

Hazardous waste: Solid waste that, due to its toxic properties, poses a hazard to humans or to the environment.

Superfund: Fund established under the Comprehensive Environmental Response Compensation and Liability Act to be used for cleaning up toxic waste dumps.

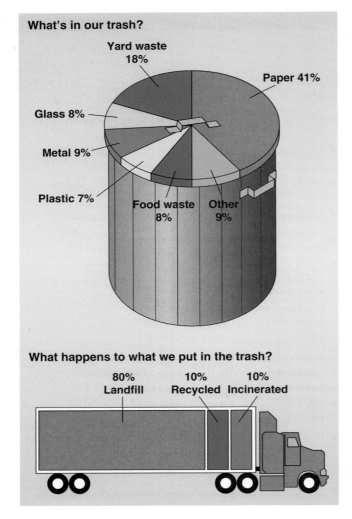

What's in our trash?

Yard waste 18%

Paper 41%

Glass 8%

Metal 9%

Plastic 7%

Food waste 8%

Other 9%

What happens to what we put in the trash?

80% Landfill   10% Recycled   10% Incinerated

FIGURE 23.6

The Composition and Disposition of our Trash

the EPA estimated that an additional $8 to $23 billion was needed to finish the cleanup.[22] By the end of the decade, the estimated funds needed to do the job exceeded $100 billion. Some estimates of the ultimate cost are as high as $500 billion.[23]

To date, 32,500 potentially hazardous waste sites have been identified across the nation. After initial investigation, 17,800 of these sites were determined to require no further action. But 1,207 sites were proposed for listing on the National Priorities List (NPL), which identifies the nation's most toxic waste sites.[24]

The large number of hazardous waste dump sites in the United States indicates the severity of our toxic chemical problem. American manufacturers generate more than 1

Ionizing radiation: Radiation produced by photons having high enough energy to ionize atoms.

ton of chemical waste per person per year (approximately 275 million tons). Three industrial groups produce most of this waste: chemicals and allied products, metal-related industries, and petroleum and coal products.[25]

The EPA and the states have undertaken a "cradle-to-grave" program to manage hazardous wastes by monitoring their generation, transportation, storage, treatment, and final disposal. To ensure that hazardous wastes being generated today do not become complex and expensive cleanup problems tomorrow, the following steps are being taken:

As the United States runs out of space to dispose of the millions of tons of solid waste generated daily, more and more communities have developed recycling programs and other strategies to reduce the amount of trash destined for local landfills.

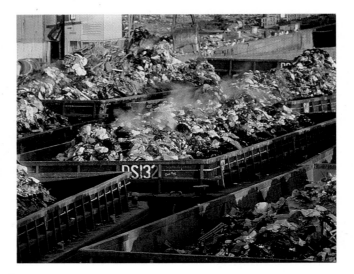

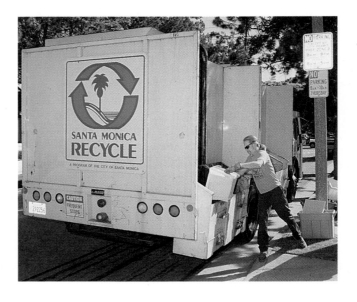

Are Minorities and the Poor More Exposed to Pollution?

Hazardous waste production and disposal continue to be pressing environmental and public health concerns because of the harm toxic substances may cause people living near hazardous waste sites and facilities. In the United States, there is clear documentation that people of color and people with lower incomes are more likely than other Americans to live and work in neighborhoods with high levels of pollution. A recent update of the United Church of Christ Commission for Racial Justice, *Toxic Wastes and Race in the United States,* found that the situation has worsened during the past six years. People of color are currently 47 percent more likely than are whites to live near a commercial toxic waste facility.

In response to growing concerns that low-income, racial, and ethnic minority groups may be disproportionately at risk from environmental problems, the Environmental Protection Agency established an Environmental Equity Workgroup in July 1990 to examine the issue. The workgroup's report, "Environmental Equity: Reducing Risk for All Communities," released in March 1992, does the following:

- It assesses the available information on environmental health effects among economic, racial, and ethnic groups and concludes that, except for blood lead levels, there are inadequate data on the subject.

- It recommends putting a new emphasis on risk assessment and risk communication, including building a better data base, to describe and explain risks that affect particular populations and communities such as inner cities.

- It also recommends a review of the EPA's outreach efforts and consultation with minority and low-income organizations.

- It suggests ways that the EPA can incorporate environmental equity into long-range planning, management, and other activities of federal and state environmental agencies.

Source: Most text adapted from U.S. Environmental Protection Agency, *Securing Our Legacy: An EPA Progress Report, 1989–1991* (EPA Publication No. 175R-92-001, 1992); figure reprinted and text just above it adapted by permission of the Center for Policy Alternatives from "Toxic Waste and Race: An Unnatural Association," in *Scientific American,* December 1994, 26.

- Many wastes are now banned from land disposal or are being treated in such a way that their toxicity is reduced before they become part of land disposal sites.

- The EPA has developed protective requirements for land disposal facilities, such as double liners, detection systems for substances that may leach into groundwater, and groundwater monitoring systems.

- Hazardous waste handlers must now clean up contamination resulting from past waste management practices as well as from current activities.

- The EPA is exploring ways to create economic incentives to encourage ingenuity in waste minimization practices and recycling.[26]

See the Multicultural Perspectives box for a summation of an EPA report on the likelihood that lower-income Americans are more exposed than other Americans to hazardous waste and other toxic substances.

WHAT DO YOU THINK?

What do you currently recycle? What are some of the reasons you do not recycle? What concerns would you have about living near a landfill or hazardous waste production or disposal site?

RADIATION

A substance is said to be radioactive when it emits high-energy particles from the nuclei of its atoms. There are three types of radiation: alpha particles, beta particles, and gamma rays. Alpha particles are relatively massive particles and are not capable of penetrating human skin. They pose health hazards only when inhaled or ingested. Beta particles are capable of slight penetration of the skin and are harmful if ingested or inhaled. Gamma rays are the most dangerous radioactive particles because they can pass straight through the skin, causing serious damage to organs and other vital structures.

Ionizing Radiation

Exposure to ionizing radiation is an inescapable part of life on this planet. **Ionizing radiation** is caused by the release of particles and electromagnetic rays from atomic nuclei during the normal process of disintegration. Some naturally occurring elements, such as uranium, emit radiation. Other radiation-producing elements, such as deuterium, develop as part of the decay process of uranium or are created by scientists in laboratories. Radiation, whether naturally occurring or human-made, can damage the genetic material in the reproductive cells of living organisms. It can also cause mutations, miscarriages, physical and mental deformities, cancer, eye cataracts, gastrointestinal illnesses, and shortened life expectancies.

Scientists cannot agree on a safe level of radiation. Reactions to radiation differ from person to person. Exposure is measured in **radiation absorbed doses, or rads** (also called roentgens). Recommended maximum "safe" dosages range from 0.5 rads to 5 rads per year. Approximately 50 percent of the radiation to which we are exposed comes from natural sources, such as building materials. Another 45 percent comes from medical and dental X-rays. The remaining 5 percent comes from computer display screens, microwave ovens, television sets, luminous watch dials, and radar screens and waves (see Table 23.5). Most of us are exposed to far less radiation than the "safe" maximum dosage per year.

Radiation can cause damage at dosages as low as 100 to 200 rads. At this level, signs of radiation sickness include nausea, diarrhea, fatigue, anemia, sore throat, and hair loss. Death is unlikely at this dosage. At 350 to 500 rads, all these symptoms become more severe, and death may result because the radiation hinders bone marrow production of the white blood cells we need to protect us from disease. Dosages above 600 to 700 rads are invariably fatal. The effects of long-term exposure to relatively low levels of radiation are unknown. Some scientists believe that such exposure can cause lung cancer, leukemia, skin cancer, bone cancer, and skeletal deformities.

Nonionizing Radiation

The lower-energy portions of the electromagnetic spectrum, ranging from lower-energy ultraviolet radiation down through infrared, radar, radio, and the electric and magnetic fields associated with many household appliances and electric power lines, are **nonionizing radiation.** Although the biological effects of ionizing radiation have been recognized for some time, we still do not know very much about the effects of certain types of nonionizing

TABLE 23.5 ■ Doses of Radiation

Source	Rads (per year)
Cosmic rays	0.45
Soil	0.15
Water, food, air	0.25
Air travel (round trip New York–London)	0.04
Medical X-rays	0.10
Nuclear power plant in vicinity	0.01
Brick structures	0.50–1.0
Concrete structures	0.70–1.0
Wooden structures	0.30–0.50

Source: Reprinted by permission from International Atomic Energy Agency, *Radiation—A Fact of Life,* 1981 ed.

radiation—in particular, the photons associated with electric and magnetic fields. Techniques for assessing radiation from many such sources are still evolving.[27]

Nuclear Power Plants

One source of radioactive emissions is nuclear power plants. At present, these plants account for less than 1 percent of the total radiation to which we are exposed. Radioactive wastes are produced not only by nuclear power plants but also by medical facilities that use radioactive materials as treatment and diagnostic tools and by nuclear weapons production facilities.

Proponents of nuclear energy believe that it is a safe and efficient way to generate electricity. Initial costs of building nuclear power plants are high, but actual power generation is relatively inexpensive. A 1,000-megawatt reactor produces enough energy for 650,000 homes and saves 420 million gallons of fossil fuels each year. In some areas where nuclear power plants were decommissioned, electricity bills tripled when power companies turned to hydroelectric or fossil fuel sources to generate electricity.

Nuclear reactors also discharge fewer carbon oxides into the air than do fossil-fuel powered generators. Advocates believe that conversion to nuclear power could help slow the global warming trend. Over the past 15 years, carbon emissions were reduced by 298 million tons, or 5 percent.[28]

All these advantages of nuclear energy must be weighed against the disadvantages. First, disposal of nuclear wastes is extremely problematic for the entire world. Additionally, the chances of a reactor core meltdown pose

---

Radiation absorbed doses (rads): Units that measure exposure to radioactivity.

Nonionizing radiation: Radiation produced by photons associated with lower-energy portions of the electromagnetic spectrum.

Meltdown: An accident that results when the temperature in the core of a nuclear reactor increases enough to melt the nuclear fuel and the containment vessel housing it.

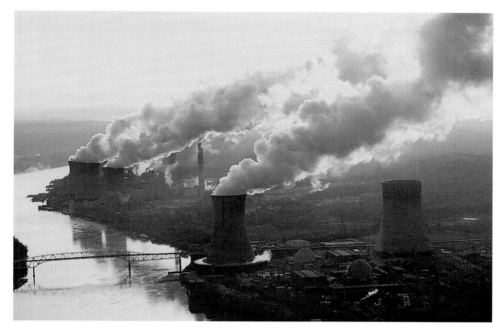

Controversy continues to surround nuclear power plants—with proponents citing the efficiency and relative safety compared with burning fossil fuels to generate power and with opponents pointing to the problems of waste disposal and the dangers of an accident or meltdown at a plant.

serious threats to a plant's immediate environment and to the world in general.

A **meltdown** occurs when the temperature in the core of a nuclear reactor increases enough to melt both the nuclear fuel and the containment vessel that holds it. Most modern facilities seal their reactors and containment vessels in concrete buildings having pools of cold water on the bottom. If a meltdown occurs, the building and the pool are supposed to prevent the escape of radioactivity.

In early 1990, the United States had 122 licensed commercial nuclear reactors on line. These plants were producing 15,000 metric tons of radioactive waste annually. This amount is estimated to climb to 40,000 tons annually by the year 2000. Opponents of nuclear energy believe

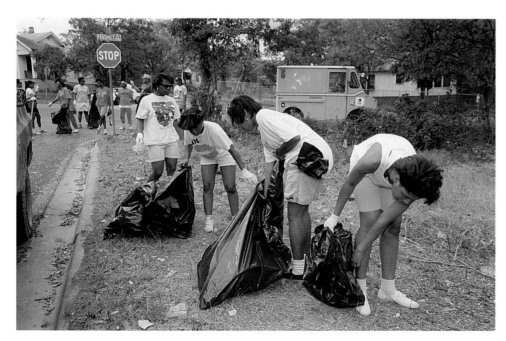

While we may feel that many of the environmental problems facing the world today are beyond our individual control, we can play a significant role in keeping our own little part of it clean, green, and beautiful.

Managing Environmental Pollution

Environmental health begins at home. One celebrant of the 1990 Earth Day stated that in order to save the planet, we will all have to overcome our inertia and make sacrifices that contribute to the good of the planet. By understanding how political and economic issues affect the environment, we can pressure corporations and elected representatives to change policies that are harmful to the environment. For example, environmentalists pressured the World Bank to stop issuing development loans that were leading to the destruction of rain forests. Discussing issues with lawmakers and making decisions at the polls are two ways you can help influence environmental policy.

Making Decisions for You

One of the biggest decisions that we make as consumers is whether to pay more for environmentally safe products. As a student on a tight budget, are you willing to pay 30 to 50 percent more for products such as safer soap and laundry detergent? If not, are you willing to buy a less environmentally friendly product? While it's not likely that you can increase your budget enough to buy all environmentally safe products, you can get a start now. Think about the products you buy: Which could you substitute for more environmentally friendly brands?

Checklist for Change: Making Personal Choices

✓ Do you vote? Do you know the difference between rhetoric and reality when it comes to environmental issues?

✓ Do you conserve water? Fix leaky faucets quickly. Run washers only with full loads. Don't overwater lawns or gardens.

✓ Do you think before you buy? Do you buy products in recyclable packaging? Do you reuse containers rather than buy new ones?

✓ Do you think before you throw household chemicals away? Make sure you use them up, give them away, or save them for a household hazardous waste collection instead. Consider nonhazardous substitutes.

✓ Do you recycle used oil? Oil dumped down storm drains or on the ground can pollute streams, killing insects, fish, and wildlife.

✓ Do you recycle tin cans, glass, newspaper, paper, plastic, and cardboard?

✓ Have you considered turning in people who litter?

✓ Have you considered walking, riding the bus, using your bike, and/or carpooling whenever possible?

✓ Are you cautious concerning the amount of fertilizers and pesticides you use? If they are overapplied, rain can wash them off lawns and carry them into lakes and streams. Always use low-phosphorous fertilizers.

✓ Do you ask yourself if you really need a product?

✓ Do you consider whether a product is practical and durable, well-made, and of timeless design?

✓ Do you buy used and rebuilt products whenever possible? Do you resell your unused items at yard or garage sales (your trash may be someone else's treasure) or donate them to charities?

✓ Do you compost leaves, clippings, and kitchen scraps?

Checklist for Change: Making Community Choices

✓ Do you work in your community to help create and enforce laws that protect drinking water and that prohibit the manufacture, use, storage, transport, or disposal of hazardous substances in your water supply area?

✓ Do you volunteer to take part in clean-up activities in your community?

✓ Does your community have a hazardous materials ordinance?

Critical Thinking

Your health teacher is leading a protest next week to the corporate headquarters of "one of the country's worst polluters." You are told not only that this company has a terrible record of both point and nonpoint source pollutants, but also that the "corporate bigwigs refuse to do anything about it." After hearing the brief appeal to join the protest, you decide it's your duty as a citizen to go. As your teacher hands out maps to the protest site, you realize that the company in question is your employer! Now you're really confused: Your company claims to have spent billions of dollars to reduce pollution and considers itself an innovator in cleaning up sites it polluted in the past. You are upset because only one side of the story is being told. Should you speak up in class?

Using the DECIDE model in Chapter 1, decide what you would do. First, decide why you are upset. Then decide what you would like to accomplish by speaking up. In addition, consider the best setting to communicate your message to your teacher (in class, during office hours, e-mail, etc.).

that there is no safe place to dispose of, contain, or store our escalating supply of nuclear waste.

Two serious nuclear accidents within seven years of one another caused a steep decline in public support for nuclear energy. The first occurred in 1979 at Three Mile Island near Harrisburg, Pennsylvania, when a mechanical failure caused a partial meltdown of one reactor core and small amounts of radioactive steam were released into the atmosphere. No loss of human life was reported, although residents in the area were evacuated. Miscarriages, birth defects, and cancer rates in the area are reported to have increased, but no public health statistics have been released.

Human error and mechanical failure were the reported causes of the April 1986 reactor core fire and explosion at the Chernobyl nuclear power plant in the Soviet Union. In just 4.5 seconds, the temperature in the reactor rose to 120 times normal, causing the explosion. Eighteen people were killed immediately, 30 workers died later from radiation sickness, and 200 other workers were hospitalized for severe radiation sickness. Soviet officials evacuated towns and villages near the plant. Some medical workers estimate that the eventual death toll from Chernobyl could top 100,000 from radiation-induced cancers.

Radioactive fallout from the Chernobyl disaster spread over most of the northern hemisphere. Milk, meat, and vegetables in Scandinavian countries were contaminated with radioactive iodine and cesium and were declared unfit for human consumption. Thousands of reindeer in Lapland were declared contaminated and were destroyed. In Great Britain, thousands of sheep had to be destroyed because they were contaminated, and three years after the disaster, sheep in the northern regions of the country were still found to be contaminated. Direct costs of the disaster totaled more than $13 billion, including lost agricultural output and the cost of replacing the power plant.[29]

Accidents at nuclear power plants are not rare occurrences. In 1985, United States plants experienced nearly 3,000 mishaps and 765 emergency shutdowns. At least 18 of the shutdowns were reported to be the result of serious accidents that could have led to reactor core damage.

What Do You Think?

How much exposure do you have to ionizing and nonionizing radiation a year? What measures could you take to reduce this exposure? Do you feel the advantages outweigh the disadvantages of nuclear power? Explain why or why not.

Summary

- Population growth is the single largest factor affecting the demands made on the environment. Demand for more food, products, and energy—as well as places to dispose of waste—places great strains on the earth's resources.

- The primary constituents of air pollution are sulfur dioxide, particulate matter, carbon monoxide, nitrogen dioxide, ozone, lead, and hydrocarbons. Air pollution takes the forms of photochemical smog and acid rain, among others. Indoor air pollution is caused primarily by woodstove smoke, furnace emissions, asbestos, passive smoke, formaldehyde, and radon. Pollution is depleting the earth's protective ozone layer, causing global warming.

- Water pollution can be caused by either point (direct entry through a pipeline, ditch, etc.) or nonpoint (runoff or seepage from a broad area of land) sources. Chemicals that are major contributors to water pollution include dioxins, pesticides, trihalomethanes, and lead.

- Noise pollution affects our hearing and produces other symptoms such as reduced productivity, reduced concentration, headaches, and tension.

- Solid waste pollution includes household trash, plastics, glass, metal products, and paper; limited landfill space creates problems. Hazardous waste is toxic; its improper disposal creates health hazards for those in surrounding communities.

- Ionizing radiation results from the natural erosion of atomic nuclei. Nonionizing radiation is caused by the electric and magnetic fields around power lines and household appliances, among other sources. The disposal and storage of radioactive wastes from nuclear power plants and weapons production pose serious potential problems for public health.

Discussion Questions

1. Explain the ways in which the expanding global population affects the environment.

2. List the primary sources of air pollution, acid rain, and indoor air pollution. What can be done to reduce each type of pollution?

3. What are the environmental consequences of global warming? What can we as U.S. citizens do to help slow the deforestation of tropical rain forests?

4. Explain point and nonpoint sources of water pollution. Discuss how water pollution can be reduced or prevented altogether. What personal actions can you as a student take?

5. List the loudest sounds you have encountered in the last week (rock concert, construction, airplanes, etc.). How many could have been avoided? What could be done to ease the strain of the unavoidable noises?

6. Given all the open land in the United States, why do you think solid waste disposal is a problem?

7. Are the advantages of nuclear power worth the risks involved with storing nuclear waste? Put another way, if you live near a nuclear power plant, would you be willing to pay two or three times as much for electricity in order to have the nuclear power plant closed? Explain why or why not.

Application Exercise

Reread the What Do You Think? scenarios at the beginning of the chapter and answer the following questions:

1. Does the United States government have the right to pressure developing countries to reduce population in return for economic help? Would it be constitutional to control our own citizens' birth rate?

2. Countries without pollution-control laws in place are able to produce goods in factories at lower prices than are countries where expensive anti-pollution laws are in effect. What incentives or disincentives could be put in place to persuade foreign companies to reduce pollution?

3. Identify key components that would need to be included in an environmental program for developing nations.

4. How much progress can be made in the fight against environmental polluters by community action? Are there alternatives that are more effective?

5. What are an industry's responsibilities to its neighbors?

Further Reading

L. Allen, ed., *Annual Editions: Environment 93/94* (Guilford, CT: Dushkin Publishing, 1993).

A collection of selected articles on environmental topics from magazines, newspapers, and journals that is updated annually. This issue includes articles about the global environment, world population, energy, pollution, resources, and the biosphere.

L. R. Brown, ed., *State of the World, 1993* (New York: Norton, 1993).

Annual publication of the Worldwatch Institute. Gives valuable insight into how well we are meeting the environmental challenges presented to us this year. New in this edition are discussions of water scarcity, energy development in the Third World, the economic costs of environmental degradation, and the new industrial revolution.

R. Caplan, *Our Earth, Ourselves* (New York: Bantam, 1990).

Caplan is executive director of the Environmental Action group. Offers summaries of environmental problems and ideas for individual action toward solving them.

The Earthworks Group, *50 Simple Things You Can Do to Save the Earth* (Berkeley, CA: Earthworks Press, 1990).

Begins with summaries of various environmental problems, such as the greenhouse effect, vanishing wildlife, acid rain, and ozone depletion. Offers 50 ideas for individual plans of action to help reduce environmental stresses. Ideas are categorized as "simple" (stop junk mail), "it takes some effort" (recycle glass), and "for the committed" (install a graywater tank).

P. H. Hynes, *Earthright* (Rocklin, CA: Prima Publishing and Communication, 1990).

A citizen's guidebook to the environment. Offers simple and positive ideas for personal participation in cleaning up the environment.

A. Nadakavukaren, *Man and Environment: A Health Perspective* (Prospect Heights, IL: Waveland Press, 1990).

Provides an overview of environmental problems affecting human health. Among the topics covered are ecological principles, population dynamics and related problems, environmental disease, pesticides, food contaminants, air pollution, water pollution, noise pollution, and solid and hazardous wastes.

U.S. Environmental Protection Agency, *EPA Journal* (Washington, DC: U.S. Government Printing Office).

Periodical published by the Office of Communications and Public Affairs six times a year. Devoted entirely to environmental areas regulated by the EPA. Often has a particular focus, such as nonpoint source pollution, recycling, or clean air legislation.

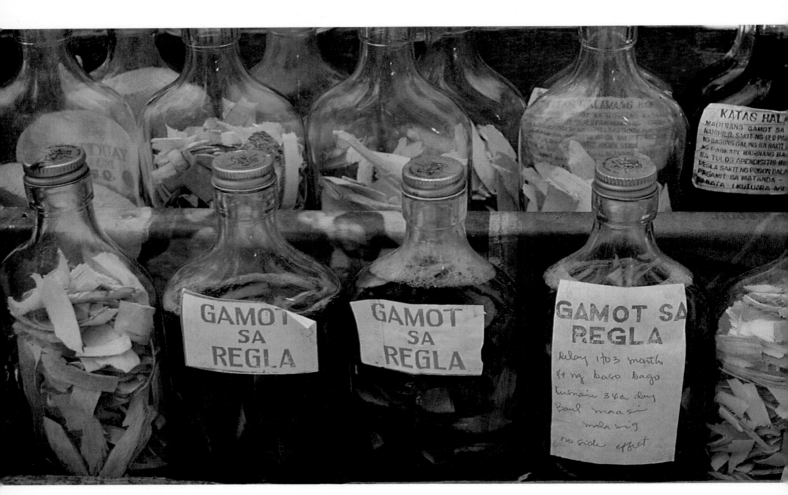

CHAPTER OBJECTIVES

◆ Discuss the methods advertisers use to attract customers.

◆ Explain when self-diagnosis and self-care are appropriate, when you should seek medical care, and how to assess health professionals.

◆ Compare and contrast allopathic and nonallopathic medicine, including the types of treatments that fall into each category.

◆ Discuss the types of health care available, including types of medical practices, hospitals, and clinics.

◆ Examine the current problems associated with our health-care system, including cost, access, and quality.

◆ Describe health insurance options, including private insurance coverage, Medicare, Medicaid, and managed care choices (HMOs and PPOs).

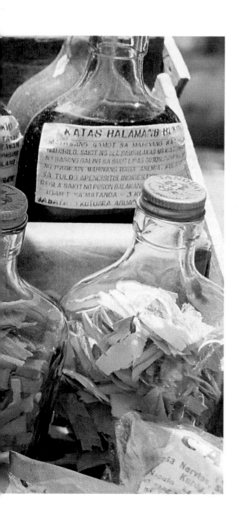

Consumerism

Selecting Health-Care Products and Services

Lisa, a recent college graduate just starting her new job but not yet insured, develops a bad cough. She knows that if she seeks treatment she will have to pay out-of-pocket, so she delays seeking care. During this delay, the cough develops into bronchitis and then pneumonia. One evening, her breathing becomes so impaired that her roommate must drive her to the emergency room. There, doctors use high-tech diagnostic and treatment techniques on Lisa, and she is required to stay overnight at the hospital to stabilize her condition.

- Who should pay for this expensive form of care? Was there a way to prevent such a sequence of events?

Roberta is a slightly older-than-average college student. She has a history of chronically painful menstrual periods and excessive bleeding. She seeks care from a gynecologist, who immediately states that she must have a hysterectomy. Because she believes that this is the most drastic option and because she has not yet had children and does not wish to go through early menopause, Roberta seeks a second opinion from the first doctor's colleague. Without giving her much of an exam, the second doctor agrees with the first, so she seeks yet another opinion—but this time from a doctor outside the original group's practice. This third doctor adamantly disagrees with the first two and suggests a more conservative treatment not involving surgery.

- Which doctor's advice should Roberta follow? Is it appropriate to seek more than one opinion or more than two? How much say should the patient have in her course of treatment? How can a consumer determine what "quality health care" is?

There are many reasons for you to be an informed health-care consumer. Most important, you have only one body, and it is no one's top priority but yours. Doing everything you can to stay healthy and to recover rapidly when you do get sick will enhance every other part of your life. Another reason to be an active health consumer is that as a citizen or resident of the United States you have no constitutional right to health care. Our society generally treats health care as a private-consumption good or service to be bought and sold rather than as a social good to which everyone is entitled. Therefore, you need to be not only informed but also assertive in order to obtain optimal care at an affordable cost. But, as you may already know, medical and health-care services are much harder to evaluate for need, availability, cost, and quality than are, say, clothing or fruit and vegetables. In addition, you may seek medical and health services in circumstances of either physical or emotional distress. Thus, your decision-making powers may be compromised and you may find yourself vulnerable when faced with the claims of inferior caregivers or products.

This chapter will help you to become more proactive in making decisions that affect your health and health care. Our health-care system is a maze of health-care providers, payers (insurance, government, and individuals), and products, and many of us find it hard to thread our way through it. Health care is the fifth-largest industry in our country, accounting for over 10 percent of our workforce, and many different companies aggressively market health products and services to the public. Even medical professionals sometimes feel overwhelmed, confused, and frustrated by the multitude of choices and lack of coordination in our system. So if you've experienced these feelings, you are not alone. However, there is much you can do to become an informed, responsible consumer of health-care products and services.

RESPONSIBLE CONSUMERISM: CHOICES AND CHALLENGES

Perhaps the single greatest difficulty that we face as health consumers is the sheer magnitude of choices available to us. If you try to select a general practitioner from the telephone book when you are sick, you may have to thumb through dozens of pages of specialists. When going to the drugstore for a bottle of cough syrup, you may have to choose from more than 30 brands, each claiming to do more for you than the brand next to it. Even trained pharmacists sometimes find it impossible to keep up with the explosion of new drugs and health-related products.

Informed health consumers are aware that there is always more to learn. Because there are so many charlatans competing for a share of the lucrative health market and because misinformation is so common, wise health consumers use every means at their disposal to ensure that they are acting responsibly in their own health choices. Check out your own knowledge in the Rate Yourself self-assessment.

Attracting Consumers' Dollars

Today's marketing specialists can identify a target audience for a given product and carefully go after it with a whole arsenal of gimmicks, subtle persuaders, and sophisticated strategies. Many advertisements present a product as a status symbol that will make you a member of the "in" crowd. In addition, many ads play on your inner fears and insecurities, causing you to wonder whether your deodorant is working, your breath is bad, or your skin is greasy. They may also convince you to purchase the socially correct product.

Other marketing strategies attempt to appeal to your hidden desires. Whatever your desires, countless products and services are available to meet them. Although some marketing tactics are obvious, others are much more subtle and difficult to discern. Perfume advertisements that depict passionate embraces and automobile ads that feature expensive sports cars with beautiful women are common. The implied message is that if you purchase a given perfume, your love life will improve, and if you buy that flashy car, attractive people will flock to you.

Many other marketing strategies revolve around "trendy" news items. A good example of this is the current concern about high cholesterol levels. Whereas food ads once focused heavily on "low calories," the heart-disease scare has prompted advertisements focusing on "low cholesterol" or "low fat."

Why Some False Claims May Seem True

People often fall victim to false health claims because they mistakenly believe that a product or provider has helped

How Good a Health Consumer Are You?

Select the response that best describes your typical health behavior. After completing this survey, total your points and assess your competence regarding health-care products and services.

1 = I never act this way
2 = I sometimes act this way
3 = I act this way most of the time
4 = I always act this way

1. When moving to a new location, I seek recommendations from friends and ask for referrals from physicians who have treated me in the past whom I respect before I get ill.　　1　2　3　4

2. I give consideration to selection of health-care services before I get sick.　　1　2　3　4

3. I schedule an interview with health professionals prior to treatment to determine if I am comfortable with them.　　1　2　3　4

4. I ask about costs of health-care procedures even if I have health insurance.　　1　2　3　4

5. I carefully assess my symptoms and go to the doctor only when necessary.　　1　2　3　4

6. I get second opinions when I am unsure of what my physician tells me.　　1　2　3　4

7. I ask my physician why a test is being given and what my options are before I allow that test to be performed.　　1　2　3　4

8. I follow recommended guidelines for health exams, inoculations, and self-care.　　1　2　3　4

9. Whenever I receive a prescription drug, I follow the directions on the bottle exactly, using all medications in the prescribed time period.　　1　2　3　4

10. I am aware of differences in prices at various pharmacies and comparison-shop whenever possible.　　1　2　3　4

11. When my peers make statements that are obviously incorrect about "health alternatives," I tactfully point out their errors.　　1　2　3　4

12. I am aware of my own body and seek medical care quickly when unusual changes occur.　　1　2　3　4

13. I attempt to obtain my health information from reputable sources rather than from tabloids.　　1　2　3　4

14. I carefully scrutinize health-related advertisements and news items.　　1　2　3　4

15. I read the labels of health products and follow instructions carefully.　　1　2　3　4

Interpreting Your Score

15–20　Health consumer skills dangerously weak

21–30　Health consumer skills below average

31–45　Health consumer skills about average, not adequate for many situations

46–60　Very good health consumer skills

Beyond Interpretation

In which five areas above do you believe you need improvement?

What can you do to improve in these areas?

---

them. This belief often arises from two conditions: spontaneous remission and the placebo effect.

Spontaneous Remission. It is commonly said that if you treat a cold, it will disappear in a week, but if you leave it alone, it will last seven days. A **spontaneous remission** from an ailment refers to the disappearance of symptoms without any apparent cause or treatment. Many illnesses, like the common cold and even back strain, are self-limiting

and will improve in time, with or without treatment. Other illnesses, such as multiple sclerosis and some cancers, are characterized by alternating periods of severe symptoms

Spontaneous remission: The disappearance of symptoms without any apparent cause or treatment.

and sudden remissions. Because of this phenomenon, people seeking profit may exploit consumers by claiming that their particular treatment, procedure, or drug cured the condition. People experiencing spontaneous remissions can easily attribute their "cure" to a treatment, drug, or provider that had no real effect on the disease or condition.

Placebo Effect. The **placebo effect** is an apparent cure or improved state of health brought about by a substance, product, or procedure that has no therapeutic value. It is not uncommon for patients to report improvements based on what they expect, desire, or were told would happen after taking simple sugar pills that they believed were powerful drugs. About 10 percent of the population is believed to be exceptionally susceptible to the power of suggestion; the remainder may be influenced in varying degrees. Those who are most susceptible may be victimized by aggressive marketing of products and services. Although the placebo effect is often harmless, it does account for the expenditure of millions of dollars on worthless health products and services every year. Ingesting megadoses of vitamin C to treat cancer is one glaring example, but there are many others ranging from weight-loss and wrinkle creams to pain-killing devices that send small shocks into the muscles. One of the key concepts in the placebo effect lies in the fact that people want to believe that these products will work. People who mistakenly use placebos when medical treatment is needed increase their risk for health problems.

ACCEPTING RESPONSIBILITY FOR YOUR HEALTH CARE

As the health-care industry has become more sophisticated about seeking your business, so must you become more sophisticated about purchasing its products and services. Apathy and ignorance are not viable options if you want care that serves your own best health interests.

You need to learn how, when, and where to enter the massive technological maze that is our health-care system without incurring unnecessary risk and expense. Acting responsibly in times of illness can be difficult, but the person best able to act in your behalf is you.

If you are not feeling well, you must first decide whether you really need to seek medical care. Estimates vary, but many sources indicate that up to 70 percent of all trips to the doctor and over one-third of all hospital

> **Placebo effect:** An apparent cure or improved state of health brought about by a substance or product that has no medicinal value.

stays are unnecessary and may even be harmful. According to a recent study, 50 percent of all emergency room visits are really not emergencies and would be better treated elsewhere.[1] On the other hand, not seeking treatment also has its dangers. Being knowledgeable about self-care and its limits is critical for responsible consumerism.

Self-Help or Self-Care

A recent concept in health consumerism is that the patient is the primary health-care provider or first line of defense in health. Patients can practice behaviors that promote health, prevent disease, and minimize reliance on the formal medical system. They can also interpret basic changes in their own physical and emotional health and treat minor afflictions without seeking professional help. Self-care consists of knowing your own body and its signals and taking appropriate action to stop the progression of illness or injury or to improve your overall health. The most common forms of self-care are:

- Diagnosis of symptoms or conditions that occur frequently but may not need physician visits (e.g., the common cold, minor abrasions).

- Breast and testicular self-examination (monthly).

- First aid for common, uncomplicated injuries and conditions.

- Checking blood pressure, pulse, and temperature.

- Home pregnancy and ovulation kits.

- Monitoring of cervical mucus for natural family planning.

- Monitoring protein, sugar, and bacteria-producing nitrites and bacteria-fighting leukocytes in the urine.

- Periodic checks for serum cholesterol.

- Home stool test kits for blood and early colon cancer detection.

- Self-help books, tapes, and videos.

- Relaxation techniques, including meditation and exercise.

When to Seek Help

Effective self-care requires understanding when you should seek professional medical attention rather than treat a condition by yourself. Surprisingly, people with diagnosed active chronic conditions get professional medical attention for only 5 percent of their episodes or flare-ups and treat the remaining 95 percent themselves.[2] Unfortunately, deciding what conditions warrant professional attention is not always easy. Generally, you should consult a physician if you experience any of the following:

- A serious accident or injury.

- Sudden or severe chest pains causing breathing difficulties.

- Trauma to the head or spine accompanied by persistent headache, blurred vision, loss of consciousness, vomiting, convulsions, or paralysis.

- Sudden high fever or recurring high temperature (over 102°F for adults and 103°F for children) and/or sweats.

- Tingling sensation in the arm accompanied by slurred speech or impaired thought processes.

- Adverse reactions to a drug or insect bite (shortness of breath, severe swelling, dizziness).

- Unexplained bleeding or loss of bodily fluid from any body opening.

- Unexplained sudden weight loss.

- Persistent or recurrent diarrhea or vomiting.

- Blue-colored lips, eyelids, or nail beds.

- Any lump, swelling, thickness, or sore that does not subside or that grows for over a month.

- Any marked change in or pain accompanying bowel or bladder habits.

- Yellowing of the skin or the whites of the eyes.

- Any symptom that is unusual and recurs over time.

- If you are pregnant.

The growing interest in self-care in the United States is fueled by Americans' desire to exercise more control over their own health and health behaviors. Higher levels of education and greater coverage of health issues in the popular media have contributed to this trend. So has a more realistic appraisal of physicians. The rising cost of professional care has also contributed to consumers' interest in self-care. With the vast array of home diagnostic devices currently available, it appears to be relatively easy for most people to take care of themselves. But a strong word of caution is in order here: Although many of these devices are valuable for making an initial diagnosis, home health tests cannot fully substitute for regular, complete examinations by a trained practitioner. The Skills for Behavior Change box offers valuable information about taking an active part in your own health care.

Assessing Health Professionals

Suppose you decide that you do need medical help. You must then identify what type of medical help you need and find out where to obtain it. Initially, selecting a doc-

For parents, knowing when to seek help for a sick child is often a challenge since young children are unable to assess their own symptoms and may not be able to describe them adequately.

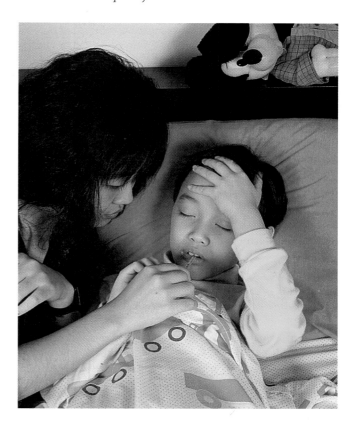

tor may seem a simple matter, yet many people have no idea how to assess the qualifications of a medical practitioner.

Knowledge of both traditional medical specialties and alternative medicine is critical to making an intelligent selection. You also need to be aware of your own criteria for evaluating a health professional. In one study,[3] when asked which factors were most important in choosing a doctor, consumers listed the following:

Willingness of doctor to explain the illness to patient	100 percent
Physician's access to a hospital of patient's choice	89 percent
Length of time to get an appointment	88 percent
Personality or appearance of the physician	84 percent
Fees	75 percent
Years of experience	73 percent
Office location	66 percent

Being Proactive in Your Health Care

Your personal involvement in your own wellness is critical. Taking a proactive approach to practicing preventive behaviors can go a long way toward giving you a long and healthy life. Sometimes, however, regardless of the steps you take to care for yourself, you still get sick. At such a time, it is important that you continue to be actively involved in your care. The more you know about your own body and about factors that can affect your health, the better able you will be to communicate complete information to your doctor. It also helps you to make informed decisions and to recognize when a certain treatment may not be right for you. The following points can help:

- Know your own and your family's medical history.
- Be knowledgeable about your condition—causes, physiological effects, possible treatments, prognosis. Don't rely on the doctor for all this information. Do some research.
- Bring a friend or relative along for medical visits to help you review what the doctor says.
- Ask the practitioner to explain the problem and possible treatments, tests, and drugs in a clear and understandable way.
- If the doctor prescribes any medications, ask for their generic names so that you can pay less for them.
- Ask for a written summary of the results of your visit and any lab tests.
- If you have any doubt about the doctor's recommended treatment, seek a second opinion.

Afterward,

- write down an accurate account of what happened and what was said. Be sure to include the names of the doctor and all other people involved in your care, the date, and the place.
- shop around drugstores for the best prices in the same way that you would when shopping for clothes.
- when filling prescriptions, ask to see the pharmacist's package inserts that list medical considerations concerning the medicines. Request detailed information about any potential drug interactions.

- have clear instructions written on the label to avoid risk to others who may take the drug in error.

Just like you, doctors are human. Their decisions are based on the best information they have available to them and may be influenced by a number of factors—workload, limited information, personal views. Therefore, in addition to following the practical steps listed above, being proactively involved in your health care also means that you should be aware of your rights as a patient. The following are the basic rights of all individuals seeking care from a health-care professional.

1. The right of informed consent. Before receiving any care, you have the right to be fully informed of what is being planned, the risks and potential benefits, and possible alternative forms of treatment, including the option of no treatment. Your consent must be voluntary and without any form of coercion. It is critical that you read any consent forms carefully and amend them as necessary before signing.

2. You have the right to know whether the treatment you are receiving is standard or experimental. In experimental conditions, you have the legal and ethical right to know if the study is one in which some people receive treatment while others do not in order to compare the results and if any drug is being used in the research project for a purpose not approved by the Food and Drug Administration (FDA).

3. You have the right to privacy, which includes the source of payment for treatment and care. It also includes protecting your right to make personal decisions concerning all reproductive matters.

4. You have the legal right to refuse treatment at any time and to cease treatment at any time during the course of care.

5. You have the right to receive care.

6. You have the right to access all your medical records and to confidentiality of your records.

7. You have the right to seek the opinions of other health-care professionals regarding your condition.

Weekend and evening office hours	66 percent
Doctor's involvement in civic organizations	37 percent
Listing in the Yellow Pages and other directories	30 percent

As this study and similar studies indicate, many people's greatest concerns when choosing a doctor have less to do with medical qualifications than with availability

and personality. While a warm and caring personality is certainly a valuable attribute, doctors who lack a good bedside manner may, in fact, be better trained and qualified than more cordial practitioners. Carefully consider the following factors about all prospective health-care providers:

- What professional educational training have they had? What license or board certification do they hold? Note that there is a difference between "board eligible" and "board certified." You want doctors who are "board certified." This title indicates that they have passed the national board examination for their specialty (e.g., pediatrics) and have been certified as competent in that specialty. In contrast, "board eligible" merely means that they are eligible to take the specialty board's exam or even that they may have failed the exam.

■ Are they affiliated with an accredited medical facility or institution? The Joint Commission on the Accreditation of Healthcare Organizations (JCAHO) requires these institutions to verify all education, licensing, and training claims of their affiliated practitioners.

■ Do they indicate clearly how long a given treatment may last, or do they keep you returning week after week with no apparent end in sight?

■ Do their diagnoses, treatments, and general statements appear to be consistent with established scientific theory and practice?

■ Do they listen to you, and appear to respect you as an individual, and give you time to ask questions?

Asking the right questions at the right time may save you personal suffering and expense. Many patients find that writing their questions down ahead of time helps them to get all their inquiries answered. You should not accept a defensive or hostile response; asking questions is your right as a patient. The Building Communication Skills box discusses finding a personal physician in more detail.

$\mathcal{W}$HAT DO YOU THINK?

If you had the choice of seeing a practitioner of your same gender or ethnicity, would you? Why? Do you think it would make a difference in how comfortable you may feel sharing personal or embarrassing but relevant health information? Have you ever had difficulty finding a practitioner with whom you are comfortable?

$\mathcal{C}$HOICES OF MEDICAL CARE

Familiarizing yourself with the various health professions and health subspecialties will help you choose the right provider for your needs. There are 687,000 physicians in the United States today. To assist you in sorting through them, Table 24.1 provides a list of types of practitioners. These professionals all subscribe to allopathic medical procedures. Most people believe that **allopathic medicine,** or traditional, Western medical practice, is based on scientifically validated methods, but you should consider the fact that only about 20 percent of all allopathic treatments have been proven clinically efficacious in scientific trials.

Many standard procedures focus on countering a patient's symptoms, not necessarily on curing the root problem. Medical practitioners who adhere to allopathic principles are bound by a professional code of ethics.

Traditional (Allopathic) Medicine

Selecting a **primary care practitioner**—a medical practitioner whom you can go to for routine ailments, preventive care, general medical advice, and appropriate referrals—is not an easy task. The primary care practitioner for most people is either a family practitioner, an internist, a pediatrician, or an obstetrician/gynecologist. Many people routinely see nurse practitioners or physician assistants who work for an individual doctor or a medical group, and others use nontraditional providers as their primary source of care. The common denominator in all these choices is continuity in services over a period of time. Having a "usual source of care" is important to the quality of care you receive.

Active participation in your own treatment is the only sensible course in a health-care environment that encourages "defensive medicine." That is, physicians will frequently order tests to rule out rare or unlikely diagnoses simply because they are worried about possible malpractice suits. Researchers have documented that this practice often leads to unnecessary tests and overtreatment. By some estimates, between 20 and 70 percent of what is done in medicine either does not improve health outcomes or creates iatrogenic disease (illness caused by the medical process itself). Informed consent refers to your right to have explained to you—in nontechnical language you can understand—all possible side effects, benefits, and consequences of a specific procedure and treatment regimen as well as available alternatives to it. It also means that you have the right to refuse a specific treatment or to seek a second or even third opinion from unbiased, noninvolved providers.[4]

The legal doctrine of informed consent gives you the right to ask:

■ What will happen if I choose not to have a particular test or treatment?

■ Can other tests be performed instead? What are their risks?

Allopathic medicine: Traditional, Western medical practice; in theory, based on scientifically validated methods and procedures.

Primary care practitioner: A medical practitioner who treats routine ailments, advises on preventive care, gives general medical advice, and makes appropriate referrals when necessary.

Finding a Personal Physician

Consider the following situation:

Mary wakes one morning with a chest cold. Within several days, the cold has worsened and she thinks she may have developed bronchitis. Mary knows she should see a doctor but she doesn't have a primary care physician, so she decides to let the cold takes its course without seeing someone. The next day, after a night of very labored breathing, Mary gives in and looks up the name of a doctor in the phone book and calls for an appointment.

Unfortunately, a great many people hesitate about seeking early care because they don't have a physician. The treatment Mary receives will probably be fine. But she will know nothing about the doctor and will be taking a chance on whether she will feel comfortable being treated by this person. Had Mary had a primary care physician, she could have called him or her up as soon as her symptoms had worsened.

One of the most important decisions a person or family has to make is choosing a primary care physician. Your physician plays a critical role in both the prevention and treatment of illnesses. When you are ill or develop symptoms that need attention, having someone to contact in whom you have confidence can relieve a great deal of anxiety. Yet, despite the importance of identifying and regularly visiting a primary care physician, a great many people wait until they are ill to seek out a doctor. Depending on the severity of the illness, waiting this long can limit a person's options. Selecting a doctor long before the development of an illness allows you the opportunity to identify and interview several doctors in order to find the one that will best fit your needs and with whom you will feel the most comfortable. The following procedure can help you with this process:

- First, consider the following questions:
  - Would you feel more comfortable with a male or female health professional?
  - Is age an important factor to you?

- Do you have a preexisting condition for which specialization may be helpful?
- Do you prefer to see primarily one physician or are you comfortable visiting a service having a team of doctors?
- Does your health plan limit your choice of doctors to a special list? If it does and you choose someone off-list, what will it cost?

- Assemble a list of names of doctors in your area. Names of potential physicians can be identified by
  - asking friends and colleagues for recommendations. These are often your best sources of information about a doctor's availability and promptness and overall general concern.
  - calling the local or county medical society, local health advocacy groups (many communities provide references as a service), or the local hospital for names of doctors accepting new patients.
  - researching medical directories at your local library. The American Medical Directory, for example, includes information about every physician who belongs to the AMA.

- Call the offices of the physicians on your list and explain that you are seeking a primary care physician. Ask the receptionist about the doctor's hospital affiliation, fees for checkups and office visits, office hours, and the kind of coverage the physician has for emergency situations that occur outside normal office hours. Identify whether the doctor participates in your health insurance plan. Take into consideration the receptionist's tone and how your questions are answered. Find out how much time is allotted for appointments (30 to 45 minutes for a routine physical is average).

- Narrow the list to two or three physicians and make appointments for brief consultations. Be prepared to pay for this time.

- While visiting with each doctor, you should find answers to the following questions:

(continued)

- How often has the doctor performed this test, surgery, or procedure, and with what proportion of successful outcome?

- Are the risks from the treatment greater than the risks from the condition?

- What are the side effects of the diagnostic tests? Can these side effects be treated or reduced?

- Does this procedure require an overnight stay at a hospital or can it be performed in a doctor's office?

- Why has this test been ordered? What is the doctor trying to find or exclude?

- Is a second opinion necessary before my insurance company will pay the costs? If not, if I request a second opinion, will my insurance cover the cost?

- Are these medications necessary? What are their possible side effects? What will happen if I decide not to take them? What alternatives are available? Is there a generic version that costs less?

- Is the doctor's educational and experiential background appropriate?

- While visiting, do you feel that he or she cares about you as a person?

- Do you feel relaxed in his or her presence?

- Does he or she make you feel rushed?

- Are you encouraged to ask questions and are answers explained clearly?

- Does the physician use a lot of medical jargon, and how do you feel about that?

- Does the doctor use a condescending tone?

- Does the physician attend to you personally or does he or she serve primarily as a "gatekeeper" to specialists?

- Do the fees seem reasonable to you?

- Develop some direct questions about treatment that will help to identify the person's philosophy on care. For example, you could ask how the physician would treat a terminally ill patient or about his or her willingness to accommodate your religious feelings.

- Once you choose a physician, get the most from your visits by maintaining an open line of communication. You can do this by

  - always being prepared for an appointment. Know your medical and family history and be very specific and detailed about any symptoms you may be experiencing.

  - being an educated patient. Expect and insist on a diagnosis explained in a way that you fully understand. Never leave your doctor's office with questions unanswered.

  - taking a proactive role in your health care. Treatment will only work if you follow it. Listen to and follow instructions, find out when you can call with follow-up questions, and be sure that the doctor reports any test results to you promptly.

  - communicating your needs to the doctor. If you have concerns about his or her communication or treatment, speak up. If the response does not meet with your satisfaction, don't be afraid to find a new doctor.

- What caused me to have this problem? What can I do to make sure it doesn't happen again?

*W*HAT DO YOU THINK?

Have you ever brought a list of questions to your practitioner's office? If you have, were your questions answered fully? Did you feel at all intimidated or rushed? Do you think patients have the right to question their practitioners' judgment or should they turn over responsibility to the practitioner?

Other Forms of Allopathic Specialties

Although Table 24.1 provides an overview of common sources of health care, it is by no means all-inclusive. Other specialists include **osteopaths,** general practitioners who receive training similar to a medical doctor's but who put special emphasis on the skeletal and muscular systems. Their treatments may involve manipulation of the muscles and joints. Osteopaths receive the degree of doctor of osteopathy (D.O.) rather than doctor of medicine (M.D.).

Much confusion exists about the roles of optometrists and ophthalmologists. An **ophthalmologist** holds a medical degree and can perform surgery and prescribe medications. An **optometrist** typically evaluates visual problems and fits glasses but is not a trained physician. If

you have an eye infection, glaucoma, or other eye condition needing diagnosis and treatment, you need to see an ophthalmologist.

Dentists are specialists who diagnose and treat diseases of the teeth, gums, and oral cavity. They attend dental school for four years and receive the title of doctor of dental surgery (D.D.S.) or doctor of medical dentistry (D.M.D.). They must also pass both state and national board examinations before receiving their licenses to practice. The field of dentistry includes many specialties. For example, **orthodontists** are specialists in the align-

Osteopath: General practitioner who receives training similar to a medical doctor's but who puts special emphasis on the skeletal and muscular systems, often using spinal manipulation as part of treatment.

Ophthalmologist: Physician who specializes in the medical and surgical care of the eyes, including prescriptions of glasses.

Optometrist: Eye specialist whose practice is limited to prescribing and fitting lenses.

Dentist: Specialist who diagnoses and treats diseases of the teeth, gums, and oral cavity.

Orthodontist: Dentist who specializes in the alignment of teeth.

TABLE 24.1 ■ Medical/Health Professionals

Allergist	A specialist who diagnoses and treats allergies.	*Nuclear medicine specialist*	A specialist who uses radioactive substances to diagnose and treat various disorders.
Anesthesiologist	A specialist who administers drugs during surgical procedures to reduce pain or induce unconsciousness.	*Obstetrician/gynecologist (OB/GYN)*	A specialist who diagnoses and treats problems of the female reproductive system.
Cardiologist	A specialist in the diagnosis and treatment of heart and blood vessel disorders.	*Oncologist*	A specialist who diagnoses and treats cancerous growths and tumors.
Dermatologist	A specialist in the diagnosis and treatment of skin disorders.	*Ophthalmologist*	A specialist who diagnoses, treats, and provides general care of eye disorders.
Family practitioner	A physician who offers routine medical service for a variety of ailments.	*Orthopedist/orthopedic surgeon*	A specialist who diagnoses, treats, or provides surgical care for bone and joint injuries and problems.
Endocrinologist	A specialist in the diagnosis and treatment of glandular disorders.	*Otolaryngologist*	A specialist who specializes in ear, nose, and throat disorders.
Exercise physiologist	A specialist in the effects of exercise on the function of body systems (nonphysician).	*Pathologist*	A specialist who examines body organs, tissues, cells, and fluids to determine disease states.
Gastroenterologist	A specialist who diagnoses and treats disorders of the stomach and intestinal tract.	*Pediatrician*	A physician who treats childhood diseases.
Geneticist	A specialist who diagnoses and treats genetic diseases.	*Physical therapist*	A specialist who rehabilitates people after impairment due to injury or disease (nonphysician).
Health educator	A specialist in the field of health education and health promotion who holds a degree in a health-related area (nonphysician).	*Physician assistant*	Health-care professional trained to assist physicians.
Hematologist	A specialist who diagnoses and treats blood-related disorders.	*Plastic surgeon*	A specialist who provides corrective surgery for irregularities of body or facial contours.
Neurologist	A specialist who diagnoses and treats diseases of the brain, nervous system, and spinal cord.	*Psychiatrist*	A physician who diagnoses and treats mental and emotional disorders.
Neurosurgeon	A specialist who is similar to a neurologist but who specializes in surgery.	*Pulmonary specialist*	A specialist who diagnoses and treats disorders of the respiratory system.
Nurse practitioner	Nurse specialist with additional training in a specified area, such as OB/GYN.	*Urologist*	A specialist who diagnoses and treats disorders of the urinary tract.

ment of teeth. **Oral surgeons** perform surgical procedures to correct problems of the mouth, face, and jaw.

Many dental patients will actually spend more time with their dental hygienists than with their dentists. Dental hygienists are responsible for cleaning and polishing teeth, taking X-rays, and teaching preventive oral care.

A health care profession that has taken on vast responsibility in a changing health-care market is nursing.

Nurses are highly trained and strictly regulated health practitioners who provide a wide range of services for patients and their families, including patient education, counseling, community health and disease prevention information, and administration of medications. Although nurses may work in HMOs, clinics, doctors' offices, student health centers, nursing homes, public health departments, schools, businesses, and other health-care settings, about two-thirds are employed in the hospital setting. There has been an increasing trend away from hospital-based employment as the demand for nurses in other settings has increased.

Nurses may today choose from several training options. There are over 2.2 million licensed registered nurses (R.N.) in the United States who have completed either a four-year program leading to a bachelor of science in nursing (B.S.N.) degree or a two-year associate degree program. More than .5 million lower-level licensed practical or vocational nurses (L.P.N. or L.V.N) have completed a one- to two-year training program, which may have been community college-based or hospital-based.

Nurse practitioners (N.P.) are professional nurses having advanced training obtained through either a master's degree program or a specialized nurse practitioner program. Nurse practitioners have the training and authority to conduct diagnostic tests and prescribe medications (in some states). They work in a variety of settings, particularly in HMOs, clinics, and student health centers. They have become an increasingly popular source of health care in recent years and command excellent salaries in the fields of pediatrics, family health, and obstetrics and gynecology. Nurses may also earn the clinical doctor of nursing degree (N.D.) or a doctorate of nursing science (D.N.S. and D.N.Sc.), or a research-based Ph.D. in nursing.

Some 25,000 physician assistants (P.A.) currently practice in the United States. Most of these are in office-based practices, including school health centers, but approximately 40 percent practice in areas where physicians are in short supply. Studies have shown that this relatively new class of midlevel practitioners may competently care for 80 percent of those seeking primary care. All physician assistants must work under the supervision of a licensed physician, but 35 states do allow physician assistants to prescribe drugs.[5]

Nonallopathic Medicine

While people in other nations consider nonallopathic medicine the "traditional" form of treatment, in the United States we tend to think of **nonallopathic medicine** as "alternative medicine." According to the new Office of Alternative Medicine (OAM) in the National Institutes of Health, nonallopathic medicine includes any medical intervention that hasn't had sufficient documentation in the United States to show that it is safe and effective; that is

generally not taught in medical schools; and that generally is not reimbursed by third-party insurance. (The intent of the office is to facilitate the evaluation of alternative medical treatments for the purpose of determining their effectiveness and to help integrate effective treatment into mainstream medical practice. It is not, however, a referral agency. In order to achieve its goals, the OAM will sponsor research, conduct grant and clinical research workshops, perform field investigations, act as a clearing house, sponsor conferences and international programs, and collaborate with the NIH institutes and with government agencies.) As the government, private payers, and consumers have begun to evaluate the costs, effectiveness, and quality of traditional health care, many have found it wanting. Thus, each year more and more people seek nonallopathic or alternative medical care from providers other than licensed medical doctors. Many nonallopathic practitioners offer effective care at reasonable prices, but because they are not all licensed or regulated, the consumer's job of verifying credentials can be even more difficult than it is in traditional medicine.

There are numerous nonallopathic alternatives. Many people turn to nonallopathic medicine only after more traditional methods have failed to improve their conditions. Because they are often "providers of last resort," these unconventional treatments may appear to produce more negative outcomes overall than does traditional medicine. This has given them a bad reputation in some quarters even though it was the failure of traditional medicine that sent many patients to nonallopathic practitioners in the first place.

A recent study published in the *New England Journal of Medicine* revealed that one in three respondents reported using at least one unconventional therapy in the past year, ranging from relaxation, chiropractic, and massage to herbal medicine, homeopathy, and acupuncture.[6] Although some alternative therapies are controversial and even dangerous, many offer significant benefits at a relatively low cost (the average is $27.60 per visit). Nearly $14 billion per year is spent on unconventional services, with most of this cost paid by the patient. Still, this sum is less than 2 percent of what we as a nation spend on all health

Oral surgeon: Dentist who performs surgical procedures to correct problems of the mouth, jaw, and face.

Nurse: Health practitioner who provides many services for patients and who may work in a variety of settings.

Nonallopathic medicine: Medical alternatives to traditional, allopathic medicine.

services. Interestingly, the users of unconventional therapies tend to have above-average incomes and education.

As with any type of therapy, you must be assertive and directly ask providers of nonallopathic medicine about their training, licensing (if relevant to their field), and affiliations. You should also ask them how many patients suffering from your complaint they have treated. The greatest danger in seeking the assistance of an alternative medical practitioner is usually that it may keep you from obtaining more efficacious conventional treatment (if any is available for your complaint).

Chiropractic Treatment. **Chiropractic medicine** has been practiced for over 100 years. Allopathic medicine and chiropractic medicine were in direct competition over a century ago.[7] Once allopathic medicine became more formally organized and entrenched in society, state medical associations exerted their power to restrict the practice of chiropractors, even though there were not many empirical studies at the time proving the safety and efficacy of allopathic medicine. The relationship between medical doctors and doctors of chiropractic has improved since the settlement of a bitter lawsuit in which a group of chiropractors successfully argued that the American Medical Association (AMA) was conspiring to eliminate the practice of chiropractic in the United States.[8] Although there have always been some medical doctors who worked collaboratively with chiropractic doctors, their number has recently increased. Many insurance companies will now pay for chiropractic treatment if a medical doctor recommends it. More than 18 million Americans now visit chiropractors each year.

Chiropractic medicine is based on the idea that a life-giving energy flows through the spine via the nervous system. If the spine is subluxated (partly misaligned or dislocated), that force is disrupted. Chiropractors use a variety of techniques to manipulate the spine back into proper alignment so the life-giving energy can flow unimpeded through the nervous system. It has been established that their treatment is effective for chronic low back pain, neck pain, and headaches. In fact, a 1990 *British Medical Journal* article reported that chiropractors were more successful in treating certain types of chronic pain than traditional doctors were. Very recently, the National Institutes of Health released findings stating that chiropractic is the preferred treatment for back-related injuries and complaints.

The typical chiropractor has had the same number of hours of training and courses as has an allopathic non-specialized physician. The average chiropractic training

program requires six years of intensive courses in biochemistry, anatomy, physiology, diagnostics, pathology, nutrition, and so forth combined with hands-on clinical training. Moreover, many chiropractors continue their training to obtain specialization certification, for instance, in women's health, gerontology, or pediatrics. Like allopathic physicians, chiropractors are licensed and regulated by the states in which they practice. You should investigate and question a chiropractor as carefully as you would a licensed medical doctor. Be sure to ask whether the chiropractor uses such controversial and unproved practices as colonic flushes, herbal medications, and diet therapies or follows standard chiropractic regimens in treatment. As with many health professionals, you may note vast differences in technique among specialists.

Acupuncture. Acupuncture is the ancient (over 2,000 years old) Chinese art of inserting fine needles at points on the skin that fall along 14 major meridians, or pathways of energy (called *qi*), that flow through the body. These points and meridians are thought to be associated with particular internal organs and bodily functions. Proponents of acupuncture believe that the vital forces of life—the yin and the yang—are restored to equilibrium when these points are stimulated. In U.S. studies, acupuncture has proved effective for treating chronic pain and for blocking acute pain briefly.[9] Some 9 to 12 million visits to acupuncturists were made last year for complaints as diverse as back and neck pain, menstrual cramps, childbirth, morning sickness, addiction, asthma, infections, and arthritis.

Acupuncturists are state-licensed and each state has specific requirements regarding training programs. Most acupuncturists have either completed a two- to three-year postgraduate program to obtain a master of traditional Oriental medicine (M.T.O.M.) degree or attended a shorter certification program either here or in Asia. Acupuncturists may be licensed in multiple areas—for example, the M.T.O.M. is also trained in the use of herbs and moxabustion (the application of a heated herbal moxa stick). Some licensed M.D.s and chiropractors have trained in acupuncture and obtained certification to use this treatment. If you decide to have acupuncture, it is very important to ascertain whether the needles the acupuncturist uses are disposable or are properly sterilized using an autoclave because needles reused without proper sterilization can transmit the AIDS virus.

Acupressure is similar to acupuncture, but does not use needles. Instead, the practitioner applies pressure to points critical to balancing yin and yang. Practitioners must have the same basic understanding of energy pathways as do acupuncturists. Acupressure should not be applied to pregnant women or to anyone having a chronic condition by an untrained person.

Herbalists and Homeopaths. Herbalists practice herbal medicine, which is based on the medicinal qualities of

---

Chiropractic medicine: A form of medical treatment that emphasizes the manipulation of the spinal column.

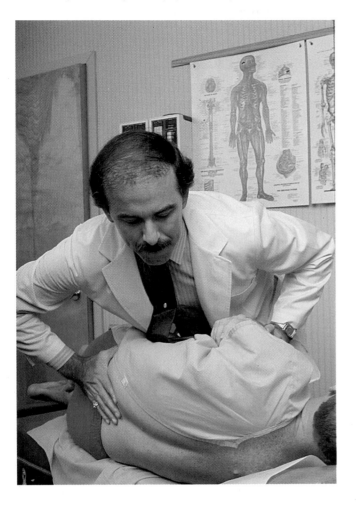

Consumers who choose unregulated forms of "alternative medicine" may be putting themselves at risk, but mandatory licensing of chiropractic and acupuncture practitioners assures consumers that standards for training and safety are being met.

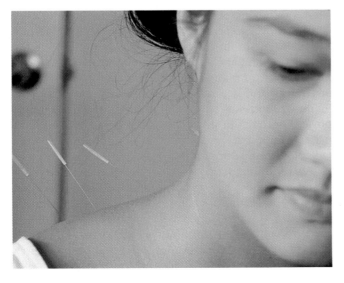

plants or herbs. Homeopaths also use herbal medicine (as well as minerals and chemicals), but at the root of their practice is the theory that the administration of extremely diluted doses of potent natural agents that produce disease symptoms in healthy persons will cure the disease in the sick. Herbal and homeopathic medicines are common in Europe and Asia, but are not nearly as accepted in the United States.

Although plants have been used for medicinal purposes for centuries and form the basis of many modern "wonder drugs," herbal medicine is not to be taken lightly. Because something is natural does not necessarily mean that it is safe. Many plants are poisonous, and others can be toxic if used in high doses. One of the greatest dangers with this kind of therapy is that practitioners who mix their own tonics do not use standardized measures. Regulation of commercially prepared herbal therapies is rather weak in the United States because they are considered foods rather than drugs, though the Food and Drug Administration is actively investigating claims made by manufacturers of herbal treatments for herpes and an herbal cleansing agent known as "colon clenz."

Some practitioners have received graduate-level training as herbalists in special programs such as herbal nutrition or traditional Oriental medicine. These practitioners have been trained in diagnosis; in mixing herbs, titrations, and dosages; and in the follow-up of patients. Unfortunately, a large number of unskilled people who do not fully understand the potential chemical interactions of their preparations are treating patients. It is therefore imperative that you carefully investigate the chemical properties of herbs yourself before you ingest them.

Naturopathy. Naturopaths believe that illness results from violations of natural principles of life in modern societies. They view diseases as the body's effort to ward off impurities and harmful substances from the environment. Naturopathic treatment uses substances and forces found in nature: water, magnets, gravity, heat, crystals and minerals, herbs, and even the sun. Practitioners argue that returning to a natural, purified state will restore health.

Although there is some validity to the belief that we could benefit from returning to a purer form of living, naturopaths often take this belief to extremes. For example, some naturopaths want to eliminate fluoridation of water and the addition of preservatives to foods, regardless of the benefits these practices have brought. Actually, bottled purified waters—a major component of some naturopathy—have not proved any safer than standard municipal water. In fact, few naturopathic claims have been substantiated. Although many naturopaths use the title "doctor," the vast majority are not M.D.s, and many have not even received a minimum of health training. Thorough training is provided at three naturopathic medical schools in the United States and Canada, and those who receive a naturopathic doctor (N.D.) degree from one of these schools have been through a four-year graduate program that emphasizes humanistically oriented family medicine. Still, the N.D. degree is not widely recognized. If you decide to be treated by a naturopath, you should be exceedingly careful about checking the practitioner's credentials.

Other Alternative Therapies. Many other therapies exist, including reflexology (zone therapy), iridology (light therapy), aromatherapy, and auramassage. Some of these may work, but they have yet to be substantiated scientifically. Others may be harmful to your health or delay you from seeking more efficacious forms of care. Until we can sort through the proliferation of new therapies, it's a good idea to follow the maxim "buyer beware."

*W*HAT DO YOU THINK?

Should people be allowed to choose any type of practitioner they want—regardless of whether the treatment they advocate has been proven safe or effective? How much should the government spend to investigate new or alternative therapies?

*H*EALTH-CARE AGENCIES, PROGRAMS, AND FACILITIES

Today many people are restricted in their choice of a health practitioner by their type of insurance coverage or lack of it. Selective contracting between insurers or employers and health providers has limited the freedom of choice that Americans used to enjoy. Two critical decisions you may have to make are (1) choosing an insurance carrier or type of plan (if you have a choice) and then (2) choosing the agency, program, or facility from which you will seek care. This section lists the most common choices.

Types of Medical Practices

In the highly competitive market for patients, many health-care providers have found it essential to combine resources into a **group practice,** which can be single- or multispecialty. Physicians share their offices, equipment, utility bills, and staff costs. Besides sharing costs, they may also share profits. Proponents of group practice maintain that it reduces unnecessary duplication of equipment and improves the quality of health care through peer review. Critics argue that group practice may limit competition and patients' access points to services.

Solo practitioners are medical providers who practice independently of other practitioners. It is hard for solo prac-

titioners to survive in today's high-cost, high-technology health-care market. Additionally, solo practitioners often have little time away from their offices, and have to trade on-call hours with other doctors. For these reasons, there are far fewer solo practices today than in the past. Most solo practitioners are doctors who established their practices years ago, have a specialty that's in high demand, or are in a rural or underserved area.

Hospitals and Clinics

Both hospitals and clinics provide a range of health-care services, including emergency treatment, diagnostic tests, and inpatient and outpatient (ambulatory) care. Your selection of a hospital or clinic will depend on your particular needs, your income, your insurance coverage, and the availability of services in your community. As the number of hospitals has decreased in recent years due to an oversupply of hospital beds, a decreasing need for inpatient care, and an increase in competition, the number of clinics has grown. In addition, we have witnessed a tremendous diversification and growth in what are known as integrated health networks. These networks run from groups of loosely affiliated health-service organizations and hospitals to HMOs that control their own very tightly joined hospitals, clinics, pharmacies, and even home health agencies.

There are several ways to classify hospitals: by profit status (nonprofit or for-profit), by ownership (private, city, county, state, federal), by specialty (children's, maternity, chronic care, psychiatric, general acute), by teaching status (teaching-affiliated or not), by size, and by whether they are part of a chain of hospitals. **Nonprofit (voluntary) hospitals** have traditionally been run by religious or other humanitarian groups. Earnings have generally been reinvested in the hospital for purposes of improving health care. These hospitals have often cared for patients whether they could pay or not.

The number of **for-profit (proprietary) hospitals** has been multiplying over the past two decades. Today they constitute over 15 percent of nongovernmental acute-care hospitals. For-profit hospitals, which do not receive tax breaks, provide far less charity care than do either nonprofit private or public hospitals.[10] Most for-profit hospitals quickly transfer indigent or uninsured patients either to public hospitals (hospitals that are heavily tax supported) or to nonprofit hospitals. This practice, known as patient dumping, was so brutal at times that in 1986 the federal government passed a law requiring that hospitals at least examine patients who arrive at their emergency rooms and medically stabilize them before transferring them to another hospital. In 1990, the federal government found it necessary to increase the fines for violations of the 1986 act because hospitals were ignoring the regulation. To get around the law, some for-profit hospitals now divert ambulances to other hospitals on Friday and Saturday nights (times when gunshot and stab wounds and accidents are most likely among the poor and uninsured) to minimize their number of uninsured and uncompensated cases.[11]

More treatments or services, including surgery, are being delivered on an **outpatient (ambulatory) care** basis (care which does not involve an overnight stay) by hospitals, traditional clinics, student health clinics, and nontraditional clinical centers. One type of ambulatory facility that is becoming common is the surgicenter—a place where minor, low-risk procedures such as vasectomies, tubal ligations, tissue biopsies, cosmetic surgery, abortions, and minor eye operations are performed. In 1982, nearly 85 percent of all surgeries in the United States involved an overnight hospital stay; by 1996, only 33 percent of surgeries will have done so.

To reduce the distance patients have to travel, many hospitals are locating satellite clinics in cities' outlying areas, sometimes in large shopping centers. A few hospitals have designated their satellites as freestanding emergency centers, or urgicenters, that function like hospital emergency rooms for uncomplicated immediate-care cases but have lower operating costs. Some consumers have begun to refer to these as "doc-in-the-box" centers.

Many hospitals and group practices now have freestanding imaging and diagnostic laboratory centers affiliated with them through either direct ownership or other profit-sharing arrangements. Significant debate surrounds this practice because research has found that when doctors own the diagnostic and laboratory services to which they refer patients, they tend to order an excessive number of tests.

Besides offering more convenient and more affordable services in a consumer-oriented environment, hospitals have also made efforts to improve the quality of care and patient outcomes. Many hospitals are now designated as trauma centers. They have helicopters available to transport patients to the hospital quickly, specialty physicians who are in-house (not just on-call) around-the-clock, and specialized diagnostic equipment. This combination of rapid transport and readily available specialty equipment and staff has dramatically reduced mortality rates for trauma patients. However, this same combination means that trauma centers are exceptionally expensive to run. In many areas, over half of all trauma patients are uninsured victims of gunshot or stabbing wounds or auto accidents who run up very large bills that go unpaid. These centers have therefore been facing extreme financial pressure.

The majority of health clinics was once located within hospitals. Today they are more likely to be independent facilities run by medical practitioners. Other health clinics are run by county health departments; these offer low-cost diagnosis and treatment for financially needy patients. Additionally, some 1,500 college campuses have student health centers that, along with county, city, or community clinics, supply low-cost family planning, sex-

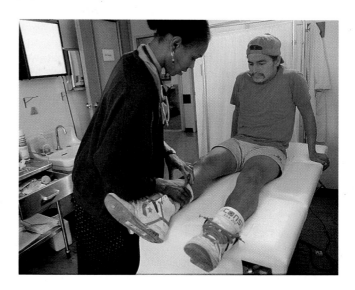

Students frequently turn to health centers, clinics, and hospital emergency rooms for treatment when needed, but those who rely solely on these settings miss out on the benefits of continuity of care by a primary care physician.

ually transmitted disease, gynecological, and vaccination services.

Consumers who are considering using a hospital or clinic should scrutinize the facility's accreditation. Accredited hospitals have met rigorous standards set by the Joint Commission on the Accreditation of Healthcare Organizations (JCAHO). If you use an institution having this form of accreditation, you have a high likelihood of obtaining quality care.

In December 1994, the JCAHO began offering performance report cards on 1,400 hospitals, nursing homes, clinics, surgical centers, home-care agencies, and mental

Group practice: A group of physicians who combine resources, sharing offices, equipment, and staff costs, to render care to patients.

Solo practitioner: Physician who renders care to patients independently of other practitioners.

Nonprofit (voluntary) hospitals: Hospitals run by religious or other humanitarian groups that reinvest their earnings in the hospital to improve health care.

For-profit (proprietary) hospitals: Hospitals that provide a return on earnings to the investors who own them.

Outpatient (ambulatory) care: Treatment that does not involve an overnight stay in a hospital.

health units. The reports, formerly kept secret, will be available for $30 each. Such reports will assist you in making side-by-side comparisons of different health-care facilities and providers by listing data on provider training, numbers of procedures, outcomes, and health status indicators of the populations they have served.[12]

Still, such information is sometimes hard for a consumer to evaluate. For example, during the early 1980s, a Boston-area hospital survey showed that Brigham and Women's Hospital had a cesarean birth rate that was markedly higher than other local hospitals'. Without further information, you may be led to believe that unnecessary cesareans were performed there. However, Brigham and Women's has a high-risk pregnancy obstetric unit and a neonatal intensive care unit that are among the best in the world. Its higher cesarean rate was thus due to the specialized populations that the hospital served.

𝒲HAT DO YOU THINK?

If you had access to a health-care report card for the hospitals in your area, would you try to switch your upcoming surgery to the hospital having the lowest complication and mortality rate? Have you ever checked on a doctor's or health-care facility's credentials or do you take it for granted that they are licensed, certified, or accredited?

𝒫ROMISES AND PROBLEMS OF OUR HEALTH-CARE SYSTEM

Ninety percent of Americans believe that our health-care system needs fundamental reform.[13] What are the problems that have brought us to this point? Cost, access, malpractice, unnecessary procedures, complicated and cumbersome insurance rules, and dramatic ranges in quality are the issues involved in typical criticisms. One of the most frequently voiced criticisms concerns lack of access to adequate health insurance: thirty percent of Americans report that someone in their household has remained in an undesirable job in order to avoid losing health benefits.[14] This phenomenon, known as job lock, affects the ability of the United States to employ workers in jobs that meet their skills and to remain competitive in the global economy.

Over 80 million people in the United States suffer from chronic health conditions that should be at least monitored by medical practitioners. Their access to care is largely determined by whether or not they have health insurance. Catastrophic or chronic illness in only 10 percent of the population accounts for 70 percent of all health expenditures. Since we cannot perfectly predict

Modern technology has vastly improved the techniques available for treating many illnesses and for saving human life, but it has also played a major role in the escalating costs of medical care now facing consumers.

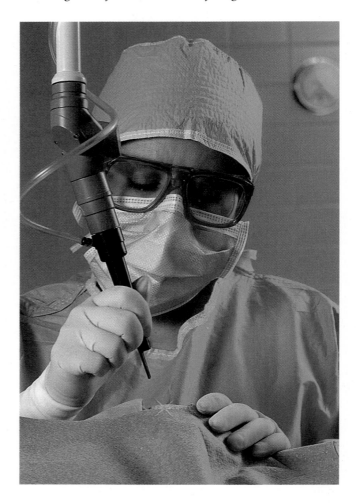

who will fall into that 10 percent, every American is potentially vulnerable to the high cost and devastating effects of such illnesses.

Cost

Both per capita and as a percent of gross domestic product (GDP), we spend more on health care than does any other nation, yet, unlike the rest of the industrialized world, we do not provide access for our entire population. In 1994, we spent approximately $1 trillion, or nearly 15 percent of our GDP on health care. This is up from 5 percent of GDP in 1960. There are a variety of theories as to why health-care costs continue to spiral upward. Most explanations are multifactorial and include at least the following: excess administrative costs, duplication of services, half-way technologies (keep people alive but don't cure them), an aging population, the technological imperative (because we have technology, we use it), an emphasis on crisis-oriented care instead of preventive care, inappropriate utilization of services by consumers (nonemergency care in emergency rooms cost $5 to 7 billion in 1993),[15] and inflationary reimbursement systems.

Our system has over 2,000 different health insurance companies, each requiring different procedures and forms. It is estimated that at least $280 billion is thrown away on administrative waste, unnecessary or even harmful care, and overpriced services.[16] Policy analysts have studied these problems for years, but the public is only starting to realize the breadth of the problem. Business is spending 61 percent of pretax profits and 108 percent of after-tax profits on health benefits for employees (compared to 20 and 36 percent, respectively, in 1970).[17] This huge expense is forcing companies to require employees to share more of the costs, to cut back on benefits, and to drop some benefits altogether. The remaining costs are largely passed on to consumers in the form of higher prices for goods and services. Figure 24.1 shows who pays for health care and into what parts of the health-care system the money goes.

Access

Your access to health care is determined by numerous factors, including the supply of providers and facilities, your health status, and your insurance coverage. Although there are 687,000 physicians in the United States, many Americans do not have adequate access to physician care or other health services because of insurance barriers or maldistribution of providers. Doctors are maldistributed by specialty and geographic area. There is an oversupply of higher-paid specialists and a shortage of lower-paid primary care physicians (family practitioners, pediatricians, internists, OB/GYNs, gerontologists). Inner cities and some rural areas face constant shortages of physicians. Subsidized community and public health clinics (sometimes mistakenly called free clinics), family planning clinics, and the 1,500 student health centers are estimated to provide sporadic care for nearly one-fifth of our population. Yet, while better than no care, these often leave large gaps in both service type and provider continuity. And even if you live in an area having an adequate supply of providers, you have no guarantee of access because other factors play a major role in whether or not you obtain care.

Quality and Malpractice

The U.S. health-care system employs several mechanisms for assuring quality services overall: education, licensure, certification/registration, accreditation, peer review, and, as a last resort, the legal system of malpractice litigation.

Some of these mechanisms are mandatory before a professional or organization may provide care, while others are purely voluntary. (Consumers should note that licensure, although state mandated for some practitioners and facilities, is only a minimum guarantee of quality.) Insurance companies and government payers may also require a higher level of quality by linking payment to whether a practitioner is board certified or a facility is accredited by the appropriate agency. In addition, most insurance plans now require prior authorization and/or second opinions as means not only to reduce costs also to but improve quality of care.

Many people believe that malpractice is a leading cause of our health-care crisis. Yet the U.S. Department of Health and Human Services estimates that the total cost of malpractice is less than 1 percent of total health outlays. However, these figures do not account for the previously

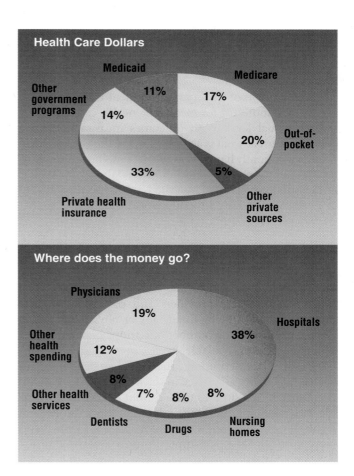

FIGURE 24.1

The charts measure how we spend our health-care dollar.

Source: Adapted from K. R. Levit, H. C. Lazenby, C. A. Cowan, and S. W. Letch, "National Health Care Expenditures, 1990," *Health Care Financing Review* 13, no. 1 (Fall 1991): 29–54; published by the U.S. Department of Health and Human Services, Health Care Financing Administration.

described practice of "defensive medicine." Defensive medicine not only costs money and places patients at additional risk, it has also changed the standards of care in that people have come to expect these extra, but unnecessary, tests and procedures.

Consumer, provider, and advocacy groups have begun to focus on the great variation in quality as a main problem in our health-care system. Although we are still relatively unsophisticated at measuring the quality of medical care, our measures are improving. Two of the most commonly used measures at the population level are infant mortality rates and life expectancy. Infant mortality rates are stated as a ratio of number of deaths of children under one year of age to number of live births. These rates permit an overall quick assessment of maternal nutrition, prenatal health, and prevalence of infant disease. Life expectancy rates provide a rough indication of how a society's lifestyle and medical care factors affect its population's health. Currently, 17 countries have lower infant mortality rates than the United States and 11 countries have higher average life expectancies. The Multicultural Perspectives box takes a look at how U.S. health care stacks up against the world.

A newer form of quality measurement uses "outcome" as the main indicator for measuring health-care quality at the individual level. With outcomes measurements, we don't look just at what is actually done to the patient but at what subsequently happens to the patient's health status or health condition. Thus, mortality rates and complication rates (such as infections) become very important statistics in assessing individual practitioners and facilities.

Detecting Fraud and Abuse in the System

Becoming knowledgeable and acting responsibly when selecting health-care providers and payers will reduce your likelihood of being financially or physically abused. Nevertheless, with the number of options in health products and services available, even the most careful consumer can be victimized. Individual states maintain boards for quality assurance in the medical system. If you find yourself in a situation you cannot deal with, remember that the Food and Drug Administration, the Federal Trade Commission, the Centers for Disease Control and Prevention, and the Consumer Product Safety Commission are responsible for protecting you and other health consumers. Unfortunately, due to their downsizing during the 1980s and early 1990s, when there was an overall deemphasis on government regulation, these agencies are often overwhelmed with complaints. But it is still their job to protect citizens from unscrupulous and ignorant health practitioners and businesses, so do not hesitate to contact them if you have suspicions about a provider, service, or product.

WHAT DO YOU THINK?

Do you believe prospective patients should have access to information about practitioners' and facilities' malpractice experience? How about their success and failure rates or outcomes of various procedures?

HEALTH INSURANCE

Insurance is built around the concept of spreading risks among a large, diverse group of people. Policyholders pay into a pool, which fills with reserves until needed. When you are sick or injured, the insurance company pays out of the pool, regardless of your total amount of contribution. For example, one of the editors who worked on this book and his wife paid premiums to an HMO for 10 years. During this time, they had only minor medical bills. However, the premature birth of their child ran up bills of over $75,000, which was substantially more than they had paid in premiums. But the HMO covered the full amount. Depending on circumstances, you may never pay for what your medical care costs or you may pay much more for insurance than your medical bills ever total. The idea is that you pay in affordable premiums so that you never have to face catastrophic bills.

Unfortunately, not everyone has health insurance. Almost 40 million Americans are uninsured at any given point in time—that is, they have no private health insurance and are not eligible for Medicare, Medicaid, or any other health program that would cover the cost of their care. The number of the uninsured has been growing since the late 1970s.[18] People lacking any type of health insurance make up nearly 17 percent of the nonelderly population, or 15 percent of the total population. Another 20 to 40 million Americans are estimated to be underinsured (at risk for spending more than 10 percent of their income on medical care because their insurance is inadequate).[19]

Contrary to the common belief that the uninsured are unemployed, 75 percent of the uninsured are either workers or the dependents of workers. One-quarter of all the uninsured are children under the age of 16. College students are one of the largest groups of the uninsured not in the labor force. This presents a difficult dilemma for both universities and students when they must seek care because most university insurance plans are designed as short-term, noncatastrophic plans having low upper limits of benefits. As a full-time student, you should consider purchasing a higher level catastrophic plan to protect yourself in the event of a rare, but very costly, illness or accident.

For the uninsured and many of the underinsured, health care may not be available through any source be-

How Good Is U.S. Health Care?

...Americans fervently believe that the U.S. has the best health care in the world. But we all need to be aware of the data in the accompanying tables, which show that in fact we have a lot of catching up to do with other nations.

If Americans get the best health care in the world, that is not reflected in our average life expectancy, which ranks behind 17 other nations. Life expectancy is not solely a function of health care, of course; factors like diet and highway fatalities push a nation's average up or down. But it is widely accepted as the best proxy....

Even though the U.S. is the world's richest nation in terms of real gross domestic product per person, we can expect shorter lives than nations with a total population of 450 million....Yet all these countries manage to spend considerably less on health care than we do. The average health expenditure per person in the 21 other nations was $1,603 a year in 1991; in the U.S. it was $2,932. Multiply the difference, $1,329, by our population of 250 million, and the total comes to $330 billion a year—a third of our total health care bill.

Why do we spend so much for less service and shorter life expectancy? A big part of the explanation is overhead, inefficiency, waste and even outright fraud. The insurance industry dominates health care in the U.S. as it does in no other country. The administrative cost of health care in this country is about 25 percent; in Canada it is about 10 percent. Average U.S. insurance company overhead is 14 percent—more than three times the overhead for Medicare and Medicaid, our much-maligned Government health programs for the elderly, poor and disabled....

Life Span, Health, and Wealth

Countries in Order of Life Expectancy	Life Expectancy at Birth, 1992, in Years	Population in Millions, 1992	Real G.D.P. per Capita, 1991	Total Expenditure on Health, % of G.D.P.	Expenditure on Health per Capita, 1991
1 Japan	78.6	124.5	$19,390	6.8	$1,771
4 Sweden	77.7	8.6	17,490	8.8	2,372
5 Spain	77.4	39.1	12,670	6.5	877
6 Greece	77.3	10.2	7,680	4.8	274
7 Canada	77.2	27.4	19,320	9.9	1,847
8 Netherlands	77.2	15.2	16,820	8.7	1,664
11 Australia	76.7	17.6	16,680	8.6	1,466
12 France	76.6	57.1	18,430	9.1	1,912
13 Israel	76.2	5.1	13,460	4.2	509
14 U.K.	75.8	57.7	16,340	6.6	1,003
17 Germany	75.6	80.2	19,770	9.1	1,782
18 U.S.	75.6	255.2	22,330	13.3	2,932
22 Ireland	75.0	3.5	11,430	8.0	886

Sources: U.N. Development Program; Organization for Economic Cooperation and Development.

Source: Excerpted from Paul Spector, "Failure, by the Numbers," *New York Times,* 24 September 1994, 19. © 1994 by The New York Times Company. Reprinted by permission. Information in table, titled "Lifespan, Health and Wealth," from U.N. Development Program; Organization for Economic Cooperation and Development.

cause of their inability to pay. Many either will not or cannot seek care from charitable providers, so they fail to receive the medical care they need. People without health-care coverage are less likely than other Americans to have their children immunized, to seek early prenatal care, to obtain annual blood pressure checks, and to seek care for serious symptoms of illness. Many experts believe that this ultimately leads to higher system costs because the conditions of these people deteriorate to a more debilitating and costly stage before they are forced to seek help.

Early Private Health Insurance

Our current health system began in the last century and its growth accelerated in the post-World War II era to its current massive, complex web. Hospitals became the engines of medicine during the middle of this century. Doctors became the drivers or conductors of this rapidly moving system. The system was fueled by a variety of funding sources but, chiefly, first by the growth of tax-exempt nonprofit private insurance companies established in the 1940s and later by the growth of for-profit insurance companies.

Health insurance originally consisted solely of coverage for hospital costs (it was called major medical), but gradually coverage was extended to routine physicians' treatment and to other areas such as dental services and pharmaceuticals. Payment mechanisms used until recently laid the groundwork for the ever-rising health-care costs of today. Hospitals were reimbursed on a cost-plus basis after services were rendered. That is, they billed for the costs of providing care plus an amount for profit. This system provided no incentive to contain costs, limit the number of procedures, or curtail capital investment in redundant equipment and facilities. Physicians were reimbursed on a fee-for-service basis determined by "usual, customary, and reasonable" fees. These were arrived at by comparing what a doctor charged for a service with what that same doctor charged last year for the service and with what other doctors in the area were charging. This system encouraged doctors to charge high fees, to raise them often, and to perform as many procedures or services as

Medicare: Federal health insurance program for the elderly and the permanently disabled.

Medicaid: Federal-state health insurance program for the poor.

Diagnosis related groups (DRGs): Diagnostic categories established by the federal government to determine in advance how much hospitals will be reimbursed for the care of a particular Medicare patient.

Resource-based relative value scale (RBRVS): A system established by the federal government that uses physician work, practice expense, and practice risk to determine in advance how much a physician will be reimbursed for the care of a particular Medicare patient.

Managed care: Cost-control procedures used by health insurers to coordinate treatment.

possible. At the same time, because most insurance did not cover routine or preventive services, consumers were encouraged to use hospitals whenever possible (the coverage was better) and to wait until illness developed to seek care instead of seeking preventive care. Consumers were also free to choose any provider or service they wished, including even inappropriate—and often very expensive—levels of care.

Private insurance companies have increasingly employed several mechanisms to control consumers' use of insurance and to limit the companies' potential losses. These mechanisms include cost-sharing (in the form of deductibles, copayments, and coinsurance), exclusions, "preexisting condition" clauses, waiting periods, and upper limits on payments. Deductibles are front-end payments (commonly $250 to $1,000) that you must make to your provider before your insurance company will start paying for any services you use. Copayments are set amounts that you pay per service received regardless of the cost of the services (e.g., $5 per doctor visit or $10 per prescription). Coinsurance is the percentage of the bill that you must pay throughout the course of treatment (e.g., 20 percent of whatever the total is). Preexisting condition clauses limit the insurance company's liability for medical conditions that a consumer had before obtaining insurance coverage (i.e., the insurance company will cover everything except "normal pregnancy" for a woman who takes out coverage when she is pregnant; however, pregnancy complications and infant care are covered). Because many insurance companies use a combination of these mechanisms, keeping track of the portion of costs you are responsible for can become very difficult.

Group plans of large employers (government agencies, school districts, or corporations, for example) generally do not have preexisting condition clauses in their plans. But smaller group plans (a group may be as small as two) often do.[20] Some plans will never cover services for preexisting conditions, while others specify a waiting period (such as six months) before they will provide coverage. All insurers set some limits on the types of services they will cover (e.g., most exclude cosmetic surgery, private rooms, and experimental procedures). Some insurance plans may also include an upper or lifetime limit, after which your coverage will end. Although $250,000 many seem like an enormous sum, medical bills for a sick child or chronic disease can easily run this high within a few years.

Medicare and Medicaid (Social Insurance versus Welfare)

After years of debate about whether we should have a national health program like those of most other industrialized countries, the U.S. government directed the system toward a less-than-universal mixed private and public approach in the 1960s. Most Americans obtained their health insurance through their employers. But this meant that two groups—the nonworking poor and the aged—were left out. To take care of these groups, in 1965 Medicare and Medicaid were established by amendments to the 1935 Social Security Act. Although enacted simultaneously, these programs were vastly different. **Medicare,** basically a federal social insurance covering 99 percent of the elderly over 65 years of age, all totally and permanently disabled people (after a waiting period), and all people with end-stage renal failure, is a universal program that covers a broad range of services except long-term care and pharmaceuticals. It currently covers 36 million people. Medicare is widely accepted by physicians and hospitals and has relatively low administrative costs.

On the other hand, **Medicaid,** covering approximately 35 million people, is a federal-state matching-funds welfare program for the categorically eligible poor (blind, disabled, aged, or receiving Aid to Families with Dependent Children). Because each state determines income eligibility levels and payments to providers, there are vast differences in the way Medicaid operates from state to state. Medicaid insurance is not widely accepted by providers because of its administrative difficulties, its slow and low payments, and the stigma attached to the program and its recipients. Medicaid currently covers less than half of all poor people in this country and very few of the working poor. Medicaid gives many people the incentive to stay on welfare because those who go to work usually lose their coverage, and the kinds of jobs they can get often provide no health insurance. Among Medicaid's many problems, then, is its failure to achieve its original goal of "mainstreaming the poor."

In order to control hospital costs, beginning in 1983 the federal government set up a prospective payment system based on **diagnosis related groups (DRGs)** for Medicare. Using a complicated formula, nearly 500 groupings of diagnoses were created to establish in advance how much a hospital would be reimbursed for a particular patient. If a hospital can treat the patient for less than that amount, it can keep the difference. However, if a patient's care costs more than the set amount, the hospital must absorb the difference (with a few exceptions that must be reviewed by a panel). This system gives hospitals the incentive to discharge patients quickly after doing as little as possible for them, to provide more ambulatory care, and to admit only patients with favorable (profitable) DRGs. Many private health insurance companies have followed the federal government in adopting this type of reimbursement. In 1992, the federal government also began basing payments to physicians who treat Medicare patients on a prospectively determined fee scale in order to control costs and to shrink the payment disparity between specialists and primary care physicians. This system, known as the **resource-based relative value scale (RBRVS)**/Medicare Fee Scale (**MFS**), uses physician work, practice expense, and practice risk (including malpractice costs), to set payments for physicians. Under RBRVS/MFS, Medicare payments to some specialists (pathologists, radiologists, thoracic surgeons, and cardiovascular surgeons) were reduced by as much as 25 to 45 percent, while payments to other doctors (family practitioners, internists, and immunologists) were raised by 20 to 50 percent. Two Blue Shield plans (in Oregon and Minnesota) have already adopted a modified version of the RBRVS/MFS, and more private insurance companies have promised to follow suit.

Last year, all levels of government combined paid 42 percent of our total health-care bill. We have now reached the point where we can no longer say that we have a truly private system—we have a mixed pluralistic system. The private health insurance market has also changed dramatically since its inception over half a century ago. See Figure 24.2 for a comparison of public/private systems among the industrialized nations.

Managed Care: New Types of Health-Care Delivery

The past 25 years have witnessed a dramatic change not only in the financing of health care, but also in the organization and delivery patterns of that care. Traditionally, insurance was not supposed to influence how care was provided. However, through a system known as **managed care,** insurance companies determine not only whether you get care, but also where, how much, and by whom. Health maintenance organizations, preferred provider organizations, and exclusive provider organizations as well as fee-for-service plans that use techniques of utilization review are all examples of managed care plans. Under managed care, your health insurance company uses various cost-control procedures to coordinate your health care. It is estimated that 88 percent of our health plans are now controlled by some form of managed care system.[21] This percentage includes privately insured, as well as people with Medicare and Medicaid coverage. Students and people that travel for a living or for a significant portion of the year, need to verify what their "out-of-area" eligibility would be under different managed care plans. The Choices for Change box discusses the move toward managed care.

Health Maintenance Organizations (HMOs). In 1973, the federal government passed the HMO Act to encourage enrollment in HMOs. Today, nearly 45 million people are enrolled in approximately 600 HMOs. An HMO is an organized health-care system that provides both financing for and delivery of comprehensive services to an enrolled population for a fixed, prepaid fee. Although virtually all HMOs employ primary care practitioners as gatekeepers to specialist care, the way they pay providers

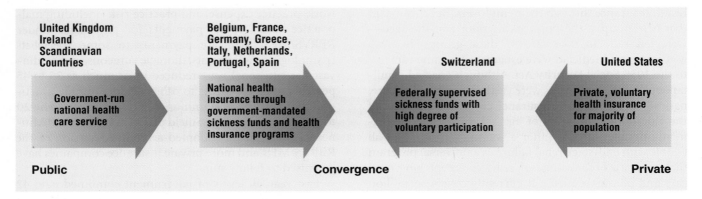

FIGURE 24.2

The Convergence of Public/Private Health-Care Systems

Source: Reprinted with permission from "European Health Issues," by Gunter Becher, which appeared in the March 1993 issue of *Employee Benefits Journal,* 38, published by the International Foundation of Employee Benefit Plans, Brookfield, WI.

can vary: some pay salaries, some pay capitation (per enrollee) fees, while some pay by fee-for-service. Research has demonstrated that HMOs save between 10 and 40 percent of traditional fee-for-service costs by providing more preventive services, more ambulatory care, and less hospitalization. The key principles of HMO management are:

■ reduced consumer administrative requirements

■ reduced utilization of services, especially of inpatient services

■ broader benefit structure, especially for preventive services

■ enhanced provider risk-sharing

■ greater management control over providers and consumers

Preferred Provider Organizations (PPOs). Patients enrolled in a preferred provider organization are given a list of "preferred providers" from which to choose practitioners. If they use these practitioners, they are reimbursed at a higher rate than if they choose to "go out of plan" and use nonpreferred providers. For example, the patient who uses a physician listed by the PPO may be reimbursed for 90 percent of the cost of services, while one who uses a nonlisted doctor may be reimbursed for only 60 percent. Physicians who belong to a PPO are reimbursed on a discounted fee-for-service basis, usually after agreeing to some form of utilization review, and may also treat non-PPO patients. Research has not demonstrated that PPOs are successful at containing costs, probably because many doctors arrange more follow-up visits than necessary to compensate for their discounted fees and because most

preferred provider plans do not exercise control over practice patterns and facilities.

*W*HAT DO YOU THINK?

Why is it important that private insurance cover preventive or lower-level care as well as hospitalization and high-technology interventions? What kinds of incentives cause you to seek early care rather than to delay care?

What Are the Options?

The United States and South Africa are currently the only industrialized nations that do not have a national health program that guarantees all citizens access to at least a basic set of health benefits. The United States has seen four major political movements supporting national health insurance during this century, but none has succeeded. Whether universal coverage will—or should—be achieved soon and through what mechanism are hotly debated topics. Many analysts believe that the recent push for health-care reform failed due to a combination of circumstances and influences: lobbying efforts by the insurance industry and the medical community; a proposed plan that was too complicated; and interest groups who felt that the plan either went "too far" or "not far enough." But some people also believe that our current system serves people well, as seen in the Health Headlines box.

One critical point must be made, though, and that is that we are paying for the most expensive system in the world without obtaining full coverage. We pay for people who don't have insurance through cost shifting that increases our premiums and taxes, and we are paying more than necessary because prevention and early treatment in

The Move to Managed Care

Over the past few years, health-care reform has been a major topic of discussion in legislative bodies, homes, and corporate board rooms. Americans have suddenly become familiar with terms such as *single payer, managed competition,* and *managed care.* While all the discussion in Washington has resulted in little legal reform, a ground swell of change has occurred. Due primarily to pressure from corporations to restrict the costs of fee-for-service medicine, this change is largely the product of a movement toward managed care.

Managed care means simply that, for a prepaid amount, a circle or network of providers manages your care. Such networks include health maintenance organizations (HMOs) and preferred provider organizations (PPOs). Managed care is designed to increase the cost-effectiveness of medical care. Under these plans, all care must be regulated by a "gatekeeper," the primary-care physician. Patients are prohibited from seeking out the services of a specialist who is not part of their managed care plan unless they are willing to pay some or all of that doctor's fee directly.

The health-care system is still in flux. Many insurance companies are initiating their own changes rather than waiting for directives from the federal government. Many companies are offering a greater selection of health-care plans, and sometime overseeing managed care plans, to demonstrate to their employees their companies' flexibility and willingness to provide more efficient service. Insurance companies are also streamlining their administration processes to better meet the needs of their clients.

The movement toward managed care is also affecting teaching hospitals across the nation. As a result, many of these hospitals have been teaming with local facilities and groups to create integrated networks that often include teaching and community hospitals, community clinics, nursing homes, and home health-care agencies.

What does all this mean for you, the health-care consumer? It means that you must do careful homework prior to selecting your health-care plan. The key to getting the most from your plan is knowing how it works and how to use it to obtain the greatest benefits.

- Choose your plan wisely. Read all the information provided carefully. If choosing among several plans, compare the information. Consider several hypothetical health-care situations and investigate which plan would best meet your needs in those situations. Health-care plans vary a great deal in their provisions for services such as mental health care, physical therapy, and preventive measures such as fitness programs. Some include provisions for vision care. The plan having the lowest copayments may not be the least expensive in the long run.

- Select your physician carefully. Remember, this person is your gatekeeper to all health services. Consider her or his location and hospital affiliation among other factors.

- See your physician soon. The sooner you meet with your physician for a general physical and meeting, the sooner you can begin your own wellness efforts.

- Read the rules of your plan. All managed care plans have guidelines that you must follow. Know what is expected of you.

- Take advantage of wellness incentives offered by your plan. Many HMOs and other managed care organizations (MCOs) offer programs designed to encourage the prevention of illness, such as smoking cessation classes, first-aid training, nutrition education, and reduced rates for membership in fitness programs.

appropriate settings are not emphasized. We also pay for much duplication of services and technologies, for practitioners who practice defensive medicine and who refer patients to their own diagnostic labs for profit reasons, and for the vast bureaucracy made inevitable by having over 1,500 private health insurance companies.

Several basic models of health-care reform, having infinite variations, can be—and have been—drawn up depending on: comprehensiveness of benefits; proportion of the population covered; financing and payment mechanisms; quality assurance and improvement measures; cost-control features; and the level at which these measures are attempted (federal, state, or local government or private enterprise). The most modest current proposals call for reforming the private insurance industry by simplifying administrative procedures and changing tax codes

to create different incentives. The most radical call for eliminating, or severely curtailing, the role of private insurers and instituting a system of universal, government-administered insurance, like that at work in Canada.

The managed competition model proposed by the Clinton administration was essentially based on an employer mandate whereby employers and the major insurance companies would still play a central role. This had appeal for those who don't wish to change the structure of the system radically or to place a great deal of power in the hands of one institution but do want to do more than merely provide incentives through the tax system. It did not appeal to those who believe that a system based on competition actually fuels costs and increases the emphasis on high technology while leaving the sickest and poorest at a severe disadvantage.

Another Side to the Health-Care Crisis

The following opinion piece from the Wall Street Journal *is written by Leslie Kaufmann, based on a 1994 study she prepared on this subject for the Alexis de Tocqueville Institution. As it shows, a number of the highly touted cases of insurance discrimination that fueled the fire of the health-care reform in 1993–1994 were actually able to resolve themselves without government intervention.*

Since announcing their health plan [in] September [1993], President Clinton and the first lady have toured the country listening to stories of hardship. They have also staged events, inviting people to various forums and town meetings to describe their experiences under the current system. Most of these folks have told variations on a single story: They "played by the rules" but got a raw deal from the insurance companies and from current government programs.

In hours of phone interviews, I have looked into more than a dozen of these cases. The most affecting of them involve people with extreme medical needs—victims, for example, of stroke or cerebral palsy. Such cases evoke sympathy less for how they are handled under the current system than for the conditions themselves, which no amount of reform can undo.

More complex are the stories intended to demonstrate the arbitrariness and inadequacy of the current system for average people with less extraordinary medical needs. Here there are some surprises. A number of the cases were resolved just months after being presented at the White House. Others look less like genuine problems on further investigation.

Take, to begin with, the question of the uninsurability of individuals with pre-existing conditions. Last September, the Clintons invited Margie Silverman, a retiree from Florida, to speak at a Rose Garden event. Mrs. Silverman's daughter "Jane," a 27-year-old teacher in California, had recently undergone a radical hysterectomy. The daughter was insured by Kaiser Permanente and wanted to move back to Florida after her surgery to be near her family. She was constrained, however, by the terms of her insurance coverage: Kaiser Permanente, an HMO, will only treat its patients in its own facilities and has none in Southern Florida. Mrs. Silverman tearfully told the president that because no other company would insure her daughter with a pre-existing condition, the family was being separated when they most needed to be together.

As it turns out, though, the Silvermans quickly found a solution to Jane's problems. The school district in Dade County, Fla., like many big employers, insures even those workers with pre-existing conditions. Less than six months after her mother's White House visit, Jane had moved to Florida, found a job in her field and become fully insured.

Suzy Somers, an independent businesswoman recovering from breast cancer, also told her story in the Rose Garden. Ms. Somers was insured by Prudential through her ex-husband's company when she was told she had cancer.

Her policy paid for her treatment, which included a mastectomy, breast reconstruction, and chemotherapy. Soon after she went into remission, however, her ex-husband's company went bankrupt. She then discovered that because of certain misrepresentations her husband had made to Prudential, her policy was being canceled. Moreover, these earlier questionable dealings deprived her of continuing coverage under COBRA, a law that normally allows people to stay on their employer's policy for 18 months if they pay the full premiums.

Ms. Somers explained to a sympathetic president that she then began a long, fruitless search for insurance: No one would consider accepting her until her cancer had been in remission for at least two years. Ms. Somers ended her presentation with these chilling words: "I would like you to know that my insurance situation remains the same, and last week I found another lump."

When I caught up with Ms. Somers four months after her White House visit, however, her problems had been resolved. First, the lump was benign. Second, she now had full insurance coverage. Blue Cross/Blue Shield had issued her a comprehensive policy at the incredibly low cost of $400 a quarter. Why did the insurance mammoth volunteer to take on such a high-risk case? "My understanding," says Ms. Somers, "is that they have had a lot of lawsuits against them involving preexisting conditions, and they just don't want to fight it anymore."

Another priority much touted by the Clintons is the need to include mental health care in any standard benefits package. When the president introduced his plan last fall, Karen Nangle was invited to the White House to tell the story of her 28-year-old daughter, Jocelyn. When Jocelyn was 16 she was diagnosed as having severe clinical depression. The costs for her medicine and therapy sessions amounted to tens of thousands of dollars a year, significantly more than was covered by the family's insurance. Eventually the Nangles, financially exhausted by their efforts, decided to retire, and Jocelyn was granted Supplementary Security Income and Medicaid coverage.

Unfortunately, the two doctors who had been working with Jocelyn—one at home in Connecticut, the other at school in Massachusetts—were not covered under Medicaid's rules. Mrs. Nangle protested the injustice of this system to the Clintons. "There is no way to describe . . . the humiliation of having to apply for assistance only to find that it is hamstringing," she told the president.

As it turns out, however, soon after her mother's trip to the White House, Jocelyn Nangle also received clearance for coverage under Medicare. Medicare, unlike Medicaid, will pay for out-of-state doctors, so Jocelyn can now see her Connecticut doctor on the government's tab. It is true that her doctor in Massachusetts was turned down as a caregiver,

(continued)

but only because a well-known specialist in chemical depression, a doctor approved by Medicaid, also practices in the area. In short, while the Nangles may not have exactly what they want from the current system, they are far from "hamstrung."

The president claims that health care reform is necessary because current medical costs are destroying the finances of many American families. To illustrate his point, he told the story of Richard Anderson in his first State of the Union address.

A few years ago Mr. Anderson was working as a parts salesman at a car dealership in Reno, Nev., where he had health-insurance coverage for himself and his wife at a cost of just over $40 a month. Then, as the president described it, Mr. Anderson "lost his job and, with it, his health insurance. Two weeks later, his wife, Judy, suffered a cerebral aneurysm. He rushed her to the hospital, where she stayed in intensive care for 21 days; the Andersons' bills were over $120,000. Although Judy recovered and Richard went back to work, the bills were too much for them and they were literally forced into bankruptcy."

The actual course of events is considerably more complicated. First, despite being fired, Mr. Anderson had the option of continuing his health insurance through COBRA. His wife was still employed, but they decided that they could not afford the investment of $240 a month even temporarily while he looked for another job. Even without insurance,

the Andersons agree that Judy got excellent care during her emergency.

Moreover, they weren't exactly "forced into bankruptcy." Washoe Medical Center maintains a fund to reimburse hardship patients. Families earning up to 150% of the poverty line can apply for a 50% reduction in the bill and set up a long-term payment plan for the rest. According to Washoe records, the Anderson were sent two applications for the fund, but they failed to use them. They chose bankruptcy instead because it was the least costly of their options and, as an added benefit, wiped out their consumer debts with J.C. Penney and MasterCard.

If the cases chosen by the Clintons are at all representative, they paint a picture very different from the one intended. They certainly don't point to a national health care crisis. Rather, they show a current system that despite its size, diversity and unwieldiness remains responsive to public pressures. Moreover, they suggest that the current system, whatever its imperfections, still serves most Americans quite well, even those with problems that seemed so hopeless when told to the president in the Rose Garden.

Source: Reprinted from Leslie Kaufman, "Crocodile Tears," *The Wall Street Journal*, 7 June 1994. Reprinted by permission of the *Wall Street Journal*. © 1994 Dow Jones & Company, Inc. All rights reserved worldwide.

Another proposal involves the federalization and incremental expansion of Medicaid. The idea is to eliminate state disparities and improve coverage gradually through progressive general tax financing. First would come federalization of Medicaid eligibility, benefits, and reimbursement to improve access for those determined eligible. Next would come a step-by-step expansion raising the age limits for children, then covering all pregnant women, then allowing "intact" poor families to obtain coverage, then increasing the income limit to incorporate the uninsured near-poor, and finally allowing the middle class to buy into the program. This type of plan could work well if reimbursements were set high enough to encourage provider participation. But it would take a long time to provide universal coverage, and it is not a likely option at this time.

Either managed competition/employer mandate or Medicaid expansion could evolve into a single-payer, tax-financed scheme that severs insurance ties from employment. This type of health insurance mechanism, perhaps similar to the Canadian model, would cover everyone—regardless of income or other factors such as health status. Even under this plan, there would be many different ways to tailor a plan specifically to the needs of the U.S. citi-

zenry. A single federal plan or a privately administered plan paid for by general tax funds or earmarked taxes could be created. Thus, all (or most) private insurers would be eliminated or would see their role limited to that of fiscal administrators. Benefits would be comprehensive and provide incentives for cost-effective care. In addition, benefits would be "portable": they would remain in effect when individuals changed jobs or moved to a different area of the country. Freedom of choice in terms of providers might actually improve in a single-payer system, given how restrictive our current private health insurance system has become. Such a plan would allow far greater control over resource and personnel planning, would improve access to preventive services, and could eliminate duplicate services and technology. Researchers have estimated that adopting a single-payer system would save upward of $120 billion annually in administrative costs—enough to provide coverage to all uninsured Americans. Claims that the Canadian system has long waiting lists have either proven entirely untrue or exaggerated: modest waits did not result in any reduction of health status.

Given the delay in realizing national health-care reform, several states have sought ways both to contain costs and to improve access for their populations. The Oregon Health Plan (OHP) has been highly publicized as a systematic "rationing" plan; however, the plan has more to it than meets the eye. The original intent of the OHP was to cover the population universally by means of several mechanisms: a Medicaid expansion, establishment of high risk/medically uninsurable and small-employer risk pools, and an employer mandate. The Medicaid expansion to cover certain uninsured people includes a prioritization of services that are deemed to be both of high priority (determined by a community consensus process) and cost-effective and a thorough integration of managed care in services provided to the Medicaid population. The Medicaid portion of the plan was implemented in 1994, but the employer mandate portion hangs tenuously on the outcome of budget restrictions, small business lobbying efforts, and a waiver requested from the federal government to exempt Oregon from the Employee Retirement Income Security Act of 1974 (ERISA).

*W*HAT DO YOU THINK?

Do you believe that health care is a right of all Americans or is it a privilege to be earned? Why or why not? Have you ever for financial reasons had difficulty accessing the health-care system?

Summary

◆ Advertisers of health-care products and services use sophisticated tactics to attract your attention and get your business. Advertising claims sometimes appear to be supported by spontaneous remission (symptoms disappearing without any apparent cause) or the placebo effect (symptoms disappearing because you think they should).

◆ Self-care and individual responsibility are key factors involved in reducing rising health-care costs and improving health status. But you need to seek medical treatment in situations that are unfamiliar to you or that are emergencies. You should assess health professionals using their qualifications, their record of treating your specific problem, and their ability to work with you.

◆ In theory, allopathic ("traditional") medicine is based on scientifically validated methods and procedures. Medical doctors, specialists of various kinds, nurses, physician assistants, and other health professionals practice allopathic medicine. Many nonallopathic

("alternative") forms of health service—including chiropractic treatment, acupuncture, herbalists and homeopaths, and naturopathy—have proven effective for a variety of ailments.

◆ Health-care providers may provide services as solo practitioners or in group practices (in which overhead is shared). Hospitals and clinics are classified by profit status, ownership, specialty, and teaching status.

◆ Problems experienced in the U.S. health-care system concern cost, access, quality and malpractice, and fraud and abuse.

◆ Health insurance is based on the concept of spreading risk. Insurance is provided by private insurance companies (who charge premiums) and the government Medicare and Medicaid programs (funded by taxes). Managed care (in the form of HMOs and PPOs) attempts to keep costs lower by streamlining administrative procedures and stressing preventive care (among other initiatives).

Discussion Questions

1. List some dubious claims made by health-care products (such as thigh-reducing creams, hair-growth tonics, muscle-building milkshakes, to name a few). Why do marketers use such claims to attempt to sell their products? Why do consumers buy such products?

2. List some conditions (resulting from illness or accident) for which you don't need to seek medical help. When would you consider each condition to be bad enough to require medical attention? How do you decide to whom and where to go for treatment?

3. What are the differences in education between M.D.s and chiropractors? Under what circumstances would you seek treatment from a nonallopathic practitioner? Which types of nonallopathic medicine seem valid to you? Which seem like quackery?

4. What are the pros and cons of group practices? Of nonprofit and for-profit hospitals? If you had health insurance, where do you believe you would get the best care? On what do you base your choice?

Managing Your Health-Care Needs

Throughout this text, we have emphasized behaviors important to keeping you healthy. But now you need to turn your attention to your potential behavior when you need medical attention. Most people wait until a problem arises to seek medical care and take the first available physician or medical facility. But by looking ahead to future needs, you can take charge of your choices and make positive moves toward getting better health care.

Making Decisions for You

As you have seen in this chapter, many health-care decisions are dictated by physicians, insurance companies, and government agencies. But many decisions still rest with you. Start by learning about your own insurance protection. What coverage do you currently have? If none, how would you pay for a medical emergency (i.e., an accident)? What coverage is available to you as a student? Once you establish your protection, find out what you have control over. Do you have your choice of physicians or hospitals? How can you best make your choices?

Checklist for Change: Making Personal Choices

✓ How long did you have to wait before getting an appointment?

✓ How long did you have to wait in the waiting room before being seen?

✓ Does the clerical staff convey their concern for you when delays occur?

✓ Are there educational materials available in the waiting areas?

✓ Are the doctor's credentials clearly displayed?

✓ Does the office accept insurance or do you have to pay now and be reimbursed by your insurer later?

✓ Does the physician treat you as if he or she is concerned about your problem?

✓ Do you feel comfortable discussing your problems with the physician?

✓ Are you confident that your doctor knows what he or she is talking about?

✓ Is the doctor willing to talk about issues such as credentials, hospital affiliations, qualifications of referrals for special problems, and fees?

✓ Are you able to understand answers to your questions? Does the doctor seem interested in whether you understand? Seem willing to answer questions? Encourage you to ask questions?

✓ Does the physician tell you why one test is being given rather than another? About risks of the test? About preparation for the tests? About what to expect concerning certain results?

✓ Is the physician willing to refer you to a nongroup specialist in a location of your choice?

✓ Does the doctor support your obtaining a second opinion, or does he or she seem irritated with such a request?

✓ If you became seriously ill and had to see a lot of this doctor, would you feel comfortable with him or her, or would you rather have someone else?

Checklist for Change: Making Community Choices

✓ What health-care services are located in your community?

✓ How long has your doctor been practicing in your community?

✓ How many hospitals are within a 30-minute drive from your home? Are any of them teaching hospitals?

✓ How will potential changes in health-care coverage affect people in your community?

✓ What percentage of people in your community don't have health insurance?

✓ What services are available in your community to help people who are under- or uninsured?

✓ What are the policies of local hospitals concerning the treatment of uninsured individuals who need care?

✓ Have you written your congressional leaders concerning your views about health-care legislation?

Critical Thinking

You and two friends decide to take advantage of a long weekend to go camping and hiking at a state park in a neighboring state. On the second morning of your trip, you're hiking along the edge of a steep, rocky ridge when one of your friends slips and falls over the side. Peering over the side, you know that after a drop of almost 150 feet your friend is seriously injured or even dead. While your other friend takes off for help, you gingerly climb down the ridge to get to your injured friend. When you get there, your friend is barely conscious. You can tell that your friend will need major surgery and extensive rehabilitation. You also know that your friend has no health insurance. As you hear help arriving, you consider exchanging identities so that your friend can immediately receive the benefits of your health insurance.

Using the DECIDE model described in Chapter 1, decide what you would do in this situation. What are the legal and ethical considerations involved in your dilemma?

5. Discuss the problems of the U.S. health-care system. If you were president, what would you propose as a solution? Which groups might oppose your plan? Which groups might support it?

6. Explain the differences between traditional insurance and managed health care. Which would you feel more comfortable with? Should insurance companies dictate rates for various medical tests and procedures in an attempt to keep prices down?

Application Exercise

Reread the What Do You Think? scenarios at the beginning of the chapter and answer the following questions:

1. Who should pay for an uninsured person who waits to get treatment? Should Lisa be required to pay for her treatment with her future earnings? Or should we all pay her bill through taxes and/or higher insurance premiums?

2. When you have a medical problem like Roberta's, how do you know if you are getting good advice? Make up a list of questions for Roberta to ask each physician. Your goal is to give her a better understanding of her diagnosis.

Further Reading

Boston Women's Health Book Collective, *The New Our Bodies, Ourselves: Updated and Expanded for the 90s* (New York: Touchstone Books, 1992).

A wonderful self-help book for women by women. Includes coverage of fertility, contraception, sexuality, relationships, nutrition, exercise, psychological health, and specific health problems.

H. J. Cornaccia and S. Barrett, *Consumer Health: A Guide to Intelligent Decisions,* 5th ed. (St. Louis: Times Mirror/Mosby, 1993).

Gives an in-depth account of major consumer health issues. Provides a needed baseline of information for anyone involved in personal health-care decision making.

P. Lee and C. Estes, *The Nation's Health,* 4th ed. (Boston: Jones and Bartlett, 1994).

Excellent survey of the varying points of view on our collective national health. Examines the whole scope of the American health-care system: its strengths, failures, and future. Extremely well-researched and accurate.

Bill Moyers, *Healing and the Mind,* Public Broadcasting Service, 1993.

Level-headed tour through the various alternative or unconventional medical practices available today.

M. Murray and J. Pizzorno, *Encyclopedia of Natural Medicine* (Rocklin, CA: Prima, 1991).

Surveys the principles of natural medicine and outlines their application through the use of herbs, vitamins, minerals, diet, and nutrition.

University of California at Berkeley, *Wellness Made Easy: 101 Tips for Better Health* (Berkeley: Health Letter Associates, 1990).

Provides useful hints on nutrition, fitness, stress management, safe travel, and self-care. All topics briefly discussed in one-paragraph sections. Based upon the *Berkeley Wellness Letter.*

S. Williams and P. Torrens, *Introduction to Health Services,* 4th ed. (New York: Wiley Medical, 1993).

Covers all the basic components of the U.S. health-care system. A wonderful introduction to the topic of how health care is organized, financed, regulated, and delivered in this country.

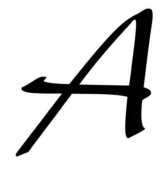

First Aid and Emergency Care

In certain situations, it may be necessary to administer first aid. Ideally, first-aid procedures should be performed by someone who has received formal training from the American Red Cross or some other reputable institution. If you do not have such training, contact your physician or call your local emergency medical service (EMS) by dialing 911 or your local emergency number. In life-threatening situations, however, you may not have time to call for outside assistance.

In cases of serious injury or sudden illness, you may need to begin first aid immediately and continue until help arrives. This appendix contains basic information and general steps to follow for various emergency situations. Simply reading these directions, however, may not prepare you fully to handle these situations. For this reason, you may want to enroll in a first-aid course.

Calling for Emergency Assistance

When calling for emergency assistance, be prepared to give exact details. Be clear and thorough, and do not panic. Never hang up until the dispatcher has all the information needed. Be ready to answer the following questions:

1. Where are you and the victim located? This is the most important information the EMS will need.

2. What has happened? Was there an accident or is the victim ill?

3. What is the victim's apparent condition?

4. What has been done to help the victim?

5. Are there any life-threatening situations that the EMS should know about (for example, fires, explosions, or fallen electrical lines)?

6. Do you know the victim's name?

7. Is the victim wearing a medic-alert tag (a tag indicating a specific medical problem such as diabetes)?

Are You Liable?

According to the laws in most states, you are not required to administer first aid unless you have a special obligation to the victim. For example, parents must provide first aid for their children, and a lifeguard must provide aid to a swimmer.

Before administering first aid, you should obtain the victim's consent. If the victim refuses aid, you must respect that person's rights. However, you should make every reasonable effort to persuade the victim to accept your help. In emergency situations, consent is *implied* if the victim is unconscious.

Once you begin to administer first aid, you are required by law to continue. You must remain with the victim until someone of equal or greater competence takes over.

Can you be held liable if you fail to provide adequate care or if the victim is further injured? To help protect people who render first aid, most states have "Good Samaritan" laws. These laws grant immunity (protection from civil liability) if you act in good faith to provide care to the best of your ability, according to your level of training. Because these laws vary from state to state, you should become familiar with the Good Samaritan laws in your state.

When Someone Stops Breathing

If someone has stopped breathing, you should perform mouth-to-mouth resuscitation. This involves the following steps:

1. Check for responsiveness by gently tapping or shaking the victim. Ask loudly, "Are you OK?"

2. Call the local EMS for help (usually 911).

3. Gently roll the victim onto his or her back.

4. Open the airway by tilting the victim's head back; placing your hand nearest the victim's head on the victim's forehead, and applying backward pressure to tilt head back and lift the chin.

5. Check for breathing (3 to 5 seconds): look, listen, and feel for breathing,

6. Give 2 slow breaths.
   - Keep victim's head tilted back.
   - Pinch the victim's nose shut.
   - Seal your lips tightly around the victim's mouth.
   - Give 2 slow breaths, each lasting 1½ to 2 seconds.

7. Check for pulse at side of neck; feel for pulse for 5 to 10 seconds.

8. Begin rescue breathing.
   - Keep victim's head tilted back.
   - Pinch the victim's nose shut.
   - Give 1 breath every 5 to 6 seconds.
   - Look, listen, and feel for breathing between breaths.

9. Recheck pulse every minute.
   - Keep victim's head tilted back.
   - Feel for pulse for 5 to 10 seconds.
   - If the victim has a pulse but is not breathing, continue rescue breathing. If there is no pulse, begin CPR.

There are some variations when performing this procedure on infants and children. For children ages 1 to 8, at step 8, give one slow breath every 4 seconds. For infants, you should not pinch the nose. Instead, seal your lips tightly around the infant's nose and mouth. Also, at step 8, you should give one slow breath every 3 seconds.

In cases in which the victim has no pulse, cardiopulmonary resuscitation (CPR) should be performed. This technique involves a combination of artificial respiration and chest compressions. You should not perform CPR unless you have received training in it. You cannot learn CPR simply by reading directions, and without training, you could cause further injury to the victim. The American Red Cross offers courses in mouth-to-mouth resuscitation and CPR as well as general first aid. If you have taken a CPR course in the past, you should be aware that certain changes have been made in the procedure. You should, therefore, consider taking a refresher course.

When Someone is Choking

Choking occurs when an object obstructs the trachea (windpipe), thus preventing normal breathing. Failure to expel the object and restore breathing can lead to death within 6 minutes. The universal signal of distress related to choking is the clasping of the throat with one or both hands. Other signs of choking include not being able to talk and/or noisy and difficult breathing. If a victim can cough or speak, do not interfere. The most effective method for assisting choking victims is the Heimlich maneuver, which involves the application of pressure to the victim's abdominal area to expel the foreign object.

The Heimlich maneuver involves the following steps: If the victim is standing or seated:

1. Recognize that the victim is choking.

2. Wrap your arms around the victim's waist, making a fist with one hand.

3. Place the thumb side of the fist on the middle of the victim's abdomen, just above the navel and well below the tip of the sternum.

4. Cover your fist with your other hand.

5. Press fist into victim's abdomen, with up to 5 quick upward thrusts.

6. After every 5 abdominal thrusts, check the victim and your technique.

7. If the victim becomes unconscious, gently lower him or her to the ground.

8. Try to clear the airway by using your finger to sweep the object from the victim's mouth or throat.

9. Give 2 rescue breaths. If the passage is still blocked and air will not go in, proceed with the Heimlich maneuver as follows:

If the victim is lying down:

10. Facing the person, kneel with your legs astride the victim's hips. Place the heel of one hand against the abdomen, slightly above the navel and well below the tip of the sternum. Put the other hand on top of the first hand.

11. Press inward and upward using both hands with up to 5 quick abdominal thrusts.

12. Repeat the following steps in this sequence until the airway becomes clear or the EMS arrives:
    a. Finger sweep.
    b. Give 2 rescue breaths.
    c. Do up to 5 abdominal thrusts.

Controlling Bleeding

External Bleeding. Control of external bleeding is an important part of emergency care. Survival is threatened by the loss of 1 quart of blood or more. There are three major procedures for the control of external bleeding: direct pressure, elevation, and use of pressure points.

DIRECT PRESSURE. The best method is to apply firm pressure by covering the wound with a sterile dressing, bandage, or clean cloth. Apply pressure for 5 to 10 minutes to stop bleeding.

ELEVATION. Elevating the wounded section of the body can slow bleeding. For example, a wounded arm or leg should be raised above the level of the victim's heart.

PRESSURE POINTS. Pressure points are sites where an artery that is close to the body's surface lies directly over a bone. Pressing the artery against the bone can limit the flow of blood to the injury. This technique should be used only as a last resort when direct pressure and elevation have failed to stop bleeding.

Knowing where to apply pressure to stop bleeding is critical (see Figure A.1). For serious wounds, seek medical attention immediately.

Internal Bleeding. Although internal bleeding may not be immediately obvious, you should be aware of the following signs and symptoms:

- Symptoms of shock (discussed later in this appendix)
- Coughing up or vomiting blood
- Blood in urine
- Black, tarlike stools
- Abdominal discomfort or pain (rigidity or spasms)

In some cases, a person who has suffered an injury (such as a blow to the head, chest, or abdomen) that does not cause external bleeding may experience internal bleeding.

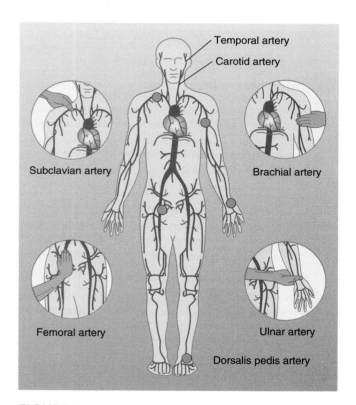

FIGURE A.1

This figure shows pressure points; the points at which pressure can be applied to stop bleeding. Unless absolutely necessary, you should avoid applying pressure to the carotid arteries, which supply blood to the brain. Also, never apply pressure to both carotid arteries at the same time.

If you suspect that someone is suffering from internal bleeding, follow these steps:

1. Have the person lie on a flat surface with knees bent.

2. Keep the victim warm. Cover the person with a blanket, if possible.

3. Do *not* give the victim any medications or fluids.

4. Send someone to call for emergency medical help immediately.

Nosebleeds. To control a nosebleed, follow these steps:

1. Have the victim sit down and lean slightly forward to prevent blood from running into the throat. Pinch the person's nose firmly closed using the thumb and forefinger. Keep the nose pinched for at least 5 minutes.

2. While the nose is pinched, apply a cold compress to the surrounding area.

3. If pinching does not work, gently pack the nostril with gauze or a clean strip of cloth. Do not use absorbent cotton, which will stick. Be sure that the ends of the gauze or cloth hang out so that it can be easily removed later. Once the nose is packed with gauze, pinch it closed again for another 5 minutes.

4. If the bleeding persists, seek medical attention.

Treatment for Burns

Minor Burns. For minor burns caused by fire or scalding water, apply running cold water or cold compresses for 20 to 30 minutes. Never put butter, grease, salt water, aloe vera, or topical burn ointments or sprays on burned skin. If the burned area is dirty, gently wash it with soap and water and blot it dry with a sterile dressing.

Major Burns. For major burn injuries, call for help immediately. Wrap the victim in a dry sheet. Do not clean the burns or try to remove any clothing attached to burned skin. Remove jewelry near the burned skin immediately, if possible. Keep the victim lying down and calm.

Chemical Burns. Remove clothing surrounding the burn. Wash skin that has been burned by chemicals by flushing with water for at least 20 minutes. Seek medical assistance as soon as possible.

Shock

Shock is a condition in which the cardiovascular system fails to provide sufficient blood circulation to all parts of the body. Victims of shock display the following symptoms:

- Dilated pupils

- Cool, moist skin

- Weak, rapid pulse

- Vomiting

- Delayed or unrelated responses to questions

All injuries result in some degree of shock. Therefore, treatment for shock should be given after every major injury. The following are basic steps for treating shock:

1. Have the victim lie flat with his or her feet elevated approximately 6 to 10 inches. (In the case of chest injuries, difficulty breathing, or severe pain, the victim's head should be slightly elevated.)

2. Keep the victim warm. If possible, wrap him or her in blankets or other material. Also, keep the victim calm and reassured.

3. Seek medical help.

Electrical Shock

Do not touch a victim of electrical shock until the power source has been turned off. Approach the scene carefully, avoiding any live wires or electrical power lines. Pay attention to the following:

1. If the victim is holding on to the live electrical wire, do not remove it unless the power has been shut off at the plug, circuit breaker, or fuse box.

2. Check the victim's breathing and pulse. Electrical current can paralyze the nerves and muscles that control breathing and heartbeat. If necessary, give mouth-to-mouth resuscitation. If there is no pulse, CPR might be necessary. (Remember that only trained people should perform CPR.)

3. Keep the victim warm and treat for shock. Once the person is breathing and stable, seek medical help or send someone else for help.

Poisoning

Of the 1 million cases of poisoning reported in the United States each year, about 75 percent occur in children under age 5, and the majority are caused by household products. Most cases of poisoning involving adults are attempted suicides or attempted murders.

You should have emergency telephone numbers for the poison control center and the local EMS ready. Many people keep these numbers on labels on their telephones. The National Safety Council recommends that you be prepared to give the following information when calling for help:

- What was ingested? Have the container of the product and the remaining contents ready so you can describe it. You should also bring the container to the emergency room with you.

- When was the substance taken?

- How much was taken?

- Has vomiting occurred? If the person has vomited, save a sample to take to the hospital.

- Are there any other symptoms?

- How long will it take to get to the nearest emergency room?

When caring for a person who has ingested a poison, keep these basic principles in mind:

1. Maintain an open airway. Make sure the person is breathing.

2. Call the local poison control center. Follow their advice for neutralizing the poison.

3. If the poison control center or another medical authority advises inducing vomiting, then do so. In general, if the victim has ingested poison within the previous 3 to 4 hours, you should induce vomiting to empty the stomach. However, never induce vomiting if the person is unresponsive, unconscious, or has swallowed acids or alkalies (such as drain and toilet cleaners, ammonia, lye, or oven cleaners) or petroleum products (such as floor polish, gasoline, lighter fluid, or paint thinner).

4. For most other ingested poisons (cosmetics, ink, rat poison, medicines, or illicit drugs), use syrup of Ipecac to induce vomiting. The recommended dose for an adult is 2 tablespoons with two or three glasses of water. For a child over the age of 1 year, the dose is 1 tablespoon with one or two glasses of water. If vomiting does not occur within 20 minutes, the dose should be repeated. Do not give more than two doses. If you do not have syrup of Ipecac, do not use other techniques or home remedies to induce vomiting. Transport the victim to the nearest health facility.

Injuries of Joints, Muscles, and Bones

Sprains. Sprains result when ligaments and other tissues around a joint are stretched or torn. The following steps should be taken to treat sprains:

1. Elevate the injured joint to a comfortable position.

2. Apply an ice pack or cold compress to reduce pain and swelling.

3. Wrap the joint firmly with a (roller) bandage.

4. Check the fingers or toes periodically to ensure that blood circulation has not been obstructed. If the bandage is too tight, loosen it.

5. Keep the injured area elevated, and continue ice treatment for 24 hours.

6. Apply heat to the injury after 48 hours if there is no further swelling.

7. If pain and swelling continue or if a fracture is suspected, seek medical attention.

Fractures. Any deformity of an injured body part usually indicates a fracture. A fracture is any break in a bone, including chips, cracks, splinters, and complete breaks. Minor fractures (such as hairline cracks) might be difficult to detect and might be confused with sprains. If there is doubt, treat the injury as a fracture until X-rays have been taken.

Do not move the victim if a fracture of the neck or back is suspected because this could result in a spinal cord injury. If the victim must be moved, splints should be applied to immobilize the fracture, to prevent further damage, and to decrease pain. Following are some basic steps for treating fractures and applying splints to broken limbs:

1. If the person is bleeding, apply direct pressure above the site of the wound,

2. If a broken bone is exposed, do not try to move it back into the wound. This can cause contamination and further injury.

3. Do not try to straighten out a broken limb. Splint the limb as it lies.

4. The following materials are needed for splinting:
   - Splint: wooden board, pillow, or rolled up magazines and newspapers
   - Padding: towels, blankets, socks, or cloth
   - Ties: cloth, rope, or tape

5. Place splints and padding above and below the joint. Never put padding directly over the break. Padding should protect bony areas and the soft tissue of the limb.

6. Tie splints and padding into place.

7. Check the tightness of the splints periodically. Pay attention to the skin color, temperature, and pulse below the fracture to make sure the blood flow is adequate.

8. Elevate the fracture and apply ice packs to prevent swelling and reduce pain.

Head Injuries

A head injury can result from an auto accident, a fall, an assault, or a blow from a blunt object. All head injuries can potentially lead to brain damage, which may result in a cessation of breathing and pulse.

For minor head injuries:

1. For a minor bump on the head resulting in a bruise without bleeding, apply ice to decrease the swelling.

2. If there is bleeding, apply even, moderate pressure. Because there is always the danger that the skull may be fractured, excessive pressure should not be used.

3. Observe the victim for a change in consciousness. Observe the size of pupils and note signs of inability to think clearly. Check for any signs of numbness or paralysis. Allow the victim to sleep, but wake him or her periodically to check for awareness.

For severe head injuries:

1. If the victim is unconscious, check the airway for breathing. If necessary, perform mouth-to-mouth resuscitation.

2. If the victim is breathing, check the pulse. If it is less than 55 or more than 125 beats per minute, the victim may be in danger.

3. Check for bleeding. If fluid is flowing from the ears or nose, do not stop it.

4. Do not remove any objects imbedded in the victim's skull.

5. Cover the victim with blankets to maintain body temperature, but guard against overheating.

6. Seek medical help as soon as possible.

Temperature-Related Emergencies

Frostbite. Frostbite is damage to body tissues caused by intense cold. Frostbite generally occurs at temperatures below 32°F. The body parts most likely to suffer frostbite are the toes, ears, fingers, nose, and cheeks. When skin is exposed to the cold, ice crystals form beneath the skin. Avoid rubbing frostbitten tissue, because the ice crystals can scrape and break blood vessels.

To treat frostbite, follow these steps:

1. Bring the victim to a health facility as soon as possible.

2. Cover and protect the frostbitten area. If possible, apply a steady source of external warmth, such as a warm compress. The victim should avoid walking if the feet are frostbitten.

3. If the victim cannot be transported, you must rewarm the body part by immersing it in warm water (100°F to 105°F). Continue to rewarm until the frostbitten area is warm to the touch when removed from the bath. Do not allow the body part to touch the sides or bottom of the water container. After rewarming, dry gently and wrap the body part in bandages to protect from refreezing.

Hypothermia. Hypothermia is a temperature-related emergency that can be prevented with proper precautions. Hypothermia is a condition of generalized cooling of the body resulting from exposure to cold temperatures or immersion in cold water. It can occur at any temperature below 65°F and can be made more severe by wind chill and moisture. The following are key symptoms of hypothermia:

- Shivering
- Vague, slow, slurred speech
- Poor judgment
- Lethargy, or extreme exhaustion
- Slowed breathing and heartbeat
- Numbness and loss of feeling in extremities

You should take the following steps to provide first aid to a victim of hypothermia:

1. Replace any wet clothing. Make sure the person is warmed evenly, using whatever sources of heat are available (blankets, heating pads, or hot water bottles). If possible, give the victim a warm bath. The temperature of the fluids or the heating sources should not exceed 110°F (43°C).

2. Give the victim hot drinks. Do not give the victim alcohol or caffeinated beverages, and do not allow the victim to smoke.

3. Do not allow the victim to exercise.

Temperature-related problems common in the summer months include heatstroke, heat exhaustion, and heat cramps. These conditions result from prolonged exertion or exposure to high temperatures and humidity.

Heatstroke. Heatstroke, the most serious heat-related disorder, results from the failure of the brain's heat-regulating mechanism (the hypothalamus) to cool the body. The following are signs and symptoms of heatstroke:

- Rapid pulse
- Hot, dry, flushed skin (absence of sweating)
- Disorientation leading to unconsciousness
- High body temperature

As soon as these symptoms are noticed, the body temperature should be reduced as quickly as possible. The victim should be immersed in a cool bath, lake, or stream. If there is no water nearby, a fan should be used to help lower the victim's body temperature.

Heat Exhaustion. Heat exhaustion results from excessive loss of salt and water. The onset is gradual, with the following symptoms:

- Fatigue and weakness
- Anxiety
- Nausea
- Profuse sweating
- Clammy skin
- Normal body temperature

To treat heat exhaustion, get the victim out of the sun. Have the victim lie down flat or with feet elevated. Replace lost fluids slowly and steadily.

Heat Cramps. Heat cramps result from excessive sweating, resulting in an excessive loss of salt and water. Although heat cramps are the least serious heat-related emergency, they are the most painful. The symptoms include muscle cramps, usually starting in the arms and legs. To relieve symptoms, the victim should drink electrolyte-rich beverages or a light saltwater solution or eat salty foods.

First-Aid Supplies

Every home, car, or boat should be supplied with a basic first-aid kit. In order to respond effectively to emergencies, you must have the basic equipment. This kit should be stored in a convenient place, but it should be kept out of the reach of children. Following is a list of supplies that should be included:

- Bandages, including triangular bandages (36 inches by 36 inches), butterfly bandages, a roller bandage, rolled white gauze bandages (2- and 3-inch widths), adhesive bandages
- Sterile gauze pads and absorbent pads
- Adhesive tape (2- and 3-inch widths)
- Cotton-tip applicators
- Scissors
- Thermometer
- Antibiotic ointments
- Syrup of Ipecac (to induce vomiting)
- Aspirin
- Calamine lotion
- Antiseptic cream or petroleum jelly
- Safety pins
- Tweezers
- Flashlight
- Paper cups
- Blanket

You cannot be prepared for every medical emergency. Yet these essential tools and a knowledge of basic first aid will help you cope with many emergency situations.

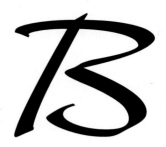

Health Resource Guide

This guide is designed to provide you with information sources on a variety of health and wellness topics. Many of these numbers are toll free; some represent national clearinghouses that may direct you in your information search or provide the most up-to-date data sources.

Computer-Based Information Services. Most of the information listed below may be available through your campus computer network through DIRLINE, an online database (through the National Library of Medicine's MEDLARS system) containing information on approximately 15,000 organizations. These organizations provide information and services directly to requesters. For information about access to DIRLINE or MEDLARS contact:

MEDLARS Management Section
National Library of Medicine
8600 Rockville Pike
Bethesda, MD 20894
800-638-8480

BRS Information Technologies
5 Computer Drive, South
Albany, NY 12205
800-235-1209

Knight-Ridder Information, Inc.
2440 El Camino Real
Mountainview, CA 94040
800-334-2564

Adoption

The Adoptive Parents' Committee, Inc.
212-304-8479

American Adoption Congress
1000 Connecticut Avenue, NW
Suite 9
Washington, DC 20036
202-483-3399

The National Adoption Center
1500 Walnut Street
Suite 701
Philadelphia, PA 19102
800-TO-ADOPT

National Council for Adoption
1930 17th Street, NW
Washington, DC 20009
202-328-1200

North American Council on Adoptable Children
970 Raymond Avenue
Suite 106
St. Paul, MN 55114
612-644-3036
fax 612-644-9848

Orphan Foundation
1500 Massachusetts Avenue
Washington, DC 20005
202-861-0762

Aging

American Association of Retired Persons (AARP)
1909 K Street, NW
Washington, DC 20049
202-872-4922

CAPS (Children of Aging Parents)
1609 Woodbourne Road
Levittown, PA 19057
215-345-5104

The National Council on the Aging
409 Third Street, SW
Suite 200
Washington, DC 20024
202-479-1200

Allergy and Asthma

American Academy of Allergy and Immunology
611 East Wells Street
Milwaukee, WI 53202
414-272-6071

American Allergy Association
PO Box 640
Menlo Park, CA 94026
415-322-1663

Asthma and Allergy Foundation of America
800-7-ASTHMA

Asthma Foundation of Southern Arizona
PO Box 30069
Tucson, AZ 85751-0069
602-323-6046

National Asthma Center
National Jewish Hospital and Research Center
800-222-5864

America Online Health Services

Better Health and Medical Forum
Keyword: BHMF

Elle Fitness & Health / Health Newsletter
Keyword: ELLE

The Gay and Lesbian Community Forum (GLCF)
Keyword: GLCF

HealthFocus
Keyword: HEALTHFOCUS

Institute of Medicine (IOM)
(affiliated with National Academy of Sciences)
Keyword: NAS

Lifetime
Keyword: LIFETIME

Longevity Magazine
Keyword: Longevity

National Alliance for the Mentally Ill (NAMI)
Keyword: NAMI

National Multiple Sclerosis Society
Keyword: NMSS

United Cerebral Palsy Association (UCPA)
Keyword: UCPA

Blood Disorders

Center for Sickle Cell Disease
2121 Georgia Avenue, NW
Washington, DC 20059
202-806-7930

Children's Blood Foundation
333 East 38th Street
New York, NY 10016
212-297-4336

Cooley's Anemia Foundation
129-09 26th Street
Suite 203
Flushing, NY 11354
800-522-7222

National Hemophilia Foundation
110 Green Street
Room 303

New York, NY 10012
212-219-8180

Sickle Cell Disease Association of America
200 Corporate Point
Suite 495
Culver City, CA 90230
800-421-8453

Cancer

American Cancer Society
1599 Clifton Road, NE
Atlanta, GA 30329-4251
800-ACS-2345

American Medical Center for Cancer Information
800-525-3777

City of Hope/Cancer and Major Disease Center
1500 East Duarte Road
Duarte, CA 91010
800-423-7119

Leukemia Society of America
2900 Eisenhower Avenue
Suite 419
Alexandria, VA 22314
703-960-1100

National Cancer Institute
Cancer Information Service
800-4-CANCER

Y-ME National Breast Cancer Organization
(for breast cancer survivors)
800-221-2141

Children's Services

ALSAC–St. Jude Children's Research Hospital
332 North Lauderdale Street
Memphis, TN 38105
901-495-3300

Child Reach
155 Plan Way
Warwick, RI 02886
800-556-7918
e-mail: usno@childreach.org

Child Welfare League of America
440 First Street, NW
Suite 310
Washington, DC 20001
202-638-2952

Children's Aid International
3550 Afton Road
San Diego, CA 92123
703-354-5809

Children's Defense Fund
25 E Street, NW
Washington, DC 20001
202-628-8787

Children's Foundation
725 15th Street, NW
Suite 505
Washington, DC 20005
202-347-3300

Children's Survival Fund
600 Eastgate
Suite B
Carbondale, IL 62901
618-549-7873
800-894-5038

Christian Children's Fund
PO Box 26484
Richmond, VA 23261-6484
804-756-2700

Council for Exceptional Children
1920 Association Drive
Reston, VA 22091-1589
703-620-3660

Healing the Children
PO Box 9065
Spokane, WA 99209
509-327-4281

Holt International Children's Services
PO Box 2880
Eugene, OR 97402
503-687-2202

International Children's Care, Inc.
PO Box 4406
Vancouver, WA 98662
800-422-7729

Johns Hopkins Children's Center
1620 McElderry Street
Reed Hall 204
Baltimore, MD 21205
410-955-8767

National Down's Syndrome Society
666 Broadway
8th Floor, Suite 810
New York, NY 10012-2317
800-221-4602

National Easter Seal Society for Crippled Children
230 Monroe Street
Suite 1800
Chicago, IL 60606-4802
312-726-6200

National Institute of Child Health and Human Development (NIH)
9000 Rockville Pike
Building 31 Room 2a-32
Bethesda, MD 20892
301-496-5133

National Runaway Switchboard
3080 North Lincoln Avenue
Chicago, IL 60657
800-621-4000

Save the Children
54 Wilton Road
Westport, CT 06880
203-226-7271

United Cerebral Palsy Association (UCPA)
1660 L Street, NW
Suite 700
Washington, DC 20036
800-USA-5UCP
Fax 202-842-3519
America Online (Keyword: UCPA)

Youth Haven, Inc.
PO Box 7007
Naples, FL 33941
813-774-2904

Consumer Issues

Auto Safety Hotline
800-424-9393

Consumer Information Center
Pueblo, CO 81009
719-948-3334

Consumer's Union of the U.S., Inc.
101 Truman Avenue
Yonkers, NY 10703
914-378-2000

Council of Better Business Bureaus
4200 Wilson Boulevard
Suite 800
Arlington, VA 22203
703-276-0100

Federal Trade Commission
202-326-2222

National Council Against Health Fraud, Inc.
PO Box 1276
Loma Linda, CA 92354
909-824-4690

U.S. Department of Health and Human Services
Office of Consumer Affairs
Food and Drug Administration
5600 Fishers Lane
Rockville, MD 20580
301-443-3170

U.S. Department of Transportation
National Highway Traffic Safety Administration
Office of Public and Consumer Affairs
400 7th Street, SW
Washington, DC 20590
202-366-9550

U.S. Postal Service
Fraud Division
Chief Postal Inspector
475 L'Enfant Plaza
Washington, DC 20260
202-268-2000

Death and Dying

Choice in Dying
200 Varick Street
10th Floor
New York, NY 10014
212-366-5540

The Grant-A-Wish Foundations of Maryland
PO Box 21211
Baltimore, MD 21228
410-242-1549
e-mail: grantawish@aol.com

The Hemlock Society
310-476-8696

Hospice Link
Hospice Education Institute
190 Westbrook Road
Essex, CT 06426-1511
800-331-1620

The Living Bank
PO Box 6725
Houston, TX 77265
800-528-2971

Make-A-Wish Foundation of America
100 West Clarendon Street
Suite 2200
Phoenix, AZ 85013
602-279-9474

Medic Alert Organ Donor Program
2323 Colorado Avenue
Turlock, CA 95382
800-334-3226
209-668-3333

National Hospice Organization
1901 North Moore Street
Suite 901
Arlington, VA 22209
703-243-5900

Organ Donor Hotline
800-24-DONOR

Starlight Foundation International
12424 Wilshire Boulevard
Suite 1050
Los Angeles, CA 90025
800-274-7827

Sudden Infant Death Syndrome Alliance
1314 Bedford Avenue
Suite 210
Baltimore, MD 21208
800-221-SIDS

Support Source
610-544-3605

Diabetes

American Diabetes Association, Inc.
PO Box 968
Framingham, MA 01701
800-342-2383
or
149 Madison Avenue
New York, NY 10016
212-725-4925

Diabetes Research Institute Foundation
3440 Hollywood Boulevard
Hollywood, FL 33021
800-321-3437

Juvenile Diabetes Foundation
120 Wall Street
19th Floor
New York, NY 10015
800-223-1138
212-889-7575

Digestive Disorders

Gluten Intolerance Group of North America
(for wheat intolerance)
206-325-6980

National Foundation For Ileitis and Colitis
Crohn's and Colitis Foundation
386 Park Avenue South
17th Floor
New York, NY 10016-8804
800-343-3637

Drug and Alcohol Abuse and Prevention

Al-Anon and Alateen
PO Box 862
Midtown Station
New York, NY 10018-0862
800-356-9996

Alcohol HOTLINE
107 Lincoln Street
Worcester, MA 01605
800-ALCOHOL

Alcoholics Anonymous
General Services Office
475 Riverside Drive
New York, NY 10115
212-870-3400
800-870-3400

American Council on Drug Education
212-758-8060
800-488-DRUG

BACCHUS and GAMMA Peer Education Network
PO Box 100430
Denver, CO 80250
303-871-3068

Center for Substance Abuse Prevention (CSAP)
Office of Substance Abuse Prevention
5600 Fishers Lane, Rockwall 2
Rm. 9d-10
Rockville, MD 20782
301-443-0365

Children of Alcoholics Foundation
555 Madison Avenue
20th Floor
New York, NY 10022
212-754-0656

Healthy Lifestyles Initiative Target
PO Box 20626
Kansas City, MO 64195
816-464-5400
800-366-6667

Join Together
441 Stuart Street
Boston, MA 02116
617-437-1500
Fax 617-437-9394

Narcotics Anonymous World Service Office
PO Box 9999
Van Nuys, CA 91409
818-773-9999

National Clearinghouse for Alcohol and Drug Information
PO Box 2345
Rockville, MD 20847-2345
301-468-2600
800-729-6686

National Cocaine HOTLINE
164 W. 74th St.
New York, NY 10023
800-COCAINE

National Council on Alcoholism
800-622-2255

National Council on Alcoholism and Drug Dependents Hope Line
800-622-2255

National Families in Action
2296 Henderson Mill Road, NE
Suite 300
Atlanta, Georgia 30345
404-934-6364

National Institute on Alcohol Abuse and Alcoholism
6000 Executive Boulevard
Suite 409
Bethesda, MD 20892-7003
301-443-3860

National Institute on Drug Abuse
5600 Fishers Lane
Room 10a-39
Rockville, MD 20857
301-443-6245
Helpline: 800-662-HELP

National PTA
330 North Walbush Avenue
Suite 2100
Chicago, IL 60611
312-670-6782

Mothers Against Drunk Driving (MADD)
511 East John Carpenter Freeway
Suite 700
Irving, TX 75062
800-438-MADD

Parents' Resource Institute for Drug Education, Inc. (PRIDE)
10 Park Plaza South
Suite 540
Atlanta, GA 30303
404-577-4500

Remove Intoxicated Drivers (RID)
PO Box 520
Schenectady, NY 12301
518-372-0034

Students Against Driving Drunk
(SADD)
PO Box 800
Marlboro, MA 01752
508-481-3568

Toughlove
PO Box 1069
Doylestown, PA 18901
215-348-7090

Eating Disorders

American Anorexia/Bulimia Association, Inc.
293 Central Park West
Suite 1-R
New York, NY 10024
212-501-8351

Anorexia Nervosa and Related Eating Disorders, Inc.
503-344-1144

Center for the Treatment of Eating Disorders
445 East Granville Road
Worthington, OH 43085
614-846-2833

Environmental Issues

Citizen's Clearinghouse for Hazardous Waste
PO Box 6806
Falls Church, VA 22040
703-237-2249

Energy Efficiency
PO Box 3048
Maryfield, VA 22116
800-428-2525
e-mail: energyinfo@delphi.com

Environmental Protection Agency (EPA)
Public Information Center
401 M Street, SW
Washington, DC 20460
202-260-2090

GreenPeace, USA
1436 U Street, NW
Washington, DC 20009
202-462-1177

Hazardous Waste Hotline
800-424-9346

National Coalition Against the Misuse of Pesticides
701 E Street, SE
Suite 200
Washington, DC 20003
202-543-5450

National Institute of Environmental Health Sciences
PO Box 12233
Research Triangle Park, NC 27709
919-541-3345

National Pesticide Information Clearinghouse
Oregon State University
Weniger Hall Room 333
Corvallis, Oregon 97331-6502
800-858-7378

National Safety Council
PO Box 558
Itaska, IL 60143-0558
800-621-7619

Nuclear Information and Resource Service
1424 16th Street, NW
Suite 601
Washington, DC 20036
202-328-0002
e-mail: nirsnet@aol.com

Public Citizen
215 Pennsylvania Avenue, SE
Washington, DC 20003
202-546-4996

Sierra Club
330 Polk Street
San Francisco, CA 94109
415-776-2211

Gay and Lesbian Services

Federation of Parents and Friends of Lesbians and Gays (Parents FLAG)
1101 14th Street, NW
Suite 1030
Washington, DC 20005
202-638-4200

The Gay and Lesbian Community Forum
America Online (Keyword: GLCF)

National Gay and Lesbian Task Force
1734 14th Street, NW
Washington, DC 20009-4309
202-332-6483

General Information Resources

Adventist Development and Relief Agency International
12501 Old Columbia Pike
Silver Spring, MD 20904
301-680-6380

American College Health Association
PO Box 28937
Baltimore, MD 21240-8937
410-859-1500

American Genetic Association
301-695-9292

American Health Care Association
1201 L Street, NW
Washington, DC 20005
202-842-4444

American Hospital Association
1 North Franklin Street, Suite 27
Chicago, IL 60606
312-422-3000

American Medical Association
515 North State Street
Chicago, IL 60610
312-464-5000

American Mental Retardation Association
444 North Capitol Street, NW
Suite 846
Washington, DC 20001
202-387-1968

Care
151 Ellis Street
Atlanta, GA 30303
404-681-2552

Center for Disease Control and
  Prevention, Public Inquiries
U.S. Public Health Service
Atlanta, GA 30333
404-639-3534

Christian Relief Services
8815 Telegraph Road
Lorton, VA 22079
703-550-2472
e-mail: crserve@access.digex.net

Church World Service
PO Box 968
Elkhart, Indiana 46515
219-264-3102

Institute of Medicine (IOM)
America Online (Keyword: NAS)

International Lifeline
PO Box 32714
Oklahoma City, OK 73123
800-456-4464

International Social Service
390 Park Avenue South
New York, NY 10016
212-532-6350

National Center for Health Statistics
6525 Belcrest Road
Hyattsville, MD 10782
301-436-8500

National Coalition for the Homeless
1612 K Street, NW
Suite 1004
Washington, DC 20006
202-775-1322

National Health Information Center
PO Box 1133
Washington DC 20013-1133
800-336-8500

National Institutes of Health
9000 Rockville Pike
Bethesda, MD 20892
301-496-4000

National Vaccine Information
  Service
512 West Maple Avenue, #216
Vienna, VA 22180
703-938-3783
fax 703-938-5768
800-909-SHOT

Pearl S. Buck Foundation Inc.
Green Hills Farm
PO Box 181

Perkasie, PA 18944
215-249-0100

Presiding Bishop's Fund for World
  Relief
815 Second Avenue
New York, NY 10017
212-867-8400

U.S. Committee for Unicef
333 East 38th Street
6th Floor
New York, NY 10016
212-686-5522

World Vision, Inc.
PO Box 1131
Pasadena, CA 91131
800-423-4200

Healthy Relationships and Sexuality

American Association of Sex
  Educators, Counselors and
  Therapists
435 North Michigan Avenue
Suite 1717
Chicago, IL 60611
312-644-0828

Factual Information Regarding Sex
  and Teens
PO Box 57
Sanford, NC 27331
919-774-9515

Information Service of the Kinsey
  Institute for Sex Research
313 Morrison Hall
Indiana University
Bloomington, IN 47405
812-855-7686

Impotence Information Center
PO Box 9
Minneapolis, MN 55440
800-843-4315

National Women's Health Network
514 10th Street, NW
Suite 400
Washington, DC 20004
202-347-1140

Sex Information and Education
  Council of the U.S.
130 West 42nd Street
Suite 3500
New York, NY 10036
212-819-9770

Women Against Pornography
PO Box 845
Times Square Station
New York, NY 10036-0845
212-307-5055

Hearing-Impaired Services

Alexander Graham Bell Association
  for the Deaf
3417 Volta Place, NW
Washington, DC 20007-2778
202-337-5220

Deafpride, Inc.
202-675-6700

International Hearing Dogs, Inc.
5901 East 89th Avenue
Henderson, CO 80640
303-287-3277

Modern Talking Picture Service,
  Inc.
4707 140th Avenue North
Suite 105
Clearwater, FL 34622
800-237-6213

National Captioning Institute
1900 Gallows Road
Suite 3000
Vienna, VA 22182
703-917-7600

Heart Disease

American Heart Association
7272 Greenville Avenue
Dallas, TX 75231
214-748-7212
800-242-8721

National Heart, Lung, and Blood
  Institute
31 Center Drive, Bldg. 31
MSC 2470
Bethesda, MD 20892-2470
301-496-4236

National Stroke Association
8480 East Orchard Road
Suite 1000
Englewood, CO 80111
800-STROKES
303-771-1700

Kidney Disease

American Kidney Fund
6110 Executive Boulevard
Suite 1010
Rockville, MD 20852
800-638-8299

National Kidney Foundation
30 East 33rd Street
New York, NY 10016
800-622-9010

Lung Disease

American Lung Association
1740 Broadway
New York, NY 10019
212-315-8700

Breath of Life
PO Box 744
Newbury Park, CA 91319-0744

Lung Line
800-222-LUNG

Miscellaneous Disorder Resources

Acne Helpline
AHC Pharmaceutical
888 West 16th Street
Newport Beach, CA 92663
800-222-SKIN

Alzheimer's Disease and Related Disorders Foundation
919 North Michigan Avenue
Suite 1000
Chicago, IL 60611
800-621-0379
e-mail: greenfld@class.org

American Cleft Palate–Cranial Facial Association
1218 Grandview Avenue
Pittsburgh, PA 15211
800-242-5338

American Liver Foundation
1425 Pompton Avenue
Cedar Grove, NJ 07009
800-223-0179

American Pain Society
5700 Old Orchard Road
Skokie, IL 60077
708-966-5595

Arthritis Foundation
1314 Spring Street, NW
Atlanta, GA 30309
404-872-7100

Autism Services Center
PO Box 507
Huntington, WV 25710-0507
304-525-8014

Cystic Fibrosis Foundation
6931 Arlington Road
Bethesda, MD 20814

800-FIGHT-CF
or 301-951-4422

Epilepsy Foundation of America
4351 Garden City Drive
Landover, MD 20785-2267
800-332-1000
310-459-3700

Huntington's Disease Society of America
800-345-4372

Lupus Foundation of America
4 Research Place
Suite 180
Rockville, MD 20850
301-670-9292
800-558-0121

Muscular Dystrophy Association
10 East 40th Street
Room 4110
New York, NY 10016
212-689-9040

Myasthenia Gravis Foundation, Inc.
61 Gramercy Park
Suite 605
New York, NY 10010
212-533-7005

National Ataxia Foundation
15500 Wayzata Boulevard
Suite 750
Wayzata, MN 55391
612-473-7666
e-mail: nbxu87a@prodigy.com

National Center for Stuttering
200 East 33rd Street
New York, NY 10016
800-221-2483
e-mail: schwrtz@is.nyu.edu

National Headache Foundation
5252 North Western Avenue
Chicago, IL 60625
800-843-2256

National Hydrocephalus Foundation
22427 South River Road
Joliet, IL 60436
815-467-6548

National Multiple Sclerosis Society
800-344-4867
America Online (Keyword: NMSS)

National Organization for Rare Disorders
100 Route 37

PO Box 8923
New Fairfield, CT 06812-8923
800-447-6673

National Parkinson Foundation
1501 NW 9th Avenue
Miami, FL 33136
800-327-4545

National Spinal Cord Injury Association
545 Concord Avenue
Suite 29
Cambridge, MA 02138
800-962-9629

National Tay-Sachs and Allied Diseases Association
2001 Beacon Street
Brookline, MA 02146
617-277-4463

PMS Access
800-222-4-PMS

Spina Bifida Information and Referral
4590 MacArthur Boulevard, NW
Suite 250
Washington, DC 20007
800-621-3141

Tourette Syndrome Association
42-40 Bell Boulevard
Bayside, NY 11361
800-237-0717

United Ostomy Association
36 Executive Park
Suite 120
Irvine, CA 92714
800-826-0826
714-660-8624

Nutrition and Weight Control

American Dietetic Boulevard
216 West Jackson Boulevard
Chicago, IL 60606-6995
312-899-0040

American Institute of Nutrition
9650 Rockville Pike
Bethesda, MD 20814
301-530-7050
e-mail: sec@ain.faseb.org

Food and Nutrition Board
National Research Council
2101 Constitution Avenue, NW
Washington, DC 20418
202-334-2000

TOPS (Take Off Pounds Sensibly)
PO Box 07360
Milwaukee, WI 53207-0360
414-482-4620

Vegetarian Resource Group
PO Box 1463
Baltimore, MD 21203
410-366-8343

Weight Watchers International, Inc.
500 North Broadway
Jericho, NY 11753
516-939-0400

Physical Fitness

President's Council on Physical Fitness and Sports
202-272-3430

Women's Sports Foundation
Eisenhower Park
East Meadow, NY 11554
800-227-3988

Pregnancy

Alan Guttmacher Institute
120 Wall Street
New York, NY 10005
212-248-1111

American College of Nurse-Midwives
818 Connecticut Avenue, NW
Suite 900
Washington, DC 20006
202-728-9860

American College of Obstetricians and Gynecologists
122 East 42nd Street
New York, NY 10168
212-351-2555

American Fertility Society
1209 Montgomery Highway
Birmingham, AL 35216-2809
205-978-5000

Association for Voluntary Surgical Contraception
79 Madison Avenue
7th Floor
New York, NY 10016
212-561-8000

Birthright
686 North Broad Street
Woodberry, NJ 08096
800-848-5683

Center for Population Options
1025 Vermont Avenue, NW
Suite 200
Washington, DC 20005
202-347-5700

Committee on Population
National Research Council
2101 Constitution Avenue, NW
Washington, DC 20418
202-334-3167

Gladney Center
2300 Hemphill Road
Fort Worth, TX 76110
800-433-2922

March of Dimes
Birth Defects Foundation
1275 Mamaroneck Avenue
White Plains, NY 10605
914-428-7100

National Abortion Federation
1436 U Street, NW
Suite 103
Washington, DC 20009
800-772-9100

National Abortion Rights Action League (NARAL)
1156 15th Street, NW
Suite 700
Washington, DC 20005
202-828-9300

National Clearinghouse for Family Planning and Reproductive Health Association
122 C Street, NW
Suite 380
Washington, DC 20001
202-628-3535

National Women's Law Center
11 DuPont Circle
Suite 800
Washington, DC 20036
202-588-5180

Orphan Foundation
1500 Massachusetts Avenue
Suite 448
Washington, DC 20005
202-861-0762

Parents Without Partners, Inc.
401 North Michigan Avenue
Chicago, IL 60611-4267
800-637-7974

Planned Parenthood Federation of America, Inc.
810 Seventh Avenue
New York, NY 10019
212-541-7800
800-829-7732

Pregnancy and Infant Loss Center
612-473-9372

Psychological Health

American Association of Suicidology
4201 Connecticut Avenue, NW
Suite 310
Washington, DC 20008
202-237-2280

American Psychiatric Association
1400 K Street, NW
Washington, DC 20005
202-682-6000

American Psychological Association
750 First Street, NE
Washington, DC 20002
202-336-5500

Biofeedback Society of America
10200 West 44th Avenue
Suite 304
Wheat Ridge, CO 80033
303-420-2902

Depression/Awareness, Recognition, Treatment (D/ART)
National Institute of Mental Health
5600 Fishers Lane
Rockville, MD 20857
301-443-4130

Mental Health Law Project
1101 15th Street, NW
Suite 1212
Washington, DC 20005
202-467-5730

National Alliance for the Mentally Ill
800-950-6264
America Online (Keyword: NAMI)

National Association for Research on Schizophrenia and Depression
60 Cutter Mill Road
Suite 200
Great Neck, NY 11021
516-829-0091
800-829-8289

National Clearinghouse for Mental Health Information
Public Inquiries Section
5600 Fishers Lane
Room 11a-21
Rockville, MD 20857
301-443-4515

National Depressive and Manic Depressive Association
730 North Franklin St.
Suite 501
Chicago, IL 60610
312-642-0049

National Foundation for Depressive Illness
800-248-4344

National Institutes of Mental Health
5600 Fishers Lane
Room 7c-02
Rockville, MD 20857
301-443-4515

National Mental Health Association
1021 Prince Street
Alexandria, VA 22314-2971
703-684-7722
800-969-6642

Recovery, Inc.
802 North Dearborn Street
Chicago, IL 60610
312-337-5661

Rape

National Coalition Against Sexual Assault
Pennsylvania Coalition Against Rape
717-232-7460

Women Against Rape (WAR)
PO Box 346
Collingwood, NJ 08108
609-858-7800

Safety and Emergency Services

American Red Cross
8111 Gatehouse Road
Falls Church, VA 22042
202-737-8300

Medic Alert Foundation
PO Box 1009
Turlock, CA 95381
800-344-3226

National Head Injury Foundation
1776 Massachusetts Avenue, NW
Suite 100
Washington, DC 20036-1904
800-444-NHIF

National Safety Council
PO Box 558
Itasca, IL 60143-0558
708-285-1121
800-621-7619

Poison Control Center
800-329-9111

Sexually Transmitted Diseases, HIV Diseases, and AIDS

American Foundation for the Prevention of Venereal Disease
799 Broadway
Suite 638
New York, NY 10003
212-759-2069

Centers for Disease Control and Prevention
1600 Clifton Road, NE
Atlanta, GA 30333
404-639-3311

National AIDS Hotline
800-342-AIDS
800-342-SIDA (Spanish)
800-AIDS-TTY (hearing impaired)

National STD Hotline
800-227-8922

Shanti Project
1546 Market Street
San Francisco, CA 94102
415-864-2273

Smoking

Action on Smoking and Health
2013 H Street, NW
Washington, DC 20006
202-659-4310

Smoking Hotline
800-TRY-TO-STOP
800-TDD-1477 (hearing impaired)

Violence and Abuse

The American Civil Liberties Union (ACLU)
132 West 43rd Street
New York, NY 10036
212-944-9800

Child Find
PO Box 277
New Paltz, NY 12561-9277
800-I-AM-LOST

Child Keepers' International
PO Box 6292
Lake Worth, FL 33466
407-586-6695

Child Welfare League of America
440 First Street, NW
Suite 310
Washington, DC 20001-2085
202-638-2952

Emerge
25 Huntington Avenue
Room 324
Boston, MA 02216
617-422-1550

Legal Resource Center for Child Advocacy and Protection
740 15th Street, NW
9th Floor
Washington, DC 20005
202-662-1720

Missing Children Help Center
410 Ware Boulevard
Suite 400
Tampa, FL 33619
813-623-5437

National Black Child Development Institute
1023 15th Street, NW
Suite 600
Washington, DC 20005
202-387-1281

National Center for Missing and Exploited Children
2101 Wilson Boulevard
Suite 550
Arlington, VA 22201
800-843-5678

National Center for the Prosecution of Child Abuse
99 Canal Center Plaza
Suite 510
Alexandria, VA 22314
703-739-0321

National Child Abuse Hotline
800-422-4453

National Child Safety Council
Missing Children Division
PO Box 1368
Jackson, MI 49204-1368
800-222-1464

National Coalition Against Domestic Violence (NCADV)
PO Box 15127
Washington, DC 20003-0127
202-638-6388
703-763-0339
303-839-1852

National Committee to Prevent Child Abuse
800-55NCPCA

National Council on Child Abuse and Family Violence
1155 Connecticut Avenue, NW
Suite 400
Washington, DC 20036
202-429-6695

National Crisis Prevention Institute
3515-K North 124th Street
Brookfield, WI 53005
800-558-8976

Office of Victims of Crime
Department of Justice
633 Indiana Avenue, NW
Washington, DC 20531
202-307-5983

Parents Anonymous
800-882-1250

Parents of Murdered Children (POMC)
100 East 8th Street
Room B 41
Cincinnati, OH 45202
513-721-5683

Runaway Hotline
3080 North Lincoln
Chicago, IL 60657
800-231-6946

Village of Child Help
PO Box 247
Beaumont, CA 92223
909-845-3155

Vision-Impaired Services

Blind Children's Center
4120 Marathon Street
Los Angeles, CA 90029
213-664-2153

Eye Bank for Sight Restoration
210 East 64th Street
New York, NY 10021
212-980-6700

Foundation for Fighting Blindness
1401 Mount Royal Avenue
4th Floor
Baltimore, MD 21230
410-225-9400

Guide Dog Foundation for the Blind
371 East Jericho Turnpike
Smithtown, NY 11787-2976
800-548-4337

Helen Keller National Center for the Deaf-Blind Youth and Adult
111 Middle Neck Road
Sands Point, NY 11050
516-944-8900

National Association for the Visually Handicapped (NAVH)
22 West 21st Street
New York, NY 10010
212-889-3141

National Center for the Blind
1800 Johnson Street
Baltimore, MD 21230
410-659-9314

Prevent Blindness America
500 East Remington Road
Schaumburg, IL 60173-5611
800-221-3004

Recordings for the Blind
609-452-0606

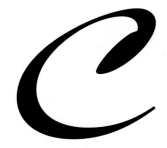
Nutritional Information

Selected Fast-Food Restaurants

We love fast food: it's convenient, delicious, and fast. The restaurants are clean, the staff friendly and courteous. As a consumer, you can depend on consistent quality, no matter which branch of your favorite restaurant you choose to patronize.

As part of a planned diet, fast food fits many lifestyles. For example, if your diet requires that you eat 65 grams of fat or less per day and you plan to have a Big Mac and large fries for dinner (total fat: 49 grams), you know that you must limit yourself to 16 grams of fat for breakfast and lunch.

You could, however, learn the nutritional content of your favorite foods, and reduce fat while still enjoying your favorite meals. Many fast-food restaurants offer nutritional information charts. From these charts you can devise eating strategies that work for you. For example,

you could plan to have your Big Mac and *small* fries for dinner and only consume 39 grams of fat. Here are some ideas for healthier eating at fast-food restaurants:

- Hold the cheese. Cheese adds 90 calories, 7 grams of fat, and over 400 mg of sodium to a Burger King Whopper.

- Order small french fries. At McDonald's the difference between a small and large order is 90 calories, 10 grams of fat, and 90 mg of sodium.

- Hold the mayonnaise. At Burger King each serving of mayonnaise contains 210 calories and 23 grams of fat.

- Order small drinks. At McDonald's a child's size drink contains 120 calories, a small drink 160, a medium 240, and a large 350.

- Look for low-fat alternatives. The McDonald's Fajita Chicken Salad (not on the chart that follows because it is so new) is 200 calories, with 7 grams of fat and 340 mg of sodium.

- Choose salad dressings carefully. McDonald's Ranch and Bleu Cheese dressings each contain 240 calories and 21 grams of fat; their Lite Vinaigrette contains only 50 calories and 2 grams of fat.

- Avoid high-fat dipping sauces. At Burger King the Ranch Dipping Sauce has 17 grams of fat, but the other sauces (A. M. Express® dip, honey, and barbecue) have *no* fat.

- Choose pizza toppings with care. Pepperoni adds 62 calories, extra cheese and pepperoni add 111 calories to two slices of Domino's pizza.

- The type of pizza you order may make a difference. The 12-inch deep dish pizza at Domino's has 14.3 more grams of fat and 216 more calories (for two slices) than the 12-inch hand-tossed.

- Consider the different fat contents in chicken sandwiches. Order Wendy's Grilled Chicken sandwich instead of the Breaded Chicken Sandwich to save 160 calories and 13 grams of fat.

- Take note of the low-fat alternatives at Kentucky Fried Chicken. The Colonel's Rotisseries Gold® Chicken quarter, with skin and wing removed by the customer, is 199 calories, with 53 calories from fat.

Eat fast foods in moderation. If a Big Mac and large fries is your reward for a good week at school, simply try cutting back on fat the other days of the week. While you may still wish to eat your favorites, a little bit of cutting back goes a long way.

Also, try some of the new low-fat alternatives that the fast-food chains are introducing. In 1995, Taco Bell launched an alternative line of products that cuts the fat by at least 50 percent. Their Light Taco Salad reduces fat by 30 grams compared to their traditional Taco Salad; hold the chips and save another 9 grams of fat.

TABLE C.1 ■ McDonald's

Menu Item	Serving Size	Calories	Calories from Fat	Total Fat (g)	% Daily Value	Saturated Fat (g)	% Daily Value	Cholesterol (mg)	% Daily Value	Sodium (mg)	% Daily Value	Carbohydrates (g)	% Daily Value	Dietary Fiber (g)	% Daily Value	Sugars (g)	Protein (g)	Vitamin A	Vitamin C	Calcium	Iron
Sandwiches																					
Hamburger	106g	270	80	9	13	3	16	30	10	530	22	35	12	2	8	6	12	2	4	15	15
Cheeseburger	122g	320	120	13	20	6	28	40	14	770	32	36	12	2	8	6	15	6	4	15	15
Quarter Pounder®	171g	420	180	20	31	8	39	70	23	690	29	36	12	2	7	7	23	4	4	15	25
Quarter Pounder® with Cheese	199g	520	260	29	45	13	63	95	32	1160	48	37	12	2	7	8	28	10	4	15	25
McLean Deluxe™	214g	340	100	12	18	4.5	22	60	20	810	34	37	12	2	9	8	24	8	15	15	25
McLean Deluxe™ with Cheese	220g	400	140	16	25	7	34	70	24	1040	44	38	13	2	9	8	26	10	15	15	25
Big Mac®	216g	510	230	26	39	9	46	75	25	930	39	46	15	3	13	8	25	6	4	20	25
Filet-O-Fish®	145g	360	150	16	25	3.5	18	35	12	710	30	41	14	1	6	6	14	2	*	10	10
McGrilled Chicken Classic	188g	250	30	3	5	0.5	3	45	16	510	21	33	11	2	8	6	24	4	8	10	15
McChicken® Sandwich	189g	490	260	29	44	5	27	50	17	800	33	42	14	2	7	6	17	2	2	15	15
French Fries																					
Small French Fries	68g	210	90	10	15	1.5	9	0	0	135	6	26	9	2	10	0	3	*	15	*	2
Large French Fries	147g	450	200	22	33	4	19	0	0	290	12	57	19	5	21	0	6	*	30	2	6
Salads																					
Chef Salad	313g	210	100	11	16	4	21	180	60	730	30	9	3	3	11	6	19	90	35	15	10
Chunky Chicken Salad	296g	160	45	5	8	1.5	6	75	25	320	13	8	3	3	13	5	23	160	50	6	8
Garden Salad	234g	80	35	4	6	1	6	140	46	60	3	7	2	3	11	5	6	60	35	6	8
Breakfast																					
Egg McMuffin®	137g	290	110	13	19	4.5	23	235	78	730	30	27	9	1	6	3	17	10	2	15	15
Sausage McMuffin®	112g	360	210	23	35	8	41	45	15	750	31	26	9	1	6	2	13	4	*	15	10
Sausage McMuffin® with Egg	163g	440	260	29	44	10	50	255	86	820	34	27	9	1	6	3	19	10	*	15	15
English Muffin	55g	140	20	2	3	0	0	0	0	220	9	25	8	1	6	1	4	*	*	10	8
Sausage Biscuit	119g	430	260	29	45	9	43	35	11	1130	47	32	11	1	5	3	10	*	*	8	15
Sausage Biscuit with Egg	170g	520	320	35	54	10	52	245	82	1200	50	33	11	1	5	3	16	6	*	10	15
Bacon, Egg & Cheese Biscuit	152g	450	250	27	42	9	44	240	79	1310	55	33	11	1	5	3	17	10	*	10	15
Biscuit	75g	260	120	13	20	3	15	0	0	640	35	32	11	1	5	2	4	*	*	6	10
Sausage	43g	170	150	16	25	5	27	35	11	290	12	0	.0	0	0	0	6	*	*	*	2
Scrambled Eggs (2)	102g	170	110	12	19	3.5	18	425	141	140	6	1	0	0	0	1	13	10	*	6	6
Hash Browns	53g	130	70	8	12	1.5	7	0	0	330	14	14	5	1	6	0	1	*	4	*	2
Hotcakes (plain)	150g	280	35	4	6	0.5	4	10	4	600	25	54	18	2	8	12	8	*	*	10	10
Hotcakes w/Syrup & Margarine (2 pats)	222g	560	120	14	21	2.5	12	10	4	750	31	100	33	2	8	43	8	8	*	10	10
Desserts/Shakes																					
Vanilla Lowfat Frozen Yogurt Cone	90g	120	5	0.5	1	0	0	5	1	85	4	24	8	0	0	16	4	*	2	15	2
Hot Fudge Lowfat Frozen Yogurt Sundae	179g	290	45	5	8	4.5	24	5	2	190	8	54	18	2	7	46	8	*	2	25	4
Baked Apple Pie	84g	290	130	15	22	3.5	19	0	0	220	9	37	12	1	4	14	3	*	45	2	6
McDonandland Cookies® (1 pkg)	56g	260	80	9	14	2	9	0	0	270	11	41	14	1	4	13	4	*	*	*	10
Chocolaty Chip Cookies (1 pkg)	56g	280	120	14	21	4	20	5	1	230	10	36	12	1	4	16	3	*	*	2	10
Vanilla Shake -- Small (16 fl oz)	480 ml	310	45	5	8	3.5	16	25	8	170	7	54	18	0	0	51	12	4	4	35	2
Chocolate Shake -- Small (16 fl oz)	480 ml	350	50	6	8	3.5	18	25	8	240	10	62	21	1	4	58	13	4	4	35	6
Strawberry Shake -- Small (16 fl oz)	480 ml	340	45	5	8	3.5	17	25	8	170	7	63	21	0	0	59	12	4	4	35	2

*Contains less than 2% of the Daily Value of these nutrients.

Source: ©1994 McDonald's Corporation. Rev. 7/94.

TABLE C.2 ■ Burger King

	Serving Size (g)	Calories	Calories from Fat	Total Fat (g)	Saturated Fat (g)	Cholesterol (mg)	Sodium (mg)	Total Carbohydrate (g)	Dietary Fiber (g)	Sugars (g)	Protein (g)	% DV* Vitamin A	% DV* Vitamin C	% DV* Calcium	% DV* Iron
Burgers															
Whopper® Sandwich	270	640	350	39	11	90	870	45	3	8	27	10	15	8	25
Whopper® with Cheese Sandwich	294	730	410	46	16	115	1300	46	3	8	33	15	15	25	25
Double Whopper® Sandwich	351	870	500	56	19	170	940	45	3	8	46	10	15	8	40
Double Whopper® with Cheese Sandwich	375	960	570	63	24	195	1360	46	3	8	52	15	15	25	40
Whopper Jr.® Sandwich	168	420	220	24	8	60	570	29	2	5	21	4	8	6	20
Whopper Jr.® with Cheese Sandwich	180	460	250	28	10	75	780	29	2	5	23	8	8	15	20
Hamburger	129	330	140	15	6	55	570	28	1	4	20	2	0	4	15
Cheeseburger	142	380	170	19	9	65	780	28	1	5	23	6	0	15	15
Double Cheeseburger	213	600	320	36	17	135	1040	29	1	5	41	8	0	20	25
Double Cheeseburger with Bacon	221	640	350	39	18	145	1220	29	1	5	44	8	0	20	25
Sandwich/Side Orders															
BK Fish Sandwich	255	720	390	43	8	60	1090	59	2	4	25	2	2	6	20
BK Broiler® Chicken Sandwich	248	540	260	29	6	80	480	41	2	3	30	4	10	4	30
Chicken Sandwich	229	700	380	43	9	60	1400	54	2	4	26	*	*	10	20
Chicken Tenders® (6 piece)	88	250	110	12	3	35	530	14	2	0	16	*	*	*	4
Broiled Chicken Salad	302	200	90	10	5	60	110	7	3	4	21	100	25	15	20
Garden Salad	215	90	45	5	3	15	110	7	3	0	6	110	50	15	6
Side Salad	133	50	25	3	2	5	55	4	2	0	3	50	20	6	2
French Fries (Medium, Salted)	116	400	180	20	5	0	240	43	3	0	5	*	4	*	6
Onion Rings	124	310	130	14	2	0	810	41	5	6	4	*	*	*	*
Dutch Apple Pie	113	310	140	15	3	0	230	39	2	22	3	*	10	*	8
Drinks															
Vanilla Shake (Medium)	284	310	60	7	4	20	230	53	1	47	9	6	6	30	*
Chocolate Shake (Medium)	284	310	60	7	4	20	230	54	3	48	9	6	*	20	10
Chocolate Shake (Medium, Syrup Added)	341	460	70	7	4	20	300	87	1	22	11	6	6	30	*
Strawberry Shake (Medium, Syrup Added)	341	430	60	7	4	20	260	83	1	47	9	6	6	30	*
Coca-Cola® Classic (Medium)	22 (fl oz)	260	0	0	0	0	@	70	0	70	0	*	*	*	*
Diet Coke® (Medium)	22 (fl oz)	1	0	0	0	0	@	<1	0	<1	0	*	*	*	*
Sprite® (Medium)	22 (fl oz)	260	0	0	0	0	@	66	0	66	0	*	*	*	*
Tropicana® Orange Juice	311	140	0	0	0	0	0	33	0	28	2	0	100	0	0
Coffee	355	5	0	0	0	0	5	1	0	0	0	*	*	*	*
Milk-2% Low Fat	244	120	40	5	3	20	120	12	0	0	8	10	4	30	*2
Breakfast															
Croissan'wich® with Bacon, Egg and Cheese	118	350	220	24	8	225	790	18	<1	2	15	8	*	15	10
Croissan'wich® with Sausage, Egg and Cheese	159	530	370	41	14	255	1000	21	<1	2	20	8	*	15	15
Croissan'wich® with Ham, Egg and Cheese	144	350	200	22	7	230	1390	19	<1	2	18	8	*	15	10
French Toast Sticks	141	500	240	27	7	0	490	60	1	11	4	*	*	6	15
Hash Browns	71	220	110	12	3	0	320	25	2	0	2	10	8	*	2
A.M. Express® Grape Jam	12	30	0	0	0	0	0	7	0	6	0	0	0	0	0
A.M. Express® Strawberry Jam	12	30	0	0	0	0	5	8	0	5	0	0	0	0	0

†= Without Dressing   @ = Depends on the water supply   * = Contains less than 2% of the daily value of this nutrient   * = Percent Daily Values (DV) are based on a 2,000 calorie diet

Source: © 1994 Burger King Corporation F6001 Issue Date: 12/94 (Revised)

TABLE C.3 ▪ Taco Bell

	Serving Size (grams)	Calories	Calorie % Reduction	Calories from Fat	Total Fat (grams)	Total Fat % Reduction	% Daily Value	Saturated Fat (grams)	% Daily Value	Cholesterol (mg)	% Daily Value	Sodium (mg)	% Daily Value	Carbohydrates (grams)	% Daily Value	Dietary Fiber (grams)	% Daily Value	Sugars (grams)	Protein (grams)	Vitamin A	Vitamin C	Calcium	Iron
Taco	78	180	--	100	11	--	17	4.5	22	30	10	280	12	11	4	1	4	0	10	35	2	8	6
Light Taco	78	140	22	50	5	55	8	1.5	8	20	7	280	12	11	4	2	8	0	11	4	0	0	0
Taco Supreme™	106	230	--	140	15	--	23	7.5	38	45	15	290	12	12	4	1	4	1	11	40	4	10	6
Light Taco Supreme™	106	160	30	50	5	67	8	1.5	8	20	7	340	14	14	5	2	8	2	13	10	4	0	0
Soft Taco	99	220	--	100	11	--	17	5.0	25	30	10	540	22	19	6	2	8	0	12	20	0	6	10
Light Soft Taco	99	180	18	50	5	55	8	2.5	12	25	8	550	23	19	6	2	8	0	13	4	0	4	6
Soft Taco Supreme®	128	270	--	140	15	--	23	7.5	36	45	15	550	23	21	7	2	8	1	13	30	4	8	10
Light Soft Taco Supreme®	128	200	26	50	5	67	8	2.5	12	25	8	610	25	23	8	2	8	2	14	10	4	4	6
Bean Burrito	198	390	--	110	12	--	18	4.0	20	5	2	1140	48	58	19	8	32	4	13	40	4	20	20
Light Bean Burrito	198	330	15	60	6	50	9	2.0	10	5	2	1340	56	55	18	8	32	1	14	30	4	10	20
Burrito Supreme®	248	440	--	170	19	--	29	8.5	42	45	15	1180	49	50	17	5	20	4	18	80	15	20	20
Light Burrito Supreme®	248	350	20	70	8	58	12.0	3	15	25	8	1300	54	50	17	4	16	3	20	60	15	8	15
7-Layer Burrito*	276	540	--	210	23	--	35	7.0	35	20	7	1160	48	65	22	10	40	3	17	35	10	10	15
Light 7-Layer Burrito	276	440	19	80	9	61	14	3.5	10	5	2	1430	60	67	22	10	40	3	19	35	8	25	25
Taco Salad	535	860	--	500	55	--	83	15.5	70	80	20	1620	68	64	21	10	40	6	32	120	45	15	30
Taco Salad*	507	700	--	370	41	--	63	13.0	65	60	20	1510	63	51	17	10	40	6	30	120	45	15	25
Light Taco Salad w/chips	507	550	21	170	19	54	29	6.0	30	50	17	1620	68	63	21	10	40	6	33	150	45	20	20
Light Taco Salad w/o chips	464	330	--	80	9	--	14	4.5	22	50	17	1610	67	35	12	10	40	6	30	120	45	10	15
Chicken Soft Taco	120	223	--	90	10	--	15	4.0	18	58	18	553	23	20	7	1	4	1	14	15	10	6	8
Light Chicken Soft Taco	120	180	19	45	5	50	8	1.0	5	30	10	570	24	26	9	1	4	1	9	15	8	4	8
Chicken Burrito	170	345	--	110	13	--	20	5.0	20	57	30	854	34	39	13	3	12	4	17	20	8	14	14
Light Chicken Burrito	170	290	16	60	6	54	9	1.5	8	30	10	900	38	45	15	2	8	2	12	20	6	6	15
Chicken Burrito Supreme	248	520	--	200	23	--	35	9.0	40	125	38	1130	44	47	16	3	12	4	27	25	10	15	50
Light Chicken Burrito Supreme	248	410	21	90	10	57	15	2.0	10	65	22	1190	50	62	21	2	8	3	18	25	8	6	15

Light=50% less fat per serving.

*% Fat reduction based on equivalent weight bases

Source: Nutritional Brochure © 1995 TACO BELL CORP. ITEM #2582

TABLE C.4 ■ Domino's Pizza

12″ HAND-TOSSED NUTRIENT	CHEESE Per 2 of 8 slices 147.4g	PEPPERONI Per 2 of 8 slices 159.4g	X-TRA CHEESE & PEPPERONI Per 2 of 8 slices 175.3g	HAM Per 2 of 8 slices 160.7g	ITALIAN SAUSAGE & MUSHROOM Per 2 of 8 slices 176g	VEGGIE* Per 2 of 8 slices 176g
Calories, kcal	344.2	406.2	455.0	361.6	402.4	360.0
Cal, from fat, kcal	90	140	170	90	120	90
Protein, g	14.8	17.5	20.9	17.2	17.5	15.2
Carbohydrates, g	50.0	50.2	50.5	50.3	52.2	51.7
Sugars, g	1.0	1.0	1.0	1.2	1.3	1.2
Dietary Fiber, g	2.4	2.5	2.5	2.4	2.9	3.0
Fat-total, g	9.5	15.1	18.8	10.2	13.9	10.4
Saturated fat, g	4.4	6.6	8.6	4.6	6.1	4.5
Cholesterol, mg	19.1	32.1	41.7	26.1	30.5	19.1
Ash, g	3.4	4.1	4.6	4.0	4.2	3.6
Water, g	68.7	71.5	79.2	78.1	87.2	93.9
Vitamin A, IU	456.9	467.6	578.7	456.5	483.0	493.5
Vitamin C, mg	2.6	2.7	2.7	2.7	3.2	12.7
Calcium, mg	277.8	282.3	411.8	279.3	286.5	285.9
Iron, mg	4.0	4.3	4.5	4.2	4.5	4.4
Sodium, mg	980.5	1179.0	1304.0	1143.0	7151.0	1028.0

12″ THIN CRUST NUTRIENT	1/3 Pizza 140.9g	1/3 Pizza 156.7g	1/3 Pizza 177.7g	1/3 Pizza 158.5g	1/3 Pizza 178.7g	1/3 Pizza 178.7g
Calories, kcal	364.3	447.1	512.3	387.7	442.3	385.7
Cal, from fat, kcal	140	210	250	150	190	150
Protein, g	16.1	19.7	24.2	19.3	19.8	16.7
Carbohydrates, g	40.1	40.4	40.8	40.5	43.1	42.5
Sugars, g	2.2	2.3	2.3	2.5	2.6	2.5
Dietary Fiber, g	1.9	2.0	2.0	1.9	2.5	2.6
Fat-total, g	15.5	23.0	28.0	16.5	21.4	16.7
Saturated fat, g	6.3	9.2	12.0	6.6	8.6	6.5
Cholesterol, mg	25.5	42.8	55.6	34.8	40.7	25.5
Ash, g	3.7	4.7	5.3	4.4	4.8	3.9
Water, g	64.2	67.8	77.8	76.5	88.5	97.5
Vitamin A, IU	567.4	582.6	731.0	567.9	603.5	617.5
Vitamin C, mg	3.5	3.5	3.5	3.6	4.2	16.9
Calcium, mg	422.3	428.4	601.1	424.3	434.0	433.3
Iron, mg	1.5	1.8	2.1	1.7	2.1	2.0
Sodium, mg	1012.0	1277.0	1443.0	1229.0	1240.0	1076.0

12″ DEEP DISH NUTRIENT	Per 2 of 8 slices 205.3 g	Per 2of 8 slices 218 g	Per 2 of 8 slices 234.9g	Per 2 of 8 slices 219.4g	Per 2 of 8 slices 235.7g	Per 2 of 8 slices 235.7g
Calories, kcal	559.7 g	621.8	670.7	577.2	618.2	575.8
Cal, from fat, kcal	210	260	300	220	250	220
Protein, g	23.5	26.2	29.6	25.9	26.2	24.0
Carbohydrates, g	63.2	63.4	63.7	63.5	65.5	65.0
Sugars, g	4.3	4.4	4.4	4.5	4.6	4.5
Dietary Fiber, g	3.2	3.2	3.2	3.2	3.7	3.7
Fat-total, g	23.8	29.4	33.1	24.5	28.9	24.7
Saturated fat, g	9.0	11.9	13.3	9.3	10.8	9.2
Cholesterol, mg	31.5	44.5	54.0	38.4	42.9	31.5
Ash, g	4.4	5.1	5.5	4.9	5.1	4.5
Water, g	92.2	95.7	104.3	102.3	112.4	119.1
Vitamin A, IU	763.9	775.3	886.6	764.3	791.0	801.5
Vitamin C, mg	3.0	3.0	3.0	3.1	3.5	13.0
Calcium, mg	451.4	455.9	585.5	452.9	460.2	459.6
Iron, mg	4.8	5.0	5.2	4.9	5.2	5.1
Sodium, mg	1184.0	1383.0	1508.0	1347.0	1356.0	1233.0

*Veggie–includes fresh mushrooms, onions, green peppers, & ripe olives.

Data based on minimal portioning requirements. Nutrient values may vary slightly by location & supplier base.

Source: ©1994 Domino's Pizza, Inc.

TABLE C.5 ■ Wendy's

NUTRITIONAL INFORMATION	Serving Size	Weight (g)	Calories	Calories from Fat	Total Fat (g)**	Saturated (g)	Cholesterol (mg)	Sodium (mg)	Total Carbohydrates (g)	Dietary Fiber	Sugars (g)	Protein (g)	Vitamin A	Vitamin C	Calcium	Iron
Sandwiches																
Plain Single	1 ea.	133	380	140	16	6	65	460	31	2	5	25	0	0	10	25
Single with Everything	1 ea.	219	420	180	20	7	70	810	37	3	9	26	6	10	10	30
Big Bacon Classic	1 ea.	287	610	290	33	13	105	1510	45	3	11	38	15	25	25	35
Jr. Hamburger	1 ea.	117	270	90	10	3	30	560	34	2	7	15	2	2	10	20
Jr. Cheeseburger	1 ea.	129	320	120	13	8	45	770	34	2	7	17	6	2	15	20
Jr. Bacon Cheeseburger	1 ea.	170	410	190	21	8	80	910	34	2	7	22	8	15	15	20
Jr. Cheeseburger Deluxe	1 ea.	179	360	150	18	8	45	840	36	3	9	18	10	10	15	20
Hamburger, Kids' Meal	1 ea.	111	270	80	10	3	30	560	33	2	7	15	2	0	10	20
Cheeseburger, Kids' Meal	1 ea.	123	320	120	13	6	45	770	33	2	7	17	6	0	15	20
Grilled Chicken Sandwich	1 ea.	177	290	60	7	1.5	55	720	35	2	8	24	4	10	10	15
Breaded Chicken Sandwich	1 ea.	208	440	160	18	3	60	840	44	2	8	28	4	10	10	15
Chicken Club Sandwich	1 ea.	220	500	200	23	5	70	1090	44	2	7	32	4	15	10	20
French Fries																
Small	3.2 oz.	91	260	120	13	2.5	0	85	33	3	0	3	0	8	2	4
Medium	4.6 oz.	130	380	170	19	4	0	120	47	5	0	5	0	10	2	6
Biggie	5.6 oz.	159	480	200	23	5	0	150	58	8	0	6	0	15	2	8
Baked Potato																
Plain	10 oz.	284	310	0	0	0	0	25	71	7	5	7	0	60	2	20
Bacon & Cheese	1 ea.	380	540	160	18	4	20	1430	78	7	5	17	10	60	20	25
Broccoli & Cheese	1 ea.	411	470	120	14	3	5	470	80	9	6	9	35	120	20	25
Cheese	1 ea.	383	570	210	23	9	30	640	78	7	5	14	15	60	40	25
Chili & Cheese	1 ea.	439	820	220	24	9	40	780	83	9	7	20	20	80	35	30
Sour Cream & Chives	1 ea.	314	380	60	6	4	15	40	74	8	6	8	30	80	8	25
Sour Cream	1 pkt.	28	60	50	6	4	10	15	1	0	1	1	4	0	4	0
Whipped Margarine	1 pkt.	14	60	60	7	1	0	110	0	0	0	0	10	0	0	0
Chili																
Small	8 oz.	227	210	60	7	2.5	30	800	21	5	5	15	8	6	8	15
Large	12 oz.	340	310	90	10	4	45	1190	32	7	8	23	10	10	10	25
Cheddar Cheese, shredded	2 T.	17	70	50	6	3	15	110	1	0	0	4	4	0	10	0
Saltine Crackers	2 ea.	8	25	5	0.5	0	0	80	4	0	0	0	0	0	0	2
Chicken Nuggets																
6 piece	6	94	280	180	20	6	50	600	12	0	N/A	14	0	0	2	4
Barbeque Sauce	1 pkt.	28	50	0	0	0	0	100	11	N/A	N/A	1	6	0	0	4
Honey	1 pkt.	14	45	0	0	0	0	0	12	0	12	0	0	0	0	0
Sweet & Sour Sauce	1 pkt.	28	45	0	0	0	0	55	11	N/A	N/A	0	0	0	0	2
Sweet Mustard Sauce	1 pkt.	28	60	10	1	0	0	140	9	N/A	N/A	1	0	0	0	0

**Total fats are comprised of many substances other than those listed.

©Copyright 1994, Wendy's International, Inc.

TABLE C.6 ■ Kentucky Fried Chicken

Amount Per Serving	Serving	Calories	Calories from Fat	Total Fat (g)	% Daily Value	Saturated Fat (g)	% Daily Value	Cholesterol (mg)	% Daily Value	Sodium (mg)	% Daily Value	Carbohydrates (g)	% Daily Value	Dietary Fiber (g)	% Daily Value	Sugars (g)	Protein (g)	Vitamin A	Vitamin C	Calcium	Iron
Colonel's Rotisserie Gold® Chicken Quarter—Breast and Wing as Served with Skin	6.2 oz	335	168	18.7	29	54	27	157	52	1104	46	1	–	–	–	–	40	<2%	<2%	<2%	<2%
(same) with skin and wing removed by customer	4.1 oz	199	53	5.9	9	1.7	9	97	32	667	28	0	–	–	–	–	37	<2%	<2%	<2%	<2%
Original Recipe® Chicken Breast	4.8 oz	360	180	20	31	5	27	115	38	870	36	12	4%	1	4%	0	33	–	–	6%	6%
Extra Tasty Crispy™ Chicken Breast	5.9 oz	470	250	28	42	7	35	80	27	930	39	25	8	1	4	0	31	–	–	4%	6%
Hot & Spicy Chicken Breast	6.5 oz	530	310	35	54	8	42	110	36	1110	46	23	8	2	9	0	32	–	–	4%	6%
Mashed Potatoes with Gravy	4.2 oz	109	45	5	8	<1	<5	<1	<1	386	16	16	5	2	8	<.1	1	–	–	–	–
Cornbread	2.0	175	58	6.4	10	1.4	7	0	0	285	12	27	9	0.7	3	10.7	2.1	0%	0	6%	4%
Corn on the Cob	5.3	222	104	12	18	2	9	0	0	76	3	27	9	8	31	4	4	4%	3%	0	2%

Source: Reprinted by permission of Kentucky Fried Chicken (KFC) Corp.

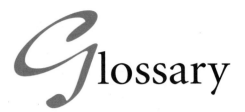

Glossary

12-step programs: Peer support groups patterned after Alcoholics Anonymous.

Abortion: The medical means of terminating a pregnancy.

Abstinence: Refraining from an addictive behavior.

Accessory glands: The seminal vesicles, prostate gland, and Cowper's glands.

Accountability: Accepting responsibility for personal decisions, choices, and actions.

Acid rain: Precipitation contaminated with acidic pollutants.

Acquired immune deficiency syndrome (AIDS): Extremely virulent sexually transmitted disease that renders the immune system inoperative.

Acquired immunity: Immunity developed during life in response to disease, vaccination, or exposure.

Adaptive response: Form of adjustment in which the body attempts to restore homeostasis.

Adaptive thermogenesis: Theoretical mechanism by which the brain regulates metabolic activity according to caloric intake.

Addiction: An unhealthy, continued involvement with a mood-altering object or activity in spite of harmful consequences.

Addictive exercisers: People who exercise compulsively to try to meet needs of nurturance, intimacy, self-esteem, and self-competency.

Adjustment: Our attempt to cope with a given situation.

Adrenocorticotrophic hormone (ACTH): A pituitary hormone that stimulates the adrenal glands to secrete cortisol.

Aerobic capacity: The current functional status of a person's cardiovascular system; measured as VO_2max.

Aerobic exercise: Any type of exercise, typically performed at moderate levels of intensity for extended periods of time (20 to 30 minutes or longer), that increases heart rate.

Afterbirth: The expelled placenta.

Ageism: Discrimination based on age.

Aggressive communicators: People who use hostile, loud, and blaming communication styles.

Aging: The patterns of life changes that occur in members of all species as they grow older.

Alcohol abuse (alcoholism): Use of alcohol that interferes with work, school, or personal relationships or that entails violations of the law.

Alcoholic hepatitis: Condition resulting from prolonged use of alcohol in which the liver is inflamed. It can result in death.

Alcoholics Anonymous: An organization whose goal is to help alcoholics stop drinking; includes auxiliary branches such as Al-Anon and Alateen.

Allergy: Hypersensitive reaction to a specific antigen or allergen in the environment in which the body produces excessive antibodies to that antigen or allergen.

Allopathic medicine: Traditional, Western medical practice; in theory, based on scientifically validated methods and procedures.

Alternative insemination: Fertilization accomplished by depositing a partner's or a donor's semen into a woman's vagina via a thin tube; almost always done in a doctor's office.

Alveoli: Tiny air sacs of the lungs.

Alzheimer's disease: A chronic condition involving changes in nerve fibers of the brain that results in mental deterioration

Amino acids: The building blocks of protein.

Amniocentesis: A medical test in which a small amount of fluid is drawn from the amniotic sac; it tests for Down's syndrome and genetic diseases.

Amniotic sac: The protective pouch surrounding the baby.

Amphetamines: Prescription stimulants not commonly used today because of the dangers associated with them.

Amyl nitrite: A drug that dilates blood vessels and is properly used to relieve chest pain.

Anabolic steroids: Artificial forms of the hormone testosterone that promote muscle growth and strength.

Anal intercourse: The insertion of the penis into the anus.

Analgesics: Pain relievers.

Androgyny: Combination of traditional masculine and feminine traits in a single person.

Anemia: Iron deficiency disease that results from the body's inability to produce hemoglobin.

Aneurysm: A weakened blood vessel that may bulge under pressure and, in severe cases, burst.

Angina pectoris: Severe chest pain occurring as a result of reduced oxygen flow to the heart.

Angiography: A technique for examining blockages in heart arteries. A catheter is inserted into the arteries, a dye is injected, and an X-ray is taken to find the blocked areas. Also called *cardiac catheterization*.

Angioplasty: A technique in which a catheter with a balloon at the tip is inserted into a clogged artery; the balloon is inflated to flatten fatty deposits against artery walls, allowing blood to flow more freely.

Anorexia nervosa: Eating disorder characterized by excessive preoccupation with food, self-starvation, and/or extreme exercising to achieve weight loss.

Antagonism: A type of interaction in which two or more drugs work at the same receptor site.

Antibiotics: Prescription drugs designed to fight bacterial infection.

Antibodies: Substances produced by the body that are individually matched to specific antigens.

Antidepressants: Prescription drugs used to treat clinically diagnosed depression.

Antigen: Substance capable of triggering an immune response.

Anxiety disorders: Disorders characterized by persistent feelings of threat and anxiety in coping with the everyday problems of living.

Appetite: The desire to eat, or a learned response that is tied to an emotional or psychological craving for food that is often unrelated to nutritional need.

Arrhythmia: An irregularity in heartbeat.

Arteries: Vessels that carry blood away from the heart to other regions of the body.

Arterioles: Branches of the arteries.

Arteriosclerosis: Characterized by deposits of fatty substances, cholesterol, cellular waste products, calcium, and fibrin in the inner lining of an artery.

Arthritis: Painful inflammatory disease of the joints.

Asbestos: A substance that separates into stringy fibers and lodges in lungs, where it can cause various diseases.

Assertive communicators: People who use direct, honest communication that maintains and defends their rights in a positive manner.

Asthma: A chronic respiratory disease characterized by attacks of wheezing, shortness of breath, and coughing spasms.

Asymptomatic: Without symptoms, or symptom-free.

Atherosclerosis: A general term for thickening and hardening of the arteries.

Atria: The two upper chambers of the heart, which receive blood.

Attitude: Relatively stable set of beliefs, feelings, and behavioral tendencies in relation to something or someone.

Autoerotic behaviors: Sexual self-stimulation.

Autoinoculation: Transmission of a pathogen from one part of the body to another.

Autonomic nervous system (ANS): The portion of the central nervous system that regulates bodily functions that we do not normally consciously control.

Autonomy: The ability to care for oneself emotionally, socially, and physically.

Background distressors: Environmental stressors that we may be unaware of.

Bacteria: Single-celled organisms that may be disease-causing.

Basal metabolic rate (BMR): The energy expenditure of the body under resting conditions at normal room temperature.

Behavioral psychology: Branch of psychology that posits that all behavior is learned through a system of punishments and rewards.

Behavioral therapy: Therapy aimed at teaching a person to change unwanted behaviors through a system of rewards and punishments.

Belief: Appraisal of the relationship between some object, action, or idea and some attribute of that object, action, or idea.

Benign: Harmless; refers to a noncancerous tumor.

Bereavement: The loss or deprivation experienced by a survivor when a loved one dies.

Beta blockers: Major type of drug used to treat angina, they control potential overactivity of the heart muscle.

Binge drinking: Drinking for the express purpose of becoming intoxicated; five drinks in a single sitting for men and four drinks in a sitting for women.

Binge eating disorder (BED): Eating disorder characterized by recurrent binge eating. However, BED sufferers do not take excessive measures to lose the weight gained during binges.

Bioelectrical impedance analysis (BIA): A technique of body fat assessment in which electrical currents are passed through fat and lean tissue.

Biofeedback: A technique involving self-monitoring by machine of physical responses to stress.

Biopsy: Microscopic examination of tissue to determine if a cancer is present.

Biopsychosocial model of addiction: Theory of the relationship among an addict's biological (genetic) nature and psychological and sociocultural influences.

Bisexual: Refers to attraction to and preference for sexual activity with people of both sexes.

Black tar heroin: A dark brown, sticky substance made from morphine.

Blood-alcohol concentration (BAC): The ratio of alcohol to total blood volume; the factor used to measure the physiological and behavioral effects of alcohol.

Body mass index (BMI): A technique of weight assessment based on the relationship of weight to height.

Body temperature method: A birth control method that requires a woman to monitor her body temperature for the rise that signals ovulation and to abstain from intercourse around this time.

Brief intervention therapy: Therapy based on the assumption that even very brief treatment, if designed properly, can be highly successful in treating addicts.

Brown fat cells: Specialized type of fat cell that affects the ability to regulate fat metabolism.

Bulimia nervosa: Eating disorder characterized by binge eating followed by inappropriate compensating measures taken to prevent weight gain.

Burnout: Physical and mental exhaustion caused by excessive stress.

Caffeine: A stimulant found in coffee, tea, chocolate, and some soft drinks.

Caffeinism: Caffeine intoxication brought on by excessive caffeine use; symptoms include chronic insomnia, irritability, anxiety, muscle twitches, and headaches.

Calendar method: A birth control method that requires mapping the woman's menstrual cycle on a calendar to determine presumed fertile times and abstaining from penis-vagina contact during those times.

Calorie: A unit of measure that indicates the amount of energy we obtain from a particular food.

Cancer: A large group of diseases characterized by the uncontrolled growth and spread of abnormal cells.

Candidiasis: Yeastlike fungal disease often transmitted sexually.

Capillaries: Minute blood vessels that branch out from the arterioles; their thin walls allow for the exchange of oxygen, carbon dioxide, nutrients, and waste products with body cells.

Carbohydrates: Basic nutrients that supply the body with the energy needed to sustain normal activity.

Carbon monoxide: An odorless, colorless gas which originates in motor vehicle emissions and cigarette smoke; it binds at oxygen receptor sites in blood.

Carcinogens: Cancer-causing agents.

Cardiovascular diseases (CVDs): Diseases of the heart and blood vessels.

Cardiovascular fitness: The ability of the heart, lungs, and blood vessels to function efficiently.

Cardiovascular system: A complex system consisting of the heart and blood vessels that transports nutrients, oxygen, hormones, and enzymes throughout the body and regulates temperature, the water levels of cells, and the acidity levels of body components.

Carpal tunnel syndrome: A common occupational injury in which the median nerve in the wrist becomes irritated, causing numbness, tingling, and pain in the fingers and hands.

Cataracts: Clouding of the lens that interrupts the focusing of light on the retina, resulting in blurred vision or eventual blindness.

Celibacy: State of not being involved in a sexual relationship.

Cellulose: Fiber, a major form of complex carbohydrates.

Cerebrospinal fluid: Fluid within and surrounding the brain and spinal cord tissues.

Cervical cap: A small cup made of latex that is designed to fit snugly over the entire cervix.

Cervical mucus method: A birth control method that relies upon observation of changes in cervical mucus to determine when the woman is fertile so the couple can abstain from intercourse during those times.

Cervix: Lower end of the uterus that opens into the vagina.

Cesarean section (C-section): A surgical procedure in which a baby is removed through an incision made in the mother's abdominal and uterine walls.

Chancre: Sore often found at the site of syphilis infection.

Chemotherapy: The use of drugs to kill cancerous cells.

Chewing tobacco: A stringy type of tobacco that is placed in the mouth and then sucked or chewed.

Child abuse: The systematic harming of a child by a caregiver, generally a parent.

Chiropractic medicine: A form of medical treatment that emphasizes the manipulation of the spinal column.

Chlamydia: Bacterially caused STD of the urogenital tract.

Chlorofluorocarbons (CFCs): Chemicals that contribute to the depletion of the ozone layer.

Cholesterol: A form of fat circulating in the blood that can accumulate on the inner walls of arteries.

Chronic bronchitis: A serious respiratory disorder in which the bronchial tubes become so inflamed and swollen that respiratory function is impaired.

Cirrhosis: The last stage of liver disease associated with chronic heavy use of alcohol during which liver cells die and damage is permanent.

Clitoris: A pea-sized organ located at the top of the labia minora.

Cloning: Replacing the nucleus of an in vitro-fertilized egg with the nucleus of a donor cell.

Cocaine: A powerful stimulant drug made from the leaves of the South American coca shrub.

Codeine: A drug derived from morphine; used in cough syrups and certain painkillers.

Codependence: A self-defeating relationship pattern in which a person is "addicted to the addict."

Cognitive stress system: The psychological system that governs our emotional responses to stress.

Cognitive therapy: Therapy aimed at teaching a person to recognize and refute the beliefs that hinder personal growth.

Cohabitation: Living together without being married.

Collateral circulation: Adaptation of the heart to partial damage accomplished by rerouting needed blood through unused or underused blood vessels while the damaged heart muscle heals.

Commercial preparations: Commonly used chemical substances including cosmetics, household cleaning products, and industrial by-products.

Common-law marriage: Cohabitation lasting a designated period of time (usually seven years) that is considered legally binding in some states.

Communication: The transmission of information and meaning from one individual to another.

Comorbidity: The presence of a number of diseases at the same time.

Complete (high-quality) proteins: Proteins that contain all of the eight essential amino acids.

Complex carbohydrates: A major type of carbohydrate which provides sustained energy.

Compulsion: Obsessive preoccupation with a behavior and an overwhelming need to perform it.

Compulsive gambler: A person addicted to gambling.

Computerized axial tomography (CAT scan): A machine that uses radiation to view internal organs not normally visible on X-rays.

Concentric muscle action: Force produced while shortening the muscle.

Conception: The fertilization of an ovum by a sperm.

Condom: A sheath of thin latex or other material designed to fit over an erect penis and to catch semen upon ejaculation.

Conflict: Simultaneous existence of incompatible demands, opportunities, needs, or goals; an emotional state that arises when the behavior of one person interferes with the behavior of another.

Conflict resolution: A concerted effort by all parties to resolve points in contention in a constructive manner.

Congeners: Forms of alcohol that are metabolized more slowly than ethanol and produce toxic by-products.

Congenital heart disease: Heart disease that is present at birth.

Conjunctivitis: Serious inflammation of the eye caused by any number of pathogens or irritants; can be caused by STDs such as chlamydia.

Contraception: Methods of preventing conception.

Contraceptive effectiveness rate: The percentage rate of women who will become pregnant in one year when the contraceptive method is used correctly.

Contraceptive sponge: A doughnut-shaped device moistened with water and placed in the vagina to block access to the uterus; the sponge is saturated with spermicide. This form of contraception is no longer available in the United States.

Coronary bypass surgery: A surgical technique whereby a blood vessel is implanted to bypass a clogged coronary artery.

Coronary thrombosis: A blood clot occurring in the coronary artery.

Cortisol: Hormone released by the adrenal glands that makes stored nutrients more readily available to meet energy demands.

Counselor: A person having a variety of academic and experiential training who deals with the treatment of emotional problems.

Crack: A distillate of powdered cocaine that comes in small, hard "chips" or "rocks."

Crank: An amphetamine-like stimulant having effects that last longer than those of crack or cocaine.

Cross reactivity: Allergic reaction to a whole family of foods.

Cross-tolerance: The development of a tolerance to one drug that reduces the effects of another, similar drug.

Cross training: Regular participation in two or more types of exercises (e.g., swimming and weight lifting).

Cunnilingus: Oral stimulation of a female's genitals.

Death: The "final cessation of the vital functions" and the state in which these functions are "incapable of being restored."

Dehydration: Abnormal depletion of body fluids; a result of lack of water.

Deliriant: Any substance that produces delirium at relatively low doses, including PCP and some herbal substances.

Delirium: An agitated mental state characterized by confusion and disorientation that can be produced by psychoactive drugs.

Delirium tremens (DTs): A state of confusion brought on by withdrawal from alcohol. Symptoms include hallucinations, anxiety, and trembling.

Denial: Inability to perceive or accurately interpret the effects of the addictive behavior.

Dentist: Specialist who diagnoses and treats diseases of the teeth, gums, and oral cavity.

Depo-Provera: An injectable method of birth control that lasts for three months.

Designer drug: A synthetic analog (a drug that produces similar effects) of an existing illicit drug.

Detoxification: The early abstinence period during which an addict adjusts physically and cognitively to being free from the influence of the addiction.

Developmental psychology: Branch of psychology that focuses on the personality's development by means of progression through developmental tasks.

Diabetes: A disease in which the pancreas fails to produce enough insulin or the body fails to use insulin effectively.

Diagnosis related groups (DRGs): Diagnostic categories established by the federal government to determine in advance how much hospitals will be reimbursed for the care of a particular Medicare patient.

Diaphragm: A latex, saucer-shaped device designed to cover the cervix and block access to the uterus; should always be used with spermicide.

Diastolic pressure: The lower number in the fraction that measures blood pressure, indicating pressure on the walls of the arteries during the relaxation phase of heart activity.

Diethylstilbestrol (DES): Type of morning-after pill containing large amounts of estrogen.

Digestive process: The process by which foods are broken down and either absorbed or excreted by the body.

Dilation and curettage (D&C): An abortion technique in which the cervix is dilated with laminaria for one to two days and the uterine walls are scraped clean.

Dilation and evacuation (D&E): An abortion technique that combines vacuum aspiration with dilation and curettage; fetal tissue is both sucked and scraped out of the uterus.

Dioxins: Highly toxic chlorinated hydrocarbons contained in herbicides and produced during certain industrial processes.

Disaccharide: A combination of two monosaccharides.

Disenfranchised grief: Grief concerning a loss that cannot be openly acknowledged, publicly mourned, or socially supported.

Distillation: The process whereby mash is subjected to high temperatures to release alcohol vapors, which are then condensed and mixed with water to make the final product.

Distress: Stress that can have a negative effect on health.

Diuretic: Drugs that increase the excretion of urine from the body.

Diverticulosis: A condition in which bulges form in the walls of the intestine; results in irritation and infection of the intestine.

Documenting: Giving specific examples of issues you are discussing.

Domestic violence: The use of force to control and maintain power over another person in the home environment; it includes both actual harm and the threat of harm.

Down's syndrome: A condition characterized by mental retardation and a variety of physical abnormalities.

Drug abuse: The excessive use of a drug.

Drug misuse: The use of a drug for a purpose for which it was not intended.

Dyathanasia: The passive form of "mercy killing" in which life-prolonging treatments or interventions are not offered or are withheld, thereby allowing a terminally ill person to die naturally.

Dying: The process of decline in body functions resulting in the death of an organism.

Dynamic stretching: Techniques that employ the repetitive, rapid stretching of muscles with no holding of the stretch at a terminal position; not recommended because of the risk of injury to muscle and/or tendon.

Dysfunctional family: A family in which the interaction between family members inhibits rather than enhances psychological growth.

Dyspareunia: Pain experienced by women during intercourse.

Eating disorder: Disorder consisting of severe disturbances in eating behavior, unhealthy efforts to control body weight, and abnormal attitudes about one's body and shape.

Eccentric muscle action: Force produced while lengthening the muscle.

Ectopic pregnancy: Implantation of a fertilized egg outside the uterus, usually in a fallopian tube; a medical emergency that can end in death from hemorrhage for the mother.

Editing: The process of censoring comments that would be intentionally hurtful or irrelevant to the conversation.

Ego: Personality force that seeks to restrain the id.

Ejaculation: The propulsion of semen from the penis.

Electrocardiogram (ECG): A record of the electrical activity of the heart.

Electroencephalogram (EEG): A device that measures the electrical activity of brain cells.

ELISA: Blood test that detects presence of antibodies to HIV virus.

Embolus: Blood clot that is forced through the circulatory system.

Embryo: The fertilized egg from conception until the end of two months' development.

Embryo freezing: The freezing of an embryo for later implantation.

Embryo transfer: Artificial insemination of a donor with male partner's sperm; after a time, the embryo is transferred from the donor to the female partner's body.

Emotional availability: The ability to give to and receive from other people emotionally without being inhibited by fears of being hurt.

Emotional health: The "feeling" part of psychosocial health. Includes your emotional reactions to life.

Emotions: Intensified feelings or complex patterns of feelings.

Emphysema: A respiratory disease in which the alveoli become distended or ruptured and are no longer functional.

Enablers: People who knowingly or unknowingly protect addicts from the natural consequences of their behavior.

Endemic: Describing a disease that is always present to some degree.

Endogenous depression: A type of depression that has a biochemical basis, such as neurotransmitter imbalances.

Endometriosis: A disorder in which uterine lining tissue establishes itself outside the uterus; it is the leading cause of infertility in the United States.

Endometrium: The mucous membrane lining the uterus.

Endorphins: Opiate-like hormones that are manufactured in the human body and contribute to natural feelings of well-being.

Environmental tobacco smoke (ETS): Smoke from tobacco products, including sidestream and mainstream smoke.

Enzymes: Organic substances that cause bodily changes and destruction of microorganisms.

Epidemic: Disease outbreak that affects many people in a community or region at the same time.

Epidermis: The outermost layer of the skin.

Epididymis: A comma-shaped structure inside the testis where sperm mature.

Epilepsy: A neurological disorder caused by abnormal electrical brain activity; can be accompanied by altered consciousness or convulsions.

Epinephrine: Also called adrenaline, a hormone that stimulates body systems in response to stress.

Episiotomy: A straight incision in the mother's perineum.

Erectile dysfunction: Also known as impotence; difficulty in achieving or maintaining a penile erection sufficient for intercourse.

Ergogenic drug: Substance that enhances athletic performance.

Erogenous zones: Areas in the body of both males and females that, when touched, lead to sexual arousal.

Esophagus: Tube that transports food from the mouth to the stomach.

Essential amino acids: Eight of the basic nitrogen-containing building blocks of protein that we must obtain from foods to ensure our personal health.

Essential hypertension: Hypertension that cannot be attributed to any cause.

Estrogens: Hormones that control the menstrual cycle.

Ethyl alcohol (ethanol): An addictive drug produced by fermentation and found in many beverages.

Eustress: Stress that presents opportunities for personal growth.

Euthanasia: The active form of "mercy killing" in which a person or organization knowingly acts to hasten the death of a terminally ill person.

Exercise metabolic rate (EMR): The energy expenditure that occurs during exercise.

Exercise training: The systematic performance of exercise at a specified frequency, intensity, and duration to achieve a desired level of physical fitness.

Exercise: Physical activity at higher-than-normal levels of exertion.

Exogenous depression: A type of depression that has an external cause, such as the loss of a loved one.

External female genitals: The mons pubis, labia majora and minora, clitoris, urethral and vaginal openings, and the vestibule of the vagina and its glands.

External male genitals: The penis and scrotum.

Fallopian tubes: Tubes that extend from the ovaries to the uterus.

Family therapy: Therapy that focuses on the problems of an entire family system rather than on those of one individual in that system.

Fats: Basic nutrients composed of carbon and hydrogen atoms; needed for the proper functioning of cells, insulation of body organs against shock, maintenance of body temperature, and healthy skin and hair.

Fellatio: Oral stimulation of a male's genitals.

Female condom: A single-use polyurethane sheath for internal use by women.

Fermentation: The process whereby yeast organisms break down plant sugars to yield ethanol.

Fertility: A person's ability to reproduce.

Fertility awareness methods (FAM): Include several types of birth control that require alteration of sexual behavior rather than chemical or physical intervention into the reproductive process.

Fertility drugs: Hormones that stimulate ovulation in women who are not ovulating; often responsible for multiple births.

Fetal alcohol effects (FAE): A syndrome describing children with a history of prenatal alcohol exposure but without all the physical or behavioral symptoms of FAS. Among its symptoms are low birth weight, irritability, and possible permanent mental impairment.

Fetal alcohol syndrome (FAS): A disorder that may affect the fetus when the mother consumes alcohol during pregnancy. Among its effects are mental retardation, small head, tremors, and abnormalities of the face, limbs, heart, and brain.

Fetus: The name given the developing baby from the third month of pregnancy until birth.

Fibrillation: A sporadic, quivering pattern of heartbeat resulting in extreme inefficiency in moving blood through the cardiovascular system.

Fibrocystic breast condition: A common, noncancerous condition in which a woman's breasts contain fibrous or fluid-filled cysts.

Flexibility: The measure of the range of motion, or the amount of movement possible, at a particular joint.

Follicle-stimulating hormone (FSH): Hormone that signals the ovaries to begin producing estrogens.

Food allergies: Overreaction by the body to normally harmless proteins, which are perceived as allergens. In response, the body produces antibodies, triggering allergic symptoms.

Food intolerance: Adverse effects resulting when people who lack the digestive chemicals needed to break down certain substances eat those substances.

Food irradiation: Treating foods with gamma radiation from radioactive cobalt, cesium, or some other source of X-rays to kill microorganisms.

Foreskin: Flap of skin covering the end of the penis; it is removed during circumcision.

Formaldehyde: A colorless, strong-smelling gas released through outgassing; causes respiratory and other health problems.

For-profit (proprietary) hospitals: Hospitals that provide a return on earnings to the investors who own them.

Freebase: The most powerful distillate of cocaine.

Fungi: A group of plants that lack chlorophyll and do not produce flowers or seeds; several varieties are pathogenic.

Gamete intrafallopian transfer (GIFT): An egg is harvested from the female partner ovary and placed with the male partner's sperm in her fallopian tube, where it is fertilized and then migrates to the uterus for implantation.

Gender: Your sense of masculinity or femininity as defined by the society in which you live.

Genderlect: The "dialect," or individual speech pattern and conversational style, of each gender.

Gender identity: Your personal sense or awareness of being masculine or feminine, a male or female.

Gender role stereotypes: Generalizations concerning how males and females should express themselves and the characteristics each possesses.

Gender roles: Expression of maleness or femaleness exhibited on a daily basis.

General adaptation syndrome (GAS): The pattern followed by our physiological responses to stress, consisting of the alarm, resistance, and exhaustion phases.

Generic drugs: Drugs marketed by their chemical name rather than by a brand name.

Genital herpes: STD caused by herpes simplex virus type 2.

German measles (rubella): A milder form of measles that causes a rash and mild fever in children and may cause damage to a fetus or a newborn baby.

Gerontology: The study of our individual and collective aging processes.

Girth and circumference measures: A method of assessing body fat that employs a formula based on girth measurements of various body sites.

Glaucoma: Elevation of pressure within the eyeball, leading to impaired vision and possible blindness.

Glycogen: The polysaccharide form in which glucose is stored in the liver.

Gonadotropin-releasing hormone (GnRH): Hormone that signals the pituitary gland to release gonadotropins.

Gonads: The reproductive organs in a male (testes) or female (ovaries).

Gonorrhea: Second most common STD in the United States; if untreated, may cause sterility.

Graded exercise test: A test of aerobic capacity administered by a physician, exercise physiologist, or other trained person; two common forms are the treadmill running test and the stationary bike test.

GRAE list: A list of drugs generally recognized as effective; they work for their intended purpose when used properly.

GRAS list: A list of drugs generally recognized as safe; they seldom cause side effects when used properly.

Greenhouse gases: Gases that contribute to global warming by trapping heat near the earth's surface.

Grief: The mental state of distress that occurs in reaction to significant loss, including one's own impending death, the death of a loved one, or a quasi-death experience.

Grief work: The process of accepting the reality of a person's death and coping with memories of the deceased.

Group practice: A group of physicians who combine resources, sharing offices, equipment, and staff costs, to render care to patients.

Habit: A repetitive behavior in which the repetition may be unconscious.

Hallucination: An image (auditory or visual) that is perceived but is not real.

Hangover: The physiological reaction to excessive drinking, including such symptoms as headache, upset stomach, anxiety, depression, diarrhea, and thirst.

Hashish: The sticky resin of the cannabis plant, which is high in THC.

Hay fever: A chronic respiratory disorder that is most prevalent when ragweed and flowers bloom.

Hazardous waste: Waste that, due to its toxic properties, poses a hazard to humans or to the environment.

Health: Dynamic, ever-changing process of trying to achieve your individual potential in the physical, social, emotional, mental, spiritual, and environmental dimensions.

Health Belief Model (HBM): Model for explaining how beliefs may influence behaviors.

Health promotion: Combines educational, organizational, policy, financial, and environmental supports to help people change negative health behaviors.

Heart attack: A blockage of normal blood supply to an area in the heart.

Heat cramps: Muscle cramps that occur during or following exercise in warm/hot conditions.

Heat exhaustion: A heat stress illness caused by significant dehydration resulting from exercise in warm/hot conditions; frequent precursor to heat stroke.

Heat stroke: A deadly heat stress illness resulting from dehydration and overexertion in warm/hot conditions; can cause body core temperature to rise from normal to 105°F to 110°F in just a few minutes.

Hepatitis: A disease in which the liver becomes inflamed, producing such symptoms as fever, headache, and jaundice.

Herbal preparations: Substances that are of plant origin that are believed to have medicinal properties.

Heroin: An illegally manufactured derivative of morphine, usually injected into the bloodstream.

Heterosexual: Refers to attraction to and preference for sexual activity with people of the opposite sex.

High-density lipoproteins (HDLs): Compounds that facilitate the transport of cholesterol in the blood to the liver for metabolism and elimination from the body.

Histamines: Chemical substances that dilate blood vessels, increase mucous secretions, and produce other allergy-like symptoms.

Holographic will: A will written in the testator's own handwriting and unwitnessed.

Homeostasis: A balanced physical state in which all the body's systems function smoothly.

Homicide: Death that results from intent to injure or kill.

Homophobia: Irrational hatred or fear of homosexuals or homosexuality.

Homosexual: Refers to attraction to and preference for sexual activity with people of the same sex.

Hormone replacement therapies (HRT): Therapies that replace estrogen in postmenopausal women.

Hospice: A concept of care for terminally ill patients designed to maximize the quality of life.

Human chorionic gonadotropin (HCG): Hormone detectable in blood or urine samples of a mother within the first few weeks of pregnancy. If increased levels of estrogen and progesterone are detected, fertilization has taken place.

Human immunodeficiency virus (HIV): The slow-acting virus that causes AIDS.

Humanistic psychology: Branch of psychology that posits that behavior is motivated by the desire to grow and achieve by making rational decisions that meet our individual needs.

Hunger: An inborn physiological response to nutritional needs.

Hydrocarbons: Chemical compounds that contain carbon and hydrogen.

Hydrostatic weighing techniques: Methods of determining body fat by measuring the amount of water displaced when a person is completely submerged.

Hymen: Thin tissue covering the vaginal opening.

Hyperglycemia: Elevated blood sugar levels.

Hyperplasia: A condition characterized by an excessive number of fat cells.

Hypertension: Sustained elevated blood pressure.

Hypertrophy: The theory that fat cells have the ability to enlarge and shrink.

Hypervitaminosis: A toxic condition caused by overuse of vitamin supplements.

Hypnosis: A process that allows people to become unusually responsive to suggestion.

Hypothalamus: An area of the brain located near the pituitary gland. The hypothalamus works in conjunction with the pituitary gland to control reproductive functions. The hypothalamus also controls the sympathetic nervous system and directs the stress response.

Hypothermia: Potentially fatal condition caused by abnormally low body core temperature.

Hysterectomy: Surgical removal of the uterus.

Hysterotomy: The surgical removal of the fetus from the uterus.

"I" messages: Ways of communicating with others by taking personal responsibility for communicating our own feelings, thoughts, and beliefs.

Ice: A potent, inexpensive stimulant that has long-lasting effects.

Id: Our unconscious desire for immediate gratification of wants and needs.

Illicit (illegal) drugs: Drugs whose use, possession, cultivation, manufacture, and/or sale are against the law because they are generally recognized as harmful.

Imagined rehearsal: Practicing through mental imagery, to become better able to perform an event in actuality.

Immunological competence: Ability of the immune system to defend the body from pathogens.

Immunotherapy: A process that stimulates the body's own immune system to combat cancer cells.

Impotence: Inability to attain or maintain an erection sufficient for intercourse.

In vitro fertilization: Fertilization of an egg in a nutrient medium and subsequent transfer back to the mother's body.

Incomplete proteins: Proteins that are lacking in one or more of the essential amino acids.

Incubation period: The time between exposure to a disease and the appearance of the symptoms.

Induction abortion: A type of abortion in which chemicals are injected into the uterus through the uterine wall; labor begins and the woman delivers a dead fetus.

Infertility: Difficulties in conceiving.

Influenza: A common viral disease of the respiratory tract.

Inhalants: Products that are sniffed or inhaled in order to produce highs.

Inhalation: The introduction of drugs through the nostrils.

Inhibited sexual desire (ISD): Lack of sexual appetite or simply a lack of interest and pleasure in sexual activity.

Inhibition: A type of interaction in which the effects of one drug are eliminated or reduced by the presence of another drug at the receptor site.

Injection: The introduction of drugs into the body via a hypodermic needle.

Insulin: A hormone produced by the pancreas; required by the body for the metabolism of carbohydrates.

Interferon: A protein substance produced by the body that aids the immune system by protecting healthy cells.

Internal female genitals: The vagina, uterus, fallopian tubes, and ovaries.

Internal male genitals: The testes, epididymides, vasa deferentia, ejaculatory ducts, urethra, and accessory glands.

Intervention: A planned confrontation with an alcoholic in which family members or friends express their concern about the alcoholic's drinking. Or any planned process of confrontation by significant others.

Intestate: The situation in which a person dies without having made a will.

Intimate relationships: "[C]lose relationships with another person in which you offer, and are offered, validation, understanding, and a sense of being valued intellectually, emotionally, and physically."

Intolerance: A type of interaction in which two or more drugs produce extremely uncomfortable symptoms.

Intramuscular injection: The introduction of drugs into muscles.

Intrauterine device (IUD): A T-shaped device that is implanted in the uterus to prevent pregnancy.

Intravenous injection: The introduction of drugs directly into a vein.

Inunction: The introduction of drugs through the skin.

Ionizing radiation: Radiation produced by photons having high enough energy to ionize atoms.

Irritable bowel syndrome (IBS): Nausea, pain, gas, or diarrhea caused by certain foods or stress.

Ischemia: Reduced oxygen supply to the heart.

Isometric muscle action: Force produced without any resulting muscle movement.

Jealousy: An aversive reaction evoked by a real or imagined relationship involving a person's partner and a third person.

Ketosis: A condition in which the body adapts to prolonged fasting or carbohydrate deprivation by converting body fat to ketones, which can be used as fuel for some brain activity.

Labia majora: "Outer lips" or folds of tissue covering the female sexual organs.

Labia minora: "Inner lips" or folds of tissue just inside the labia majora.

Laxative: Medications used to soften stool and relieve constipation.

Leach: A process by which chemicals dissolve and filter through soil.

Leachate: A liquid consisting of soluble chemicals that come from garbage and industrial waste that seeps into the water supply from landfills and dumps.

Lead: A metal found in the exhaust of motor vehicles powered by fuel containing lead and in emissions from lead smelters and processing plants.

Learned behavioral tolerance: The ability of heavy drinkers to modify their behavior so that they appear to be sober even when they have high BAC levels.

Learned helplessness: Pattern of responding to situations by giving up because you have always failed in the past.

Leukoplakia: A condition characterized by leathery white patches inside the mouth.

Leveling: The communication of a clear, simple, and honest message.

Limerence: The quality of sexual attraction based on chemistry and gratification of sexual desire.

Loss of control: Inability to predict reliably whether any isolated involvement with the addictive object or behavior will be healthy or damaging.

Low sperm count: A sperm count below 60 million sperm per milliliter of semen; it is the leading cause of infertility in men.

Low-density lipoproteins (LDLs): Compounds that facilitate the transport of cholesterol in the blood to the body's cells.

Lupus: A disease in which the immune system attacks the body, producing antibodies that destroy or injure organs such as the kidneys, brain, and heart.

Luteinizing hormone (LH): Hormone that signals the ovaries to release an egg and to begin producing progesterone.

Lysergic acid diethylamide (LSD): Psychedelic drug causing sensory disruptions; also called *acid.*

Macrominerals: Minerals that the body needs in fairly large amounts.

Magnetic resonance imaging (MRI): A device that uses magnetic fields, radio waves, and computers to generate an image of internal tissues of the body for diagnostic purposes without the use of radiation.

Mainstream smoke: Smoke that is drawn through tobacco while inhaling.

Malignant: Very dangerous or harmful; refers to a cancerous tumor.

Malignant melanoma: A virulent cancer of the melanin (pigment-producing portion) of the skin.

Managed care: Cost-control procedures used by health insurers to coordinate treatment.

Marijuana: Chopped leaves and flowers of the *cannabis indica* or *cannabis sativa* plant (hemp); a psychoactive stimulant that intensifies reactions to environmental stimuli.

Masturbation: Self-stimulation of genitals.

Measles: A viral disease that produces symptoms including an itchy rash and a high fever.

Medicaid: Federal-state health insurance program for the poor.

Medicare: Federal health insurance program for the elderly and the permanently disabled.

Meditation: A relaxation technique that involves deep breathing and concentration.

Meltdown: An accident that results when the temperature in the core of a nuclear reactor increases enough to melt the nuclear fuel and the containment vessel housing it.

Menarche: The first menstrual period.

Menopause: The permanent cessation of menstruation.

Mental health: The "thinking" part of psychosocial health. Includes your values, attitudes, and beliefs.

Mescaline: A hallucinogenic drug derived from the peyote cactus.

Metastasis: Process by which cancer spreads from one area to different areas of the body.

Methadone maintenance: A treatment for people addicted to opiates that substitutes methadone, a synthetic narcotic, for the opiate of addiction.

Middle-old: People aged 75 to 84.

Migraine: A condition characterized by localized headaches that result from alternating dilation and constriction of blood vessels.

Minerals: Inorganic substances that aid physiological processes.

Miscarriage: Loss of the fetus before it is viable; also called spontaneous abortion.

Modeling: Learning specific behaviors by watching others perform them.

Monogamy: Exclusive sexual involvement with one partner.

Monosaccharide: A simple sugar that contains only one molecule of sugar.

Mons pubis: Fatty tissue covering the pubic bone in females; in physically mature women, the mons is covered with coarse hair.

Morbidity: Illness rate.

Morning-after pill: Drugs taken within three days after intercourse to prevent fertilization or implantation.

Morphine: A derivative of opium; sometimes used by medical practitioners to relieve pain.

Mortality: Death rate.

Mourning: The culturally prescribed behavior patterns for the expression of grief.

Multifactorial disease: Disease caused by interactions of several factors.

Municipal solid waste: Includes such wastes as durable goods, nondurable goods, containers and packaging, food wastes, yard wastes, and miscellaneous wastes from residential, commercial, institutional, and industrial sources.

Muscular endurance: A muscle's ability to exert force repeatedly without fatiguing.

Muscular strength: The amount of force that a muscle is capable of exerting.

Mutant cells: Cells that differ in form, quality, or function from normal cells.

Myocardial infarction (MI): Heart attack.

Narcotics: Drugs that induce sleep and relieve pain; primarily the opiates.

Natural immunity: Immunity passed to a fetus by its mother.

Negative consequences: Physical damage, legal trouble, financial ruin, academic failure, family dissolution, and other severe problems associated with addiction.

Neoplasm: A new growth of tissue that serves no physiological function, resulting from uncontrolled, abnormal cellular development.

Neurotransmitters: Biochemical messengers that exert influence at specific receptor sites on nerve cells.

Nicotine: The stimulant chemical in tobacco products.

Nicotine poisoning: Symptoms often experienced by beginning smokers; they include dizziness; diarrhea; lightheadedness; rapid, erratic pulse; clammy skin; nausea; and vomiting.

Nicotine withdrawal: Symptoms including nausea, headaches, and irritability, suffered by smokers who cease using tobacco.

Nitrogen dioxide: An amber-colored gas found in smog; can cause eye and respiratory irritations.

Nitrous oxide: The chemical name for "laughing gas," a substance properly used for surgical or dental anesthesia.

Nonallopathic medicine: Medical alternatives to traditional, allopathic medicine.

Nonassertive communicators: Individuals who tend to be shy and inhibited in their communication with others.

Nonionizing radiation: Radiation produced by photons associated with lower-energy portions of the electromagnetic spectrum.

Nonpoint source pollutants: Pollutants that run off or seep into waterways from broad areas of land.

Nonprofit (voluntary) hospitals: Hospitals run by religious or other humanitarian groups that reinvest their earnings in the hospital to improve health care.

Nonsurgical embryo transfer: In vitro fertilization of a donor egg by the male partner's (or donor's) sperm and subsequent transfer to the female partner's or another woman's uterus.

Nonverbal communication: All unwritten and unspoken messages, both intentional and unintentional.

Norplant: A long-lasting contraceptive that consists of six silicon capsules surgically inserted under the skin in a woman's upper arm.

Nurse: Health practitioner who provides many services for patients and who may work in a variety of settings.

Nurturing through avoidance: Repeatedly seeking the illusion of relief to avoid unpleasant feelings or situations, a maladaptive way of taking care of emotional needs.

Nutrients: The constituents of food that sustain us physiologically: proteins, carbohydrates, fats, vitamins, minerals, and water.

Nutrition: The science that investigates the relationship between physiological function and the essential elements of foods we eat.

Obesity: A weight disorder generally defined as an accumulation of fat beyond that considered normal for a person's age, sex, and body type.

Obsession: Excessive preoccupation with an addictive object or behavior.

Obsessive-compulsive disorder (OCD): A disorder characterized by obsessive thoughts or habitual behaviors that cannot be controlled.

Old-old: People aged 85 and over.

Oncogenes: Suspected cancer-causing genes present on chromosomes.

Oncologists: Physicians who specialize in the treatment of malignancies.

One repetition maximum (1RM): The amount of weight/resistance that can be lifted/moved one time, but not twice; a common measure of strength.

Open relationship: A relationship in which partners agree that there can be sexual involvement outside the relationship.

Ophthalmologist: Physician who specializes in the medical and surgical care of the eyes, including writing prescriptions for glasses.

Opium: The parent drug of the opiates; made from the seedpod resin of the opium poppy.

Optometrist: Eye specialist whose practice is limited to prescribing and fitting lenses.

Oral contraceptives: Pills taken daily for three weeks of the menstrual cycle which prevent ovulation by regulating hormones.

Oral ingestion: Intake of drugs through the mouth.

Oral surgeon: Dentist who performs surgical procedures to correct problems of the mouth, jaw, and face.

Organically grown: Foods that are grown without use of pesticides or chemicals.

Orthodontist: Dentist who specializes in the alignment of teeth.

Osteoarthritis: A disease characterized by degeneration of joint cartilage and irritation of surrounding bone and soft tissue.

Osteopath: General practitioner who receives training similar to a medical doctor's but who puts special emphasis on the skeletal and muscular systems, often using spinal manipulation as part of treatment.

Osteoporosis: A disease characterized by low bone mass and deterioration of bone tissue.

Outpatient (ambulatory) care: Treatment that does not involve an overnight stay in a hospital.

Ovarian follicles (egg sacs): Areas within the ovary in which individual eggs develop.

Ovaries: Organs that produce eggs and female sex hormones.

Over-the-counter (OTC) drugs: Medications that can be purchased in pharmacies or supermarkets without a physician's prescription.

Overload: A condition in which we feel overly pressured by demands made on us.

Overuse injuries: Injuries that result from the cumulative effects of day-after-day stresses placed on tendons, muscles, and joints.

Ovulation: The point of the menstrual cycle at which a mature egg ruptures through the ovarian wall.

Ozone: A gas formed when nitrogen dioxide interacts with hydrogen chloride.

Panic attack: The sudden, rapid onset of disabling terror.

Pap test: A procedure in which cells taken from the cervical region are examined for abnormal cellular activity.

Parasympathetic nervous system: Part of the autonomic nervous system responsible for slowing systems stimulated by the stress response.

Particulates: Nongaseous air pollutants.

Pathogen: A disease-causing agent.

Pelvic inflammatory disease (PID): Term used to describe various infections of the female reproductive tract. PID can cause infertility.

Penicillin: Antibiotic used to fight a variety of bacterially caused ailments.

Penis: Male sexual organ designed for releasing sperm into the vagina.

Peptic ulcer: Damage to the stomach or intestinal lining, usually caused by digestive juices.

Perineum: The area between the vulva and the anus.

Periodontal diseases: Diseases of the tissue around the teeth.

Personal control: Belief that your internal resources can allow you to control a situation.

Pesticides: Chemicals that kill pests.

Peyote: A cactus with small "buttons" that, when ingested, produce hallucinogenic effects.

Phencyclidine (PCP): A deliriant commonly called *angel dust.*

Phobia: A deep and persistent fear of a specific object, activity, or situation that results in a compelling desire to avoid the source of the fear.

Photochemical smog: The brownish-yellow haze resulting from the combination of hydrocarbons and nitrogen oxides.

Physical fitness: A set of attributes related to the ability to perform normal physical activity.

Pinch test: A method of determining body fat whereby a fold of skin just behind the triceps is pinched between the thumb and index finger to determine the relative amount of fat.

Pituitary gland: A gland located deep within the brain; controls reproductive functions.

Placebo effect: An apparent cure or improved state of health brought about by a substance or product that has no medicinal value.

Placenta: The network of blood vessels that carries nutrients to the developing fetus and carries wastes away; it connects the umbilical cord to the uterus.

Plaque: Cholesterol buildup on the inner walls of arteries, causing a narrowing of the channel through which blood flows; a major cause of atherosclerosis.

Plateau: That point in a weight-loss program at which the dieter finds it difficult to lose more weight.

Platelet adhesiveness: Stickiness of red blood cells associated with blood clots.

Pneumonia: Bacterially caused disease of the lungs.

Point source pollutants: Pollutants that enter waterways at a specific point.

Polychlorinated biphenyls (PCBs): Toxic chemicals that were once used as insulating materials in high-voltage electrical equipment.

Polydrug use: The use of multiple medications or illicit drugs simultaneously.

Polysaccharide: A complex carbohydrate formed by the combination of long chains of saccharides.

Positive reinforcement: Presenting something positive following a behavior that is being reinforced.

Positron emission tomography (PET scan): Method for measuring heart activity by injecting a patient with a radioactive tracer that is scanned electronically to produce a three-dimensional image of the heart and arteries.

Postpartum depression: The experience of energy depletion, anxiety, mood swings, and depression that women may feel during the postpartum period.

Power: The ability to make and implement decisions.

Preconception care: Medical care received prior to becoming pregnant that helps a woman assess and address potential maternal health.

Prejudice: A negative evaluation of an entire group of people that is typically based on unfavorable and often wrong ideas about the group.

Premature ejaculation: Ejaculation that occurs prior to or almost immediately following penile penetration of the vagina.

Premenstrual syndrome (PMS): A series of physical and emotional symptoms that may occur in women prior to their menstrual periods.

Preorgasmic: In women, the state of never having experienced an orgasm.

Prescription drugs: Medications that can be obtained only with the written prescription of a licensed physician.

Prevention: Actions or behaviors designed to keep you from getting sick.

Primary care practitioner: A medical practitioner who treats routine ailments, advises on preventive care, gives general medical advice, and makes appropriate referrals when necessary.

Primary prevention: Actions designed to stop problems before they start.

Progesterone: Hormone secreted by the ovaries; helps keep the endometrium developing in order to nourish a fertilized egg; also helps maintain pregnancy.

Proof: A measure of the percentage of alcohol in a beverage.

Prostaglandin inhibitors: Drugs that inhibit the production and release of prostaglandins associated with arthritis or menstrual pain.

Prostate gland: Gland that secretes nutrients and neutralizing fluids into the semen.

Prostate-specific antigen (PSA): An antigen found in prostate cancer patients.

Proteins: The essential constituents of nearly all body cells. Proteins are necessary for the development and repair of bone, muscle, skin, and blood, and are the key elements of antibodies, enzymes, and hormones.

Protooncogenes: Genes that can become oncogenes under certain conditions.

Protozoa: Microscopic, single-celled organisms.

Psilocybin: The active chemical found in psilocybe mushrooms; it produces hallucinations.

Psychedelics: Drugs that distort the processing of sensory information in the brain.

Psychiatrist: A licensed physician who specializes in treating mental and emotional disorders.

Psychoactive drugs: Drugs that have the potential to alter mood or behavior.

Psychoanalyst: A psychiatrist or psychologist having special training in psychoanalysis.

Psychodynamic therapy: Therapy that allows a person to express emotions dramatically; release comes through catharsis.

Psychological hardiness: A personality characteristic characterized by control, commitment, and challenge.

Psychologist: A person with a Ph.D. degree and training in psychology.

Psychoneuroimmunology (PNI): Science of the interaction between the mind and the immune system.

Psychosocial health: The mental, emotional, social, and spiritual dimensions of health.

Puberty: The period of sexual maturation.

Pubic lice: Parasites that can inhabit various body areas, especially the genitals; also called "crabs."

Quasi-death experiences: Losses or experiences that resemble death in that they involve separation, termination, significant loss, a change of personal identity, and grief.

Rabies: A viral disease of the central nervous system often transmitted through animal bites.

Radiation absorbed doses (rads): Units that measure exposure to radioactivity.

Radiotherapy: The use of radiation to kill cancerous cells.

Radon: A naturally occurring radioactive gas resulting from the decay of certain radioactive elements.

Rape: Sexual penetration without the victim's consent.

Raynaud's syndrome: A disease in which exposure to cold temperatures produces exaggerated constriction of the small arteries in the extremities, causing fingers and toes to go numb, turn white, and then turn deep purple.

Rebound effects: Severe withdrawal effects experienced by users of stimulants, including depression, nausea, and violent behavior.

Receptor sites: Specialized cells to which drugs can attach themselves.

Recreational drugs: Legal drugs that contain chemicals that help people to relax or socialize.

Relapse: The tendency to return to the addictive behavior after a period of abstinence.

Resistance exercise program: A regular program of exercises designed to improve muscular strength and endurance in the major muscle groups.

Resource-based relative value scale (RBRVS): A system established by the federal government that uses physician work, practice expense, and practice risk to determine in advance how much a physician will be reimbursed for the care of a particular Medicare patient.

Respite care: The care provided by substitute caregivers to relieve the principal caregiver from his or her continuous responsibility.

Resting metabolic rate (RMR): The energy expenditure of the body under BMR conditions plus other daily sedentary activities.

Retarded ejaculation: The inability to ejaculate once the penis is erect.

Reticular formation: An area in the brain stem that is responsible for relaying messages to other areas in the brain.

Rh factor: A blood protein related to the production of antibodies. If an Rh-negative mother is pregnant with an Rh-positive fetus, the mother will manufacture antibodies that can kill the fetus, causing miscarriage.

Rheumatic heart disease: A heart disease caused by untreated streptococcal infection of the throat.

Rheumatoid arthritis: A serious inflammatory joint disease.

RICE: Acronym for the standard first-aid treatment for virtually all traumatic and overuse injuries: rest, ice, compression, and elevation.

Rickettsia: A small form of bacteria that live inside other living cells.

Route of administration: The manner in which a drug is taken into the body.

RU-486: A steroid hormone that induces abortion by blocking the action of progesterone. Testing in the United States began in late 1994.

Saliva: Fluid secreted by the salivary glands; enzymes in the fluid aid in the breakdown of certain foods for digestion.

Satiety: The feeling of fullness or satisfaction at the end of a meal.

Saturated fats: Fats that are unable to hold any more hydrogen in their chemical structure; derived mostly from animal sources; solid at room temperature.

Schizophrenia: A mental illness with biological origins that is characterized by irrational behavior, severe alterations of the senses (hallucinations), and, often, an inability to function in society.

Scleroderma: A disease in which fibrous growth of connective tissue underlying the skin and body organs hardens and makes movement difficult.

Scrotum: Sac of tissue that encloses the testes.

Seasonal affective disorder (SAD): A type of depression that occurs in the winter months, when sunlight levels are low.

Secondary hypertension: Hypertension caused by specific factors, such as kidney disease, obesity, or tumors of the adrenal glands.

Secondary prevention: Intervention early in the development of a health problem.

Secondary sex characteristics: Characteristics associated with gender but not directly related to reproduction, such as vocal pitch, degree of body hair, and location of fat deposits.

Sedatives: Central nervous system depressants that induce sleep and relieve anxiety.

Self-deliverance: A positive action taken to provide a permanent solution to the long-term pain and suffering for the individual and his or her loved ones faced with terminal illness.

Self-disclosure: The process of revealing one's inner thoughts, feelings, and beliefs to another person.

Self-efficacy: Belief in your ability to perform a task successfully.

Self-esteem: Sense of self-respect or self-confidence.

Self-nurturance: Developing individual potential through a balanced and realistic appreciation of self-worth and ability.

Semen: Fluid containing sperm and nutrient fluids that increase sperm viability and neutralize vaginal acid.

Seminal vesicles: Storage areas for sperm where nutrient fluids are added to them.

Senility: A term associated with loss of memory and judgment and orientation problems occurring in a small percentage of the elderly.

Serial monogamy: Monogamous sexual relationship with one partner before moving on to another.

Set: The total internal environment, or mindset, of a person at the time a drug is taken.

Setpoint theory: A theory of obesity causation that suggests that fat storage is determined by a thermostatic mechanism in the body that acts to maintain a specific amount of body fat.

Setting: The total external environment of a person at the time a drug is taken.

Sexual abuse of children: Sexually suggestive conversations; inappropriate kissing; touching; petting; oral, anal, or vaginal intercourse; and/or other kinds of sexual interaction between a child and an adult or an older child.

Sexual assault: Any act in which one person is sexually intimate with another person without that other person's consent.

Sexual aversion disorder: Type of desire dysfunction characterized by sexual phobias and anxiety about sexual contact.

Sexual dysfunction: Problems associated with achieving sexual satisfaction.

Sexual fantasies: Sexually arousing thoughts and dreams.

Sexual harassment: Any form of unwanted sexual attention.

Sexual identity: Our recognition of ourselves as sexual creatures; a composite of gender, gender roles, sexual preference, body image, and sexual scripts.

Sexual orientation: Attraction to and interest in members of the opposite sex, the same sex, or both sexes in emotional, social, and sexual situations.

Sexually transmitted diseases (STDs): Infectious diseases transmitted via some form of intimate, usually sexual, contact.

Shaping: Using a series of small steps to get to a particular goal gradually.

Sickle cell anemia: Genetic disease commonly found among African Americans; results in organ damage and premature death.

Sidestream smoke: The cigarette, pipe, or cigar smoke breathed by nonsmokers; also called *secondhand smoke.*

Simple sugars: A major type of carbohydrate which provides short-term energy.

Sinoatrial node (SA node): Node serving as a form of natural pacemaker for the heart.

Situational inducement: Attempt to influence a behavior by using situations and occasions that are structured to exert control over that behavior.

Skinfold caliper test: A method of determining body fat whereby folds of skin and fat at various points on the body are grasped between thumb and forefinger and measured with calipers.

Slow-acting viruses: Viruses having long incubation periods and causing slowly progressive symptoms.

Small intestine: Muscular, coiled digestive organ; consists of the duodenum, jejunum, and ileum.

Snuff: A powdered form of tobacco that is sniffed and absorbed through the mucous membranes in the nose or placed inside the cheek and sucked.

Social bonds: Degree and nature of our interpersonal contacts.

Social death: An irreversible situation in which a person is not treated like an active member of society.

Social learning theory: Theory that people learn behaviors by watching role models—parents, caregivers, and significant others.

Social supports: Structural and functional aspects of our social interactions.

Social worker: A person with an M.S.W. degree and clinical training.

Socialization: Process by which a society identifies behavioral expectations to its individual members.

Soft-tissue roentgenogram: A technique of body fat assessment in which radioactive substances are used to determine relative fat.

Solo practitioner: Physician who renders care to patients independently of other practitioners.

Spermatogenesis: The development of sperm.

Spermicides: Substances designed to kill sperm.

Spontaneous remission: The disappearance of symptoms without any apparent cause or treatment.

Staphylococci: Round, gram-positive bacteria, usually found in clusters.

Static stretching: Techniques that gradually lengthen a muscle to an elongated position (to the point of discomfort) and hold that position for 10 to 30 seconds.

Sterilization: Permanent fertility control achieved through surgical procedures.

Stillbirth: The birth of a dead baby.

Stomach: Large muscular organ that temporarily stores, mixes, and digests foods.

Strain: The wear and tear our bodies and minds sustain as we adjust to or resist a stressor.

Streptococci: Round bacteria, usually found in chain formation.

Stress: Our mental and physical responses to change.

Stressor: A physical, social, or psychological event or condition that causes us to have to adjust to a specific situation.

Stroke: A condition occurring when the brain is damaged by disrupted blood supply.

Subcutaneous injection: The introduction of drugs into the layer of fat directly beneath the skin.

Sudden infant death syndrome (SIDS): Death that occurs without apparent cause in babies under two years of age; some cases may be associated with tobacco use by the mother during pregnancy.

Sulfur dioxide: A yellowish-brown gaseous by-product of the burning of fossil fuels.

Superego: Personality force that serves as our conscience.

Superfund: Fund established under the Comprehensive Environmental Response Compensation and Liability Act to be used for cleaning up toxic waste dumps.

Suppositories: Mixtures of drugs and a waxy medium designed to melt at body temperature that are inserted into the anus or vagina.

Sympathetic nervous system: Branch of the autonomic nervous system responsible for stress arousal.

Sympathomimetics: Drugs found in appetite suppressants that affect the sympathetic nervous system.

Synergism: An interaction of two or more drugs that produces more profound effects than would be expected if the drugs were taken separately.

Synesthesia: A (usually) drug-created effect in which sensory messages are incorrectly assigned—for example, hearing a taste or smelling a sound.

Syphilis: One of the most widespread STDs; characterized by distinct phases and potentially serious results.

Systolic pressure: The upper number in the fraction that measures blood pressure, indicating pressure on the walls of the arteries when the heart contracts.

Tai chi: An ancient, Chinese form of exercise widely practiced in the West today that promotes balance, coordination, stretching, and meditation.

Tar: A thick, brownish substance condensed from particulate matter in smoked tobacco.

Target heart rate: Calculated as a percentage of maximum heart rate (220 minus age); heart rate (pulse) is taken during aerobic exercise to check if exercise intensity is at the desired level (e.g., 70 percent of maximum heart rate).

Temperature inversion: A weather condition occurring when a layer of cool air is trapped under a layer of warmer air.

Teratogenic: Causing birth defects; may refer to drugs, environmental chemicals, X-rays, or diseases.

Tertiary prevention: Treatment and/or rehabilitation efforts.

Testator: A person who leaves a will or testament at death.

Testes: Two organs, located in the scrotum, that manufacture sperm and produce hormones.

Testosterone: The male sex hormone manufactured in the testes.

Tetrahydrocannabinol (THC): The chemical name for the active ingredient in marijuana.

Thanatology: The study of death and dying.

Theory of Reasoned Action: Model for explaining the importance of our intentions in determining behaviors.

Therapy: One of over 250 types of treatment designed to help people overcome their personal problems.

Thrombolysis: Injection of an agent to dissolve clots and restore some blood flow, thereby reducing the amount of tissue that dies from ischemia.

Thrombus: Blood clot.

Thyroid gland: A two-lobed endocrine gland located in the throat region that produces a hormone that regulates metabolism.

Tolerance: Phenomenon in which progressively larger doses of a drug or more intense involvement in a behavior is needed to produce the desired effects.

Total body electrical conductivity (TOBEC): Technique using an electromagnetic force field to assess relative body fat.

Toxic shock syndrome (TSS): A potentially life-threatening disease that occurs when specific bacterial toxins are allowed to multiply unchecked in wounds or through improper use of tampons or diaphragms.

Toxins: Poisonous substances produced by certain microorganisms that cause various diseases.

Trace minerals: Minerals that the body needs in only very small amounts.

Tranquilizers: Central nervous system depressants that relax the body and calm anxiety.

Trans-fatty acids: Fatty acids that are produced when polyunsaturated oils are hydrogenated to make them more solid.

Transient ischemic attacks (TIAs): Mild form of stroke; often an indicator of impending major stroke.

Transition: The process during which the cervix becomes nearly fully dilated and the head of the fetus begins to move into the birth canal.

Traumatic injuries: Injuries that are accidental in nature; they occur suddenly and violently (e.g., fractured bones, ruptured tendons, and sprained ligaments).

Trichomoniasis: Protozoan infection characterized by foamy, yellowish discharge and unpleasant odor.

Triglyceride: The most common form of fat in the body; excess calories consumed are converted into triglycerides and stored as body fat.

Trimester: A three-month segment of pregnancy; used to describe specific developmental changes that occur in the embryo or fetus.

Trust: The degree of confidence felt in a relationship.

Tubal ligation: Sterilization of the female that involves the cutting and tying off of the fallopian tubes.

Tuberculosis (TB): A disease caused by bacterial infiltration of the respiratory system.

Tumor: A neoplasmic mass that grows more rapidly than surrounding tissues.

Ulcerative colitis: An inflammatory disorder that affects the mucous membranes of the large intestine, producing bloody diarrhea.

Unsaturated fats: Fats that do have room for more hydrogen in their chemical structure; derived mostly from plants; liquid at room temperature.

Urethral opening: The opening through which urine is expelled.

Urinary incontinence: The inability to control urination.

Uterus (womb): Hollow, pear-shaped muscular organ whose function is to contain the developing fetus.

Vaccination: Inoculation with killed or weakened pathogens or similar, less dangerous antigens in order to prevent or lessen the effects of some disease.

Vacuum aspiration: The use of gentle suction to remove fetal tissue from the uterus.

Vagina: The passage in females leading from the vulva to the uterus.

Vaginal intercourse: The insertion of the penis into the vagina.

Vaginismus: A state in which the vaginal muscles contract so forcefully that penetration cannot be accomplished.

Vaginitis: Set of symptoms characterized by vaginal itching, swelling, and burning.

Validating: Letting your partner know that although you may not agree with his or her point of view, you still respect the fact that he or she thinks or feels that way.

Variant sexual behavior: A sexual behavior that is not engaged in by most people.

Vas deferens: A tube that transports sperm toward the penis.

Vasectomy: Sterilization of the male that involves the cutting and tying of both vasa deferentia.

Vasocongestion: The engorgement of the genital organs with blood.

Vegetarian: A term with a variety of meanings: vegans avoid all foods of animal origin; lacto-vegetarians avoid flesh foods but eat dairy products; ovo-vegetarians avoid flesh foods but eat eggs; lacto-ovo-vegetarians avoid flesh foods but eat both dairy products and eggs; pesco-vegetarians avoid meat but eat fish, dairy products, and eggs; semivegetarians eat chicken, fish, dairy products, and eggs.

Veins: Vessels that carry blood back to the heart from other regions of the body.

Venereal warts: Warts that appear in the genital area or the anus; caused by the human papilloma viruses (HPVs).

Ventricles: The two lower chambers of the heart, which pump blood through the blood vessels.

Very low calorie diets (VLCDs): Diets with a caloric value of 400 to 700 calories.

Violence: Refers to a set of behaviors that produce injuries, as well as the outcomes of these behaviors (the injuries themselves).

Virulent: Said of organisms able to overcome host resistance and cause disease.

Viruses: Minute parasitic microbes that live inside another cell.

Vitamins: Essential organic compounds that promote growth and reproduction and help maintain life and health.

Vulva: The female's external genitalia.

Wellness: The achievement of the highest level of health possible in each of several dimensions.

Western blot: More precise test than the ELISA to confirm presence of HIV antibodies.

Withdrawal: A method of contraception that involves withdrawing the penis from the vagina before ejaculation. Also called "coitus interruptus."

Withdrawal: A series of temporary physical and biopsychosocial symptoms that occurs when the addict abruptly abstains from an addictive chemical or behavior.

Workaholic: A person who gradually becomes emotionally crippled and addicted to control and power in a compulsive drive to gain approval and success.

Xanthines: The chemical family of stimulants to which caffeine belongs.

Yoga: A variety of Indian forms of exercise widely practiced in the West today that promote balance, coordination, flexibility, and meditation.

Young-old: People aged 65 to 74.

Yo-yo diet: Cycles in which people repeatedly gain weight, then starve themselves to lose weight. This lowers their BMR, which makes regaining weight even more likely.

References

CHAPTER 1

1. World Health Organization, "Constitution of the World Health Organization," *Chronicles of the World Health Organization,* Geneva, Switzerland, 1947.
2. René Dubos, *So Human the Animal* (New York: Scribners, 1968), 15.
3. Department of Health and Human Services, *Healthy People 2000: National Health Promotion and Disease Prevention Objectives for the Year 2000* (Washington, D.C.: Government Printing Office, 1990).
4. Ibid.
5. Lisa Miller, "Medical Schools Put Women in Curricula," *Wall Street Journal,* 24 May, 1994, B1, B7.
6. Elizabeth Austin, "Women in Focus," *Shape,* September 1994, 46–47.
7. Carol Tavris, *The Mismeasure of Woman* (New York: Touchstone, 1992), 99.
8. Ibid.
9. Miller, op cit., B1, B7.
10. M. DiMatteo, *The Psychology of Health, Illness, and Medical Care: An Individual Perspective* (Pacific Grove, CA: Brooks/Cole 1994), 101–103.
11. Edward P. Sarafino, *Health Psychology* (New York: John Wiley & Sons, 1990), 189–191.
12. George D. Bishop, *Health Psychology* (Needham Heights, MA: Allyn and Bacon, 1994), 84–86.
13. A. Ellis and M. Bernard, *Clinical Application of Rational Emotive Therapy* (New York: Plenum, 1985).
14. P. Watson and R. Tharp, *Self-Directed Behavior: Self Modification for Personal Adjustment* (Pacific Grove, CA: Brooks/Cole, 1993), 13.
15. *The Stanford DECIDE Drug Education Curriculum,* Garfield Company, CA.

CHAPTER 2

1. National Mental Health Association, *Mental Health,* (Alexandria, VA: National Mental Health Association, 1988), 3–4; W. Menninger, "Emotional Maturity," in *A Psychiatrist for a Troubled World: Selected Papers of William Menninger,* ed. Bernard H. Hall (New York: Viking, 1967), 789–807.
2. Richard Lazarus, *Emotion and Adaptation* (New York: Oxford Press, 1991).
3. Christine Ritter, "Social Supports, Social Networks, and Health Behaviors," in *Health Behavior: Emerging Research Perspectives,* ed. David Gochman. (New York: Plenum, 1988).

4. Lester Lefton, *Psychology,* Fifth Edition (Boston: Allyn and Bacon, 1994), 626.
5. A. O'Connell and V. O'Connell, *Choice and Change: Psychology of Holistic Growth, Adjustment, and Creativity* (Englewood Cliffs, NJ: Prentice Hall, 1992).
6. C. G. Jung, *Man and His Symbols,* ed. Aniela Jaffe (Garden City, NY: Doubleday, 1963).
7. Ibid., 65.
8. Martin Seligman, *Learned Optimism* (New York: Knopf, 1990).
9. Excerpted by permission from the *University of California at Berkeley Wellness Letter,* July 1992, 3–4. © Health Letter Associates, 1992.
10. D. Grady, "Think Right, Stay Well," *American Health,* xi (1992): 50–54.
11. Ibid., 50–54.
12. Bernie Siegel, *Love, Medicine, and Miracles* (New York: HarperCollins, 1988).
13. Grady, op. cit., 50–54.
14. Ibid., 50–54.
15. Ibid., 50–54.
16. Ibid., 50–54.
17. Lydia Temoshock, *The Type C Connection* (New York: Random House, 1989).
18. Adapted by permission of the author from Kathryn Rose Gertz, "Mood Probe: Pinpointing the Crucial Differences between Emotional Lows and the Gridlock of Depression," *Self,* November 1990, 165–168, 204.
19. G. Terence Wilson, Peter Nathan, K. Daniel O'Leary, and Lee Anna Clark, *Abnormal Psychology* (Boston: Allyn and Bacon, 1996), from chapter 7.
20. Ibid.
21. Lefton, op. cit., 480–482.
22. Ibid., 480–482.

CHAPTER 3

1. Hans Selye, *Stress without Distress* (New York: Lippincott, 1974), 28–29.
2. Charles Morris, *Understanding Psychology* (Englewood Cliffs, NJ: Prentice Hall, 1993), 471–473.
3. Walter Schafer, *Stress Management for Wellness,* 2nd ed. (New York: Harcourt Brace, Jovanovich, 1992),
4. R. Ader and S. Cohen, "Psychoneuroimmunology: Conditioning and Stress," *Annual Review of Psychology* 44 (1993): 53–85.
5. N. Cohen, D. Tyrrell, and A. Smith, "Negative Life Events, Perceived Stress, Negative Affect, and Susceptibility to the Com-

mon Cold," *Journal of Personality and Social Psychology* (1993): 64 (131–140).

6. Ader and Cohen, op. cit., 53–85.

7. Ibid., 59.

8. Selye, op. cit., 28–29.

9. Thomas Holmes and Richard Rahe, "The Social Readjustment Rating Scale," *Journal of Psychosocial Research* (1967): 213–217.

10. Ibid., 214.

11. Richard Lazarus, "The Trivialization of Distress," *Preventing Health Risk Behaviors and Promoting Coping with Illness,* ed. J. Rosen and L. Solomon (Hanover, NH: University Press of New England, 1985), 279–298.

12. Lester Lefton, *Psychology* (Boston: Allyn and Bacon, 1994), 471.

13. Ibid., 471.

14. R. C. Kessler, K. S. Kendler, A. C. Heath, M. C. Neale, and L. J. Eaves, "Social Support, Depressed Mood, and Adjustment to Stress: A Genetic Epidemiological Investigation," *Journal of Personality and Social Psychology* 62 (1992): 257–272.

15. Charles Morris, op. cit., 447–448.

16. Meyer Friedman and Ray H. Rosenman, *Type A Behavior and Your Heart* (New York: Knopf, 1974).

17. R. Ragland and R. Brand, "Distrust, Rage May Be Toxic Cores That Put Type A Person at Risk," *Journal of the American Medical Association* 261 (1989): 813, 814.

18. Philip L. Rice, *Stress and Health* (Monterey, CA: Brooks/Cole, 1992), 471.

19. Ibid.

20. Robert Eliot, *Is It Worth Dying For?* (New York: Bantam, 1984), 225.

CHAPTER 4

1. Daniel J. Canary and Michael J. Cody, *Interpersonal Communication* (New York: St. Martin's, 1994), 33.

2. G. Terence Wilson, Peter Nathan, K. Daniel O'Leary, and Lee Anna Clark, *Abnormal Psychology* (Boston: Allyn and Bacon, 1996), chapter 10.

3. George D. Bishop, *Health Psychology: Integrating Mind and Body* (Boston: Allyn and Bacon, 1994), 216–217.

4. Don Colburn, "Domestic Violence," *Washington Post,* Health Section, 28 June 1994, 10, 12.

5. John S. Caputo, Harry C. Hazel, and Colleen McMahon, *Interpersonal Communication* (Boston: Allyn and Bacon, 1994), 100.

6. Brian Luke Seaward, *Managing Stress* (Boston: Jones and Bartlett, 1994), 224.

7. John S. Caputo et al., op. cit., 100.

8. Peter G. Northouse and Laurel L. Northouse, *Health Communication: A Handbook for Health Professionals* (Englewood Cliffs: Prentice Hall, 1985), 57.

9. Tomina Toray, "Communicating Effectively: A Key to Interpersonal Health," in Rebecca J. Donatelle and Lorraine G. Davis, *Access to Health,* 3rd ed. (Englewood Cliffs, NJ: Prentice Hall).

10. John S. Caputo et al., op. cit., 183.

11. Mary Ellen Guffy, *Business Communication: Process and Products* (Belmont, CA: Wadsworth, 1994), 38.

12. Ibid., 38.

13. Ibid., 41.

14. M. Beard, *Interpersonal Relationships* (Dubuque, IA: Kendall/Hunt, 1989), N. Coupland, H. Giles, and W. Wieman, *Miscommunication and Problematic Talk* (London: Sage, 1991), and Tomina Toray, op. cit.

15. Daniel Goleman, "Marriage: Research Reveals Ingredients of Happiness," *New York Times,* 16 April 1985, C1, C4.

16. Deborah Tannen, *You Just Don't Understand: Women and Men in Conversation* (New York: Ballantine, 1990).

17. Tomina Toray, op. cit.

18. Carol Gilligan, *In a Different Voice: Psychological Theory and Women's Development* (Cambridge, MA: Harvard University Press, 1982).

19. John S. Caputo et al., op. cit., 302.

20. Ibid., 302.

21. Deborah Tannen, op. cit.

22. C. Morris, *Understanding Psychology* (Englewood Cliffs, NJ: Prentice Hall, 1993).

23. Ibid.

24. Tannen, op. cit.

25. M. Brenton, *Sex Talk* (New York: Stein and Day, 1972), J. Gottman, C. Notarius, and H. Markman, *A Couple's Guide to Communication* (Champaign, IL: Research Press, 1976).

CHAPTER 5

1. Janet D. Woititz, *Struggle for Intimacy* (Pompano Beach, FL: Health Communications, 1985).

2. Sharon S. Brehm, *Intimate Relationships* (New York: McGraw-Hill, 1992), 4–5.

3. E. Berscheid, M. Snyder, and A. M. Omoto, "The Relationship Closeness Inventory: Assessing the Closeness of Interpersonal Relationships," *Journal of Personality and Social Psychology* 57 (1989): 792–807.

4. R. A. Baron and D. Byrne, *Social Psychology* (Boston: Allyn and Bacon, 1994), 311–312, 342.

5. J. Dunn, "Siblings and Development," *Current Directions in Psychological Science* 1 (1992): 6–11.

6. F. Klagsbrun, *Mixed Feelings: Love, Hate, Rivalry and Reconciliation in Brothers and Sisters* (New York: Bantam 1992).

7. R. A. Baron and D. Byrne, op. cit., 308.

8. G. E. Kennedy, "Grandchildren's Reasons for Closeness with Grandparents," *Journal of Social Behavior and Personality* 6 (1991): 692–712.

9. R. A. Baron and D. Byrne, op. cit., 309.

10. J. Turner and L. Rubinson, *Contemporary Human Sexuality* (Englewood Cliffs, NJ: Prentice Hall, 1993), 457.

11. Dan McAdams, *Intimacy: The Need to Be Close* (New York: Doubleday, 1989), 87–91.

12. J. Turner and L. Rubinson, op. cit., 457.

13. G. Levinger, "Can We Picture Love?" in *The Psychology of Love,* ed. R. J. Sternberg and M. Barnes (New Haven: Yale University Press, 1988), 139–159.

14. E. Hatfield, "Passionate and Companionate Love," in *The Psychology of Love,* ed. R. J. Sternberg and M. Barnes (New Haven: Yale University Press, 1988), 191–217.

15. R. A. Baron and D. Byrne, op. cit., 318.

16. E. Hatfield and G. W. Walster, *A New Look at Love* (Reading, MA: Addison Wesley, 1981).

17. Helen Fisher, *Anatomy of Love: The Natural History of Monogamy, Adultery, and Divorce* (New York: Norton, 1993).

18. A. Toufexis and P. Gray, "What is Love? The Right Chemistry," *Time,* 1993, 47–52.

19. Ibid., 51.

20. Ibid., 49.

21. Helen Fisher, op. cit.

22. E. Hatfield, *Love, Sex, and Intimacy: Their Psychology, Biology, and History* 1993.

23. Deborah Tannen, *You Just Don't Understand: Women and Men in Conversation* (New York: Ballantine, 1990).

24. M. McGill, *The McGill Report on Male Intimacy* (New York: Holt, Rinehart and Winston, 1985), 87–88.

25. J. Caputo, H. Hazel, and C. Mahon, (Boston: Allyn and Bacon, 1994), 214.

26. Lillian Rubin, *Intimate Strangers* (New York: Harper and Row, 1983).

27. S. Hendricks and C. Hendricks, *Liking, Loving, and Relating*, 2nd ed. (Pacific Grove, CA: Brooks/Cole, 1992).

28. R. Landerman, M. Swartz, and L. George, "The Long-Term Effects of Childhood Exposure to Parental Drinking" (paper presented at the annual meeting of the American Public Health Association, Mental Health session, Washington, DC, 1992). See also A. Diaz, F. Yancovitz, N. Showers, and I. Epstein, "Predictors and Psychological Consequences of Disclosure of Incest by Female Adolescents" (paper presented at the annual meeting of the American Public Health Association, Mental Health session, Washington, DC, 1992).

29. M. Klausner and B. Hasselbring, *Aching for Love: The Sexual Drama of the Adult Child* (New York: Harper and Row, 1990).

30. Sharon S. Brehm, op. cit., 263.

31. U.S. Census Bureau, *Statistical Abstract of the United States* (Washington, DC: U.S. Government Printing Office, 1994).

32. N. Glenn and C. Weaver, "The Changing Relationship of Marital Status to Reported Happiness," *Journal of Marriage and Family* 50 (1988): 317–324. See also W. Wood, N. Rhodes, and M. Whelan, "Sex Differences and Positive Well-Being: A Consideration of Emotional Style and Marital Status," *Psychological Bulletin* 106 (1989): 249–264.

33. U.S. Census Bureau, op. cit.

34. R. Friedman and J. Downey, "Homosexuality," *New England Journal of Medicine* 33 (1994): 923–928.

35. D. Olson and J. DeFrain, *Marriage and Family* (Mountain View, CA: Mayfield, 1994), 104.

36. N. Glenn and C. Weaver, op. cit., 318; W. Wood et al., op. cit., 249–252; Sharon S. Brehm, op. cit., 20–23.

37. Oregon Department of Labor, *Fact Sheet* (Women's Health Conference, Women in the Workplace session, Portland, Oregon, March 1994).

CHAPTER 6

1. R. Crooks and K. Baur, *Our Sexuality* (Redwood City, CA: Benjamin/Cummings, 1993), 60–61.

2. "Sexuality and Aging: What It Means to Be Sixty or Seventy or Eighty in the '90s," *Mayo Clinic Health Letter*, February 1993.

3. E. Schoen, G. Anderson, C. Bohon, F. Hinman, R. Poland, and E. Wakeman, "Report of the Task Force on Circumcision," *Pediatrics* 84 (1989), 388–391.

4. R. C. Friedman and J. I. Downey, "Homosexuality," *JAMA* 331 (1994), 923–930.

5. J. S. Turner and L. Rubinson, *Contemporary Human Sexuality* (Englewood Cliffs, NJ: Prentice Hall, 1993), 251.

6. I. G. Sarason and B. R. Sarason, *Abnormal Psychology*, 6th ed. (Englewood Cliffs, NJ: Prentice Hall, 1989).

7. Martin Weinberg, *Society and the Healthy Homosexual* (New York: Anchor, 1973).

8. Centers for Disease Control, "The HIV/AIDS Epidemic: The First 10 Years," *Morbidity and Mortality Weekly Report* 40 (1991), 357–358.

9. A. Bell, M. S. Weinberg, and S. K. Hammersmith, *Sexual Preference: Its Development in Men and Women* (Bloomington: Indiana University Press, 1981).

10. Simon LeVay, "A Difference in Hypothalamic Structure between Heterosexual and Homosexual Men," *Science*, 253:1034.

11. N. Bailey and R. Pillard, "Are Some People Born Gay?" *New York Times,* 17 December 1991, 13.

12. R. C. Friedman and J. I. Downey, op. cit., 923–930.

13. Dorothy Tennov, *Love and Limerence* (Chelsea, MI: Scarborough House, 1989), 45–50.

14. J. H. Gagnon and W. Simon, "The Sexual Scripting of Oral-Genital Contact," *Archives of Sexual Behavior,* 16:1–25.

15. Alex Comfort, *The Joy of Sex* (New York: Simon and Schuster, 1972), 14.

16. R. O'Carroll, "Sexual Desire Disorders: A Review of Controlled Treatment Studies," *The Journal of Sex Research* 28 (19): 607–624.

17. Robert J. Crane, Darwin Goldstein, and Inigo de Tejada, "Impotence," *New England Journal of Medicine,* 14 December 1989, 1648–57.

18. C. Darling and J. Davidson, "Enhancing Relationships: Understanding the Feminine Mystique of Pretending Orgasm," *Journal of Sex and Marital Therapy* 12 (19):182–196.

CHAPTER 7

1. Centers for Disease Control, *Contraceptive Options: Increasing Your Awareness* (Washington, DC: NAACOG, 1990).

2. University of Southern California School of Medicine, "Noncontraceptive Health Benefits," *Dialogues in Contraception* 3 (1990): 2.

3. D. E. Greydanus and R. B. Shearin, *Adolescent Sexuality and Gynecology* (Philadelphia: Lea & Febiger, 1990), 107.

4. P. Silva and K. E. Glasser, "Update on Subdermal Contraceptive Implants," *The Female Patient* 17 (1992): 34–45.

5. Ibid.

6. Boston Women's Health Collective, *The New Our Body, Ourselves* (New York: Simon and Schuster, 1984), 218.

7. R. Lacayo, "Abortion: The Future Is Already Here," *Time,* 4 May 1992, 28.

8. D. A. Grimes and R. J. Cook, *The New England Journal of Medicine,* 8 October 1992, 1041–44; "Pop Council Wins RU-486 Rights, but Abortion Pill Still Years from Release," *Family Planning World,* May/June 1993, 1,6; "New, Improved and Ready for Battle," *Time,* 14 June 1993, 48–51; Andrea Sachs, "The Abortion Pills on Trial," *Time,* 5 December 1994, 45–46.

9. K. Schmidt, "The Dark Legacy of Fatherhood," *U.S. News and World Report,* 14 December 1992, 94–95.

10. U.S. Department of Health and Human Services, *The Health Benefits of Smoking Cessation: A Report of the Surgeon General,* 1990.

11. American College of Obstetricians and Gynecologists, "Nutrition During Pregnancy," *Patient Education Pamphlet (AP001),* April 1992,

12. D. Hall and D. Kaufmann, "Effects of Aerobic and Strength Conditioning on Pregnancy Outcomes," *American Journal of Obstetrics and Gynecology* 157 (1987): 1199–1203.

13. J. D. Forrest, "Contraceptive Needs through Stages of Women's Reproductive Lives," *Contemporary OB/GYN* (Special Issue on Fertility) (1988): 12–22.

14. Gregory Goyert et al., "The Physician Factor in Cesarean Births," *New England Journal of Medicine* 320 (1989): 706.

15. University of Southern California of Medicine, *Dialogues in Contraception* 3 (1991): 2.

CHAPTER 8

1. J. Beary, (Ph.D. diss., Oregon State University, 1994).

2. M. Boyle and G. Zyla, *Personal Nutrition* (St. Paul, MN: West, 1991), 340.

3. Hass, *Staying Healthy with Nutrition* (Berkeley: Celestial Arts, 1992), 31.

4. Janet Christian and Janet Gregor, *Nutrition for Living,* 4th ed. (Benjamin Cummings, 1994), 129.

5. Ibid., 129.

6. R. B. Kanarck and R. Kaufman, *Nutrition and Behavior* (New York: Van Nostrand Reinhold, 1991).

7. *University of California Wellness Letter,* April 1992, 4–6.

8. R. Mensink and M. Katan, "Effect of Dietary Trans-Fatty Acids on High-Density and Low-Density Lipoprotein and Cholesterol Levels in Healthy Subjects," *New England Journal of Medicine,* 16 August 1990.

9. G. Ruoff, "Reducing Fat Intake with Fat Substitutes," *American Family Physician* 43 (1991): 1235–42.

10. F. Mattson, "A Changing Role for Dietary Monounsaturated Fatty Acids," *Journal of American Dietetic Association* (1989): 387–391.

11. Walter Willet and Albert Ascherio, "Trans-Fatty Acids: Are the Effects Only Marginal?" *American Journal of Public Health* 84 (1994): 722–724.

12. Janet Christian and Janet Gregor, op. cit., 56.

13. Haas, op cit., 165.

14. Haas, op. cit., 470–471; J. Solonen et al., "Iron and Your Heart," *Circulation,* September 1992.

15. Bonnie Liebman, "A Meat and Potatoes Man," *Nutrition Action Healthletter* 27, no. 5 (1995): 6–7.

16. L. Katzenstein, "Food Irradiation: The Story behind the Scare," *American Health,* 60–80.

17. "The Brave New World of Food Irradiation," *University of California at Berkeley Wellness Letter,* May 1992, 1–2.

18. A. Hechtt, "Preventing Food-Borne Illnesses," *FDA Consumer Magazine.*

19. "Diagnosing Food Allergies," *University of California at Berkeley Wellness Letter,* May 1992, 7.

20. Ibid., 7.

21. Ibid., 7.

22. Ibid., 7.

23. Claire Renzetti and Daniel Curran, *Women, Men, and Society* (Boston: Allyn and Bacon, 1995), 476.

CHAPTER 9

1. Philip Elmer-Dewitt, "Fat Times," *Time,* 16 January 1995, 60.

2. Ibid., 60.

3. M. Lavery et al., "Long-Term Follow-up of Weight Status of Subjects in a Behavioral Weight Control Program," *Journal of the American Dietetic Association* 89 (1989): 1259–64; J. Schlosber, "The Demographics of Dieting," *American Demographics* 9 (1987): 35–62.

4. N. Schneider-Wood, R. Donatelle, and T. Wood, "Effectiveness of Selected Components in Behavioral Weight-Loss Interventions: A Metaanalysis" (thesis, Oregon State University, 1992).

5. F. Katch and W. McArdle, *Introduction to Nutrition, Exercise, and Health,* 4th ed. (Philadelphia: Lea & Febiger, 1992), 53.

6. American Dietetic Association, "Position of the American Dietetic Association: Nutrition for Physical Fitness and Athletic Performance of Adults," *Journal of the American Dietetic Association* 87 (1987): 933–939.

7. W. Sheldon, S. Stevens, and W. Tucker, *The Varieties of Human Physique* (New York: Harper and Row, 1940), 104.

8. A. Stunkard, *Psychiatric Update: American Psychiatric Association* (New York: Harper and Row, 1985), 87.

9. Claude Bouchard et al., "The Response to Long-Term Overfeeding in Identical Twins," *New England Journal of Medicine* 322 (1990):1477–88.

10. Ibid.

11. Albert Stunkard et al., "The Body-Mass Index of Twins Who Have Been Raised Apart," *New England Journal of Medicine* 322 (1990):1483–87.

12. P. Jaret, "The Way to Lose Weight," *Health,* January/February 1995, 52–59.

13. Ibid., 55.

14. F. Katch and W. McArdle, op. cit., 77.

15. Philip Elmer-DeWitt, op. cit., 61.

16. Ibid., 61.

17. Ibid., 61.

18. S. Lichman et al., "Discrepancy between Self-Reported and Actual Caloric Intake and Exercise in Obese Subjects," *New England Journal of Medicine* 327 (1992):1894–97.

19. Kelly Brownell, "Comments on the Latest Study on Yo-Yo Diets by Steven N. Blair of the Institute for Aerobics Research in Dallas" (paper presented at the annual research meeting of the American Heart Association, Monterey, CA, January 1993).

20. Philip Elmer-DeWitt, op. cit., 64.

21. Oprah Winfrey, introduction, Rosie Daley, *In the Kitchen with Rosie* (New York: Alfred A. Knopf, 1994), xi.

22. M. Boyle and G. Zyla, *Personal Nutrition* (St. Paul, MN: West Publishing, 1991), 21.

23. J. Robison et. al., "Obesity, Weight Loss, and Health," *Journal of the American Dietetic Association* 93 (1993):448.

24. Ibid., 448.

25. Simone French and R. Jeffery, "Consequences of Dieting to Lose Weight: Effects on Physical and Mental Health," *Health Psychology* 13, no. 3 (1994):195–212; G. Wilson, "Relation of Dieting and Voluntary Weight Loss to Psychological Functioning and Binge Eating," *Annals of Internal Medicine* 119 (1993):727–730.

26. Simone French and R. Jeffrey, op. cit., 195–96.

27. L. Lissner et. al., "Variabilities in Body Weight and Health Outcomes in the Framingham Study," *New England Journal of Medicine* 324 (1991):1839–44; ibid., 197–98.

28. J. Horm and K. Anderson, "Who in American Is Trying to Lose Weight," *Annals of Internal Medicine* 119 (1993):672–676; and ibid., 203.

29. American Psychiatric Association, *Diagnostic and Statistical Manual of Mental Disorders,* 4th ed. (Washington, D.C.: American Psychiatric Association, 1994), 539–540.

30. G. Terrence Wilson, Peter Nathan, K. Daniel O'Leary, and Lee Anna Clark, *Abnormal Psychology* (Boston: Allyn and Bacon, 1996).

31. Ibid.

32. Ibid.

33. Ibid.

CHAPTER 10

1. B. A. Dennison, J. H. Straus, E. D. Mellits, et al., "Childhood Physical Fitness Tests: Predictor of Adult Physical Activity Levels?" *Pediatrics* 82 (1988): 324–330; K. E. Powell and W. Dysinger, "Childhood Participation in Organized School Sports and Physical Education As Precursors of Adult Physical Activity," *American Journal of Preventive Medicine* 3 (1987): 276–281.

2. U.S. Department of Health and Human Services, *Healthy People 2000: National Health Promotion and Disease Prevention Objectives* (DHHS [PHS] Publication no. 91-50213) (Washington, DC: U.S. Government Printing Office, 1991).

3. R. Gates, "Fitness is Changing the World: For Women," *IDEA Today,* July–August 1992, 58.

4. DHHS, op. cit.

5. C. J. Caspersen, K. E. Powell, G. M. Christianson, "Physical Activity, Exercise, and Physical Fitness: Definitions and Distinctions for Health-Related Research," *Public Health Report* 100 (1985): 126–131.

6. L. Kravitz and R. Robergs, "To Be Active or Not to Be Active," *IDEA Today,* March 1993, 47–53.

7. T. Baranowski, C. Bouchard, O. Bar-Or, et al., "Assessment, Prevalence, and Cardiovascular Benefits of Physical Activity and Fitness in Youth," *Medicine and Science in Sports and Exercise* 24 no. 6, supplement (1992): S237–S247.

8. L. Bernstein et al., "Adolescent Exercise Reduces Risk of Breast Cancer in Younger Women," *Journal of the National Cancer Institute,* September 1994.

9. T. Baranowski et al., op. cit.

10. G. S. Berenson, C. A. McMahon, A. W. Voors, et al., *Cardiovascular Risk Factors in Children: The Early Natural History of Atherosclerosis and Essential Hypertension* (New York: Oxford University Press, 1980).

11. A. Lubell, "Can Exercise Help Treat Hypertension in Black Americans?" *The Physician and Sportsmedicine,* September 1988, 165–168.

12. V. H. Heyward, *Advanced Fitness Assessment and Exercise Prescription,* 2nd ed. (Champaign, IL: Human Kinetics Publishers, 1991).

13. W. L. Haskell, A. S. Leon, C. J. Caspersen, et al., "Cardiovascular Benefits and Assessment of Physical Activity and Physical Fitness in Adults," *Medicine and Science in Sports and Exercise* 24, no. 6, supplement (1992): S201–S220.

14. Ibid.

15. W. H. Ettinger, Jr. and R. F. Afable, "Physical Disability from Knee Osteoarthritis: The Role of Exercise As an Intervention," *Medicine and Science in Sports and Exercise* 26 (1994): 1435–1440.

16. P. A. Kovar, J. P. Allegrante, C. R. MacKenzie, et al., "Supervised Fitness Walking in Patients with Osteoarthritis of the Knee: A Randomized, Controlled Trial," *Annals of Internal Medicine* 116 (1992): 529–534; D. T. Felson, Y. Zhang, J. M. Anthony, et al., "Weight Loss Reduces the Risk of Symptomatic Knee Osteoarthritis in Women: The Framingham Study," *Annals of Internal Medicine* 116 (1992): 535–539.

17. B. L. Drinkwater, "Does Physical Activity Play a Role in Preventing Osteoporosis?" *Research Quarterly for Exercise and Sport* 65 (1994): 197–206.

18. H. M. Frost, "Skeletal Structural Adaptations to Mechanical Usage (SATMU)—1. Redefining Wolff's Law: The Bone Remodeling Problem," *The Anatomical Record* 226 (1990): 403–413.

19. B. L. Drinkwater, op. cit.

20. American College of Sports Medicine, *Guidelines for Exercise Testing and Prescription,* 4th ed. (Philadelphia: Lea and Febiger, 1991).

21. National Institutes of Health, "Consensus Development Conference Statement on Diet and Exercise in Non-Insulin-Dependent Diabetes Mellitus," *Diabetes Care* 10 (1987): 639–644.

22. S. P. Helmrich, D. R. Ragland, and R. S. Paffenbarger, Jr., "Prevention of Non-Insulin-Dependent Diabetes Mellitus with Physical Activity," *Medicine and Science in Sports and Exercise* 26 (1994): 824–830.

23. S. N. Blair, H. W. Kohl III, R. S. Paffenbarger, et al., "Physical Fitness and All-Cause Mortality: A Prospective Study of Healthy Men and Women," *JAMA* 262 no. 17 (1989): 2395–2401.

24. E. R. Eichner, "Infection, Immunity, and Exercise: What to Tell Patients?" *Physician and Sportsmedicine,* January 1993, 125–135.

25. D. C. Nieman, "Exercise, Immunity and Respiratory Infections," *Sports Science Exchange,* August 1992.

26. D. C. Nieman, L. M. Johanssen, J. W. Lee, et al., "Infectious Episodes in Runners Before and After the Los Angeles Marathon," *Journal of Sports Medicine and Physical Fitness* 30 (1990): 316–328.

27. E. R. Eichner, op. cit.

28. Ibid.

29. Ibid.

30. R. Gates, op. cit., 58.

31. C. J. Casperson et al., op. cit.

32. T. Baranowski et al., op. cit.

33. American College of Sports Medicine, op. cit.

34. E. T. Howley, and D. B. Franks, *Health Fitness Instructor's Handbook,* 2nd ed. (Champaign, IL: Human Kinetics Books, 1992).

35. B. Stamford, "Tracking Your Heart Rate for Fitness," *Physician and Sportsmedicine,* March 1993.

36. Ibid.

37. US Centers for Disease Control and Prevention and American College of Sports Medicine, "Summary Statement: Workshop on Physical Activity and Public Health," *Sports Medicine Bulletin* 28 no. 4 (1993): 7.

38. G. A. Klug and J. Lettunich, *Wellness: Exercise and Physical Fitness* (Guilford, CT: Dushkin, 1992).

39. P. D. Wood, "Physical Activity, Diet, and Health: Independent and Interactive Effects," *Medicine and Science in Sports and Exercise* 26 (1994): 838–843.

40. S. J. Hartley-O'Brien, "Six Mobilization Exercises for Active Range of Hip Motion," *Research Quarterly for Exercise and Sport* 51 (1980): 625–635.

41. R. A. Schmidt, *Motor Control and Learning,* 2nd ed. (Champaign, IL: Human Kinetics, 1988).

42. P. A. Sienna, *One Rep Max: A Guide to Beginning Weight Training* (Indianapolis: Benchmark, 1989).

43. Ibid.

44. H. G. Knuttgen, and W. J. Kraemer, "Terminology and Measurement in Exercise Performance," *Journal of Applied Sport Science Research* 1 (1987): 1–10.

45. W. J. Kraemer, "Involvement of Eccentric Muscle Action May Optimize Adaptations to Resistance Training," *Sports Science Exchange,* November 1992.

46. P. A. Sienna, op. cit.

47. W. L. Westcott, "Muscular Strength and Endurance," *Personal Trainer Manual—The Resource for Fitness Instructors* (San Diego: American Council on Exercise, 1991), 235–274.

48. D. M. Brody, "Running Injuries: Prevention and Management," *Clinical Symposia* 39 (1987).

49. Ibid.

50. J. C. Erie, "Eye Injuries: Prevention, Evaluation, and Treatment," *Physician and Sportsmedicine,* November 1991, 108–122.

51. J. G. Stock and M. F. Cornell, "Prevention of Sports-Related Eye Injury," *American Family Practice,* August 1991, 515–520.

52. R. C. Wasserman and R. V. Buccini, "Helmet Protection from Head Injuries among Recreational Bicyclists," *American Journal of Sports Medicine* 18 (1990): 96–97.

53. J. Andrish and J. A. Work, "How I Manage Shin Splints," *Physician and Sportsmedicine,* December 1990, 113–114.

54. D. M. Brody, op. cit.

55. American Academy of Orthopedic Surgeons, *Athletic Training and Sports Medicine,* 2nd ed. (Park Ridge, IL: AAOS, 1991).

56. Ibid.

57. B. Q. Hafen and K. J. Karren, *Prehospital Emergency Care and Crisis Intervention,* 4th ed. (Englewood Cliffs, NJ: Prentice-Hall, 1992).

58. J. S. Thornton, "Hypothermia Shouldn't Freeze out Cold-Weather Athletes," *Physician and Sportsmedicine,* January 1990, 109–113.

CHAPTER 11

1. R. Prussin, P. Harvey, and T. F. DeGeronimo, *Hooked on Exercise: How to Understand and Manage Exercise Addiction* (Park Ridge, IL: Parkside, 1992), 13–14.

2. H. F. Doweiko, *Concepts of Chemical Dependency* (Pacific Grove, CA: Brooks/Cole, 1993), 9.

3. C. Nakken, *The Addictive Personality* (Center City, MN: Hazelden, 1988), 23.

4. V. Johnson, *Intervention: Helping Someone Who Doesn't Want Help* (Minneapolis, MN: Johnson Institute, 1986), 16–35.

5. A. Washton and D. Boundy, *Willpower's Not Enough: Recovering from Addictions of Every Kind* (New York: HarperCollins, 1990), 7.

6. K. Blum and J. E. Payne, *Alcohol and the Addictive Brain* (New York: The Free Press, 1991), 186.

7. J. Kinney and G. Leaton, *Loosening the Grip: A Handbook of Alcohol Information* (St. Louis: C. V. Mosby, 1991), 75–80.

8. Ibid., 89.

9. J. D. Hawkins and R. F. Catalano, *The Social Development Strategy* (Report from the Oregon State Office of Alcohol and Drug Abuse Programs, 1991), 186.

10. W. A. Payne, D. B. Hahn, and R. R. Pinger, *Drugs: Issues for Today* (St. Louis: C. V. Mosby, 1991), 28.

11. B. Yoder, *The Resource Recovery Book* (New York: Simon & Schuster, 1990), 156.

12. J. R. Wilson and J. A. Wilson, *Addictionary* (New York: Simon & Schuster, 1992), 166.

13. R. Custer and H. Milt, *When Luck Runs Out: Help for Compulsive Gamblers and Their Families* (New York: Facts On File Publications, 1985), 233.

14. B. Yoder, op. cit., 246.

15. R. Custer and H. Milt, op. cit., 245.

16. A. Washton and D. Boundy, op. cit., 14.

17. Ibid., 14.

18. B. Yoder, op. cit., 259.

19. B. Klinger, *Workaholics: The Respectable Addiction* (New York: Simon & Schuster, 1991), 6.

20. A. Washton and D. Boundy, op. cit., 15.

21. B. Yoder, op. cit., 259.

22. C. Nakken, op. cit., 21.

23. A. Washton and D. Boundy, op. cit., 14.

24. P. Mellody, *Facing Codependence* (New York: Harper & Row, 1989), 4.

25. Ibid., 160.

26. S. Forward, *Obsessive Love: When Passion Holds You Prisoner* (New York: Bantam Books, 1991), 123.

27. P. Mellody, op. cit., 22.

28. J. R. Wilson and J. A. Wilson, op. cit., 167.

29. J. Christopher, *SOS Sobriety* (Buffalo, NY: Prometheus Books, 1992), 24–25.

30. B. G. Reed, "Developing Women-Sensitive Drug Dependence Treatment Services: Why So Difficult?" *Journal of Psychoactive Drugs,* April/June 1987, 151–164.

31. S. Wilsnack, R. Wilsnack and A. Klassen, *Epidemiological Research on Women's Drinking 1978–1984* (Research Monograph No. 16, U.S. Department of Health and Mental Health Administration, National Institute on Alcohol and Alcoholism, 1986).

32. M. E. Heinemann, *Treatment Considerations—A Response* (Research Monograph No. 16, U.S. Department of Health and Mental Health Administration, National Institute on Alcohol and Alcoholism, 1986).

33. Marsha Vannicelli, *Treatment Considerations* (Research Monograph No. 16, U.S. Department of Health and Mental Health Administration, National Institute on Alcohol and Alcoholism, 1986).

CHAPTER 13

1. C. Presley and P. Meilman, *Alcohol and Drugs on American College Campuses: A Report to College Presidents* (Carbondale, IL: Southern Illinois University Press, 1992), 3–8.

2. L. D. Johnson, P. M. O'Malley, and J. G. Bachman, *Drug Use among American High School Seniors, College Students, and Young Adults, 1975–1990,* vol. 11 (Rockville, MD: NIDA, 1991).

3. L. Eigen, *Alcohol Practices, Policies, and Potentials of American Colleges and Universities* (1991), 6.

4. P. C. Burda and A. C. Vaux, "Social Drinking in Supportive Contexts among College Males," *Journal of Youth and Adolescence* 17 (1988): 165–171.

5. H. Wechsler, "Health and Behavioral Consequences of Binge Drinking in College," *JAMA* 272 (1994): 1672–1677.

6. Ibid.

7. C. Presley and P. Meilman, op. cit., 9.

8. National Institute on Alcohol Abuse and Alcoholism, *Apparent Per Capita Consumption: National, State and Regional Trends, 1977–1987* (Surveillance report No. 13, 1989).

9. U.S. Department of Health and Human Services, *Proceedings of the Surgeon General's Workshop on Drunk Driving,* December 14–16, 1988 (1989).

10. H. Wechsler, op. cit.

11. R. D. Moore and T. A. Pearsons, "Moderate Alcohol Consumption and Coronary Heart Disease: A Review," *Medicine* 65 (1986):242–67; Y. Okamota et al., "Role of Liver in Alcohol-Induced Alteration of High Density Lipoprotein Metabolism," *Journal of Laboratory Clinical Medicine* 111 (1988):484–485.

12. W. C. Willett et al., "Moderate Alcohol Consumption and the Risk of Breast Cancer," *New England Journal of Medicine* 316 (1987):1174–80.

13. "Update: Alcohol-Related Traffic Fatalities—United States, 1982–1993," *Morbidity and Mortality Weekly* 43, no. 47 (1994): 862.

14. National Highway Traffic Safety Administration, 1993.

15. L. Eigen, op. cit., 25.

16. National Highway Traffic Safety Administration, 1993.

17. "Update: Alcohol-Related Traffic Fatalities—United States, 1982–1993," *Morbidity and Mortality Weekly* 43, no. 47 (1994):862.

18. U.S. Department of Health and Human Services, op. cit.

19. F. K. Goodwin and E. M. Gause, "Alcohol, Drug Abuse, and Mental Health Administration," *Prevention Pipeline* 3 (1990): 19.

20. S. I. Benowitz, "Studies Help Scientists Home in on Genetics of Alcoholism," *Science News,* 29 September 1984, 17.

21. Kenneth Blum et al., "Allelic Association of Human Dopamine D2 Receptor Gene in Alcoholism," *AMA* 262 (1990):2055–59.

22. Ray and Ksir, *Drugs, Society, and Human Behavior* (St. Louis: Times Mirror/Mosby, 1990).

23. Do It Now Foundation, *Children of Alcoholics.* 1989.

24. Black, *It Will Never Happen to Me* (New York: Ballantine, 1981), 194.

25. Ray and Ksir, op. cit., 153.

26. U.S. Department of Health and Human Services, *Seventh Special Report to the U.S. Congress on Alcohol and Health* (1990) 22.

27. J. Kinney and G. Leaton, *Loosening the Grip: A Handbook of Alcohol Information,* 4th ed. (St. Louis: Times Mirror/Mosby, 1991).

28. Ibid.

29. L. Timnick, "A Sobering Finding, No Social Drinks for the Alcoholic," *Social Resources Issues* 3 (1982): Article 2.

CHAPTER 14

1. Centers for Disease Control, *Reducing the Health Consequences of Smoking: 25 Years in Progress—A Report of the Surgeon General,* DHHS Publication No. (CDC) 89-8411 (Rockville, MD: U.S. Department of Health and Human Services, 1989).

2. Centers for Disease Control, *Morbidity and Mortality Weekly Report* 41 (1994).

3. G. Berger, *Smoking Not Allowed* (New York: Franklin Watts, 1987), 91.

4. L. White, *Merchants of Death* (New York: William Morrow, 1988), 172.

5. U.S. Department of Health and Human Services, *Smoking, Tobacco, and Cancer Program: 1985–1989 Status Report,* September 1990.

6. *Smoking and Health: National Health Status Report* (Rockville, MD: U.S. Department of Health and Human Services, 1992).

7. J. R. Difranza and J. Richards, Jr., "RJR Nabisco's Cartoon Camel Promotes Camel Cigarettes to Children," *AMA* 266 (1991):3149–53.

8. "Comparison of the Cigarette Brand Preference of Adult and Teenaged Smokers—United States, 1989, and 10 U.S. Communities, 1988 and 1990," *Morbidity and Mortality Weekly* 41 (1992): 172.

9. American Cancer Society, 1990.

10. L. Brown, ed., *The State of the World, 1990* (New York: Norton, 1990), 100–102.

11. American Cancer Society, *Smoking,* 1986.

12. *Cancer Facts and Figures,* 1994, 20.

13. Ibid., 11.

14. "Study Links Smoking to Pancreatic Cancer," *Science News,* 22 October 1994, 261.

15. M. Samuels and N. Samuels, *The Well Adult* (New York: Summit, 1988), 140.

16. G. Teel, "Smoking Adds a Decade," *Circulation,* 15 December 1994.

17. C. Sears, "Three More Reasons Not to Smoke," *American Health,* June 1990, 42.

18. "Cigarettes and Cervical Cancer," *Health Action Managers,* 25 April 1989, 3.

19. National Institutes of Health, *Smokeless Tobacco or Health,* Monograph 2, May 1993, 3.

20. *Postgraduate Medicine,* 1991, Patient Notes.

21. R. D. Tollison, *Cleaning the Air: Perspectives on Environmental Tobacco Smoke* (Lexington, MA: Lexington Books, 1988), 7.

22. Environmental Protection Agency, *Secondhand Smoke Report,* 1993.

23. P. Hilts, "Wide Peril Is Seen in Passive Smoking," *The New York Times,* 9 May 1990, A25.

24. K. Steenland, "Passive Smoking and the Risk of Heart Disease," *AMA* 267 (1992): 94–99.

25. P. Hilts, op. cit., A25.

26. R. D. Tollison, op. cit., 7.

27. M. Dewey, *Smoke in the Workplace* (Toronto: N.C. Press, 1986), 14.

28. Centers for Disease Control, *Morbidity and Mortality Weekly* 41 (1992): 2.

29. "The Butt Stops Here," *Time,* 58.

30. "Nicotine Patches Seen to Help Smokers Quit," *Boston Globe,* 23 June 1994, 3.

31. "Grounds for Breaking the Coffee Habit?" *Tufts University Diet and Nutrition Newsletter* 7 (1990): 4.

32. Ibid., 6.

33. "Caffeine, Conception: No Correlation," *Science News,* 10 February 1990, 92.

CHAPTER 15

1. S. Gust and M. Welsh, "Research on Prevalence, Impact, and Treatment of Drug Abuse in the Workplace," *Drugs in the Workplace: Research and Evaluation Data* (NIDA Research Monograph 91, 1989).

2. U.S. Department of Justice, *Drugs and Crime Data,* May 1992, 1.

3. U.S. Department of Health and Human Services, *National Household Survey on Drug Abuse: Population Estimates 1993* (October 1994), 17.

4. National Institute on Drug Abuse, *National Survey Results on Drug Use from the Monitoring the Future Study, 1975–1993, College Students and Young Adults,* vol. 11 (1994), 150.

5. B. Moore, "NIDA Surveys Continuing Drop in Drug Use," *ADAMHA News,* March-April 1991.

6. NIDA Notes 5, Winter 1991, p. 2.

7. *Drug Abuse Update,* Spring 1991.

8. National Institute on Drug Abuse Statistical Series, *Annual Data Report,* 1989.

9. National Institute on Drug Abuse, *NIDA Capsules,* April 1989, 18–19.

10. Ibid.

11. M. S. Gold, *800 Cocaine* (Toronto: Bantam Books, 1984), 1–3.

12. National Institute on Drug Abuse Statistical Series, *Annual Data Report,* 1989.

13. M. A. Learner, "The Fire of Ice," *Newsweek,* 27 November 1989, 37–38.

14. Ibid.

15. National Institute on Drug Abuse, *NIDA Capsules: Marijuana Update,* May 1989, 12–14.

16. U.S. Department of Justice, *Drugs and Crime Data,* May 1992, 1.

17. U.S. Department of Health and Human Services, *National Household Survey on Drug Abuse: Population Estimates 1993* (October 1994), 107.

18. *The New York Times,* 11 March 1992.

19. National Institute on Drug Abuse, *NIDA Capsules: Marijuana Update,* May 1989, 12–14.

20. *Drug Abuse Update,* Summer 1992, 7.

21. "Acid Use among Teens Grows at Alarming Rate," *Western Center News,* March 1992, 4.

22. Ibid., 4.

23. "Update on the Drug Enforcement Administration," *Drug Abuse Update*, Spring 1992, 10.

24. National Institute on Drug Abuse, *NIDA Capsules: Designer Drugs*, August 1989, pp. 17–21.

25. Ibid.

26. Ibid.

27. K. Liska, *Drugs and the Human Body, with Implications for Society*, 3rd ed. (New York: Macmillan, 1990), 306–307.

28. "Special K," *Drug Abuse Update*, Spring 1992, 8.

29. "The History of Synthetic Testosterone," *Scientific American*, February 1995, 80.

30. *Patient Care*, 15 August 1990, 129–140.

31. "Americans Spend Billions on Illicit Drugs," *Drug Abuse Update*, Fall 1991, 10.

32. "Homegrown," *Insight*, 44–52.

33. D. Dusek and D. A. Girdano, *Drugs: A Factual Account* (New York: McGraw-Hill, 1993), 247.

34. J. Sherida, "An Evaluation of Drug Testing in the Workplace," *Drugs in the Workplace* (NIDA Research Monograph 91, 1989), 198.

35. R. Tricker and D. L. Crook, *Athletes at Risk: Drugs and Sport* (Dubuque, IA: Wm. C. Brown, 1990), 47.

CHAPTER 16

1. American Heart Association, *Heart and Stroke Facts 1995* (Dallas, TX: American Heart Association, 1995), 1.

2. Ibid., 1.

3. Ibid., 1.

4. Ibid., 1.

5. Ibid., 27.

6. Ibid., 2.

7. American Heart Association, *Heart and Stroke Facts: 1995 Statistical Supplement* (Dallas, TX: American Heart Association, 1995), 2.

8. American Heart Association, op. cit., 2.

9. Ibid., 2.

10. Ibid., 2.

11. Ibid., 3.

12. Ibid., 3.

13. Ibid., 4.

14. Ibid., 32.

15. Ibid., 19.

16. Ibid., 20.

17. American Heart Association, Twentieth Science Writers Conference, January, 1993.

18. American Heart Association, Monterey Meeting, January, 1993.

19. H. M. Krumbols et al., "Lack of Association Between Cholesterol and Coronary Heart Disease Mortality and Morbidity and All-Cause Mortality in Persons Older than 70 Years," *JAMA*, 2 November 1994, 1335–1340.

20. L. Katzenstein, *American Health*, June 1992.

21. American Heart Association, *Heart and Stroke Facts 1995*, 20.

22. Ibid., 20.

23. Ibid., 21.

24. Ibid., 21.

25. R. Eliot, "Changing Behavior: A New Comprehensive and Quantitative Approach" (keynote address at the annual meeting of the American College of Cardiology on stress and the heart, Jackson Hole, WY, July 3, 1987).

26. American Heart Association, *Silent Epidemic: The Truth about Women and Heart Disease* (1995), 2.

27. *JAMA*, 18 January 1995,

28. *Heart and Stroke Facts 1995*, 12.

29. Ibid., 12.

30. National Heart, Lung, and Blood Institute, *Heart Memo: The Cardiovascular Health of Women* 5.

31. L. A. Green and M. T. Ruffin, "A Closer Examination of Sex Bias in the Treatment of Ischemic Cardiac Disease," *Journal of Family Practice*, October 1994, 331–336.

32. *Heart and Stroke Facts 1995*, 10.

33. New Study- Effectiveness of Bypass vs Aggressive Use of Medications.

34. J. E. Willard, R. A. Lange, and D. L. Hillis, "The Use of Aspirin in Ischemic Heart Disease," *New England Journal of Medicine* 327 (1992): 175–179.

35. *Heart and Stroke Facts 1995*, 10.

CHAPTER 17

1. American Cancer Society, *Cancer Facts & Figures—1994* (Atlanta: American Cancer Society, 1995), 1.

2. Ibid., 1.

3. Ibid., 18.

4. T. G. Krontirus, "The Emerging Genetics of Human Cancer," *New England Journal of Medicine* 309 (1983), 404; and A. G. Knudson, "Genetics of Human Cancer," *Annual Review of Genetics* 20 (1986): 23.

5. American Cancer Society, op. cit., 21.

6. Ibid., 20.

7. Ibid., 23.

8. Ibid., 20.

9. Ibid., 12.

10. Ibid., 9.

11. Ibid., 9.

12. National Cancer Institute statistics, in "Breast Cancer Risk," *Health*, May/June 1994, 14.

13. American Cancer Society, op. cit., 10.

14. Ibid., 10.

15. Ibid., 10; and K. C. Allison, "Eat To Beat Cancer," *American Health*, October 1993, 72–78.

16. American Cancer Society, op. cit., 10.

17. Leslie Bernstein, Brian E. Henderson, Rosemarie Hanisch, Jane Sullivan-Halley, and Ronald K. Ross, "Physical Exercise and Reduced Risk of Breast Cancer in Young Women," *Journal of the National Cancer Institute* 86, no. 18, 21 September 1994, 1403–1408.

18. American Cancer Society, op. cit., 9.

19. Ibid., 9.

20. Ibid., 10–11.

21. Ibid., 11.

22. Ibid., 11–12.

23. Ibid., 15.

24. Ibid., 15.

25. Ibid., 15–16.

26. Ibid., 16.

27. Harvey A. Risch, Meera Jain, Loraine D. Marrett, and Geoffrey R. Howe, "Dietary Fat Intake and Risk of Epithelial Ovarian Cancer," *Journal of the National Cancer Institute* 86, no. 18, 21 September 1994, 1409–1415.

28. American Cancer Society, op. cit., 16.

29. Ibid., 12–13.

30. Ibid., 13.
31. Ibid., 13.
32. Ibid., 12.
33. Ibid., 14.
34. Ibid., 14.
35. Ibid., 14.
36. Ibid., 21.
37. Ibid., 2.
38. Ibid., 2.
39. Ibid., 3.
40. Ibid., 2.

CHAPTER 18

1. H. Sheldon, *Boyd's Introduction to Human Disease* (Philadelphia: Lea and Febiger, 1992).
2. T. Shulman, J. Phair, and H. Sommers, *The Biological and Clinical Basis of Infectious Disease* (Philadelphia: W. B. Saunders, 1992); and A. Benenson, *Control of Communicable Diseases in Man* (Washington, DC: American Public Health Association, 1990).
3. T. Shulman et al., op. cit., 322; and H. Sheldon, op. cit., 406.
4. Centers for Disease Control, *Mortality and Morbidity Weekly,* April 1993.
5. "Sexually Transmitted Disease in the 1990s," *STD BULLETIN* 11 (1992): 3–9; and S. Aral and K. Holmes, "Sexually Transmitted Diseases in the AIDS Era," *Scientific American* 264 (1991): 62–69.
6. "PID: Guidelines for Prevention, Detection, and Management," *Clinical Courier* 10 (1992): 1–5.
7. P. Marchbanks, N. Lee, and H. Peterson, "Cigarette Smoking as a Risk Factor for PID," *American Journal of Obstetrics and Gynecology* 162 (1990): 639–644, J. Kahn, C. Walker, and A. Washington, "Diagnosing Pelvic Inflammatory Disease," *Journal of the American Medical Association* 226 (1991): 2594–2604, and "Sexually Transmitted Diseases in the 1990's," op. cit., 8.
8. "Sexually Transmitted Diseases in the 1990's," op. cit., 7.
9. E. Hook and C. Marra, "Acquired Syphilis in Adults," *New England Journal of Medicine* 326 (1992): 1060–67, and S. Aral and K. Holmes, op. cit., 65.
10. "Sexually Transmitted Diseases in the 1990's," op. cit., 7.
11. Lawrence K. Altman, "AIDS Is Now the Leading Killer of Americans From 25 to 44," *The New York Times,* 31 January 1995, C7.
12. "AIDS Spreading at Lower Rate, Report by Disease Center Says," *The New York Times,* 3 February 1995, A17.
13. Lawrence K. Altman, op. cit., C7.
14. Ibid., C7.
15. "AIDS Spreading at Lower Rate . . . ," op. cit., A17.
16. Gerald J. Stine, *AIDS UPDATE, 1994–1995* (Englewood Cliffs, NJ: Prentice Hall, 1995), 213.
17. "1993 Revised Classification System for HIV Infection and Expanded Surveillance Case Definition for AIDS Among Adolescents and Adults," *Mortality and Morbidity Weekly* 41 (1993), 1–19.
18. Gerald J. Stine, op. cit., 212.
19. Ibid., 198.
20. Ibid., 198.
21. K. Castro and J. Ward, "Aids Trends Among Hispanics in the U.S.," *American Journal of Public Health* 83 (1993): 504–510.
22. Gerald J. Stine, op. cit., 204.
23. Ibid., 203.
24. Ibid., 203.
25. Gerald J. Stine, *Acquired Immune Deficiency Syndrome: Biological, Medical, Social and Legal Issues* (Englewood Cliffs, NJ: Prentice Hall, 1993), 125–146.
26. Ibid., 132–133.
27. Ibid., 125.
28. Ibid., 147–148

CHAPTER 19

1. "Asthma Update: Parts I & II," *Harvard Health Letter,* 1991.
2. J. Allen, "Oh, My Aching Head," *Life,* 1994, 66–76.
3. Ibid., 70.
4. Ibid., 70.
5. Ibid., 72.
6. Carol Tavris, *The Mismeasure of Woman* (New York: Touchstone, 1992), 139–142.
7. H. Sheldon, *Boyd's Introduction to the Study of Diseases,* 11th ed. (Philadelphia: Lea and Febiger, 1993), 503.
8. *Bureau of Labor Statistics Bulletin,* 1993, and National Council on Compensation Insurance, Yearly report, 1993.
9. R. J. Donatelle, S. Hall, and E. Eyler, "The Failure of Low Back Pain Programs in the Workplace," submitted for publication, 1995.
10. New Study of Back Pain Treatment.
11. A. J. Barsky, "The Paradox of Health," *New England Journal of Medicine* 318 (1988): 414–418.
12. Brownson, Remington, Davis. *Chronic Disease Epidemiology and Control* (Washington, DC: APHA, 1993).

CHAPTER 20

1. B. Hayslip and P. Panek, *Adult Development and Aging* (New York: Harper and Row), 1992, 21.
2. Program Resources Department, American Association of Retired Persons, and the Administration on Aging, U.S. Department of Health and Human Services, *Profile of Older Americans* (1992), 1–2.
3. Ibid., 1.
4. Ibid., 2.
5. Ibid., 10.
6. Ibid., 14.
7. National Osteoporosis Foundation, *Physicians Resource Manual on Osteoporosis: A Decision-Making Guide,* 2nd ed. (National Osteoporosis Foundation, 1991), and National Dairy Council, "Calcium and Osteoporosis: New Insights," *Dairy Council Digest* 63 (1992): 1–6.
8. National Dairy Council, op. cit., 1, National Dairy Council, "Conference Report," *American Journal of Medicine* 90 (1991): 107, and U.S. Department of Health and Human Services, Public Health Service, National Institutes of Health, *Osteoporosis Research, Education, and Health Promotion* (NIH Publication No. 91-3216, September 1991).
9. U.S. Department of Health and Human Services, op. cit., 2.
10. National Dairy Council, "Calcium and Osteoporosis," 2.
11. Ibid., 2.
12. U.S. Department of Health and Human Services, op. cit., 2.
13. Ibid., 4–6.
14. National Dairy Council, "Calcium and Osteoporosis," 3, and Food and Nutrition Board, *Subcommittee on the 10th Edition of the FDA's Recommended Dietary Allowances,* 10th ed. (Washington, DC: National Academy Press, 1989).
15. Ibid., 6.
16. U.S. Department of Health and Human Services, op. cit., 21–25.

17. Ibid., 6.
18. Ibid., 7.
19. A. Ferrini and R. Ferrini, *Health in the Later Years* (Madison, WI: Brown and Benchmark, 1993), 280.
20. Ibid., 281.
21. Ibid., 283.
22. Ibid., 243.
23. L. Palinkas, D. Wingard, and C. Barrett, "Chronic Illness and Depression Symptoms in the Elderly: A Population-Based Study," *Journal of Clinical Epidemiology,* 43 (1990): 1131–1141.
24. Gina Kolata, "Researchers Discover Simple Eyedrop Test to Detect Alzheimer's," *New York Times,* 11 November 1994.
25. Ibid.
26. C. Holzer et al., "Antecedents and Correlates of Alcohol Abuse and Dependence in the Elderly," in *Nature and Extent of Alcohol Abuse and Dependence in the Elderly,* ed. G. Maddox et al. (New York: Springer, 1986).
27. National Center for Health Statistics, *Provisional Data from the National Health Interview Study,* May 1989 (Hyattsville, MD: Public Health Service, 1991), and A. Ferrini and R. Ferrini, op. cit., 249.
28. A. Ferrini and R. Ferrini, op. cit., 249, and R. Moore et al., "Prevalence, Detection, and Treatment of Alcoholism in Hospitalized Patients," *AMA,* 1989, 403–407.
29. A. Ferrini and R. Ferrini, op. cit., 250.
30. J. Busby, A. Campbell, M. Borrie, and G. Spears, "Alcohol Use in a Community-Based Sample of Subjects Aged 70 Years and Older," *Journal of the American Geriatrics Society* 36 (1988): 301–305.
31. N. Watts et al., "Intermittent Cyclical Etidronate Treatment of Postmenopausal Osteoporosis," *New England Journal of Medicine* 323 (1990): 73–80.
32. T. Brubaker and K. Roberto, "Family Life Education for the Later Years," *Family Relations,* 1993, 213.

CHAPTER 21

1. *Oxford English Dictionary,* (Oxford: Oxford University Press, 1969), 72, 334, 735.
2. President's Commission for the Study of Ethical Problems in Medicine and Biomedical and Behavioral Research, *Deciding to Forgo Life-Sustaining Treatment* (New York: Concern for Dying, 1983), 9.
3. Ad Hoc Committee of the Harvard Medical School to Examine the Definition of Brain Death, "A Definition of Irreversible Coma," *JAMA,* 205 (1968), 377.
4. Lewis R. Aiken, *Dying, Death, and Bereavement,* 3rd ed. (Boston: Allyn and Bacon, 1994), 4.
5. D. Lester and D. M. Becker, "College Students' Attitudes toward Death Today as Compared to the 1930's," *Omega,* 26, no. 3 (1992–93): 219–222.
6. Elisabeth Kübler-Ross, *On Death and Dying* (New York: Macmillan, 1969), 113.
7. Robert J. Kastenbaum, *Death, Society, and Human Experience,* 5th ed. (Boston: Allyn and Bacon, 1995), 95.
8. K. J. Doka, ed., *Disenfranchised Grief: Recognizing Hidden Sorrow* (Lexington, MA: Lexington Books, 1989).
9. Kastenbaum, op. cit., 336–337.
10. Kastenbaum, op. cit., 325–326.
11. Ibid., 337.
12. Ibid., 330.
13. Ibid., 330.

14. J. B. Kamerman, *Death in the Midst of Life* (Englewood Cliffs, NJ: Prentice Hall, 1988), 126.
15. The term *quasi-death experience* was coined by J. B. Kamerman; see ibid., 71.
16. C. M. Parkes, *Bereavement* (New York: International Universities Press, 1972), 6.
17. "Last Rights: Why a 'Living Will' Is Not Enough," *Consumer Reports on Health,* September 1993, 5, 9.
18. M. F. Leming and G. E. Dickenson, *Understanding Death, Dying, and Bereavement,* 2nd ed. (New York: Holt, Rinehart and Winston, Dryden Press, Saunders College Publishing, 1990).

CHAPTER 22

1. David Zucchio, "Today's Violent Crime Is an Old Story with a New Twist," *San Jose Mercury News,* 21 November 1994, transmitted via America Online.
2. Elaine Shannon, "Crime: Safer Streets, Yet Greater Fear," *Time,* 2 February 1995, transmitted via America Online.
3. Centers for Disease Control and Prevention/National Center for Health Statistics, "Advanced Report: Final Mortality," *Monthly Vital Statistics Report,* 8 December 1994.
4. M. Rosenberg and M. Fenley, eds., *Violence in America: A Public Health Approach* (New York: Oxford University Press, 1991), 15.
5. Ibid.
6. A. Matthews, "Campus Crime 101," *Eugene Register Guard,* March 1993, 2B.
7. Ibid., 4B.
8. P. Wolfe, "Stopping the Violence," *Community Safety Quarterly* 5 (1992): 15.
9. N. West, "Crimes against Women," *Community Safety Quarterly* 5 (1992): 1.
10. G. Terrence Wilson, Peter Nathan, K. Daniel O'Leary, and Lee Anna Clark, *Abnormal Psychology* (Boston, MA: Allyn and Bacon, 1996).
11. M. A. Straus and R. Gelles, eds., *Physical Violence in American Families: Risk Factors and Adaptations to Violence in 8,145 Families* (New Brunswick, NJ: Transaction, 1993), 101–201.
12. G. Terrence Wilson et al., op. cit.
13. N. West, op. cit., 2–3.
14. P. Wolfe, op. cit., 15.
15. A. Joerger and L. McClellan, "Why Men Batter: Why Women Stay," *Community Safety Quarterly* 5 (1992): 22–23.
16. N. West, op. cit., 3.
17. M. A. Straus and R. Gellis, op. cit.
18. H. Pan, P. Neidig, and K. O'Leary, "Physical Aggression in Early Marriage: Pre-relationship and Relationship Effects," *Journal of Consulting and Clinical Psychology.*
19. G. Terrence Wilson et. al., op. cit.
20. Ibid.
21. Ibid.
22. E. Newberger, "Child Sexual Abuse," in M. Rosenberg and M. Fenley, op. cit., 85.
23. Ibid., 53.
24. Marjorie Whittaker, "The Continuum of Violence against Women: Psychological and Physical Consequences," *Journal of American College Health* 40 (1992): 155.
25. D. Finkelhor, "Child Sexual Abuse," in M. Rosenberg and M. Fenley, op. cit., 25.
26. Ibid., 86.
27. N. West, "Children: The Invisible Victims of Domestic Violence," *Community Safety Quarterly* 5 (1992): 20.

28. Marjorie Whittaker, op. cit., 152.
29. Alan Berkowitz, "College Men as Perpetrators of Acquaintance Rape and Sexual Assault: A Review of Recent Literature," *Journal of American College Health,* 40 (1992): 175.
30. Ibid.
31. National Victims Center, 1992.
32. J. Baier, M. Rosenzweig, and E. Shipple, "Patterns of Sexual Behavior, Coercion, and Victimization of University Students," *Journal of College Student Development* 32 (1991): 310–322.
33. M. Koss, "Rape: Scope, Impact, Interventions, and Public Policy Responses," *American Psychologist* 48 (1993): 1062–1069.
34. J. Baier et al., op. cit., 178.
35. M. Koss, C. Gidycz, and N. Wisneiwski, "The Scope of Rape: Incidence and Sexual Aggression and Victimization in a National Sample of Higher Education Students," *Journal of Counseling Clinical Psychology* 55 (1987): 162–170.
36. Alan Berkowitz, op. cit., 177.
37. Ibid., 178.
38. Marjorie Whittaker, op. cit., 153–154.
39. R. Brannon and D. David, *The Forty-Nine Percent Majority* (Reading MA: Addison-Wesley, 1976), 47.
40. Alan Berkowitz, op. cit., 178.
41. Ibid., 175.
42. Ibid., 176.
43. Ibid., 176.
44. D. Benson, C. Charlton, and F. Goohart, "Acquaintance Rape on Campus: A Literature Review," *Journal of American College Health* (1992): 157.
45. G. Terrence Wilson et al., op. cit.
46. D. Benson et al., op. cit., 158.
47. Marjorie Whittaker, op. cit., 151.
48. Center for Research on Women at Wellesley College and the Legal Defense and Education Fund of the National Organization of Women.
49. A. Matthews, op. cit., 4B.
50. T. Schneider, "Rape Prevention," *Community Safety Quarterly* (1992): 8–13.
51. Ibid., 12.
52. Ibid., 13.
53. Ibid.

CHAPTER 23

1. U.S. Environmental Protection Agency, *Securing Our Legacy: An EPA Progress Report, 1989–1991* (EPA Publication No. 175R-92-001, 1992).
2. R. Caplan, *Our Earth, Ourselves* (New York: Bantam, 1990), 247.
3. Ibid., 248.
4. M. Lowe, "Shaping Cities," in *State of the World, 1992,* ed. Lester Brown (New York: Norton, 1992).
5. Lester Brown, "The Illusion of Progress," in *State of the World, 1990,* ed. Lester Brown (New York: Norton, 1990), 11.
6. Ibid., 10–11.
7. W. Reilly, "The New Clean Air Act: An Environmental Milestone," *EPA Journal* 17 (1991): 2–10.
8. L. Wegman, "Air Toxics: The Strategy," *EPA Journal* 17 (1991): 32–33.
9. Lester Brown, "A New Era Unfolds," in *State of the World, 1993,* ed. Lester Brown (New York: Norton, 1993), 107.
10. H. F. French, "Clearing the Air," in *State of the World, 1990,* op. cit., 109.

11. L. Pringle, *Rain of Troubles* (New York: Macmillan, 1988), 78.
12. U.S. Environmental Protection Agency, *A Citizen's Guide to Radon,* 2nd ed. (Washington, DC: U.S. Department of Health and Human Services, 1992), 21.
13. Lester Brown, "A New Era Unfolds," op. cit., 111.
14. H. F. French, "Clearing the Air," op. cit., 110.
15. A. Nadakavukaren, *Man and Environment: A Health Perspective* (Prospect Heights, IL: Waveland, 1990), 412–414.
16. R. Griffin, Jr., "Introducing NPS Water Pollution," *EPA Journal* 17 (1991): 6–9.
17. J. Naar, *Design for a Livable Planet* (New York: Harper and Row, 1990), 68.
18. A. Nadakavukaren, op. cit., 183.
19. Ibid., 447.
20. "New Lead Rules for Water," *Science News* 139 (1991): 308, and USEPA, *Securing Our Legacy,* op. cit., 3.
21. U.S. Environmental Protection Agency, *Characterization of Municipal Solid Waste in the United States: 1990 Update* (EPA Publication No. 530-SW-90-042A, 1990).
22. J. M. Moran, M. Morgan, and J. H. Wiersma, *Introduction to Environmental Science,* 2nd ed. (New York: W. H. Freeman, 1986), 49.
23. R. Caplan, op. cit., 248.
24. U.S. Environmental Protection Agency, *Meeting the Environmental Challenge: EPA's Review of Progress and New Directions in Environmental Protection* (EPA Publication No. 21K-2001, 1990), 7.
25. A. Nadakavukaren, op. cit., 415.
26. USEPA, *Meeting the Environmental Challenge,* op. cit., 4.
27. D. W. Moeller, *Environmental Health* (Cambridge, MA: Harvard University Press, 1992), 31.
28. C. Flavin, "Slowing Global Warming," in *State of the World, 1990,* op. cit.
29. J. Naar, op. cit., 69.

CHAPTER 24

1. L. C. Baker and L. S. Baker, "Excess Cost of Emergency Department Visits for Nonurgent Care," *Health Affairs* Winter 1994, 162–180.
2. K. J. Egan and W. J. Katon, "Responses to Illness and Health in Chronic Pain Patients and Healthy Adults," *Psychosomatic Medicine* 49 (1987): 470–481.
3. H. J. Cornaccia and S. Barrett, *Consumer Health: A Guide to Intelligent Decisions,* 4th ed. (St. Louis: Times Mirror/Mosby, 1989), 48.
4. G. Annas, *The Rights of Patients: The Basic ACLU Guide to Patient Rights,* 2nd ed. (Chicago: Southern Illinois University Press, 1989), 105, and J. A. Robertson, *The Rights of the Critically Ill* (New York: Bantam, 1983), 32–77.
5. National Commission on Certification of Physician Assistants, Inc., 2845 Henderson Mill Rd., NE, Atlanta, GA 30341.
6. D. M. Eisenberg et al., "Unconventional Medicine in the U.S.: Prevalence, Costs, and Patterns of Use," *New England Journal of Medicine,* 28 January 1993, 246–252.
7. P. Starr, *The Social Transformation of American Medicine* (New York: Basic Books, 1982), 127, 229.
8. J. Drawbridge, "Medical Report: The Chiropractic Cure," *Glamour,* April 1993, 61–62.
9. A. Toufexis, "Dr. Jacob's Alternative Mission: A New NIH Office Will Put Unconventional Medicine to the Test," *Time,* 1 March 1993, 43–44, 64–66.
10. S. Sofaer, T. G. Rundall, and W. L. Zeller, "Restrictive Reimbursement Policies and Uncompensated Care in California's

Hospitals" (paper presented at the APHA Annual Conference, Boston, 1988).

11. C. Hafner, "California's Uninsured: The Problem and Proposed Solutions," *Journal of Ambulatory Care Management* 14 (1991): 28–36, and C. Hafner-Eaton, "Patterns of Hospital and Physician Utilization among the Uninsured," *Journal of Health Care for the Poor and Underserved* 5, no. 4 (1994): 297–315.

12. Associated Press, "Health Care Report Cards Coming," *San Jose Mercury News,* 28 October 1994,

13. M. D. Smith et al., "Taking the Public's Pulse on Health Reform," *Health Affairs,* Summer 1992, 125–133.

14. E. Eckholm, "Health Benefits Deter Job Switching," *New York Times,* 26 September 1991, A1, A12.

15. L. C. Baker and L. S. Baker, op. cit., 162–180.

16. Consumers Union, "Wasted Health Care Dollars," *Consumer Reports,* July 1992, 435–449, and C. Hafner-Eaton, "When the Phoenix Rises, Where Will She Go?: The Women's Health Agenda," in *Health Care Reform in the 1990s,* ed. P. Vailliancourt Rosenau (Thousand Oaks, CA: Sage, 1994).

17. R. Fein, "Health Care Reform," *Scientific American,* November 1992, 46–53.

18. C. Hafner-Eaton, "When the Phoenix Rises, Where Will She Go?" op. cit.

19. T. Bodenheimer, "Uninsurance in America," *New England Journal of Medicine,* 327, no. 4 (1992): 274–278.

20. Ibid.

21. A. R. Kovner, *Jonas' Health Care Delivery in the United States,* 5th ed. (New York: Springer, 1995).

Index

Food
  allergies to, 224–225
  organic, 225
  See also Nutrition
Food industry, 242
Food intolerance, 225
Food irradiation, 223
Food labeling, 201, 214, 222
Food Guide Pyramid, 197, 199, 200
Food-borne illness, 223–224, 466
Footwear, choosing, 280, 281
For-profit hospitals, 628, 629
Foreskin, 140
Formaldehyde, as environmental hazard, 596
FRAMES, brief intervention therapy, 303–304
France, aging population in, 526
Free radicals, and cancer, 439
Freebase cocaine, 391
Friendship
  compared with love, 111, 121
  cross-cultural aspects of, 121
  ingredients of, 109
  success at, 110
Fructose, 204
FSH, 136, 137
Functional age, 524
Functional death, 544–545
Funerals, 556–557
  attitudes toward, 557
  costs of, 558
  stress related to, 557–558
Fungi, 472, 473
Furnace emissions, 596

Gallbladder disease, 508–509
Gambling, addiction to, 298
Gamete intrafallopian transfer, 187
Gamma hydroxybutyrate, 402
Gang violence, 572–573
  protection against, 573
GAS. *See* General adaptation syndrome
Gasoline, as environmental hazard, 601–602
GASP (Group Against Smokers' Pollution), 373
Gastroenterologist, 624
Gastroesophageal reflux, 508
Gay, defined, 142
Gay partnership, as committed relationship, 119
Gender
  as barrier to communication, 87
  bereavement and, 552
  cancer and, 437
  communication differences and, 99–102
  death rates and, 15
  defined, 132, 133
  depression and, 51
  eating disorders and, 257
  feelings and, 100
  health and, 12, 14–15
  heart disease and, 424–425
  medications and, 322–323
  nutrition and, 217–218
  obesity and, 244–245
  osteoporosis and, 530
  physiology and, 14
  psychosocial health and, 53
  relationships and, 113–115
  roles, 123
  stress and, 72–73
  suicide and, 53
  weight and, 235
Gender identity, defined, 132, 133
Gender role stereotypes, defined, 132, 133
Gender roles, defined, 132, 133
Gender-specific disorders, 504–506
Genderlect, 99

General adaptation syndrome
  defined, 64
  phases of, 64–67
General urinary tract infections, 483–484
Generic drugs, 315, 324
Genetic mutation theory of aging, 529
Geneticist, 624
Genital herpes, 484
  prevention of, 485
  treatment of, 484–485
Genital warts, 482–483
Genitals
  external female, 134, 135
  external male, 138
  internal female, 136
  internal male, 138
German measles, 472, 473
  vaccination against, 475
Germany, aging population in, 526
Gerontology, defined, 524
GHB (gamma hydroxybutyrate), 402
Giardiasis, 473
Gidjingali people, view of emotions, 49
GIFT (gamete intrafallopian transfer), 187
  ethics of, 199
Girth and circumference measures, 237
Glaucoma
  defined, 531
  therapeutic use of marijuana for, 394
Global warming, 509
Glucose, 204
Glycogen, 206
GnRH, 136, 137, 506
Goals
  setting, 30
  stress related to, 68
Gonadotropin-releasing hormone, 136, 137, 506
Gonadotropins, 132
Gonads, defined, 132
Gonorrhea, 480, 481
Gossypol, 165
Graded exercise test, 270
GRAE list, 326, 327, 328
GRAS list, 326, 327, 328
Graves' disease, characteristics of, 515
Greece
  aging population in, 526
  bereavement in, 555
Greenhouse gases, 598, 599
Grief
  aspects of, 551
  defined, 550, 551
  disenfranchised, 548
  for infant or child, 552
  manifestations of, 550
  stages of, 550
Grief work, 551
Groundwater contamination, 601
Group Against Smokers' Pollution, 373
Group practice, 628, 629
Group sex, 146
Group therapy, for addiction, 306
Gynelotrimin, deregulation of, 325

Habit
  defined, 293
  distinguished from addiction, 292–293
Haemophilus influenzae type B, vaccination
    against, 475
Hallucination, 397
Hangover, 346, 347
Hantavirus, 467
Hardening of the arteries, 208
  exercise to prevent, 265
Harris method of childbirth, 182
Harvests, affected by environment, 591

Hashish, 393
Hassles, as stressor, 68
Hate crime, 571–572
  prevention of, 572
Hay fever, defined, 498
Hazardous waste, 604–607
HBM (Health Belief Model), 20–22
HCG, 136, 137
  as marker for pregnancy, 177
HDLs (high-density lipoproteins), 208, 209, 418
  exercise and, 265
Head, age-related changes in, 530–531
Head and neck rotation, 79
Headaches, 501
  types of, 502–503
Health
  behaviors to improve, 16–17
  checklists of, 8–11
  continuum of, 6
  definitions of, 4
  dimensions of, 5
  importance of, 16
  information about, 21
  mental. *See* Mental health
  preventive aspects of, 12
  promotion of, 7–10, 12, 87
  psychosocial. *See* Psychosocial health
Health bashing, 10, 12
Health Belief Model, 20–22
Health care
  access to, 630, 631
  assessing practitioners of, 619–621, 622–623
  choices of, 621–628, 641
  costs of, 630–631
  elderly and, 526–527
  fraud and abuse in, 632
  proactive involvement in, 620
  quality of, 631–632
  reform of, 637–640
  report card on, 633
  responsibility for, 618
  seeking help, 618–619
Health educator, 624
Health insurance
  group, 634
  HMOs, 635–636
  importance of, 632–633
  options in, 636–640
  overhead of, 633
  PPOs, 636
  private, 634
Health maintenance organizations, 635–636
Health Management Resources weight-loss plan,
    253
Healthy People 2000, 7–12, 87
  evaluation of, 13–14
  goals of, 7
Hearing, age-related changes in, 531
Hearing-impaired, communicating with, 532
Heart
  age-related changes in, 531
  alcohol effects on, 347
  anatomy of, 412
Heart attack, 413, 414–415
  first aid for, 415
Heart disease
  alcohol and, 346, 347
  aspirin and, 14–15
  caffeine and, 380
  cost of, 410
  diagnosis of, 426
  diet and, 207, 218
  exercise to prevent, 264, 421–422
  facts about, 411
  health care for, 425, 428
  incidence of, 13, 14, 410

barriers to, 115–117
characteristics of, 106–107
developing, 126
forming, 108–113
gender and, 113–115
need for, 107
in relationships, 122
types of, 107–108
Intolerance, drug, 322
Intramuscular injection, of drugs, 317
Intrauterine device. *See* IUD
Intravenous injection, of drugs, 317
Intrinsic rewards, 25
Inunction, of drugs, 317–318
Iodine
fetal deficiency of, 175
as nutrient, 215
Ionizing radiation, 606, 607–608
Iridology, 628
Iron
fetal deficiency of, 175
as nutrient, 215, 216–217
Irradiation, of food, 223
Irregular heartbeat. *See* Arrhythmia
Irritable bowel syndrome
defined, 506
described, 506–507
Ischemia, 414
ISD (inhibited sexual desire), 148, 149
Isometric muscle movement, 276, 277
Italy, aging population in, 526
IUD
effectiveness of, 159
risk of, 184
use of, 163–164
IVF (in vitro fertilization), 187
ethics of, 188

Japan, aging in, 526
Jealousy, 116–117
Jejunum, 200, 201
Jenny Craig weight-loss plan, 253
Jock itch, 472
Joints, age-related changes in, 529–530

Kaposi's sarcoma, 486, 487
Kenya, AIDS in, 486
Ketamine, illegal use of, 400–401
Ketosis, 254, 255
Kidney, cancer of, incidence of, 446
Killer T-cells, 474
Kissing, 145

L-dopa, sexual effects of, 151
Labia majora, 136
Labia minora, 136
Labor, 181–182
Lacto-ovo-vegetarians, 218
Lacto-vegetarians, 218
Lactose, 205
Lactose intolerance, 508
Lamaze method of childbirth, 182
Land pollution
by hazardous waste, 604–607
by solid waste, 604
Landfills, as polluter, 601
Laparoscopy, 166–167
risk in, 184
Laryngeal cancer, incidence of, 446
Laser surgery, 482
Late syphilis, 481
Latent syphilis, 481
Laughing gas, 401
Laughter
expressing emotion by, 77
importance of, 47

Laxatives, 328, 329
drug interactions of, 321
side effects of, 329
Lay midwives, 174
LDLs (low-density lipoproteins), 208, 209, 418
exercise and, 265
Leach, defined, 596
Leachate, 600, 601
Lead
as environmental hazard, 591, 594, 596,
602–603
incidence of poisoning, 14
Learned behavior tolerance, 342
Learned helplessness, defined, 40, 41
Leboyer method of childbirth, 182–183
Legal age, 524
Legionnaire's disease, 468
Lesbian, defined, 142
Lesbian partnership, as committed relationship,
119
Leukemia, 445, 453
incidence of, 446
Leukoplakia, 372, 373
Leveling, 100
LH, 136, 137
Librium, 324
drug interactions of, 319
Lice, 482, 483
Licensed practical nurse, 625
Licensed vocational nurse, 625
Life expectancy, 633
improvements in, 13
Life-support technology, 546
Light therapy, 628
Liking, features of, 111
Limerence, 144, 145
Lipids. *See* Fats
Lipoprotein analysis, 420–421
Listening, 92
active, 96
barriers to, 92, 93
improving skills in, 92–93
self-assessment of, 93
Liver, alcohol effects on, 347
Living will, 560, 561–562
Local death, 544
Loneliness, coping with, 128
Longevity, exercise and, 266–267
Loss of control, 294, 295
Love
characteristics of, 109
chemical aspects of, 111–113
compared with friendship, 111, 121
compared with infatuation, 112
cross-cultural aspects of, 121
defined, 110
distinguished from limerence, 144
Love Canal, 604–605
Love, Medicine, and Miracles (Siegel), 47
Low back pain, 512
prevention of, 512–513, 514
risk factors for, 512
Low sperm count, 186, 187
Low-birth-weight infants, 13, 14
Low-density lipoproteins, 208, 209
exercise and, 265
LSD, 397–399
sexual effects of, 151
Lung cancer, 445–446
diet and, 217
family history of, 437
incidence of, 446
smoking and, 368, 369, 434
Lungs, age-related changes in, 531
Lupus erythematosus, 510, 511–512
gender and, 12

Luteinizing hormone, 136, 137
Luxembourg, aging population in, 526
Lyme disease, 466
depression in, 50
Lymphocytes, types of, 474
Lymphomas, 445
incidence of, 446
Lysergic acid diethylamide. *See* LSD

Macrominerals, 211
Macrophages, 474
MADD (Mothers Against Drunk Driving), 349
Magnesium, as nutrient, 215
Magnetic resonance imaging, 52, 457
Mainlining, 396
Mainstream smoke, 373
Malaria, 473
Malay, view of emotions, 49
Males. *See* Men
Malignant, defined, 436
Malignant melanoma, 450–451
Malpractice, 631–632
Managed care, 634, 635–636
Managed care organizations, 637
Manganese, as nutrient, 216
Manipulative reinforcement, 25
MAO inhibitors, tyramine and, 315
Marijuana
adolescent use of, 13, 14
and driving, 394–395
effects of, 393, 394
medical use of, 394
and pregnancy, 394
preparations of, 393–394
sexual effects of, 151
user profile, 386–387
Marriage
age at, 117
as committed relationship, 117–119, 122
common-law, 119
and divorce, 122, 126, 127
Masculinity, politics of, 134
Massage, stress reduction using, 80
Mast cells, 499
Masturbation, 144, 145
MCOs (managed care organizations), 637
MDMA, 400
Measles, 472, 473
incidence of, 14
vaccination against, 475
Medicaid, 632, 633, 634–635
expansion of, 639
Medical education, gender gap in, 15
Medical profession, communication with, 88–90
Medicare, 632, 633, 634–635
Medicine
allopathic, 621–625
nonallopathic, 625–628
types of practices and facilities, 628–630
Medifast weight-loss plan, 253
Meditation
defined, 80
stress reduction using, 80
Melanoma, 450–451
incidence of, 446
Meltdown, 608–609
Memory
age-related changes in, 532–533
improving, 534
Memory B-cells, 474
Memory T-cells, 474
Men. *See also* Gender
attitudes toward women, 579, 581
conversational style of, 113
intimacy style of, 113–114
jealousy in, 116–117

Obstetrician-gynecologist, 174, 624
OCD (Obsessive-compulsive disorder), 51
Office of Research on Women's Health (ORWH), 12
Oil, as environmental hazard, 601
Old-old, defined, 524, 525
On Death and Dying (Kübler-Ross), 547
Oncogenes, 436, 437
Oncologists, 436, 437
One repetition maximum (1RM), 275
   determining, 277–278
Open relationship, 116, 117
Operant conditioning, for nicotine addiction, 376
Ophthalmologist, 623, 624
Opiates, 395
   birth defects from, 175
   drug interactions of, 319
   effects of, 395
Opium, 394, 395
Optifast weight-loss plan, 253
Optometrist, 623
Oral cancer, 453
   tobacco chewing and, 372
Oral contraceptives, 158–160
   drug interactions of, 320, 321
   effectiveness of, 159
   male, 164–165
   proper use of, 323
   risk of, 184
Oral ingestion, of drugs, 316–317
Oral surgeon, 624, 625
Oral-genital stimulation, 145
Oregon Health Plan (OHP), 640
Organ donation, 558
Organ transplant, donor of, 545
Organically grown food, 225
Orgasm, 140, 141, 142
   disorders of, 149
Orthodontist, 623–624, 625
Orthopedist, 624
ORWH (Office of Research on Women's Health), 12
Osteoarthritis, 265–266, 510
Osteopath, 623
Osteoporosis, 529
   exercise to prevent, 264, 266, 267
   gender and, 12
OTC preparations. *See* Over-the-counter drugs
Otolaryngologist, 624
Outercourse, 157
Outpatient care, 629
Ovarian cancer
   family history of, 437
   incidence of, 446
   prevention of, 451–452
   risk of, 451
Ovarian follicles, 136, 137
Ovaries, 136, 137
Over-the-counter drugs, 314–315, 536
   deregulation of, 325
   economics of, 324–325
   precautions for use of, 329–330
   side effects of, 329
   types of, 325–328
   using, 329–330
Overload
   defined, 68
   described, 69
Overload principle, 275
Overmedicating, 328
Overpopulation, 590–592
Overuse injuries, 280, 281–282
   treatment of, 283
Ovo-vegetarians, 218
Ovulation, 136, 137
Oxytocin, 111, 112, 113

Ozone, as environmental hazard, 591, 594
Ozone layer, depletion of, 597–598

Pain, 474–475
Panadol, 327
Pancreas, 506
   alcohol effects on, 348
Pancreatic cancer, 453
   incidence of, 446
Panic attacks, 52
   defined, 53
Pantothenic acid, characteristics and RDA of, 212
Pap smears, 14
Paraguard, 163
Paraphrasing, 93, 96
Parasites, 473
Parasympathetic nervous system
   defined, 67
   role in GAS, 66
Parenting, 124
Parkinson's disease, characteristics of, 515
Particulates, as environmental hazard, 592, 593
Partnering, 109. *See also* Love
Partnering scripts, 120
Passionate love, 110
Passive immunity, 475
Pathogens, 464, 465
   routes of invasion of, 466, 468–473
Pathologist, 624
Patient dumping, 628
Patient-doctor communication, 88–90
PBBs (polybrominated biphenyls), as
   environmental hazard, 602
PCBs (polychlorinated biphenyls), as
   environmental hazard, 602
PCP (drug), 400, 401
PCP (type of pneumonia), 486, 491
PDR (*Physicians' Desk Reference*), 328
PEA (phenylethylamine), 112, 113
Pediatrician, 624
Pedophilia, 146
Peer pressure, 23, 28
Pelvic inflammatory disease, 186, 187, 479–480
   chlamydia and, 477
Penicillin, 468, 469
   drug interactions of, 323, 346
Penis, 138, 139
   cancer of, 140
PEPAP, designer drug, 400
Peptic ulcer, 508, 509
Pergonal, 187
Perineum, 136, 181
Periodontal diseases, 469
Personal control, defined, 40
Personality
   aspects of, 41–42
   development of, 42–43
   self-description of, 44
   Type A vs. Type B, 72
Pertussis, vaccination against, 475
Pesco-vegetarians, 218
Pesticides
   carcinogenicity of, 438
   as environmental hazard, 602
PET (positron emission tomography) scan, 52, 426
Petroleum products, as environmental hazard, 601–602
Pets, influence on psychosocial health, 41
Peyote, 399
Phencyclidine, 400, 401
Phenobarbital, 324
   drug interactions of, 319
Phenylethylamine (PEA), 112, 113
Phenylpropanolamine, 328
Philippines, tobacco use in, 364

Phobias, 52
   defined, 53
Phosphorus, as nutrient, 215
Photochemical smog, 594
Physical activity, defined, 264
Physical fitness
   benefits of, 264–269
   components of, 268
   defined, 269
   improving, 268–279
   injuries, 279–284
   managing, 289
   planning for, 285–286
Physical health, 5
   checklist of, 8
   influence on psychosocial health, 46
   reducing stress by improving, 78
Physical inertia, and osteoporosis, 530
Physical therapist, 624
Physician assistant, 624, 625
Physicians' Desk Reference, 328
PID (pelvic inflammatory disease), 186, 187, 479–480
   chlamydia and, 477
Pill, the. *See* Oral contraceptives
Pima people, obesity among, 240
Pinch test, 237
Pinworms, 473
Pituitary
   defined, 132, 136
   role in puberty, 137
Placebo effect, 618
Placenta, 178
Placidyl, drug interactions of, 346
Plantar fasciitis, 281–282
Plaque, 208, 209, 414
Plastic surgeon, 624
Plateau, 241
Plateau phase, 140, 141
Platelet adhesiveness, 368–369
PMS (premenstrual syndrome), 53, 504–505
Pneumocystis carinii pneumonia (PCP), 486, 491
Pneumonia, 468
PNI (psychoneuroimmunology), defined, 63–64
Podophyllin, 482
Point source pollutants, 600
Poison ivy, oak, and sumac, 500
Polio, vaccination against, 475
Politics, as barrier to communication, 87
Pollution
   air, 593–599
   land, 604–607
   noise, 603
   poverty and, 607
   radiation, 607–611
   water, 599–603
Polybrominated biphenyls, as environmental hazard, 602
Polychlorinated biphenyls, as environmental hazard, 602
Polydrug use, 318–319
Polynesia, attitudes toward obesity in, 233
Polysaccharide, 204, 205
Polyunsaturated fats, 208
Pondimin, 324, 393
Poppers, 401
   sexual effects of, 151
Population
   growth of, 590–592
   urban, 593
Portugal, aging population in, 526
Positive affirmations, 26
Positive reinforcement, 24, 25
Positive thinking, 46
Positron emission tomography, 52, 426
Possessional reinforcement, 25

PHOTO CREDITS

Chapter 1: 2 Bachmann/The Image Works. 5 David Coleman/ Stock Boston. 7 Robert Daemmrich/Tony Stone Worldwide. 18 Brian Bailey/Tony Stone Worldwide. 20 Prettyman/Photo Edit. 24 Richard Clintsman/Tony Stone Worldwide. 27 Elena Dorfman/ Offshoot Stock.

Chapter 2: 32 Terry Vine/Tony Stone Worldwide. 36 Lori Adamski Peek/Tony Stone Worldwide. 45 Mark Richards/Photo Edit. 48 David Young-Wolff/Photo Edit. 50 Acey Harper/Reportage Stock. 54 Cleo/Photo Edit. 55 AP Wide World Photo.

Chapter 3: 60 John Running. 63 Ben Barnhart/Offshoot Stock. 66 David Young-Wolff/Photo Edit. 71 Bruce Ayres/Tony Stone Worldwide. 74 Doug Menuez/Reportage Stock. 77 Jennings/The Image Works.

Chapter 4: 84 John Henley/The Stock Market. 88 AP Wide World Photo. 91 Bob Daemmrich/Stock Boston. 94 David Young-Wolff/Photo Edit. 99 Elena Rooraid/Photo Edit. 102 R. Lord/The Image Works.

Chapter 5: 104 Renee Lynn/Tony Stone Worldwide. 107 Robert Brenner/Photo Edit. 114 Capital Features/The Image Works. 115 M. Greenlar/The Image Works. 116 Cary Wolinsky/Tony Stone Worldwide. 117 Joel Rogers/Offshoot Stock. 125 Owen Franken/Stock Boston.

Chapter 6: 130 W. Hill/The Image Works. 133 John Curtis/ Offshoot Stock. 134 Bill Gillette/Stock Boston. 142 Michael Newman/Photo Edit. 143 Lisa Quinones/Black Star. 150 Elena Dorfman/Offshoot Stock.

Chapter 7: 154 Michel Tcherevkoff/The Image Bank. 156 Charles Thatcher/Tony Stone Worldwide. 174 Bruce Ayres/Tony Stone Worldwide. 176 Julie Marcotte/Stock Boston. 179 (Top) Claude Edelman/Photo Researchers. 179 (Center) Petit Format-Nestle/ Photo Researchers. 179 (Bottom) Petit Format-Nestle/ Photo Researchers. 181 Tom McCarthy/Photo Edit. 183 John Eastcott & Yva Momatiuk/The Image Works. 184 Myrleen Ferguson Cate/Photo Edit.

Chapter 8: 192 Mark Lewis/Tony Stone Worldwide. 195 J. Da Cunha-Petit Format/Photo Researchers. 202 A. Neste. 206 B. Daemmrich/The Image Works. 207 Matthew Klein/Photo Researchers. 217 Tony Freeman/Photo Edit. 221 Will & Deni McIntyre/Photo Researchers. 225 J. Sohm/The Image Works.

Chapter 9: 230 David Madison/Tony Stone Worldwide. 234 Carlos Henderson/Shooting Star. 236 David Young-Wolff/Photo Edit. 237 Elena Dorfman/Offshoot Stock. 240 Rick Friedman/Black Star. 244 Frank Siteman/Tony Stone Worldwide. 256 Biophoto Associates/Photo Researchers.

Chapter 10: 262 Anthony Neste. 266 Robert E. Daemmrich/Tony Stone Worldwide. 269 Bob Daemmrich/Stock Boston. 272 David R. Frazier/Tony Stone Worldwide. 278 Steve Leonard/Tony Stone Worldwide. 285 (Top) Jean Francois Causse/Tony Stone Worldwide. 285 (Bottom) A. Neste.

Chapter 11: 290 Goldberg/Monkmeyer Press Photo. 300 David De Lossy/The Image Bank. 306 Ken Whitmore/Tony Stone Worldwide.

Chapter 12: 312 R. Campillo/The Stock Market. 317 Mark Clarke/ Photo Researchers. 323 James Prince/Photo Researchers. 326 Courtesy of Johnson & Johnson. 328 Kagan/Monkmeyer Press Photo.

Chapter 13: 334 Timothy Shonnard/Tony Stone Worldwide. 336 Jeff Isaac Greenberg/Photo Edit. 338 Nik Kleinberg/Stock Boston. 342 Photo Researchers. 344 J. Pickerell/The Image Works. 349 Tony Freeman/Photo Edit. 352 Le Duc/Monkmeyer Press Photo. 356 Mary Kate Denny/Photo Edit.

Chapter 14: 360 Evan Agostini/Liaison International. 362 David Young-Wolff/Photo Edit. 368 Michael Newman/Photo Edit. 371 Courtesy of The American Cancer Society. 372 Tony Freeman/Photo Edit. 374 Tony Freeman/Photo Edit. 376 Mark C. Burnett/Stock Boston. 379 Ed Kashi.

Chapter 15: 384 Jeffrey L. Rotman/Peter Arnold Inc. 386 Michael Newman/Photo Edit. 395 Earl Young/Tony Stone Worldwide. 398 Michael Newman/Photo Edit. 402 Greg Weiner/Liaison International. 405 Bonnie Kamin.

Chapter 16: 408 Courtesy of Health Corp. 413 Dorothy Greco/The Image Works. 421 Lisa Quinones/Black Star. 427 Jay Thomas/International Stock.

Chapter 17: 432 Roy Morsch/The Stock Market. 447 Stacy Pick/Stock Boston. 451 Myrleen Ferguson/Photo Edit. 454 Elena Dorfman/Offshoot Stock. 455 Dennis Brack/Black Star. 458 James W. Kay.

Chapter 18: 462 Vanessa Vick/Photo Researchers. 468 Dr. Tony Brain & David Parker, Science Photo Library/Photo Researchers. 469 Jon Levy/Liaison International. 484 Steven J. Nussenblatt/Custom Medical Stock Photo. 488 (Top) Okonewski/The Image Works. 488 (Bottom) Chris Bjormberg/Photo Researchers. 491 Viviane Moos/The Stock Market.

Chapter 19: 496 Bonnie Kamin. 499 A. Neste. 500 (Top) Michael Gadomski/Photo Researchers. 500 (Center) Renee Lynn/Photo Researchers. 500 (Bottom) Scott Camazine/Photo Researchers. 502 Elena Dorfman/Offshoot Stock. 513 James A. Martin/Offshoot Stock. 516 Mark Richards/Photo Edit.

Chapter 20: 520 Christopher Bissell/Tony Stone Worldwide. 524 Dan Bosler/Tony Stone Worldwide. 527 S. Gazin/The Image Works. 528 Ed Kashi. 533 (Top) Joe Monroe/Photo Researchers. 533 (Bottom) Dennis Brack/Black Star. 538 Peter Menzel/Stock Boston.

Chapter 21: 542 Tim Crosby/Liaison International. 546 Michael Townsend/Tony Stone Worldwide. 551 Lawrence Migdale/Tony Stone Worldwide. 552 Michael Grecco/Stock Boston. 554 Spencer Grant/Stock Boston. 559 Alexander Tsiaras, Science Source/Photo Researchers. 560 Mark Richards/Photo Edit. 562 John Hilary/Black Star.

Chapter 22: 566 Shumsky/The Image Works. 568 Reinstein/The Image Works. 572 Mark Richards/Photo Edit. 573 Robert Yager/ Tony Stone Worldwide. 575 (Top) Todd Bigelow/Black Star. 575 (Bottom) Robert Daemmrich/Tony Stone Worldwide. 578 Jacques Chenet/Woodfin Camp and Associates. 584 Ellie Herwig/Stock Boston.

Chapter 23: 588 David Woodfall/Tony Stone Worldwide. 590 John McDermott/Tony Stone Worldwide. 595 Will & Deni McIntyre/Photo Researchers. 599 William Thomas/Tony Stone Worldwide. 606 (Top) Jim Sully/The Image Works. 606 (Bottom) David Young-Wolff/Photo Edit. 609 (Top) Martin Rogers/ Tony Stone Worldwide. 609 (Bottom) B. Daemmrich/The Image Works.

Chapter 24: 614 Alain Evrard/Photo Researchers. 619 Esbin-Anderson/The Image Works. 627 (Top) Art Stein, Science Source/Photo Researchers. 627 (Bottom) W. Hill Jr./The Image Works. 629 Andy Levin/Photo Researchers. 630 Mulvehill/The Image Works.